SABISTON

ESSENTIALS

OF *SURGERY*

SABISTON
ESSENTIALS
OF SURGERY

Second Edition

DAVID C. SABISTON, JR., M.D.

James B. Duke Professor of Surgery
Chairman of the Department of Surgery
Duke University Medical Center
Durham, North Carolina

H. KIM LYERLY, M.D.

Assistant Professor of Surgery and Pathology
Duke University Medical Center
Durham, North Carolina

W. B. SAUNDERS COMPANY
A Division of Harcourt Brace & Company
Philadelphia   London   Toronto   Montreal   Sydney   Tokyo

W. B. SAUNDERS COMPANY
A Division of Harcourt Brace & Company

The Curtis Center
Independence Square West
Philadelphia, PA 19106

Library of Congress Cataloging-in-Publication Data

Sabiston essentials of surgery / [edited by] David C. Sabiston, Jr.,
  H. Kim Lyerly. — 2nd ed.
        p.   cm.
    Rev. ed. of: Essentials of surgery. 1987.
    Includes bibliographical references and index.
    ISBN 0-7216-5019-8
    1. Surgery.   I. Sabiston, David C.,   II. Lyerly, H.
Kim.   III. Title: Essentials of Surgery.
    [DNLM: 1. Surgery.   WO 100 S116 1994]
RD31.E75   1994
617 — dc20
DNLM/DLC
                                                93–33972

SABISTON ESSENTIALS OF SURGERY   ISBN 0-7216-5019-8

Copyright © 1994, 1987 by W. B. Saunders Company.   International Edition 0-7216-5334-0

Printed in the United States of America.

Last digit is the print number: 9   8   7   6   5   4   3   2   1

This text is dedicated to medical students everywhere who continually stimulate their teachers with incisive questions and dialogue, and who engender in them the enthusiasm necessary to remain abreast of the field.

The Editors

CONTRIBUTORS

N. Scott Adzick, M.D.
Associate Professor of Surgery and Pediatrics, University of California, San Francisco, School of Medicine, San Francisco, California
Wound Healing

Paul M. Ahearne, M.D.
Senior Surgery Resident, Department of Surgery, Duke University Medical Center, Durham, North Carolina
Pancreatic Pseudocysts

Dana K. Andersen, M.D.
Professor of Surgery and Medicine, Chief, Section of General Surgery, The University of Chicago, Chicago, Illinois
The Pancreas

Mark P. Anstadt, M.D.
Senior Assistant Resident, Department of Surgery, Duke University Medical Center, Durham, North Carolina
Cardiac Assist Devices and the Artificial Heart

Erle H. Austin, III, M.D.
Professor of Surgery, University of Louisville School of Medicine, Chief of Cardiothoracic Surgery, Kosair Children's Hospital, Louisville, Kentucky
Truncus Arteriosus, Transposition of the Great Arteries, Aortic, Pulmonary, Mitral, and Tricuspid Valve Disease

Timothy J. Babineau, M.D.
Instructor in Surgery, Harvard Medical School, Boston, Massachusetts
The Liver

James M. Becker, M.D.
Associate Professor of Surgery, Chief, Division of General and Gastrointestinal Surgery; Associate Professor of Surgery, Harvard Medical School; Chief, Division of General and Gastrointestinal Surgery, Brigham and Women's Hospital, Boston, Massachusetts
The Acute Abdomen

Albert Bothe, Jr., M.D.
Associate Professor of Surgery, Harvard Medical School; Associate Chairman, Department of Surgery, New England Deaconess Hospital, Boston, Massachusetts
The Liver

Larry C. Carey, M.D.
Professor and Chairman, Department of Surgery, University of South Florida; Chief of Surgery, Tampa General Hospital, Tampa, Florida
The Spleen

Orlo H. Clark, M.D.
Chief of Surgery, Department of Surgery, Mount Zion Medical Center, University of California, San Francisco, San Francisco, California
The Pituitary and Adrenal Glands

Bryan M. Clary, M.D.
Research Fellow, Department of General and Thoracic Surgery, Duke University Medical Center, Durham, North Carolina
The Colon and Rectum

Thomas A. D'Amico, M.D.
Chief Resident in Surgery, Department of Surgery, Duke University Medical Center, Durham, North Carolina
Carcinoma of the Lung

R. Duane Davis, Jr., M.D.
Assistant Professor of Surgery, Department of Surgery, Duke University Medical Center, Durham, North Carolina
The Mediastinum; Coronary Artery Disease and Ventricular Aneurysms

J. Michael DiMaio, M.D.
Research Fellow, Department of Surgery, Duke University Medical Center, Durham, North Carolina
Surgical Aspects of the Acquired Immunodeficiency Syndrome

James M. Douglas, Jr., M.D.
Assistant Professor of Surgery, Duke University Medical Center, Durham, North Carolina
Diagnostic Thoracoscopy; Benign Tumors of the Trachea and Esophagus, Including Bronchial Adenomas; Surgical Disorders of the Pericardium

David L. Dunn, M.D., Ph.D.
Professor of Surgery, University of Minnesota, Minneapolis, Minnesota
Surgical Infections and Antibiotics

André Duranceau, M.D.
Professor of Surgery, Université de Montréal; Division of Thoracic Surgery, Hôtel-Dieu de Montréal, Montreal, Quebec, Canada
The Esophagus

Mark N. Feinglos, M.D., C.M.
Professor of Medicine, Duke University Medical Center, Durham, North Carolina
Surgical Aspects of Diabetes Mellitus

T. Bruce Ferguson, Jr., M.D.
Associate Professor of Surgery, Washington University School of Medicine, St. Louis, Missouri
Surgical Procedures for Cardiac Arrhythmias, Pacemakers, Cardiac Arrest, and Management of the Patient with Heart Disease

Stephen J. Ferzoco, M.D.
Resident in Surgery, Harvard Medical School, Brigham and Women's Hospital, Boston, Massachusetts
The Acute Abdomen

Mitchell P. Fink, M.D.
Associate Professor of Surgery, Harvard Medical School; Director, Division of Trauma and Surgical Critical Care, Beth Israel Hospital, Boston, Massachusetts
Trauma

J. William Gaynor, M.D.
Assistant Professor of Surgery, Duke University Medical Center, Durham, North Carolina
Patent Ductus Arteriosus, Coarctation of the Aorta, Interruption of the Aortic Arch, Aortopulmonary Window, Anomalies of the Aortic Arch, Pulmonary Artery Sling, Atrial Septal Defects, and Ventricular Septal Defects

Gregory S. Georgiade, M.D.
Associate Professor of Surgery, Associate, Division of Plastic and Reconstructive Surgery, Duke University Medical Center, Durham, North Carolina
Reconstructive and Aesthetic Breast Surgery

Donald D. Glower, Jr., M.D.
Assistant Professor of Surgery, Duke University Medical Center, Durham, North Carolina
Aortic, Mitral, and Tricuspid Valve Disease and Hypertrophic Cardiac Myopathy

John P. Grant, M.D.
Associate Professor of Surgery, Duke University Medical Center, Durham, North Carolina
Nutrition in Surgical Patients

Charles S. Greenberg, M.D.
Associate Professor, Department of Medicine, Division of Hematology-Oncology, Duke University Medical Center, Durham, North Carolina
Blood Transfusions and Disorders of Surgical Bleeding

Richard F. Grossman, M.D.
Resident in Surgery, Research Fellow in Endocrine Surgery, University of California, San Francisco, San Francisco, California
The Pituitary and Adrenal Glands

John W. Hallett, Jr., M.D., F.A.C.S.
Director of Surgical Education, Associate Professor of Surgery, Mayo Medical School, Rochester, Minnesota
The Arterial System

John B. Hanks, M.D.
Professor of Surgery, University of Virginia Medical School; Chief, Division of General Surgery, University of Virginia Health Sciences Center, Charlottesville, Virginia
Principles of Operative Surgery

Robert C. Harland, M.D.
Assistant Professor of Surgery, Duke University Medical Center, Durham, North Carolina
Transplantation

J. Michael Henderson, M.B., Ch.B, F.R.C.S.
Chairman, Department of General Surgery, The Cleveland Clinic Foundation, Cleveland, Ohio
Portal Hypertension

David N. Herndon, M.D.
Jesse H. Jones Professor of Surgery, University of Texas Medical Branch; Chief of Staff, Shriners Burns Institute, Galveston, Texas
Burns

Ronald C. Hill, M.D.
Associate Professor of Surgery, West Virginia University School of Medicine, Morgantown, West Virginia
Pulmonary Infections; The Pleura and Empyema; Bronchiectasis

Stefanie S. Jeffrey, M.D.
Assistant Professor of Surgery, Stanford University School of Medicine, Stanford, California
The Pituitary and Adrenal Glands

Patrick D. Kenan, M.D.
Associate Professor of Otolaryngology—Head and Neck Surgery, Duke University Medical Center, Durham, North Carolina
Tracheostomy and its Complications

Scott E. Langenburg, M.D.
Research Fellow, Department of Surgery, University of Virginia Medical School; Resident, Department of Surgery, University of Virginia Health Sciences Center, Charlottesville, Virginia
Principles of Operative Surgery

Maggie C. Lee, B.S.
Fourth-Year Medical Student, Duke University Medical Center, Durham, North Carolina
The Small Intestine

Bruce J. Leone, M.D.
Associate Professor of Anesthesiology; Director, Anesthesiology Cardiopulmonary Research Laboratory, Duke University Medical Center, Durham, North Carolina
Anesthesia

L. Scott Levin, M.D.
Assistant Professor, Division of Orthopaedic, Plastic, and Reconstructive Surgery; Assistant Professor of Surgery, Duke University Medical Center, Durham, North Carolina
Fractures and Dislocations; The Skin

W. Marston Linehan, M.D.
Head, Urologic Oncology Section, Surgery Branch, National Cancer Institute; Associate Professor of Surgery, Uniformed Services University of Health Sciences School of Medicine, Bethesda, Maryland
The Urogenital System

H. Peter Lorenz, M.D.
Senior Resident in Surgery, University of California, San Francisco, San Francisco, California
Wound Healing

H. Kim Lyerly, M.D.
Assistant Professor of Surgery and Pathology, Duke University Medical Center, Durham, North Carolina
Surgical Aspects of the Acquired Immunodeficiency Syndrome; Principles of Surgical Oncology; Soft Tissue Sarcomas; Tumor Markers; The Breast; Surgical Disorders of the Thyroid; The Colon, and Rectum

Samuel M. Mahaffey, M.D.
Assistant Professor, Department of General and Cardiothoracic Surgery, Division of Pediatric Surgery, Duke University Medical Center, Durham, North Carolina
Pediatric Surgery

James R. Mault, M.D.
Senior Assistant Resident, General and Cardiothoracic Surgery, Department of Surgery, Duke University Medical Center, Durham, North Carolina
Extracorporeal Membrane Oxygenation

Richard L. McCann, M.D.
Professor of Surgery, Chief, Section of Vascular Surgery, Duke University Medical Center, Durham, North Carolina
Disorders of the Lymphatic System

Diana B. McNeill, M.D.
Assistant Professor, Division of Endocrinology, Department of Medicine, Duke University Medical Center, Durham, North Carolina
Surgical Aspects of Diabetes Mellitus

Jonathan L. Meakins, M.D., D.Sc.
Professor, McGill University; Surgeon-in-Chief, Royal Victoria Hospital, Montréal, Quebec, Canada
Shock: Causes and Management of Circulatory Collapse

Peter Metrakos, M.D.
Resident in General Surgery, Royal Victoria Hospital, Montréal, Quebec, Canada
Shock: Causes and Management of Circulatory Collapse

Jon F. Moran, M.D.
Professor and Chairman, Department of Cardiothoracic Surgery, University of Kansas Medical Center, Kansas City, Kansas
Surgical Treatment of Pulmonary Tuberculosis

Sean J. Mulvihill, M.D.
Associate Professor of Surgery, University of California, San Francisco, San Francisco, California
The Biliary System

James G. Norman, M.D.
Assistant Professor of Surgery, University of South Florida, Tampa, Florida
The Spleen

Jeffrey A. Norton, M.D.

Professor of Surgery; Chief of Endocrine and Oncologic Surgery, Washington University School of Medicine, St. Louis, Missouri

The Multiple Endocrine Neoplasias; The Parathyroid Glands

Albert D. Pacifico, M.D.

John W. Kirklin Professor of Surgery; Director, Division of Cardiothoracic Surgery, The University of Alabama at Birmingham School of Medicine, Birmingham, Alabama

Disorders of Pulmonary Venous Connection, Tetralogy of Fallot, Double Outlet Right Ventricle, Tricuspid Atresia

Theodore N. Pappas, M.D., F.A.C.S.

Associate Professor of Surgery, Duke University Medical Center; Chief of Surgical Services, Durham V.A. Medical Center, Durham, North Carolina

The Small Intestine

Walter J. Pories, M.D.

Professor and Chairman, Department of Surgery, East Carolina University School of Medicine, Greenville, North Carolina

The Surgical Approach to Morbid Obesity

Scott K. Pruitt, M.D.

Research Fellow, Department of Surgery, Duke University Medical Center, Durham, North Carolina

Acute Renal Failure in Surgical Patients

William J. Richtsmeier, M.D., Ph.D.

Professor and Chief, Division of Otolaryngology—Head and Neck Surgery, Duke University Medical Center, Durham, North Carolina

Otolaryngology: Head and Neck Surgery

Wallace P. Ritchie, Jr., M.D., Ph.D.

Professor and Chairman, Department of Surgery, Temple University School of Medicine, Philadelphia, Pennsylvania

The Stomach and Duodenum

David B. Roos, M.D.

Clinical Professor of Surgery, University of Colorado Health Sciences Center, Denver, Colorado

Thoracic Outlet Syndrome

Randi L. Rutan, R.M., B.S.N.

Research Nurse and Clinical Data Coordinator, Shriners Burn Institute and the University of Texas Medical Branch, Galveston, Texas

Burns

David C. Sabiston, Jr., M.D.

James B. Duke Professor of Surgery; Chairman of the Department of Surgery, Duke University School of Medicine, Durham, North Carolina

Historical Aspects of the Origin and Development of Modern Scientific Surgery; Appendicitis; Hernias; Pulmonary Embolism; Carcinoma of the Lung; Congenital Deformities of the Chest Wall; The Mediastinum; Coronary Artery Disease and Ventricular Aneurysms

Worthington G. Schenk, III, M.D.

Associate Professor of Surgery, University of Virginia Medical Center, Charlottesville, Virginia

Venous Disorders

Richard L. Scher, M.D.

Assistant Professor, Division of Otolaryngology—Head and Neck Surgery, Duke University School of Medicine, Durham, North Carolina

Otolaryngology: Head and Neck Surgery

Bruce D. Schirmer, M.D.

Associate Professor of Surgery, University of Virginia Health Sciences Center, Charlottesville, Virginia

Principles of Preoperative Preparation of the Surgical Patient

James A. Schulak, M.D.

Professor of Surgery, Case Western Reserve University School of Medicine; Director of Transplantation, University Hospitals of Cleveland, Cleveland, Ohio

Surgical Complications

Lewis B. Schwartz, M.D.

Chief Resident in Surgery, Duke University Medical Center, Durham, North Carolina

Pulmonary Embolism

G. Tom Shires, III, M.D.

Professor of Surgery, University of Texas-Southwestern Medical Center, Dallas, Texas

Management of Fluid and Electrolytes

Thomas F. Slaughter, M.D.

Assistant Professor, Department of Anesthesiology, Duke University Medical School, Durham, North Carolina

Blood Transfusions and Disorders of Surgical Bleeding

Craig L. Slingluff, Jr., M.D.

Assistant Professor, Department of Surgery, Division of Surgical Oncology, University of Virginia Health Sciences Center, Charlottesville, Virginia

Malignant Melanoma

Peter K. Smith, M.D.
Associate Professor of Surgery, Duke University Medical Center; Assistant Professor of Biomedical Engineering, Duke University Medical Center, Durham, North Carolina
Pulmonary Function

Wiley W. Souba, M.D., Sc.D.
Professor of Surgery, Harvard Medical School; Chief, Division of Surgical Oncology, Massachusetts General Hospital, Boston, Massachusetts
Homeostasis: Bodily Changes in Trauma and Surgery

Glenn Steele, Jr., M.D., Ph.D.
The William V. McDermott Professor of Surgery, Harvard Medical School; Chairman, Department of Surgery, New England Deaconess Hospital, Boston, Massachusetts
The Liver

Dennis A. Turner, M.D.
Assistant Professor, Departments of Surgery (Neurosurgery) and Neurobiology, Duke University Medical Center, Durham, North Carolina
Neurosurgery

Henry L. Walters, III, M.D.
Assistant Professor of Surgery, Department of Cardiovascular Surgery, Children's Hospital of Michigan, Wayne State University School of Medicine, Detroit, Michigan
Disorders of Pulmonary Venous Connection, Tetratology of Fallot, Double Outlet Right Ventricle, Tricuspid Atresia

J. Paul Waymack, M.D., Sc.D.
Associate Professor of Surgery, University of Texas Medical Branch, Galveston, Texas
Burns

Samuel A. Wells, Jr., M.D.
Professor and Chairman, Department of Surgery, Washington University School of Medicine, St. Louis, Missouri
The Multiple Endocrine Neoplasias; The Parathyroid Glands

Christina Weltz, M.D.
Senior Resident in Surgery, Duke University Medical Center, Durham, North Carolina
The Breast

PREFACE

To study the phenomena of disease without books is to sail an uncharted sea; while to study books without patients is not to go to sea at all.

Sir WILLIAM OSLER

The reception of the first edition of ESSENTIALS OF SURGERY has provided a strong stimulus to extensively revise and update this text. It is now clear that medical students do indeed require a *compact* yet *thorough* textbook to fulfill the requirements of the surgical courses in medical school. It is also well recognized that students require a text that includes the surgical specialties as well as general surgery. For this reason, the fields of cardiothoracic surgery, neurosurgery, plastic and maxillofacial surgery, orthopedics, otolaryngology, and urology are covered in the current edition.

The policy of selecting authoritative contributors has continued in this edition, and fifty-four new authors have been added. Many new topics appear in this edition, including *Surgical Aspects of Diabetes Mellitus, Melanoma, Tumor Markers, The Surgical Approach to Morbid Obesity, Diagnostic Thoracoscopy, Benign Tumors of the Trachea and Esophagus, Acute Renal Failure in Surgical Patients, Soft Tissue Sarcomas, The Multiple Endocrine Neoplasias, Portal Hypertension, Tracheostomy and Its Complications,* and *Extracorporeal Membrane Oxygenation.*

Emphasis has been placed on a *full* presentation of these subjects, including the major historical points, clinical features, and the basic scientific aspects of each disorder. The latter include integrated discussions of the anatomic, pathologic, physiologic, pharmacologic, biochemical, and immunologic features of each surgical disorder. The era of *molecular medicine* has moved rapidly ahead and is now an integral part of essentially all surgical problems. The role of molecular biology is particularly applicable to the fields of transplantation, oncology, endocrine disorders, surgical infections and antibiotics, and immunodeficiency states, and in each instance, these important advances further solidify the scientific basis of medicine. This rapidly emerging field has been appropriately integrated throughout the text.

The parent of this edition, *TEXTBOOK OF SURGERY: The Biological Basis of Modern Surgical Practice,* is recommended as the definitive resource for more complete and detailed descriptions of surgical problems. This text is three times the size of ESSENTIALS OF SURGERY, with extensive coverage of details as well as additional illustrations and bibliographies on each subject. Although it is primarily written for surgical residents and practicing surgeons, it is also useful to medical students seeking more extensive coverage of specific subjects.

Finally, ESSENTIALS OF SURGERY has been written with the specific goal of providing medical students a concise text that is sufficiently detailed to fulfill the requirements of surgical courses in medical schools.

DAVID C. SABISTON, JR., M.D.
H. KIM LYERLY, M.D.

ACKNOWLEDGMENTS

The Editors are well aware of their invaluable colleagues who have made this second edition of *ESSENTIALS OF SURGERY* a reality. The contributors were carefully selected for their knowledge and impact upon the subjects in their chapters. Each has given a full commitment to a commentary of highest quality with full realization of the challenge to provide descriptions of surgical disorders, always bearing the medical student firmly in mind. Individually and collectively, they deserve much praise for their contributions.

Special recognition is due Lisette Bralow, Vice President and Editor-in-Chief of Medical Books at W. B. Saunders Company, who has been an invaluable and close advisor throughout all phases of the preparation of this text. Her keen knowledge and persuasive abilities have meant much in the final product, and her genuine and continuing interest in this effort is gratefully acknowledged. It would be difficult to over-praise Tzipora Sofare, our Editorial Assistant, who possesses unmatched abilities, unique insights, and a very commendable compulsion for perfection, which she applied in the production of this text from beginning to end.

To Faith Voit, Associate Developmental Editor, and Joan Sinclair, Production Manager, we owe special thanks for their committed interest and selective attention to those special features of publication in the production of a final work which in its quality and appearance has exceeded our highest expectations. We also are most grateful to Berta Steiner, President of Bermedica Production, Ltd., and her staff for their praiseworthy efforts in the meticulous production of this text.

Finally, to the entire staff of the W. B. Saunders Company, we owe our continuing appreciation for their continuing tradition of maintaining excellence in medical publication.

DAVID C. SABISTON, JR., M.D.
H. KIM LYERLY, M.D.

CONTENTS

49
THE HEART

1
HISTORICAL ASPECTS OF THE ORIGIN AND DEVELOPMENT OF MODERN SCIENTIFIC SURGERY

DAVID C. SABISTON, Jr., M.D.

Only the man who is familiar with the art and science of the past is competent to aid in its progress in the future.

THEODOR BILLROTH

The development of surgery is of much significance in understanding its art and science as currently practiced. The reason is straightforward, since surgical history provides a basis for an appreciation of the evolution of this increasingly important field of medical science. The more significant and landmark achievements considered to be necessary for all medical students will be reviewed. Although ancient medicine holds an interest for historians and archeologists as evidenced by the earliest of known medical writings, these are seldom directly associated with the contemporary practice of clinical surgery. However, there were some notable descriptions of disease in the ancient writings including the definition of inflammation by Celsus, the Roman medical encyclopedist of the first century AD. In defining inflammation, he said: "Now the characteristics of inflammation are four: redness and swelling, with heat and pain." In the second century, the works of Galen attracted much attention, as did his doctrine that disease is controlled by the "four humors." Surprisingly, this concept was accepted for centuries but became outmoded and was discarded during the Middle Ages.

PIONEERS IN SURGERY

The field of surgery is much indebted to the first of the scientific anatomists, Andreas Vesalius (Fig. 1). He began detailed and accurate dissections of human anatomy while a medical student, and his careful descriptions and realistic illustrations completely changed the former emphasis on Galenical anatomy, which was based primarily on animal dissections. The day following his graduation as a doctor of medicine at the University of Padua, Vesalius was made a full Professor on the basis of his scholarly work in anatomic dissection. Within 4 months, his first atlas of anatomy, *De Humani Corporis Fabrica*, was published and became widely used. With this single work, he corrected many errors that had been used for a thousand years in Galen's anatomic reproductions.

A discovery that was to greatly affect the subject of physiology was that of William Harvey (Fig. 2), who established the principles of the circulation. He demonstrated that when the heart contracts in systole, blood from the right ventricle flows through the pulmonary artery and into the lung. The blood then passes into the left atrium and ventricle to the systemic circulation. Although he could not demonstrate the capillaries, Harvey proposed that anastomoses must be present between the arteries and veins to make possible his concept of a complete circulation.

Fielding H. Garrison, the noted medical historian, selected three surgeons whom he considered the greatest of all time. They were Ambroise Paré, John Hunter, and Joseph Lister (Fig. 3). Paré was a French

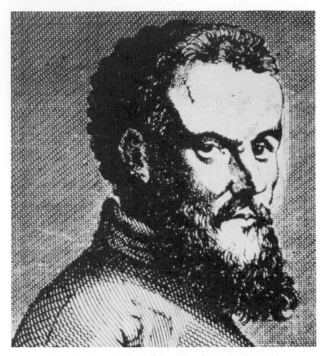

Figure 1. Andreas Vesalius (1514–1564).

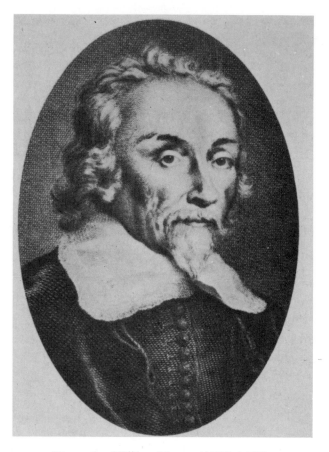

Figure 2. William Harvey (1578–1657).

military surgeon who had a keen observing mind and who reintroduced the ancient use of the ligature to control hemorrhage. He is also known for a classic controlled clinical experiment when, during the Battle of Denonvilliers (1552), he treated two injured soldiers with similar wounds as they lay side by side in a tent near the field of battle. The first soldier's wound was managed by the standard method of the day; that is, routine cauterization with boiling oil. The second soldier was managed by débridement, cleansing, and the application of a clean dressing. Paré later commented that he spent a restless night, being convinced that the second patient would do very poorly. However, his wisdom was demonstrated the following morning when he found the second patient to be essentially without systemic symptoms, whereas the former had a high fever, tachycardia, and disorientation. When Paré was congratulated on this quite successful new method, he very humbly replied: "Je le pansay, Dieu le guarit" ("I dressed him, God healed him"), a quotation that can be found today inscribed on Paré's statue in Paris.

John Hunter was a brilliant teacher of anatomy and surgery who will be remembered for his introduction of the *experimental method*. He systematically used animals to develop surgical techniques prior to their use in humans. A very thoughtful surgeon, and among the first to be scientifically oriented, his philosophy and practice are best summarized in his response to a question from his friend and colleague, Edward Jen-

ner, the discoverer of the smallpox vaccination. When the latter was speculating with ideas concerning hibernation in hedgehogs, Hunter simply said, "I think your solution is just, but why think? Why not try the experiment?" Hunter devised a number of operations and was particularly interested in arterial aneurysms. Following a life filled with contributions to anatomy,

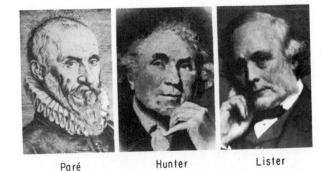

Pare   Hunter   Lister

Figure 3. Ambroise Paré (1510–1590), John Hunter (1728–1793), and Joseph Lister (1827–1912).

physiology, surgical pathology, as well as clinical surgery, there is little wonder that Garrison said of him: "With the advent of John Hunter, surgery ceased to be regarded as a mere technical mode of treatment, and began to take its place as a branch of scientific medicine, firmly grounded in physiology and pathology."

It is of considerable interest that throughout the advances in medicine, the basic sciences frequently have been the source of discoveries and principles subsequently applied to clinical problems. A brilliant example is the work of Louis Pasteur (1822–1895), the originator of the germ theory of disease. In the mid-19th century, Pasteur was the first to show that fermentation and putrefaction were caused by living organisms, and he reasoned that the formation of pus in infected wounds had a similar pathogenesis. In 1867, Lister published the first of a series of papers introducing the concept of *antiseptic surgery*. The principles were based upon destruction of all living organisms—primarily, bacteria—which might come into contact with the patient's tissues during the surgical procedure. Careful cleansing of the patient's skin and the surgeon's hands and the use of sterile drapes surrounding the operative field and sterilized instruments and suture material formed the basis of antiseptic surgery. Lister's concepts and practice spread throughout the world. It is Lister, more than any other, to whom primary credit should be given for the ultimate expansion in the number and types of operations. When these procedures became safe for the patient, with a sharp reduction in postoperative infection, the surgical management of a host of disorders became widely adopted.

THE DEVELOPMENT OF ANESTHESIA

The introduction of *anesthesia* was a major achievement that created the potential for many new, difficult, and much needed surgical procedures. As a medical student in 1799, Humphrey Davy prepared and inhaled large quantities of nitrous oxide and noted its analgesic effect. In experiments upon himself, he noted that headache and toothache "always diminished after the first four or five inspirations." He then summarized his findings saying, "As nitrous oxide in its extensive effects appears capable of destroying physical pain, it may be probably used with advantage during surgical operations."

Crawford W. Long of Georgia was the first to use ether as an inhalation anesthetic in 1842 with the excision of a lipoma of the neck. He used this technique in eight subsequent operations and carefully recorded them in his journal, but unfortunately did not publish these observations at the time.

In 1846, William T.G. Morton (Fig. 4) administered ether to a patient operated upon by John Collins Warren at the Massachusetts General Hospital, which proved such a dramatic success that it was immediately published. It was this contribution that prompted Warren to say at the end of the procedure to those present: "Gentlemen, this is no humbug!" Shortly thereafter, use of ether anesthesia spread rapidly around the world. The impact of general anesthesia is clearly demonstrated by the use of chloroform in 1847 for Queen Victoria during childbirth, giving rise to the term "chloroform á la reine" (for the Queen).

ROENTGENOGRAPHY

A monumental discovery was that of Röntgen (Fig. 5) with the introduction of the x-ray in 1895. From that time forth, refinements in radiography, including the use of contrast agents in the gastrointestinal tract and in arteriography, have greatly expanded the diagnostic potentials in this field. In addition, roentgen-guided radiography for needle biopsy, dilatation of vascular obstructions, and drainage of abscesses has been equally impressive.

DEVELOPMENT OF SURGICAL TRAINING PROGRAMS

Following the introduction of scientific principles to the discipline of surgery, emphasis began to be placed on the proper training of surgeons. The original pat-

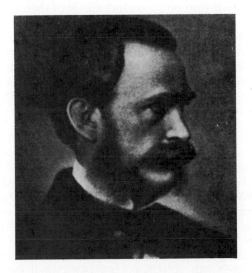

Figure 4. William T. G. Morton (1819–1868).

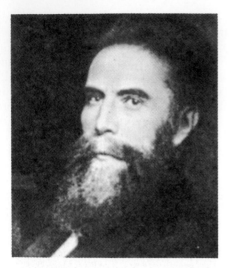

Figure 5. Wilhelm K. Röntgen (1845–1923).

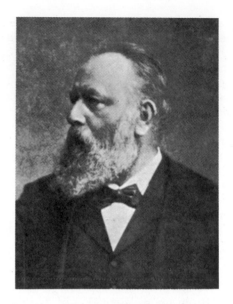

Figure 6. Theodor Billroth (1829–1894).

terns of surgical training programs were established in Europe during the latter half of the 19th century, particularly in the university clinics of Germany, Austria, and Switzerland. It was there that the surgical giants, all powerful in their respective fields, established the principle of progressive training over a period of years culminating in the position of Chief Resident. Most agree that the father of modern surgical training programs was Bernhard von Langenbeck, an exceedingly gifted and skillful clinical surgeon. He was also a master teacher who surrounded himself with a group of bright trainees and taught them with much thoroughness. He was Chief of Surgery at the famed Charité, the teaching hospital of the University of Berlin. When Langenbeck's pupils completed his training program, they were called to other major universities and clinics throughout Europe to assume chairs of their own. His most notable pupil was Theodor Billroth (Fig. 6), who became Professor of Surgery at the University of Zurich and later at the University of Vienna, where he was Chief Surgeon to the world renowned Allegemeines Krankenhaus. He was the first to resect successfully a part of the alimentary tract when, in 1881, he performed a gastrectomy with anastomosis of the end of the remaining stomach to the duodenum.

The development of the surgical residency training programs in the United States is clearly related to the Langenbeck-Billroth school, because William S. Halsted (Fig. 7), the Professor at the newly opened Johns Hopkins University School of Medicine and Hospital, had been deeply impressed by the Langenbeck plan during his travels to Germany, Switzerland, and Austria just prior to his appointment in Baltimore. Halsted, generally regarded as the most outstanding surgeon in North America, regularly visited the major European clinics in the latter half of the 19th century.

He became deeply impressed with the progressive system of surgical training and was completely devoted to the concept that highly selected, bright young trainees should begin as interns and gradually progress through the residency with increasing responsibility. He agreed with Langenbeck that upon completion of the program, the trainee should have essentially the same abilities as the teachers in the program. Thus, many of Halsted's trainees were appointed directly to prestigious academic chairs immediately upon completion of the training program.

Halsted's specific concepts of surgical training ap-

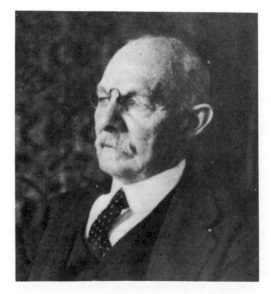

Figure 7. William S. Halsted (1852–1922).

pear in his essay, "The Training of a Surgeon." He said:

> It was our intention originally to adopt as closely as feasible the German plan, which in the main, is the same for all principal clinics . . . every facility and the greatest encouragement is given each member of the staff to do work in *research*.

In this address delivered at Yale in 1904, Halsted stressed:

> The assistants are expected in addition to their ward and operating duties to prosecute original investigations and to keep in close touch with the work in surgical pathology, bacteriology, and so far as possible physiology . . . . Young men contemplating the study of surgery should early in life seek to acquire knowledge of the subjects fundamental to the study of their profession.

Halsted stated further:

> We need a system, and we shall surely have it, which will produce not only surgeons but surgeons of the highest type, men who will stimulate the youths of our country to study surgery and devote their energies and their lives to raising the standard of surgical science.

Halsted's astonishing success in the training of surgeons was later duplicated by others including his successor at Johns Hopkins, Alfred Blalock (Fig. 8), and by other master teachers and investigative surgeons including Wangensteen at the University of Minnesota, Graham at Washington University and Barnes Hospital, and Ravdin and Rhoads (Fig. 9) at the University of Pennsylvania. These gifted teachers produced many trainees who subsequently became professors of surgery and chairmen of departments.

In his Presidential Address at the American Surgical Association in 1956, Blalock emphasized his views on the significance of research in saying:

> The only way an interested person can determine whether or not he has an aptitude in research is to give it a trial . . . . My point is that he should not shy away from it because of a misconception and fear that he does not have originality. As a medical student, I felt pity for the investigator, but later this changed to admiration and envy.

MAJOR DEVELOPMENTS IN GENERAL SURGERY

The first successful laparotomy was performed in rural Kentucky on Christmas Day 1809 by Ephraim McDowell (Fig. 10), who had trained in Edinburgh under some of the finest teachers of the time. McDowell removed a huge ovarian tumor in a patient who recovered uneventfully and lived for many years. He

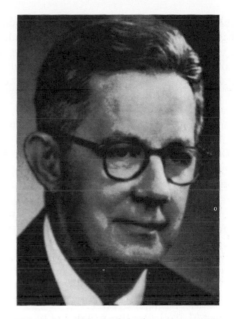

Figure 8. Alfred Blalock (1899–1964).

later removed 11 other ovarian tumors with only one death. Other major advances in abdominal surgery were made by Billroth, with the first gastric resection in 1881, and by Karl Langenbuch, with the first cholecystectomy in 1882. In 1886, Reginald Fitz described the clinical findings and symptoms of acute appendicitis, and shortly thereafter McBurney and others developed the appropriate surgical techniques to safely remove the inflamed appendix.

Hernia has been described through the centuries, and it is remarkable that surgical correction became

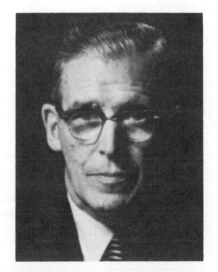

Figure 9. Jonathan Rhoads (1907–   ).

achievable only a century ago. While a number of procedures were attempted during the 19th century, it remained for Bassini and Halsted to simultaneously but independently devise an anatomically designed operation that was at the time termed "the radical cure of inguinal hernia." These two surgical pioneers contributed greatly to marked improvement in long-term results following their procedures, and the principles of their operations remain in practice today.

In 1900, Karl Landsteiner first detected the presence of agglutinins and isoagglutinins in blood and found that blood could be typed into four groups. Although blood transfusions had been previously administered, success had been marred by many fatal reactions. When the ability to type blood was demonstrated, its use gradually became widespread and made possible many extensive surgical procedures not previously feasible. For his notable work, Landsteiner was awarded the Nobel Prize.

The development of surgery of the thyroid gland was pioneered by Theodor Kocher (Fig. 11) who in 1895 described 1000 thyroidectomies for goiter. At the time of his death in 1917, he had performed 5000 thyroidectomies with a mortality of only 0.11 per cent. He also noted that following total thyroidectomy, hypothyroidism was frequent and that administration of thyroid extract was followed by a return of normal metabolism. For these contributions, Kocher became the first surgeon to be awarded the Nobel Prize in 1909.

The development of surgical procedures on the parathyroid glands was initiated by Mandl of Vienna in 1925 with removal of the first parathyroid tumor in a patient with advanced osteitis fibrosus cystica. Following these landmark achievements, many other dates became significant as new procedures were successfully performed (Table 1).

Many specific contributions to surgery have had an extraordinary impact upon the field. The concepts of fluid and electrolyte balance have their scientific origin in the early observations of Claude Bernard who, in 1859, published a series of lectures entitled "Liquids of the Organism." In these major contributions, he emphasized the significance of the *milieu intérieur*, which he proposed was the physiologic state that allowed an organism to exist independently. These concepts were furthered in subsequent years, primarily by Cannon, who introduced the term "homeostasis." *The Metabolic Care of the Surgical Patient*, a monograph by Francis D. Moore, remains the standard reference in this important field. Another major contribution made in the late 1960s was the introduction of total parenteral alimentation following the notable experimental and clinical work of Dudrick and Rhoads. They showed experimentally that in paired canine littermates, one receiving normal alimentation by mouth

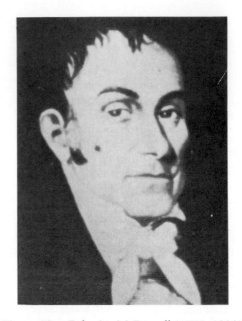

Figure 10. Ephraim McDowell (1771–1830).

and the other receiving its total caloric intake intravenously, both animals developed normally and had similar weights when grown. This extraordinary contribution greatly altered the management and future course of many patients with severe nutritional problems, particularly those with enteric fistulas who had losses of large amounts of fluids and nutritive elements with a high morbidity and mortality rate.

The introduction of *chemotherapy* and *antibiotics* has greatly altered the course of many surgical pro-

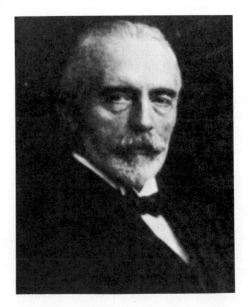

Figure 11. Theodor Kocher (1841–1917).

cedures. Ehrlich is due initial credit for introducing a chemotherapeutic agent, salvarsan ("606"), in the management of syphilis. In 1935, Domagk introduced Prontosil, a sulfonamide, and for the first time an agent was available that immediately attacked bacteria, with dramatic clinical results for susceptible organisms. In 1929, Fleming had noted the antibacterial properties of certain molds, especially *Penicillium notatum*. Florey and Chain found methods to produce penicillin in amounts necessary for clinical use in 1944. For this monumental achievement, these three workers shared the Nobel Prize in 1945. The *hormonal* control of neoplastic disease was demonstrated

by Huggins (Fig. 12) in 1940 when he showed that antiandrogenic management by orchiectomy or the administration of estrogen caused the regression of disseminated carcinoma of the prostate. For this work, as well as studies of serum enzymes and protein chemistry and the role of the adrenal gland in controlling metastases from neoplastic disease, he was awarded the Nobel Prize in 1966.

DEVELOPMENT OF VASCULAR AND CARDIOTHORACIC SURGERY

Modern vascular surgery was initiated when Alexis Carrel (Fig. 13) demonstrated that it was possible to successfully join the two ends of a divided blood vessel with careful surgical technique, fine needles, and carefully selected suture materials. This contribution led to primary healing of vessels without infection or thrombosis. Prior to his experimental and clinical work, there had not been a successful vascular anastomosis, previous attempts having ended in either thrombosis or infection. Carrel was also the first to transplant tissues and organs using his careful technique of vascular surgery. He clearly predicted the scientific basis for the forthcoming field of transplantation, and for all of these landmark achievements, he was awarded the Nobel Prize in physiology and medicine in 1912.

The first use of a saphenous vein to replace an artery was by Goyannes in Madrid in 1906. After correction of a popliteal arterial aneurysm, he restored vascular continuity using the patient's saphenous vein. Subsequent workers, especially DeBakey, demonstrated the feasibility of using *plastic arterial substitutes* with prolonged durability and consistent clinical success. In the

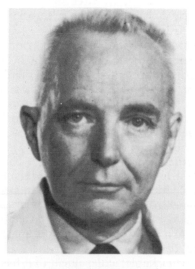

Figure 12. Charles B. Huggins (1901–   ).

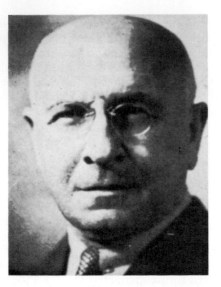

Figure 13. Alexis Carrel (1873–1944).

1896 edition of Paget's *Surgery of the Chest*, one finds the following statement:

> Surgery of the heart has probably reached the limits set by Nature to all surgery: no new method, and no new discovery, can overcome the natural difficulties that attend a wound to the heart. It is true that "heart suture" has been vaguely proposed as a possible procedure, and has been done on animals; but I cannot find that it has ever been attempted in practice.

For this reason, it is of special interest that in the same year, 1896, Ludwig Rehn first successfully closed a stab wound to the heart in a 22-year-old male who had been unconscious for a period of 3 hours prior to operation. Rehn controlled hemorrhage from a wound in the right ventricle with three silk sutures. This historic patient recovered, and the event marked the beginning of cardiac surgery.

Rudolph Matas first described his innovative endoaneurysmorrhaphy in the treatment of arterial aneurysms. This represented the first definitive management of these lesions with restoration of the circulation.

In 1925, Souttar of London was the first to introduce a finger into the left atrial appendage, accomplishing a splitting of a stenotic mitral valve in a patient with rheumatic valvar disease. This was not repeated until 1946, when Bailey and then Harken began the procedure again with much success. Closure of a patent ductus arteriosus was first successfully achieved by Gross in 1938, and coarctation of the aorta was corrected with end-to-end anastomosis by Crafoord in 1944.

Another remarkable achievement that has had a tremendous impact on the field of cardiovascular surgery was the introduction of cardiac catheterization by Forssmann in 1929. This pioneering work later became a routine diagnostic procedure when Cournand and Richards demonstrated its usefulness in the diagnosis of many forms of heart disease. These workers were awarded the Nobel Prize in 1956.

The treatment of congenital cyanotic heart disease was greatly augmented by Blalock in 1944, when he performed the first successful procedure for the tetralogy of Fallot. The subclavian artery was anastomosed to the pulmonary artery to improve blood flow to the lungs in patients with obstructive lesions in the pulmonary arterial circuit. The use of hypothermia in cardiac surgery permitted temporary interruption of the circulation, an approach stimulated by the early work of Bigelow, who showed in the experimental animal that the circulation could be safely interrupted for a period of 10 minutes or more at reduced temperatures without the damaging effects of cerebral hypoxia. This technique was applied successfully in the closure of an atrial septal defect by Lewis and Varco in 1952. The next notable achievement in this field was that of Gibbon, who developed extracorporeal circulation. This monumental advance began with laboratory experiments in 1931 and was systematically pursued by this dedicated investigator and his wife until 1953, when the heart-lung machine was first successfully employed in the closure of an atrial septal defect using the pump oxygenator to substitute for the heart and lungs while the defect was being corrected. Shortly thereafter and using this technique, Lillehei and also Kirklin successfully corrected ventricular septal defects, the tetralogy of Fallot, and many other congenital cardiac defects.

An abdominal aortic aneurysm was first corrected surgically by DuBost in Paris in 1951. In the same year, the first plastic arterial grafts were introduced experimentally by Voorhees and Blakemore. The first successful implantation of a prosthetic cardiac valve was achieved by Starr in 1960. DeBakey added much to the development of plastic arterial grafts and the operative techniques in removing extensive aneurysms of the thoracoabdominal aorta.

The surgical management of myocardial ischemia is now widespread. The first use of the saphenous vein bypass graft to the coronary circulation was in 1962. It was the application of this technique in a series of patients by Favaloro and Johnson that demonstrated its usefulness, and the procedure has now become the most common cardiac surgical procedure performed in the United States. It has been responsible for complete relief of anginal pain as well as a significant extension of life.

TRANSPLANTATION

The experimental work establishing the feasibility of transplantation of tissues and organs was done by

Carrel and associates at the turn of the century. The first successful long-term renal transplant was achieved by Murray in 1954. In 1963, Starzl successfully implanted a liver, and in 1964 the first lung transplant was made by Hardy. Najarian achieved a pancreatic transplant in 1966, and this entire field has now become a very important one throughout the world. The long-term survival of organ transplants has been significantly advanced with the introduction of agents to suppress rejection, including Imuran, steroids, antilymphocyte globulin, and, more recently, cyclosporine. Barnard, in 1967, was the first to successfully transplant the human heart, and this is now an everyday procedure. A combination heart-lung transplant was performed by Reitz in 1982, and this feat represents another distinctive advance in an ever-increasing field. The development of antirejection agents including azathioprine, steroids, antilymphocyte globulin, and cyclosporine have greatly advanced this entire field. Currently, attention is being directed toward *xenotransplantation*, with the hope that transplants from animals to humans may become successful.

SUMMARY

It becomes clear in retrospect that many advances in surgery have been dependent upon previous discoveries. While the recent leaders in the field have expanded its horizons in ways previously not thought possible, much yet remains for the future. It is certain that the incorporation of fundamental biologic principles will bring significant advances. An example is rapid progress being made in oncology with development of antitumor agents and the increasing understanding of the genetics and molecular biology of cell division and development of neoplasms. Much interest is now being directed to the development of cancer vaccines.

Finally, the student should continuously recall the fact that intellect and new ideas alone are not enough;

rather, they must be combined with a committed and productive effort. The words of Sir William Osler, Regius Professor of Medicine at Oxford, speak brilliantly to this point. In replying to the medical students of the day who asked him to give them the reason for his extraordinary success in medicine, Osler simply replied:

> It seems a bounden duty on such an occasion to be honest and frank, so I propose to tell you the secret of life as I have seen the game played, and as I have tried to play it myself. . . . This I propose to give you in the hope, yes, in the full assurance that some of you at least will lay hold upon it to your profit. Though a little one, the master-word looms large in meaning. [WORK] It is the open sesame to every portal, the great equalizer in the world, the true philosopher's stone, which transmutes all the base metal of humanity into gold. The stupid man among you it will make bright, the bright man brilliant, and the brilliant student steady. With the magic word in your heart all things are possible, and without it all study is vanity and vexation. The miracles of life are with it . . . to the youth it brings hope, to the middle-aged confidence, to the aged repose. . . . It is directly responsible for all advances in medicine during the past twenty-five centuries.

REFERENCES

Blalock A: The Nature of discovery. Presidential address to the American Surgical Association. Ann Surg *144*:3, 1956.

DeBakey ME: Presidential address to the Southern Surgical Perspective. Ann Surg *213*:499–531, 1991.

Halsted WS: The training of the surgeon. Bull Johns Hopkins Hosp *15*:267, 1904.

Meade RH: An Introduction to the History of General Surgery. Philadelphia, WB Saunders Company, 1968.

Ravitch MM: A Century of Surgery: The History of the American Surgical Association, Vols. 1 and 2. Philadelphia, JB Lippincott Company, 1981.

Sabiston DC Jr: A continuum in surgical education: Presidential Address to the Society of University Surgeons. Surgery *66*:1, 1969.

Wangensteen OH, Wangensteen SD: The Rise of Surgery From Empiric Craft to Scientific Discipline. Minneapolis, University of Minnesota Press, 1978.

2

HOMEOSTASIS: Bodily Changes in Trauma and Surgery

WILEY W. SOUBA, M.D., Sc.D.

Incorporated into the body's armamentarium of protective mechanisms is a complex and complicated set of well-regulated defense responses that are initiated within moments of injury or insult. These responses are involuntary but essential for survival. They are designed to maintain body homeostasis at a time when key physiologic processes are threatened, and are initiated by various components of the response to injury such as volume loss, tissue damage, fear, and pain. Later factors that reinitiate or perpetuate these responses include invasive infection and starvation. The events are generally related to the severity of injury; that is, the greater the insult, the more pronounced the specific response. Incorporated into the human genome are genes, which encode the synthesis of key hormones, and peptides, which allow the body to respond to such insults with remarkable resilience. From an evolutionary standpoint these biologic responses are the result of a process that favors survival of the fittest in the struggle to survive and preserve the species. From a teleologic standpoint, they are designed to benefit the organism, enhance recovery, and assure a relatively speedy return to health. In this chapter, the adaptive and homeostatic responses that occur after surgery and trauma are discussed.

INJURY: ELECTIVE VERSUS ACCIDENTAL

Whether the body is injured accidentally or within the carefully monitored confines of an operating room, the responses to such trauma are remarkably similar. However, it is apparent to the student of surgery that such settings are also different in ways that influence the extent and magnitude of the stress response (Table 1). Accidental injury is unplanned and uncontrolled; tissues are torn, ripped, bruised, and contaminated. The associated volume loss may be substantial, leading to tissue underperfusion which, if prolonged, causes cellular deterioration and death in tissues that may have not been initially traumatized. Pain, excitement, and fear are generally heightened and uncontrolled. As a consequence, the magnitude of the physiologic responses to major accidental injury is considerable.

In contrast, the "elective" tissue trauma that is inflicted within the confines of an operating room is calculated, planned, and monitored. Although elective surgery causes pain, often interrupts food intake, and is often associated with the removal of an organ or tissue, the perioperative management of elective surgical patients is often designed to attenuate such changes. Patients are seen prior to surgery by anesthesiologists and surgeons and evaluated to determine the need for preoperative nutritional support or additional medical consultation. Hydration prior to operation is common as is the administration of prophylactic antibiotics and drugs that relieve anxiety and fear. In the operating theater, the surgical site is "prepped" in a sterile manner to minimize contamination, and numerous physiologic responses (i.e., blood pressure, pulse, urine output) are continually monitored. Blood and blood products are invariably available. During the operation, tissues are carefully dissected and incised to minimize tissue trauma; tissues are reapproximated with care when possible. Appropriately selected pharmacologic agents are used to block undesirable cardiovascular responses, and specific techniques such as epidural anesthesia or patient-con-

TABLE 1. DIFFERENCES BETWEEN ELECTIVE SURGERY AND ACCIDENTAL INJURY

Perturbation	Elective Operation	Accidental Injury (Trauma)
Tissue damage	Minimal; tissues are dissected with care and reapproximated	Can be substantial; tissues usually torn or ripped; débridement necessary
Hypotension	Uncommon; preoperative hydration employed and fluid status is carefully monitored intraoperatively	Fluid resuscitation often not immediate; blood loss can be substantial, leading to shock
Pain/fear/anxiety	Generally can be alleviated	Generally present
Infectious complications	Uncommon; prophylactic antibiotics often administered	More common due to contamination, hypotension, and tissue devitalization
Overall stress response	Controlled and of lesser magnitude; starvation better tolerated	Uncontrolled; proportional to the magnitude of the injury; malnutrition poorly tolerated

trolled anesthesia are effective in minimizing postoperative pain. As a consequence, the physiologic responses to elective surgery are generally of a lesser magnitude than those seen with major accidental injury. Even major operations such as aortic aneurysmectomy, liver resection, and pancreaticoduodenectomy can be done with minimal morbidity and mortality.

The body responds to these insults in a remarkable manner (Fig. 1). For example, when the body is injured, blood flow is redistributed to preferentially provide oxygen and nutrients to vital organs, the clotting cascade is set into motion at the site of injury, and renal mechanisms are initiated that maintain acid-base balance and blood volume. White blood cells invade injured tissues and release chemotactic substances and growth factors that promote healing and repair. Amino acids stored in muscle are exported so they can be used by other organs for protein synthesis. The liver uses these precursors for the synthesis of acute-phase proteins, and the wound uses them for the synthesis of collagen. Unless the injury is incompatible with life or unless the patient develops multiple organ failure from invasive infection, most patients recover fully and lead productive lives.

SPECIFIC COMPONENTS OF THE INJURY RESPONSE THAT INITIATE HOMEOSTATIC RESPONSES AND ADJUSTMENTS

Volume Loss and Tissue Underperfusion

Several important responses occur following reduction of the circulating blood volume. The body immediately attempts to compensate in order to maintain adequate organ perfusion. Pressure receptors in the aortic arch and carotid artery and volume (stretch) receptors in the wall of the left atrium detect the fall in blood volume and immediately respond by signaling the brain. Heart rate and stroke volume, the two determinants of cardiac output, increase. Afferent nerve signals are also initiated that stimulate the release of

both antidiuretic hormone (ADH) and aldosterone. Antidiuretic hormone is produced by the posterior pituitary gland, is a response to hypotonicity, and functions to increase water reabsorption in the kidney. Aldosterone is produced via the renin-angiotensin system, which is activated when the juxtaglomerular apparatus in the kidney is stimulated by a fall in pulse pressure. Aldosterone increases renal sodium reabsorption and thereby serves to conserve intravascular water. These mechanisms are only partially effective, and severe hemorrhage, in the absence of adequate resuscitation, often leads to a prolonged low-flow state. Under these circumstances, oxygen delivery is inadequate to meet tissue demands, and the cell is forced to switch to anaerobic metabolism, which leads to lactic acidosis. Eventually, cell function deteriorates, resulting in the local and systemic release of toxic products, which can cause hypotension and organ dysfunction.

Tissue Damage

Injury of body tissues appears to be the most important factor that sets the stress response into motion. Hypovolemia and malnutrition may act synergistically with tissue destruction, but in and of themselves hypovolemia and starvation do not initiate a hypermetabolic/hypercatabolic response unless they cause infection or tissue injury. For example, prolonged underperfusion may lead to ischemia, cellular death, and the release of toxic products that can initiate the "stress" response. Afferent neural pathways from the wound signal the hypothalamus that injury has occurred; tissue destruction is generally sensed in the conscious patient as pain. Efferent pathways from the brain are immediately triggered and stimulate a number of responses designed to maintain homeostasis.

Pain and Fear

Pain and fear are definite components of the stress response. Both lead to excessive production of the catecholamines that prepare the body for the "fight-or-flight" response.

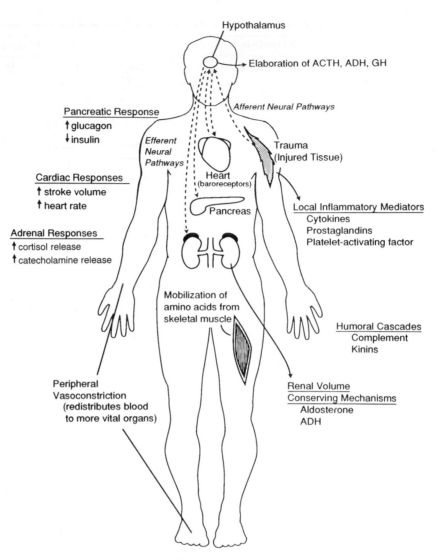

Figure 1. Homeostatic adjustments that are initiated after injury.

Lack of Nutrient Intake and the Consequences of Malnutrition

The metabolic response to injury and surgery causes an increased energy expenditure. In many patients undergoing surgery, nutrient intake is inadequate for a period of time (1 to 5 days) following operation. If energy intake is less than expenditure, oxidation of body fat stores and erosion of lean body mass occurs, with the resultant loss of weight. Body glycogen stores are limited and are depleted within 24 to 36 hours. Consequently, glucose, which is required by the central nervous system and by white blood cells, must be synthesized de novo. Amino acids, which are released principally by skeletal muscle, are the major gluconeogenic precursors. Most injured patients can tolerate a loss of 15 per cent of their weight prior to injury without a significant increase in the risks of surgery. When weight loss exceeds 15 per cent of body weight, the complications of undernutrition interact with the stress process and may impair the body's ability to respond appropriately to the injury and to inhibit responses to added complications such as infection.

A major impact of nutritional support in the trauma patient is to match the energy and nitrogen expenditure that occurs following injury and to aid host defense. In contrast to injured patients, the catabolic and hypermetabolic responses that occur after elective operations are of a lesser magnitude because there is less tissue destruction and the neurohormonal/inflammatory response is less intense. Consequently, well-nourished patients undergoing major operations do not require nutritional support postoperatively unless it is anticipated that food intake will be precluded for more than 7 days.

Invasive Infection

The major complication observed in surgical patients is infection. Most patients, particularly those in the intensive care units, are exposed to a variety of infectious agents. The normal barrier defense mechanisms are disrupted by multiple indwelling catheters, nasotracheal and nasogastric tubes, and breakdown of skin and mucous membrane. Infection alone initiates catabolic responses that are similar to (but not the same as) those described following injury in non-infected patients. Both processes cause fever, hyperventilation, tachycardia, accelerated gluconeogenesis, increased proteolysis, and lipolysis, with fat utilized as the principal fuel. Inflammatory cells release a variety of soluble mediators that aid host resistance and wound repair. Undernutrition may compromise the available host defense mechanism and thereby increase the likelihood of invasive sepsis, multiple organ system failure, and death.

BODY COMPOSITION CHANGES THAT OCCUR AFTER INJURY AND OPERATION

Total body mass is comprised of an aqueous component and a nonaqueous component. The nonaqueous portion is comprised of bone, tendons, and mineral mass as well as adipose tissue, while the aqueous phase contains the body cell mass, which is comprised of skeletal muscle, intra-abdominal and intra-thoracic organs, skin, and circulating blood cells. Also contributing to the aqueous portion is interstitial fluid and the intravascular volume. Total body water in the average-sized (70-kg) adult male makes up approximately 55 to 60 per cent (~40 L) of total body mass. Of this 40 L, some 22 L are intracellular, 14 L are interstitial fluid, and the plasma volume is approximately 3 to 3.5 L. Following injury or surgery, changes in body composition are common. These changes are characterized by a loss of lean body mass (often most apparent clinically as a decrease in leg circumference), a loss of body fat, and expansion of the extracellular fluid compartment (Fig. 2). The extracellular fluid compartment enlarges and salt is retained, while the functional, actively metabolizing body mass is diminished.

The body contains fuel reserves that it can mobilize and utilize during times of starvation or stress (Table 2). By far the greatest energy component is fat, which

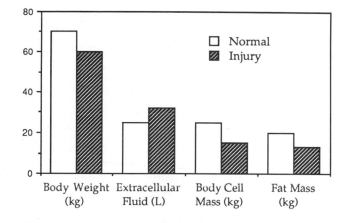

Figure 2. Changes in body composition characteristic of injury. The catabolic response results in an overall decrease in total body weight because the catabolic response results in a reduction in lean body mass and fat mass. The extracellular fluid space is expanded because of the renal conserving mechanisms that are initiated. As recovery begins, a spontaneous diuresis occurs and a gradual anabolic state begins.

is calorically dense and, when oxidized, provides about 9 cal/gm. Body protein comprises the next largest mass of utilizable energy, but amino acids yield, on the average, only about 4 kcal/gm. Unlike fat reserves, body protein is not a storage form of energy but serves as structural and functional components of the body. Loss of body protein, if severe, is associated with functional consequences. Following injury, proteolysis is accelerated to generate amino acids to support gluconeogenesis. In the long run, a chronic catabolic state can lead to erosion of body protein stores such that susceptibility to infection is increased, wound healing is impaired, and outcome is unfavorably impacted. Glucose is stored in the body as glycogen in the liver and in skeletal muscle. Glycogen stores are small and become rapidly depleted in stressed patients. Since tissues such as the brain, peripheral nervous system, circulating blood cells, and healing wounds require glucose, de novo synthesis is required in the injured patient.

TABLE 2.   FUEL RESERVES OF A HEALTHY (70-KG) ADULT MALE

Energy Source	kg	kcal Value
Fat	14	125,000
Protein		
Skeletal muscle	6	24,000
Other	6	24,000
Glycogen		
Muscle	0.15	600
Liver	0.075	300
Free glucose	0.02	80

HOMEOSTASIS FOLLOWING ELECTIVE OPERATIVE PROCEDURES

Physiologic and Endocrine/Metabolic Changes

Tissue trauma, initiated when the surgeon's scalpel incises the patient's skin at the start of a surgical procedure, signals the hypothalamus via afferent pathways that injury has occurred. The brain responds by activating the sympathetic nervous system. A characteristic early response to surgery is stimulation of the adrenal medulla via the sympathetic nervous system with elaboration of epinephrine. Norepinephrine, produced in peripheral nerve endings, is also secreted in increased amounts in surgical patients. These catecholamines rise during, and remain elevated following, elective operative procedures. In addition, the excitement, pain, fear, and hypovolemia that may accompany the surgical procedure are also potent stimulators of the sympathetic nervous system. Such responses can be modified with the use of local anesthesia, which eliminates pain locally, or with general anesthesia, which modulates responses centrally. Other pharmacologic agents also modulate cardiovascular responses and renal responses. Urinary catecholamines may be elevated for 24 to 48 hours after operation, after which they generally return to normal. These hormones increase cardiac output, redistribute blood flow, and stimulate hepatic glycogenolysis and gluconeogenesis.

Another early consequence of a surgical procedure is the rise in levels of circulating cortisol that occurs in response to a sudden release of adrenocorticotropic hormone (ACTH) from the anterior pituitary gland. Activation of the pituitary gland occurs when afferent nervous signals from the operative site reach the hypothalamus to initiate the stress response. The rise in ACTH stimulates the adrenal cortex to elaborate cortisol and other glucocorticoid hormones. Cortisol mobilizes amino acids from skeletal muscle that provide substrates for wound healing and serve as precursors for the hepatic synthesis of acute-phase proteins or new glucose. The glucocorticoid hormones remain elevated for approximately 24 to 36 hours after a major operation.

The ability to excrete a water load after elective surgical procedures is restricted. Aldosterone is a potent stimulator of renal sodium retention, whereas ADH stimulates renal tubular water reabsorption. The usual postoperative patient concentrates urine even in the presence of adequate hydration. Hence, weight gain secondary to salt and water retention is usual following operation. Edema occurs to a varying extent in all surgical wounds, and this accumulation is proportional to the extent of tissue dissection, the length of the operation, and the amount of fluid the patient receives intraoperatively. Administration of sodium-containing solutions during operation replaces this functional volume loss as extracellular fluid redistributes in the body. This "third-spaced" fluid eventually returns to the circulation as the wound edema subsides and diuresis commences 2 to 4 days following the operation.

Pancreatic islet cell production of hormones that regulate glucose metabolism is also altered by surgery. Insulin elaboration is diminished, and glucagon concentrations increase resulting in a decrease in the circulating insulin/glucagon ratio. This response may be related to increased sympathetic activity or to the rise in levels of circulating epinephrine, which is known to suppress insulin release. The rise in glucagon and the corresponding decrease in insulin stimulate hepatic glucose production.

Most, even those undergoing major operative procedures, recover uneventfully. In most situations, aside from pain control and hydration, relatively little patient care is necessary, and intervention may even be meddlesome. This observation attests to the wonderful capacity of the body to recover from injury on its own. Because the injury response is such a powerful one and is essential for survival, current techniques of postoperative care minimize, but do not reverse, the catabolic responses that were incorporated into the human genome at a time when hospitals did not exist.

Stages of Surgical Convalescence

Surgical convalescence (i.e., the body's recovery from operative stress) has been categorized into four stages. The first stage is termed the "adrenergic-corticoid phase," since it corresponds to the time when adrenal secretion of epinephrine and cortisol is enhanced. This phase represents a period of catabolism initiated by the circulating hormonal environment in combination with a period of inadequate nutrition. The patient goes into negative nitrogen balance and may actually gain weight secondary to fluid retention. The second phase, a turning point from catabolism and anabolism, is referred to as the "corticoid-withdrawal phase" because it is characterized by a spontaneous sodium and free-water diuresis, a positive potassium balance, and a reduction in nitrogen excretion. In general, in the absence of postoperative complications, this phase starts 3 to 6 days after an abdominal operation, often concomitant with the commencement of oral feedings. This transitional phase usually lasts only 1 to 2 days. Should the patient develop a complication such as wound dehiscence, pneumonia, or an anastomotic disruption, the adrenergic-corticoid phase can be reinitiated, leading to further body catabolism.

In the absence of a complication, the corticoid-withdrawal phase gives way to a prolonged period of "early anabolism" characterized by positive nitrogen balance and weight gain. Protein synthesis is increased as a result of sustained enteral feedings and an increasing level of activity, and this change is related to the return of lean body mass and muscular strength. The positive nitrogen balance is usually in the range of 2 to 4 gm of nitrogen per day in the average adult, a range representing a daily gain of 60 to 120 gm of lean tissue. The total amount of nitrogen ultimately gained equals the amount lost, but the rate of gain is much slower than the rate of initial loss.

The fourth and final phase of surgical convalescence is "late anabolism," the hallmark of which is much slower weight gain. During this period, the patient is in nitrogen equilibrium but in positive carbon balance, which results from the deposition of body fat.

HOMEOSTASIS FOLLOWING TRAUMA

Characteristic Early Responses

Accidental injury is followed by a well-described pattern of physiologic responses. The events are generally related to the severity of injury; that is, the greater the insult, the more pronounced the specific response. In the 1930s, Cuthbertson studied patients with long-bone fractures and described the time course for many of the posttraumatic responses. Two distinct periods were identified, an early "ebb" or shock phase and a later "flow" phase of injury. The ebb phase was usually brief in duration (12 to 24 hours) and occurred immediately following injury. Blood pressure, cardiac output, body temperature, and oxygen consumption were reduced. These events were frequently associated with hemorrhage, resulting in hypoperfusion and lactic acidosis. With restoration of blood volume, ebb-phase alterations gave way to more accelerated responses characteristic of the flow phase of injury.

The flow phase is characterized by hypermetabolism, increased cardiac output, increased urinary nitrogen losses, altered glucose metabolism, and accelerated tissue catabolism. The flow-phase responses to accidental injury are similar to those seen following elective operation. In contrast to elective surgical stress, the response to injury is usually more intense and extends over a long period of time. For example, injured patients often have an impaired ability to excrete a water load because of the heightened elaboration of aldosterone and ADH. The retention of large quantities of sodium and water that may occur during fluid resuscitation causes a dramatic increase in body weight, which may rise 10 to 20 per cent over the patient's weight before injury. During recovery, the edema fluid reenters the vascular compartment and the

salt and water load is gradually excreted by the kidneys. Although sodium and water retention may occur following elective operation, the magnitude and subsequent events (fluid mobilization followed by volume expansion and diuresis) are much less dramatic than in injured patients.

Characteristics of the Flow Phase of the Injury Response

$BMR = 4.8 \ (O_2 \text{cons}/\text{min}) = \sim 1440 \text{ kcal/d}$

Hypermetabolism

Hypermetabolism is defined as an increase in basal metabolic rate (BMR) above that predicted on the basis of age, sex, and body size. Metabolic rate is usually determined by measuring the exchange of respiratory gases and by calculating heat production from oxygen consumption and carbon dioxide production. A simple formula that can be used to determine metabolic rate (kilocalories per unit time) for a particular patient multiplies oxygen consumption (liters per unit time) by 4.8. For example, the average-sized male consumes about 200 to 225 ml of oxygen per minute at rest. This is equivalent to consuming about 300 L of oxygen per day. Multiplying 300 by 4.8 yields a basal metabolic rate of approximately 1440 kcal/day. This figure does not include the additional energy expenditure associated with activity. In trauma patients, the degree of hypermetabolism (increased oxygen consumption) is generally related to the severity of the injury. Elective surgical patients have a 5 to 15 per cent increase in metabolic rate, whereas the metabolic needs of patients with multiple injuries increase by more than 50 per cent. Patients with severe burn injury have resting metabolic rates that may reach twice basal levels. As a consequence of this hypermetabolism, trauma patients usually develop a 1° to 2°C elevation in body temperature, which represents an upward shift in the thermoregulatory set point of the hypothalamus. Such a fever is not indicative of infection and rarely needs to be treated.

Altered Glucose Metabolism

An elevation of the fasting blood sugar level is characteristic of injury, and the degree of hyperglycemia generally parallels the severity of stress in the ebb phase. This has been referred to as the "pseudodiabetes of stress." Later, during the flow phase, insulin concentrations are normal or elevated; yet, hyperglycemia persists. This phenomenon suggests an alteration in the relationship between insulin sensitivity and glucose disposal. Hepatic gluconeogenesis rates are increased, and much of the new glucose synthesized by the liver arises from precursors (lactate, pyruvate, and amino acids) released from peripheral tissues. Most of this additional glucose is consumed by the wound and by the kidneys. These alterations in glucose metabolism have a profound impact on the handling of exogenously administered glucose contained in enteral or parenteral feedings. When a glucose infusion is administered, normal individuals demonstrate a progressive increase in glucose disposal with time; whereas injured patients maintain a constant glucose disposal. The quantity of insulin elaborated in injured patients is greater than in control subjects; nonetheless, rising insulin concentrations fail to increase glucose clearance in these patients.

Other studies in trauma patients have demonstrated a failure to suppress hepatic glucose production during glucose infusion or insulin administration. In normal individuals, both of these perturbations inhibit hepatic glucose production. Glucose uptake by uninjured skeletal muscle of trauma patients is less than that observed in control subjects. Thus, profound insulin insensitivity is a characteristic feature of injured patients. The liver is also a resistant tissue, and lipolysis is not attenuated in trauma patients after glucose administration. The cause of this marked insensitivity to insulin is unknown; however, similar effects are observed when counterregulatory hormones are infused into normal subjects. Glucose infusions to trauma patients should not exceed 5 to 6 mg/kg/min.

Alterations in Protein Metabolism

A diminished protein economy is characteristic of trauma patients. Extensive urinary nitrogen losses occur, and negative nitrogen balance develops. Negative nitrogen balance occurs if the breakdown rate increases and protein synthesis remains the same, or if the breakdown rate remains the same and the rate of synthesis decreases. The use of isotopically labeled, nonradioactive amino acids allows protein synthesis and breakdown rates to be measured in trauma patients. Such studies have shown that synthesis is diminished in normal individuals if protein intake is restricted. In contrast, such adaptations do not occur in injured patients (Table 3). Protein breakdown is increased in spite of a diminished food intake, and urinary nitrogen losses are accelerated (Fig. 3). Feeding such patients attempts to elevate protein synthetic rates with the goal of matching rates of protein catabolism. Thus, trauma accelerates nitrogen turnover. In unfed patients, breakdown rates exceed synthesis and negative balance results. Providing exogenous calories and nitrogen increases synthesis, and, when adequate nutrients are provided, the rate of protein synthesis approaches the rate of protein degradation and the magnitude of negative nitrogen balance is reduced.

Skeletal muscle is the origin of the majority of the

TABLE 3. METABOLIC DIFFERENCES BETWEEN THE RESPONSE TO SIMPLE STARVATION AND TO INJURY

	Simple Starvation	Severe Injury
Basal metabolic rate	↓	↑↑
Presence of mediators	—	+++
Major fuel oxidized	Fat	Mixed
Ketone body production	+++	±
Hepatic ureagenesis	+	+++
Negative nitrogen balance	+	+++
Gluconeogenesis	+	+++
Muscle proteolysis	+	+++
Hepatic protein synthesis	+	+++

nitrogen that is lost in the urine following extensive injury. Only recently has it been appreciated that the composition of amino acid efflux does not reflect the composition of muscle protein. Alanine and glutamine comprise 50 to 60 per cent of amino acids released, whereas each makes up only about 6 per cent of muscle protein. Oxidation of branched-chain amino acids by skeletal muscle is accelerated following injury. These amino acids donate their nitrogen group to support the biosynthesis of glutamine, and alanine is increased.

Glutamine is utilized by the gastrointestinal tract as a principal energy source. It is also extracted by the kidney, where it contributes ammonium groups for ammonia generation, a process that excretes acid loads. The gut enterocytes convert glutamine primarily to ammonia and alanine and these two substances are released into the portal venous blood. This ammonia is then removed by the liver and is converted to urea; the alanine may also be removed by the liver and may serve as a gluconeogenic precursor. Following elective surgical stress, glutamine consumption by the bowel and the kidney is accelerated, a reaction that appears to be regulated by the increased elaboration of the glucocorticoids. Glutamine is also required by endothelial cells, fibroblasts, and cells of the immune system (Fig. 4). Hence, glutamine and alanine are important participants in the transfer of nitrogen from skeletal muscle to visceral organs; however, their metabolic pathways favor the production of urea and ammonia, both of which are lost from the body.

Alterations in Fat Metabolism

Stored triglyceride is mobilized and is oxidized at an accelerated rate in injured patients. Lipolysis is poorly attenuated following glucose administration, possibly because of continuous stimulation of the sympathetic nervous system, which favors breakdown of triglycerides. Although the mobilization and oxidation of free fatty acids are accelerated in injured subjects, ke-

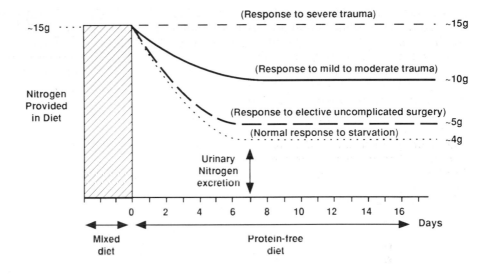

Figure 3. Urinary nitrogen losses following simple starvation, postoperative starvation, and postinjury starvation. The hormonal/inflammatory environment associated with injury prevents the normal adaptive responses to starvation from occurring. Consequently, nitrogen losses remain high leading to a significant loss of lean body mass in the absence of nutritional support.

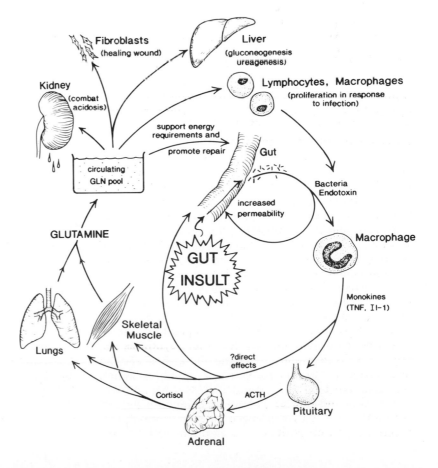

Figure 4. The interorgan glutamine cycle. The cycle can be initiated by local and/or systemic gut insults that cause an increase in bowel permeability and bacterial translocation. Bacteria and endotoxins stimulate macrophages to release cytokines that activate the pituitary/adrenal axis. The release of cortisol accelerates muscle and lung glutamine release and enhances intestinal glutamine uptake. Simultaneously, glutamine supports renal ammoniagenesis, hepatic gluconeogenesis, and lymphocyte and endothelial proliferation in response to bacterial invasion. If the cycle persists, or if the patient is unable to take oral feedings or remains glutamine deficient, a prolonged catabolic state develops.

tosis during brief starvation is blunted, and the accelerated protein catabolism persists. If unfed, severely injured patients rapidly deplete their fat and protein stores.

Mediators of the Injury Response

The response to operative stress (elective injury) or accidental injury (trauma) is comprised of two components: a neurohormonal arm and an inflammatory arm. These pathways work together to determine the magnitude of the response. The principal hormones involved are the catecholamines, the corticosteroids, and glucagon. The inflammatory component of injury involves the local elaboration of cytokines and the systemic activation of humoral cascades involving complement, eicosanoids, and platelet-activating factor. These mediators promote wound healing by stimulating angiogenesis, white cell migration, and ingrowth of fibroblasts. During elective surgical procedures, the local inflammatory response is confined to the wound and significant amounts of these mediators do not gain access to the systemic circulation. Following accidental injury in which there is massive tissue destruction or prolonged hypotension leading to cell injury, these substances may be produced locally in the wound in excessive amounts resulting in "spillover" into the systemic circulation. In addition, cells in other tissues (such as Kupffer cells in the liver) may become activated to produce these mediators. Such responses can lead to a systemic response in which these mediators cause detrimental effects such as hypotension and organ dysfunction. In this capacity, much work has focused on the beneficial and detrimental effects of cytokines.

Counterregulatory Hormones

Following moderate to severe injury, a marked rise is noted in the production and circulating level of the counterregulatory hormones glucagon, glucocorticoids, and epinephrine. During the ebb phase of injury, the sympathoadrenal axis helps maintain the pressure-flow relationships necessary for an intact cardiovascular system. With the onset of hypermetabolism, characteristic of the flow phase, these and other hormones exert a variety of metabolic effects. Glucagon has potent glycogenolytic and gluconeogenic effects on the liver, which signal the hepatocytes to make new glucose from hepatic glycogen stores and gluconeogenic precursors. Cortisol mobilizes amino acid from skeletal muscle and increases hepatic gluconeogenesis. The catecholamines stimulate hepatic glycolysis and gluconeogenesis and increase lactate production from peripheral tissues (skeletal muscle).

Catecholamines also increase metabolic rate and stimulate lipolysis. The level of growth hormone is elevated, even in the presence of hyperglycemia, and thyroid levels are reduced to low-normal concentrations. Infusion of counterregulatory hormones into normal subjects reproduces many of the metabolic alterations that are characteristic of injury.

Cytokines

Although the classic counterregulatory hormones of stress play an important role in mediating the body's response to injury and surgery, they exert their influence largely via endocrine mechanisms. Other mediators, peptide compounds known collectively as cytokines that are produced both at the site of injury by endothelial cells and by diverse immune cells throughout the body, also occupy a pivotal position in the stress response (Table 4). Cytokines differ from classic endocrine hormones in that they are produced by a variety of cell types and have the capacity to exert the majority of their tissue effects locally via direct cell-to-cell communications ("networking") in a paracrine manner. In addition to specific target tissue effects, cytokines stimulate production of other cytokines leading to important cascades that both amplify and diversify the effects of the proximal cytokine. Cytokines

TABLE 4. SOME BIOLOGIC ACTIVITIES OF CYTOKINES

Immune/inflammatory	Stimulate release of neutrophils from bone marrow
	Activate monocytes, eosinophils and neutrophils
	Initiate neutrophil margination/transendothelial migration
Metabolic	Stimulate:
	Release of amino acids from skeletal muscle
	Hepatic uptake of amino acids
	Hepatic protein synthesis
	Lipolysis
	Release of ACTH
	Inhibit:
	Lipoprotein lipase activity
	Fatty acid synthesis
Other effects	Stimulate proliferation of fibroblasts
	Increase vascular permeability
	Stimulate microvascular angiogenesis
	Inhibit vascular tone
Clinical manifestations	Leukocytosis
	Cachexia
	Negative nitrogen balance
	Hyperlipidemia
	Hypotension, organ failure, death

can also stimulate their own production locally, amplifying activity in an autocrine manner. Occasionally, when produced in excess, cytokines may act as hormones and "spill over" into the systemic circulation and become detectable in the bloodstream. Under these circumstances, cytokines produce systemic responses via endocrine mechanisms.

Those cytokines that have been studied most extensively and appear to play the most important role in the injury response are tumor necrosis factor-α (TNF-α, cachectin), interleukin-1 (IL-1), interleukin-2 (IL-2), interleukin-6 (IL-6), and interferon-γ (IFN-γ). Originally it was thought that the primary influence of cytokines was on immune cell function. It is now clear that cytokines are key regulators of the metabolic response to injury. These polypeptide signals, produced by the organism in response to tissue injury or necrosis, bacteremia or endotoxemia, induce many of the adverse responses following severe injury. The production of cytokines is likely to be greatest when the injury is most severe. Under these circumstances local cytokine production may gain access to the systemic circulation and trigger detrimental response such as hypotension and organ dysfunction. Tissue injury and necrosis produced by higher concentrations of TNF-α is mediated by effects on the microvasculature that produce an intense inflammatory reaction that leads to ischemic and hemorrhagic necrosis.

The most powerful stimulus for release of TNF-α by macrophages is endotoxin from the cell walls of gram-negative bacteria. TNF-α is considered to be the primary mediator of the systemic effects of endotoxin, producing anorexia, fever, tachypnea, and tachycardia at low doses; and hypotension, organ failure, and death at higher doses. TNF-α acts through binding with specific receptors present on most tissues; high-affinity TNF-α receptors have been identified on nearly all cells. TNF-α is produced primarily by macrophages, but lymphocytes, Kupffer cells, and a number of other cell types have been identified as sources of TNF-α. In healthy humans, plasma levels of TNF-α are quite low, generally ranging from 0 to 35 pg/ml. Concentrations in tissues are likely to be higher. In animal models, stimulation of TNF-α–producing cells with endotoxin induces both transcription and translation of the protein within minutes, with detection in serum after 20 minutes. In both humans and animals, TNF-α levels peak between 90 minutes and 2 hours after injection of endotoxin.

TNF-α causes release of neutrophils from bone marrow and regulates neutrophil chemotaxis, superoxide production, degranulation, and release of lysozyme. TNF-α stimulates proliferation of fibroblasts and elicits production of other cytokines. These cytokine–cytokine interactions act synergistically to effect a number of biologic processes such as hematopoiesis, immune cell activation, and acute-phase responses. TNF-α is an endogenous pyrogen, acting directly on hypothalamic neurons. It also activates the hypothalamic-pituitary axis, producing elevated levels of ACTH and cortisol. TNF-α causes proteolysis and release of amino acids from skeletal muscle contributing to the negative nitrogen balance and muscle wasting seen after injury and infection. Concurrently, it has a stimulatory effect on amino acid uptake by the liver and redirection of hepatic protein synthesis. Administration of TNF-α to animals causes decreased lipoprotein lipase activity and elevation in plasma levels of triglycerides and free fatty acids.

IL-1, like TNF-α, has a variety of proinflammatory activities. A single low dose of IL-1 causes fever, neutrophilia, hypozincemia, increased hepatic acute-phase protein synthesis, decreased albumin synthesis, anorexia, sleep, and release of ACTH, glucocorticoids, and insulin in vivo. At higher doses, IL-1 induces hypotension, leukopenia, tissue injury, and death in a manner characteristic of septic shock. IL-1 induces many of the same biologic effects as TNF-α, and the combined effect of these two cytokines is often greater than the effect of either alone. Each of these cytokines also induces the elaboration of the other so that it is unlikely that either is present systemically without the other.

IL-6 is now recognized as the primary mediator of altered hepatic protein synthesis known as the acute-phase protein synthetic response. Glucocorticoid hormones augment the cytokine effects on acute-phase protein synthesis. Elevated levels of IL-6 are found in the circulation of patients with infections, trauma, and cancer.

IL-2 is responsible for signaling T lymphocyte proliferation. IL-2 receptors are not present on quiescent T cells, but are expressed within hours of the cells' being activated by an antigen. Binding of IL-2 with the receptor on T cells causes clonal expansion of T cells activated by the specific antigen. IL-2 markedly enhances the cytolytic activity of natural killer cells. When administered to humans both alone and with autologous lymphokine-activated killer cells, IL-2 has marked tumoricidal activity.

Interferons are a family of proteins that were originally identified for their ability to inhibit viral replication in infected cells. IFN-γ is a type II interferon, totally unrelated in structure and function to the type I interferons, which have antiviral properties. IFN-γ is produced only by T lymphocytes and natural killer cells, induced by specific antigens or mitogens. It is one of the major cytokines capable of activating macrophages, enhancing both antigen presenting and processing, as well as cytocidal activity. IFN-γ is synergistic with TNF-α, and the primary mechanism for this effect appears to be the ability of IFN-γ to upregulate the number of TNF-α receptors on various cell types.

IF CYTOKINES HAVE DETRIMENTAL EFFECTS, WHY DO THEY EXIST?

The genes that regulate cytokine biosynthesis are likely to be conserved because they have important beneficial roles that confer a survival advantage following injury. In general, cytokines exert a number of beneficial effects under the majority of circumstances that appear to outweigh the detrimental effects seen in extreme pathophysiologic states. These beneficial effects are briefly discussed below.

Mobilization of Amino Acids and Stimulation of Acute-Phase Protein Synthesis

Cytokines act in conjunction with other mediators to promote mobilization of amino acids from skeletal muscle. This response provides key nutrients to support cellular metabolism at a time when the animal generally cannot acquire food because of the associated immobility and anorexia. These precursors support energy requirements in other tissues and support the acute-phase protein response in the liver. Cytokines, particularly TNF-α, IL-1, and IL-6, are the primary regulators of the hepatic acute-phase protein synthetic response. The glucocorticoid hormones augment the response. Early observations on the effects of TNF-α and IL-1 on hepatic protein synthesis demonstrated a stimulation of protein synthesis and subsequent elevation in the elaboration of the acute-phase proteins. IL-6 is now recognized as the cytokine primarily responsible for the alteration in hepatic protein synthesis recognized as the acute-phase response. The primary metabolic component of the acute-phase response is a qualitative alteration in hepatic protein synthesis, with a resulting alteration in plasma protein composition. Characteristically, proteins that act as serum transport and binding molecules (albumin, transferrin) are reduced in quantity, and acute-phase proteins (fibrinogen, C-reactive protein) are increased (Table 5). Acute-phase proteins are elaborated, in part, for the purpose of reducing the systemic effects of tissue damage. While the true physiologic role of many of the acute-phase proteins remains unclear, many act as antiproteases, opsonins, or coagulation and wound-healing factors, and they likely inhibit the generalized tissue destruction that is associated with the local initiation of inflammation. For example, increases in fibrinogen enhance thrombus formation, while antiproteases reduce tissue damage caused by proteases released by dead or dying cells. C-reactive

TABLE 5.   THE ACUTE-PHASE PROTEIN RESPONSE

Proteins	Function
Decreased	
Albumin	Transport
Transferrin	Transport
Increased	
C-reactive protein	Scavenger function, opsonin
Serum amyloid A	Apolipoprotein
Fibrinogen	Enhance thrombus formation
α₁-acid glycoprotein	Antiproteases; reduce tissue
α₂-macroglobulin	damage due to proteases
α₁-antitrypsin	released by dead or dying cells
Ceruloplasmin	Oxygen scavenger, transport
Complement factor C3	Opsonin
Haptoglobin	Binds and removes hemoglobin
	released by erythrocyte lysis

protein has been hypothesized to have a scavenger function. This acute-phase response confers a significant survival advantage following injury and infection.

Elevation in White Blood Cell Count

Leukocytosis is recognized by an elevated circulating white blood cell count (WBC), with an increase in the proportion of immature cells. This phenomenon has been attributed, in part, to the release of neutrophils and their precursors into the circulation from the bone marrow. It has recently been recognized that the elevated level of cytokines in the presence of sepsis and inflammation may be responsible for the appearance of the elevated WBC. Both TNF-α and IL-1 produce an increase in the number and immaturity of circulating neutrophils. Release of neutrophils is apparently due to a direct action on the bone marrow. TNF-α and IL-1 are chemotactic for neutrophils that form a defense perimeter and destroy invading bacteria.

Hypoferremia

Serum iron and zinc levels are reduced in septic patients, an event that is cytokine mediated. The decrease in serum iron is probably important in protecting the host against various bacteria. The reduction of iron can inhibit the growth rate of microorganisms that have a strict requirement for iron as a growth factor. Both TNF-α and IL-1 have been shown to mediate hypoferremia, hypozincemia, and other alterations in trace-element metabolism.

Localization of the Wound/Inflammatory Site

Localization or containment of tissue injury may be an important response designed to minimize systemic effects from the inflammation at the trauma site. This is accomplished by vasodilation, migration of neutrophils and monocytes to the wound, initiation of the coagulation cascade, and proliferation of endothelial cells and fibroblasts in later stages of wound healing. These effects function to confine the insult as much as possible and activate defense mechanisms to minimize adverse systemic effects, such as cardiovascular collapse and subsequent organ failure. Cytokines are involved in all of these functions. The wound becomes an organ of cytokine production in which local metabolism is controlled in part by cytokines.

Fever/Subjective Discomfort

Fever is the systemic response to invading microorganisms and their toxins that is elicited by changes in the microenvironment of the anterior hypothalamus. Fever has both beneficial and detrimental effects on the body, but it is generally believed that the generation of fever by endogenously produced substances has adaptive value and imparts a survival advantage on the organism. Fever induced by the injection of cytokines in humans is associated with symptoms of malaise, myalgias, headaches, and joint pain. These constitutional symptoms are likely beneficial, since they encourage the "sick" animal to seek shelter, safety, and rest and to avoid additional stressful situations. Energy is conserved, and a quiescent state is achieved with all efforts focused on combating the inflammatory process, healing the wound, and restoring homeostasis.

Gut Mucosal Barrier Dysfunction as a Mediator of the Stress Response

Although the intestinal tract is generally viewed as an organ of digestion and absorption, it also protects the host from intraluminal bacteria and their toxins. The maintenance of an intact brush border and intercellular tight junctions prevents the movement of toxic substances into the intestinal lymphatics and circulation. Gut immune function is the term applied to the structural and functional characteristics of the gastrointestinal tract that make it resistant to the entry of infectious or toxic agents into the systemic circulation. This function is a combination of nonimmunologic processes (physical factors, intestinal flora) and the local mucosal immune system function. Immune factors include the secretion of secretory IgA (S-IgA) and the function of macrophages and lymphocytes in the Peyer's patches, mesenteric lymph nodes, and lamina propria of the intestinal mucosa. These groups of cells of the immune system within the gastrointestinal tract are known collectively as the gut-associated lymphoid tissue (GALT). Maintenance of a gut mucosal barrier

that effectively excludes luminal bacteria and toxins requires an intact epithelium and normal mucosal immune mechanisms.

Bacterial translocation is the process by which microorganisms migrate across the mucosal barrier and invade the host. The most extensive work on bacterial translocation has been done in animal models, where the number and pathogenicity of the endogenous flora can be precisely controlled and the microorganism that invades the host can be carefully quantified. There are generally three principal mechanisms that promote bacterial translocation: (1) altered permeability of the intestinal mucosa (as caused by hemorrhagic shock, sepsis, distant injury, or administration of cell toxins); (2) decreased host defense (secondary to glucocorticoid administration, immunosuppression, or protein depletion); and (3) an increased number of bacteria within the intestine (as caused by bacterial overgrowth, intestinal stasis, or the feeding of bacteria to experimental animals). A number of retrospective and epidemiologic studies have associated infection in specific patient populations with bacterial invasion from the gut. These reports suggest that bacterial invasion occurs in patients after injury, multiorgan system failure, or severe burns, and in persons with cancer after undergoing chemotherapy. Nonmetabolizable markers of known size, such as lactulose or mannitol, have also been used to determine permeability. These studies have demonstrated an increase in mucosal permeability in normal volunteers receiving endotoxin and in infected burn patients. Because many of the factors that facilitate bacterial translocation occur simultaneously in surgical patients and their effects may be additive or cumulative, patients in an intensive care unit may be extremely vulnerable to the invasion of enteric bacteria or to the absorption of their toxins. Such patients do not generally receive enteral feedings, and current parenteral therapy causes gut atrophy. Methods currently used to support critically ill patients neither facilitate repair of the intestinal mucosa nor maintain gut barrier function.

METHODS OF MODIFYING OR ATTENUATING THE CATABOLIC RESPONSE TO INJURY AND SURGERY

Nutrition Support: Enteral Feedings

Enteral nutrition is superior to parenteral nutrition. Whenever feasible, injured patients requiring nutritional support should be fed enterally rather than intravenously. The trophic effects of luminal nutrition are well documented even if relatively small amounts of nutrients are provided. Several well-designed clinical studies have demonstrated that trauma patients nourished enterally have a reduction in the incidence of major complications compared to patients receiving total parenteral nutrition in the immediate postinjury period. The mechanisms by which enteral feedings exert a beneficial effect are likely to be multifactorial and include (1) maintenance of gut mucosa barrier function, (2) enhanced production of trophic gut hormones, and (3) maintenance of the immune system.

Tissue-Specific Nutrients

It is now clear that the composition of the diet as well as the route of delivery plays an important role in maintaining organ structure and function. It has been suggested that certain nutrients may be required in increased amounts following injury. Those substances that have received the most attention are glutamine, arginine, ω-3 fatty acids, and dietary nucleotides. Arginine has potent immunomodulatory properties and has been shown to augment macrophage and natural killer cell activity. Arginine is a nonessential component of the diet for healthy adults, indicating that the endogenous synthetic pathways provide adequate amounts of this amino acid. In critically ill patients, arginine may be semiessential, since supplemental dietary arginine may improve weight gain, nitrogen retention, wound healing, and immune function.

Although glutamine is the most abundant amino acid in the body, its concentration in whole blood and tissues decrease significantly during critical illness, leading to a state of marked glutamine depletion. Several well-designed human studies have shown that glutamine-enriched nutrition can improve muscle protein synthesis, improve nitrogen balance, prevent the redistribution of body water that occurs after a standard catabolic stress, and shorten hospital stay.

Cytokine Blockade

As our knowledge of how the injury response is regulated at the cellular and molecular level increases and as we better understand the negative systemic effects of cytokines (hemodynamic collapse, multiple organ failure, and death), the possibilities of neutralizing some of the undesirable effects of cytokines as a therapeutic modality in treating critical illness may become a reality. To date, most methods of modifying the effects of cytokines on target tissues have focused on the use of anticytokine antibodies and specific cytokine receptor antagonists. The impetus for such investigations derived from work demonstrating that administration of TNF-α to animals causes sepsis and that TNF-α levels in septic humans were correlated with outcome. Several animal studies have demonstrated that anti-TNF-α monoclonal antibodies confer

significant protection against the effects of sepsis, but only if given before the septic challenge. Several potential problems may be associated with such therapy in patients. First, pretreatment with anticytokine antibodies may be difficult to implement in the clinical setting. Second, treatment with the antibody is likely to block beneficial responses as well as deleterious ones. For example, pretreatment with an anti-TNF-α antibody diminishes the endotoxin-induced hepatic amino acid transport by 50 to 60 per cent. It is tempting to speculate that such an effect may decrease the availability of key precursors for acute-phase protein synthesis. Of considerable concern are other preclinical trials that have shown that the use of neutralizing antibodies to TNF-α worsen outcome.

Use of the IL-1 receptor antagonist may be another strategy that can be employed in septic patients. It binds to the IL-1 receptor with similar affinity as IL-1 but with no agonist activity. Pretreatment of animals made septic either by administering killed *Escherichia coli* or endotoxin attenuates hypotension and decreases mortality. These studies demonstrate that IL-1 blockade must be maintained for at least 24 hours for beneficial effects to occur. Preliminary studies indicate that treatment of septic animals with antibodies against IL-6 and IFN-γ may be useful. Using antibodies and receptor agonists synergistically may also be a worthwhile strategy. It is anticipated that researchers will eventually be able to selectively block the deleterious effects of excessive cytokines and preserve their beneficial effects.

Growth Factors

Specific growth factors that may promote healing have been implicated in a number of physiologic processes including growth, tissue repair, and regeneration. In burn patients, topical application of epidermal growth factor can accelerate the healing of donor sites. Likewise, studies in the 1970s demonstrated that short courses of growth hormone (GH) promoted nitrogen retention following thermal injury. More recently, the safety and efficacy of long-term exogenous recombinant GH administration has been demonstrated. Growth hormone stimulates protein synthesis during hypocaloric feedings and increases retention of sodium and potassium by the kidney. The potential synergistic effects of specialized nutrition in combination with GH may play a role in the management of the critically injured patient.

Other Methods of Modulating the Stress Response

Several other methods of modifying the physiologic and biochemical responses to injury have been studied in an effort to reduce the magnitude of the stress of operations and to provide insight into mechanisms that regulate these responses. A variety of human studies have shown that many postoperative responses can be ablated following denervation of the wound. These studies suggest that regional anesthetic techniques block afferent signals from the wound and interrupt sympathetic nervous efferent signals to the adrenal gland and possibly to the liver. Epidural anesthesia can suppress hyperglycemia and hypercortisolism and improve nitrogen balance. Large doses of morphine given prior to the skin incision have been shown to diminish the usual rise in plasma ACTH, cortisol, GH, and glucose in patients undergoing aortic valve replacement. These reports indicate that central nervous system blockade interrupts afferent signals stimulated by operative procedures.

Several investigators have studied stress responses in sympathectomized animals by blocking the efferent limb of the neuroendocrine reflex response. Propranolol has been shown to improve postoperative nitrogen balance and decrease muscle protein breakdown. Administration of propranolol to burned children decreased cardiac work without affecting wound healing or mortality. Cyclooxygenase inhibitors such as aspirin and ibuprofen attenuate the symptoms and endocrine responses that occur with critical illness without altering cytokine elaboration. For example, pretreat-ment with ibuprofen can attenuate the undesirable systemic symptoms associated with the inflammatory response. No doubt, patient care strategies in the future will use combination therapies designed to minimize the undesirable consequences of the body's response to critical illness and simultaneously accelerate wound healing, immune function, and recovery.

REFERENCES

Bessey PQ, Watters JM, Aoki TT, Wilmore DW: Combined hormonal infusion simulates the metabolic response to injury. Ann Surg 200:264, 1984.

Cannon WB: The Wisdom of the Body. New York, WW Norton and Company, 1939.

Cuthbertson DP: The disturbance of metabolism produced by bone and non-bony injury, with notes on certain abnormal conditions of bone. Biochem J 24:1244, 1930.

Fong Y, Lowry SF: Cytokines and the cellular response to injury and infection. In Wilmore DW et al (eds): Care of the Surgical Patient (Critical Care). Scientific American, 1992, Trauma Section, Chapter 7.

Jiang ZM, He GZ, Zhang SY, Wang XR, Yang NF, Zhu Y, Wilmore DW: Low-dose growth hormone and hypocaloric nutrition attenuate the protein catabolic response after major operation. Ann Surg 210:514, 1989.

Moore FD: The Metabolic Care of the Surgical Patient. Philadelphia, WB Saunders Company, 1959.

Souba WW: Glutamine: A key substrate for the splanchnic bed. Ann Nutrition 11:285–308, 1991.

Wilmore DW: The Metabolic Management of the Critically Ill. New York, Plenum Medical Book Company, 1977.

3

SHOCK: Causes and Management of Circulatory Collapse

PETER METRAKOS, M.D.   JONATHAN L. MEAKINS, M.D., D.Sc.

Shock is a clinical syndrome that occurs when tissues are inadequately perfused due to insufficient cardiovascular perfusion or increased metabolic demand. When the mismatch between cardiac output and metabolic requirements is great enough, the patient is said to be in shock, because the cardiovascular system does not adequately support the metabolic needs of the patient. Shock is not simply low blood pressure. Low blood pressure is hypotension, which may accompany the state of shock, but it is an insufficient criterion as a definition for shock. Classification and treatment begin with the recognition that the shock state may be present. The response to therapy is useful in determining the diagnostic classification, as similar findings may be present in all types of shock except for high-output septic shock and neurogenic shock.

HISTORY

The understanding of shock has largely followed observations made during war. Until the late 19th century, toxins were considered very important in the pathogenesis of shock. This was the reason that venesection (bleeding) was used as therapy prior to the mid-1800s. The significance of an altered intravascular volume became recognized at the beginning of this century, and low blood pressure was thought to be a cause of shock. Toxins were thought to be significant until World War II, when measurements of blood volume and its correction were recognized as crucial. The importance of volume replacement after trauma be-

came apparent in Korea with the high incidence of renal failure and its prevention. Later, in Vietnam, overly aggressive resuscitation lead to the discovery of adult respiratory distress syndrome, and improved resuscitation led to the saving of many lives that would have been otherwise lost. This then led to the description of clinical syndromes associated with multiple organ dysfunction or failure. Further descriptions of shock followed, including *hypovolemic, septic, cardiogenic,* and *neurogenic* shock with their variants.

CLASSIFICATION

Shock can be classified into two broad categories: (1) *decreased circulating volume* or *decreased preload,* and (2) *compromised cardiac function.* The three subgroups of shock within the context of decreased preload are *hypovolemic, septic,* and *neurogenic.* Within the category of compromised cardiac function, the two subgroups are *cardiac compressive shock* and *cardiogenic shock.* The expected findings in the different forms of shock are summarized in Table 1.

SHOCK DUE TO DECREASED PRELOAD

Hypovolemic Shock

The causes of hypovolemic shock can be hemorrhagic or nonhemorrhagic and include the loss of intravascular volume by internal or external hemor-

TABLE 1. CHARACTERISTICS OF SHOCK STATES*

	Cardiogenic Shock	Cardiac Compressive Shock	Hypovolemic or Traumatic Shock			Low-Output Septic Shock	High-Output Septic Shock	Neurogenic Shock
			Mild	Moderate	Severe			
Skin perfusion	Pale	Pale	Pale	Pale	Pale	Pale	Pink	Pink
Urine output	Low	Low	Normal	Low	Low	Low	Low	Low
Pulse rate	High	High	Normal	Normal	High	High	High	Low
Blood pressure	Normal	Low	Normal	Normal	Low	Low	Low	Low
Mental status	Anxious	Anxious	Normal	Thirsty	Anxious	Anxious	Anxious	Anxious
Neck veins	Distended	Distended	Flat	Flat	Flat	Flat	Flat	Flat
Oxygen consumption	Low	Low	Low	Low	Low	Low	Low	Low
Cardiac index	Low	Low	Low	Low	Low	Low	High	Low
Cardiac filling pressures	High	High	Low	Low	Low	Low	Low	Low
Systemic vascular resistance	High	High	High	High	High	High	Low	Low

*From Holcroft JW: Shock In Wilmore DW, Brennan MF, Harken AH, Holcroft JW, Meakins JL (eds): Care of the Surgical Patient, vol 1. Critical Care. A Publication of the Committee on Pre- and Postoperative Care, American College of Surgeons. New York, Scientific American, Inc, 1989, with permission.

rhage, by the loss of fluid into the alimentary tract, as in bowel obstruction; by dehydration secondary to vomiting or diarrhea; or by reactive fluid loss seen in patients with pancreatitis, trauma, and major burn.

Diagnosis: Clinical Evaluation

The signs and symptoms of hypovolemic shock depend on the degree of depletion of intravascular volume and its duration, and the compensatory reactions to hypovolemia, as manifested progressively by: (1) signs of adrenergic nerve discharge to the skin which will be pale, cold, and clammy; (2) oliguria; (3) hypotension and electrocardiographic (ECG) signs of myocardial ischemia; and (4) neurologic signs and symptoms. The clinical findings in shock correlate with its severity and the order in which the various involved organs are compromised following redistribution of blood flow. Flow to the skin is reduced first, then to the viscera and kidneys, and lastly flow to the heart and brain (Table 2).

Patients in *mild shock* have lost less than 20 per cent of the circulating blood volume and have adrenergic nerve discharge that constricts cutaneous blood vessels causing pale, cool skin. However, blood pressure remains normal in the supine position and urine output may be normal or decreased but with a high specific gravity. These patients also may complain of cold and thirst. When a patient has lost 20 to 40 per cent of the circulating blood volume, *moderate shock* is present accompanied by oliguria and often restlessness. Blood pressure in the supine position usually is not reduced, although a postural drop is expected. *Severe shock* is present when more than 40 per cent of the blood volume has been lost. Patients in this state have decreased urinary output, decreased blood pressure,

possible ECG changes consistent with myocardial ischemia, and are usually agitated, restless, or obtunded solely on the basis of hypovolemia. Older patients show more myocardial ischemia, whereas younger patients show central nervous system changes.

Patients with evidence of adrenergic discharge to the skin, indicating mild shock, require careful attention to detect progressing hypovolemia. The most sensitive indicator of intravascular volume is urinary output, making insertion of an indwelling catheter necessary for reliable monitoring. Serial hematocrits should be done. Adequate fluid resuscitation sufficient to restore organ perfusion, urinary output, and blood pressure have a dilutional effect on the hematocrit. Therefore, as the patient is resuscitated with fluids the hematocrit falls. Postural blood pressures should be followed

TABLE 2. STAGES OF HYPOVOLEMIC SHOCK*

Peripheral venous constriction
 Poor capillary filling
  Pallor
   Peripheral cooling
    Oliguria
     Increased pulse rate
      Thirst
       Increased respiratory rate
        Hypotension
         Trunk cooling
          Agitation
           Decreased pain sensation
            Loss of deep tendon reflexes
            Acidotic breathing
             Deep pallor
              Loss of consciousness
               Death

*From Holcroft JW, Trunkey DD. Shock. In Polk IIC Jr, Stone IIII, Gardner B (eds): Basic Surgery. Norwalk, CT, Appleton-Century-Crofts, 1983, with permission.

carefully, and a decrease of the systolic blood pressure of 10 mm Hg or more lasting 30 seconds or longer indicates hypovolemia.

Patients who are inebriated with alcohol may not have the pale cool skin from adrenergic discharge or a decrease in urinary output. Alcohol induces a generalized vasodilation that can override the effects of the adrenergic nervous system and also inhibits vasopressin secretion, allowing a hypovolemic patient to maintain a good urinary output. Because of the generalized vasodilation of alcoholic intoxication, these patients may experience a fall in blood pressure with only mild to moderate shock.

A traumatized patient with altered mental status should be assessed for hypovolemia even if there is obvious head injury. Correction of the hypovolemia often corrects the abnormalities in mental status. Hemodynamic instability should not be ascribed to a head injury, as most patients with head injuries and hypotension are hypotensive because they are hypovolemic and should be thoroughly examined for sites of hemorrhage.

Treatment

The principles in the treatment of hypovolemic shock are the same whether the shock is due to volume losses of hemorrhagic or nonhemorrhagic origin. The most common form of shock seen by surgeons is hypovolemic shock due to hemorrhage from the gastrointestinal tract or trauma. The principles apply to fluid loss from the gastrointestinal tract, pancreatitis, a burn wound, or any cause of hypovolemia.

Airway and breathing problems should be addressed first to ensure adequate ventilation and oxygenation. Once intravenous lines are inserted and fluid resuscitation is well underway, hemorrhagic shock is best treated by identifying the source of bleeding and taking the appropriate action for its control. External bleeding can usually be controlled with external compression, but internal bleeding usually requires surgical control.

Fluid Resuscitation

Volume loss must be corrected immediately once the diagnosis has been made. Intravenous fluid should be administered simultaneously as preparations are made to control the bleeding. Intravenous fluids are best given through large-bore catheters (16-gauge or larger) placed percutaneously in a peripheral or central vein. On occasion in severe hypovolemia, a saphenous vein cutdown at the ankle is required. A crystalloid solution with an electrolyte composition approximating that of plasma should be used for the initial resuscitation of patients with all forms of shock except car-

diogenic shock. Most centers use lactated Ringer's solution, but the solution can be acetated Ringer's or normal saline supplemented with an ampule of bicarbonate for each liter. The lactate, acetate, or bicarbonate buffers the hydrogen ion that leaves the tissues when perfusion is reestablished (*reperfusion*). To replace blood loss, crystalloid solutions should be given in a ratio of 3:1 or 4:1 with packed cells because they quickly equilibrate within the interstitial and intravascular spaces.

Colloid solutions such as albumin, hydroxyethyl starch, or dextran compounds may be useful when it is impossible to infuse large amounts of resuscitative fluids. Colloid solutions provide a larger intravascular expansion than the equivalent amount of isotonic crystalloid, but the effect of the colloid is transient because severe shock is accompanied by disruption of the microvascular endothelium. Colloid leaks out of the vascular space into the interstitium within 1 or 2 hours, and the fluids are also in the interstitium. Albumin should not be used, and glucose should not be given with crystalloid unless the patient is thought to be in hypoglycemic shock from an insulin reaction. Rapid administration of glucose, even as a 5 per cent solution, can induce an osmotic diuresis, compounding the basic intravascular depletion and confusing the clinical management by eliminating urinary output as an index of the adequacy of resuscitation.

Administration of fluid helps resuscitate patients in hemorrhagic shock but also serves as a diagnostic test to detect continuing bleeding. Two to 3 L of fluid given over 5 to 15 minutes resuscitates patients with arrested hemorrhage, and the need for administration of more fluid indicates continuing bleeding. Such hemorrhage usually requires surgical control.

If the patient is to be taken to the operating room soon, administration of blood should be withheld if possible until just before the induction of anesthesia. A young patient can tolerate hematocrits as low as 15, as long as the blood volume is kept normal by the administration of fluid. If blood is administered prematurely, before surgical control of the hemorrhage, at least a portion of it will be lost through bleeding. Rapid replacement after control of hemorrhage with the freshest blood available leads to the most efficient use of blood products and the least risk of transfusion complications.

At times, blood must be given before surgical intervention, and fully cross-matched blood is optimal. Type-specific blood, which can be obtained within a few minutes from most blood banks, may be given if cross-matched blood is not available or if the urgency dictates, as it has a negligible risk of transfusion reaction in the massively injured patient. These patients have little of their own blood remaining in the vascular space after resuscitation, and clinically evident reactions are rare. If type-specific blood is not available, O-negative blood can be given. However, its administration depletes a valuable blood bank resource that is better used in obstetric bleeding. Administration of more than 3 U complicates typing of blood after the initial resuscitation. A hematocrit of 20 per cent after resuscitation is usually adequate if control of hemorrhage is assured, although the generally accepted level is 25 per cent. Patients with coronary artery disease should be transfused to hematocrits of approximately 30 to 35 per cent, because their hearts do not have the reserve to tolerate even transient episodes of ischemia.

When faced with traumatic shock, temporary measures include pneumatic antishock trousers at the scene or in the emergency room. The antishock trousers are controversial, and their use should probably be restricted to immobilization of pelvic fractures to help control hemorrhage. Occlusion of the descending thoracic aorta through an anterolateral thoracotomy is occasionally useful in the resuscitation of patients with very serious hemorrhage from abdominal or pelvic injuries. The occlusion should be brief and no longer than 15 minutes to avoid spinal cord and renal damage.

Nonhemorrhagic hypovolemic shock is treated with the same goals as those for hemorrhagic shock, except that blood transfusion is usually not necessary. In true hypovolemic shock, the kidneys are the preferred organs to monitor as an indicator of vital organ perfusion. A urinary output of between 0.5 and 1 ml/kg/hr ensures that resuscitation is adequate, but less is an indication of circulatory inadequacy and the need for infusion of more volume. If volume requirements appear excessive or coexistent medical conditions are present, a Swan-Ganz catheter should be placed in the pulmonary artery to determine left-sided filling pressures. If low, the pulmonary artery wedge pressure should be raised gradually by infusion of balanced salt crystalloid to 13 to 15 mm Hg, with the effect on cardiac output and urinary output continuously monitored.

Septic Shock

Sepsis is defined as clinical evidence of infection and of a systemic response to the infection (including tachypnea, hyperthermia, and leukocytosis), together with insufficient cardiovascular support and increased metabolic demands. Septic shock has become a growing clinical problem, and its incidence has increased 20-fold over the past 25 years. Any organism capable of being a pathogen can cause septic shock, and gram-negative rods are the most frequent cause. It is also possible to have a septic shock–like state without infection.

Diagnosis

The clinical hemodynamic syndrome associated with septic shock is not constant. Patients may have either a high cardiac output (*hyperdynamic*) or a low cardiac output (*hypodynamic*) state. Systemic infection can lead to a state of septic shock with initial manifestations of hyperventilation, respiratory alkalosis, and warm and dry extremities caused by diversion of blood flow to the skin through the opening of cutaneous arteriovenous shunts because of the body's attempt to dissipate heat. This diversion causes a decreased blood flow to other parts of the body, including the kidneys, and patients become oliguric. The circulatory system is unable to hold volume within the vascular space, and hypovolemia follows. Because of the hypovolemia and hypermetabolism, the cardiovascular system enters into a hyperdynamic state, with the cardiac output being at least doubled and systemic vascular resistance falling as a result of the peripheral vasodilation. This is termed *early* or *high-output septic shock.*

As the septic shock progresses, usually by lack of recognition, hypoperfusion of the vital organs causes blood to be diverted from the skin and subcutaneous tissue to the vital organs, causing a decrease in skin temperature, which patients perceive as cold and which produces shaking chills. This vasoconstriction, which is required to maintain blood pressure and splanchnic perfusion, compromises the body's ability to dissipate heat and leads to another rapid rise in body temperature. In the terminal phase of sepsis, inflammatory mediators disrupt the microvascular endothelium, leading to hypovolemia and a marked decrease in the cardiac output (i.e., low-output or late septic shock).

Treatment

Early recognition of sepsis and definitive treatment of the infection is essential with administration of appropriate antibiotics and surgical drainage. Gram-negative bacteria most commonly cause septic shock. Circulatory resuscitation must be prompt, and large volumes of fluid may be needed to correct the hypovolemia causing shock and hypotension. At this time, the patient should be placed in a monitored bed with a Swan-Ganz catheter to monitor filling pressures and cardiac output. Adequate oxygen delivery is essential. The two components that need to be maximized to achieve clinical success are maintenance of a proper blood oxygen content and cardiac output. To maximize oxygen content, blood should be given to maintain the hemoglobin at approximately 12 gm and the oxygen saturation should approach 100 per cent, utilizing mechanical ventilation if necessary. After maximizing the oxygen content, if the desired oxygen delivery is not achieved, the cardiac output can be increased by the use of inotropic agents, such as dopamine or dobutamine. Oxygen delivery to the tissues is a function of hemoglobin, oxygen content, and cardiac output.

Cytokine Response

The endocrine response to injury has been well described and includes increased levels of catecholamines and glucocorticoids. Recently, certain protein mediators, *cytokines*, have been identified that appear to have a significant role in the cardiovascular response and in metabolic alterations to injury and infection. It is also likely that the acute exaggerated production of some cytokines may generate the hemodynamic manifestations of septic shock and that excessive chronic production may be responsible for the debilitating tissue wasting of cachexia. A large number of cytokines have been identified, and the number is increasing daily. The five cytokines that have been studied most extensively include tumor necrosis factor-α (TNF-α), interleukin-1 (IL-1), interleukin-2 (IL-2), interleukin-6 (IL-6), and interferon-γ (IFN).

Tumor necrosis factor-α exerts potent effects on metabolism that promote mobilization of nitrogenous and carbonaceous substrates from peripheral muscle, inducing peripheral wasting and mobilizing lipid stores for transport to splanchnic tissues, where the synthesis of hepatic proteins with roles as protease inhibitors, local immune modulators, and scavengers for trace minerals and free radicals are important in the response to injury and/or infection. A sudden increase in the secretion of TNF-α may be responsible, in part, for the clinical setting of collapse, shock, and death in the patient with severe infection.

As with TNF-α, IL-1 induces skeletal muscle wasting in vivo and is a principal inducer of hepatic acute-phase proteins, which are important in immune and coagulation functions. IL-2 is predominantly an immunostimulant that induces T-cell proliferation in vitro, and these effects may be protective in the injured patient.

IL-6 has two functions, the first being that of immunostimulation, as it enhances differentiation of lymphocytes, stimulates proliferation of B cells and the production of immunoglobulins by these cells, and activates T cells. It also has been identified as an interferon with the ability to induce an antiviral state. The second function is enhancement after injury of acute-phase protein synthesis (C-reactive protein, serum amyloid A, fibrinogen, antitrypsin, A1-antichymotrypsin, and haptoglobin).

The principal effect of IFN is immunologic. It also has antiviral activity and provides some protection against bacteria, fungi, and parasites.

Cytokines are produced by cells of both myeloid and nonmyeloid origin. For example, TNF-α can be produced by pulmonary macrophages, Kupffer cells, peritoneal macrophages, and endothelial cells. The ability of many different tissues to make cytokines is an important characteristic that differentiates cytokine mediators from the classic hormones. This means that cytokines produced locally can exert an autocrine and paracrine influence. There is also evidence that cytokine production is increased at tissue sites near the injury. This local production of cytokines may be clinically more important than absolute cytokine serum levels, as these levels generally correlate poorly with the clinical outcome.

The release of cytokines may involve a cascade, as cytokines are potent stimuli for the release of other mediators. In a primate model of bacteremia, administration of antibodies specific for TNF-α can block the release of classic hormones such as cortisol and epinephrine, as well as the release of cytokines IL-1B and IL-6. Release of an early mediator such as TNF-α apparently triggers the release of the complete complement of cytokines that combine to elicit the host responses.

As knowledge of the effects of this cytokine cascade increases, the possibility of modulating the cytokine response to injury may evolve. This ability may allow for the beneficial qualities to be enhanced and the detrimental effects to be reduced. Thus far, five strategies have been employed: (1) preventing injurious stimuli from reaching the sources of cytokine production, (2) decreasing cytokine production, (3) neutralizing cytokines, (4) increasing cytokine clearance, and (5) modulating effector cell responses to cytokines(s).

When a pathologic process or injury is present, the most important part of the treatment plan is removal of the source of injury. Traditional treatments of excision, drainage, and antibiotic administration for abscesses or excision of tumors abolish noxious stimuli that can elicit or propagate a host cytokine response. Removal of the noxious stimuli (source control) often reverses the hypermetabolic state associated with the injury infection. In clinical infections, toxins released even from killed bacteria may cause a cytokine response sufficient to produce a detrimental biologic response. Lipopolysaccharide (LPS), one of the most potent bacterial toxins, is an important trigger of the cytokine cascade. Prophylactic administration of antibodies to LPS not only attenuates cytokine responses, but also reduces the mortality from subsequent experimental bacterial infection. Two prospective, randomized clinical trials using these antibodies to treat severe infection have suggested some efficacy.

An attractive approach is to neutralize the cytokines, and this can be done by using anticytokine antibodies or by the use of natural cytokine antagonists. Neutralizing antibodies have been produced for many of the cytokines, but those for TNF-α have been the most extensively tested for their role in treating septic shock. Anti–TNF-α antibodies have been shown to be protective in rodents, rabbits, and primates against mortality during overwhelming bacteremia. The major obstacle with this therapy is that the cytokine antibodies are likely to be administered after the physiologic effects of cytokines have already begun. It is necessary to determine the amount of time after initiation of the mediator cascade that the delivery of cytokine antibodies can affect clinical outcome and whether beneficial effects can also be blocked. Blockade of cytokine-soluble receptors and binding proteins may achieve the effect of cytokine antibodies. These proteins are natural inhibitors of cytokine activity by competing with cell surface receptors for the binding of cytokines. TNF-α and IL-1 receptor antagonists are the best characterized of these proteins. Whether such agents are important clinically is the subject of much current and intensive research.

Neurogenic Shock

Neurogenic shock is caused by the loss of vasomotor control that can cause a severalfold expansion of the venous capacitance bed with peripheral pooling and inadequate ventricular filling. They, in a sense, bleed into their intravascular space.

Diagnosis

The shock state produced is similar to that in patients with warm septic shock. The skin is pink, warm, and well perfused. The blood pressure is low and urinary output is low to normal. The heart rate is usually rapid but may be slow when the adrenergic nerves to the heart are blocked. A patient with this clinical presentation with evidence of neurologic injury, or known to have had a regional anesthetic agent or an autonomic nerve blocker, can be diagnosed as having neurogenic shock. Heat loss in these patients can be a major problem, and many patients are hypothermic on initial presentation.

Treatment

The therapy is directed toward restoration of cardiac filling by infusing balanced saline solution. If the patient does not respond appropriately to fluid resuscitation, a vasoconstrictor should be given to restore venous tone, ventricular diastolic volumes, and cardiac output.

SHOCK DUE TO COMPROMISED CARDIAC FUNCTION

The etiology of shock in this group involves the heart and is classified under two headings either cardiac compressive shock or cardiogenic shock. Distended neck veins are characteristic in these patients. The nature of compromised cardiac function must be identified because treatment requires different interventions.

Cardiac Compressive Shock

Cardiac compressive shock usually occurs in injured patients but can develop in noninjured patients with abdominal distention and diaphragmatic elevation, in those on positive-pressure ventilation, or in those developing tamponade secondary to infection, or with uremia or malignancy. A central venous pressure or right atrial pressure of 15 cm H_2O or more, measured at end-expiration with the patient breathing spontaneously, excludes pure hypovolemic, traumatic, septic, and neurogenic shock and confirms the presence of either cardiogenic or cardiac compressive shock with an increased preload.

While distended neck veins can confirm cardiac compressive shock, their absence does not exclude it, because the patient may simultaneously be hypovolemic. If cardiac compressive shock is present, the neck veins do not remain flat for long due to the hypovolemia, as all trauma patients in shock should be given a fluid bolus of 30 ml/kg as part of the initial therapy.

Treatment

The treatment of cardiac compressive shock consists of fluid administration to increase ventricular filling pressures and correction of the underlying mechanical cause of shock. In a traumatized patient, the cause is usually hemorrhagic tamponade or a tension pneumothorax. A tension pneumothorax should be decompressed either by the immediate insertion of a chest tube or a 14-gauge needle in the second intercostal space in the midclavicular line. Acute pericardial tamponade in an unstable patient should be treated by a left anterolateral thoracotomy, with decompression of the tamponade and surgical control of the underlying problem. In a stable patient (traumatized or not), a pericardiocentesis is performed by inserting a needle to the left of the xiphoid process and directing it longitudinally upward and posteriorly, at a 45-degree angle, toward the vertebral column with removal of the pericardial fluid. When blood is encountered, it should also be aspirated. Withdrawal of 50 ml of blood or fluid should return cardiovascular dynamics toward

Rx
1. heart rate (arrhythmia)
2. filling pressures (NS or furosemide)
3. ↓ SVR (nitroglycerin or N-pusside)
4. maximize contractility (dobutamine)
β-blocker if mI (esmolol)
?intra-aortic balloon pump

normal. Failure of the patient to respond after 50 ml has been aspirated suggests that the blood was withdrawn from the heart rather than the pericardial sac. Nonbloody fluid should be sent for culture and cytology.

The treatment of cardiac compression caused by mechanical ventilation requires volume expansion combined with adjustment of the ventilator. In patients with a Swan-Ganz catheter, fluid resuscitation and ventilator adjustments should be treated to produce the highest cardiac output with the lowest filling pressures and the least compromise of pulmonary support.

Cardiogenic Shock

Cardiogenic shock is defined as shock arising from primary cardiac causes that include arrhythmias, myocardial failure (most often following myocardial infarction), valvular dysfunction, and elevated pulmonary or systemic arterial resistance.

Diagnosis

Patients in cardiogenic shock present with distended neck veins and a positive hepatojugular reflex and, frequently, orthopnea, dyspnea, and anxiety. Placement of a Swan-Ganz catheter is likely to produce decreased cardiac index with normal filling pressures. If the cardiac index is decreased along with decreased filling pressures, the diagnosis of cardiogenic shock should only be made after the filling pressures are optimized and the cardiac index remains low. The clinical findings of cardiogenic shock are associated with discharge of the sympathetic adrenergic nervous system and the release of angiotensin and vasopressin. These findings include pale, cool skin and low urinary output, and in severe cases, the systemic arterial blood pressure is also low. If the right heart is failing, the neck veins are distended, whereas with left heart failure, rales and a gallop rhythm are present. If chronic heart failure is present, the heart is enlarged.

Treatment

Treatment should proceed with the identification and correction of hemodynamically compromising arrhythmias, with optimization of the filling pressure and reduction of elevated vascular resistance. Myocardial contractility should be maximized with a reduction in excessive myocardial oxygen consumption. Mechanical assistance to the heart and/or operative correction of anatomic abnormalities may be required.

Optimization of the heart rate is the first treatment of cardiogenic shock, and this varies with age and status of the coronary arteries. A rapid heart rate is tolerated in young patients with compliant large arteries and minimal myocardial oxygen demands, but may not be tolerated in older patients, especially those with stenotic coronary artery disease. The limited time for perfusion of the coronary arteries with a rapid heart rate in a patient with coronary artery disease may be a significant problem. A patient with normal coronary arteries can maintain a heart rate equal to the difference of 220 and the patient's age in years multiplied by three fourths, for an indefinite period of time. In the presence of coronary artery disease, the rate should not exceed this number minus 30. The definitive test for assessing whether the heart rate is too fast is observation for signs or symptoms of ischemia.

Life-threatening bradycardias should be cardioverted, and more stable patients should be treated with chronotropic agents. All tachyarrhythmias that create hemodynamic instability should be cardioverted. If a patient with a tachyarrhythmia is stable, a full 12-lead ECG should be done to further characterize the arrhythmia (Fig. 1).

If cardiogenic shock persists after correction of the ventricular rate and arrhythmias, the next therapeutic maneuver is to optimize the ventricular end-diastolic volumes. The optimal ventricular end-diastolic volume is determined by monitoring the responses of the heart to alterations in filling pressure. The end-diastolic volume can be either increased by infusing a balanced salt solution or decreased by administering furosemide for diuresis. Frequently, optimal filling pressures are neither obvious nor consistent, and change as the problem resolves or progresses.

Once the heart rate and filling pressures have been optimized, attention is given to reduction of the elevated vascular resistance usually present. An isoproterenol drip can be used, but caution should be exercised due to secondary tachycardia and arrhythmias. If filling pressures are normal or elevated, a nitroglycerin drip can be used, dilating the vessels responsible for systemic resistance, as well as the venules and small veins. If nitroglycerin is not successful or the filling pressures are low to normal at the beginning, a sodium nitroprusside drip can be begun, as it exerts its maximal effect on the systemic arterioles. However, it breaks down to thiocyanate and cyanide, and these levels should be measured periodically when therapy is prolonged.

Obstruction of the pulmonary vasculature by an embolus, tension pneumothorax, or by large tidal volume positive-pressure ventilation can produce right-sided cardiac failure. The treatment is directed toward the underlying mechanical problem; that is, anticoagulation, lytic therapy or, rarely, pulmonary embolectomy or insertion of a chest tube for tension pneumothorax. Adjustment of the ventilator for

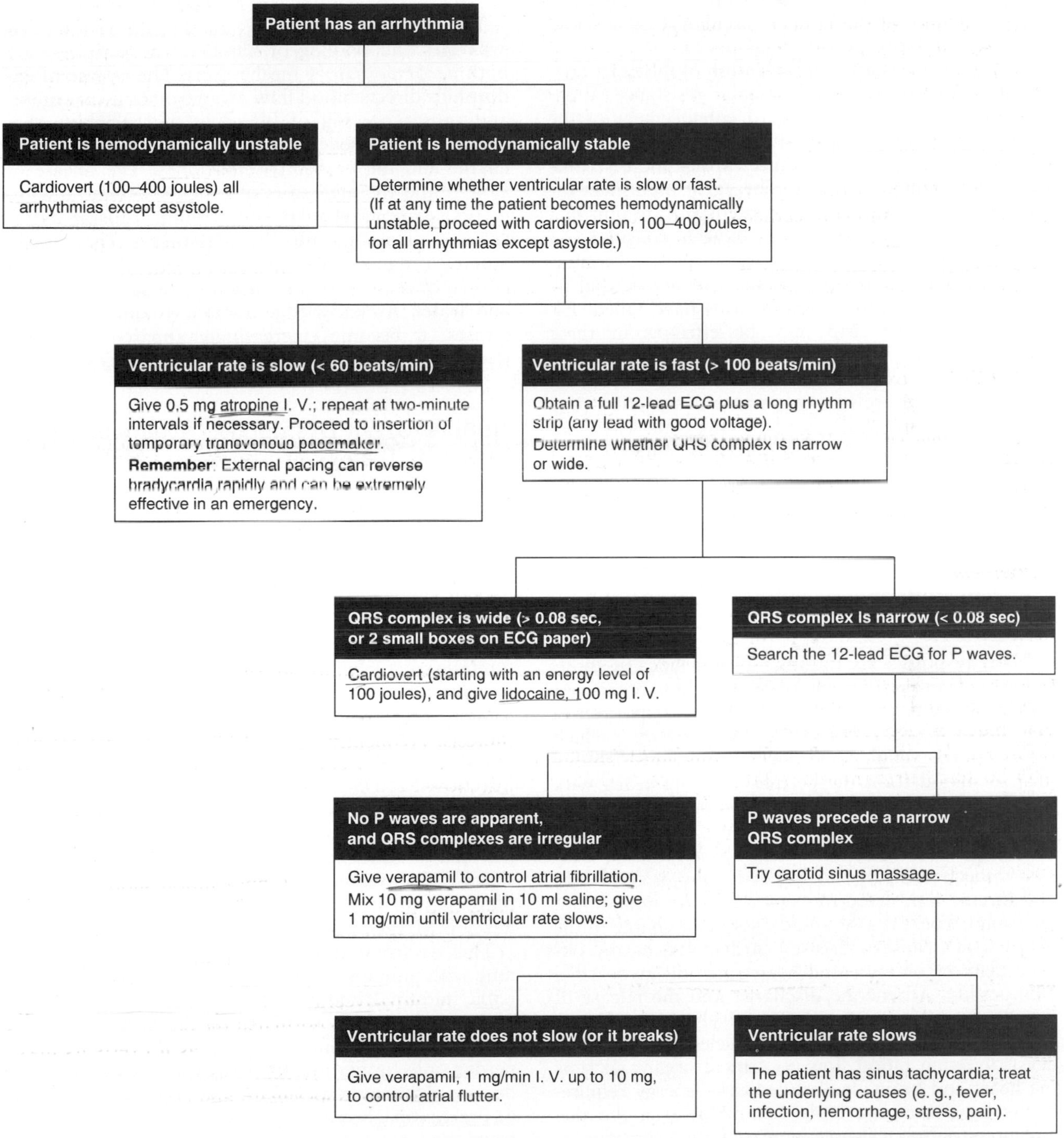

Figure 1. Algorithm for treatment of arrhythmias. (From Harken AH: Cardiac arrhythmias. *In* Wilmore DW, Brennan MF, Harken AH, Holcroft JW, Meakins JL [eds]: Care of the Surgical Patient, vol 1. Critical Care. A Publication of the Committee on Pre- and Postoperative Care, American College of Surgeons. New York, Scientific American, Inc, 1989, with permission.)

compression of the pulmonary vasculature by positive-pressure ventilation is also necessary.

If shock persists after optimization of the heart rate, end-diastolic volumes, and vascular resistance, attention should be directed toward enhancement of the myocardial contractility by inotropic agents. The goal of this approach is to maximize cardiac indices while minimizing filling pressures. The agent used most often in surgical patients in the intensive care unit is a *dobutamine drip*. Myocardial oxygen consumption should be reduced by a β-blocker in patients continuing with symptoms or ECG signs of myocardial ischemia after the other interventions have failed. Esmolol used as a drip may be effective in these situations.

Mechanical circulatory assistance can be helpful in patients with severe left ventricular dysfunction. Use of an intra-aortic balloon pump augments coronary filling and increases cardiac output in patients with cardiogenic shock.

RESPONSE TO SHOCK

Compensatory and Decompensatory Mechanisms

Many responses are initiated during shock in an attempt to maintain perfusion of important organ systems required to maintain life. The most important of these mechanisms is the *adrenergic discharge*, which constricts the venules and small veins with displacement of blood from the periphery to the heart, with increases in end-diastolic volume, stroke volume, the cardiac index, and delivery of oxygen to tissues. This same adrenergic discharge also promotes a decompensatory mechanism by causing distention of capillaries and forcing fluid from the vascular space into the interstitium. There is also an adrenergic discharge to the heart, which causes increased cardiac indices and oxygen delivery by increased heart rate and myocardial contractility. Adrenergic discharge and the release of vasopressin and angiotensin selectively constrict arterioles in the skin, fat, skeletal muscles, gut, and kidneys, diverting blood flow to critical organs such as the heart and brain. It also decreases energy requirements by conserving body heat. However, the disadvantage is that it causes increased input impedances with hindrance of ventricular emptying.

The release of aldosterone and vasopressin stimulates the kidneys to conserve salt and water from the glomerular filtrate. The release of epinephrine, cortisol, and glucagon increases the extracellular glucose concentration, and extracellular osmolality draws water from the intracellular space to the extracellular space.

The release of endorphins dilating the venules and arterioles and pooling of blood in the periphery are both *decompensatory* mechanisms. The release of endorphins directs blood flow away from critical organs, and causes pooling of blood in the periphery that counteracts the beneficial effects of the adrenergic discharge and the vasoactive hormones. The release of TNF-α and the mediators of coagulation and inflammation disrupts venular endothelium, causing extravasation of plasma into the interstitium. These mediators also damage the function of the cell membrane with intracellular sequestration of sodium, chloride, and water. As knowledge about cytokine release increases, it becomes increasingly apparent that this release produces major adverse consequences.

Multiple Organ Dysfunction Syndrome and Molecular Biology of Shock

The immediate goal in treating shock is the restoration of hemodynamic stability, and often this resuscitation is only the beginning of the patient's illness. Some survivors of resuscitation may succumb subsequently to the serial dysfunction and/or failure of multiple organ systems despite aggressive medical and surgical intervention. This organ failure, once termed multiple organ failure (MOF) or multiple organ system failure (MOSF), is now termed *multiple organ dysfunction syndrome* (MODS). It has become the major cause of death in critically ill patients. Although initially proposed as a sign of occult or uncontrolled infection, MODS has been documented to occur after a number of diverse noninfective clinical conditions, including mechanical and thermal trauma, severe hematomas, ischemic reperfusion, pancreatitis, and shock. Whatever the etiology of the injury, if the condition is sufficiently severe or persists, the patient may develop MODS.

This syndrome follows a predictable course, beginning with pulmonary dysfunction and followed by hepatic, intestinal, and renal failure, usually in this order and none of which is related to the primary disease process. These patients are hypermetabolic, with a hyperdynamic circulation, increased cardiac output, and decreased systemic vascular resistance. As the number of organs that become dysfunctional or fail increases from one to four, the mortality progressively increases from 30 per cent to 100 per cent. There is a lag phase of days to weeks between the initial inciting events and the development of organ dysfunction. Although there is lack of consensus on the definition of organ dysfunction, some general guidelines concerning the time and the magnitude of the problem are shown in Table 3.

The cytokine response for MODS is the same as that

TABLE 3. RECOGNITION AND ASSESSMENT OF ORGAN SYSTEM DYSFUNCTION*

Organ System	Indicators of Dysfunction	Degree of Dysfunction		
		Mild	*Moderate*	*Severe*
Respiratory	PaO_2, FIO_2, PaO_2/FIO_2 PEEP, number of days on ventilator, peak airway pressure, use of high-frequency ventilation or ECMO	PaO_2/FIO_2 >250	PaO_2/FIO_2 150–250	PaO_2/FIO_2 <150
Renal	Creatinine level, creatinine clearance, BUN, need for dialysis to regulate serum potassium and bicarbonate	Creatinine < 150 μmol/L	Creatinine 150–300 μmol/L	Creatinine > 300 μmol/L; need for dialysis
Hepatic	Bilirubin, albumin, cholesterol, ALT, AST, γ-glutamyltransferase, alkaline phosphatase, ammonia	Bilirubin < 30 μmol/L	Bilirubin 30–80 μmol/L; elevation of transaminases or alkaline phosphatase to >2 times normal values	Bilirubin > 80 μmol/L; elevation of serum ammonia
Gastrointestinal	Stress-related mucosal ulceration and bleeding, mucosal acidosis, failure of pH regulation, volume of NG drainage, ileus, diarrhea, intolerance of enteral feeding, acalculous cholecystitis, pancreatitis	NG drainage < 30 ml/24 hr; diarrhea in response to enteral feeding	NG drainage 300–1000 ml/ 24 hr; visible blood in drainage fluid	NG drainage > 1000 ml/24 hr; upper GI bleeding necessitating transfusion, acalculous cholecystitis, pancreatitis
Cardiac	Supraventricular arrhythmias, elevated PAWP and mean pulmonary arterial pressure, reduced ventricular stroke work index, requirement for inotropes or vasopressors to maintain adequate mean arterial pressure	Development of supraventricular tachycardias with HR < 140 beats/min and no fall in mean arterial pressure	PAWP 16–20 mm Hg; requirement for dopamine or dobutamine at dosage of < 10 μg/kg/min to maintain satisfactory cardiac output and PAWP	Requirement for vasopressors (e.g., dopamine, epinephrine, norepinephrine, phenylephrine) to maintain mean arterial pressure >80 mm Hg
Central nervous system	Glasgow Coma Scale score, especially on components reflecting level of consciousness	Glasgow Coma Scale score 13–14	Glasgow Coma Scale score 10–12	Glasgow Coma Scale score ≤ 9
Hematologic	Thrombocytopenia, elevated PT and PTT elevated fibrin degradation products	Platelet count > 60,000/mm³	Platelet count 20,000– 60,000/mm³; mild elevation of PT or PTT in absence of anticoagulation	Platelet count < 20,000/mm³, DIC
Metabolic/ endocrine	Insulin requirements, levels of T_4 and reverse T_3	Insulin requirements ≤ 1 U/ hr	Insulin requirements 2–4 U/hr	Insulin requirements ≥ 5 U/hr

Table continued

TABLE 3. RECOGNITION AND ASSESSMENT OF ORGAN SYSTEM DYSFUNCTION* (*Continued*)

Organ System	Indicators of Dysfunction	Degree of Dysfunction		
		Mild	*Moderate*	*Severe*
Immunologic	Impaired DTH responsiveness, reduced in vitro lymphocyte proliferation, infection with ICU pathogens (e.g., *S. epidermidis*, *Candida*, *Pseudomonas*, enterococci)	Reduced DTH reactivity	Cutaneous anergy	Cutaneous anergy, recurrent infection with ICU pathogens
Wound healing	Wound infection, impaired formation of granulation tissue, wound dehiscence	Wound infection	Impaired formation of granulation tissue	Decubitus ulcers, wound dehiscence

*From Marshall JC, Meakins JL: Multiorgan failure. *In* Wilmore DW, Brennan MF, Harken AH, Holcroft JW, Meakins JL (eds): Care of the Surgical Patient, vol 1. Critical Care. A Publication of the Committee on Pre- and Postoperative Care, American College of Surgeons. New York, Scientific American, Inc, 1989, with permission.

Abbreviations: ECMO = extracorporeal membrane oxygenation, ALT = alanine aminotransferase, AST = aspartate aminotransferase, BUN = blood urea nitrogen, NG = nasogastric, PAWP = pulmonary arterial wedge pressure, PT = prothrombin time, PTT = partial thromboplastin time, HR = heart rate, ICU = intensive care unit.

for septic shock. MODS appears to be an uncontrolled inflammatory response that activates multiple inflammatory effector cells, including macrophages, neutrophils, and lymphocytes, and the humoral protein cascades such as the coagulation, complement, prostaglandin, kinin, and cytokine systems.

The best treatment for MODS is prevention. Therefore, each component, including infection, inadequate tissue perfusion, and a persistent inflammatory state, should be treated aggressively. Early definitive surgical intervention with the removal of necrotic tissue, the drainage of abscesses, and the control of peritoneal soilage is often effective in preventing intensification of MODS. Further treatment is primarily supportive and includes fluid and electrolyte therapy, nutrition support, mechanical ventilation, hemodialysis, and the use of inotropic and pressor agents. Further options presently under investigation include the use of agents that block endotoxin and/or the cytokines, antioxidants, and monoclonal antibodies directed at neutrophils.

At the cellular and molecular levels, an injury is the stimulus that initiates a series of events leading to the synthesis of certain proteins. Mediators and modulators are released by a variety of cells in response to the injury. These mediators bind to cellular receptors, and through a process termed *signal transduction* certain genes are expressed by synthesizing corresponding proteins. These proteins are secreted into the circulation and affect sites other than where they were synthesized. Many patterns of stress gene expression have been identified; principally, the hepatic acute-phase response and the heat shock response.

The *acute-phase reactants* are proteins synthesized in the liver and secreted into the bloodstream to protect the organism from the cause of shock or the consequences of shock and resuscitation. Examples of acute-phase proteins include the procoagulant fibrinogen, which is usually double the normal plasma concentration within 3 to 4 days after injury, and plasma proteinase inhibitors (e.g., A1-chymotrypsin), which modulate the destructive effects of neutrophil-derived or other proteinases that are elevated three- to fivefold within days of injury.

The *heat shock response* is a conserved cellular response to selected environmental stresses, including hypoxia and reoxygenation, which is exactly what happens with shock. The decreased tissue perfusion that occurs with shock corresponds to a state of hypoxia at the cellular level and a state of reoxygenation when the resuscitation occurs. The heat shock gene expression includes the synthesis of new mRNA coding for about 30 new proteins that constitutes an intracellular salvage and repair mechanism for damaged macromolecules and is fundamental to intracellular homeostasis during physiologic stress. In contrast to the liver-specific acute-phase genes, changes in expression of heat shock genes occur in many organs that have sustained severe metabolic stress. Also contrary to the acute-phase genes, hepatic expression of the genes of major heat shock has not been observed universally in response to shock.

REFERENCES

Holcroft JW, Blaisdell FW: Shock. *In* Sabiston DC Jr (ed): Textbook of Surgery: The Biological Basis of Modern Surgical Practice, ed 14. Philadelphia. WB Saunders Company, 1991, pp 34–56.

Shires GT, Cunningham JN, Backer CRF, Reeder SF, Illner H, Wagner IY, Maher J: Alterations in cellular membrane function during hemorrhagic shock in primates. Ann Surg *176*:288, 1972.

Simeone FA: Shock, trauma, and the surgeon. Ann Surg *158*:759, 1963.

Wiggers CJ: Physiology of Shock. New York, Commonwealth Fund Publications, 1950.

Wilmore DW, Brennan MF, Harken AH, Holcroft JW, Meakins JL (eds): Care of the Surgical Patient, vol 1. Critical Care, A Publication of the Committee on Pre- and Postoperative Care, American College of Surgeons. New York, Scientific American, Inc, 1989.

4

MANAGEMENT OF FLUID AND ELECTROLYTES

G. Tom Shires, III, M.D.

Management of fluid and electrolyte abnormalities is a fundamental aspect of medicine. In health, fluid and electrolyte homeostasis is achieved by a balance of oral intake and the sum of renal, gastrointestinal, and insensible losses. Surgical illnesses, in particular, profoundly disrupt this ability to defend the status quo by impairing oral intake, producing pathologic external losses, and by deranging the internal distribution of water and solute between body compartments. Consequently, the approach to fluid and electrolyte management of the surgical patient must be based on knowledge of the various body fluid compartments and the normal mechanisms that maintain them.

ANATOMY OF BODY FLUID COMPARTMENTS

Water is the major constituent of total body weight. In normal health, it varies with age, sex, physical activity, and body composition. Using isotope dilution techniques to measure total body water, the average normal value for young adults is 60 per cent of body weight for males and 50 per cent of body weight for females. The water content of different tissues varies widely, from 10 per cent for fat to over 70 per cent for skin and muscle. The lean, muscular individual has a greater percentage of body water, reflecting a higher percentage of muscle mass. The lower mean percentage of total body water in females reflects the larger proportion of adipose tissue as a percentage of body weight.

Age is inversely related to body water. At birth, 75 to 80 per cent of body weight of the newborn is body water. By the end of the first year of life, total body water has fallen to approximately 65 per cent , where it remains through childhood. Hormonal effects in adolescence stimulate an increase in muscle mass in males and alterations in fat distribution in females. In addition, there is a gradual decline of total body water with age, falling to almost 50 per cent in males and 45 per cent in females by the seventh decade. Total body water in humans is partitioned between two main anatomic spaces.

The intracellular fluid is contained within cells, while the extracellular fluid is further partitioned between the intravascular space and the interstitial extravascular space between cells. The largest component of body water is the intracellular fluid volume, which comprises 30 to 40 per cent of body weight (Fig. 1). This again varies with body composition, being higher in males and lean individuals with a greater percentage of muscle mass and smaller in average females with a smaller muscle mass and proportionally larger fat content.

The extracellular fluid compartment totals 20 per cent of the body weight. A variety of substances have been used to measure the volume of the extracellular space. Small molecules that equilibrate rapidly tend to slightly overestimate the true extracellular fluid compartment, while large molecules such as inulin and mannitol tend to underestimate the extracellular space due to a slower diffusion into this compartment. The 20 per cent of body weight represented by extracellular fluid is further divided into the intravascular or plasma volume and the extracellular extravascular fluid, the interstitial fluid. The plasma volume is approximately 5 per cent of body weight in normal humans, while the interstitial space contains the other 15 per cent of body weight.

This interstitial fluid is further characterized by a rapidly equilibrating component and a slow equilibrating component. The slow or nonfunctional component is less than 10 per cent of the total interstitial fluid and is found primarily in joint and cerebrospinal fluids. Most of the interstitial fluid is composed of a functional space between cells and capillary membranes and is crucial to the to-and-fro movement of substances between cells and the blood stream.

ELECTROLYTE COMPOSITION OF BODY FLUID COMPARTMENTS

The differences in ionic composition between the intracellular and extracellular fluid are shown in Figure 2. These electrolytes are expressed in terms of the number of electrical charges per unit volume, or milliequivalents (mEq) per liter. This unit of expression is important in that the number of milliequivalents of anions is balanced by the same number of milliequivalents of cations within a compartment. The plasma contains a substantial component of anionic circulating proteins, which is reflected in a lower chloride and bicarbonate composition to maintain an electroneutral environment, relative to the interstitial fluid.

The major differences in ionic composition between the intracellular and extracellular fluids are maintained by the semipermeable cell membrane. Because this membrane is permeable to water, the osmotic pressures between compartments are equal. An alteration in the osmotic pressure in either compartment promotes a redistribution of water to maintain net osmotic equilibrium. For example, a decrease in extracellular sodium concentration due to the administration of free water would promote a transfer of water from this extracellular space to the intracellular fluid. Alterations in the extracellular fluid (ECF) volume by the administration of isotonic fluid would not change the concentration of extracellular ions, causing no movement of free water between spaces. Unlike water movement, the transcellular distribution of ions is maintained by an energy-dependent, active transport process. The primary cations involved are sodium and potassium, with the active transport of sodium in exchange for potassium by sodium potassium ATPase producing the almost inverse relationship of intracellular sodium to potassium, relative to the ECF, as shown in Figure 2.

FLUID AND ELECTROLYTE HOMEOSTASIS

The maintenance of a stable fluid and electrolyte environment is fundamental to normal physiologic

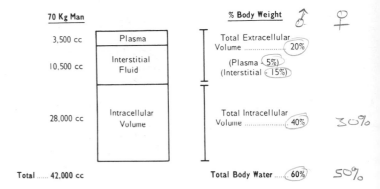

Figure 1. Functional compartments of body fluids. (From Shires GT, Canizaro PC: Fluid and electrolyte management of the surgical patient. *In* Sabiston DC Jr [ed]: Textbook of Surgery: The Biological Basis of Modern Surgical Practice, ed 14. Philadelphia, WB Saunders Company, 1991, p 58, with permission.)

and biochemical functions in normal humans. The daily intake of salt and water via the oral route is modulated by the gastrointestinal tract, the kidneys, and pulmonary and cutaneous losses to maintain homeostasis in the face of varied physiologic demand.

Pathophysiologic states, particularly severe surgical illnesses, impair the ability of these organ systems to respond to altered demands. Water balance is maintained primarily by alterations in renal excretion of

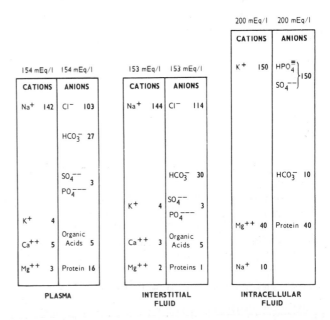

Figure 2. Chemical composition of body fluid compartments. (From Shires GT, Canizaro PC: Fluid and electrolyte management of the surgical patient. *In* Sabiston DC Jr [ed]: Textbook of Surgery: The Biological Basis of Modern Surgical Practice, ed 14. Philadelphia, WB Saunders Company, 1991, p 58, with permission.)

free water. The normal average oral intake of 2000 to 2500 ml replaces obligate insensible loss, via the lungs and skin, of 600 to 900 ml/day. The remainder is excreted as urine, with a minimal volume of 500 to 800 ml of urine per day required to excrete the acidic and nitrogen by-products of metabolism.

Insensible water gain is derived from the water of oxidation, produced when carbohydrates are metabolized. Another potential source is the water of solution, which is cellular water liberated by the catabolic destruction of cells when the hypermetabolic state is not met by exogenous sources of substrate, yielding excessive catabolism.

Insensible water losses are primarily from the skin. The capacity for insensible losses may be exceeded during thermal stress and lead to a sensible loss, sweat production. The normal insensible loss via the lung, approximately 25 per cent of insensible losses at rest, may be increased by hyperventilation, particularly by tracheostomy, which obviates the humidifying effects of the oral and nasal pharynx (Table 1).

The daily sodium intake in normal humans varies widely, reflecting dietary customs more than physiologic need. In the United States, excess salt intake usually leads to natriuresis to prevent sodium retention, beyond the normal extrarenal sodium losses of 100 to 200 mEq/day via the skin as sweat, urine, and stool. The wide variation in salt intake is managed by the remarkable ability of the normal kidney to vary sodium excretion from over 100 mEq/L of urine to less than 1 mEq/L of urine. Because insensible fluid losses from the skin and lungs are sodium free, the daily loss of sodium in healthy patients may approach zero in the setting of normal renal function and avid sodium conservation (Table 2).

PATHOPHYSIOLOGY OF FLUID ALTERATIONS

Disturbances of fluid balance may be characterized by changes in the isotonic fluid *volume*, in osmotically active *concentrations*, and in physiologically important yet osmotically insignificant nonsodium ion *composition*.

The volume of the extracellular fluid is altered by gains or losses of isotonic sodium-containing solutions. Volume expansion may be produced by the exogenous administration of saline solution, which freely distributes throughout the extracellular fluid spaces. The losses of isotonic fluid from the functional extracellular fluid space may be produced by external losses, such as intestinal fluid or blood, or by internal redistribution of isotonic fluid in response to a burn wound, the edema of peritonitis or a traumatic injury.

The concentration of sodium ions reflects the tonic-

ity of the body fluid compartments across semipermeable membranes. Water passes freely between the intracellular and extracellular spaces and equilibrates between them until isosmolarity is achieved. Consequently, the addition of free water or excess sodium ion produces these transcellular shifts, altering the concentration of osmotically active particles as a result.

Although other ions are present in insufficient concentrations to exert significant osmotic effects, alterations in composition may have profound physiologic effects. The potassium and hydrogen ion concentrations in particular may exert significant influence on a variety of biologic processes without significantly changing the osmotic environment of the extracellular fluid compartment. Although changes in volume, concentration, and composition are frequently concurrent and may be interrelated, appropriate therapeutic decisions must be based on assessing each of these disorders.

Alterations in Volume

The most common fluid and electrolyte disorder in the acutely ill patient is an extracellular fluid deficit. Alterations in gastrointestinal function both preoperatively and postoperatively may lead to pathologic losses of gastrointestinal fluids. As shown in Table 3, the composition of gastrointestinal secretions suggests that most losses are isotonic if they originate distal to the pylorus. Even vomiting frequently causes reflux through the pylorus and may not always lead to the classic hypochloremic hypokalemic state that occurs in gastric outlet obstruction. Internal losses may occur by the movement of fluid into a nonfunctional "third space" in response to infection and inflammation. Peritonitis, bowel obstruction, extensive soft-tissue injury, and burn wounds are all causes of sequestration of extracellular fluid that produces contraction of the functional extracellular space.

Although laboratory tests indicating hemoconcentration and an elevated blood urea nitrogen (BUN) to creatinine ratio may reflect established volume contraction, clinical examination remains the basis of diagnosis. As shown in Table 4, the clinical signs are relatively nonspecific until profound volume contraction occurs. Nevertheless, a high index of suspicion based on the clinical setting should lead to appropriate intervention in the acutely ill.

Volume excess usually occurs in the setting of renal failure or excessive intravenous fluid administration. As noted in Table 4, the early signs may be subtle and are primarily cardiovascular. In the absence of central venous pressure or Swan-Ganz catheter measurements, patients with poor cardiac reserve may abruptly decompensate and develop pulmonary

TABLE 1. WATER EXCHANGE (60- to 80-kg man)*

	Average Daily Volume (ml)	Minimal (ml)	Maximal (ml)
H₂O Gain—Routes			
Sensible			
Oral fluids	800–1500	0	1500/hr
Solid foods	500–700	0	1500
Insensible			
Water of oxidation	250	125	800
Water of solution	0	0	500
H₂O Loss—Routes			
Sensible			
Urine	800–1500	300	1400/hr (diabetes insipidus)
Intestinal	0–250	0	2500/hr
Sweat	0	0	4000/hr
Insensible			
Lungs and skin	600–900	600–900	1500

*From Shires GT, Canizaro PC: Fluid and electrolyte management of the surgical patient. *In* Sabiston DC Jr [ed]: Textbook of Surgery: The Biological Basis of Modern Surgical Practice, ed 14. Philadelphia, WB Saunders Company, 1991, p 69, with permission.

edema. However, the end-organ failure associated with prolonged inadequate perfusion supports vigorous resuscitation in younger patients, as minor transient volume overload is usually well tolerated and easily treated.

Alterations in Concentration

Unlike volume changes, laboratory measurement of the sodium ion concentration easily demonstrates alterations in serum sodium, which reflect body osmolarity. As shown in Table 5, the signs of hyponatremia may be subtle, and usually are inapparent until severe hyponatremia occurs. Hyponatremia most often follows an inappropriate intake of free water in the presence of concurrent pathologic sodium losses.

Hypernatremia is also manifest by cardiovascular and central nervous system responses. The loss of free water may occur via burns and large open wounds, hypotonic sweating in response to fever, and hyperventilation with nonhumidified air. In the absence of iatrogenic hypernatremia, most often occurring in the pediatric population, hypernatremia rarely develops as an isolated abnormality.

Abnormalities of both volume and concentration may develop concomitantly. A patient with abnormal gastrointestinal losses may drink water alone, causing hyponatremia and concurrent volume deficit. Hypernatremia may be accompanied by an ECF volume deficit as well, as in the setting of obligate free water losses from an osmotic diuresis such as glycosuria.

Alterations in Composition

Changes in physiologically important concentrations in potassium, calcium, and magnesium may cause no change in osmolarity, yet may have profound effects on body function. Alterations in acid-base balance also represent a compositional abnormality. The pH of body fluids is maintained within a narrow range, to provide an appropriate milieu for vital enzyme systems. Because the by-products of metabolism produce a large daily acid load, an efficient system for both buffering and excreting this proton excess is necessary to maintain a narrow pH range. Acids are rapidly buffered by their conversion to the appropriate salt by protein and phosphate buffers in the intracellular space and the bicarbonate-carbonic acid system

TABLE 2. SODIUM (SALT) EXCHANGE (60- to 80-kg man)*

Sodium Exchange	Average	Minimal	Maximal
Sodium gain			
Diet	50–90 mEq/day	0	75–100 mEq/hr (oral)
Sodium loss			
Skin (sweat)	10–60 mEq/day†	0	300 mEq/hr
Urine	10–80 mEq/day	<1 mEq/day‡	110–200 mEq/L§
Intestine	0–20 mEq/day	0	300 mEq/hr

*From Shires GT, Canizaro PC: Fluid and electrolyte management of the surgical patient. *In* Sabiston DC Jr [ed]: Textbook of Surgery: The Biological Basis of Modern Surgical Practice, ed 14. Philadelphia, WB Saunders Company, 1991, p 70, with permission.
†Depending on the degree of acclimatization of the individual.
‡With normal renal function.
§With renal salt wasting.

TABLE 3.   COMPOSITION OF GASTROINTESTINAL SECRETIONS*

	Volume (ml/24 hr)	Na (mEq/L)	K (mEq/L)	Cl (mEq/L)	HCO₃⁻ (mEq/L)
Salivary	1000 (500–2000)	10 (2–10)	26 (20–30)	10 (8–18)	30
Stomach	1500 (100–4000)	60 (9–116)	10 (0–32)	130 (8–154)	—
Duodenum	200 (100–2000)	140	5	80	—
Ileum	1800 (100–9000)	140 (80–150)	5 (2–8)	104 (43–137)	30
Colon	200	60	30	40	—
Pancreas	1000 (500–2500)	140 (113–185)	5 (3–7)	75 (54–95)	115
Bile	800 (300–1200)	145 (131–164)	5 (3–12)	100 (89–180)	35

*From Shires GT, Canizaro PC: Fluid and electrolyte management of the surgical patient. *In* Sabiston DC Jr [ed]: Textbook of Surgery: The Biological Basis of Modern Surgical Practice, ed 14. Philadelphia, WB Saunders Company, 1991, p 67, with permission.

in the extracellular space. The acids may be rapidly eliminated by carbon dioxide excretion by the lung and, slowly, by renal excretion. Respiratory compensation occurs within minutes, controlled by a central mechanism that alters minute ventilation. Unlike respiratory compensation, metabolic compensation of acid-base disorders by the kidney is slow, requiring hours to days to achieve.

The causes of primary respiratory and metabolic acid-base abnormalities are outlined in Table 6. Primary disturbances in one buffering system may be compensated by secondary changes in the other sys-

TABLE 4.   EXTRACELLULAR FLUID VOLUME*

	Deficit		Excess	
	Moderate	*Severe*	*Moderate*	*Severe*
CNS	Sleepiness Apathy Slow responses Anorexia Cessation of usual activity	Decreased tendon reflexes Anesthesia of distal extremities Stupor Coma	None	None
Gastrointestinal	Progressive decrease in food consumption	Nausea, vomiting Refusal to eat Silent ileus and distention	*At Operation:* Edema of stomach, colon, lesser and greater omenta, and small bowel mesentery	
Cardiovascular	Orthostatic hypotension Tachycardia Collapsed veins Collapsing pulse	Cutaneous lividity Hypotension Distant heart sounds Cold extremities Absent peripheral pulses	Elevated venous pressure Distention of peripheral veins Increased cardiac output Loud heart sounds Functional murmurs Bounding pulse High pulse pressure Increased pulmonary second sound Gallop	Pulmonary edema
Tissue signs	Soft, small tongue with longitudinal wrinkling Decreased skin turgor	Atonic muscles Sunken eyes	Subcutaneous pitting edema Basilar rales	Anasarca Moist rales Vomiting Diarrhea
Metabolism	Mild decrease of temperature, 97–99°F	Marked decrease of temperature, 95–98°F	None	None

*From Shires GT, Canizaro PC: Fluid and electrolyte management of the surgical patient. *In* Sabiston DC Jr [ed]: Textbook of Surgery: The Biological Basis of Modern Surgical Practice, ed 14. Philadelphia, WB Saunders Company, 1991, p 60, with permission.

TABLE 5.   ACUTE CHANGES IN OSMOLAR CONCENTRATION*

| | Hyponatremia (Water Intoxication) | | Hypernatremia (Water Deficit) | |
	Moderate	*Severe*	*Moderate*	*Severe*
CNS	Muscle twitching Hyperactive tendon reflexes Increased intracranial pressure (compensated phase)	Convulsions Loss of reflexes Increased intracranial pressure (decompensated phase)	Restlessness Weakness	Delirium Maniacal behavior
Cardiovascular	Changes in blood pressure and pulse secondary to increased intracranial pressure		Tachycardia Hypotension (if severe)	
Tissue signs	Increased salivation, lacrimation Watery diarrhea "Fingerprinting" of skin (sign of intracellular volume excess)		Decreased saliva and tears Dry and sticky mucous membranes Red, swollen tongue Flushed skin	
Renal	Oliguria progressing to anuria		Oliguria	
Metabolic	None		Fever	

*From Shires GT, Canizaro PC: Fluid and electrolyte management of the surgical patient. *In* Sabiston DC Jr [ed]: Textbook of Surgery: The Biological Basis of Modern Surgical Practice, ed 14. Philadelphia, WB Saunders Company, 1991, p 61, with permission.

tem. Acidosis is the most frequently encountered abnormality in the untreated, critically ill patient. Respiratory acidosis may follow any process that impairs minute ventilation, while metabolic acidosis is caused by intravascular volume contraction or cardiac dysfunction with resulting hypoperfusion. Alkalosis is more common in the critically ill resuscitated patient who has maintained normal renal and pulmonary function. Respiratory alkalosis most often follows excessive mechanical ventilation or the hyperventilatory response to hypoxia, pain, and the hypermetabolic state. Metabolic alkalosis in this setting is frequently due to the renal response to hypovolemia. The kidney attempts to defend volume by sodium reabsorption, causing increased regeneration of bicarbonate. Hypo-

kalemia and hypochloremia also impair the renal excretion of bicarbonate. Excess intravenous administration of sodium bicarbonate or excess buffer in massive transfusion may produce metabolic alkalosis.

The treatment of acid-based disorders is directed toward correction of the underlying abnormality. The variety of conditions causing hypoventilation (Table 6) are usually promptly diagnosed by radiography and physical examination. Correction of any mechanical etiologies and institution of mechanical ventilation should be done promptly. Hyperventilation with respiratory alkalosis is a common finding in critical illness that may cause increased renal excretion of bicarbonate in compensation. Severe alkalosis may be more difficult to treat than hypoventilation, as the un-

TABLE 6.   ACIDOSIS-ALKALOSIS*

	Defect	Common Causes	$\dfrac{BHCO_3}{H_2CO_3} = \dfrac{20}{1}$	Compensation
Respiratory acidosis	Retention of CO_2 (decreased alveolar ventilation)	Depression of respiratory center by morphine CNS injury Pulmonary disease—emphysema, pneumonia	↑Denominator Ratio less than 20:1	Renal Retention of bicarbonate, excretion of acid salts, increased ammonia formation Chloride shift into red cells
Respiratory alkalosis	Excessive loss of CO_2 (increased alveolar ventilation)	Hyperventilation; emotional disturbances, severe pain, assisted ventilation, encephalitis	↓Denominator Ratio greater than 20:1	Renal Excretion of bicarbonate, retention of acid salts, decreased ammonia formation
Metabolic acidosis	Retention of fixed acids or loss of base bicarbonate	Diabetes, azotemia, lactic acid accumulation, starvation Diarrhea, small bowel fistulas	↓Numerator Ratio less than 20:1	Pulmonary (rapid): increased rate and depth of breathing Renal (slow): as in respiratory acidosis
Metabolic alkalosis	Loss of fixed acids Gain of base bicarbonate Potassium depletion	Vomiting or gastric suction with pyloric obstruction Excessive intake of bicarbonate Diuretics	↑Numerator Ratio greater than 20:1	Pulmonary (rapid): decreased rate and depth of breathing Renal (slow): as in respiratory alkalosis

*From Shires GT, Canizaro PC: Fluid and electrolyte management of the surgical patient. *In* Sabiston DC Jr [ed]: Textbook of Surgery: The Biological Basis of Modern Surgical Practice, ed 14. Philadelphia, WB Saunders Company, 1991, p 62, with permission.

derlying causes, including injury to the central nervous system and the hypermetabolic state, are less amenable to correction. Care should be taken to avoid hypokalemia in response to potassium entering cells to replace hydrogen ion losses, precipitating cardiac arrhythmia.

The treatment of metabolic acidosis is also directed at the underlying disorder. Either the retention or production of excess acid or the pathologic loss of bicarbonate produces a lower pH. As shown in Table 7, the etiology may be predicted by assessing the anion gap, determined by subtracting the sum of chloride and bicarbonate from the serum sodium concentration. Normal anion gap acidosis tends to follow more chronic conditions. In surgical patients, acute circulatory failure with hypoperfusion leading to lactic acidosis is a common cause of elevated anion gap acidosis. Renal dysfunction secondary to shock further widens the anion gap by the retention of sulfuric and phosphoric acids. Exogenous sodium bicarbonate does not restore a normal pH in the patient with circulatory failure. However, volume resuscitation restores adequate circulatory function and rapidly clears the endogenous lactate load. At this point, severe metabolic alkalosis may develop if excess sodium bicarbonate has been administered during resuscitation.

Potassium Metabolism

Potassium is the major intracellular cation, with a concentration of 150 mEq/L of cell water. Although 98 per cent of the body potassium is located in the intracellular space, the plasma potassium concentra-

TABLE 7. CAUSES OF METABOLIC ACIDOSIS*

Causes	Mechanisms
Normal Anion Gap	
Diarrhea, small bowel fistula, ureterosigmoidostomy	Loss of HCO_3^-
Proximal renal tubular acidosis	Decreased tubular reabsorption of HCO_3^-
Distal renal tubular acidosis	Decreased acid excretion
Acid administration (NH_4Cl, HCl)	Increased acid load
"Dilutional" acidosis	Volume expansion with HCO_3^- free fluids
Elevated Anion Gap	
Shock (inadequate perfusion)	Increased lactic acid
Diabetes, starvation, alcohol intoxication	Increased ketoacids
Uremia	Retention of sulfuric and phosphoric acids
Ingestion of methanol, ethylene glycol, aspirin	Conversion to formic, oxalic, and salicylic acids

*From Shires GT, Canizaro PC: Fluid and electrolyte management of the surgical patient. *In* Sabiston DC Jr [ed]: Textbook of Surgery: The Biological Basis of Modern Surgical Practice, ed 14. Philadelphia, WB Saunders Company, 1991, p 64, with permission.

tion must be maintained within a narrow range to maintain normal cardiovascular, neuromuscular, and gastrointestinal function. The plasma potassium concentration is a poor measure of total body potassium. Alterations in the patient's volume status, acid-base balance, and glucose metabolism, particularly with severe injury and hypermetabolism, influence plasma potassium concentrations.

Hypokalemia is more common than hyperkalemia in the surgical patient. Hypokalemia may exist with low, normal, or high total body potassium content. Alkalosis promotes increased renal potassium loss, as hydrogen ions are conserved preferentially over potassium in exchange for sodium ions, leading to kaliuresis. Hypokalemia may also further the degree of metabolic alkalosis. Urinary hydrogen ion excretion paradoxically increases when the intracellular potassium decreases, becoming less available for sodium exchange. In addition, any increase in the distal tubular delivery of sodium, either from volume expansion or proximal loop diuretics, increases the renal tubular excretion of potassium ions.

The major source of extrarenal potassium losses is gastrointestinal secretion. Vomiting, diarrhea, high-output fistulas, and colonic villous adenomas may produce significant losses of potassium, despite the relatively low potassium concentration in these fluids. Any etiology of hypokalemia may be magnified by the inappropriate use of potassium-free fluids as intravenous replacement.

The signs and symptoms of hypokalemia are the result of abnormalities of cardiac, skeletal, and smooth muscle function. Vomiting and ileus may be accompanied by a generalized weakness, muscle cramps, and hyporeflexia. Most characteristic are the ECG changes of low voltage with flat T waves and ST segment depression. U waves may appear as serum potassium falls below 3.0 mEq/L, or higher in patients with alkalosis or digitalis effect.

The treatment of hypokalemia requires the administration of potassium in addition to attention to the underlying cause. It is frequently associated with volume contraction and a depletion of total body potassium as in the patient with vomiting from pyloric obstruction. The loss of large volumes of sodium, chloride, and hydrogen ions leads to hypochloremic hypokalemic metabolic alkalosis. The severe potassium depletion that occurs is a result of both the direct loss of potassium by vomiting and the kaliuresis, outlined above, caused by volume depletion and alkalosis. In the patient with normal renal function, potassium may be replaced either by the oral or parenteral route. To prevent even transient hyperkalemia, no more than 40 mEq/hr should be administered, and the patient should be monitored.

The clinical signs of hyperkalemia are similar to those in hypercalcemia. Again, the ECG findings are the most characteristic, with peaked T waves, a shortened Q-T interval, and widened QRS. Eventually, the T waves may disappear with heart block, causing diastolic cardiac arrest. The normal body defense against hyperkalemia involves the acute movement of potassium into cells, augmented by insulin, with renal excretion following over the ensuing 6 hours. Even in the presence of decreased total body potassium, acute acidosis is a common cause of hyperkalemia by promoting movement of intracellular potassium into the extracellular space in response to cellular uptake of hydrogen ions. Iatrogenic hyperkalemia may occur with continued administration of potassium in the setting of occult renal insufficiency.

Hyperkalemia should be treated by correcting the elevated plasma potassium level and reversing the underlying mechanism. Exogenously administered potassium should be withheld and the cardiac effects reversed by the administration of 1 ml of 10 per cent calcium gluconate under ECG monitoring. Because infusion of calcium counteracts the myocardial effect of potassium without changing serum potassium levels, serum potassium levels should also be lowered by the administration of bicarbonate, glucose, and insulin, thus lowering extracellular levels by driving potassium into the intracellular space. The administration of 50 gm of glucose with 10 to 20 U of regular insulin, accompanied by 45 mEq of sodium bicarbonate in the acidotic patient, allows time to eliminate the excess potassium from the body. With normal renal function, the withholding of potassium administration and volume expansion alone may be sufficient. In patients with renal insufficiency, peritoneal dialysis or hemodialysis may be necessary for life-threatening hyperkalemia. Finally, cation-exchange resins may be given orally or by enema to promote potassium losses in the stool.

INTRAVENOUS THERAPY OF FLUID AND ELECTROLYTES

The composition of commonly available parenteral fluids is shown in Table 8. Given the normal serum concentrations and a knowledge of the measured or expected losses, the proper choice of parenteral fluids should permit the maintenance of normal volume, composition, and concentration without depending on renal compensation. Lactated Ringer's solution is an inexpensive and effective replacement for extracellular fluid volume deficits and most gastrointestinal losses that originate distal to the pylorus. Although the solution is slightly hyponatremic and hyperchloremic, the lactate, used instead of bicarbonate, is promptly metabolized to bicarbonate. The lactate is used simply to produce a more stable form of base substrate in solution during storage. Normal saline (0.9 per cent

TABLE 8. COMPOSITION OF PARENTERAL FLUIDS: ELECTROLYTE CONTENT (mEq/L)*

Solution	Cations				Anions	
	Na	K	Ca	Mg	Cl	HCO$_3$
Extracellular fluid	142	4	5	3	103	27
Lactated Ringer's	130	4	2.7		109	28†
0.9% sodium chloride (saline)	154				154	
D$_5$/0.45% sodium chloride	77				77	
M/6 sodium lactate	167					167†

*From Shires GT, Canizaro PC: Fluid and electrolyte management of the surgical patient. *In* Sabiston DC Jr [ed]: Textbook of Surgery: The Biological Basis of Modern Surgical Practice, ed 14. Philadelphia, WB Saunders Company, 1991, p 71, with permission.
†Present in solution as lactate, which is converted to bicarbonate.

sodium chloride) is hypernatremic and hyperchloremic. However, it may be used for the initial correction of both the extracellular fluid volume and the chloride deficits induced by vomiting. Maintenance fluids for patients who are unable to take anything by mouth are frequently administered as 0.45 per cent saline and 5 per cent dextrose. This solution provides free water for insensible losses and a moderate amount of sodium to allow renal adjustment of serum sodium levels without requiring maximal sodium reabsorption.

The administration of fluid-containing colloidal substances such as albumin or dextran continues to be advocated for fluid resuscitation. A lower total volume of resuscitative fluid may be required, as colloids are transiently retained in the intravascular space. The presumed benefit of avoiding postresuscitation pulmonary dysfunction was based on the incorrect assumption that the oncotic gradient between the pulmonary capillaries and the lung interstitium could be manipulated by the administration of colloids. In addition, colloid solutions are more expensive, may depress the production of immunoglobulins and albumin, and may further compromise the extracellular fluid volume deficit, particularly during shock.

Multiple studies have attempted to address these clinically relevant issues. Prospective, randomized clinical trials have usually shown no differences in survival rates or the incidence of pulmonary failure. A recent meta-analysis of colloid versus crystalloid and fluid resuscitation concluded that crystalloid is superior to colloid in the trauma setting. In addition, there is little clinical evidence that crystalloid resuscitation to appropriate hemodynamic end-points can be improved by the addition of oncotically active substances.

The preoperative evaluation and treatment of fluid disturbances should minimize the deleterious effects of the neurohormonal response to stress and the hemodynamic consequences of anesthesia and blood loss. A combination of bedside clinical assessment and laboratory tests should ascertain preexisting disorders of volume, concentration, and composition. The most frequent abnormality in surgical patients is extracellular fluid volume deficit. Because the signs may be subtle and the laboratory findings minimal, a high index of suspicion should lead to appropriate correction. A variety of preoperative maneuvers, including restriction of oral intake, bowel preparation, and radiologic procedures that may induce osmotic diuresis can lead to a subtle volume deficit. In the emergency patient, burns, crush injury, peritonitis, bowel obstruction with associated edema, and shock may all lead to "third-space" losses with internal redistribution of extracellular fluid into a nonfunctional compartment.

There are no clinically available bedside laboratory methods to quantify these deficits. However, the adequacy of hemodynamic function may be assessed by measurement of blood pressure, pulse, skin perfusion, alterations in the sensorium, and hourly urinary output. The classic tissue signs that may be useful in estimating the degree of pediatric dehydration are of little use when there is acute and rapid loss of fluid, at which time cardiovascular signs predominate.

Fluid replacement should be initiated and altered according to clinical response of the patient. The rate of fluid administration should vary with the severity of the fluid deficit and the cardiac status. Isotonic solutions may be infused at rates greater than 1000 ml/hr in otherwise healthy individuals. Excessive rates of administration may transiently expand the intravascular volume without complete restitution of the extracellular fluid deficit, causing a temporary increase in urinary output. In addition, elderly patients with cardiovascular disease may require a slower reexpansion of the extracellular fluid volume. In this setting, more sophisticated measures of cardiac function and intravascular volume may be necessary. Assessment of the central venous pressure and pulmonary capillary wedge pressure maximizes the rate of safe resuscitation without causing acute pulmonary edema in the setting of extracellular fluid volume contraction.

Following adequate volume replacement, the intraoperative management of fluids is simplified and hypotension and cardiovascular collapse may be avoided during anesthetic induction. Fluid losses during operation consist of blood and extracellular fluid losses, both from direct losses into operative field and from internal redistribution of fluid into the nonfunctional third space. Edema in the operative field, including trauma to the intestine and the surgical wound, may be extensive. The requirement to replace these losses is proportional to the extent of operative trauma, the duration of the procedure, and the preexisting surgical condition that may be producing ongoing losses. In elective surgical procedures, several studies have shown these losses to require between 500 and 1200 ml/hr of crystalloid replacement.

Blood loss may be measured during the operative procedure to guide transfusion therapy. With modern component therapy, packed red blood cells may be given to ensure adequate oxygen-carrying capacity. It now appears that hemoglobin concentrations below 10 gm/dl per cent are well tolerated by most patients. However, blood replacement should be started as values fall below this range in the setting of ongoing blood loss, hemodynamic instability, or preexisting cardiopulmonary disease. Fresh frozen plasma and other asanguineous components of whole blood should not be given for volume resuscitation alone, but should be given for indications discussed in Chapter 6.

In the recovery room, the patient's intraoperative course and total volume administration should be reviewed, in addition to the vital signs, the urine output, and available hemodynamic monitoring. "Routine" maintenance fluids should not be ordered in this setting, as fluid requirements vary widely between patients. Following extensive procedures or resuscitation from shock, frequent reevaluation of the patient's volume status, including an hourly urinary output of greater than 0.5 ml/kg/hr is often necessary to properly assess these fluid requirements. In the later postoperative period, the replacement and measurement of sensible losses and estimated insensible losses forms an initial basis for estimating fluid requirements. As noted above, in the absence of fever or hypermetabolism, the insensible losses average 600 to 900 ml of water per day. In addition, approximately 1000 ml/day is given to replace the obligate urinary excretion of the products of metabolism. Although the normal kidney avidly conserves sodium, if only 5 per cent dextrose and water is administered, it is reasonable to provide some amount of salt for renal losses. In the absence of pathologic losses or surgical complications, the determination of serum electrolytes is usually unnecessary in the early postoperative period. The amount of administered potassium should approximate 40 mEq/day, in addition to appropriate replacement for measured gastrointestinal losses. The administration of diuretics and spontaneous postoperative diuresis may increase the potassium requirements in otherwise stable patients who may develop occult hypokalemia.

REFERENCES

Kokko JP, Tannen RL (eds): Fluids and Electrolytes, ed 2. Philadelphia, WB Saunders Company, 1990.

Maxwell MH, Kleeman CR, Narins RG (eds): Clinical Disorders of Fluid and Electrolyte Metabolism, ed 4. New York, McGraw-Hill, 1987.

Moss GS, Gould SA: Plasma expanders: An update. Am J Surg *155*: 425, 1988.

Oh MS, Carroll HJ: Disorders of sodium metabolism: Hypernatremia and hyponatremia. Crit Care Med 20(1):94, 1992.

Williams ME: Hyperkalemia. Crit Care Clin 7:155, 1991.

Velanovich V: Crystalloid versus colloid fluid resuscitation: A meta-analysis of mortality. Surgery *105*:65, 1989.

5

PRINCIPLES OF PREOPERATIVE PREPARATION OF THE SURGICAL PATIENT

BRUCE D. SCHIRMER, M.D.

An important aspect of the practice of surgery is the decision-making process involved in evaluating the indications and urgency of an operation, and *experience* is the great instructor in developing these skills. Once the decision to perform an operation is made, the surgeon must focus on proper preparation of the patient.

PREOPERATIVE COMMUNICATION

The doctor–patient relationship is best established by good communication, and it is essential that the surgeon devote time preoperatively to establish a relationship that will serve to reassure each patient and family during a time of worry and stress. Their concerns should also be paramount in the surgeon's mind, and discussion should continue until the surgeon is satisfied that they understand the indications, the procedure, and the attendant risks of the proposed procedure.

ASSESSING OPERATIVE RISK

Factors considered in assessing perioperative risk include those related to the general health of the patient, the specific disease, the current condition of the patient, and the proposed operation. The American Association of Anesthesiologist's Physical Status Scale is shown in Table 1. Postoperative mortality correlates well with these classifications, as does anesthesia-related mortality. Death rates range from 0.01 per cent

(category 1) to 18 per cent (category 4). Anesthetic and surgical mortalities double in categories 1, 2, and 3 if the procedures are performed emergently, and patients in categories 4 and 5 have no increased risk in the emergency setting. Mortality rates for specific procedures vary from institution to institution based on experience and the number of cases done. The decision to perform an operation and its urgency are directly related to the therapeutic benefit likely to be obtained versus the operative risk. Knowledge of the natural history of a disease is very important. Similarly, the timing of the operation can often be significant in influencing ultimate outcome.

FLUIDS AND ELECTROLYTES

The proper intravascular volume is always important, and ensuring adequate tissue perfusion as well as correction of acid-base or electrolyte disturbances are paramount considerations even in the most emergent of operations. Only efforts to maintain the circulation and ventilation have greater priority in preparing the patient for an operation.

The most common preoperative disorder in this setting is *intravascular volume depletion*, which often follows the patient's disease process, through hemorrhage, vomiting, or diarrhea. Tachycardia, hypotension, oliguria, increased urinary osmolality, and decreased urine sodium concentration confirm the diagnosis. Hydration with fluid appropriate to replace the specific losses is indicated. Transfusion of blood products is necessary to restore significant blood loss while isotonic saline solutions are given for less severe volume depletion. In emergent resuscitation from hypovolemic shock, immediate infusion of Ringer's lactate is recommended as both a resuscitative measure and a means of estimating intravascular blood loss (based on blood pressure responses). Adequate hydration is achieved when intravascular volume is sufficient to assure good organ perfusion. A urinary output of more than 30 ml/hr in adults or 1 ml/kg/hr in children ensures adequate renal perfusion. Measurement of central venous or even pulmonary capillary wedge pressure may be required to maintain optimal levels of hydration in patients with compromised cardiopulmonary function.

Excessive intravascular volume is characterized by pulmonary edema. These conditions, unless very acute, are accompanied by overexpansion of the extracellular component of body fluid, common causes including renal failure, congestive heart failure, and cirrhosis. In renal failure, the intravascular and extracellular compartments are equilibrated and total body water and sodium overload are present. Careful monitoring of intake and output, the daily weight, and maintenance of a dialysis schedule are indicated in the preoperative preparation of patients in renal failure. In congestive heart failure, the decrease in cardiac output results in increased hydrostatic pressure within capillaries causing a net shift of water to the interstitial space and an effective loss of intravascular volume. This is interpreted by the kidneys as a condition requiring retention of excess sodium and water, and therapy consists of restriction of salt and water and use of loop diuretics such as furosemide. Cirrhosis also represents a condition of excess body retention of sodium and water in the extracellular space. Increased portal pressure secondary to increased splanchnic blood volume causes transudate of water and sodium to the peritoneal cavity as ascites, and optimal treatment is achieved by restriction of water and potassium-sparing diuretics.

ELECTROLYTE ABNORMALITIES

Hyponatremia

The serum sodium content is usually the initial marker used to detect abnormalities of sodium and water metabolism. In many patients, relative hyponatremia is more a manifestation of a *water balance excess than sodium deficit*. Hyponatremia and decreased total body sodium can occur when losses of sodium via excess gastrointestinal, renal, or other causes cause a sodium deficit greater than water deficit. Treatment is repletion of intravascular volume with isotonic saline and a high-sodium diet. Hyponatremia and hypotonicity more commonly occur following disorders causing increased total body water greater than total body sodium and urinary sodium content less than 10 mEq/L. Congestive heart failure, cirrhosis, and renal failure may cause such hyponatremia. Severe hyponatremia and hypotonicity may become life threatening with cerebral edema. In symptomatic patients, administration of small amounts of hypertonic saline and potent diuretics is indicated. Patients with hyponatremia but normal total body sodium content have accompanying hypotonicity due to increased total body water, and edema is absent. The syndrome of inappropriate antidiuretic hormone secretion (SIADH) most commonly causes this condition, in which patients have excess total body water and a high urine sodium concentration and osmolality. The treatment is water restriction.

Hypernatremia

Hypernatremia may occur in the settings of normal, decreased, or increased total body sodium. Rarely, it may be from iatrogenic causes. Diabetes insipidus is an example of hypernatremia with normal total body sodium. The renal concentrating mechanism is impaired due to lack of ADH and accompanying polydipsia, polyuria; and hypotonic urine; and vasopressin is indicated for treatment. Hypotonic fluid loss can cause hypernatremia and hypertonicity with decreased total body sodium. Prolonged nasogastric suctioning or severe vomiting may cause these findings, and therapy is restoration of intravascular volume.

Hypokalemia

Hypokalemia is usually associated with decreased total body potassium stores, the most common cause being chronic use of diuretics. In these settings the relative plasma hypokalemia may reflect a large total body potassium deficit. Other common causes for hypokalemia include gastrointestinal losses from vomiting or diarrhea and renal tubular acidosis. Preoperative correction of hypokalemia is especially important in patients with a history of cardiac disease, because

TABLE 1. CLASSIFICATION OF PHYSICAL STATUS*†

Category 1	Healthy
Category 2	Mild systemic disease
Category 3	Severe systemic disease limiting activity
Category 4	Incapacitating systemic disease
Category 5	Moribund

*From American Society of Anesthesiologists: Classification of physical status. Anesthesiology 24(1):111, 1963, with permission.

†In event of emergency operation, the category number is preceded with an E.

postoperative cardiac arrhythmias, particularly atrial fibrillation, are increased with hypokalemia. Potassium chloride is the agent of choice for correcting metabolic alkalosis and hypokalemia from excessive diuretics or gastrointestinal losses. If renal potassium wasting has led to metabolic acidosis, potassium bicarbonate is effective. Oral administration safely allows intake of the large quantities of potassium necessary to correct the deficit. Should intravenous supplementation of potassium be necessary, the safe limit is 20 mEq/hr.

Hyperkalemia

Serum potassium can be elevated due to increased potassium intake, decreased renal excretion, cell death, and hypoaldosteronism. The most important clinical condition involving hyperkalemia is acute renal failure. It is unwise to proceed with an operation unless potassium can first be effectively removed. Hemodialysis and peritoneal dialysis are the best options, the former being indicated in the acute setting. Preoperative hyperkalemia is treated based on the levels of serum potassium. If the potassium is in the 6.5-mEq/L range, simple measures to remove potassium such as the administration of Kayexalate resins are recommended. If the level exceeds 6.5 mEq/L, emergent therapy is indicated, including intravenous calcium gluconate to reverse the cardiac effects of hyperkalemia. Sodium bicarbonate or glucose and insulin shift potassium ions to the intracellular space, and therapy to shift potassium ions is followed with measures to remove potassium.

ACID-BASE DISTURBANCES

Metabolic Alkalosis

Metabolic alkalosis can be caused by excess alkali (such as intravenous sodium bicarbonate or citrate infused with banked blood) or loss of acid (following nasogastric suctioning). The treatment of metabolic alkalosis begins by ensuring that the kidney can excrete an adequate bicarbonate load. Replacement of intravascular and extracellular volume counteracts *contraction* alkalosis. Other requirements of the nephron for excreting bicarbonate include adequate available chloride and potassium for exchange. Expansion of extracellular fluid volume is followed by potassium chloride (KCl) administration. In severe cases, acid administration using 0.1N HCl in 5 per cent D5W may be given up to 0.2 mEq/kg/hr by a central vein.

Metabolic Acidosis

Metabolic acidosis is classified according to anion gap. *Normal anion gap* causes of metabolic acidosis (where $[Na] - [Cl] + [HCO_3] < 4$) include renal disease leading to bicarbonate loss (renal tubular acidosis), certain drugs (acetazolamide), ileal loop with stasis, diarrhea, or pancreatic fistula. *High anion gap* causes include diabetic ketoacidosis, lactic acidosis, toxins (salicylate, methanol), and uremia. Treatment of normal anion gap acidosis is conservative and involves treating the etiologic agent where possible. High anion gap acidosis also requires treatment of the offending condition, and dialysis may be required to remove drugs or to correct uremia. Shock and tissue hypoperfusion must be corrected if producing lactic acidosis. Sodium bicarbonate therapy may be necessary in an emergent situation (cardiopulmonary arrest).

BLEEDING DISORDERS AND TRANSFUSIONS

Bleeding Disorders

The best preoperative screening procedure for bleeding disorders is a careful history. Patients with a history of prolonged bleeding after dental procedures, hematoma formation and intra-articular bleeding after trauma, or easy bruisability warrant consideration for screening for bleeding disorders. Prothrombin time (PT), activated partial thromboplastin time (aPTT), platelet count, and bleeding time are sensitive enough to detect significant surgical bleeding disorders in over 95 per cent of cases. A history of aspirin ingestion is of concern preoperatively because aspirin irreversibly effects platelet aggregation for the life of the affected platelets (7 to 10 days), and bleeding time is prolonged in these patients. Hemophilia is suggested by a family history. If factor VIII (hemophilia A) or factor IX (hemophilia B) levels are present at less than 25 per cent of normal, intraoperative or postoperative surgical bleeding may result. Prophylaxis for hemophilia is administration of cryoprecipitate containing factor VIII to raise levels to 80 per cent of normal or to obtain a VIII:C ratio of 80 to 100 (U/dl). The cryoprecipitate is normally given 2 hours prior to operation as a loading dose and continued every 12 hours for 1 to 2 weeks following operation.

Liver disease, especially cirrhosis, is the most common cause of prolonged prothrombin time. Patients with vitamin K malabsorption may also manifest a prolonged PT. Such patients should receive parenteral vitamin K preoperatively. Patients requiring anticoagulants, either heparin or Coumadin, warrant special consideration. Because anticoagulation is required in the postoperative period due to the danger of thromboembolic events, it is best not to fully reverse anticoagulation for long periods of time. Operations on the central nervous system, liver, and eye require full anticoagulant reversal at the time of operation. For other major procedures, titrating the anticoagulation to the lower end of the therapeutic range may be sufficient. This is facilitated by converting patients on Coumadin to heparin because adjustments in anticoagulation from heparin are made more rapidly. Parenteral vitamin K or the infusion of fresh frozen plasma are the recommended means of reversing anticoagulation from Coumadin or heparin preoperatively.

Patients with Underlying Blood Disorders

Patients with underlying blood disorders such as anemia, thrombocytopenia, leukemia, and polycythemia warrant special considerations in their preoperative preparation. Anemia may increase the risk of operation in some patients with hemoglobin levels less than 10 gm/dl by compromising maximal oxygen delivering capacity. Preoperative transfusions may be indicated in selected anemic patients, and they are optimally given at least 24 hours prior to operation, allowing adequate time for the body to reaccumulate normal levels of 2,3-diphosphoglycerate (DPG).

Sickle cell anemia is associated with significant surgical morbidity, and conditions that precipitate sickle cell crisis, such as hypothermia, infections, acidosis, and dehydration, are to be avoided. Administration of oxygen 24 hours prior to surgery is recommended, as is preoperative exchange transfusion to lower the hemoglobin S level to less than 30 per cent. Patients with polycythemia vera have an increased risk of perioperative complications from hemorrhage. It is recommended that phlebotomy and myelosuppressive agents be used to maintain the hematocrit at less than 52 per cent in these patients for several months prior to elective procedures. Patients with leukemia and granulocytopenia ($<1000/mm^3$) are at increased risk for infection, and antibiotics are indicated prophylactically in such patients. Patients with leukemia with platelet counts below 50,000 may be supplemented with immediate preoperative transfusion of platelets.

Transfusions

The availability of an adequate supply of crossmatched blood is a prerequisite for all major elective surgical procedures. In an emergency, transfusion for resuscitation purposes may proceed with type-specific or even O-negative blood, depending on the urgency of the situation. Transfusions have a defined risk of complications that include a 1 per cent incidence of transfusion or allergic reactions, an approximate 1 per cent incidence of transmission of clinically apparent hepatitis, and very rarely, transmission of the human immunodeficiency virus (HIV). The incidence of transmission of hepatitis from transfusions may be as high as 10 per cent, as most patients never manifest themselves clinically. Hepatitis C accounts for 90 per cent of cases of transfusion-associated hepatitis. Recent estimates of hepatitis transmission via transfusion range from 3 to 8 per cent.

PROPHYLAXIS OF POSTOPERATIVE DEEP VEIN THROMBOSIS

An estimated 2.5 million cases of deep vein thrombosis occur annually, with over 600,000 episodes of pulmonary embolism and 200,000 deaths. Approximately 15 per cent of all deaths in acute care hospitals follow pulmonary embolism, especially following *routine* surgical procedures such as cholecystectomy and herniorrhaphy. Prophylactic techniques for prevention of deep vein thrombosis include mechanical techniques and chemical techniques. The position recommended for prophylaxis of deep vein thrombosis is shown in Figure 1 and is as effective as elastic stockings or aspirin in reducing the incidence of deep vein thrombosis. Heparin given in a dose of 5000 U subcutaneously 2 hours preoperatively and then at 8- to 12-hour intervals postoperatively has been shown in some trials to decrease the incidence of postoperative deep vein thrombosis and pulmonary embolism. Of significance

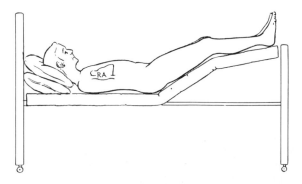

Figure 1. Correct position for lower extremities in prophylaxis of pulmonary embolism. Note the additional break at the knees. It is important that the level of the veins in the lower extremities be above the mean level of the right atrium (RA). (From Sabiston DC Jr: Pulmonary embolism. *In* Sabiston DC Jr [ed]: Davis-Christopher Textbook of Surgery, ed 13. Philadelphia, WB Saunders Company, 1986, p 1742, with permission.)

are the complications of low-dose heparin therapy, including an increased incidence of wound hematoma. Most failures of low-dose heparin therapy occur following operations that greatly stimulate iliac and femoral vein thrombosis, such as hip replacements. Dextran is occasionally used with possible benefit as a prophylactic agent.

PREOPERATIVE NUTRITION

The nutritional status of the patient is an important preoperative consideration. Patients may be classified into three categories regarding nutritional status:

1. Those who have had little starvation (weight loss <10 per cent body weight) and can tolerate several days of intravenous glucose as the only caloric source without adverse effect on morbidity or mortality.

2. Those suffering starvation from their disease (such as an obstructing carcinoma of the gastrointestinal tract) who have lower than normal basal metabolic rates and must be restarted on full calorie support slowly, with attention for hypophosphatemia, hypokalemia, and hypomagnesemia (the refeeding syndrome).

3. Those with hypermetabolic states, such as burns or sepsis, who require greater than average caloric intake to meet daily energy requirements.

The latter group should receive adequate calories and protein to maintain visceral proteins and body weight and to minimize the hypermetabolic state and acute-phase reaction of the stress of injury. Weight gain is not a goal in this state. Methods used to assess nutritional status include monitoring of weight loss and measurement of biochemical, immunologic, and anthropometrical parameters.

Malnutrition has adverse effects on the ability to withstand the stresses of injury and operation. The negative nitrogen balance of severely hypermetabolic patients may rapidly deplete visceral organ mass and strength. Poor pulmonary toilet; atelectasis, depletion of serum proteins causing sodium retention, water retention, and edema; and poor wound healing may ensue. Malnutrition reduces immune competence, with greater risk for postoperative infection. Preoperative nutritional supplementation in certain nutritionally depleted patients significantly reduces postoperative complications.

Considerations in Nutritional Support

Whenever possible, if the gastrointestinal tract is functional, *enteric* feeding is the preferred route of nutritional support. Enteral feedings avoid the risk of intravenous catheter–related problems such as sepsis or thrombosis. The cost is substantially less for supplements by enteral nutrition compared to parenteral nutrition. Recent studies have shown a decreased risk of postoperative complications in patients in whom postoperative enteral feeding is begun soon after operation. Enteral feedings also may be important in limiting the phenomenon of translocation as a factor in sepsis and the hypermetabolic state. *Total parenteral nutrition* is indicated in the perioperative setting when an extended nonfunctional gastrointestinal tract prevents adequate enteral nutritional intake. Central venous access, usually by the subclavian approach, is required, and meticulous care of the catheter site is essential. Low institutional infection rates of the latter complication have been achieved by specially trained personnel. Formulas are modified to each patient's requirements but include amino acid solutions and dextrose, as well as additives such as vitamins, heparin, insulin, albumin, and electrolytes as indicated. Isotonic fat solutions can be administered simultaneously or separately.

INFECTIOUS COMPLICATIONS

Wound infection and postoperative sepsis are primarily related to the risk factors for infection present at the time of operation. These factors include the host's defense mechanisms, the environment in which infection occurs, and the microorganisms producing the infection. The host response to injury is a major factor in survival, contributing to the syndrome of multiorgan failure in settings where severe injury and sepsis lead to a high incidence of mortality. The measures that improve or normalize host defense mechanisms, limit the environmental exposure to high-risk pathogenic organisms, and reduce the degree of tissue contamination with such organisms serve to decrease the incidence of postoperative infection. Humoral and cellular immunity, as well as phagocytic cell function, can be adversely influenced by preoperative disease states or treatment. Immunosuppressive drugs, glucocorticoids, and radiation therapy inhibit host defense mechanisms against infection. Anergy is associated with a high incidence of postoperative sepsis and death.

The duration of preoperative hospitalization should be minimized to limit replacement of the patient's endogenous skin flora with nosocomial organisms. Preoperative hair removal may also affect surgical infection rates, and a lower incidence of wound infection occurs when either clippers or depilatory cream is used rather than razor shaving, while some studies suggest that the removal of hair is unnecessary. Preoperative showering with hexachlorophene soap may also decrease wound infection. It should be stressed that proper surgical technique, including asepsis, gentle handling of tissue, hemostasis, irrigation, débridement of devitalized tissue, assurance of good blood supply to the wound and areas of operation, and delayed primary closure of contaminated wounds, is the factor *most* responsible for maintaining a low postoperative infection rate. Assuming these measures are followed, additional improvement in decreasing infection rates can be achieved only in certain cases through the appropriate use of perioperative prophylactic antibiotics. Prophylactic antibiotics are indicated when the risk of morbidity from infection secondary to the operation outweighs the possible adverse problems of drug reaction, emergence of resistant bacteria, or where a wound infection would be life threatening.

Wound infections are directly correlated with the type of operation and the number of bacteria present in the operative field, and the categories established to define these risks of wound infection are shown in Table 2. Antibiotics are only indicated in clean surgical cases where infection would be catastrophic, in association with placement of a prosthesis or foreign body, or in those instances where a second infection exists elsewhere in the body. Prophylactic use of antibiotics is usually indicated in *clean-contaminated* cases and always in *contaminated* surgical operations. In the contaminated cases, antibiotics are considered treatment for the condition.

The choice of antibiotic depends on the contaminating organism most likely to be encountered in each procedure, as the drug must be effective against the majority of bacteria likely to cause the infection. The timing of administration of prophylactic antibiotics is important. Overwhelmingly, studies show that if prophylactic antibiotics are to be most effective they must be administered parenterally preoperatively to produce adequate tissue and blood levels at the time of operation. The duration of administration should not exceed 48 to 72 hours.

Preoperative measures that decrease the contamination from bowel flora at the time of colorectal procedures include: (1) mechanical intestinal cleansing, usually with a large volume of orally administered purgatives such as a polyethylene-glycol-based liquid, (2) poorly absorbed oral antibiotics given between 8 and 24 hours prior to operation, and (3) prophylactic systemic antibiotics. Postoperative wound infection rates decrease from 30 to 40 per cent in patients given mechanical bowel preparation, to 8 to 10 per cent in patients receiving both mechanical and oral antibiotic bowel preparation. Parenteral antibiotics (cephalosporins) are effective in reducing the incidence of wound infection in patients undergoing colorectal operation to about 25 per cent of the incidence seen in patients receiving only mechanical bowel preparation. Parenteral antibiotics with oral antibiotics may not necessarily lead to a further decrease in infectious complications.

PREOPERATIVE CONSIDERATIONS BY ORGAN SYSTEMS

Cardiovascular

Perioperative myocardial infarction is the leading cause of operative mortality for most thoracic and abdominal operations. Identification of high-risk patients is important, since the incidence of cardiovascular complications in the general population undergoing general anesthesia is only 0.2 per cent. The most important factors in preoperatively predicting cardiac risks from noncardiac surgery can be estimated from a thorough history, physical examination, and the electrocardiogram. The most important factor in the history is documentation of a myocardial infarction occurring within the previous 6 months. Recurrent myocardial infarction occurs in 30 per cent of patients undergoing surgery within 3 months of a myocardial infarction, 15 per cent at 3 to 6 months, and 5 per cent of patients thereafter. Preoperative significant risk factors are summarized in Table 3. Based on these risk factors, patients were grouped into classes with the following mortality and complication rates:

1. Class I (0 to 5 points), with 0.2 per cent cardiac deaths and 0.7 per cent complications.

TABLE 2. CATEGORIES OF SURGICAL OPERATIONS BASED ON DEGREE OF BACTERIAL CONTAMINATION

Category	Description
Clean	Procedures in which aseptic technique is maintained and inflammation is not encountered and the alimentary, respiratory, genitourinary, or oropharyngeal cavities or systems are not entered
Clean-contaminated	Procedures in which the above-mentioned cavities or systems are entered but in which contamination is minimal
Contaminated	Procedures involving serious breaks in aseptic technique, serious contamination from an entered hollow viscus, or where inflammation but not purulence exists in the operative field
Dirty	Procedures involving purulence or gross infection in the wound, gross inflammation and contamination from a previously perforated viscus, or traumatic wounds greater than 6 hours old or containing a large amount of foreign material or devitalized tissue

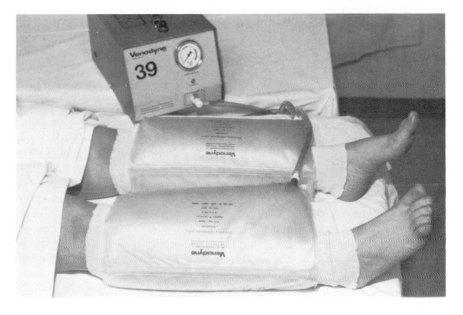

Figure 2. Intermittent pneumatic compression device with compression sleeve covering lower leg. (From Persson AV, Davis RJ, Villavicencio JL: Deep venous thrombosis and pulmonary embolism. Surg Clin North Am 71[6]:1195–1210, 1991, with permission.)

2. Class II (6 to 12 points), with 2 per cent deaths and 5 per cent complications.

3. Class III (13 to 25 points), with 2 per cent deaths and 11 per cent complications.

4. Class IV (26 or more points), with 56 per cent deaths and 22 per cent complications.

The risk of surgical procedure with significant cor-

TABLE 3. PREOPERATIVE SIGNIFICANT RISK FACTORS*

Criteria	Points
History	
Age >70 years	5
MI in previous 6 months	10
Physical examination	
S₃ gallop or JVD	11
Important valvular aortic stenosis	3
Electrocardioram	
Rhythm other than sinus or PACs on last ECG	7
>5 PVC/min at any time before surgery	7
General Status	3
PO₂ <60 or PCO₂ >50 mm Hg	
K+ C3.0 or HCO₃ <20 mEq/L	
BUN >50 or creatinine >3.0 mg/dl	
Signs of chronic liver disease, +SGOT	
Bedridden from noncardiac causes	
Operation	
Intraperitoneal, intrathoracic, or aortic operation	3
Emergency operation	4
Total possible	53

*From Goldman L, et al: N Engl J Med 297:848, 1977, with permission.
Abbreviations: MI = myocardial infarction, JVD = jugular venous distention, PAC = premature atrial contraction, ECG = electrocardiogram, PVC = premature ventricular contraction, BUN = blood urea nitrogen, SGOT = serum glutamic-oxaloacetic transaminase.

onary artery disease can be decreased if the patient first undergoes myocardial revascularization. Noninvasive screening of all patients at increased risk for coronary artery disease is recommended, using exercise tolerance tests, radionuclide angiography, and stress thallium scanning. Correction of congestive heart failure is strongly recommended prior to operation, as uncontrolled failure is associated with a 20 per cent cardiac mortality as contrasted with 5 per cent if congestive failure is controlled.

Preoperative cardiac arrhythmias are associated with an increased risk of perioperative cardiac death. Preoperative prophylaxis for ventricular ectopy, with lidocaine being the drug of choice, is given to patients who have either an ischemic event within 48 hours preceding operation or a history of symptomatic ventricular arrhythmias. Supraventricular arrhythmias occur frequently in those patients undergoing major vascular, intra-abdominal, and especially thoracic (up to 30 per cent) operations. Digitalis is recommended only for patients at high risk of developing supraventricular arrhythmias. Patients with valvular heart disease have a lessened ability to compensate hemodynamically for miscalculations in fluid therapy or drug therapy and require more careful perioperative monitoring of hemodynamic parameters. In general, stenotic valvular disease is more difficult to manage than regurgitant disease. Patients with significant aortic stenosis have a decreased ability to increase blood flow across the stenotic valve and tolerate vasodilation poorly. Consequently, spinal anesthesia is usually contraindicated.

Other valvular lesions, though not associated with as high an operative mortality, require similar hemodynamic considerations. Patients with mitral stenosis tolerate volume overload poorly. Therefore, mild hypovolemia is preferred to fluid overload. Chronic atrial fibrillation is often present, and anticoagulation is indicated in such patients. They also may benefit from prophylactic digitalis therapy. Aortic and mitral regurgitation are hemodynamic problems only when left ventricular function is consequently compromised. Patients with prosthetic heart valves require perioperative management of anticoagulant therapy, and the incidence of hemorrhagic complications is 13 per cent. Antibiotic prophylaxis is always indicated for patients with prosthetic valves and significant in those with other valvar disease who undergo any surgical procedure in which bacteremia is a possibility.

Pulmonary

Pulmonary complications occur in an estimated 5 to 7 per cent of operations, and the incidence is approximately doubled in abdominal operations, tripled in cigarette smokers, and quadrupled in patients with chronic obstructive pulmonary disease. Respiratory insufficiency is the direct cause of approximately 25 per cent of all postoperative mortalities and contributes to death in an additional 25 per cent. Static lung volumes are usually decreased in the postoperative period, and the magnitude of decrease is directly related to the site of the incision and the extent of pain. Tracheobronchial ciliary function is also decreased after operation, and these alterations promote atelectasis, which is the most common postoperative pulmonary complication.

Risk Factors

Cigarette smoking is associated with the development of a variety of respiratory diseases in addition to promoting postoperative atelectasis. Smoking severely affects mucociliary clearance in the respiratory tract and creates more viscous and copious secretions. The patient should be encouraged to stop smoking at least 4 weeks prior to operation. Obesity, prolonged duration of the procedure, and preoperative symptoms of chronic obstructive pulmonary disease are also associated with increased perioperative pulmonary complications.

Preoperative Screening Tests

The history and physical examination are usually sufficient to identify risk factors and signs of pulmonary dysfunction. A preoperative chest film is usually indicated in patients over age 40, those with planned thoracic procedures, and those with significant risk factors for pulmonary complications. Preoperative arterial blood gas determination is an accurate prognostic test for pulmonary problems in the perioperative period and is indicated prior to contemplated pulmonary resection. Pulmonary function tests are helpful in assessing postoperative risks from pulmonary problems, and patients with pulmonary function levels significantly below predicted levels should be assessed for functional improvement following bronchodilators. Pulmonary function tests can also predict respiratory adequacy following major thoracic or cardiac procedures. An MMV of greater than 50 per cent predicted or an FEV_1 of greater that 2 L is considered adequate functional reserve. In patients with marginal pulmonary function contemplating lung resection, the extent to which the diseased lung is contributing to effective ventilatory function can be accurately estimated by radionuclide ventilation and perfusion lung scanning.

Endocrine

Certain specific problems of endocrine dysfunction are either sufficiently common or sufficiently dangerous to warrant special enumeration. In general, for states of endocrine insufficiency such as *hypothyroidism*, the preoperative preparation involves confirmation of endocrine insufficiency followed by replacement therapy. If the clinical picture of excess hormone secretion is confirmed biochemically, steps should be taken preoperatively to ablate the hormonal excess.

Diabetes mellitus is not a risk factor for surgical procedures when it is well controlled at the time of operation. The goals of preoperative and perioperative management are maintenance of a relative state of mild hyperglycemia, avoidance of excess hyperglycemia, and avoidance of dangerous hypoglycemia. The serum blood glucose is the best parameter to monitor the patient's insulin requirements. The potentially fatal complication of intraoperative hypoglycemia must always be avoided; therefore, a constant infusion of intravenous fluids containing glucose is maintained throughout anesthesia. Type II diabetics may require little if any insulin in the perioperative period. In patients with type I diabetes, insulin therapy should be based on maintaining the blood glucose in the 150- to 250-mg/dl range. For type I diabetics, one half the usual morning dose of insulin given as regular insulin subcutaneously on call usually prevents excess hyperglycemia.

Hyperthyroidism

Preoperative recognition of hyperthyroidism is important to avoid the consequences of intraoperative thyroid storm, which can be fatal if not properly treated. Propranolol is effective against the cardiovascular collapse associated with thyroid storm and is used as a perioperative prophylactic agent for hyperthyroid patients. Propylthiouracil (PTU), an effective inhibitor of T_4 synthesis, is the main agent used to treat hyperthyroidism pharmacologically.

Adrenal Insufficiency

The most common adrenal cortical abnormality in the preoperative setting is secondary adrenal insufficiency due to glandular suppression in patients taking daily exogenous glucocorticoids. Primary adrenal insufficiency results from primary adrenal failure, or Addison's disease. Replacement steroid therapy for patients with primary or secondary adrenal insufficiency is essential at the time of surgical stress to prevent potentially fatal acute adrenal insufficiency. Patients taking supraphysiologic doses of steroids (>7.5 mg/day of prednisone) for more than 1 week are susceptible to adrenal suppression for up to 1 year thereafter. The adrenocorticotropic hormone (ACTH) stimulation test is a good predictor of adrenal adequacy in response to stress. An intravenous drip of hydrocortisone at 10 mg/hr or doses of 100 mg every 8 hours provides adequate replacement for patients undergoing major operative procedures. Replacement therapy is tapered by approximately 20 per cent per day once operative stress is resolved.

Gastrointestinal

The foremost concern preoperatively with respect to the gastrointestinal system is the ability to sustain the patient's nutritional requirements.

Liver Function

A history of alcoholism, jaundice, or upper gastrointestinal bleeding or physical findings of liver disease such as ascites suggest significant liver impairment. Hepatic insufficiency can be further quantified by laboratory evaluation. Biochemical and radiologic studies usually characterize the etiology of most causes of hepatic insufficiency and cholestasis. Patients with liver disease require a preoperative check of PT. The liver synthesizes clotting factors II, V, VII, and X. Significant hepatocellular damage is necessary before inadequate clotting factor synthesis results in prolongation of the PT. Hypoalbuminemia of less than 3.5 mg/dl suggests either starvation or chronic hepatic insufficiency.

Child and Turcotte described a classification of patients with cirrhosis based on criteria described in Table 4. Child's class A patients have adequate hepatic reserve to tolerate anesthesia and elective procedures

TABLE 4. CLASSIFICATION OF PATIENTS WITH CIRRHOSIS*

Class	Encephalopathy	Serum Albumin (mg/dl)	Ascites	Serum Bilirubin (mg/dl)
A	No	>3.5	No	<2.0
B	Mild	3.0–3.5	Mild	2.0–3.0
C	Yes	<3.0	Marked	>3.0

*From Child CG (ed): The Liver and Portal Hypertension. Philadelphia, WB Saunders Company, 1964, p 50, with permission.

with minimal additional risk. However, the operative mortality for emergency shunt procedures (for upper gastrointestinal bleeding) for patients in the Child's B and C categories is estimated to be 20 to 30 per cent and 40 to 50 per cent, respectively. Operative morbidity and mortality are also excessive in patients with acute alcoholic hepatitis who have an approximate 50 per cent mortality without operation and, therefore, only emergency procedures should be performed. Acute viral hepatitis is also a contraindication to all but emergency operations. Chronic carriers of hepatitis B have no excessive risk from operation, but the operating team must be aware of the danger of hepatitis transmission and take appropriate precautions. A preoperative course of corticosteroids may cause a remission in chronic active hepatitis.

Nervous System

Cerebrovascular Disease

In patients with extracranial cerebrovascular occlusive disease, intraoperative hypotension, anoxia, or increased blood viscosity can exacerbate preexistent compromised cerebral perfusion and result in stroke. Elective procedures are contraindicated for 6 to 8 weeks in patients who have sustained a frank stroke or intracerebral hemorrhage. Patients with preoperative transient ischemic attacks (TIAs) have a 37 per cent chance of developing a stroke during noncarotid surgery. Therefore, surgical repair of patients with TIAs and proven significant carotid stenosis or ulcerated plaque is indicated prior to other major surgery, except possibly concurrent coronary bypass. Noninvasive means of estimating carotid occlusive disease are generally good screening procedures, and angiography can be done to confirm the degree of disease. Patients with asymptomatic carotid bruits probably have no excess risk of neurologic deficit following elective procedures.

Seizure Disorders

Patients with seizure disorders must be assessed for the adequacy of control of the disorders on the current medical regimens. If a reliable history of good control is obtained, it can be ascertained that the patient has no additional risk for the morbidity that comes from perioperative seizures. If, however, no such documentation is available, either measurement of serum levels of anticonvulsants or a period of observation is advisable.

Alcoholism

Alcoholics are predisposed to *delirium tremens* as a serious neurologic complication of chronic alcoholism caused by the acute withdrawal from alcohol. The mild symptoms of restlessness and anxiety associated with mild alcohol withdrawal states can progress to hallucinations, fever, disorientation, and rarely, death. Treatment with sedatives, usually of the benzodiazepine family, is indicated as is postponement of contemplated elective surgical procedures. Thiamine deficiency in chronic alcoholics may be manifested as Wernicke's syndrome and can be prevented by the routine administration of 100 mg of thiamine intramuscularly.

Myasthenia Gravis

Myasthenia gravis is an example of the preoperative considerations for the patient with a myopathy. The measures taken when this disorder is present include providing adequate ventilatory support in the immediate postoperative period; careful attention to muscle relaxants, anticholinesterase drugs, or other medications particularly affecting muscle strength; and steroid coverage for patients on maintenance prednisone. The dose of anticholinesterase agent is reduced usually by about half on the day prior to operation. Use of competitive muscular blocking agents such as pancuronium is contraindicated.

Renal

The majority of problems concerning preoperative preparation with respect to renal function have been addressed in the previous sections on fluids and electrolytes. Patients with renal insufficiency or failure pose several special dilemmas in the preoperative period. Diagnostic tests using contrast dye convey a special risk to patients with marginal renal function. Hydration is essential in these patients to minimize further deterioration in renal function. Patients requiring chronic dialysis must have this incorporated into their treatment plan.

TABLE 5. PREOPERATIVE SUMMARY CHECKLIST

Consent obtained
Preoperative orders
  NPO
  Urinary voiding on call
  Preoperative skin preparation
  Possible preoperative antibiotics
  Steroids?
  Cardiac medications
  Other medications patient usually takes
  Preoperative sedative
  IV fluids
Pertinent x-rays available (including chest)
Blood (blood products prn) in bank
Preoperative lab results
  CBC
  Urinalysis
  Electrolytes, BUN, creatinine
  Possible coagulation studies
  Possible other chemistries/enzymes
Possible preoperative ECG
Special medical problems requiring consultation
Allergies

Abbreviations: NPO = nothing by mouth, IV = intravenous, CBC = complete blood count, BUN = blood urea nitrogen, ECG = electrocardiogram.

CONCLUSIONS

A useful checklist of common orders that apply to many patients' preoperative preparation is shown in Table 5. It is simply a suggestion; it is neither a comprehensive guideline nor to be used as a substitute for the careful individual attention that must be given to each patient. The maximal benefit of surgical therapy is achieved when an operation appropriate to correct the existing pathologic condition is performed correctly and at an indicated time in the disease process. Thorough preoperative preparation of the patient is mandatory to avoid problems at the critical time of operation, and appropriate consultation with the anesthesiologist should be obtained well in advance of a surgical procedure. The plan of the operation and the expected pathologic findings should be clear, as should be plans if possible alternative findings are encountered. Optimal surgical results occur when the surgical team has thoroughly prepared the patient for the procedure and when the team is fully prepared to perform the proposed surgical procedure.

REFERENCES

Clarke JS, Condon RE, Bartlett JG, et al: Preoperative oral antibiotics reduce septic complications of colorectal operations: Results of a prospective, randomized, double-blind clinical study. Ann Surg 186:251–259, 1977.

Cruse PJ, Foord R: The epidemiology of wound infection: A 10-year prospective study of 62, 939 wounds. Surg Clin North Am *60*: 27–40, 1980.

Lewin I, Lerner AG, Green SH, et al: Physical class and physiologic status in the prediction of operative mortality in the aged sick. Ann Surg *174*(2): 217–231, 1971.

MacLean LD: Host resistance in surgical patients. J Trauma *19*: 297–304, 1979.

Rombeau JL, Barot LR, Williams CE, Mullen JL: Preoperative total parenteral nutrition and surgical outcome in patients with inflammatory bowel disease. Am J Surg *143*:139–143, 1982.

Wolfe WG, Sabiston DC Jr: Pulmonary embolism. *In* Major Problems in Clinical Surgery, vol 25. Philadelphia, WB Saunders Company, 1980, pp 96–111.

6

BLOOD TRANSFUSIONS AND DISORDERS OF SURGICAL BLEEDING

THOMAS F. SLAUGHTER, M.D.   CHARLES S. GREENBERG, M.D.

The hemostatic system utilizes plasma proteins, platelets, and endothelial cells to initiate blood coagulation and to arrest bleeding. Vascular injury initiates a complex series of reactions that leads to the transformation of blood from the liquid state into a gel-like clot. Pathologic defects in this system may cause either bleeding or thrombosis. This chapter focuses on the normal physiology of coagulation, pathologic defects of hemostasis, and transfusion medicine.

BIOCHEMISTRY AND PHYSIOLOGY OF HEMOSTASIS

Platelet Adhesion

Under normal conditions, platelets do not adhere either to endothelium or to other platelets. Following tissue injury, however, exposure of adhesive molecules present in the subendothelial matrix provides platelet binding sites. A variety of proteins participate in platelet adhesion including collagen, vitronectin, fibronectin, and von Willebrand factor (vWF). Von Willebrand factor plays a particularly important role in platelet adhesion. This large multimeric protein present in plasma, platelets, and the subendothelial matrix acts as a bridge linking platelet surface glycoproteins (GP) with subendothelial adhesive molecules. Under conditions of high shear rate, as found in arteries and the microvasculature, vWF binds to the platelet surface GPIb. Quantitative and qualitative disorders of the vWF protein account for the most frequent inheritable bleeding disorder—von Willebrand's disease. Platelet adhesion represents the primary event in the process of hemostasis. As platelets spread over a damaged endothelial surface and undergo adhesion, a complex series of metabolic events is triggered, leading to the process of platelet aggregation.

Platelet Aggregation

During the process of adhesion, stimulation of the platelet GPIb receptor by vWF or exposure of platelet surface receptors to agonists such as thrombin, adenosine 5'-diphosphate (ADP), or collagen causes platelet activation and subsequent aggregation. Just as with platelet adhesion, aggregation must precede formation of a stable platelet plug. Platelet activation and aggregation are characterized by the release of intracellular storage granule contents, phospholipase cleavage of membrane phospholipids, mobilization of intracellular calcium, and exposure of various protein receptors on the platelet surface.

The platelet release reaction appears analogous to secretory processes in other cells. Upon platelet activation, storage granules fuse with the cell membrane, releasing their contents. Alpha granules contain proteins active in coagulation, including factor V, vWF, fibrinogen, fibronectin, thrombospondin, and platelet-derived growth factor. Dense bodies comprise the other major platelet storage site and contain serotonin, ADP, and adenosine 5'-triphosphate (ATP). Potent stimulators of the release reaction include thrombin, collagen, epinephrine, and ADP. Specific receptors for these proteins have been characterized on the platelet surface.

Intracellular 3′,5′-cyclic adenosine monophosphate (cAMP) concentrations contribute to the regulation of platelet aggregation. Compounds that increase cAMP concentration (i.e., prostacyclin and dipyridamole) inhibit platelet aggregation, whereas those that lower cAMP concentration (ADP and epinephrine) stimulate platelet aggregation. Platelet membrane receptors are coupled to adenylate cyclase, the enzyme that synthesizes cAMP. Second messengers other than cAMP have been described linking membrane receptors with secretory processes. Similar systems may exist within the platelet. Several platelet agonists stimulate phospholipase A_2–mediated generation of arachidonate, leading to the production of prostaglandin endoperoxides and thromboxane A_2.

Recently, the cleavage of inositol-containing phospholipids by phospholipase C has been demonstrated to generate second messengers for platelet activation. Production of 1,2-diacylglycerol and 1,4,5-inositol trisphosphate (IP_3) by phospholipase C cleavage of phosphatidylinositol 4,5-bisphosphate (PIP_2) is associated with both the thrombin-mediated platelet release reaction and platelet aggregation. Diacylglycerol functions within the cell membrane to activate protein kinase C. Protein kinase C phosphorylates molecules essential to platelet secretion. IP_3 binds to specific calcium channel proteins of the endoplasmic reticulum, causing the release of calcium into the cytosol. Mobilization of calcium appears essential for both platelet secretion and aggregation.

The final common pathway for platelet aggregation involves fibrinogen. Upon platelet activation, the platelet membrane GPIIb/IIIa undergoes a conformational change to become an active fibrinogen receptor. Fibrinogen acts as the bridge to link adjacent platelets into stable aggregates. Absence of GPIIb/IIIa causes a severe bleeding disorder known as Glanzmann's thrombasthenia.

Despite the important contribution of platelets to primary hemostasis, the platelet plug is incapable of providing a stable hemostatic barrier in the absence of fibrin formation. The platelet acts as a specialized phospholipid surface upon which the process of plasma-mediated coagulation may be accelerated. During the process of platelet activation, anionic phospholipids are exposed on the platelet surface. These phospholipids provide binding sites for plasma coagulation protein complexes, thereby localizing hemostatic reactions and accelerating the kinetics of thrombin and fibrin formation.

Blood Coagulation Factors, the Coagulation Cascade, and Thrombin Generation

Although platelet adhesion and aggregation comprise the primary response to vascular injury, fibrin formation mediated by thrombin is essential to formation of a stable clot. Formation of thrombin occurs through a series of precise proteolytic cleavages of plasma proteins. Inactive plasma proteins (zymogens) are converted to active serine proteases, culminating in the formation of fibrin. The plasma proteins responsible for generating thrombin have been assigned roman numerals based upon their order of discovery (Table 1). As the inactive proteins are converted to serine proteases, their active form, they are designated by an "a" following the roman numeral. Activated serine proteases function in the cascade of reactions leading to thrombin formation. Factors V and VIII function as essential cofactors in the coagulation cascade, but they do not function as enzymes to directly convert inactive coagulation proteins into serine proteases. Since the early 1960s, two pathways have been described for the formation of thrombin. The plasma proteins described by the intrinsic and extrinsic pathways (the coagulation cascade) are responsible for initiating and amplifying thrombin formation (Fig. 1). A small stimulus at the first step of the cascade is catalytically amplified at each successive step, resulting in the rapid formation of large amounts of thrombin.

The intrinsic pathway of coagulation is initiated by contact of the plasma proteins factor XII, prekallikrein, and high-molecular-weight kininogen with a negatively charged surface, such as glass. The name for this pathway originated from the observation that all components necessary for clot formation through this pathway are present in plasma. Formation of the contact activation complex causes the activation of factor XI to XIa. Factor XIa then activates factor IX. Both the intrinsic and extrinsic pathways culminate in the formation of factor Xa. The intrinsic pathway generates factor Xa by the formation of an enzyme complex consisting of factors IXa, X, VIII, and calcium on a phospholipid surface. Factor VIII acts as an essential cofactor in this reaction as evidenced by the severe bleeding disorder occurring in its absence—hemophilia A. The phospholipid surface, most often provided by platelets, optimizes the conformation of the enzyme components in the "tenase complex" so as to maximize product formation. In the absence of a phospholipid surface, this reaction fails to generate adequate factor Xa to propagate the cascade.

The extrinsic pathway of coagulation provides an alternative mechanism for the generation of factor Xa and thrombin. Tissue factor, a constitutively expressed phospholipoprotein of the subendothelium, must be present for activation of the extrinsic pathway. Tissue factor is concentrated in the adventitia surrounding blood vessels, but does not circulate in the plasma. Monocytes and vascular endothelial cells may be induced to express tissue factor by exposure to bacterial lipopolysaccharide, interleukin-1, thrombin, tumor necrosis factor, complement activation products, or im-

TABLE 1.   COAGULATION PROTEINS

Protein	Plasma Level (mg/dl)	Effective* Hemostatic Level	Replacement Product	Half-Life (Days or Hours)	Function
Fibrinogen	180–360	100 mg/dl	Cryoprecipitate	4 days	Forms the fibrin clot
Prothrombin (factor II)	10.0	20–40%	Plasma	2–3 days	Produces thrombin and activates fibrinogen; factors V, VIII, and XIII; platelets; and protein C
Factor V	2.0	25%	Plasma	1 day	Cofactor for factor Xa activation of prothrombin
Factor VII	0.1	10–20%	Plasma	6 hours	Activates factors IX and X
Factor VIII:C (antihemophilic factor)	0.1	25%	Purified factor VII or cryoprecipitate	8–12 hours	Cofactor for factor IXa activation of factor X
Factor VIII:vWF (von Willebrand factor)	2.0	25%	Cryoprecipitate	1 day	Mediates platelet adhesion
Factor IX	1.0	20%	Plasma Purified factor IX	1 day	Activates factor X
Factor X	1.0	25%	Plasma	1–2 days	Activates prothrombin
Factor XI	0.5	15–25%	Plasma	2–3 days	Activites factor IX
Factor XII	2.0	<10%	Not necessary	—	Activates factor XII and prekallikrein
Factor XIII (fibrin-stabilizing factor)	1.0	5%	Cryoprecipitate	4 days	Covalently cross-links fibrin monomers to each other and α_2-plasmin inhibitor to fibrin

*Values expressed as percentage of the normal coagulant activity.

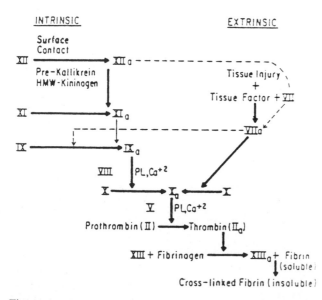

Figure 1. Intrinsic and extrinsic pathways of blood coagulation. The extrinsic pathway initiates thrombin formation after tissue injury exposes tissue factor. The intrinsic pathway amplifies and propagates the hemostatic process initiated by the extrinsic pathway. The platelet phospholipid surface provides an assembly site for the prothrombinase complex and thereby accelerates the formation of thrombin. Soluble fibrin is generated by thrombin and stabilized to an insoluble form by factor XIIIa.

mune complexes. Factor VII circulates in plasma as an inactive protein. Under normal conditions, tissue factor is not exposed to factor VII in the plasma. Following an injury to the vasculature, tissue factor exposure to factors VII and VIIa causes the formation of an active factor VIIa–tissue factor complex. This complex binds with factors IX and X on a phospholipid surface to generate the active enzymes IXa and Xa, respectively.

The intrinsic and extrinsic pathways merge upon formation of factor Xa. Factor Xa forms an enzyme complex with prothrombin, factor V, and calcium on a phospholipid surface. This "prothrombinase complex" is similar to the "tenase complex" and the factor VIIa–tissue factor–factor X complex described earlier, in that phospholipids provided by the platelet surface are essential to maximize the reaction rate and to overcome intrinsic anticoagulant protective mechanisms (Fig. 2).

Although the intrinsic and extrinsic pathways provide a convenient means of describing the cascade of reactions leading to hemostasis, many interactions exist between the two pathways. Factor VIIa is capable of converting factor IX to factor IXa. Factor Xa may also activate factor VII. Factor XIIa has been demonstrated in vitro to convert factor VII to factor VIIa. Thrombin, a product of both pathways, feeds back to

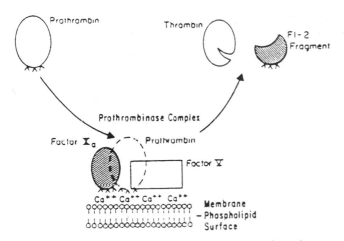

Figure 2. Formation of thrombin by the prothrombinase complex. The phospholipid surface of platelets provides an assembly site for the prothrombinase complex, an enzyme activation complex consisting of factor Xa, cofactor V, calcium, and prothrombin. Soluble prothrombin is cleaved by the prothrombinase complex to form thrombin. The prothrombin phospholipid binding site containing the γ-carboxyglutamic acid residues is released with the activation fragment F1.2 upon thrombin formation. (From Mosher DF: In MacKinney AA [ed]: Pathophysiology of Blood. New York, John Wiley & Sons, Inc., 1984, with permission.)

amplify its own formation by activating protein cofactors necessary for both pathways—factors V and VIII. In addition, thrombin in combination with a polyanionic cofactor effectively activates factor XI.

The physiologic importance of the intrinsic pathway for hemostasis appears limited, since persons with congenital deficiencies of factor XII, high-molecular-weight kininogen, or prekallikrein do not experience excessive bleeding. In contrast, individuals with deficiencies of factors XI, VIII, or IX may suffer from severe disorders of hemostasis. This suggests that the importance of the intrinsic pathway may occur in the amplification rather than the initiation of thrombin formation. Recent investigations support a revised model for in vivo coagulation. Following injury to the vessel wall, tissue factor present in the subendothelium is exposed to factors VII and VIIa in plasma. The factor VIIa–tissue factor complex leads to generation of both factors Xa and IXa. Shortly after initiation of coagulation through the extrinsic pathway, however, tissue factor pathway inhibitor (TFPI) complexes with the factor VIIa–tissue factor–factor Xa complex, causing the shutdown of thrombin production through the extrinsic pathway. At this point propagation of the hemostatic response relies upon amplification of factor Xa production through factor IXa and the intrinsic pathway. This model explains the fact that patients with hemophilia bleed despite a normal extrinsic pathway of coagulation. In the absence of factor VIII, the

patient with hemophilia A is unable to amplify the hemostatic response once TFPI shuts down the production of factor Xa through the factor VIIa–tissue factor pathway.

Factors Regulating Thrombin Formation

Thrombin represents the key regulatory step in hemostasis. Mechanisms for the downregulation of thrombin activity are essential to prevent fibrin formation downstream from the site of vascular injury. Antithrombin III (AT-III) is the major physiologic inhibitor of thrombin. This protein belongs to the family of serine protease inhibitors (serpins), and it inhibits factors IXa and Xa in addition to thrombin. The presence of heparin induces a conformational change in AT-III that greatly accelerates the inhibitory action toward thrombin (Fig. 3). The endothelial cell surface possesses endogenous anticoagulant activity in the form of heparin-like glycosaminoglycans (heparan sulfate) that also accelerate the activity of AT-III. After formation of the AT-III–protease complex, heparin is released to catalyze the formation of additional AT-III–protease complexes. The circulating AT-III–protease complexes are cleared by the liver.

The protein C–thrombomodulin system provides further limitation of thrombin activity. Protein C circulates as an inactive zymogen in plasma. As thrombin forms, it binds to thrombomodulin on the endothelial surface, forming a complex capable of activating protein C. Activated protein C, in the presence of its cofactor, protein S, proteolyzes the essential cofactors Va and VIIIa. In addition, any thrombin bound to thrombomodulin becomes inactivated and unable to convert fibrinogen to fibrin. Tissue factor pathway inhibitor is a recently characterized protein capable of regulating the activation of coagulation through the extrinsic pathway. Tissue factor pathway inhibitor forms a quaternary complex with the factors Xa, VIIa, and tissue factor, thereby blocking thrombin formation through the extrinsic pathway. Tissue factor pathway inhibitor circulates in plasma bound to lipoproteins. Heparin administration induces in vivo release of TFPI—most likely from the endothelium. Platelets release significant amounts of TFPI upon activation. They may act to concentrate TFPI and to downregulate the hemostatic process at sites of thrombin formation and platelet aggregation.

Fibrin Formation and Stabilization

Conversion of fibrinogen into a network of stable fibrin strands occurs through the action of thrombin

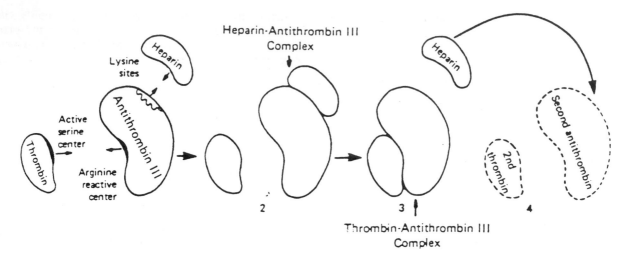

Figure 3. The mechanism of action of heparin and antithrombin III (AT-III). Heparin binds to a lysine residue on AT-III forming the heparin/AT-III complex (*panel 2*). A conformational change in AT-III exposes an arginine group that covalently binds thrombin and other serine proteases involved in hemostasis (factors IXa, Xa, XIa) (*panel 3*). Upon formation of the AT-III–serine protease complex, the heparin is released to catalyze additional AT-III molecules (*panel 4*). (Modified from Rosenberg RD: Heparin-antithrombin system. *In* Colman RW, Hirsh J, Marder VJ, Salzman WW [eds]: Hemostasis and Thrombosis: Basic Principles and Clinical Practice. Philadelphia, JB Lippincott Company, 1982, with permission.)

and factor XIII. Thrombin proteolytically releases fibrinopeptides A and B from the fibrinogen molecule, producing fibrin monomers. The fibrin monomers assemble in a staggered overlapping configuration, producing a protofibril. The protofibrils increase in size by forming long rows of fibrin strands. Fibrin strands then associate with each other to form a branching network of fibers and the fibrin gel. Blood coagulation factor XIII binds to fibrin and is converted by thrombin to factor XIIIa. Factor XIIIa covalently cross-links adjacent fibrin monomers to each other. Factor XIIIa also cross-links α_2-antiplasmin, the major inhibitor of plasmin, to the clot. Factor XIIIa cross-linked fibrin is both mechanically stronger and more resistant to lysis by plasmin. Factor XIIIa may also facilitate wound healing, since factor XIII–deficient patients experience an increased incidence of wound dehiscence and abnormal scar formation.

Digestion of Fibrin by the Fibrinolytic System

Initiation of the hemostatic process simultaneously activates the fibrinolytic system. The balance between hemostasis and fibrinolysis localizes the thrombotic process to the site of vascular damage. Plasmin is the enzyme responsible for degradation of fibrin. Plasmin is derived from a plasma precursor, plasminogen. During fibrin formation, plasminogen binds to fibrin and is incorporated into the clot. Plasminogen remains inactive until cleavage by a plasminogen activator. The two primary plasminogen activators are tissue-type plasminogen activator (t-PA), produced by the endothelium, and urokinase, produced by both the endothelium and urinary tract. A variety of stimuli produce endothelial release of plasminogen activator including physical exercise, venous occlusion, adrenaline, vasopressin, and thrombin. The presence of fibrin greatly accelerates the conversion of plasminogen to plasmin by t-PA. This important mechanism acts to localize fibrinolysis to regions of fibrin formation and active thrombosis.

Inhibitors of the fibrinolytic system form an additional means of localizing fibrin degradation. Free plasmin in the circulation is rapidly inhibited by α_2-antiplasmin. Once bound to fibrin, plasmin is protected from inactivation by α_2-antiplasmin. Under conditions in which the binding capacity of α_2-antiplasmin is exceeded, α_2-macroglobulin may also function as an inhibitor of plasmin. Specific inhibitors of plasminogen activators have been identified. Plasminogen activator inhibitor type 1 (PAI-1), produced primarily by endothelial cells, is released as an acute-phase reactant. Elevated PAI-1 activity has been implicated in the early morning peak incidence of myocardial infarctions. In addition, PAI-1 activity appears to play a role in the fibrinolytic shutdown occurring after surgery.

LABORATORY EVALUATION OF THE SURGICAL PATIENT WITH A DISORDER OF HEMOSTASIS

Assessment for abnormalities of hemostasis or thrombosis has become a routine part of the preoperative evaluation. The practice of screening all preoperative patients for laboratory abnormalities of coagulation has not proven cost effective. Despite the ability to measure quantitative and qualitative abnormalities for many aspects of clot formation, no tests currently available allow measurement of the platelet–endothelial cell interaction that is essential to in vivo coagulation. This remains the major limitation of coagulation testing. A detailed clinical history remains the most effective technique for identifying patients with either inherited or acquired disorders of coagulation.

Details elicited during the patient's history and physical examination may necessitate a more detailed laboratory evaluation prior to proceeding with surgery. Is there a family history of bleeding? Has there been excessive bleeding following prior surgery? Is there a history of frequent nosebleeds? Was nasal packing required? Has spontaneous bleeding occurred into joints or muscles? Is there bleeding from the gums? Do excessive bleeding or bruising occur following aspirin ingestion?

Preoperative evaluation of hemostasis most often includes the measurement of platelet function, thrombin formation, and fibrin formation (Table 2). The bleeding time offers a simple and rapid test of both platelet adhesion and platelet aggregation. The bleeding time is performed by inflating a blood pressure cuff to 40 mm Hg and using a commercial lancet to make a standardized 1-mm incision on the forearm. The time to

TABLE 2. COMMON COAGULATION LABORATORY TESTS AND THEIR RELATIONSHIP TO COAGULATION REACTIONS

Laboratory Test	Coagulation Reaction
Bleeding time	Platelet adhesion and aggregation
Platelet aggregometry	Platelet release and aggregation
Prothrombin time (PT)	Thrombin generation via extrinsic pathway
Activated partial thromboplastin time (aPTT)	Thrombin generation via intrinsic pathway
Thrombin clotting time	Fibrin formation
Reptilase time	Fibrin formation
Fibrin(ogen) split products	Fibrin and fibrinogen degradation

cessation of bleeding represents the bleeding time. Normal bleeding times do not exceed 10 minutes. Both quantitative and qualitative platelet defects prolong the bleeding time. Platelet counts less than 100,000/mm^3 may cause a prolonged bleeding time. Aspirin commonly prolongs the bleeding time by several minutes. Prolongation of the bleeding time should be further assessed by tests of platelet aggregation.

Platelet aggregometry assesses platelet aggregation in response to an agonist. Platelet-rich plasma from the patient is incubated with a platelet agonist (i.e., ADP, epinephrine, collagen). The suspension is stirred as changes in light transmission through the platelet suspension are recorded. Increases in light transmission correspond with platelet aggregation.

The prothrombin time (PT), activated partial thromboplastin time (aPTT), and thrombin time quantitate both thrombin and fibrin formation. The time required to clot platelet-poor plasma after the addition of tissue factor, calcium, and phospholipid is known as the prothrombin time. This test monitors thrombin formation by the extrinsic pathway of coagulation, and provides a means of monitoring the therapeutic anticoagulation achieved with warfarin. Thrombin generation via the intrinsic pathway is measured by the aPTT, which measures the time to clot formation after mixing platelet-poor plasma with a negatively charged substance (ellagic acid or celite). Clot formation occurs following the formation of factor XIIa in the intrinsic pathway. Anticoagulation with heparin is monitored with the aPTT.

The thrombin time provides a sensitive measure of fibrin formation. This test is performed by adding thrombin to platelet-poor plasma and measuring the time required for formation of a fibrin gel. Thrombin clotting times are prolonged by inhibitors of thrombin-mediated cleavage of fibrinogen (heparin, fibrin degradation products, dysfibrinogenemia) or inhibitors of fibrin monomer polymerization (monoclonal immunoglobulins, fibrin degradation products, or dysfibrinogenemia). The thrombin time may also be prolonged by fibrinogen concentrations less than 80 mg/dl or greater than 400 mg/dl. Clinically significant bleeding may occur in patients with mild factor deficiencies despite normal preoperative coagulation tests. The PT and aPTT remain normal until coagulation factor concentrations decrease below 30 per cent. Patients with mild hemophilia A or B may go undetected unless a careful history detects the hemorrhagic tendency. Von Willebrand's disease, factor XIII deficiency, and α_2-antiplasmin deficiency are important inheritable bleeding disorders that may not be detected by the PT, aPTT, or thrombin time.

The patient with a prolonged aPTT but no history of bleeding represents a common preoperative dilemma. Initially, the abnormal test must be confirmed and a mixing study should be performed. One part of normal plasma is mixed with one part of the patient's plasma; the 1:1 mixture should produce a normal aPTT. Normal plasma contains at least a 50 per cent concentration of the coagulation factors. Even if the patient's plasma was totally deficient in an intrinsic pathway coagulation protein, there would be adequate concentrations of coagulation factors in the 1:1 mixture to normalize the aPTT. Correction of the aPTT with a 1:1 mixture implies the deficiency of an intrinsic pathway coagulation factor. In the absence of a history of bleeding, the most common cause for a prolonged aPTT that corrects is a deficiency in either factor XII, prekallikrein, or high-molecular-weight kininogen.

Failure of the aPTT to correct with the 1:1 mixture implies the presence of an inhibitor to either thrombin or fibrin formation. The most common inhibitor to be detected with the aPTT is the lupus anticoagulant, an immunoglobulin molecule that binds the artificial phospholipids used in the aPTT assay. The lupus anticoagulant delays clotting in vitro by inhibiting assembly of the prothrombinase complex on phospholipid surfaces in the assay. Lupus anticoagulant does not inhibit assembly of the prothrombinase complex on the platelet surface in vivo; therefore, it does not cause a bleeding disorder. Paradoxically, lupus anticoagulant may increase the risk of venous thromboses. Additional causes of an abnormal mixing study include dysfibrinogenemia and heparin therapy.

The fibrinolytic system becomes activated concomitant with thrombin formation. Laboratory evidence that plasminogen has been converted to plasmin may be obtained indirectly by measurement of plasmin-derived fibrin and fibrinogen degradation products. The presence of fibrin(ogen) degradation products indicates the presence of plasmin in the circulation. Recently, a latex agglutination assay has been developed to quantitate the fragment D-dimer that is released into plasma during plasmin-mediated degradation of cross-linked fibrin. This assay provides the capability to measure fibrin-specific degradation products.

MANAGEMENT OF HEMOSTATIC DISORDERS IN SURGICAL PATIENTS

Hemostatic disorders may be categorized by defects in one of the steps leading to hemostasis, as follows: (1) disorders of platelets, (2) disorders of thrombin formation, (3) disorders of fibrin formation, (4) disorders of fibrinolysis, and (5) thrombotic disorders.

Disorders of Platelets

Thrombocytopenia accounts for the majority of platelet disorders in the perioperative period. The risk of spontaneous hemorrhage increases at platelet concentrations less than 20,000/mm^3. Under conditions of ongoing hemorrhage, higher platelet concentrations are needed for hemostasis. Platelet concentrations on the order of 100,000/mm^3 are generally recommended prior to proceeding with elective surgery. The ability of platelets to adhere and aggregate declines at lower platelet concentrations; however, there are exceptions to this rule. Patients with immunologic destruction of platelets, such as immune thrombocytopenic purpura (ITP), sustain a population of young hemostatically active platelets. On the other hand, platelet concentrations in excess of 100,000/mm^3 do not assure adequate hemostatic activity. Qualitative disorders of platelet function may occur as a result of drug exposure, uremia, or an intrinsic platelet defect.

The first question that needs to be addressed in evaluating the thrombocytopenic patient is whether the bone marrow is adequately producing platelets. If the platelet count has decreased more than 25 per cent over 24 hours in the absence of blood loss, then platelet consumption rather than decreased marrow production is likely. The bone marrow aspirate and biopsy provide the most direct methods for assessing platelet production.

Surgery alone rarely causes thrombocytopenia, although platelet consumption increases during active bleeding. Drug toxicity commonly causes enhanced platelet destruction. Heparin and cimetidine are two of the most commonly cited agents associated with drug-induced thrombocytopenia. Antibodies directed against the drug or a drug–platelet complex coats the platelets, resulting in their removal by the reticuloendothelial system. Heparin-induced thrombocytopenia may lead paradoxically to life-threatening arterial thromboses. Discontinuation of the heparin usually leads to a resolution of the thrombocytopenia.

Qualitative platelet defects may cause abnormal hemostasis despite normal platelet numbers in the circulation. Defects involving platelet adhesion, aggregation, and the release reaction have been associated with bleeding disorders (Table 3). Aspirin-mediated interference with the arachidonate pathway may produce abnormalities in platelet aggregation for as long as 1 week following a single dose.

Disorders of Thrombin Generation

The severity of symptoms associated with disorders of thrombin generation usually lead to diagnosis prior to surgery. Patients with severe hemophilia A (factor VIII deficiency) or hemophilia B (factor IX deficiency) often describe a history of spontaneous hemorrhage into joints and muscles. Deficiencies of factor XI may go undetected until the challenge of surgery. Highly purified plasma protein concentrates are available for

TABLE 3. CLINICAL DISORDERS OF HEMOSTATIS AND THEIR EFFECT ON BLOOD COAGULATION REACTIONS

Coagulation Reaction	Clinical Disorders
Platelet adhesion	von Willebrand's syndrome
	Bernard-Soulier disease
Platelet release reaction	Storage pool disease
Platelet aggregation	Aspirin ingestion
	Glanzmann's thrombasthenia
Thrombin generation	Hemophilia A and B
	Liver disease
	Vitamin K deficiency
Fibrin formation	DIC syndrome
Clot stabilization	Factor XIII deficiency
Fibrin digestion	α_2-Plasmin inhibitor deficiency
Regulation of thrombin formation	Antithrombin III deficiency
	Protein C deficiency

Abbreviation: DIC = disseminated intravascular coagulation.

congenital deficiencies of coagulation factors VIII and IX.

Vitamin K deficiency associated with antibiotic therapy and malabsorption is a frequent complication in the surgical patient. Factors II, VII, IX, and X require vitamin K during synthesis for the carboxylation of glutamic acid residues. Carboxylated glutamic acid residues are essential for the binding of coagulation factors to phospholipid membranes. As discussed earlier, the association of coagulation factors with phospholipid membranes accelerates the rate of thrombin formation, allowing normal hemostasis to occur. Vitamin K may be repleted by subcutaneous injection; however, 1 to 2 days are necessary for the liver to synthesize functional vitamin K–dependent coagulation factors. Administration of fresh frozen plasma may be used in the emergent situation to rapidly replete functional coagulation factors.

Disorders of Fibrin Formation

Uncontrolled activation of coagulation resulting in fibrin formation in the microcirculation leads to the syndrome of disseminated intravascular coagulation (DIC). Concomitant activation of fibrinolysis counters the fibrin formation; however, plasma coagulation factors are rapidly depleted. Also, fibrin(ogen) fragments interfere with clot formation and platelet function, contributing to diffuse bleeding. Many conditions are capable of initiating DIC including hypotension, septicemia, tissue necrosis, and transfusion reactions. Prolongation of the PT and the aPTT in the presence of thrombocytopenia, hypofibrinogenemia, and elevated fibrin(ogen) degradation fragments characterize the laboratory abnormalities of DIC.

Therapy of DIC should be directed at the stimulus that initiated activation of coagulation; this means treating the underlying disease. However, continued bleeding may require transfusion of blood products for thrombocytopenia (platelet concentrate), a low fibrinogen concentration (cryoprecipitate), or a deficiency of coagulation factors (fresh frozen plasma). The occurrence of arterial or venous thrombi may necessitate heparin therapy to prevent further embolization and thrombosis.

Both congenital and acquired disorders of fibrinogen have been described. Qualitatively abnormal fibrinogen molecules (dysfibrinogenemia) may lead to either a bleeding or a thrombotic tendency. Hepatic disease has been associated with both quantitative and qualitative defects of fibrinogen. Dysfibrinogenemic patients with a bleeding tendency may require replacement therapy with cryoprecipitate prior to surgery.

Disorders of the Fibrinolytic System

Failure to regulate the fibrinolytic system can lead to bleeding disorders. Primary disorders of fibrinolysis in the absence of thrombosis are rare. Patients with malignancy occasionally develop tumors that generate large amounts of plasminogen activator. Surgery of the urinary tract and prostate may release excessive concentrations of urokinase into the circulation. A disseminated fibrinolytic state commonly occurs during liver transplantation. Antifibrinolytic drugs (i.e., ε-aminocaproic acid) interfere with plasminogen binding to fibrin and have proven somewhat effective in the prevention of fibrinolysis. Aprotinin, a potent inhibitor of plasmin, is currently undergoing clinical trials as an antifibrinolytic agent during coronary artery bypass grafting (CABG) surgery.

Thrombotic Disorders in Surgical Patients

Surgical patients are at particular risk of thrombotic complications in the postoperative period. Prolonged immobility associated with decreased venous circulation appear to be the major predisposing factors. Several plasma proteins have thus far been determined to aid in the prevention of thrombotic complications, as follows: (1) AT-III, (2) protein C, and (3) protein S. Congenital or acquired deficiencies of these proteins cause a lifelong history of recurrent thromboses. Acquired AT-III deficiency may occur secondary to massive thrombosis, the DIC syndrome, heparin therapy, liver disease, or protein-losing disorders of the kidney and gastrointestinal tract.

TRANSFUSION THERAPY IN THE SURGICAL PATIENT

Increasing public awareness of transfusion-associated infections has led to renewed interest in the pathophysiology and treatment of anemia. The topic of transfusion medicine is of particular relevance to surgeons and anesthesiologists because over two thirds of blood products are administered in the perioperative period.

Pathophysiology of Blood Loss

The pathophysiologic consequences of blood loss are dependent upon both the extent and rate of blood loss. Normovolemic hemodilution is well tolerated by the healthy adult. In contrast, the rapid loss of blood without intravascular volume replacement rapidly leads to shock. In the healthy adult, the rapid loss of 10 to 15 per cent of the circulating blood volume causes a compensatory vascular contraction with little or no adverse consequences. Once 30 per cent of the blood volume has been lost, most patients develop signs of shock characterized by apprehension, dyspnea, hypotension, cool skin, tachycardia, and decreased urinary output. These symptoms result from a decreasing cardiac output and peripheral vasoconstriction that redirects blood from the peripheral tissues to the heart, brain, and other central organs. After 50 per cent of the circulating blood volume has been lost, decreasing perfusion of vital organs coupled with increasing lactic acidosis in the peripheral tissue leads to decreasing cardiac output and death due to circulatory shock.

As opposed to these clear limits for acute intravascular volume depletion, the limits of hemodilution in the setting of normovolemia have not been defined in humans. Delivery of oxygen to peripheral tissues is the product of cardiac output and arterial oxygen content. In order to maintain oxygen delivery in the setting of a decreasing hematocrit, either the cardiac output must increase or the oxygen extraction ratio of tissues and organs must improve. Under normal conditions the brain and heart function at an oxygen extraction ratio of 60 to 70 per cent. Clearly, these tissues are highly dependent upon increasing blood flow to maintain oxygenation following hemodilution.

Several compensatory mechanisms assist in maintaining oxygen delivery at lower hematocrits. Blood viscosity is reduced at lower hematocrits, resulting in increased perfusion. The decreased viscosity increases preload and afterload to the heart, producing increases in stroke volume and cardiac output. In addition, increased concentrations of plasma 2,3-bisphosphoglycerate (2,3-BPG) shift the oxygen-hemoglobin dissociation curve to the right, reflecting improved delivery of oxygen to the tissues. These mechanisms are highly effective at maintaining tissue oxygenation under conditions of normovolemic hemodilution.

Recent investigations have demonstrated the capacity of healthy adults to tolerate moderate reductions in hematocrit with no adverse effects. Historically, a hematocrit of 30 per cent was considered optimal in the perioperative period; however, healthy, young patients undergoing elective surgery without major blood loss appear to tolerate hematocrits in the 24 to 27 per cent range without adverse effect. Clearly, older patients or those unable to compensate for the effects of anemia continue to require higher hematocrits. For example, patients with coronary artery disease or limited ventricular function might not be capable of compensating for anemia with an increased cardiac output. A hematocrit in excess of 30 per cent would be advisable in this compromised population.

Transfusion of Erythrocytes

Replacement of oxygen carrying capacity constitutes the only indication for transfusion of red blood cells. Synthetic crystalloid and colloid products are available for the repletion of intravascular volume, obviating the need for blood products in this setting. Erythrocytes are available primarily in two forms, packed red blood cells (PRBC) and whole blood. Whole blood is available on only a limited basis, as most units of blood are fractionated to provide plasma and platelet concentrates. The transfusion of whole blood is useful when both improved oxygen delivery and intravascular volume are required; for example, as in trauma. Packed red blood cells are obtained by the centrifugation of whole blood to remove all but 50 ml of plasma. The transfusion of 1 U of PRBCs raises the hematocrit by approximately 3 per cent. Stored whole blood progressively loses plasma coagulation factor activity with time. Platelet activity is lost within 24 hours of storage.

Prior to transfusion, donor red blood cells must undergo compatibility testing with recipient serum. The four major blood types consist of A, B, AB, and O. The Rh(D) antigen comprises an additional RBC antigen present in 85 per cent of the population. Red cell membranes contain antigens corresponding to the blood group of the patient. In the absence of a particular antigen, the patient's serum contains antibodies to that antigen. For example, patients of blood group O express antibodies to blood groups A and B. Blood type is determined by mixing the patient's red cells with antisera to the different blood types and then measuring agglutination. The blood type is further confirmed by measuring agglutination after mixing the patient's serum with red blood cells containing the A and B antigens. After determination of the patient's blood type, an antibody screen is performed by incubating the patient's serum with a sample of cells containing the most common RBC antigens. If agglutination occurs at this step, the patient's serum is further screened with a panel of specific red cell antigens. The final step prior to transfusion involves the crossmatch of donor red cells with recipient serum. The crossmatch detects clerical errors in the typing of blood as well as rare antibodies to the donor red cells. The crossmatch typically requires 60 minutes for completion. In emergent situations, a type, antibody screen, and abbreviated crossmatch detect 99.96 per cent of significant antibodies, with extremely little risk of a serious transfusion reaction.

Transfusion of Platelets

Platelet transfusions are indicated in the bleeding patient with either thrombocytopenia or a qualitative defect of platelet function. The prophylactic transfusion of platelet concentrates is only indicated for profound thrombocytopenia (<20,000/mm³). Platelet concentrates are prepared by the centrifugation of fresh whole blood with resuspension of the platelets in 50 ml of plasma. Platelet concentrates are stored at 25°C for up to 5 days. Platelet concentrates are initially infused at a dose of 1 U/10 kg body weight (a total of 7 to 8 U/dose). In the absence of a consumptive process of alloimmunization, each unit of transfused platelets may be expected to raise the platelet count by approximately 10,000/mm³ within 1 hour of the transfusion. Antibodies may develop to the human leukocyte antigens (HLA) on random donor platelets. In these immunized patients, transfusion of random donor platelets does not increase the platelet count. This situation necessitates the use of single-donor HLA-matched platelets obtained by plateletpheresis of an appropriate donor.

Transfusion of Plasma Products

Transfusion of fresh frozen plasma (FFP) is indicated for the replacement of coagulation factor deficiencies in the absence of more specific component therapy. Fresh frozen plasma may also be used for the rapid reversal of warfarin anticoagulation. Fresh frozen plasma is prepared by the centrifugation of fresh whole blood. The supernatant is stored at −20°C to preserve the activity of coagulation factors V and VIII. There is no role for the administration of FFP as a volume expander or as a prophylactic means of preventing bleeding during massive blood transfusion. Most coagulopathies associated with massive transfusion occur after 1 to 1.5 blood volume exchanges and are due to dilutional thrombocytopenia. If time allows, coagulation testing should always be obtained prior to the treatment of a coagulopathy.

Cryoprecipitate is prepared by freezing plasma to −90°C and then slowly warming it to 4°C. A gelatinous precipitate enriched in fibrinogen, factor VIII, factor XIII, and von Willebrand factor remains. Cryoprecipitate may be useful in the bleeding patient with a fibrinogen concentration less than 100 mg/dl. More commonly, cryoprecipitate is used as a topical hemostatic agent (i.e., fibrin glue). Development of virally inactivated factor concentrates has reduced the applicability of cryoprecipitate in the therapy of hemophilia and von Willebrand's disease.

Complications of Transfusion Therapy

Transfusion-associated disease transmission remains foremost among the fears of the public. Donor exclusion criteria and immunologic testing for infectious agents have been highly successful in reducing the risks associated with transfusion. In addition, hepatic transaminases are measured as additional markers for hepatic infection. Non-A, non-B hepatitis remains the most frequent infectious complication of blood transfusion. Current estimates for the transfusion of an HIV-positive unit of blood range from 1 in 61,000 to 1 in 153,000. Following transfusion of an HIV-positive unit of blood, 90 per cent of recipients acquire the infection.

Metabolic complications are a frequent and often overlooked consequence of blood transfusions. Failure to administer blood through a warmer may lead to hypothermia. Decreases in core temperature produce shivering and increase oxygen consumption. In addition, hypothermia may interfere with normal hemostasis. The development of rapid-infusion devices has increased the risk of symptomatic citrate intoxication and hyperkalemia. Citrate acts as an anticoagulant in stored blood. Rapid infusion of citrate may lead to hypocalcemia and impaired myocardial contractility. During storage, PRBCs leach potassium into the plasma. Potassium-induced cardiac dysrhythmias have been associated with the rapid infusion of PRBCs.

The transfusion of blood products may cause a wide range of immunologically mediated complications ranging from the rare but serious hemolytic reaction, to the frequent but benign febrile reaction. Acute hemolytic reactions most frequently occur following transfusion of an incompatible blood type. Antigen–antibody complexes form leading to activation of the complement system and lysis of RBCs. Free hemoglobin collects in the renal tubules causing renal failure. Activation of coagulation may cause DIC. The most frequent signs of an acute hemolytic reaction include hemoglobinuria, DIC, hypotension, hemolysis, and renal failure. If signs of an acute hemolytic reaction occur, the transfusion must be stopped. The unit of blood in question is returned to the transfusion service along with a fresh blood sample from the patient for retyping. Therapy of a hemolytic reaction is primarily supportive. Aggressive hydration is recommended to maintain urine output. Delayed hemolytic reactions may occur in patients who have been previously transfused. Alloimmunization to donor red cell antigens causes lysis of RBCs, expressing those antigens during subsequent transfusions. Delayed hemolytic reactions are usually associated with less morbidity and mortality than acute reactions.

REFERENCES

Broze GJ: Why do hemophiliacs bleed? Hosp Pract 27:71–86, 1992.

Collen D, Lijnen HR: Basic and clinical aspects of fibrinolysis and thrombolysis. Blood 78:3114–3124, 1991.

Crosby ET: Perioperative haemotherapy: I. Indications for blood component transfusion. Can J Anaesth 39:695–707, 1992.

Crosby ET: Perioperative haemotherapy II: Risks and complications of blood transfusion. Can J Anaesth 39:822–837, 1992.

Furie B, Furie BC: Molecular and cellular biology of blood coagulation. N Engl J Med 326:800–806, 1992.

George JN, Shattil SJ: The clinical importance of acquired abnormalities of platelet function. N Engl J Med 324:27–39, 1991.

Stehling L: Trends in transfusion therapy. Anesth Clin North Am 8: 519–531, 1990.

7

NUTRITION IN SURGICAL PATIENTS

JOHN P. GRANT, M.D.

To meet the energy needs in times of decreased caloric intake, the body resorts to autocannibalism. Although body fat is expendable, this is not true of the protein reserves. Most protein mobilization occurs from the muscle mass, yet significant mobilization of protein from vital organs may also occur. Progressive malnutrition causes decreased skeletal and respiratory muscle function, marked intestinal malabsorption and dysmotility, depressed hepatic microsomal enzyme function and protein synthesis, loss of renal concentrating ability and inability to excrete acid and certain drugs, impaired cardiac function, and depressed humoral and cellular immune responses. Clinical studies have demonstrated morbidity and mortality to be increased in patients with low serum concentrations of albumin or transferrin, impaired delayed-type hypersensitivity skin test reactions, recent weight loss, and various combinations of these changes. Optimal patient care requires that adequate nutritional support be provided not only to treat malnutrition but, just as importantly, to prevent malnutrition.

To gain maximal benefits from nutritional intervention, it is important to initiate support as early as possible. During periods of moderate to severe stress, body losses of 10 to 15 gm/day of nitrogen are common. With initiation of nutritional support, one can expect 3 to 5 gm positive nitrogen balance per day at best. For each day delay in initiating nutritional support, therefore, up to 3 to 5 days may be required just to catch up, with additional time required to replenish prior losses. In addition, it is very difficult to replenish malnourished patients during chemotherapy, stress, or following extensive surgery. Often one can only maintain the status quo, and optimally, the status quo

should be the best possible. However, urgent medical or surgical care should not be postponed for nutritional care. If other treatment is urgent, nutritional support should be provided along with the medical or surgical care.

INDICATIONS FOR NUTRITIONAL SUPPORT

Although all agree that in some clinical settings nutritional support is necessary and in some it is not useful, the decision whether to provide nutritional support requires judgment based on experience, careful evaluation, and application of ethical principles. Support may be administered *enterally* or *intravenously*. The indications for support are shown in Tables 1 and 2.

DETERMINATION OF METABOLIC REQUIREMENTS

Caloric Needs

The caloric needs of hospitalized patients vary considerably based on age, sex, and weight; and emotional, psychological, and physical stress. A simple bedside estimate of caloric needs, derived from clinical experience, can be obtained from body weight and the degree of presumed stress (Table 3). To more accurately determine energy needs, Long et al. modified the Harris-Benedict equation for basal metabolic rate, which is based on age, sex, weight, and height, cor-

TABLE 1. ENTERAL NUTRITION

Clinical Settings Where Enteral Nutrition Should be Part of Routine Care

1. During transition to an oral diet. Enteral nutrition allows use of the gastrointestinal tract with tapering and discontinuance of intravenous feedings. Many suggest administration of enteral feedings only at night while the patient sleeps to assist in recovery of oral intake.
2. When malnutrition is not present but oral intake is less than 50 per cent of required for 7 to 10 days.
3. When there is moderate to severe malnutrition and oral intake is not adequate to meet all nutritional needs.
4. During major stress. Major stress is associated with an accelerated metabolic rate. Failure to meet energy and nitrogen needs is associated with rapid loss of lean body mass, impairment of the healing process, reduced resistance to infection, and a poorer prognosis. If oral intake is not adequate to meet all nutritional needs, and if the gastrointestinal tract has satisfactory function, enteral tube feeding should be instituted.
5. Short-bowel syndrome. Optimal treatment of patients following massive small-bowel resection includes administration of both intravenous nutrition, to assure adequate nutrient intake, and oral or enteral feeding solutions to stimulate gut adaptation. If 3 or 4 feet of bowel can be salvaged at the time of surgery, many patients can sustain adequate nutrition entirely via the gastrointestinal tract.
6. Enterocutaneous fistula. Enterocutaneous fistulas often close spontaneously if given ample time and adequate nutritional support. As fistula output appears not to be related to the probability of fistula closure, enteral feedings are fully satisfactory. Patients with fistulas in the proximal gastrointestinal tract should be fed via an access distal to the fistula site. If biliary or pancreatic secretions are lost in the fistula, use of partially digested formulas low in fat may be necessary to optimize absorption. If fistula output increases dramatically with initiation of feeding, a significant proportion of nutrients may be lost and intravenous feeding may become necessary.

Clinical Settings Where Enteral Nutrition is Likely to be of Value

1. With the postoperative patient when an oral diet is not resumed within 5 to 7 days of surgery.
2. During radiation therapy and chemotherapy. The severity of radiation and chemical enteritis may be reduced by administration of a low-residue, elemental diet.
3. During decreased oral intake associated with acute liver and renal failure, with specialized formulas to minimize hepatic encephalopathy or uremia.

Clinical Settings Where Enteral Nutrition is of Indeterminate Value

1. Immediate postoperative period. It is probably preferable to wait for 3 to 5 days following operation for the acute endocrine response to diminish.
2. Intensive chemotherapy. This is often associated with stomatitis, anorexia, nausea and vomiting, and diarrhea resulting in inadequate voluntary oral intake. Selected patients with mild symptoms may tolerate enteral feedings, all others require intravenous nutrition.

TABLE 1. ENTERAL NUTRITION *(Continued)*

Clinical Settings Where Enteral Nutrition is of No Value

1. Mechanical obstruction of the intestine.
2. Intestinal hypomotility or ileus.
3. Acute enteritis.
4. Severe acute pancreatitis.
5. Shock or intestinal ischemia.
6. When the prognosis does not warrant aggressive nutritional support or when aggressive nutritional support is not desired by the patient or legal guardian.

recting for activity and stress (Table 4). The most accurate estimate of energy needs, however, is obtained by indirect calorimetry using a Metabolic Cart. In this method, carbon dioxide production and oxygen consumption are measured in expired gases, and caloric expenditure is calculated using the formula:

$$kcal/min = 3.941 \ V_{O_2} + 1.106 \ V_{CO_2}$$

One must be careful not to initiate nutritional support too rapidly in malnourished patients or patients with cardiac disease because the caloric and fluid load may induce congestive heart failure. In malnourished patients, it is best to begin caloric support based on the patient's current weight, slowly increasing support until a weight gain of approximately 0.2 to 0.4 kg/day is observed.

Nitrogen Requirements

Caloric and nitrogen requirements are interrelated. Increasing caloric support decreases the need for nitrogen to achieve nitrogen balance, and increasing nitrogen intake reduces the calories required. The optimal ratio of calories to nitrogen in the hospitalized patient remains to be determined. Currently utilized calorie/nitrogen ratios range from 100:1 to 200:1. To determine the adequacy of nitrogen support, a nitrogen balance study can be performed (Table 5). Neutral nitrogen balance should maintain body protein mass, whereas 2 to 3 gm positive nitrogen balance per day restores the nitrogen mass. During periods of stress and sepsis, nitrogen utilization and protein synthesis may be severely impaired and positive nitrogen balance may be impossible to achieve. The goal in this setting is to minimize nitrogen loss. Recommended daily nitrogen supplementation in the unstressed adult patient is 0.128 gm/kg/day (0.8 gm protein/kg/day). With mild stress, the recommendation is 0.24 gm nitrogen/kg/day (1.5 gm protein/kg/day); with moderate stress, 0.32 gm nitrogen/kg/day (2.0 gm protein/kg/day); and with severe stress, up to 0.4 gm nitrogen/kg/day (2.5 gm protein/kg/day).

TABLE 2. INTRAVENOUS NUTRITION

Clinical Settings Where Intravenous Nutrition Should be Part of Routine Care

1. When oral intake is inadequate and enteral feedings are not tolerated in malnourished patients, whether or not stress is present. In well-nourished, nonstressed patients, intravenous feeding can be deferred for 7 to 10 days, in hopes of recovery of an oral diet. If stress is present, however, support should be initiated early.
2. Short-bowel syndrome. If less than 4 feet of small bowel remain after surgery, most patients cannot absorb adequate nutrients for survival from either an oral diet or enteral feedings. Intravenous feeding should begin within 48 to 72 hours of surgery. If less than 3 feet of small bowel is preserved, most patients require lifelong supplemental or total intravenous nutritional support in the home.
3. Acute pancreatitis. Studies show little effect on the clinical course of acute pancreatitis; however, it is relatively easy to maintain nutritional status.
4. High-output enterocutaneous fistulas when enteral feedings are not adequately absorbed.
5. Septic patients and in patients with body burns. In these two settings, intravenous feeding is essential to meet the needs of accelerated metabolism.

Clinical Settings Where Intravenous Nutrition is Likely to be of Value

1. Inflammatory bowel disease. Medically intractable Crohn's disease may respond to a course of bowel rest and intravenous nutrition. Similar beneficial response has been reported in mild disease using elemental enteral diets. Although effective in acute flares, nutritional support has no impact on the natural history of Crohn's disease. Patients with ulcerative colitis benefit from intravenous nutrition and bowel rest only with respect to maintenance or recovery of normal nutritional status. There is no effect on disease activity or need for surgery.

Clinical Settings Where Intravenous Nutrition is of Indeterminate Value

1. Immediate postoperative period. Although improved metabolic balance has been observed, no impact on patient outcome has been reported.
2. Mild stress in a well-nourished patient where the gastrointestinal tract is expected to recover within 7 to 10 days.

Clinical Settings Where Intravenous Nutrition is of No Value

1. When the expected duration of therapy is less than 5 days.
2. When operation is urgently needed such as for drainage of abscesses or exploration for small-bowel obstruction.
3. Profound shock, severe sepsis with hypotension, or multiple organ failure. These clinical conditions severely interfere with nutrient utilization and make nutritional support ineffective. Attention should be directed toward correcting the major problem, then toward nutritional support.
4. Intravenous nutrition should not be given to the terminally ill when all other therapy has been ceased.

Fluid Requirements

Fluid requirements during nutritional support are increased compared to those when 5 per cent dextrose is given. In an anabolic state, intracellular water and water of fat oxidation are no longer released. In ad-

TABLE 3. CALORIC NEEDS BASED ON STRESS

Level of Stress	UUN	Caloric Needs
None	0–5 gm	28 kcal/kg/day
Mild	5–10 gm	30 kcal/kg/day
Moderate	10–15 gm	35 kcal/kg/day
Severe	>15 gm	40 kcal/kg/day

Abbreviation: UUN = urine urea nitrogen.

dition, as new cells are formed, new intracellular water is necessary. To assure adequate fluid supplementation, basic fluid requirements should be calculated based on body weight or surface area, measured fluid losses should be replaced, estimated insensible and third-space losses should be replaced, and an additional 300 to 400 ml of fluid should be added to provide for anabolism. Care must be taken to make adjustments for patients with congestive heart failure, renal failure, excessive fluid and pulmonary edema, and those receiving humidified air.

Electrolyte Requirements

Requirements for the extracellular electrolytes, sodium and chloride, are not increased with intravenous nutrition. Due to infusion of phosphate, routine daily maintenance calcium should be given, ranging between 0.2 and 0.3 mEq/kg/day. Requirements for the intracellular electrolytes potassium, phosphorous, and magnesium are markedly increased in the anabolic state compared to infusion of 5 per cent dextrose due to the lack of mobilization of intracellular electrolytes and to the formation of new intracellular fluid with new cell formation. Maintenance potassium requirements range from 1.0 to 1.5 mEq/kg/day, phospho-

TABLE 4. CALCULATION OF ACTUAL ENERGY REQUIREMENTS*

AEE (men) = $(66.47 + 13.75 \text{ W} + 5.0 \text{ H} - 6.76 \text{ A}) \times$ (activity factor) $\times$ (injury factor)

AEE (women) = $(655.10 + 9.56 \text{ W} + 4.85 \text{ H} - 4.68 \text{ A}) \times$ (activity factor) $\times$ (injury factor)

Activity Factor	Use
Confined to bed	1.2
Out of bed	1.3

Injury Factor	24-hour UUN	Use
Minor OR	0–5 gm	1.2
Skeletal trauma	5–10 gm	1.3
Major sepsis	10–15 gm	1.6
Severe burn	>15 gm	2.1

*Modified from Long CL, Schaffel N, Geiger JW, Schiller WR, Blakemore WS: Metabolic response to injury and illness: Estimation of energy and protein needs from indirect calorimetry and nitrogen balance. JPEN 3:452–456, 1979, with permission.

Abbreviations: AEE = actual energy expenditure, W = weight in kg, H = height in cm, A = age in years, UUN = urine urea nitrogen.

TABLE 5. CALCULATION OF NITROGEN BALANCE

Nitrogen balance = (dietary protein intake ÷ 6.25) − TUN^a −
5 mg N/kg^b − 12 mg N/kg^c
where a = total urinary nitrogen excreted over 24 hours by
Kjeldahl technique,*
b = estimated insensible nitrogen losses (add any
measurable losses from other sources),
c = estimated nitrogen losses from the gastrointestinal tract.

*If the macro-Kjeldahl nitrogen assay is unavailable, a fairly accurate estimate of TUN losses can be obtained by adding 2 to 3 gm nitrogen to the total urinary urea nitrogen to account for other nitrogen-containing waste products in the urine.
Abbreviations: TUN = total urinary nitrogen.

rous requirements range from 13 to 20 mmol per 1000 kcal (varies based on serum phosphorous concentration and glucose administration), and magnesium requirements range between 0.3 and 0.45 mEq/kg/day. In addition to maintenance requirements, existing electrolyte deficiencies must be recognized and replaced or a rapid fall in serum potassium, phosphorous, or magnesium may occur.

Fatty Acid Requirements

Arachidonic acid, linoleic acid, and linolenic acid cannot be synthesized by the human body and are therefore considered essential in the diet. These fatty acids are necessary for cell membrane structure and for synthesis and action of the prostaglandin system. A minimum of 1 to 2 per cent of total caloric intake should be in the form of essential fatty acids to meet nutritional requirements.

Trace Element and Vitamin Requirements

All fat-soluble and water-soluble vitamins must be provided on a daily basis. In addition, copper, manganese, chromium, zinc, and selenium are essential trace elements.

SOLUTION FORMULATION

Caloric Sources

Calories in enteral or intravenous feeding formulations can be given as either carbohydrate or fat. Enteral formulas mainly utilize corn starch and syrup, maltodextrin, sucrose, and soy polysaccharides. Intravenous dextrose solutions are available in concentrations from 5 to 70 per cent ranging from 0.17 to 2.42 kcal/ml. Intravenous fat emulsions are available in 10 and 20 per cent concentrations containing 1.1 to 2.0 kcal/ml. In nonstressed patients, fat appears to be as useful as glucose in sparing nitrogen. In the critically ill or stressed patient, however, both glucose and fat are less efficient. Stress reduces glucose utilization to approximately 5 to 6 mg/kg/min. Giving more glucose or supplementing with large amounts of insulin does not improve net protein synthesis or nitrogen balance. Similarly, use of increasing amounts of long-chain fatty acids has not been shown to improve nitrogen retention. Alternative fuels for use during stress are under investigation, including medium-chain triglycerides, fish oils, branched-chain amino acids, and glutamine. Until these other substrates are proven and become commercially available, it is suggested that 15 to 20 per cent of calories be given as long-chain fatty acids with the remainder given as glucose, adjusting each based on clearance from the blood.

Nitrogen Sources

Nitrogen in enteral feeding products is derived mainly from beef, soy, whey, lactalbumin, egg albumin, or casein. Nitrogen in intravenous solutions is derived from synthetic crystalline amino acids. Depending on the respective nitrogen source, various electrolytes are present that must be taken into consideration in compounding formulas.

Other Requirements During Nutritional Support

If the patient is diabetic or if intolerance to carbohydrate is observed, insulin may be required. During enteral support, it must be given intramuscularly or subcutaneously. During intravenous support, it should be added to the nutrition solution. Only monocomponent insulin should be used. Insulin supplementation should not be increased to above 50 to 70 U/day due to concern over downregulation of the insulin receptors and suppression of pyruvate dehydrogenase with stimulation of fat synthesis. If glucose intolerance persists, carbohydrate administration should be reduced and consideration given to infusion of more fat. Because albumin is an important transport protein and acts as a scavenger of toxic metabolic by-products, it is frequently given intravenously when serum concentrations fall below 2.5 gm/dl. In the presence of adequate caloric support, the half-life of exogenous albumin ranges between 10 and 15 days, and serum concentrations can be corrected. Up to 37.5 gm of albumin can be administered daily until serum albumin increases to above 3.0 gm/dl. Brown et al. evaluated the amount of albumin needed to increase serum albumin concentrations in 35 adult patients with hypoalbuminemia receiving intravenous nutrition. They added 12.5 gm albumin per liter of nutrition solution and measured the average increase in serum concentrations over time. They found the following relationship:

$$y = 0.33 + 0.003x \ (r=.82)$$

Where

y = change in serum albumin concentration in gm/dl

x = amount of exogenous albumin given in grams.

For example, to raise the serum albumin from 2.0 to 3.0 gm/dl, the formula would calculate as follows:

$$1.0 = 0.33 + 0.003 \ x$$
$$x = 223 \ gm \ albumin \ required.$$

If albumin is added to the nutrient solution at 12.5 gm/day, 18 days would be required to raise the serum albumin. If given at 25 gm/day, 9 days would be required. For the most part, the patients studied were not stressed, and requirements in intensive care patients may be even greater. It must be recognized that intravascular albumin equilibrates slowly with the large extravascular pool (over 3 to 5 days), and if replenishment is accomplished rapidly with 37.5 gm/day of albumin infused, the serum albumin may not immediately reach equilibration with the body pool. In this case, the initial serum albumin concentration decreases slowly and additional albumin may be needed to achieve the desired goal. Repeated infusions of albumin may be necessary in the stressed patient, even after repletion, as the result of depressed hepatic albumin synthesis. If, however, albumin synthesis is near normal, further albumin supplementation after repletion should not be necessary.

The impact of albumin administration to a malnourished patient who is not given adequate nutritional support contrasts with the response just described. In this setting, albumin is rapidly broken down as a caloric substrate, and little if any increase in serum albumin concentrations are realized.

PATIENT MONITORING DURING NUTRITIONAL SUPPORT

Weight should be measured two to three times a week. Weight gain should not exceed 0.4 kg/day, more rapid gain reflecting fluid overload. Temperature, pulse, and blood pressure should be taken two to three times per day to aid in early detection of fluid overload, congestive heart failure, and sepsis. Urine should be tested for glucose every 6 hours initially, and at least once or twice a day thereafter to monitor for diabetes. Glucosuria may also occur 12 to 24 hours before obvious clinical sepsis, due to release of catecholamines. Potassium, phosphorous, magnesium, and blood glucose should be monitored daily or every other day during initiation of nutritional support. After advancement to full support, depending on stability, monitoring should continue twice a week for the next several weeks and weekly thereafter. Serum calcium, sodium, chloride, blood urea nitrogen (BUN), prothrombin time, white blood count, liver enzymes, bilirubin, and albumin should be monitored weekly.

ENTERAL NUTRITION

When possible, the gastrointestinal tract should be used for nutritional support. Enteral nutrition is less costly, not associated with the potential risk of catheter-related sepsis, and associated with fewer metabolic and mechanical complications. Furthermore, the atrophic changes of the gastrointestinal tract associated with bowel rest and intravenous feeding are avoided when nutrients are delivered via the gastrointestinal tract. Interest has particularly focused on the amino acid glutamine that is absent from current intravenous nutrient solutions but present either as glutamate, glutamic acid, or glutamine in most enteral products. Glutamine, a primary fuel of the gastrointestinal tract, is necessary for maintenance of normal gut anatomy and physiology. This property is important in the treatment of critically ill patients where intravenous nutrition may lead to breakdown of the gut mucosal barrier with translocation of bacteria or bacterial toxins through the gut wall into the portal blood leading to visceral injury and the multiple organ failure syndrome.

Stomach

When there is adequate gastric function with respect to motility and emptying, the stomach is the preferred route for nutrient administration. Intubation of the stomach with tubes passed through the nose is the least invasive of all access techniques for nutrient delivery, easily established at the patient's bedside, and maintained with minimal care. Endoscopically or surgically placed gastrostomy tubes provide more permanent access. Nutrient solutions can be administered continuously or intermittently and can be of any composition (blenderized, predigested, or elemental) and of nearly any osmolality. Except for the mechanical function of chewing and mixing with oral enzymes, nutrients are processed in a normal manner with respect to mixing with digestive enzymes and exposure to absorptive surfaces. Furthermore, delivery into the stomach allows administration of nearly all drugs and food supplements. Ideal patients for gastric feeding include those with difficulty swallowing such as with cerebrovascular accidents, tumors of the oropharyngeal area, or disease of the esophagus ranging from neuromuscular disorders, to partial obstructions with benign or malignant tumors.

Jejunum

Some patients cannot be safely fed by stomach, but can be fed enterally if access can be obtained to the proximal small bowel. Candidates include those patients at risk for reflux and pulmonary aspiration, those with gastroparesis, and those with gastroesophageal fistulas, pancreatitis, or intractable nausea and vomiting. Nasojejunal tubes can be passed endoscopically or fluoroscopically, or jejunostomy tubes can be placed during abdominal surgery. Care must be taken in nutrient administration to avoid dumping syndromes from rapid administration or excessive osmolality. In addition, great care must be exercised in administration of all drugs into the jejunum to assure compatibility with the nutrient solution, adequate absorption, and avoidance of dumping due to high osmolality.

INTRAVENOUS NUTRITION

As all intravenous nutrition solutions are hypertonic, they must be administered through central venous catheters. The most common access route is the superior vena cava via a subclavicular approach. With proper technique, serious complications of vascular access should occur in less than 1 per cent of patients. Such complications include pneumothorax, arterial laceration, hemothorax, mediastinal hematoma, brachial plexus injury, air or catheter embolism, and hydrothorax. For most patients, nutrient solutions should be initiated at approximately 2000 ml/day. After the first 24 to 48 hours, the infusion should be advanced to the final rate. In general, solutions should hang at room temperature for no more than 24 hours to minimize risks of bacterial overgrowth. Intravenous nutrition should be infused with an electronic device, either a controller or peristaltic pump. Gravity administration, although possible, requires greater effort to maintain constant infusion and is no longer advocated. The accuracy of the volumetric pump is rarely required for safe intravenous nutrition except in infants. When discontinuing the nutrition solution, the rate should be halved for 24 hours before stopping. If the solution must be suddenly interrupted, a 5 per cent dextrose solution should be started at the same rate to prevent hypoglycemia. Administration of 10 per cent dextrose is not necessary.

COMPLICATIONS OF NUTRITIONAL SUPPORT

Septic Complications

Catheter-related sepsis during intravenous nutrition occurs in 3 to 5 per cent of patients. Primary catheter sepsis is defined as a septic episode in which no other source is found and which resolves upon removal of the central venous catheter. Secondary catheter infections develop on the catheter due to seeding from another site. Removal of the catheter may not alter the septic course, but until the catheter is removed, treatment of the primary infection is ineffective. If a serious septic condition is present, a blood culture should be drawn through the catheter and from a peripheral vein and the catheter should be removed. If the clinical condition is not urgent and the diagnosis of catheter-related sepsis not obvious, a blood culture should be drawn through the catheter and from a peripheral vein with continuation of intravenous nutrition until culture results are available. If the blood drawn through the catheter is sterile, the catheter can be left in place. If the culture is positive with a negative peripheral culture, the catheter should be removed. If the patient spikes a high fever with shaking chills while waiting for culture results, the central catheter should be removed. Some recommend exchanging the catheter over a guidewire with culture of the catheter tip when catheter-related sepsis is suspected. Although considered valuable by some, the risk of sepsis due to catheter exchange may outweigh potential benefits of catheter salvage. If intravenous nutrition is still required after an episode of catheter-related sepsis, appropriate antibiotics should be given for at least 3 to 5 days before a new catheter is placed.

Altered Glucose Homeostasis

Serum glucose concentrations during nutritional support should rarely exceed 200 mg/dl, with no more than 1 per cent glucosuria. Patients experiencing stress; those at the extremes of age; and those with malnutrition, diabetes, and sepsis often have compromised glucose tolerance. If hyperglycemia with glucosuria greater than 2 gm/dl of urine is permitted to continue, a vigorous osmotic diuresis can lead to the syndrome of hyperglycemic, hyperosmotic, nonketonic acidosis, with an associated mortality approaching 40 to 50 per cent. Optimal therapy is prevention. If glucose intolerance develops, the following should be considered as potential causes:

1. Drug interference with the urine glucose test. A serum glucose should be obtained whenever in doubt. Also, certain drugs may effect glucose metabolism,

TABLE 6.   METABOLIC COMPLICATIONS DURING NUTRITIONAL SUPPORT*

B. **None**
C. **Elevated Triglyceride** (>400 mg/dl)
D. **Hypophosphatemia** (<2.3 mg/dl)
   Symptomatic: 1. Symptoms usually do not occur until [P] < 1.0 mg/dl
   2. Marked and progressive weakness of muscles of extremities and neck, mastication, respiration
   3. Circumoral and peripheral paresthesias
   4. Mental obtundity
   5. Hyperventilation
E. **Hyperphosphatemia** (>4.3 mg/dl)
   Symptomatic: 1. Metastatic calcifications in soft tissue
F. **Hypokalemia** (<3.2 mEq/L)
   Symptomatic: 1. Paralytic ileus, muscular weakness, possible paralysis, nausea and vomiting
   2. Atrial and ventricular premature contractions, ECG changes with flat T waves, U waves
   3. Hyperglycemia
G. **Hyperkalemia** (>4.8 mEq/L)
   Symptomatic: 1. Diarrhea, muscular weakness, intestinal colic
   2. Ventricular arrhythmias, ECG changes with peaked T waves, prolonged PR interval, cardiac arrest

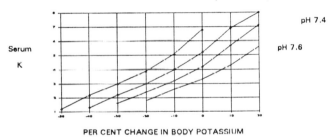

PER CENT CHANGE IN BODY POTASSIUM

H. **Hyponatremia** (<135 mEq/L)
   Symptomatic: 1. Symptoms due to marked overhydration, rarely due to sodium loss
   2. Altered mental status
   3. Nausea, vomiting, convulsion
I. **Hypernatremia** (>145 mEq/L)
   Symptomatic: 1. Thirst
   2. Oliguria, apathy, stupor
   3. Hyperosmolar coma, hypotension, death
J. **Hypochloremia** (<98 mEq/L)
   Symptomatic: 1. Metabolic alkalosis with acidic urine
K. **Hyperchloremia** (>108 mEq/L)
   Symptomatic: 1. Metabolic acidosis with alkalotic urine
L. **Hypomagnesemia** (<1.6 mEq/L)
   Symptomatic: 1. Usually occur when [Mg] <1.0 mEq/L
   2. Digitalis toxicity
   3. Positive Trousseau's and Chvostek's signs or overt tetany
   4. Muscle fasciculations, tremors, spasticity, hyporeflexia, ataxia, muscular weakness
   5. Depression, irritability, psychotic behavior, apathy
   6. Nausea and vomiting
   7. Increased losses of urinary potassium

M. **Hypermagnesemia** (>2.2 mEq/L)
   Symptomatic: 1. Hypotension, nausea, vomiting between 3 and 5 mEq/L
   2. Drowsiness, hyporeflexia, muscular weakness (5–10 mEq/L)
   3. Coma and respiratory arrest (12–15 mEq/L)
   4. Cardiac arrest (>25 mEq/L)
N. **Hyperammonemia** (>40 mg/dl)
O. **Hypoglycemia** (<75 mg/dl)
   Symptomatic: 1. Tingling sensations in extremities and mouth
   2. Posterior occipital headache, cold clammy skin, nausea
   3. Thirst, dizziness, rapid pulse, altered mental status
   4. Infrequently, convulsions, central nervous system damage
P. **Hyperglycemia** (>200 mg/dl)
   Symptomatic: 1. Osmotic diuresis
   2. Dehydration with hyperglycemic, hyperosmolar, nonketotic acidosis
Q. **Glucosuria** (>3 + spill in urine)
   Symptomatic: 1. Osmotic diuresis
R. **Copper Deficiency** (<80 µg/dl)
   Symptomatic: 1. Anemia
   2. Leukopenia (especially neutropenia)
T. **Zinc Deficiency** (<75 µg/dl)
   Symptomatic: 1. Diarrhea (early sx, can be severe, responds quickly to Rx)
   2. Apathy and depression (fairly early)
   3. Alopecia, paranasal, periorbital, and perioral dermatitis (this occurs late in disease)
   4. Altered taste, smell, and appetite
U. **Hyperbilirubinemia** (>1.2 mg/dl)
   Symptomatic: 1. Pruritis
V. **Elevated SGOT** (>35 IU)
W. **Elevated SGPT** (>35 IU)
X. **Elevated Alk Phosphatase** (>110 U)
Y. **Acidosis** (pH <7.35 or CO_2 <21)
Z. **Alkalosis** (pH >7.45 or CO_2 >30)
1. **Hypocalcemia** (<8.7 mg/dl)
   Symptomatic: 1. Positive Trousseau's and Chvostek's signs or overt tetany
   2. Muscle spasm, paresthesias, weakness, seizures
   3. Depression, irritability, psychotic behavior, apathy
   4. Nausea and vomiting
   5. Arrhythmias, bradycardia, hypotension
2. **Hypercalcemia:** (>10.2 mg/dl)
   True Ca = serum Ca + [0.8 (4 – Alb)]**
3. **Hypoalbuminemia** (<2.5 gm/L)
   Symptomatic: 1. Diarrhea
   2. Fat embolism
   3. Anasarca
4. **Volume Overloading** (all occurrences symptomatic)
   1. Pulmonary edema
   2. Congestive heart failure not due to other causes
   3. Altered mental status

*From Grant JP: Total Parenteral Nutrition. Curr Prac Surg 3:38, 1991, with permission.

such as corticosteroids, certain diuretics, phenytoin, and phenothiazines.

2. A bolus infusion of the nutrition solution.

3. Glucosuria, hyperglycemia, and hyperkalemia may occur 12 to 24 hours before other signs of stress or sepsis.

4. Finally, if none of the above are present, a prediabetic state may be present and insulin supplementation may be necessary. Occasionally chromium deficiency may be present causing insulin resistance.

Mineral and Electrolyte Abnormalities

Deficiency or excess of minerals and trace elements during nutritional support can cause numerous clinical symptoms (Table 6) and should be avoided by careful planning and monitoring.

Other

Essential fatty acid deficiency can occur as early as 7 days after initiation of fat-free nutritional support. Clinical symptoms include a dry, flaky skin, increased red blood cell fragility with anemia, and decreased prostaglandin production with decreased intraocular pressure. Elevated liver function tests are frequently observed when glucose is the main caloric substrate. When 15 to 20 per cent of the caloric support is given as fat and when overfeeding is avoided, the incidence is greatly reduced. Rarely is hepatotoxicity clinically significant. Liver enzyme abnormalities have been reported mainly with intravenous nutrition and tend to resolve when intravenous nutrition is discontinued. Elevation of BUN occurs in most patients receiving nutritional support. Usually, elevations are minimal. Occasionally, however, BUN may reach 50 to 60 mg/dl. In patients with compromised renal function, nitrogen loading must be adjusted to avoid excessive elevations in the BUN, or dialysis must be instigated. Lethargy may occasionally be observed upon initiation of nutritional support. The cause of the lethargy, which may progress to a semicomatose state, is unknown. There is no specific therapy, and symptoms usually diminish after 6 to 10 days. An occasional patient has a hypercatabolic response to initiation of nutritional support. As caloric loading increases, there is an increase in heart rate and sometimes body temperature. Typically it is associated with hypokalemia, hypophosphatemia, and hypomagnesemia—a syndrome referred to as the refeeding syndrome. When apparent, nutritional support should be reduced by half and then gradually increased over a period of 5 to 10 days until full nutritional support is achieved.

REFERENCES

Alexander JW, Boyce ST, Babcock GF, Gianotti L, Peck MD, Dunn DL, Pyles T, Childress CP, Ash SK: The process of microbial translocation. Ann Surg 212:496–512, 1990.

American Society of Parenteral and Enteral Nutrition: Guidelines for use of total parenteral nutrition in the hospitalized adult patient. JPEN 10:441–445, 1986.

American Society of Parenteral and Enteral Nutrition: Guidelines for use of enteral nutrition in the hospitalized patient. JPEN 11: 435–439, 1987.

Brown RO, Bradley JE, Luther RW: Response of serum albumin concentrations to albumin supplementation during central total parenteral nutrition. Clin Pharm 6:222–226, 1987.

Burke JF, Wolfe RR, Mullany CJ, Mathews DE, Bier DM: Glucose requirements following burn injury. Ann Surg 190:274–285, 1979.

Grant JP: Vascular access for total parenteral nutrition: Techniques and complications. In Grant JP (ed): Handbook of Total Parenteral Nutrition, ed 2. Philadelphia, WB Saunders Company, 1992, pp 107–138.

Long CL, Schaffel N, Geiger JW, Schiller WR, Blakemore WS: Metabolic response to injury and illness: Estimation of energy and protein needs from indirect calorimetry and nitrogen balance. J Parenter Enter Nutr 3:452–456, 1979.

8
SURGICAL ASPECTS OF DIABETES MELLITUS

DIANA B. McNEILL, M.D.   MARK N. FEINGLOS, M.D., C.M.

Diabetes mellitus is an abnormality of carbohydrate metabolism that causes hyperglycemia due to either complete lack of insulin secretion from the beta cells of the pancreas (type I diabetes), or from increased cellular resistance to insulin and abnormal insulin release from the beta cells (type II diabetes). The prevalence of diabetes in the American population is approximately 6 per cent of those age 40 or older, or 14 million Americans. Many ultimately require some type of surgical treatment, and because careful control of blood glucose is an important factor in determining a successful surgical outcome, it is essential to understand the basic concepts of diabetes management in the perioperative setting.

CLASSIFICATION

Characteristics of the different types of diabetes are outlined in Table 1. Type I diabetes, also known as insulin-dependent diabetes (IDDM), usually is diagnosed prior to age 30, although a second peak of presentation occurs from ages 50 to 60. Type I diabetes accounts for 10 per cent of all known diabetic patients. The initial clinical presentation is usually acute and may be accompanied by marked hyperglycemia, dehydration, and/or diabetic ketoacidosis. Type I diabetes is caused, for unknown reasons, by autoimmune destruction of the pancreatic beta cells. All patients with type I diabetes require insulin for management. When caloric intake is insufficient, hypoglycemia can occur. However, without insulin, even in the absence of caloric intake, endogenous glucose and ketone production can cause hyperglycemia and ketosis.

Type II, or non–insulin-dependent diabetes (NIDDM), the most common type of diabetes, is generally found in adults over age 30, although a subset of this type of diabetes called maturity-onset diabetes of youth (MODY) is found in teenagers and young adults. Patients with type II diabetes are not insulin dependent (they do not ordinarily develop ketoacidosis), and 80 per cent are overweight (>20 per cent over ideal body weight). Such patients can usually control their blood glucose with a simple carbohydrate, fat-restricted diet, exercise, weight loss, and, in some cases, an oral hypoglycemic agent. Ultimately, insulin therapy may be required in certain patients to achieve satisfactory glucose control. Insulin is often required temporarily in times of stress, such as severe illness or surgery.

DIAGNOSIS

The diagnosis of diabetes is made in one of three ways: (1) unequivocal elevation of plasma glucose to greater than 200 mg/dl at any time with symptoms of diabetes, (2) fasting plasma glucose values greater than 140 mg/dl on two occasions, or (3) fasting plasma glucose less than 140 mg/dl and a 75-gm glucose tolerance test with a 2-hour value greater than 200 mg/dl and one intervening value greater than 200 mg/dl. Stress of an acute illness such as surgery may transiently elevate plasma glucose due to release of the counterregulatory hormones (catecholamines, cortisol, and growth hormone), which promote glucose production and decrease glucose clearance, leading to hyperglycemia. Patients may require treatment for hy-

75

TABLE 1.   CLASSIFICATION OF DIABETES MELLITUS

Type I	Type II
Insulin-dependent (IDDM, previously called juvenile-onset diabetes)	Non–insulin-dependent (NIDDM, previously called adult-onset diabetes)
20% of all diabetes	80% of all diabetes
Onset in childhood, adolescence, although second peak in middle age	Onset after age 30, although diagnosis at adolescence known (maturity-onset diabetes of youth [MODY])
Usually nonobese	80% of patients obese
Dependent on exogenous insulin	Not dependent on insulin; can be treated with diet, exercise, and oral hypoglycemic agent; for optimal control, some patients require insulin
Positive islet cell antibodies at diagnosis	High or normal insulin levels; insulin resistance common
Ketosis prone	Non–ketosis prone
Acidosis prone	

Secondary Diabetes
Pancreatic diabetes
   Cystic fibrosis, hemochromatosis, pancreatic insufficiency, pancreatectomy
Hormonal excess
   Acromegaly, Cushing's syndrome
Drug induced
   Corticosteroids, thiazides, niacin

perglycemia, but glycemic control improves with resolution of the stress. Patients with this presentation have impaired glucose tolerance and not diabetes. Transient use of steroids may also cause marked glucose intolerance, and require insulin support.

COMPLICATIONS

Table 2 illustrates the acute and chronic complications associated with diabetes. Hyperglycemia leads to increased susceptibility to infection. In fact, 5 to 10 per cent of diabetic patients who undergo surgery may develop postoperative wound infections. Decreased

TABLE 2.   COMPLICATIONS OF DIABETES

Acute
  Hypoglycemia
  Ketosis
  Increased susceptibility to infection
  Hyperosmolar coma
  Dehydration
Chronic
  Macrovascular disease
    Cerebral vascular disease
    Coronary artery disease
    Peripheral vascular disease
  Microvascular disease
  Retinopathy
  Nephropathy
    Hypertension
    Renal failure
  Neuropathy
    Autonomic
    Gastroenteropathy
    Peripheral
    Orthostatic hypotension

leukocyte chemotaxis and loss of phagocytic function of the leukocytes in the presence of hyperglycemia have been implicated as the causal factors. There are also some reports of decreased wound tensile strength in poorly controlled diabetic patients. The major "long-term" complications of diabetes reflect the microvascular, macrovascular, and neural changes seen in states of chronic hyperglycemia. There is a threefold greater incidence of atherogenesis in the diabetic patient compared to that in the general population. Hyperinsulinemia, hyperlipidemia, and hyperglycemia contribute to this dramatic increase. Coronary artery disease, peripheral vascular disease, and cerebrovascular disease all increase surgical morbidity and mortality. Hypertension occurs in 40 per cent of patients with diabetes, and these patients require close attention perioperatively. Diabetes is the most frequent cause of end-stage renal disease and dialysis dependence. Close attention to fluid status and contrast dye exposure may prevent worsening renal azotemia. The diabetic patient's neurologic status is of importance, particularly if anesthesia is administered. Autonomic neuropathy may compromise the cardiac or pulmonary response to anesthesia and may also cause impaired recovery from hypoglycemia. Urinary retention and diabetic gastroenteropathy may slow postoperative recovery.

PERIOPERATIVE MANAGEMENT

A perioperative evaluation is essential for every diabetic patient and must focus on the type and duration of diabetes, treatment regimen (Table 3 reviews the types of insulin preparations that may be seen), and

TABLE 3. TYPES OF INSULIN*†

TABLE 3. TYPES OF INSULIN*†

Types	Onset (hours)	Peak (hours)	Duration (hours)
Short-acting			
Regular	0.25–1	2–4	5–8
Semilente	0.25–1	4–6	8–12
Intermediate			
NPH	2–4	6–10	12–24
Lente	2–4	6–10	12–24
Long-acting			
PZI	3–4	14–20	24–36
Ultralente	3–4	14–20	24–36

*Data from Schade DS, Santiago JV, Skyler JS, Rizza RA: Intensive Insulin Therapy. Princeton, Medical Examination Publishing Co, 1983, with permission.
†Above insulin preparations available as beef, pork, semisynthetic human (Novolin, Novo-Nordisk), or biosynthetic human (Humulin, Eli Lilly) insulin.
Abbreviations: NPH = neutral protamine Hageman, PZI = protamine zinc insulin.

complications. Many successful treatment regimens may be used in the perioperative management of the diabetic patient. It is essential to have a rational plan for the changing requirements of the diabetic patient in the perioperative state, not only with respect to insulin management, but also nutritional needs. Sufficient calories should be provided to prevent ketosis (600 to 800 kcal/day; 125 ml/hr of a 5 per cent dextrose solution provides approximately 600 kcal/day), and it must be remembered that the body's need for insulin is not determined only by the caloric intake, especially in a patient with type I diabetes and no endogenous insulin. Insulin should never be omitted for any prolonged period in such patients.

Following are some suggestions for the management of the diabetic surgical patient. All patients with type I diabetes and insulin-requiring type II diabetes require insulin perioperatively. Often, patients using oral hypoglycemic agents are more safely managed during lengthy surgery with insulin therapy. The basal insulin secretory rate of the normal pancreas is 0.5 to 1.0 U/hr. The use of a basal dose of insulin, given as short-acting insulin before meals and bedtime, or every 6 hours in a patient who is not eating, approximates normal pancreas function. The use of sliding-scale insulin alone in the insulin-requiring patient assures that unacceptable hyperglycemia will occur before insulin therapy is initiated. Estimate of the basal insulin needs of the patient can be made based on previous outpatient daily insulin requirements and diabetic control. For example, if a patient had a total daily outpatient requirement of 24 U/day, a reasonable basal insulin regimen might be 4 to 6 U of regular insulin every 6 hours. The use of a supplemental scale of short-acting insulin with the basal dose often prevents marked hyperglycemia in an acutely ill patient. The supplemental insulin scale should be appropriate to the total basal insulin dosage (e.g., 5 per cent of the total daily dose for the first incremental supplement, increasing by an additional 5 per cent for each 50-mg/dl increase in glucose). Supplementation should begin at the level of glucose deemed unacceptable for the particular patient, often 200 to 250 mg/dl. For the above patient, 1 additional U of regular insulin might be given for a glucose of 200 to 249, 2 U for glucose of 250 to 299, and so forth.

A continuous, intravenous (IV) insulin infusion is a safe, physiologic method of perioperative insulin delivery when used by experienced personnel. Frequent blood glucose monitoring is mandatory. The half-life of a dose of IV insulin is 7 to 10 minutes. Thus, an IV insulin infusion allows easy titration for both hyperglycemia and hypoglycemia. Table 4 illustrates typical IV insulin orders. Note that plastic IV tubing can bind insulin and that at least 50 ml of the insulin solution should be run through the tubing before starting the infusion. Postoperatively, it is important to infuse the IV insulin through a separate line, because a number of frequently used agents, such as dopamine, can inactivate insulin. Because of the very short half-life of IV insulin, subcutaneous insulin should be restarted at least 1 hour before the IV is discontinued to prevent acute deterioration of glucose control.

Elective surgical procedures in diabetic patients are best done early in the morning. Blood glucose should be monitored frequently in insulin-requiring patients who are fasting for a short surgical procedure. An intravenous glucose solution should be started 2 to 3 hours before surgery (D5 1/2 NS at 125 ml/hr), and the total morning dose of neutral protamine Hagedorn (NPH) or Lente insulin given on call to the operating room. Supplemental regular insulin can be used postoperatively if needed, with the patient's outpatient regimen resumed at supper or the next day if oral intake is good. If the patient remains fasting or has poor oral intake, basal regular insulin given every 6 hours beginning at a dosage of 0.3 U/kg in four divided dosages is appropriate. A supplemental insulin scale based on the total daily dosage, as previously outlined, should also be used. If surgery is delayed or canceled, insulin therapy must be continued throughout the day to prevent marked hyperglycemia in the insulin-requiring patient. Patients taking oral hypoglycemic agents should have their medication held on the morning of surgery. Intravenous or subcutaneous regular insulin can be used, as outlined above, if necessary. The oral agent can be resumed when the patient is eating well.

POSTOPERATIVE GUIDELINES

The diabetic patient has increased postoperative morbidity and mortality compared to the nondiabetic patient due to vascular complications, infection, and delayed wound healing. Close attention to the chang-

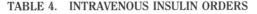

TABLE 4. INTRAVENOUS INSULIN ORDERS

1. Patent intravenous access without use for other medications, particularly dopamine.
2. Regular insulin, 25 U in 250 ml 0.9% saline (1 U/10 ml).
3. Bedside BG monitoring every hour, recorded on a flow sheet.
4. Intravenous infusion of 5% dextrose in water at 125 ml/hr. Reevaluate fluids if fluid restriction necessary, or patient receiving other dextrose support (i.e., tube feedings).
5. Begin intravenous infusion at 1 to 2 U regular insulin per hour or at a dosage 50% of outpatient insulin dosage every 24 hours.
6. Adjust every hour per algorithm; sample algorithm below.

Blood Glucose	Insulin Drip
<80 mg/dl	Decrease by 2 U
81–100 mg/dl	Decrease by 1 U
101–200 mg/dl	No change
201–250 mg/dl	Increase by 1 U
251–300 mg/dl	Increase by 2 U
301–350 mg/dl	Increase by 3 U

If BG decreases by more than 100 mg/dl in 1 hour, decrease insulin drip by 1 to 2 U or 25% of current dose.
If hypoglycemia (BG <60 mg/dl) occurs, stop insulin drip and recheck BG in 30 minutes. Restart drip at 2 to 4 U less than previous dose when glucose is <100 mg/dl.
Algorithm should be reevaluated frequently, and scale adjusted as needed.

Abbreviation: BG = blood glucose.

ing status of the diabetic patient is essential. When the insulin-requiring patient is ready to be converted to a discharge regimen (no evidence of infection, stable nutrition), 80 per cent of the 24-hour insulin requirement may be converted to either twice daily NPH (60 per cent of total daily dose given before breakfast, 40 per cent of daily dose before supper), or two injections of mixed regular and NPH insulin daily (80 per cent of the previous 24-hour insulin dose divided as two thirds in the morning and one third before supper; the morning dose is one third regular insulin and two thirds NPH, while the supper dose is one half regular insulin, one half NPH insulin). These are common insulin regimens; some patients require more complex therapy. It may be valuable to review the patient's previous home insulin regimen. Ideally, the patient should be stabilized on his final insulin regimen for at least 24 hours before discharge.

EMERGENCIES

Patients may present in diabetic ketoacidosis due to an acute surgical problem, and it is preferable to delay surgery in this life-threatening situation until the acidosis and insulin deficiency are corrected. Ketoacidosis may mimic an acute surgical abdomen. It may also appear in postoperative diabetic patients as a result of serious infection or inadvertent omission of insulin (insulin should never be stopped because of poor caloric intake). An appropriate initial insulin regimen is 0.1 U regular insulin per kilogram per hour following a 0.1-U regular insulin per kilogram loading dose. Close attention to fluid status and electroyte balance, particularly potassium, is essential. These patients are often severely dehydrated and initially require aggressive

fluid support. Once the ketoacidosis has resolved, there is often a marked decrease in insulin requirement.

Hypoglycemia may occur in the diabetic patient perioperatively. Normally, either 10 gm of carbohydrate given orally (e.g., 4 oz juice, cola), or 20 ml of 50 per cent glucose solution increases the glucose sufficiently. If the patient is unable to take oral calories and no intravenous access is available, 1 mg glucagon may be given intramuscularly with resolution of the hypoglycemia within 10 minutes. Glucose values should be rechecked 15 to 30 minutes after a low glucose reading. Subsequent insulin dosages should not be held; counterregulatory hormones released as a result of the hypoglycemia and the calories given as treatment for the low glucose cause marked rebound hyperglycemia if not controlled with insulin.

SUMMARY

Millions of patients with diagnosed and undiagnosed diabetes undergo one or more surgical procedures during their lifetime. The goal of management is to maintain the glucose as close to normal as safely possible. This can be achieved by careful blood glucose monitoring and the use of an individualized, rational plan of insulin or oral hypoglycemic management perioperatively. Concurrent care by the surgeon and diabetes team is often desirable for patients with complex medication requirements. Improved perioperative diabetes care may lead to decreased morbidity from infection, decreased mortality from diabetic complications, and an uneventful postoperative recovery for the diabetic patient.

REFERENCES

Gavin LA: Perioperative management of the diabetic patient. Endocrinol Metab Clin North Am *21*:457, 1992.

Hirsh IB, Hunt TK: Role of insulin in management of surgical patients with diabetes mellitus. Diabetes Care *13*:980, 1990.

McMurray JF: Wound healing with diabetes mellitus: Better glucose control for better healing in diabetes. Surg Clin North Am *64*:769, 1984.

Schade DS: Surgery and diabetes. Med Clin North Am *72*:1531, 1988.

Schade DS, Santiago JV, Skyler JS, Rizza RA: Intensive Insulin Therapy. Princeton, Medical Examination Publishing Co, 1983.

Shuman CR: Controlling diabetes during surgery. Diabetes Spectrum *2*:263, 1989.

9
ANESTHESIA

BRUCE J. LEONE, M.D.

Gentlemen, this is no humbug.

JOHN COLLINS WARREN

These words of John Collins Warren, Chief Surgeon at the Massachusetts General Hospital, uttered in the ether dome on October 16, 1846, ushered in the modern era of anesthesia. Warren's comment was occasioned by William Morton's administration of an ether anesthetic to a patient upon whom Warren removed a congenital venous malformation of the neck. Warren had previously remarked, when Horace Wells had attempted a nitrous oxide anesthetic 4 years earlier, that anesthesia was indeed "humbug." Since Crawford Long's experiences with ether anesthesia in 1842 were not documented by publication, Morton's demonstration firmly established the concept of painless surgery in medicine.

Anesthesia quickly progressed throughout the world, with such innovators as John Snow, John Clover, and James Young Simpson furthering the science of anesthesia. Snow used the first systematic approach to the induction and maintenance of anesthesia, and he introduced anesthesia to the royalty of England by administering chloroform to Queen Victoria during the birth of Prince Leopold, popularizing the technique as anesthesia *à la reine*. The introduction of local anesthetics toward the turn of the century introduced the concept of regional anesthesia as an option in patients undergoing peripheral surgical procedures. The organization of the first anesthesia departments and the application of physics to anesthesia administration greatly enhanced the safety and stature of anesthesia. More recent advances in pharmacology and physiology in the past two decades have served to make anesthesia extremely safe, even with devastating systemic diseases.

MODERN TECHNIQUES

Unlike early anesthetics, modern anesthesia can be administered by a variety of techniques using several approaches to render the patient insensible to pain. The classical method of administering inhalational anesthesia is still practiced, particularly in pediatric patients. In adult patients, however, the use of an appropriate induction agent prior to the administration of an inhalational anesthetic provides for a more rapid, smooth induction of anesthesia. However, many times an adjuvant is used, particularly a narcotic or benzodiazepine adjuvant, to provide a smoother, more hemodynamically stable anesthetic, as well as to afford the patient some degree of postoperative pain relief. Regional anesthesia has had a resurgence, as technical advances in equipment and increased interest in pain relief have developed.

REGIONAL ANESTHESIA

Regional anesthesia, first performed for ocular surgery in the late 19th century, has become increasingly popular. After a period when general anesthesia enjoyed almost complete prominence, regional anesthesia has had a resurgence. Familiarization with anatomic landmarks; development of new, specific needles and catheters; and the synthesis of new, more effective, and less toxic local anesthetics have brought regional anesthesia into the mainstream of anesthetic practice. Furthermore, the lack of marked cardiovascular or metabolic effects, coupled with the ability to monitor the patient's neurologic status by allowing the patient to remain conscious during surgery, gives regional anesthesia specific advantages in certain surgical procedures.

Peripheral Blocks

Many surgical procedures, in particular those involving the distal extremities, can be effectively performed under regional anesthesia. A knowledge of the peripheral nervous system and sensory innovation of the extremities is necessary for effective peripheral nerve block anesthesia. This type of anesthesia can be used most effectively in the critically ill patient requiring a peripheral procedure. The virtual absence of hemodynamic and metabolic effects, coupled with its short duration, makes it an ideal procedure in patients who are otherwise unstable.

Intravenous Bier Block

Several peripheral regional anesthetic techniques may be used. The oldest method is intravenous peripheral anesthesia, commonly known as a Bier block. This technique involves circulatory isolation of a limb, usually the arm, and administration of a local anesthetic, usually lidocaine, intravenously. The volume of the venous system in the extremity determines the volume of anesthetic to be used. A pressurized tourniquet is applied to the proximal portion of the extremity, and the local anesthetic is infused in the most distal area of the venous system of the extremity. This block is usually effective for approximately 1 to 2 hours. The block is generally limited by tourniquet pain or ischemic pain of the limb, as the limb is totally isolated from its blood supply.

The Bier block has several important uses and advantages as well as some significant disadvantages. A Bier block is a short-duration anesthesia to be applied in essentially an outpatient setting for procedures involving the extremities and requires a minimal amount of training as well as a minimal amount of equipment for its effective application. One disadvantage of this technique occurs when the tourniquet is deflated and the anesthetic is released from the venous system of the extremity into the general circulation, because the use of large doses of local anesthetic then may cause systemic toxicity when released into the central circulation, as manifested by changes in central nervous system and significant cardiovascular depression.

Plexus Blocks

As regional anesthesia has progressed, so has the popularity of performing anesthetic blocks on major nerve trunks; the arm is particularly accessible to major plexus nerve block. The brachial plexus, passing through the axillary sheath, is a defined anatomic space within which the major nerve trunk to the arm is contained. This plexus can be anesthetized quite easily at the midaxillary level with a relatively low, nontoxic dose of local anesthetic. In fact, this plexus can be continuously blocked for hours by insertion of a catheter into the axillary sheath and constant infusion of local anesthetic agent.

Lower extremity plexus blocks are technically more difficult but, if applied correctly, yield adequate anesthesia with the advantage of the lack of significant hemodynamic changes. These are particularly useful in lower extremity procedures in unstable patients. The lower extremity block requires more precise knowledge of anatomic structures, with several injection sites to adequately anesthetize the three major nerve trunks coursing through the pelvic area to the lower extremity. In general, this technique is seldom used, but it can be of significant advantage in specific instances. More peripheral nerve blocks, such as an ankle block, may be extremely useful when metatarsal or distal surgery is performed on the foot or ankle. This block can be easily applied, provides a dense nerve block distal to the metatarsals, and may be combined with a longer acting anesthetic for prolonged pain relief.

Neuraxis Blocks

Central neuraxis injection of local anesthetics are being used more frequently as techniques have improved and understanding of local anesthetic effects has increased. The achievement of adequate sedation while maintaining consciousness makes local anesthesia a preferred method by some patients. Synthesis of newer local anesthetic compounds, coupled with increased knowledge of the pharmacokinetics, pharmacodynamics, and toxicity of local anesthetics has caused safer, more widely accepted neuraxis anesthesia. Once primarily relegated to obstetric applications, neuraxis anesthesia is now used in a variety of surgical procedures that were once thought to require general anesthesia.

Spinal Anesthesia

Initially used as part of the management of difficult labor in obstetrics, spinal anesthesia has experienced a resurgence in popularity. Further interest in the use of spinal anesthesia has resulted in broader applications of this technique in a variety of clinical situations. Newer equipment and a greater understanding of pharmacokinetics and hemodynamic changes associated with spinal anesthesia have caused more widespread use of regional anesthesia; in particular, spinal anesthesia. Spinal anesthesia offers the ability to perform relatively invasive surgical procedures with virtually no pain to the patient with the advantage of the patient being lightly sedated. Careful attention to management of spinal anesthesia can ameliorate the cardiovascular changes with which it is associated (Table 1).

Spinal anesthesia is generally indicated for procedures involving the lower abdomen and the lower extremities. More recent use of spinal anesthesia has resulted in a wide variety of different agents, not limited to local anesthetics, being delivered into the subarachnoid space for the purpose of alleviating pain both intraoperatively and postoperatively. Newer uses of neuraxis delivery systems include microcatheters designed to deliver a constant low dose of local anesthesia or opiates with greater control of anesthesia and/or analgesia for prolonged periods of time. Thus, the previous limiting factor of the relatively short duration of spinal anesthesia due to metabolism and/or dissipation of the local anesthesia agents can now be circumvented with the use of a continuous infusion apparatus. This offers the prospect of prolonged spinal anesthetic techniques for high-risk patients in whom management with prolonged general anesthetics may be relatively contraindicated. Additionally, the infusion of opiates postoperatively in the neuraxis may aid in postoperative pain management.

Epidural Anesthesia

Epidural techniques involve delivery of local anesthetics and opiates to the potential space between the dura and epidural fat layer in the central neuraxis. This potential space can be entered with relative ease and a catheter inserted for repetitive dosing or continuous infusion of local anesthetics. Unlike spinal anesthesia, which has effects on the central neuraxis and conduction, epidural anesthetics affect the nerve roots emerging from the dura in the specific segmental areas in proximity to the tip of the epidural catheter. Thus, epidural anesthesia is a more regional neuraxis block

as compared to spinal anesthesia in that epidural anesthesia affects a certain segmental region associated with the exiting nerve trunk. The more segmental nature of epidural anesthesia, in general, causes a far more controlled neuraxis blockade associated with less sympathetic effects and fewer hemodynamic effects (Table 1). Local anesthetic drugs as well as opiates can be infused into the epidural space without significant complications, and epidural anesthesia offers the added advantage of regionalized pain relief. Because of this specific property, epidural anesthesia as a method of postoperative pain relief has grown remarkably in popularity in the past decade.

Complications of Neuraxis Anesthesia

Complications associated with spinal and epidural anesthesia are related to the techniques used and the dose administered. Technique-related complications include inadvertent puncture of the surrounding structures, unfamiliarity with the technique of epidural or spinal anesthesia, and postoperative headache from mild leakage of cerebral spinal fluid through the dural puncture. Postoperative headache can also occur after inadvertent spinal puncture with the larger epidural needle during a technically difficult epidural catheter insertion. With the advent of newer microcatheter techniques, long-term spinal anesthesia has been utilized in many cases. However, there have been recent reports of cauda equina syndrome associated with prolonged local anesthetic infusions through spinally placed microcatheters. The exact mechanism of this complication has not been elucidated, yet it is highly possible that toxicity associated with high concentrations of local anesthesia due to inadequate displacement of the local anesthetics infused throughout the neuraxis may ultimately damage the caudal nerve roots and result in cauda equina syndrome. Additionally, marked hemorrhagic complications, particularly in patients with bleeding diatheses or undergoing concurrent heparin therapy, have been reported with neuraxis techniques. In several large series of studies, however, appropriate technique and vigilance has resulted in no increase in hemorrhagic complications during neuraxis anesthesia in patients with bleeding disorders. Appropriately applied neuraxis anesthesia can be an extremely safe, comfortable experience and is at least as safe as general anesthesia in surgical patients.

GENERAL ANESTHESIA

General anesthesia was the first technique applied, as rendering a patient insensible to pain was thought

TABLE 1.   COMPARISON OF SPINAL AND EPIDURAL REGIONAL ANESTHESIA

Type of Block	Spinal Anesthesia Total	Epidural Anesthesia Segmental
Cardiovascular effects	++	+
Systemic toxicity	Rare	Potential*
Local toxicity	Possible	Rare
Prolonged use	Occasional	Frequent
Postoperative use	Rare	Common

*If injected intravenously.

initially to require some form of "controlled coma." While regional anesthetic techniques are becoming increasingly popular, the majority of anesthetics administered involve general anesthesia. The first anesthetics developed were volatile or inhaled anesthetics that consisted of the vapors inhaled from liquid-phase chemicals possessing an adequate vapor pressure to produce a concentration sufficient for anesthesia. Development of the first anesthetic, ether vapor, was quickly followed by investigation of other vapor anesthetics, including halothane, enflurane, and isoflurane.

Concurrent with the development of regional anesthetics, the development of intravenous anesthetics awaited the understanding of intravenous therapy and germ theory. Interest in intravenous anesthesia in the early part of the 20th century culminated in the introduction of intravenous barbiturates to clinical anesthesia practice in the mid-1930s. This revolutionized the induction of anesthesia, as a smooth and comfortable induction was now possible. During the past 25 years, the increasing effort placed on finding alternatives to volatile anesthetic agents has led to the development of more specific intravenous anesthetic agents.

Volatile Anesthetics and Nitrous Oxide

Currently, three volatile anesthetic agents are clinically available, with several other agents being actively developed. The three agents are halothane, enflurane, and isoflurane, and all produce similar effects, although there are significant differences in their cardiovascular, hepatic, renal, and cerebral effects. The concentrations of anesthetic vapor that produce anesthesia vary with the individual patient and with the drug used. In order to standardize the nomenclature for these different anesthetic agents, a system was developed according to the minimum alveolar concentration (MAC). The MAC is defined as that concentration at which 50 per cent of patients do not respond to a surgical stimulus. Each of these volatile agents has differing cardiovascular effects, and all are direct myocardial depressants and cause mild to moderate vasodilation. Additionally, all cause mild bronchodilation and alter pulmonary blood. Halothane causes clinically significant myocardial depression with increased sensitivity of the myocardium to epinephrine and a tendency to precipitate arrhythmias (Table 2). Enflurane appears not to sensitize the myocardium to catecholamines as much as halothane, but is more active in producing atrial arrhythmias. Isoflurane is more reliable in preventing atrial arrhythmias with an equal or lesser effect in sensitizing the myocardium to epinephrine. However, tachycardia and hypotension may occur due to its peripheral vascular effects.

If these general anesthetics are administered prop-

TABLE 2. COMPARISON OF VOLATILE ANESTHETIC AGENTS

	Halothane	Enflurane	Isoflurane
Potency (MAC)	0.79%	1.67%	1.12%
Catecholamine sensitization	+++	+	+
Atrial arrhythmias	++	+++	+/−
Vasodilation	+	+	+++
Bronchodilation	+++	++	++
Respiratory drive	↓	↓	↓
Muscular relaxation	+	+	+
Hepatic metabolism	20%	2%	0.2%

Abbreviation: MAC = minimum alveolar concentration.

erly, associated complications are rare. The significant cardiovascular effects are dose related, and all are metabolized to some extent, with halothane being metabolized as much as 20 per cent, enflurane metabolized 2 per cent, and isoflurane metabolized 0.2 per cent. The substantial metabolism of halothane may cause ligands that may autoimmunize the patient and cause fulminant hepatic necrosis and subsequent hepatic failure, an extremely uncommon but devastating occurrence associated with halothane anesthesia. Moreover, although there are reports of autoimmunization occurring in the pediatric population, it appears to be associated with passage through puberty to adulthood. Due to the lesser metabolism of enflurane and isoflurane, there are rare reports of this "halothane hepatitis" associated with enflurane and isoflurane.

Nitrous oxide has been used as an anesthetic for many years and, unlike other volatile anesthetics, cannot be used as a *sole* agent to induce a surgical plane of anesthesia. It is, however, an excellent adjuvant to other volatile anesthetics. Target volatile anesthetic concentrations are achieved significantly faster with the addition of nitrous oxide, due to enhanced uptake from the alveoli. Occasionally, patients may experience a paradoxic central nervous system activation effect with nitrous oxide, although this response is rare, apparently idiosyncratic, and involves synaptic activation associated with nitrous oxide. Discontinuation of nitrous oxide promptly reverses this effect.

The cardiovascular effects of nitrous oxide have been intensely studied, and although it was originally thought to have few cardiovascular effects, recent data suggest that it is a mild sympathetic stimulant that possesses minor myocardial depressant properties. These effects are exacerbated in the presence of significant coronary artery disease with myocardial ischemia, as the sympathetic effects worsen myocardial ischemia and magnify the depressant effects of nitrous oxide on the heart. The resulting decrease in myocardial performance is more pronounced but frequently not physiologically significant, although there are reports of profound cardiovascular collapse associated with the introduction of nitrous oxide to the anesthetic technique in patients with cardiovascular disease.

Intravenous Anesthesia

Modern anesthetic induction techniques are almost exclusively intravenous. The introduction of ultra-short-acting barbiturates, such as thiopental, in the mid-1930s forever changed anesthesia. The ability to quickly induce anesthesia allowed a more stable anesthetic level to be quickly obtained. Considering the propensity of enflurane and isoflurane to cause laryngospasm significant enough to preclude controlled ventilation, the importance of barbiturates for induction of anesthesia cannot be overstated.

Development of other intravenous anesthetic agents quickly followed. Morphine sulfate, used primarily as a postoperative pain management agent, was also rapidly incorporated into intraoperative use and frequently used as both an intravenous anesthetic adjuvant and for postoperative pain control. Fentanyl and sufentanil are potent purified derivatives of morphine and constitute the main narcotic adjuvants used in current anesthetic practice. Their pharmacokinetics and pharmacodynamics are more completely characterized as compared to morphine, and thus these opiates are more predictable in their responses. Fentanyl and sufentanil are virtually devoid of the cardiovascular effects seen with anesthetic doses of morphine sulfate. Alfentanyl, a derivative of fentanyl, is a shorter acting narcotic with minimal duration (>2 hours). Further development of shorter acting narcotics is being pursued intensely (Table 3).

Narcotics, however, are poor amnestics. A patient's recall of surgical procedures is far more common during a technique employing only nitrous oxide and narcotics as compared to a technique employing other amnestic agents. The benzodiazepines were originally developed as an anxiolytic class of drugs in the 1960s. It quickly became apparent that these agents are excellent amnestics and could be used effectively in anesthesia. Currently, benzodiazepines are extensively used in anesthetic management, as these agents are virtually devoid of cardiovascular effects and produce a dense anterograde and limited retrograde amnesia. The benzodiazepines lorazepam, diazepam, and midazolam are all available in intravenous form and, when combined with a narcotic for analgesic management, produce an excellent cardiovascularly stable anesthetic.

Midazolam has a relatively short half-life (2 to 4 hours) and is water soluble, allowing relatively little pain on injection and relatively early dissipation of its amnestic effects. Lorazepam has an intermediate (6 to 8 hours) pharmacokinetic half-life and, therefore, may be more suitable for intermediate-duration surgical an-

TABLE 3.　NARCOTICS

	Morphine	Fentanyl	Sufentanil
Potency (nominal)	1	70	700
Half-life (hours)	2–4	2–4	2–3
Cardiovascular effects	++*	0	0
Bronchoconstriction	++*	0	0

*Due to histamine release.

esthesia. However, lorazepam's relatively unpredictable pharmacodynamics make this agent less desirable in situations where predictable complete emergence from anesthesia is necessary. Diazepam used in lower doses does not cause dense amnesia as compared to midazolam, yet in higher doses diazepam is an excellent amnestic. However, diazepam has a prolonged pharmacokinetic elimination half-life (12 to 36 hours), which may cause prolonged postoperative amnestic effects (Table 4).

Other classes of agents are also used for both intravenous anesthetic induction and maintenance. Ketamine is a phencyclidine derivative with dissociative and analgesic properties. When combined with an anxiolytic (such as a benzodiazepine), ketamine can produce excellent anesthesia with excellent analgesia. Furthermore, the lack of development of significant tolerance to ketamine makes this agent an ideal choice for patients needing repetitive procedures (e.g., burn patients). Ketamine causes significant sympathetic activation resulting in hypertension and tachycardia, yet it can be used safely in patients with significant cardiovascular disease, provided adequate monitoring and vigilance are present. Etomidate is virtually devoid of any cardiovascular effects and dissipates relatively quickly, making it a suitable alternative to barbiturates as an induction agent. However, the development of abnormalities in steroidogenesis and alterations in the feedback loop of the adrenopituitary axis and the development of a form of iatrogenic Cushing's syndrome with etomidate have limited the use of this agent to single-dose induction. This endocrinologic effect of long-term etomidate use appears to follow depletion of vitamin C. Repletion of vitamin C and careful management may mitigate these effects. Finally, the introduction of propofol, a steroid-based anesthetic

TABLE 4.　BENZODIAZEPINES

	Diazepam	Lorazepam	Midazolam
Anterograde amnesia	++	+++	+++
Retrograde amnesia	+	+	++
Solubility	Lipid*	Lipid*	Water
Formulations (U.S.)	IV, PO	IV, PO	IV
Elimination half-life (hours)	20–50	11–22	1.7–2.6

*Results in pain with intravenous injection.
Abbreviations: IV = intravenously, PO = orally.

agent, is of great interest. Propofol has a rapid onset and disappearance of action, with little residual anesthetic effects after approximately 1 hour. It has been used with great success in same-day surgery and may have antiemetic properties in the postoperative period. Propofol can be used as a sedative as well, with a constant infusion at sedative levels providing excellent amnesia and anesthesia. However, propofol has significant cardiovascular effects and must be used with caution and appropriate monitoring in patients with significant cardiovascular disease. Nevertheless, with careful cardiovascular monitoring during administration, it can be used effectively to provide an adequate degree of sedation in patients with cardiovascular disease undergoing invasive procedures with relatively few cardiovascular and other effects.

Muscular Relaxation

The pioneering anesthesiologist Sir Robert Macintosh pronounced neuromuscular blocking agents the single greatest advance in anesthesia. The ability to control muscular tone has provided greater control of airway management and of a quiet, stable operative field, which has made possible the performance of more delicate surgical procedures in the absence of involuntary movement of the patient.

Several compounds are now available for achievement of neuromuscular paralysis. All involve direct blockade of neurotransmitter response at the molecular neuromuscular junction (Table 5). These agents have far less cardiovascular response, are more predictably metabolized than older agents, and are nondepolarizing muscle relaxants because they do not induce a membrane depolarization with resultant relaxation after tetanus. Agents can be chosen for optimizing duration of action, absence of cardiovascular effects, or site of metabolic degradation (hepatic, renal, or plasma elimination). Optimization of general anesthetic technique involves matching the patient's physiologic status and reserve to surgical and postoperative needs. Ability to provide adequate muscular

relaxation during the surgical procedure greatly enhances patient care and safety.

Subspecialties

As surgical management has become more precise and as further knowledge of disease processes has been gained, expert knowledge and familiarity with medical and surgical management of specific patient subpopulations has been necessary for proper anesthetic management. Thus, anesthesia has developed subspecialties to complement the surgical and medical management of these compound patients. Several areas of such subspecialization are cardiac anesthesia, obstetric anesthesia, pediatric anesthesia, thoracic and vascular anesthesia, intensive care, and pain management (both acute and chronic). Although in-depth examination of all of these subspecialties is beyond the scope of this chapter, the relatively unique aspects of intensive care and pain management deserve some further discussion, as these areas of subspecialization have not been classically considered when anesthesia is discussed as a specialty.

Intensive care therapy requires a firm knowledge of physiology, pharmacology, and surgical procedures. The anesthesiologist is uniquely qualified in this arena, due to the obligate study of pathophysiology and pharmacology and the experience in management of ventilation and physiologic monitoring connected with the field of anesthesiology. Acting in concert with surgical and medical subspecialties, anesthesiology brings depth and dimension to the intensive care management of patients. This new subspecialty is beginning to be embraced by increasing numbers of specialists and is a required facet of training in the 1990s. Moreover, many medical centers and hospitals are recognizing the true benefit of this involvement in intensive care therapy.

Pain management has frequently been a frustrating experience for both patients and physicians. Anesthesiologists have brought a wealth of technical and management expertise to pain management and are obviously well equipped to manage acute pain. Management of chronic pain may involve different strategies and mechanisms. A multidisciplinary approach involving anesthesiology, surgery, and other specialties has proven highly successful in pain management.

REFERENCES

Barash PG, Cullen BF, Stoelting RK (eds): Clinical Anesthesia. New York, JB Lippincott Company, 1989.
Miller RD (ed): Anesthesia, ed 3. New York, Churchill Livingstone, 1990.

TABLE 5. NEUROMUSCULAR BLOCKING (PARALYTIC) AGENTS

	Pancuronium	Vecuronium	Atracurium
Rate effects	Tachycardia	None	None
Vascular tone	Slight ≠	None	Dilation
Side effects	Sympathetic tone enhanced	None	Histamine release
Relative potency	1	4	0.9
Time to full recovery	>4 hours	75–120 minutes	60–90 minutes

10
WOUND HEALING: The Biological and Clinical Essentials

H. PETER LORENZ, M.D.   N. SCOTT ADZICK, M.D.

Wound healing occurs with a sequential cascade of overlapping processes leading to restoration of tissue integrity. *Primary* intention healing occurs in closed wounds, which are wounds in which the edges are approximated (e.g., a skin incision closed with sutures). *Secondary* intention healing occurs when the wound edges are not apposed (e.g., an open punch skin biopsy wound). Contraction occurs with open wounds and enhances closure by approximating normal tissue over the defect. Contraction is distinct from contracture, which is the loss of tissue mobility due to a shrinking scar. Both open and closed wounds heal with the same basic repair processes. The amount of tissue injury and degree of contamination influence the length and quality of healing. Small, clean, closed wounds heal quickly with little scar formation, whereas large, open, dirty wounds heal slowly with significant scar. Recent insights into the basic molecular events involved in tissue repair hold promise to facilitate clinical wound healing.

REPAIR PROCESS

The overlapping processes of wound repair are conceptually defined as inflammation, epithelialization, granulation, and fibroplasia.

Inflammation

Inflammation is the first stage of wound healing. After tissue injury, vessels immediately constrict, and platelets aggregate and degranulate. Thromboplastic tissue products are exposed, and the coagulation and complement cascades are initiated. The coagulation mechanisms lead to activation of prothrombin to thrombin, which converts fibrinogen to fibrin, and then fibrin is polymerized into stable clot. As thrombus is formed, hemostasis in the wound is achieved. After the transient vasoconstriction, local small vessels dilate secondary to the effects of kinins, complement components, and prostaglandins. An efflux of white blood cells (first neutrophils, later monocytes) and plasma proteins enter the wound. The early neutrophil infiltrate scavenges cellular debris, foreign material, and bacteria. Activated complement fragments attract neutrophils and aid in the killing of bacteria. Monocytes infiltrate later and differentiate into macrophages that are crucial in the process of tissue repair. Macrophages not only continue to consume tissue and bacterial debris, but also secrete multiple growth factors. These peptide growth factors activate and attract local endothelial cells, fibroblasts, and epithelial cells to begin their respective repair functions. Depletion of monocytes and macrophages causes a severe alteration in wound healing with poor débridement, delayed fibroblast proliferation, and inadequate angiogenesis.

Granulation

Granulation tissue is characterized by its beefy red appearance, which is a consequence of endothelial cell division and migration to form a rich bed of new capillary networks (angiogenesis) at the site of the wound. Fibroblasts migrate into the wound using the newly deposited fibrin and fibronectin matrix as a scaffold. Fibroblasts proliferate and synthesize new extracellular matrix. Thus, the directed growth of vascular endothelial cells occurs simultaneously with fibroplasia during granulation tissue formation, stimulated by platelet and activated macrophage products. Granulation is most prominent in wounds healing by secondary intention.

The initial wound matrix is provisional and is composed of fibrin and the glycosaminoglycan (GAG), hyaluronic acid. Because of its large water or hydration shell, hyaluronic acid provides a matrix that enhances cell migration. Adhesion glycoproteins, including fibronectin, laminin, and tenascin, are present throughout the early matrix and facilitate cell attachment and migration. Integrin receptors on cell surfaces bind to the matrix GAGs and glycoproteins. As fibroblasts enter and populate the wound, they utilize hyaluronidase to digest the provisional hyaluronic acid–rich matrix, and larger, sulfated GAGs are deposited. Concomitantly, collagens are deposited by fibroblasts onto a fibronectin and GAG scaffold in a disorganized array. Collagen types I and III are the major fibrillar collagens comprising skin extracellular matrix. Type III collagen is initially predominant in wounds compared to normal skin, but as the wound matures, type I collagen is deposited in increasing amounts. The majority of collagen is type I in both wounds and normal skin.

Epithelialization

Within hours after injury, morphologic changes in keratinocytes at the wound margin are evident. In skin wounds, the epidermis thickens, and marginal basal cells enlarge and migrate over the wound defect. Once a cell begins migrating, it does not divide until epidermal continuity is restored. Fixed basal cells in a zone near the cut edge of the wound continue to divide, and their daughter cells flatten and migrate over the wound matrix as a sheet. Cell adhesion glycoproteins, such as tenascin and fibronectin, provide a "railroad track" to facilitate epithelial cell migration over the wound matrix. Keratinocytes lay down laminin and type IV collagen as part of their basement membrane. The keratinocytes then become columnar and divide as the layering of the epidermis is established, thus reforming a barrier to further contamination and moisture loss. Interestingly, keratinocytes can respond to foreign body stimulation with migration as well. Sutures in skin wounds provide tracts along which these cells can migrate. Subsequent epithelial thickening and keratinization produces fibrotic reactions, cysts, and/or sterile abscesses centered on the suture.

Fibroplasia

Ultimately, the outcome of mammalian wound healing is scar formation. Scar is defined morphologically as the lack of tissue organization compared to surrounding normal tissue architecture. Disorganized collagen deposition plays a prominent role in scar. New collagen fibers secreted by fibroblasts are present as early as 3 days after wounding. As the collagenous matrix forms, densely packed fibers fill the wound site. The balance of collagen synthesis and degradation favors collagen deposition. The wound remodels slowly over months to form a mature scar. The initially dense capillary network and fibroblast infiltrate regresses until relatively few capillaries and fibroblasts remain. Wounds become stronger with time, and the wound tensile strength increases rapidly from 1 to 6 weeks after wounding. Thereafter, tensile strength increases at a slower pace and has been documented to increase up to 1 year after wounding in animal studies (Fig. 1). However, the tensile strength of wounded skin, at best, only reaches approximately 80 per cent that of unwounded skin. The final result of repair is scar, which is brittle, less elastic than normal skin, and does not contain any epidermal appendages such as hair follicles or sweat glands. The major benefit of repair by scar is the relatively rapid re-formation of tissue integrity.

GROWTH FACTORS: REGULATORS OF REPAIR

Growth factors play a prominent role in the regulation of wound healing. These polypeptides are released by a variety of activated cells at the wound site (Fig. 2). They act in either a paracrine or autocrine manner to stimulate or inhibit protein synthesis by cells in the wound. They also chemoattract new cells to the wound. A myriad of growth factors are present in wounds, many have overlapping functions, and their various biologic effects are only beginning to be unraveled. Platelet-derived growth factor (PDGF) is released from platelet alpha granules immediately after injury. PDGF attracts neutrophils, macrophages, and fibroblasts to the wound and serves as a powerful mitogen. Macrophages, endothelial cells, and fibroblasts also synthesize and secrete PDGF, which stimulates fibroblasts to synthesize a new extracellular matrix, predominantly noncollagenous components such as GAGs and adhesion proteins. PDGF also increases the amount of fibroblast-secreted collagenase, indicating a role for this cytokine in tissue remodeling.

Transforming growth factor-beta (TGF-β) directly stimulates collagen synthesis and decreases extracellular matrix degradation by fibroblasts. It is released from platelets and macrophages at the wound. In addition, TGF-β is released from fibroblasts and acts in an autocrine manner to further stimulate its own synthesis and secretion. TGF-β also chemoattracts fibro-

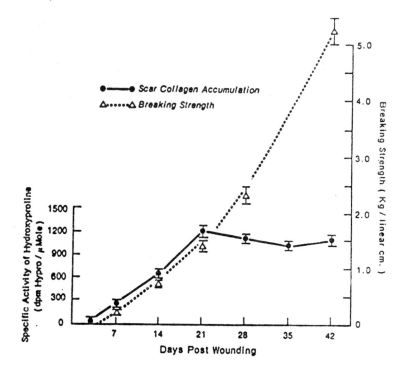

Figure 1. Comparison of scar collagen accumulation and breaking strength of rat skin wounds. Scar remodeling is demonstrated by the increase in wound breaking strength without any change in wound collagen accumulation by 21 days after injury. (From Madden JW, Peacock EE Jr: Biology of collagen during wound healing. Ann Surg *174*: 517, 1971, with permission.)

blasts and macrophages to the wound. Through these mechanisms, TGF-β can augment fibrosis at the wound site. Angiogenesis is stimulated by acidic and basic fibroblast growth factors (aFGF and bFGF, respectively). Both endothelial cells and macrophages produce aFGF and bFGF. These growth factors are bound by heparin and the GAG heparan sulfate in the extracellular matrix. The basement membrane serves as a storage depot for bFGF, which is released upon degradation of the heparin components of the basement membrane. The FGFs stimulate endothelial cells to divide and form new capillaries. They also chemoattract endothelial cells and fibroblasts. Epithelialization is directly stimulated by at least two growth factors: epidermal growth factor (EGF) and keratinocyte growth factor (KGF). EGF is released by keratinocytes to act in an autocrine manner, whereas KGF is released by fibroblasts to act in a paracrine manner to stimulate keratinocyte division and differentiation.

Multiple other growth factors affect wound repair. For example, insulin-like growth factor type 1 (IGF-1) stimulates collagen synthesis by fibroblasts, and IGF-1 functions synergistically with PDGF and bFGF to facilitate fibroblast proliferation. Interferon-γ has been shown to downregulate collagen synthesis. The various interleukins mediate inflammatory cell functions at the wound site.

Surgeons may soon have the ability to enhance repair by adding or deleting growth factors from healing wounds. Investigators have accelerated healing rates in normal wounds by adding exogenous TGF-β, PDGF, or bFGF. Addition of these same growth factors has also augmented repair in animal models of impaired wound healing conditions such as diabetes, chronic steroid use, or chemotherapy. Further studies are needed to determine the precise growth factor combination that is optimal for specific wound types before clinical application is appropriate.

CLINICAL FACTORS AFFECTING WOUND HEALING

Nutrition

The precise calorie requirements for optimal wound healing have not been defined. Large injuries such as burns greatly increase metabolic rate, while smaller injuries such as isolated fractures do not increase nutritional requirements. Protein depletion impairs wound healing if recent weight loss exceeds 15 to 25 per cent of body weight. Wound dehiscence risk is increased in hypoalbuminemic patients, signifying the detrimental effect of chronic malnutrition on repair. Vitamin C (ascorbic acid) deficiency causes scurvy. In these patients, wound healing is arrested during fibroplasia. Normal amounts of fibroblasts are present in the wound, but they produce an inadequate amount of collagen. Vitamin C is necessary for hydroxylation of

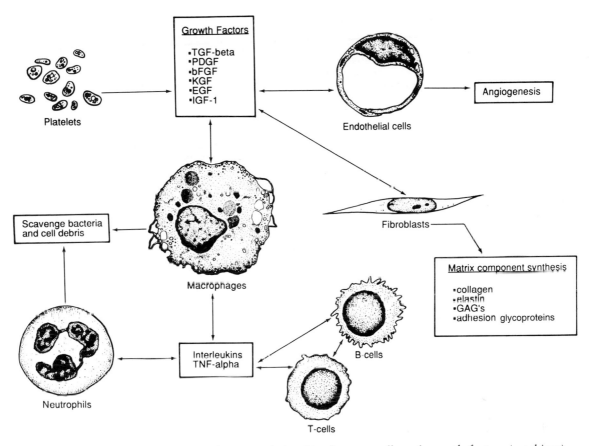

Figure 2. Schematic of the complex interrelationships between cells and growth factors (cytokines) involved in wound repair. Growth factors regulate each cell type involved in wound healing.

proline and lysine residues. Without hydroxyproline, newly synthesized collagen is not transported out of cells, and without hydroxylysine, collagen fibrils are not cross-linked.

Vitamin A (retinoic acid) requirements increase during injury. Severely injured patients require supplemental vitamin A to maintain normal serum levels. Vitamin A also partially reverses the impaired healing in chronically steroid-treated patients. Vitamin B_6 (pyridoxine) deficiency impairs collagen cross-linking. Vitamin B_1 (thiamine) and vitamin B_2 (riboflavin) deficiencies cause syndromes associated with poor wound repair. Trace metal deficiencies such as zinc and copper have been implicated with poor wound repair, since these divalent cations are cofactors in many important enzymatic reactions. Zinc deficiency is associated with poor epithelialization and chronic, nonhealing wounds.

Oxygen, Anemia, Perfusion

Wounds require adequate oxygen delivery to heal well. Ischemic wounds heal poorly and have a much greater risk of infection. Wound ischemia occurs secondary to a variety of factors: occlusive vascular disease, vasoconstriction, and hypovolemia. Excessive suture tension causes local wound ischemia and wound healing complications. Conversely, increased oxygen delivery at the wound improves wound healing. Experimentally, collagen synthesis by fibroblasts is increased with supplemental oxygen. Anemia in the normovolemic patient is not detrimental to wound repair as long as the hematocrit is greater than 15 per cent, because oxygen content in blood does not affect wound collagen synthesis. However, increasing the PO_2 in blood to levels high above 100 per cent hemoglobin saturation allows more oxygen to diffuse to the relatively poorly vascularized wound edge, which upregulates collagen synthesis. Tissue perfusion is the ultimate determinant of wound oxygenation and nutrition. To optimize wound repair, those factors leading to wound ischemia should be prevented. Sutures should not be placed too tightly. The patient should be kept warm, pain should be well controlled to prevent vasoconstriction, and hypovolemia should be avoided.

Diabetes Mellitus and Obesity

Wound healing is impaired in diabetic patients by mechanisms that are unknown, but healing is enhanced somewhat if glucose levels are well controlled. Obesity interferes with repair independently of diabetes. Obese patients with diabetes have impaired wound healing independent of glucose control and insulin therapy. Poor wound perfusion and necrotic adipose debris probably contribute to impaired healing in both diabetic and nondiabetic obese patients.

Corticosteroids

Pharmacologic steroid use impairs healing, especially when given in the first 3 days after wounding. Steroids reduce wound inflammation, collagen synthesis, and contraction.

Chemotherapy and Radiation Therapy

Both radiation and chemotherapeutic agents have their greatest effects on dividing cells. The division of endothelial cells, fibroblasts, and keratinocytes is impaired in irradiated tissue, which slows wound healing. Irradiated tissue usually has some degree of residual endothelial cell injury and endarteritis, which causes atrophy, fibrosis, and poor tissue repair. Chemotherapeutic agents are not administered until at least 5 to 7 days postoperatively in order to prevent impairment of the initial healing events.

Infection

Wound contamination by bacteria causes clinical wound infection and delays healing if greater than 10^5 organisms per milligram tissue are present. Infected wounds are erythematous, tender, and commonly have drainage. The patient may be febrile, and immediate wound opening with removal of suture and débridement is essential. Antibiotic is administered to treat the surrounding cellulitis.

FETAL WOUND HEALING

Unlike the adult, the fetus heals skin wounds with regenerative-type repair and not with scar formation. The epidermis and dermis are restored to a *normal* architecture in which the collagen matrix pattern in the wound is reticular and unchanged from unwounded dermis. The wound hair follicle and sweat gland patterns are normal. In contrast, adult tissue injury due to several disease processes causes scar and fibrosis. Examples include pulmonary fibrosis, hepatic fibrosis, keloids, intraperitoneal adhesions, and burn wound contractures. An understanding of the biology of scarless fetal wound repair may help surgeons develop therapeutic strategies to avert scar and fibrosis.

REFERENCES

Adzick NS, Longaker MT (eds): Fetal Wound Healing. New York, Elsevier Scientific Press, 1992.

Barbul A, Pines E, Caldwell M, Hunt TK (eds): Growth Factors and Other Aspects of Wound Healing: Biological and Clinical Indications. New York, Alan R. Liss, Inc, 1988.

Clark RAF, Henson PM (eds): The Molecular and Cellular Biology of Wound Repair. New York, Plenum Press, 1988.

Cohen IK, Diegelmann RF, Lindblad WJ (eds): Wound Healing: Biochemical and Clinical Aspects. Philadelphia, WB Saunders Company, 1992.

11
BURNS

J. PAUL WAYMACK, M.D., Sc.D.   RANDI L. RUTAN, R.N., B.S.N.
DAVID N. HERNDON, M.D.

Each year, 2.5 million Americans suffer a burn injury, and of these, 100,000 require hospitalization, with 10,000 eventually ending in death. Fortunately, the number of burn injuries and deaths continues to decrease annually due to burn prevention and awareness programs as well as improvements in burn care. With improved techniques in resuscitation, operative excision and grafting procedures, infection control, and metabolic and nutritional support, burn injuries that 50 years ago would have been considered incompatible with survival, are now being treated successfully.

PATHOPHYSIOLOGY

Of the four types of burn injuries, *thermal, electrical, chemical*, and *radiation*, thermal injuries are by far the most common. Both thermal injury and chemical injury cause a coagulation necrosis of tissues that come in immediate contact with either the heat or cold source. The tissue surrounding the zone of coagulation necrosis possesses a moderate degree of vascular injury that causes decreased perfusion of the tissue. This is termed the zone of *stasis* and can progress to thrombosis and necrosis unless an adequate postperiod resuscitation is achieved. Electrical injuries normally have an entrance and exit site. With direct current, the electrons pass from the entrance to the exit site, whereas with alternating current, the electrons fluctuate back and forth between the two sites. Electrical injuries cause damage not only to the skin at the entrance and exit sites, but also to all tissue in the conduction pathway between the entrance and exit sites. The damage can be far below the skin and not readily apparent on physical examination. Radiation injuries may involve all the tissues of the body.

Severe burn injuries cause many physiologic alterations, including the development of total body edema, which follows changes in postburn microvascular permeability caused by the release of various cytokines from the burn. Unless the injury is properly treated, hypotension and shock ensue from intravascular volume loss. Burn injuries also cause a hypermetabolic disturbance. The resting metabolic rate of burn patients increases in proportion to the size of the burn and can cause severe protein catabolism and malnutrition if not properly supported. The hypermetabolic response appears related to alterations in hypothalamic control of metabolism, which is again due, in part, to the cytokines released from the burn wound as well as signals to the afferent neural pathways.

Burn patients are at significant risk for developing infectious complications, and the reasons for this are threefold. First, the burn injury causes the loss of the normal skin barrier to invasion by microorganisms. A concomitant inhalation injury is frequently present in these patients and predisposes to pulmonary infection. Recurrent episodes of bacterial translocation from demonstrated increase in intestinal permeability following episodes of mesenteric vasoconstriction may serve as a source for recurrent infection. Finally, severe burn injury causes an impairment of the patient's immune system, which decreases the burn victim's ability to control microorganisms that gain access to the burn wound, pulmonary tissue, or intestinal tract.

INITIAL THERAPY

The therapy for burn injury begins at the scene with control of the burning process. For flame burns, the patient should be placed on the ground and either rolled or covered with fire resistant material. With chemical burns, the contaminated area should be profusely irrigated with (but not submerged in) water. With electrical injuries, the electrical source should be removed from contact with the patient without risk of electrical injury to the rescuer. Once stabilized, the burn victim should be transported immediately to the nearest medical facility. Upon arrival in the emergency room, the basic features of trauma management should be followed. Specifically, an adequate airway should be assured, and adequate breathing and an acceptable circulatory status should be established. A thorough search for concomitant injuries should also be performed. It is then essential to diagram the size of the burn to plan subsequent fluid resuscitation. The percentages of body surface area comprised by the various extremities and torso are shown in Figure 1. It should be noted that in small children the head accounts for a disproportionate part of the total body surface area (TBSA).

Once the burned body surface area is established, plans are made for appropriate fluid resuscitation. This should be initiated by placement of one or two large-bore intravenous catheters. For adults, the volume of resuscitation required in the first 24 hours following burn injury can be calculated by multiplying the patient's weight in kilograms times the percentage of TBSA burn times 2 to 4 ml. Lactated Ringer's is the resuscitation fluid of choice, and one half of this volume should be given in the first 8 hours following injury, a quarter during the second 8 hours, and a quarter during the third 8 hours. Additional fluid is usually required for patients with concomitant inhalation burns, abdominal or long-bone injury, delayed resuscitation, or who are intoxicated. This equation provides merely an estimate of the volume of lactated Ringer's that is required in the first 24 hours to maintain adequate perfusion of tissues. The optimal goal is to maintain a urine output of 0.5 to 1.0 ml/kg/hr, and the rate of fluid resuscitation should be adjusted to achieve this goal.

The formula for resuscitating children is different (i.e., 5000 ml/m^2 of body surface area burned plus 2000 ml/m^2 of body surface area). Infants lack adequate carbohydrate stores and require lactated Ringer's with 5 per cent dextrose as the resuscitating fluid. Half of this volume should be given during the first 8 hours following burn injury, a quarter during the second 8 hours, and a quarter during the third 8 hours. As in adults, this equation should be used as an estimate of the fluid required. The optimal goal is to maintain a urine output of 1.0 to 1.5 ml/kg/hr. After fluid resuscitation is initiated, attention is directed to the placement of a Foley catheter to measure urine output and a nasogastric tube to prevent gastric distention, which can cause vomiting and aspiration pneumonia. A complete history and physical examination is obtained, with routine blood tests.

Of particular importance is the pulmonary examination, as flame burns in a closed space are associated with an increased risk for an inhalation injury. Inhalation injury has been shown to markedly increase the mortality rate in burn patients, and is caused by toxic fumes damaging the mucosal lining of the respiratory tract, predisposing to the development of bacterial pneumonias and possible septic death. The diagnosis of inhalation injury can be made by one of two techniques: (1) fiberoptic bronchoscopy can be performed at the bedside, or (2) a ventilation perfusion scan can be obtained. Each of these techniques is quite accurate for the diagnosis of inhalation injury. However, bronchoscopy is preferred, since the patient does not leave the intensive care unit (ICU) for this test. Management of inhalation injury is supportive.

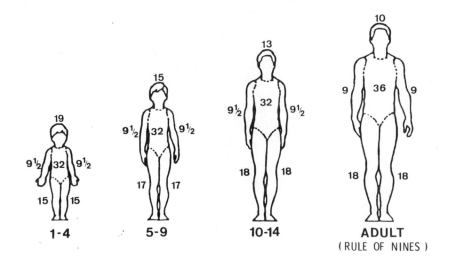

Figure 1. It is essential that an appropriate estimate of the size of the burn be made to calculate fluid replacement for adequate resuscitation. Although the "rule of nines" is appropriate for the adult, children have a different distribution of body surface area. These adjustments must be made to ensure that younger burn victims are not under- or overresuscitated. (From Eichelberger M [ed]: Pediatric Trauma. St. Louis, Mosby Year Book, 1993, with permission.)

During the initial 48 hours following burn injury and resuscitation, burned extremities are at risk for developing severe edema, which can compromise the circulation. It is essential that all extremities be sequentially examined on an hourly basis. To decrease the amount of edema, all burned extremities should be *elevated* above the level of the heart. If there is loss of arterial pulsations or the development of neurologic findings, relief of the pressure may be achieved by making an incision through the necrotic burned tissue along the medial and lateral aspects of the involved extremities, down to viable fat. Diagrams of the placement of escharotomy incisions (escharotomies), using the electrocautery are shown in Figure 2. Since burned tissue is generally insensate, only intravenous sedation is required. It should be emphasized that when escharotomies are performed on extremities, anterior compartmental pressures should be measured to determine the necessity of fasciotomy. Severe edema of the chest wall with circumferential burns can cause a similar problem. In this instance, the pressure prevents adequate expansion of the thorax and can cause pulmonary problems. A chest escharotomy relieves the chest constriction.

WOUND CARE

Once the burn patient has been stabilized, attention is given to the burn wound. The wound is gently débrided with a soap-and-water solution. A second assessment of the depth and extent of the burn wound can then be made. Superficial second-degree burns are painful and cause blistering. Deeper second-degree burns are erythematous and painful to touch. Second-degree burns heal by reepithelialization without surgery. In contrast, full-thickness (third-degree) burn injuries are white or gray in color, insensate, leathery to touch, and require excision and skin grafting for timely and cosmetically acceptable closure. Once the burn wounds have been cleansed and inspected, a topical agent is essential to decrease the degree of colonization of the wound and to prevent the development of infections. In the United States, three topical antimicrobial agents are widely utilized for burn wound care. These are silver nitrate, mafenide acetate, and silver sulfadiazine.

Silver nitrate solution must be applied to dressings frequently to prevent drying. Although silver nitrate possesses excellent antibacterial properties, its major drawbacks include its hypotonicity and sodium leeching from the burned tissues, which cause electrolyte abnormalities. Additionally, it has very poor penetration into the eschar. Finally, everything that is touched by silver nitrate is permanently stained black by it, including linens or other surfaces that touch the patient. Mafenide acetate (Sulfamylon) is an 11 per cent cream that provides excellent gram-positive and gram-negative bacterial coverage. Additionally, it provides excellent wound penetration and is able to maintain low levels of bacterial colonization and decrease bacterial counts in deeply colonized wounds. Mafenide

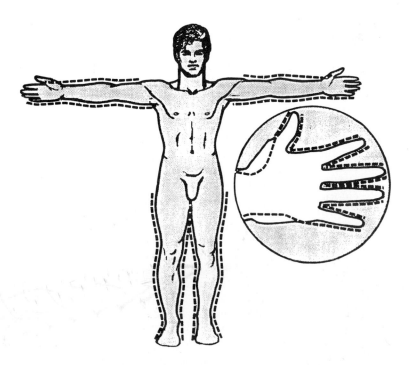

Figure 2. Escharotomies should be performed when the distal circulation is compromised due to the inelasticity of the eschar. They may be performed at the bedside following sedation and are made with the electrocautery or a scalpel along the medial and lateral aspects of the involved area. Care should be taken to preserve the hand and digits when performing escharotomies, as superficial nerves, tendons, and blood vessels can be easily damaged. (From Eichelberger M [ed]: Pediatric Trauma. St. Louis, Mosby Year Book, 1993, with permission.)

acetate has two major side effects: (1) it causes extreme pain upon application to second-degree burns; and (2) it inhibits carbonic anhydrase and thereby can cause the loss of bicarbonate in the urine, leading to a metabolic acidosis. Silver sulfadiazine, the most commonly used antimicrobial agent in the United States, has excellent gram-positive, gram-negative, and fungal coverage, and causes no pain following application. Silver sulfadiazine's major drawback is its inability to penetrate eschar. Nystatin is a useful agent to mix with silver sulfadiazine (1:1) and alternate with mafenide acetate to prevent overgrowth of *Candida* organisms. Nystatin 5 ml orally every 4 hours is also used to prevent *Candida* organism overgrowth of the esophagus and stomach.

METABOLIC SUPPORT

Severe burn injuries cause a marked hypermetabolic response that is characterized by a loss of body mass and an increase in the resting metabolic rate, nitrogen loss, oxygen consumption, lipolysis, and glucose flow. A prolonged continuous febrile response also accompanies the hypermetabolic response and is caused by the resetting of the central body core temperature 2°C above normal by the hypothalamus and is associated with a concomitant increase in basal metabolic rate. The increase in metabolic rate may exceed twice the normal rate in patients with burns exceeding 40 per cent TBSA.

It is essential to provide adequate calories and protein to these patients to prevent protein depletion with its associated poor wound healing and immune suppression. Determination of the optimal nutritional requirements of the burn patient can be made using one of two techniques; the first being measurement of resting metabolic energy expenditure by indirect calorimetry with oxygen consumption and carbon dioxide production. An approximation of caloric repletion requirements can be made by 1.4 times the resting energy expenditure (REE). Second, an estimation of the patient's nutritional requirements can be made by utilizing one of a number of formulas. For adults, the Curreri formula is frequently used in calculating the daily caloric requirements in kilocalories to be equal to 25 times the body weight in kilograms plus 40 times the percentage TBSA burned. This formula tends to overestimate the caloric requirements in small children with large burns. For these patients caloric requirements should be equal to 1500 kcal/m² of body surface area plus 1500 kcal/m² of burned skin. Protein requirements are also increased in burn patients, and the calorie/nitrogen ratio should be approximately 100:1, as opposed to the 125 to 150:1 ratio achieved with normal diets.

Because the patient may not be able to consume adequate quantities of calories and protein by mouth, it becomes necessary to supplement the nutritional support of the patient through either intravenous or enteral tube feedings. Intravenous supplementation has been shown to be associated with an extremely high complication rate and is not indicated except in the most dire circumstances. In contrast, enteral tube feedings are well tolerated, especially if a soft, flexible feeding tube is passed under fluoroscopic control into the distal duodenum or proximal jejunum. Once the tube is positioned, feedings can be given with little risk of subsequent reflux into the stomach, with resultant vomiting and aspiration. If the patient suffers from ileus with reflux into the stomach, a nasogastric tube positioned with the feeding tube can be attached to suction to maintain the stomach empty while the tube feedings into the duodenum or jejunum continue.

Some studies have suggested that the administration of enteral feedings early in the postburn period may blunt the hypermetabolic response and that early enteral feeding may decrease the incidence of bacterial translocation (i.e., the passage of enteral bacteria through the intestinal wall and into the systemic circulation). With these potential benefits, it is prudent to initiate enteral feedings as soon as possible and clearly within 24 hours of injury. It is possible to decrease intravenous fluids while concomitantly increasing the volume of enteral feedings so that the patient's fluid requirements are entirely met by the enteral route (Fig. 3).

STRESS ULCERS

Risk of stress ulcerations of the upper gastrointestinal tract is of major concern in severely burned patients. These are termed Curling's ulcers and can produce severe hemorrhage. Etiologic factors in the development of these ulcers include decreased mucosal vascular perfusion and gastric acid production. The development of hemorrhage from a Curling's ulcer is associated with a high morbidity and mortality. Thus, it is preferable to prevent development of such ulcers, and this is possible through the use of antacids to neutralize acid and maintain a gastric pH in excess of 4, or H₂ blockers to decrease acid production with maintenance of a pH over 4.

INFECTION

In patients suffering severe burn injuries who survive the initial 24 hours following burn injury, the principal cause of death is infection. The location of most infections has recently shifted from the burn

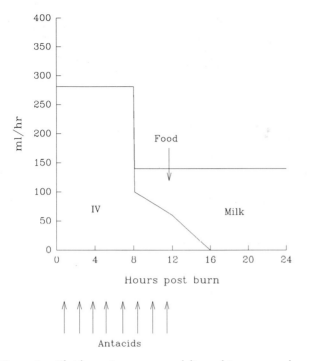

Figure 3. Fluid requirements are delivered intravenously at the outset. This diagram depicts the fluid requirements of a child with 1.0 m² body surface area and 50 per cent body surface burn. Within 6 hours, bland, nutritive fluids can be gradually introduced enterically and advanced as intravenous rates are reciprocally reduced, thus gradually delivering the bulk, if not all, of the fluid requirements at the end of the initial 24 hours following burn.

wound to the lungs, especially in patients with inhalation injuries. The routine use of parenteral antibiotics in an attempt to prevent the development of infections is not indicated, as it merely causes the development of antibiotic-resistant organisms. Rather, antibiotics should be utilized to treat newly diagnosed infections. The one exception is the use of perioperative prophylactic antibiotics, and they should be initiated immediately prior to surgery. The optimal postoperative period of coverage with prophylactic antibiotics has not been established. In the absence of objective data, the duration of postoperative coverage with antibiotics ranges from a single preoperative dose, to continued administration for the initial 48 hours postoperatively.

Antibiotics should be given when a diagnosis of infection is made, and bacteria or yeast should be grown from a sputum specimen obtained by bronchoscopy or suctioning through an endotracheal tube to be certain. The sputum should be obtained in as sterile a manner as possible, and if the patient is intubated, a suction tube should be placed in a sterile manner down the endotracheal tube, to obtain sputum. If the patient is not intubated, fiberoptic bronchoscopy should be performed to obtain the sputum. In addition to performing a culture, a Gram stain of the sputum to examine for the presence of bacteria or yeast should be done. Finally, it is also important to obtain a white blood cell count of the sputum, as sputum that contains bacteria but no white blood cells is highly suspicious for being a contaminated specimen. It is therefore essential to note the presence of in excess of 15 to 20 white blood cells per high-power field (WBC/HPF) on examination of the sputum to confidently predict the presence of an infection in the pulmonary tract. Additionally, it is important to note the presence of an infiltrate on chest film. The combination of an infiltrate on chest film, and sputum that contains in excess of 15 to 20 WBC/HPF and which demonstrates, by culture or Gram stain, the presence of bacteria or yeast can be considered diagnostic of a pneumonia. If microorganisms and greater than 15 to 20 WBC/HPF are noted in the specimen but no infiltrate is found on chest film, the diagnosis of bronchitis is made. Intravenous antimicrobial therapy is begun immediately to treat the pulmonary infection. Additionally, vigorous pulmonary toilet should be emphasized.

Burn wound infection is suspected when the patient has systemic signs of sepsis and a local sign of burn wound infection (Table 1). When the diagnosis of burn wound infection is considered, a biopsy of the burn wound should be obtained immediately. It should be examined both histologically and by quantitative culture, and if greater than 10^5 microorganisms per gram of tissue are found, it is indicative of infection. However, this test requires 24 to 48 hours to complete. Histologic examination of the biopsy can normally be completed within 6 hours of obtaining the specimen. If microorganisms are identified invading viable tissue, a diagnosis of a burn wound infection is established. When a wound infection is diagnosed, aggressive therapy is begun immediately. This includes the use of systemic antibiotics, subeschar injection of antibiotics, and surgical excision of the infected burn wound as soon as the patient is stabilized.

SURGICAL THERAPY

When infectious complications are prevented, all partial thickness burn injuries eventually heal by re-epithelialization. In contrast, full-thickness burns require surgical therapy for closure. This is accomplished by excising the burn wound, either tangentially or fascially. With tangential excision, multiple passes are made with a dermatome until viable bleeding tissue is obtained. With fascial excision, either a scalpel or electrocautery is used to remove all burned tissue and fat down to viable muscle fascia. Tangential ex-

TABLE 1. LOCAL SIGNS OF BURN WOUND INFECTION

Conversion of partial thickness injury to full-thickness injury
Black or violaceous discoloration
Separation of eschar
Discoloration of subeschar tissue
Edema or violaceous discoloration of unburned skin and wound markings
Centrifugal advancement of subcutaneous edema tumor necrosis

cision produces a greater operative blood loss, but provides a better cosmetic result than does fascial excision. Blood loss can be further decreased if the excision is performed within the first 24 hours following injury, when the edema and local wound mediators exert a local vasoconstrictive effect. After the excision is completed, obtaining hemostasis of the excised wound is important and is best obtained by a combination of topical hemostatic agents and electrocautery. The two most frequently used topical hemostatic agents are epinephrine and thrombin. Epinephrine acts by causing local vasoconstriction of transected capillaries, venules, and arterioles. Thrombin causes conversion of fibrinogen to fibrin, leading to the initiation of the clotting process.

After adequate hemostasis is obtained, the burn wound should be grafted. A graft of unburned skin between 0.005 inch and 0.016 inch in depth is usually taken. In patients with large burn injuries, it may be necessary to mesh the skin graft to allow expansion of the tissue so that it may cover a greater area. In patients with very large burns, it is important to obtain thin grafts and widely mesh them. These widely meshed grafts, as well as areas for which insufficient donor sites are available, should be covered with a cadaveric allograft (Fig. 4). This facilitates both maximal coverage of the burn wound and the most rapid healing of the donor site, permitting rapid reharvesting of the same donor site for subsequent coverage of other burned areas. In contrast, patients with small burns should have skin grafts harvested at approximately 0.016 inch and the graft should not be meshed; rather, it should be applied as a sheet, which provides a superior cosmetic result. Following placement, skin grafts are secured with either staples or sutures, and a moist dressing containing an antimicrobial agent is applied over the skin grafts. The donor sites are covered with either scarlet-red gauze or a synthetic dressing such as Biobrane. Unless evidence of sepsis is present, the dressings should be removed at 72 hours and the grafts inspected. Thereafter, dressings should be reapplied daily until the grafts have become adherent and revascularized.

REHABILITATION

Once the entire burn wound has been successfully closed by either reepithelialization or skin grafting, attention is focused on minimizing the amount of scarring. There is no clear evidence demonstrating the efficacy for the use of pharmacologic agents in decreasing the amount of scarring. Instead, pressure garments are utilized to decrease the amount of scarring following closure of the burn wound. A commonly used pressure garment is made of a tightly fitting elastic material that is manufactured to the patient's body shape and size. The pressure exerted by these garments on the healed burn wounds, healed skin graft, and donor sites is able to markedly decrease the severity of scarring. It is necessary to wear these garments for 23 hours daily for 1 to 2 years following the burn injury to obtain the best results.

Severe burn injuries can cause permanent disability due to the scarring process. Hypertrophic burn scars

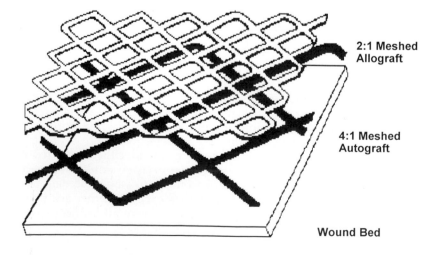

2:1 Meshed Allograft

4:1 Meshed Autograft

Wound Bed

Figure 4. The widely meshed autograft should be overlaid with narrowly meshed cadaveric allograft rotated 90 degrees. Wounds for which insufficient donor sites are available should be similarly covered with cadaveric allograft alone, which is replaced as donor sites heal and can be reharvested. (Diagram from Alexander JW, MacMillan BG, Law E: Treatment of severe burns with widely meshed skin autograft and meshed skin allograft overlay. J Trauma 21[6]:434, 1981, with permission.)

lack the elasticity of normal skin and can interfere with joint motion. Correction of this problem may require complex reconstructive surgery. It is therefore desirable to prevent the occurrence of the contracture, which is best accomplished with a combination of pressure garments and splints in combination with an active physical and occupational therapy program. Joints, when not in use, should be splinted in a position to maximally oppose the wound contracture forces. Active motion should be encouraged in all joints, and passive motion should be utilized for all joints at risk, provided the involved tendons and ligaments are viable. The use of passive motion in joints with necrotic tendons and ligaments can cause rupture of those tendons and ligaments and is contraindicated.

CONCLUSIONS

Burn injuries cause a number of physiologic alterations that place the patient at risk for serious compli

cations. With the use of aggressive resuscitation, nutritional support, infection control, and surgical therapy, the burn patient can overcome these challenges and achieve full recovery.

REFERENCES

Davies JWL: Physiologic Responses to Burning. London, Academic Press, 1982.

Herndon DN, Curreri PW, Abston S, Rutan TC, Barrow RE: Treatment of burns. Curr Probl Surg 24(6):341–397, 1987.

Shirani KZ, Pruitt BA Jr, Mason AD Jr: The influence of inhalation injury and pneumonia on burn mortality. Ann Surg 205(1):82–87, 1987.

Waymack JP, Herndon DN: Nutritional support of the burned patient. World J Surg 16:80–86, 1992.

Waymack JP, Pruitt BA Jr: Burn Wound Care. In Thompkins RK, Balch CM, Cameron JL, Langer B, Mannick JA, Sheldon FG, Shires GT, Welch CE (eds): Advances in Surgery, vol 23. Chicago, Year Book Medical Publishers, Inc, 1990, pp 261–289.

Wilmore DW, Long JM, Mason AD Jr, et al: Catecholamines: A mediator of the hypermetabolic response to thermal injury. Ann Surg 180:653–659, 1974.

12
PRINCIPLES OF OPERATIVE SURGERY

SCOTT E. LANGENBURG, M.D.   JOHN B. HANKS, M.D.

ANTISEPSIS

Historical Aspects

In Greek, antisepsis means "against putrefaction." By practicing aseptic technique, surgeons can expect low infection and mortality rates when compared to those of practitioners of surgery in the 18th and 19th centuries. In 1847, Semmelweis noted that the large discrepancy in puerperal mortality between two hospital wards was based mainly on the difference in aseptic techniques employed, such as hand washing and clothing and linen changes. A simple change of technique caused a substantial decrease in postpartum deaths. Twenty years later, Joseph Lister published his principles of antiseptic technique with careful scrubbing of the hands and arms; and use of sterile gloves, instruments, and drapes, based on the then-recent discovery of microorganisms by Pasteur. These basic principles of antiseptic technique have been maintained ever since.

Aseptic Procedures

The fundamental components of aseptic procedures are the environment (operating room), the patient, the participants, and the instruments. The operating room is designed to provide minimal bacterial or viral contamination within this separate environment and with rules concerning individuals entering the operating room and their attire. The doors to the operating suites remain closed, and traffic through them is limited. The operating rooms are equipped with air filters, positive pressure ventilation, and laminar flow.

The patients should be meticulously prepared for operation with the recognition that skin is the most common source of bacteria that cause wound infections. Hair is not shaved unless it has the potential to interfere with the procedure, and it is definitely not shaved the evening before operation, owing to increased infection rates arising in small lacerations. Skin preparation for elective procedures is begun with an antibacterial shower on the night before or the day of the operation. In the operating room, the skin is prepared with iodophor compounds (Betadine) or chlorhexidine; detergent compounds are used for those with skin sensitivity to iodine. These compounds are applied to the area of the planned incision and expanded outward in increasing circles.

Two important factors contributing to wound infections are the type of case (clean, clean-contaminated, contaminated) and the immune status of the patient. Surgeons and other operating room personnel participate in prevention of contamination by covering the hair and wearing face masks, shoe covers, sterile impermeable gowns, and sterile gloves. The hands and arms are scrubbed to the elbow using iodophor or chlorhexidine solutions for 3 to 5 minutes. Universal precautions to protect personnel are used when handling or when exposed to blood or body fluids (Table 1). This includes the aforementioned techniques, as well as the use of protection of the eyes with side shields. Once sterilized equipment is opened, it remains on sterile tables or in the operative field. Surgical equipment that is reusable is cleaned, double-wrapped in paper or cotton that is permeable to steam (but not to microorganisms), and sealed with heat-sensitive tape. The equipment is then sterilized with either

TABLE 1. UNIVERSAL PRECAUTIONS

1. Gloves must be worn for contact with blood, body fluids, mucous membranes, broken or cut skin, or human tissue of any patient. Gloves must also be worn when performing procedures like vascular access (venipuncture) or when suctioning a patient.
2. If hands or other skin surfaces have direct contact with blood or body fluids, the area must be washed immediately with soap and water. If eyes, mouth, or nose are splashed with blood or body fluids, they must be irrigated (flushed) with large amounts of water. If blood or a body fluid splashes into a skin cut, skin puncture, or skin lesion, the area should be washed, first with soap and water, then with 70 per cent isopropyl alcohol. The Health Service must be notified.
3. Do not eat or drink, apply cosmetics or lip balm, or handle contact lenses in potential exposure areas.
4. Wear fluid-resistant gowns or plastic aprons if soiling with blood or body fluids is likely.
5. A mask and eye protection must be worn if spraying, splashing, or splattering of blood or body fluids is possible (i.e., when suctioning, in operating room, performing postmortem exams).
6. Use CPR masks for resuscitation to minimize the need for mouth-to-mouth resuscitation.
7. Handle sharp instruments with care to prevent accidental cuts or punctures and discard all sharp items immediately by placing them in a puncture-resistant needle box or a puncture-resistant contaminated-materials container. Never recap or bend disposable needles.
8. Clean blood or body fluid spills promptly with water and bleach (9:1).
9. All patient specimens may be infectious and must be handled with gloves.
10. Cover any skin wound on yourself with a waterproof dressing before beginning to work.
11. Any material or items contaminated with blood, body fluids, or human tissue must be put into a contaminated-materials container.

steam, dry heat, or gas. Steam sterilization is more effective than dry heat; therefore, dry heat or gas sterilization should only be utilized when the equipment would be damaged by repeat exposure to steam (i.e., reusable equipment made of plastics or other polymers). Gas sterilization is performed by placing the equipment in heat-sensitive, tape-sealed plastic bags and sterilizing for 12 hours with ethylene oxide.

SURGICAL TECHNIQUE

Surgical technique includes incisions, ligation of bleeding vessels, and sutures, as well as aspects such as gentle handling and dissection of tissue, careful hemostasis, and effective team cooperation. Dissection is accomplished by either a blunt or sharp technique, blunt dissection being performed by manipulating tissue with the hands or with instruments, and sharp dissection by either a scalpel or scissors.

Wounds heal in three ways: (1) *primary* intention, when the tissue edges are approximated immediately after the surgical procedure; (2) *secondary* intention, when the wound is left open and healing occurs through growth of granulation tissue and epithelialization; and (3) *third* intention, or delayed primary closure, when a potentially contaminated wound is left open until evidence of infection has disappeared and the wound is closed primarily. Clean surgical wounds are allowed to heal by primary intention performed with either suture, surgical tape, or metal staples.

Wound closure with suture is performed with either cutaneous or subcuticular (dermal) sutures. Cutaneous sutures, the most common type used for closure, are usually placed with a synthetic, monofilament suture made of nylon or polypropylene. Monofilament sutures are least damaging to the tissues and permit easy wound care. They are able to stretch without breaking. There are also no interstitial spaces that can harbor bacteria. *Subcuticular* closures are usually performed with absorbable sutures with minimal tissue reactivity (polyglycolic acid or polyglactin); however, nonabsorbable, monofilaments may be used, especially a continuous suture that can be removed later. After suturing, surgical tapes are also added to optimally approximate the skin edges. This type of closure is utilized when patient follow-up is limited, for children, to avoid suture removal, and for wounds that must be covered with casts.

Surgical tape is commonly used with subcuticular suture closures, but may also be used alone in linear wounds with minimal static or dynamic tension. Ideal locations for this type of closure are on the face and abdomen. Sites not well managed with tape include the extremities, axilla, and palms and soles of the foot due to the moisture from secretions and high skin tension. Surgical staples are commonly used to close wounds by disposable devices and contain unformed, stainless steel staples that form an incomplete rectangle when inserted.

Suture Removal

Timing is important in removal of sutures to ensure both adequate wound strength and a good cosmetic result. The ability of a wound to heal with sufficient tensile strength depends largely on its blood supply. Several other factors contribute to the wound's inability to heal promptly, including increased skin tension, poor nutritional status of the patient, and prior radiation therapy, chemotherapy, or use of steroids. Guidelines for suture removal by anatomic site are shown in Table 2. When sutures are removed, the wound edges should be reinforced with sterile surgical tape.

TABLE 2. GUIDELINES FOR SUTURE REMOVAL

Anatomic Location	Removal Days
Eyelid	2–3
Face	4–5
Neck	3–5
Scalp	7
Trunk	6–14
Extremities	10–21
Joints	14

Special Wounds

Several wounds require care differing from that of uncomplicated surgical wounds. These include contaminated wounds, skin ulcers (pressure ulceration or toxic ulceration), and skin grafts (graft and donor sites). Contaminated wounds result from contact with feces, saliva, purulent exudate, soil, or other foreign material, or they are wounds for which treatment has been delayed longer than 6 hours. When these wounds are closed primarily, the infection rate is usually above 20 per cent. Therefore, open wound management and delayed primary closure is the best management. Delayed primary closure allows the wound to gain resistance to infection, thus allowing an uncomplicated closure. Open wounds are managed by packing the wound with sterile gauze and covering it with a sterile dressing. The wound is left undisturbed for several days, at which time the wound edges can be approximated if clean. The wound should be followed carefully for appearance of fever.

Skin ulcerations often require care, before skin grafting or flaps can be completed, that consists of frequent dressing changes, two or three times daily, with large saline-moistened mesh gauze covered by dry gauze. This large moist gauze dries between dressing changes and facilitates débridement of nonviable tissue. As the wound heals, capillaries develop, and a beefy red granulation tissue appears. Once the wound is well granulated, it can be covered with a skin graft or flap.

SUTURE

Selection of Suture Material

In ancient Egypt, wounds were closed with animal sinews, horsehair, or vegetable fibers. Silk was used by Galen in the second century AD, and absorbable sutures were introduced by Physick in 1806. Today, suture material is available in many different forms, absorbable or nonabsorbable, braided or monofilament, natural or synthetic, and dyed or undyed (Table 3). An ideal suture is one with a small diameter and great tensile strength, low tissue reactivity, good knot-holding capability to hold knots securely, with minimal effect on the resistance of the wound to infection. Multifilament sutures have the greatest amount of reactivity and infection potential; monofilaments have the least. The advantage of monofilaments is that they do not damage the tissue as they pass through it. However, once tied, they do have a greater tendency to untie and cut through the tissue.

Absorbable Sutures

Absorbable sutures are absorbed by the body and eventually disappear. The rate at which this occurs varies with the composition of the suture. Common sutures include the following.

Polyglactin

Polyglactin is a braided, synthetic suture with a high tensile strength, and is usually absorbed in 60 days.

Polyglycolic Acid

Similar to polyglactin, this suture is absorbed by hydrolysis in approximately 60 to 90 days, is one of the least reactive absorbable sutures, and disturbs the wound defenses the least.

TABLE 3. SUTURE TYPES

Synthetic
  Absorbable (braided)
    Polyglactin (Vicryl)
    Coated polyglactin (Vicryl)
    Polyglycolic acid (Dexon)
    Coated polyglycolic acid (Dexon)
  Absorbable (monofilament)
    Polydioxanone (PDS)
    Polyglyconate (Maxon)
  Nonabsorbable (braided)
    Nylon (Surgilon, Nurolon)
    Polyester (Dacron, Ethibond, Mersilene, Ti-cron)
  Nonabsorbable (monofilament)
    Nylon (Dermalon, Ethilon)
    Polypropylene (Prolene, Surgilene)
    Stainless steel
    Silver wire
    Iron alloy (Flexon)

Natural
  Absorbable (monofilament)
    Gut
    Chromic gut
  Nonabsorbable (braided)
    Silk
    Cotton

Polydioxanone

This suture is a synthetic, monofilament suture with excellent tensile strength, but is somewhat difficult to handle and to tie. It has the advantage of not being braided, thereby decreasing the risk of bacteria entering the interstices and escaping phagocytosis.

Polyglyconate

This is another monofilament, absorbable suture.

Catgut

Catgut is made from the intestine of cattle or sheep and derives its name from a musical instrument called a kitte, which has fine gut for its strings. *Plain* catgut absorbs in approximately 10 days; *chromic* catgut is catgut that has been treated by chromium salts and absorbs in 20 days. Catgut is very reactive in human tissue and is useful for tying off subcutaneous vessels and closing the skin in sites where local organisms are apt to cause later infection, such as in the scrotum and perineum.

Nonabsorbable Sutures

Nylon

Nylon suture is made of synthetic polyamides and is available in either a monofilament or braided variety. It possesses low tissue reactivity and causes minimal damage to wound defense. Degraded and absorbed in about 2 years, nylon is commonly used for both percutaneous and subcuticular skin closure.

Polypropylene

This monofilament suture is derived from polyolefins and has characteristics similar to monofilament nylon—minimal tissue reaction, excellent in small sizes for microsurgery, and smooth tissue passage. However, polypropylene has been shown to retain its tensile strength several years after use in vascular anastomoses. This suture, in addition to being used for skin closure, is used commonly in vascular procedures to create anastomoses. Care must be taken not to handle monofilament suture with instruments because instruments weaken the suture and may lead to suture breakage.

Polyester

Polyester sutures are braided and utilized commonly in cardiothoracic surgery and for fascial closures.

Silk

One of the oldest sutures, silk is derived from the silkworm, is treated with polybutilate and braided, and is a durable suture with good tensile strength. It loses its strength with time due to the degradation that occurs in vivo.

Stainless Steel

Wire is utilized commonly to provide a great amount of strength with minimal tissue reactivity. The strength of a wire closure is necessary, for example, in reapproximating the sternum after a median sternotomy. This suture is very difficult to handle and, with time, it frequently fatigues, leading to fracture. Stainless steel sutures also interfere with computer-assisted tomography and magnetic resonance imaging.

STAPLING DEVICES

In addition to stapling devices for the skin, several internal stapling devices are available: TA, GIA, EEA, and LDS. These instruments are descendants of the early devices created by Hultl in 1908, Von Petz, and Friedrich of Ulm in 1934. The instruments used currently closely resemble those developed by Ravitch in 1958, but are now available in reloadable or disposable units.

GIA Instruments

GIA instruments are used to create intestinal anastomoses with serosal apposition by placing two double-staggered rows of staples and simultaneously dividing tissue between the staggered rows. This instrument is used for resection of tissues, such as lung-wedge resections, in addition to anastomosis creation. The use of stapling is much faster than handsewn anastomoses. Some advocate use of an additional hand-sewn layer to reinforce the staple line.

TA Instruments

TA instruments, which place a linear, everting (mucosa to mucosa) double line of staggered staples, come in three lengths, 30, 55, and 90 mm, (TA30, TA55, and TA90). The staples are available in three sizes, 3.2 (vascular cartridge), 3.5, and 4.8 mm. The 3.2-mm vascular cartridge is utilized to close vessels in pneumonectomy and lobectomy procedures.

EEA Instruments

The EEA instrument is utilized to create end-to-end and end-to-side inverting anastomoses. The device fires a circle of staples and cuts a central ring of tissue through apposed ends of bowel. Commonly used in esophageal and rectal surgery, this device allows surgeons to perform lower resections and primary end-to-end anastomoses in sphincter-sparing rectal carcinoma resections.

SURGICAL ADHESIVES

Fibrin Glue

Fibrin glue (or fibrin sealant) is a topical biologic adhesive. It consists of two separate solutions which, when combined, imitate the final stages of coagulation. The first component is a solution of concentrated human fibrinogen with factor XIII, fibronectin, and plasminogen; the second component is bovine thrombin and calcium chloride. These are applied to the operative site simultaneously in a 1:1 ratio and cause thrombin conversion of fibrinogen to fibrin monomers, forming a clot that facilitates hemostasis and tissue sealing. The initial stability of the clot is due to hydrogen bond formation, but with activation of factor XIII by thrombin, the fibrin monomers' cross-linkages are further stabilized. The clot is completely absorbed during wound healing without foreign body reaction or extensive fibrosis.

The fibrinogen component of fibrin glue can be obtained from either pooled fresh frozen plasma (FFP), single-donor FFP, or from autologous donation. The risk of transmission of viral disease is minimized by single-donor FFP and virtually eliminated by autologous donation. The thrombin and calcium chloride solution is commercially available. Fibrin glue has found many applications in several surgical disciplines, including facilitation of hemostasis on raw or traumatized surfaces, dural patching and closure, skin grafting, and procedures on the middle ear.

Cyanoacrylate

This compound has been widely used in the fixation of the articulating surfaces of artificial joints. It has the propensity to delay healing, increase infection rate, and loosen with time in fixation of artificial joints.

Drains

Penrose drains are composed of soft, thin-walled latex and are used to evacuate blood, pus, or serum from a body cavity, permitting obliteration of the dead space. These drains should be placed dependently to function properly and are brought out of the wound through a separate stab incision adjacent to the wound. This decreases the risk of infection, wound dehiscence, and hernias. Penrose drains are becoming less frequently used, as they represent an "open" drain and are subject to infection.

Closed Suction Drain

In contrast to Penrose drains, closed suction drains (e.g., Jackson-Pratt, Hemovac) are firm, multiholed conduits made of silicon or polyvinyl chloride. They do not require dependent drainage because they have a collapsed Silastic bulb for drainage collection that is placed under negative pressure. Penrose and closed suction drains are either removed all at once when drainage has decreased or in a stepwise manner. The latter technique is felt to break down some of the fibrin deposition that forms within 24 hours of drain placement and allow further drainage.

Foley Catheters

Foley catheters are rubber tubes with a dilatable balloon at the tip that is usually placed into the urinary bladder to alleviate distention and quantify urine output. They are routinely used during and after long operating room procedures and in critically ill patients for urinary drainage. Despite insertion with sterile technique, the main risk of catheterization is urinary tract infection. The infection rate is as high as 10 per cent when left indwelling and about 1 per cent for a single insertion for catheterization with immediate removal in ambulatory patients. *Escherichia coli* is the most common pathogen. Appropriate-sized Foley catheters can also be used as duodenal, jejunal, or cecal enteric tubes as well as for abscess drainage.

Chest Tubes

Chest tubes are drains placed into the intrapleural space to evacuate blood, pus, air, or effusion. They are attached to a closed suction receptacle system that allows variance of suction pressure and quantification of output. Chest tubes, as well as the other drains, must be kept clean and dressed with a dry dressing at the point of skin entry.

SPECIAL INSTRUMENTS

Electrocautery

Electrocautery, designed by Bovie and popularized by Harvey Cushing, is an electric current in a configuration of alternating sine wave with a frequency of 20,000 Hz that is utilized to incise or coagulate tissue. The electrocautery functions in three different ways: cutting, coagulation, and a blend of both cutting and coagulation. The cutting mode utilizes a continuous current that is excellent for cutting but does not provide good hemostasis. The coagulation mode provides intermittent, short bursts of current with long gaps between bursts. The slower current delivery provides excellent hemostasis but is less efficient for cutting. The coagulation and cutting settings can be adjusted and blended to provide optimal hemostasis and dissection in different types of tissue. Electrocautery can also be either unipolar or bipolar, with unipolar being more common. Unipolar electrocautery requires a ground, but bipolar does not. Bipolar electrocautery is commonly used in delicate neurosurgical or plastic surgery procedures. The advantage of electrocautery is the speed with which dissection can be done while maintaining hemostasis. Disadvantages include poor depth control, inability to feel the tissue, muscle stimulation, tissue devitalization, and the danger of explosion of gases from anesthesia or from the bowel.

Lasers

The term laser is an acronym for light amplification by stimulated emission of radiation, and light is used as a source of energy for coagulation and cutting. The light is monochromatic, and the energy is expressed as a function of wavelength in nanometers. It must be noted that laser technology is another technique of tissue manipulation, and many techniques can be as efficient and possibly safer than laser surgery.

Argon Laser

Argon lasers emit a blue-green beam of light of 488 to 514 nm that transfers energy to red cell hemoglobin, produces heat, and creates a superficial thermal injury. Argon lasers are utilized in treatment of intraocular hemorrhage, in hepatic surgery, for tissue fusion at vascular anastomoses, and for thermal arterial recanalization. Advantages of the argon laser are the speed of effect, decrease in tissue reaction compared to suture hemostasis, and reduction of intimal hyperplasia at the site of a vascular anastomosis.

Carbon-Dioxide Laser

The carbon-dioxide laser causes a transfer of energy that causes boiling of intracellular water and cell explosion. The result of this process is steam production and carbonization of tissue. The carbon-dioxide laser is used for large surgical excisions because of its advantage of decreased blood loss, but its use is limited by the increased susceptibility to wound infection.

Nd:YAG Laser

The neodymium:yttrium-aluminum-garnet (Nd:YAG) laser has the greatest degree of forward penetration, carbon dioxide having an intermediate amount, and argon having the least. It produces its effect with destructive coagulation using a 1060-nm wavelength light beam. Nd:YAG lasers are utilized in the tracheobronchial tree and paranasal sinuses, with a flexible quartz fiber passed via fiberoptic endoscopes.

Tunable Dye Laser

These lasers have a wavelength of 577 nm and have been utilized in the treatment of cutaneous port-wine stains.

CUSA Knife

The Cavitron ultrasonic surgical aspirator (CUSA) is an ultrasound probe that selectively fragments and aspirates tissue of high water, low collagen content, such as tumors and liver parenchyma, while sparing adjacent blood vessels and nerves. The CUSA knife has been used in ophthalmologic procedures (cataract aspiration), neurosurgery (tumor removal), general and urologic operations (splenic, hepatic, prostate, and renal resection), and cardiovascular procedures (exposure of imbedded coronary arteries and dissection of the internal mammary artery). Felt to allow improved visibility, reduced tissue injury, and reduced blood loss when compared to the scalpel or electrocautery, it may also have applications intraperitoneally through laparoscopic instruments.

REFERENCES

Coit DG, Sclafani L: Care of the surgical wound. American College of Surgeons: Care of the Surgical Patient. Vol 2, Elective Care. New York, Scientific American, Inc, 1990.
Dougherty SH, Simmons RL: The biology and practice of surgical drains, Parts I & II. Curr Probl Surg 29 (8,9), 1992.
Edgerton MT: The Art of Surgical Technique. Williams & Wilkins Company, Baltimore, MD, 1988.
Edlich RF, Rodeheaver GT, Thacker JG, et al: Fundamentals of Wound Management in Surgery: Technical Factors in Wound Management. South Plainfield, NJ, Chirurgecom, Inc, 1977.

13
SURGICAL INFECTIONS AND ANTIBIOTICS

DAVID L. DUNN, M.D., Ph.D.

Infection remains a significant cause of postoperative morbidity and mortality despite major advances in the treatment of surgical patients. An historical review demonstrates that the epidemiology of surgical infections has changed considerably. For example, prior to the implementation of the antiseptic techniques advanced by Lister, the incidence of significant postoperative infections was greater than 50 per cent and was associated with high mortality. Infection in the surgical wound was thought to be a natural, unavoidable process, hence the term "laudable pus." Although the occurrence of infections in surgical patients has been reduced substantially, this complication remains a *significant* problem. Factors that assuredly contribute to the continued presence of serious postoperative infections include the application of sophisticated technology (invasive monitoring technology, anesthesia, and metabolic support), which facilitates performance of surgical procedures in severely injured, elderly, debilitated, or immunosuppressed patients. The ability to sustain failing organ systems in the intensive care unit setting and the use of increasingly complex surgical procedures have further increased this problem. Although the occurrence of infectious events now can be predicted with considerable accuracy for a group of individuals undergoing a certain type of operative intervention, it remains difficult to ascertain in advance whether a specific patient will develop a serious infection. Herein lies one of the most difficult problems facing the surgeon, because intervention in the form of aseptic technique and administration of prophylactic antimicrobial agents must anticipate the infectious event itself to be most effective. In addition, due to the serious impact many surgical infections exert upon outcome, surgeons must expedite the diagnosis and treatment of the infections that occur. Currently, the approach used to treat infectious events should combine several different modalities, including surgical intervention, antimicrobial agents, and intensive care.

Host-Microbial Interactions

The development of infection requires the presence of microbes and their adherence to host tissues, following which proliferation, local invasion, and widespread dissemination may occur. Two reservoirs of potential microbial pathogens have been identified that consist of the autochthonous (endogenous) microflora of the patient and the external environment. Infections in surgical patients can be caused by microbes derived from either or both sources. While many microbes within the external environment can become pathogens, most areas of the body possess a characteristic endogenous microflora that is capable of providing the initial inoculum for infection. Typically, this occurs when the barriers that separate sterile areas of the body from those that contain such microflora are disrupted. Thus, the skin possesses an endogenous microflora that consists of gram-positive organisms such as *Staphylococcus* and *Streptococcus* species, although in areas of the body below the umbilicus, gram-negative bacteria such as *Escherichia coli* are not uncommon. Not surprisingly, traumatic lacerations and many superficial surgical wound infections are caused by these microbes, although heavy contamination from environmental sources can also occur. Many other areas of the body also possess a microflora that becomes established soon after birth and remains relatively constant thereafter. For example, large numbers of many different microbes can be found throughout the gastrointestinal tract. At the proximal (oropharynx) and distal (colorectum) ends, large numbers of aerobic and anaerobic bacteria can be isolated. While the acidity and rapid peristalsis of the stomach largely preclude entry of organisms of the oropharynx into the upper gastrointestinal tract, in the distal small bowel, significant numbers of microbes appear (10^5 to 10^8 microbes per gram of enteric contents). In the distal colon, as many as 10^{11} to 10^{12} microbes per gram of enteric contents may be encountered. These organisms consist of both aerobes and anaerobes, although the latter predominate by a ratio of 100 to 300:1. Under normal circumstances, the epithelial and endothelial layers of the body prevent entry of these microbes into the sterile areas of the body. Should these barriers be disrupted, this endogenous microflora provides the initial inoculum that may lead to infection.

The ability of bacteria to *adhere* to mammalian cells is a prerequisite to the development of local infection. Many different organisms possess the ability to bind to the host cell membrane, and this process generally requires interaction between microbial receptors for host cell membrane saccharide residues. This process allows microbes to remain and proliferate within the host milieu, a process that simultaneously triggers activation and recruitment of local, regional, and systemic host defenses. Microbial division occurs based upon the ability of a specific organism to utilize nutrients within the host tissues. Not infrequently, microorganisms exhibit specific mechanisms by which growth is enhanced, host defenses are diminished or nullified, or adverse effects are directly exerted upon the host. These mechanisms are termed microbial virulence factors and assume many different forms. Examples of these factors include the release from the bacterial cell wall or secretion into the host environment of highly deleterious compounds such as gram-negative bacterial lipopolysaccharide (endotoxin) or clostridial or staphylococcal exotoxins, inhibition of leukocyte phagocytosis by the capsule of many different gram-negative and gram-positive bacteria, secretion of compounds such as siderophores by bacteria and fungi that serve to bind and acquire iron (a critical nutrient for microbial growth in iron-poor environments), and microbial synergy (a process by which two or more organisms enhance the growth and toxicity of one another) that occurs between certain aerobes and anaerobes during polymicrobial infections. Causation of infection (i.e., *pathogenicity*) is a relative term that is highly dependent upon microbial virulence factors, the number of infecting organisms (initial *inoculum*), and the status of host defenses. Some organisms grow

rapidly and produce overwhelming infection in normal individuals (e.g., *Neisseria meningitidis, Clostridium perfringens*), while others are more likely to produce infection only when depression of host defenses exists (e.g., *Candida, Aspergillus* species). The impact of a particular type of microbe upon the host is highly dependent upon growth in a certain environment, activity in conjunction with other microbes, toxin production, and the potency of host defenses. Thus, microbial virulence and pathogenicity are relative terms that are, in fact, based upon many different situational variables.

Surgical patients possess many different types of defense mechanisms that prevent the development of infection. Without these mechanisms operant, even individuals not undergoing surgery would suffer from a continual series of serious infectious events. Surgical patients are unique in the sense that the surgeon often breaches host defenses to conduct the operation, and this predisposes the patient to infection. The body possesses many different types of defense against infection, and comparative zoologic studies indicate that these defenses have evolved over millions of years to act alone and in concert to prevent microbial invasion. The primary host defenses against infection are simple but extremely effective physical barriers that prevent entry of microbes into the sterile confines of the body. These consist of the epithelial and endothelial layers of the body (e.g., skin and mucous membranes of the respiratory, gastrointestinal, and genitourinary tracts). Ancillary host defenses also exist at these barrier sites that serve to maintain a balance so that the endogenous microflora do not proliferate excessively. Sebaceous gland secretion of fatty acids and skin desquamation maintain relatively constant numbers of skin microbes, while respiratory epithelial ciliary action and coughing serve to expel invading microbes of environmental or oropharyngeal origin. Bacterial–bacterial interactions, a limited number of enterocyte bacterial adhesion sites and enterocyte shedding, and gut peristalsis all act to prevent overgrowth of intestinal microbes. Anaerobic bacteria, in particular, act to prevent overgrowth and invasion of gram-negative aerobic pathogens, a phenomenon termed *colonization resistance*.

The microbes that do enter the sterile confines of the body encounter several different types of host defenses. Primarily, many different types of proteins exist that are capable of binding to invading microbes. Fibronectin and fibrinogen can bind to gram-positive bacterial cell walls, and the polymerization of fibrinogen to fibrin acts to trap and sequester large numbers of bacteria. Antibody (immunoglobulin [Ig]) is present at mucosal surfaces in the form of secretory IgA and within the bloodstream and extracellular tissue spaces as IgG and IgM. This natural antibody may exhibit binding activity directed against various types of bacteria, probably due to the presence of low-grade exposure to these microbes without the development of infection. Significant, repeated exposure to microbial antigens leads to secretion of large amounts of high-affinity IgG capable of binding to invading microbes and microbial toxins. Immunoglobulin acts in several ways to promote host survival, including: (1) microbial lysis, (2) enhancement of phagocytosis, and (3) microbial toxin neutralization.

Microbial lysis is accomplished when antibody of the IgM and certain IgG classes binds to and cleaves the Clqrs protein components of the classic pathway. The complement cascade is then triggered such that a sequential series of protein cleavage steps occurs, eventuating in the formation of a membrane attack complex (C6-9) that is deposited upon the microbial cell wall. This complex provokes membrane disruption and osmotic lysis. Many microbial cell wall products are capable of activating the alternate or properdin pathway of complement activation directly without the requirement for Ig binding. The classic and alternate pathways of complement activation both share the above-mentioned final common pathway leading to microbial lysis.

During complement activation, a series of cleavage steps takes place, the by-products of which are also important effectors of host defense. Cleavage of C3 produces C3b that acts as an opsonin for phagocytic cells, while C3a and C5a serve to markedly increase vascular permeability in the area of infection. C5a and C5b67 function as chemoattractants for phagocytic leukocytes (polymorphonuclear leukocytes [PMNs] and macrophages). These processes provoke the inflammatory response at the site of infection. An influx of extracellular fluid and cellular components then occurs, and serum proteins, including additional complement components, fibrinogen, albumin, and Ig, then enter the local tissue site. Although tissue macrophages act in an efficient manner to phagocytize and kill invading microbes, their number is finite and thus their activity in composite is limited. A large influx of PMNs can be observed, however, beginning 1.5 to 3 hours after the onset of infection. This is caused by the presence of chemotactic stimuli such as the above-mentioned complement components, but compounds in the bacterial cell wall such as N-formylated-methionine–containing peptides also act as chemoattractants. Macrophage metabolic activity does increase, however, in response to the presence of many different compounds in the microbial cell wall, Ig, and complement such that enhanced phagocytosis and killing of microbes occurs. Macrophage secretion of cytokines—such as tumor necrosis factor-α (TNF-α), interleukin-1β, (IL-1β), and interleukin-6 (IL-6)—may serve to increase the activity of other phagocytic cells within the local environment. Microbial growth is then pitted against containment in the form of microbial phagocytosis and killing, direct microbial lysis, and toxin neutralization. Lack of containment of infection at the local tissue level may lead to the occurrence of systemic infection with dissemination of infection to distant sites. Systemic host defenses consist of macrophages present in organs of the reticuloendothelial system (RES) (Kupffer cells in the liver, splenic and alveolar microphages), PMNs, monocytes, Ig, and complement within the systemic circulation. The outcome of these contravening processes is determined by the number and virulence of invading microbes versus the potency of local and systemic host defenses.

Certain regions of the body possess unique host defense mechanisms that act in conjunction with the aforementioned defenses. Both the pleural and the peritoneal cavities exhibit the ability to directly remove microbes via lymphatic clearance. In contradistinction, the subcutaneous tissue is unable to directly clear microbial pathogens. Within the peritoneal cavity, invading microbes are initially attacked by resident macrophages and removed by translymphatic absorption via diaphragmatic lymphatic structures. Stomata on the undersurface of the diaphragm lead to lacunae that, in turn, drain into larger lymphatic vessels within the thoracic cavity that empty into the thoracic duct. Bacteria injected into the peritoneal cavity reach the systemic circulation within a short period of time (5 to 10 minutes), and although this process may serve to remove bacteria from the normally sterile peritoneal cavity, large numbers of transported microbes may overwhelm systemic RES clearance mechanisms and provoke systemic sepsis. Even within the peritoneal cavity, however, other host defenses remain operant. Thus, an influx of PMNs occurs accompanied by an inflammatory fluid rich in fibrinogen, Ig, and complement facilitating phagocytosis accompanied by killing of microbes as well as microbial sequestration. This latter process is probably a rather primitive host defense mechanism and is associated with containment that leads to abscess formation and more chronic types of infection.

Clinical Recognition of Infection

The surgeon must be prepared to diagnose the occurrence of infections due to many different etiologies. Most surgical infections, however, center around those that occur at a site of trauma where physical host defense barriers have been breached and invading microbes have entered the body. This may be the result of an accident or a planned surgical procedure that entails an incision and entry into a body cavity. The presentation of infection may be subtle or blatant, and this depends on the above-mentioned factors concerning both the host and invading microbes. The most common presenting signs and symptoms of infection are due to the local inflammatory response to infection and consist of local edema and erythema surrounding the site of infection. The presence of purulent material is pathognomonic for the presence of bacterial and some fungal infections, although this may not occur in the setting of immunosuppression and severe leukopenia. Spread of infection in highly visible areas of the body is often associated with cellulitis and lymphangitis and evidence of systemic infection as denoted by fever and elevation of the white blood cell count (WBC). A differential demonstrates a predominance of PMNs, and these cells are found in great numbers at the site of local infection as well. More severe infections lead to the presence of systemic manifestations that are now grouped together as the *septic response* or *sepsis syndrome*. This process can be caused by many different types of microorganisms, although it has been best characterized for systemic sepsis due to gram-negative bacteremia. The manifestations of this syndrome consist of fever, elevated cardiac index, decreased systemic peripheral vascular resistance, and disordered substrate metabolism at the tissue and cellular levels in mild to moderate cases; and metabolic acidosis, hypoxemia, hypotension, single and sequential multiple organ failure (MOF), and death can occur in more severe cases. The sequence of MOF has been well characterized, and generally hepatic, renal, and pulmonary dysfunction and failure precede patient demise.

The severity of infection is determined by many different host and microbial factors. Although these factors are very difficult to characterize in a specific patient, their influence upon outcome has been precisely evaluated in experimental animal models of infection. These factors consist of: (1) status of host defenses (local and systemic), (2) type(s) and virulence of invading microorganism, and (3) inoculum size of invading microbes. Most breaches of host physical barriers are indeed associated with microbial invasion as a prelude to infection. However, infection rarely occurs in this setting in normal individuals because host defenses act to efficiently eradicate microorganisms. Extremely large numbers of a single type of microbe may provoke significant infection, and smaller numbers of several different microbial species that are able to act synergistically to promote their growth or smaller numbers of a single, highly virulent organism can produce serious infection. Extremely virulent infections also can occur due to low-virulence organisms in immunocompromised individuals, and in this patient population, infections due to highly virulent microbes are associated with high lethality rates.

BACTERIAL INFECTIONS

Diagnostic Microbiologic Tests

Once the presence of infection at a specific site is suspected, specimens of potentially infected material should be obtained for performance of Gram stain and bacterial and fungal culture. The purpose of these tests is to determine the types of microbial pathogens that have caused the infection, and this information serves to direct appropriate antimicrobial therapy. A Gram stain is performed by first drying the specimen on a microscope slide, staining with a basic vital dye (crystal violet) that is taken up by bacterial cell walls, following which, stain fixation with iodine-potassium-iodide solution and destaining with ethanol-acetone takes place. A second counterstain (safranin red) is then applied to the specimen, and microscopic observation is performed. Gram positive organisms such as *Staphylococcus* species possess a thick cell wall structure that resists destaining and therefore appear dark blue, while gram-negative microbes destain and are then counterstained red. This simple test can provide rapidly a great deal of information regarding the nature of the infection (i.e., whether it is monomicrobial or polymicrobial, gram-negative, gram-positive, or both). The presence of microbes upon 1000X magnification Gram stain analysis indicates that approximately 10^5 microbes per cubic millimeter were present in the specimen. Most surgical infections such as secondary bacterial peritonitis, necrotizing soft tissue infections, and many wound infections are polymicrobial in nature, and this is readily ascertained at the time of the procedure.

Culture analysis is available within 24 to 48 hours for most bacterial and some fungal organisms (*Candida* species), while many other fungi and acid-fast bacteria require much longer periods of time for growth. Detection of growth in initial culture samples assuredly depends on the size of the inoculum and growth characteristics of the microbial species present. Nonetheless, this information will not be available immediately, hence the necessity of empiric antimicrobial therapy for most surgical patients who develop serious infections. Once available, culture results can be used to more precisely direct antimicrobial therapy. Most modern clinical microbiology laboratories provide information about the specific types of microorganisms present at the site of infection and their sensitivity to a panel of different antimicrobial agents. This process is often largely automated and provides data regarding the minimal inhibitory concentration (MIC) of various antimicrobial agents required to prevent the growth of a particular microbe that has been isolated. This information is used to determine the relative resistance or sensitivity of that microbe to an antimicrobial agent based upon known, achievable serum levels of the antibiotic. Performance of quantitative cultures to determine the precise types and numbers of microbes may be indicated in the assessment of patients who have suffered severe burns, those with necrotizing soft tissue infections, and in those individuals with open surgical wounds in whom delayed primary closure is being considered, but is rarely indicated for most types of infections (e.g., subcutaneous or intra-abdominal abscesses). Unfortunately, precise measurement of the factors that determine the occurrence of infection (status of host defenses, initial inoculum, microbial virulence factors) are not readily quantifiable in the clinical setting. Reliance is therefore placed upon crude indicators that include the types of microorganisms present within the established infection, MICs of these organisms to various antimicrobial agents, and temporal observation of the clinical course of the patient during treatment.

Principles of Antibacterial Agent Therapy

Many different classes of antibacterial agents are currently available, and care must be taken in selecting among them to provide appropriate therapy. A number of issues should be considered when deciding whether to initiate therapy and what type(s) of agents to administer. Perhaps foremost, one should determine the optimal means to establish the diagnosis prior to instituting antimicrobial agent therapy. Because antimicrobial agents are frequently administered as empiric therapy to seriously ill surgical patients, blood, urine, sputum, or specimens at the site of local infection should be obtained for cultural analysis immediately prior to therapy. Although the majority of patients do well based upon a multimodality approach of surgical intervention and administration of antibiotics, culture and sensitivity results often prove invaluable in those individuals (10 to 20 per cent) who do not respond to the initial regimen. Second, the initial regimen should be selected to encompass a spectrum of activity directed against the pathogens most likely to be present. Concurrently, attempts to avoid the selection of toxic agents or extremely costly agents should be made, provided equally efficacious substitutes exist. Third, a finite course of antimicrobial agent therapy should be decided on based on the pathophysiology observed at the time of surgery. Prolonged courses of antibacterial agents should be avoided, and reassessment of the need for additional antimicrobial agent therapy should take place at the end of this interval and be based upon objective criteria such as ongoing fever (>100.5°F orally) or leukocytosis (WBC >10,000/mm³). Lastly, the antimicrobial agent regimen should not be drastically altered based solely on culture and sensitivity reports in a patient who is obviously responding well to therapy and who is re-

covering apace. Such changes should be reserved for those individuals who exhibit evidence of ongoing infection in whom a site of recurrent or a secondary site of local or systemic infection has been excluded, and who demonstrate organisms outside of the spectrum of the prescribed antimicrobial agent regimen upon analysis of initial or subsequent culture results (Table 1).

β-Lactam Agents

Four classes of β-lactam agents have been identified: penicillins, cephalosporins, monobactams, and carbapenems. The antibacterial activity of all of these agents is derived from the similarity of the β-lactam ring to the D-alanyl-D-alanine component of peptidoglycan that forms a significant structural component of both gram-negative and gram-positive bacterial cell walls. Binding to transpeptidation enzymes that synthesize peptidoglycan leads to inhibition of cell wall synthesis, cell elongation, and cell lysis. Penicillin G is the prototype compound, the basic chemical β-lactam ring structure being similar but not identical among all four classes of these agents. This compound exhibits in vitro activity primarily against gram-positive bacteria such as *Streptococcus* species, spirochetes, and a variety of other organisms. Semisynthetic penicillins (e.g., methicillin and nafcillin) exert activity against a wider variety of *Streptococcus* and *Staphylococcus* species. While ampicillin lacks extensive staphylococcal activity, activity against *Streptococcus fecalis* (enterococcus) and some gram-negative bacteria occurs. Carbenicillin and ticarcillin are both penicillin derivatives termed carboxypenicillins that exert activity against gram-negative aerobic bacteria. Acylampicillins (piperacillin, azlocillin, and mezlocillin) are ampicillin derivatives that possess a spectrum of activity

TABLE 1. STANDARD PRECEPTS OF SURGICAL ANTIMICROBIAL THERAPY

1. Establish the diagnosis by obtaining specimens of potentially infected material for:
   Gram stain
   Bacterial and fungal culture
2. Direct empiric therapy against those pathogens most likely to be present
3. Avoid toxic agents if less toxic and equally efficacious alternative agents exist
4. Avoid extremely expensive agents if less expensive and equally efficacious alternative agents exist
5. Decide upon the duration of therapy at the time of implementation
6. Reassess the need for ongoing therapy based upon:
   Overall clinical course of the patient
   Presence of fever (>100.5°F orally)
   Presence of leukocytosis (WBC >10,000 cells/mm³)
7. Do not alter antimicrobial agent therapy based solely upon culture results

that encompasses gram-negative facultative aerobes such as *E. coli* and *Pseudomonas aeruginosa*, as well as some anaerobes. Based on their being derived from ampicillin, these drugs also exhibit excellent activity against *S. fecalis*. The capacity of many gram-positive and some gram-negative bacteria to secrete β-lactamase enzymes is responsible for the lack of activity of some of these agents against these types of microorganisms. For that reason, ampicillin, ticarcillin, and piperacillin have been combined with β-lactamase inhibitors (clavulanate, sulbactam, or tazobactam). This serves to extend the spectrum of activity of these agents such that more effective gram-positive and gram-negative aerobic and potent anaerobic activity is concomitantly observed.

Three classes of cephalosporins have been described (first, second, and third). In general, first-generation cephalosporins exert excellent activity against gram-positive bacteria such as common strains of *S. aureus* (e.g., cephalothin and cefazolin). Staphylococcal strains that are resistant to methicillin, however, are almost invariably resistant to first-generation cephalosporins as well. These agents possess little gram-negative aerobic and no anaerobic activity. Second-generation cephalosporins (e.g., cefamandole) demonstrate slightly lessened gram-positive bacterial activity, but generally have much better gram-negative aerobic activity. Selected agents in this group possess good to excellent anaerobic activity (e.g., cefoxitin and cefotetan). Third-generation cephalosporins (e.g., cefotaxime, cefoperazone, ceftizoxime) exhibit variable degrees of gram-positive bacterial activity but generally represent excellent anti–gram-negative aerobic agents. In this category as well, selected agents can be demonstrated to have good to excellent anaerobic activity (e.g., moxalactam and ceftriaxone). Certain third-generation cephalosporins possess excellent activity against *P. aeruginosa* (e.g., ceftazidime).

Monobactams have a spectrum of activity directed against solely gram-negative aerobic bacteria. No activity against gram-positive bacteria or anaerobes has been observed. Aztreonam is the only agent currently available. Carbapenems are extremely broad-spectrum antibacterial agents that demonstrate activity against some gram-positive bacteria, most gram-negative aerobic isolates, including *P. aeruginosa*, and anaerobes. Imipenem is the only currently available carbapenem, and this drug was combined with cilistatin to prevent degradation by renal tubular epithelial enzymes. In vitro studies demonstrate that imipenem-cilistatin exhibits antianaerobic activity comparable to metronidazole and ticarcillin-clavulanate.

Aminoglycosides

Aminoglycosides exert considerable activity against gram-negative aerobic bacteria by interfering with bacterial protein synthesis and a second, poorly understood mechanism. Little activity against gram-positive or anaerobic microbes has been observed. A series of these agents has been isolated (gentamycin, tobramycin, amikacin, netilmicin, sisomicin), all of which possess considerable ototoxicity and nephrotoxicity. For that reason, many investigators believe that administration of these drugs should take place only under carefully controlled circumstances in which drug level and serum creatinine values are closely monitored. Because the activity of these agents is limited to gram-negative aerobic isolates, many suitable alternatives exist. Thus, therapy with third-generation cephalosporins, acylampicillins, monobactams, or quinolones can be considered in place of an aminoglycoside.

Glycopeptides

Vancomycin and teicoplanin are glycopeptide antibiotics that possess activity against gram-positive bacteria, more potent than that of most other agents. They interfere with gram-positive peptidoglycan cell wall synthesis at a different enzymatic step than penicillins. Their spectrum of activity includes both *S. fecalis* and methicillin-sensitive and -resistant *S. aureus* and *epidermidis*, as well as gram-positive anaerobic cocci. Although vancomycin-resistant gram-positive strains have been reported, they are extremely rare. This antibiotic may be given orally as an alternative to oral metronidazole for the treatment of antibiotic-induced *C. difficile* colitis.

Quinolones

Quinolones (nalidixic acid, norfloxacin, ciprofloxacin) are antibiotics that exert activity against gram-negative aerobic bacteria, based upon their ability to inhibit DNA gyrase. Some of these agents exhibit a slight degree of gram-positive activity (ciprofloxacin), and only selected agents that are not yet commercially released demonstrate anaerobic activity. Although most of the second- and third-generation cephalosporins are not available in an oral formulation, the contrary is true for the quinolones. Agents such as ciprofloxacin are available in both intravenous and oral formulation, both of which provide excellent serum levels after administration.

Other Agents

Erythromycin is a macrolide drug that has activity against gram-positive bacteria, and is often used to treat such infections in patients allergic to β-lactam agents. Clindamycin exhibits good activity against anaerobes and some gram-positive activity. Tetracyclines continue to represent good anaerobic agents, but their use in surgical patients has been largely superseded by more effective drugs. Similarly, chloramphenicol no longer represents a first-line drug for anaerobic infections, due to relatively high resistance rates. All of these drugs act to inhibit different aspects of bacterial ribosomal protein synthesis. Trimethoprim-sulfamethoxazole acts upon a variety of gram-negative aerobic bacteria and may represent the drug of choice for the occasional resistant gram-negative isolate (e.g., *Xanthomonas* species) as well as more unusual infections observed in immunosuppressed patients such as those caused by *Pneumocystis carinii* and *Nocardia asteroides*. This combination agent inhibits microbial synthesis by blocking two steps in folinic acid synthesis, a compound that is necessary for nucleic acid synthesis. Metronidazole provides excellent anaerobic activity, although no gram-positive or gram-negative aerobic activity is observed. Its mechanism of action has not been precisely defined.

Antibacterial Prophylaxis and the Epidemiology of Wound Infections

Although the surgical wound is typically considered to comprise the skin and subcutaneous tissue where the incision is made, this definition has proven to be rather limiting. Current thinking dictates that the surgical wound should encompass the entire operative field. The skin and subcutaneous tissue represents the superficial portion, while the body cavity that is entered (e.g., the peritoneum) comprises the deep surgical wound. Wound infections can thus be categorized as occurring at either location or both. Wound infections are caused by the presence of contaminating microbes that may be derived from the environment (operating surgeon and assistants, surgical instruments, lavage fluid, ambient environment) or the patient (autochthonous microflora). The development or absence of wound infection is based on the quantity and virulence of contaminating microbes and the ability of local wound host defenses to combat invasion. Related factors that predispose patients to the development of postoperative wound infections include debilitation (old age, inanition); immunodepression (diabetes, uremia, chemotherapeutic and immunosuppressive drugs); blood loss and prolonged operating time; and the presence of blood, necrotic tissue, foreign bodies, or hypoxia within the wound environment. Not infrequently, these types of infections are associated with significant morbidity and mortality, as the infection may not remain localized such that systemic sepsis occurs. Some wound infections may occur prior to or concurrent with necrotizing soft tissue infections and wound dehiscence as well. Because of the demonstra-

ble morbid nature of wound infections, a large amount of effort has been directed toward their prevention.

One of the most difficult problems concerning the prevention of wound infections is that it is impossible to predict their occurrence in a specific patient. Composite data, however, has been accumulated in studies involving large numbers of individuals, providing information concerning their potential risk of development. Surgical patients are currently categorized based upon the potential degree of contamination of the wound at the time of surgery into three classes (I, II, and III). Class I cases are termed *clean* and comprise those operations in which only skin microflora and/or exogenous microbes are likely to contaminate the wound. Examples of such surgical procedures include herniorrhaphy, thyroidectomy, and skin or subcutaneous tissue biopsies. Class II cases (*clean-contaminated*) consist of procedures such as elective colonic resection, complex biliary tract procedures, abdominal or vaginal hysterectomy, or oropharyngeal operations in which a hollow viscus or region of the body that contains an endogenous microflora is entered and also include procedures during which substantial breaks in sterile technique occur, either of which could introduce significant numbers of microorganisms into the operative field. Traumatic wounds without large amounts of contamination are also grouped in this category, particularly if a delay between wounding and medical attention occurs. Class III procedures (*contaminated*) constitute those in which a large amount of contamination assuredly is present (e.g., colectomy for an obstructing lesion of the colon with spillage of intestinal contents; traumatic, neglected wounds with substantial contamination; and surgical procedures performed for drainage of purulent, necrotic material). It is important to note that at the time of surgery, the actual degree of contamination cannot be ascertained nor can the specific contaminating microbes be determined. Thus, these classes represent guidelines that indicate the likelihood of the presence of contamination and, therefore, the probability of the development of wound infection. Class I, II, and III operative procedures are associated with wound infection rates of approximately 1 to 2 per cent, 3 to 7 per cent, and 8 to 35 per cent, respectively (Table 2).

Many studies have indicated that it is possible to minimize the occurrence of wound infections, all of which revolve around techniques to reduce the amount of wound contamination (Table 3). Surprisingly, airborne contamination of wounds from the environment contributes little to the pathogenesis of wound infections. This is because the modern-day operating room environment employs ventilation systems that limit exogenous microbial contamination, often via positive-pressure air exchange combined with fil-

TABLE 2. CLASSIFICATION OF SURGICAL WOUNDS WITH REGARD TO THE RISK OF DEVELOPMENT OF INFECTION

Class	Definition	Examples	Risk of Infection
I (Clean)	Operations involving skin microflora only without breaks in sterile operative technique	Herniorraphy, thyroidectomy	~1–2%
II (Clean-contaminated)	Region of body entered that may contain low numbers of endogenous microflora	Oropharyngeal procedures; vaginal or abdominal hysterectomy	~3–7%
	Region of body entered that normally contains large numbers of endogenous microflora that have been reduced in number	Elective colon resection after mechanical bowel preparation and administration of intraluminal antimicrobial agents	
	Minor breaks in sterile operative technique		
III (Contaminated)	Unprepared region of body entered that contains large numbers of endogenous microflora	Resection of obstructed, necrotic bowel	~8–35%
	Operation upon a grossly infected area of the body	Surgical drainage of intra-abdominal abscess	
	Traumatic, neglected wounds		
	Major breaks in sterile operative technique		

tration. With the exception of certain orthopedic procedures during which prosthetic joints are inserted, more sophisticated laminar airflow systems do not reduce the rate of wound infections for routine types of operations. Most infections, therefore, arise due to inoculation of the wound via endogenous microflora or due to often unavoidable and frequently unrecognized breaks in the sterile technique through which operating room personnel inadvertently contaminate the wound. Every attempt must be made to adhere to standardized sterile techniques in the operating room

TABLE 3. CAUSATIVE FACTORS OF AND TECHNIQUES THAT SERVE TO PREVENT WOUND INFECTION

Causative Factors	Prophylactic Measures
Exogenous microbial contamination	Avoid breaks in sterile surgical technique
	Wound infection surveillance
Endogenous microbial contamination	Preoperative antiseptic showers and scrubs
	Mechanical bowel preparation plus use of intraluminal antimicrobial agents
	Systemic antimicrobial agents
Skin shaving	Hair clipping
Tissue necrosis	Meticulous operative technique
Presence of foreign bodies	Wound irrigation, avoid excessive use of braided suture
Tissue hypoxia	Maintain adequate perfusion and oxygenation
Wound hematomas	Meticulous hemostasis
Blood loss and hypotension	Meticulous hemostasis, hemodynamic monitoring
Immunosuppression	Consider reduction in exogenous immunosuppression
Debilitation	Nutritional repletion in selected cases

that include the wearing of proper apparel (e.g., masks, head coverings), restricting traffic to only necessary personnel, and meticulous intraoperative technique to avoid the risk of exogenous contamination of the wound.

Several types of techniques are employed to reduce the impact of skin microflora. Avoidance of shaving the patient's skin hours in advance of, and probably even immediately prior to, the operative procedure diminishes the rate of wound infection. The severalfold increase in the rate of wound infections that has been observed when patients undergo prior shaving of the operative site is related to disruption of the normal epithelial barrier of the skin that facilitates subsequent overgrowth of skin microflora. This can be avoided by clipping of hair-bearing structures coupled with the use of antiseptic scrubbing of the area. One or two preoperative showers using an antiseptic agent plus direct application of such an agent to the planned site of incision also markedly reduces the number of skin microorganisms. These simple procedures followed by antiseptic scrubbing of the region of the planned incision in the operating room immediately prior to the time of incision and scrubbing of the surgeon's hands and lower arms reduce the rate of wound infection. Any one of a number of antiseptic agents can be used for these procedures. Most commonly, either povidone-iodine or chlorhexidine-containing preparations are employed to scrub the patient's skin for 5 to 7 minutes prior to placement of sterile drapes. Surgeons should scrub the hands and arms for 5 to 7 minutes initially on a given day of surgery and for at least 3 to 4 minutes prior to every subsequent case. Scrub suits should be changed, and a prolonged scrub similar to the initial one should be performed prior to any operation that follows a Class III type operation.

Reduction of the number of microbes in a hollow viscus that is entered to perform an operative procedure also reduces the incidence of wound infection. For example, the use of mechanical preparation of the large bowel to remove fecal contents plus oral ingestion of antimicrobial agents significantly reduces the rate of wound infection following elective colonic resection. Because the microflora of the large bowel consists of both aerobes and anaerobes, oral agents with activity directed against both types of organisms have been shown to be more effective than agents directed solely against one or the other. This form of prophylaxis serves to reduce the absolute numbers of microbes that contaminate the surgical wound, as evidenced by the results of several studies in which the precise number and types of microbes present within the bowel lumen at the time of resection could be correlated with the frequency of wound infection. Thus, combined administration of a regimen of oral antimicrobial agents that possess activity against aerobes and anaerobes reduces the quantity of these microbes within the gut lumen and reduces the frequency of wound infection. Currently, mechanical preparation of the bowel by ingestion of a nonabsorbable polyethylene glycol–containing lavage preparation is combined with administration of three doses each of oral erythromycin and neomycin. Although administration of a single dose of an intravenous antimicrobial agent is often added to this regimen, this has not been unequivocally demonstrated to further reduce wound infection rates.

Many initial clinical studies failed to demonstrate that intravenous antimicrobial agents reduce wound infection rates, an observation that can be attributed to inclusion of widely diverse groups of patients, some of whom received the agent hours prior to or during an operation rather than immediately prior to the procedure. Experimental studies, however, provided support for the contention that there was a "golden period" during which the effect of prophylactic antibiotics was maximized. This period occurred when antibiotics were administered before inoculation of experimental wounds with *S. aureus* and diminished when administration after inoculation took place. This effect occurs on the basis of microbial growth during the early stages of the development of infection, a process that is more readily controlled when bacterial numbers are small such that antimicrobial agents act in concert with host defenses as the latter are recruited to the site of microbial invasion. An identical effect was subsequently demonstrated in the clinical setting by the performance of well-designed clinical trials. Although in the vast majority of clinical cases, the actual bacterial inoculum size is not known, prophylactic antimicrobial agents must be administered immediately prior to the time of incision such that high serum and, thus, high wound tissue drug levels are present. Typically, this is readily accomplished by administering

the agent at the time of induction of anesthesia. Not surprisingly, neither additional postoperative doses of a prophylactic antimicrobial agent nor institution of antimicrobial agent therapy (should prophylaxis be neglected) serve to reduce the rate of wound infection.

The administration of prophylactic systemic antimicrobial agents has been demonstrated to reduce the frequency with which wound infections occur after clean-contaminated and some contaminated types of operations. This has been best demonstrated for operations performed for penetrating gastrointestinal trauma, various types of hysterectomy, and gangrenous or perforated appendicitis. These agents should be administered immediately prior to all Class II and Class III procedures. Their efficacy in most types of clean surgery (Class I) remains controversial, primarily due to low rates of wound infections in this group of patients (~1 to 2 per cent) and has not been unequivocally demonstrated. Patients undergoing clean surgery during which prosthetic material is inserted (vascular prosthetic graft, cardiac valve replacement, joint prosthesis) represent a subgroup of individuals in whom prophylaxis should be administered because even superficial wound infections frequently are associated with concurrent prosthetic device infection. Should the latter event occur, removal of the prosthetic material is often necessary. Controversy also exists concerning the type of prophylactic antimicrobial agent to administer for different types of procedures. The problem concerns the inability to precisely ascertain whether or not a particular patient will develop an infection based upon the inability to quantitate host defenses and to define whether or not a significant bacterial inoculum is present in the wound at the time of surgery. In addition, several types of endogenous microflora derived from either epithelial sites, endothelial sites, or both can contribute to the initial inoculum. In general, an antimicrobial agent directed against the microflora most likely to be present should be administered. Thus, if a decision is made to administer a prophylactic antimicrobial agent prior to clean surgery, a single dose of a first-generation cephalosporin with excellent antistaphylococcal activity would be appropriate. This might occur in certain groups of patients that are suspected to be at higher risk for the development of wound infection, such as immunosuppressed, diabetic, and elderly individuals undergoing Class I surgical procedures, although this remains unsubstantiated. Should prosthetic material be inserted, use of either a first-generation cephalosporin or vancomycin is indicated.

Patients undergoing clean-contaminated procedures in whom endogenous microflora may contaminate the wound may benefit from the prophylactic administration of an agent directed against those microbes. For example, prior to elective colonic resection or exploration for suspected penetrating gastrointestinal trauma or perforation, administration of an antibiotic that exhibits activity against both aerobes and anaerobes would be appropriate. Selected second-generation cephalosporins and certain penicillin derivatives combined with a β-lactamase inhibitor are suitable for this purpose and are relatively inexpensive. These agents possess satisfactory antistaphylococcal activity to concurrently prevent those wound infections that may occur on the basis of skin microflora contamination without the need to add a second agent. Topical antibiotics (e.g., a first-generation cephalosporin) can be placed in solution and used to lavage the surgical wound during the operation and are sometimes placed in the form of powder into the superficial wound immediately prior to closure. Although this form of prophylaxis is conceptually sound, inexpensive, and carries little risk, it has not been demonstrated to provide added benefit when combined with the use of systemic antimicrobial agent prophylaxis.

Patients undergoing contaminated operations (Class III) should also receive intravenous antimicrobial agents. With these patients, however, consideration should be given to avoidance of wound infection via the techniques of delayed primary wound closure or healing of the wound by secondary intention. Delayed primary wound closure is accomplished by leaving the skin and subcutaneous portions of the wound open and packed with gauze. An antibiotic-containing solution can be used to impregnate the dressing if the surgeon desires, although povidone-iodine–containing solutions probably should not be used because they may inhibit fibroblast ingrowth and wound healing. Skin approximation sutures may be placed at the time of initial operation and left untied, or they may be placed at the time of delayed primary closure. Adhesive dressings also may serve to facilitate skin closure, obviating the need for suture closure, particularly in shallow wounds. Prior to closure, the wound should remain undisturbed for approximately 5 days unless fever or evidence of erythema or purulence develops. Should this occur during the intervening period of time, the wound should be examined immediately. If the wound exhibits granulation tissue and no evidence of purulence or erythema on the fifth postoperative day, closure can be accomplished. Quantitative cultures also can be used to determine whether wound closure can be undertaken. If a wound tissue biopsy reveals more than 10^5 microbes per gram of tissue, delayed primary closure should not be performed because the risk of wound infection remains high. Unfortunately, the 24- to 48-hour period and the expense of performing quantitative cultures has led to limited use in the clinical setting. It should be noted, however, that although the use of the technique of delayed primary closure appears to reduce the rate of wound in-

fection, late wound infections can still occur and patients should be monitored closely for the development of this process.

Heavily infected wounds should not be closed but should be allowed to heal by secondary intention, a process in which granulation tissue fills in the wound space and epithelialization occurs over a period of weeks to months, depending on the size and depth of the open area of the wound. Although this process leaves a wound that is often not cosmetically optimal, the occurrence of a wound infection following a contaminated procedure in which the wound is closed can be associated with an even less desirable cosmetic appearance, and the potential morbid sequelae of more prolonged wound management and hospitalization, wound dehiscence, necrotizing fasciitis, and systemic sepsis. A variety of intriguing techniques have been promulgated to reduce the rate of wound infection after closure of contaminated wounds. These include the use of application of antibiotic powder into the wound prior to closure, closed suction irrigation systems using an irrigant containing an antimicrobial agent, and administration of systemic antimicrobial agents. However, when their efficacy has been tested in controlled trials with rigorous wound infection surveillance, none of these techniques has been demonstrated to reduce the rate of infection in contaminated wounds that are closed. Heavily contaminated traumatic wounds often require débridement of necrotic tissue and removal of foreign bodies, and patients should also receive tetanus toxoid vaccination if they have not been vaccinated for more than 10 years. Patients who have never been vaccinated should receive tetanus immune globulin and vaccination at separate injection sites to prevent the development of tetanus caused by toxin secretion by *C. tetani*, a common soil microorganism. Two additional vaccinations should subsequently be administered.

Surveillance of wound infections has been demonstrated to be an effective means of reducing infection rates. Several studies have shown that observation of the problem itself serves to alter clinical practice so that wound infections occur less frequently. Although surgeons are capable of observing the incidence of wound infection, an independent, unbiased observer such as a nurse clinician trained in this area with the capacity to declare whether or not a wound infection has occurred provides the best surveillance system. Because only 30 to 50 per cent of wound infections occur during hospitalization, an effective surveillance program also must include postoperative observation of events for at least 60 to 90 days in the outpatient setting, either via clinic follow-up visits, phone calls, or electronic or written correspondence with patients and referring physicians. Without such measures, wound infection rates are invariably underreported, and surgeons assume that wound infections have not occurred.

The surgeon is often asked to perform noncardiac procedures in patients with valvular heart disease or prosthetic heart valves. When such patients undergo routine dental and upper respiratory procedures they should receive oral amoxicillin, or oral erythromycin if they are allergic to penicillin agents. Prophylaxis in those patients who undergo clean surgery can be accomplished by intravenous administration of ampicillin, although use of semisynthetic penicillins (e.g., nafcillin) or a first-generation cephalosporin may be more appropriate in light of the skin flora that would provide the infecting inoculum. It should be noted, however, that it is not entirely clear that such procedures provoke transient bacteremia. Oropharyngeal manipulation during intubation for the purpose of general anesthesia is a sufficient reason to administer such prophylaxis. Procedures involving the gastrointestinal and urogenital tracts have a higher probability of involving *S. fecalis*. Patients undergoing these types of operations should receive ampicillin plus an aminoglycoside as prophylaxis. Although anaerobic endocarditis is rare, common sense would dictate the addition of an antianaerobic agent (clindamycin or metronidazole, or replacing ampicillin with an acylampicillin) to this regimen to achieve appropriate wound infection prophylaxis as well. Patients allergic to penicillin should receive vancomycin in place of the β-lactam component of this type of prophylactic regimen.

Treatment of Bacterial Infection

The primary modality by which surgical infections are treated is via removal of infected, necrotic tissue and drainage of purulent material. This form of therapy is termed *source control* and must assume precedence over all other forms of therapy. Without effective eradication of the source of infection, antimicrobial agents generally exert limited efficacy. Appropriate care of the infected surgical patient also includes fluid resuscitation, hemodynamic monitoring and support, nutritional repletion, and administration of antimicrobial agents directed against causative pathogens. With the advent of large numbers of readily available antimicrobial agents, appropriate antimicrobial agent therapy has become exceedingly complex.

Intra-abdominal Infections

Infections that occur within the confines of the abdominal cavity are categorized as primary, secondary, or tertiary peritonitis (Table 4). Primary peritonitis represents infection within the confines of the peritoneal cavity that does not involve perforation of a hol-

TABLE 4. CLASSIFICATION OF MICROBIAL PERITONITIS

Class	Definition	Pathogens
Primary	No viscus perforation Increased frequency in patients with increased amounts of peritoneal fluid (cirrhosis with ascites, peritoneal dialysis)	Monomicrobial Gram-negative or gram-positive bacteria, or fungi
Secondary	Viscus perforation Endogenous microflora provide initial inoculum	Polymicrobial Gram-negative aerobes and anaerobes Gram-positive aerobes and anaerobes
Tertiary	Prior viscus perforation and secondary microbial peritonitis Normally low-virulence or highly resistant microbes (probably those selected out by initial treatment regimen)	Polymicrobial *Staphylococcus epidermidis* *Candida albicans* *Pseudomonas aeruginosa*

low viscus. This process can occur in patients who develop ascites or who are undergoing peritoneal dialysis. Presumably, direct or hematogenous contamination of microbial pathogens occurs and leads to infection within the normally sterile peritoneal fluid. This type of peritonitis is caused by a single type of microorganism. Gram-negative bacteria such as *E. coli* and gram-positive microbes such as *Streptococcus* and *Staphylococcus* species are causative agents of this disease process.

Secondary bacterial peritonitis occurs subsequent to perforation of a hollow viscus within the peritoneal cavity. In virtually all cases, the initial inoculum is polymicrobial, being derived from the endogenous microflora present within the organ that is disrupted. Subsequently, the growth of certain microbes occurs and is counteracted by local and recruited peritoneal host defenses. An initial stage of fibrinopurulent peritonitis occurs after which time survival is associated with complete resolution of infection in some individuals, while abscess formation and chronic sepsis occur in others.

Secondary bacterial peritonitis is a polymicrobial infection, most studies indicating that an average of four to five organisms can be isolated from the established infection, with a slight preponderance of anaerobes being present. Organisms such as *Bacteroides fragilis* and other *Bacteroides* species (*B. distasonis, B. thetaiotaomicron, B. melaninogenicus*), *Eubacteria* species, and *Peptostreptococcus* and *Peptidostreptococcus* species are the most common anaerobic isolates, while *E. coli, Enterobacter* and *Klebsiella* species, *S. fecalis,* and other aerobes are frequently cultured as well. Interestingly, these bacteria represent only a small fraction of the various types of microbes that constitute the initial inoculum, a simplification process that is incompletely understood. Synergistic interactions among aerobes and anaerobes have been demonstrated in experimental animal models of secondary bacterial peritonitis and probably occur clinically as well.

Despite appropriate surgical intervention and antimicrobial agent therapy, approximately 10 to 15 per cent of patients who suffer secondary bacterial peritonitis may develop some type of recurrent intra-abdominal sepsis. An intra-abdominal abscess may develop in some individuals, producing fever, abdominal pain, and systemic sepsis due to bacteremia. Ultrasonographic or computerized tomographic radiographic studies should be obtained if this diagnosis is suspected. Use of these modalities is associated with a greater than 95 per cent diagnostic accuracy rate, and percutaneous sampling of potentially infected fluid collections can take place (Fig. 1). Should evidence of infection be present (purulent material aspirated or positive Gram stain), percutaneous drainage in which a drainage catheter is inserted via ultrasonic or computerized tomographic visualization is very effective therapy in more than 90 per cent of cases. Failure of percutaneous drainage catheter therapy is associated with the following factors: (1) unrecognized abscesses, (2) incomplete abscess drainage of complex, multiloculated collection, (3) fungal abscesses, (4) pancreatic abscesses, and (5) communication with a hollow viscus such that ongoing contamination occurs. Lack of clinical improvement after percutaneous drainage of an intra-abdominal abscess mandates that surgical exploration be considered.

A small number of patients who survive the initial episode of secondary bacterial peritonitis may develop recurrent infection without abscess formation, leading to a more indolent, chronic form of disease that is termed tertiary peritonitis. Patients who develop this disease process are unable to sequester infection within the peritoneal cavity and do not form abscesses. This process is associated with the presence of normally low-virulence microorganisms such as *S. epidermidis* and *C. albicans* that are probably selected out on the basis of their being insensitive to those agents used to treat secondary bacterial peritonitis. Gram-negative aerobic bacteria such as *P. aeruginosa* that are highly resistant to many different antibiotics may be cultured at this juncture as well.

Antibacterial agent treatment of primary bacterial peritonitis should be based on initial Gram stain and subsequent culture and sensitivity reports. In most patients, therapy with one agent is sufficient. Cure may require removal of prosthetic material (e.g., a peritoneal dialysis catheter), although this is probably dependent upon the severity of the infection. In contradistinction, antibiotic therapy of secondary bacterial

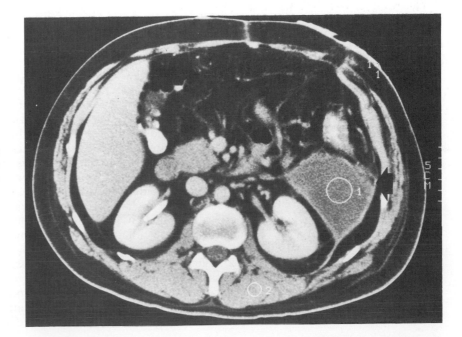

Figure 1. Computerized tomographic scan of the abdomen demonstrating the presence of an intra-abdominal abscess.

peritonitis is based on the knowledge that aerobic gram-negative bacilli and anaerobic microbes will be present in the vast majority of patients. Therapy is, therefore, empiric and should be altered only to a limited degree based on initial Gram stain results and subsequently after culture and sensitivity reports are available. The antimicrobial agent component of the treatment of secondary bacterial peritonitis has undergone considerable evolution over the past decade. Clinical trials have been performed in three groups of patients that consist of those who have developed (1) gangrenous or perforated appendicitis, (2) penetrating abdominal trauma involving perforation of the gastrointestinal tract, and (3) established secondary bacterial peritonitis. Recommendations based upon these studies can be extended to all patients who develop secondary bacterial peritonitis and are twofold: (1) it is necessary to direct antimicrobial agent therapy against both the aerobic and anaerobic components of the infection, and (2) this can be accomplished with similar efficacy using a variety of dual- or single-agent regimens.

Dual-agent regimens typically consist of the administration of either clindamycin or metronidazole as an anaerobic agent with any one of a number of aminoglycosides, all of which possess efficacy against gram-negative aerobes. This type of regimen has become the standard regimen to which other regimens must be compared. Ampicillin is often added to such a regimen to treat *S. fecalis*, and although support for this concept has been generated in experimental models, it remains to be proven in clinical trials. Because the use of aminoglycosides is associated with nephrotoxicity and the need for monitoring of drug levels, substitution of either an acylampicillin, a second- or third-generation cephalosporin, or a monobactam in place of the aminoglycoside portion of the regimen can be considered, especially in those individuals who exhibit renal dysfunction. Because of the weak gram-positive activity of these latter two groups of agents, they should be used only with clindamycin and not metronidazole. A number of single agents possess a spectrum of activity directed against both aerobes and anaerobes and provide similar efficacy for the treatment of secondary bacterial peritonitis. Selected second- or third-generation cephalosporins with anaerobic activity, acylampicillins, or drugs that combine either ampicillin or ticarcillin with a β-lactamase inhibitor such as clavulanate or sulbactam can be used for mild to moderate disease in normal patients who have not been previously hospitalized, while a carbapenem agent should be used in patients who acquire disease in the hospital setting, particularly those who are immunosuppressed or who exhibit renal dysfunction (Table 5). Treatment of tertiary peritonitis requires administration of antimicrobial agents directed against

TABLE 5. SELECTION OF ANTIMICROBIAL AGENTS FOR THE TREATMENT OF SECONDARY BACTERIAL PERITONITIS*

Mild to moderate intra-abdominal infection
1. Second- or third-generation cephalosporin with antianaerobic activity
   or
2. Ampicillin or ticarcillin + β-lactamase inhibitor
   or
3. Monobactam + clindamycin ± ampicillin
   or
4. Second- or third-generation cephalosporin + clindamycin or metronidazole

Severe intra-abdominal infection without renal dysfunction†
1. Carbapenem
   or
2. Aminoglycoside + clindamycin or metronidazole ± ampicillin

Severe intra-abdominal infection with renal dysfunction†
1. Carbapenem
   or
2. Monobactam + clindamycin ± ampicillin
   or
3. Second- or third-generation cephalosporin + clindamycin or metronidazole

*Adapted from Sawyer MD, Dunn DL: Antimicrobial therapy of intra-abdominal sepsis. Infect Dis Clin North Am 6:545–570, 1992, with permission.
†Includes mild to moderate peritonitis in immunosuppressed patients and hospital-acquired peritonitis in otherwise normal patients.

identified pathogens. Often, this requires the use of vancomycin and amphotericin B. Repeated surgical exploration may be helpful in patients with this disease process and probably in those individuals who develop secondary bacterial peritonitis with high degrees of contamination. Repeated laparotomy, open packing of the abdomen, and use of mesh closure with or without a zipper to facilitate reexploration may assist in the care of these patients, but have not been demonstrated unequivocally to be efficacious.

Skin and Soft-Tissue Infections

Infections of the skin, subcutaneous tissue, and underlying fascia not infrequently require surgical intervention. Cellulitis is often caused by the introduction of gram-positive bacteria such as *Streptococcus* or *Staphylococcus* species into the superficial skin structures and is denoted by the presence of erythema without purulence, although subcutaneous abscesses also can form. Treatment consists of administration of a first-generation cephalosporin, a semisynthetic penicillin, or vancomycin, coupled with surgical incision and drainage if an abscess is present. Most simple subcutaneous abscesses resolve solely with surgical drainage. More serious, necrotizing soft-tissue infections occur sporadically and require prompt surgical intervention and administration of antimicrobial agents. Two factors usually are necessary for the development of these severe infections: (1) a debilitated host (diabetic, elderly, debilitated, immunosuppressed individuals), and (2) the introduction of one or more virulent organisms into the soft tissue. These infections, however, do occur occasionally in normal individuals. Although *C. perfringens C. welchii, C. novyi,* and *C. septicum* can cause severe, necrotizing soft-tissue infections (clostridial myonecrosis, gas gangrene), this remains a relatively rare cause of the disease process. More commonly, several organisms acting in concert produce a polymicrobial, synergistic infection that spreads rapidly within the soft tissue. Typically, these consist of a facultative *Streptococcus* and a gram-negative aerobic rod, although strict anaerobes can also participate. Highly virulent gram-negative aerobes such as *P. aeruginosa* and certain *Streptococcus* species such as *S. pyogenes* can cause monomicrobial infections of this type as well.

These infections are often difficult to diagnose, because the disease process extends in the deep soft tissues of the trunk or extremity without causing extensive external skin changes. Eventually, however, the skin in the affected region develops a bronze hue, blebs may form, and crepitus in the soft tissue can be detected due to gas-forming organisms (a process by no means unique to clostridial infection). Hypesthesia of the involved area, disorientation of the patient, or sudden shock may be the only overt initial clinical signs of the disease process. Fulminant disease with rapid extension of infection to uninvolved areas is common, such that this type of infectious disease constitutes a surgical emergency. Should skin changes not occur and crepitus be undetectable, computerized tomography may assist in establishing the diagnosis, although this test should not be obtained if it causes undue delay in establishing the diagnosis and instituting treatment (Fig. 2). Limited exploration of the suspected region can take place in the intensive care unit or operating room to determine whether or not infection is present. Incision through the skin typically exposes necrotic soft tissue, fascia, and occasionally myonecrosis, as well as a thin, grayish exudate rather than true pus. A Gram stain often reveals the presence of numerous organisms, and specimens for culture of aerobes, anaerobes, and fungi should be obtained. Treatment consists of excision of infected, necrotic tissue (frequently involving amputation of an extremity) and administration of antimicrobial agents directed against gram-negative, gram-positive, and anaerobic bacteria. A regimen of vancomycin, plus either a third-generation cephalosporin, a monobactam, or an aminoglycoside agent, plus clindamycin or metronidazole should be administered, and high-dose penicillin G should be given until clostridial infection has been excluded. In addition, repeated débridement should take place on a daily basis to ensure control over the infection. Hyperbaric oxygen therapy has not been demonstrated to be of added benefit to the above regimen. The mortality of this disease process is greater than 50 per cent even after prompt diagnosis and therapy.

Nosocomial Infections and Systemic Sepsis

Infections that occur in the hospital environment are termed *nosocomial infections.* These infections are common in all patients, including those individuals undergoing surgical procedures. Common types of nosocomial infections include urinary tract infection, pneumonia, wound infections, and septicemia. This latter process is defined as the presence of microorganisms (bacteria or fungi) in the systemic circulation due to lack of containment of infection at the local tissue site of infection and is associated with high lethality rates. Although it can occur without a specific site of infection being identified, the above-mentioned local sites represent common sources, and indwelling intravenous catheters are etiologic as well. Indwelling devices such as urinary and arterial or venous access catheters as well as endotracheal tubes should be expeditiously removed to prevent the development of these types of infections. Although septicemia can occur without significant sequelae, in many patients it is associated with the occurrence of sepsis syndrome and appears to be most pronounced during gram-negative bacteremic events. It should be noted, however, that inflammation caused by disease processes such as severe pancreatitis can also produce similar findings. Sepsis syndrome is associated with a mortality rate of approximately 40 per cent, independent of the etiologic microorganism. Several studies have indicated that gram-negative bacterial sepsis is associated with a 10 to 20 per cent mortality rate in normal individuals, while a greater than 50 per cent lethality may occur in immunocompromised patients. Polymicrobial septicemia due to several types of bacteria or gram-negative bacteria plus *Candida* species may lead to greater than 70 per cent mortality. Unfortunately, the lethality of this disease process has not significantly changed over the last decade despite judicious use of antimicrobial agents, intensive care, and metabolic support.

Current evidence indicates that the host response to infection plays a major role with regard to outcome. Invading microbes trigger the release of a variety of secondary host mediators, such as the macrophage cytokines, leukotrienes, platelet activating factor, and release of leukocyte lysosomal enzymes. Many of these substances have been demonstrated to exert deleterious effects upon the host. In particular, bacterial cell wall compounds such as gram-negative bacterial endotoxin cause an enormous surge in the synthesis and secretion of macrophage cytokines such as TNF-α, fol-

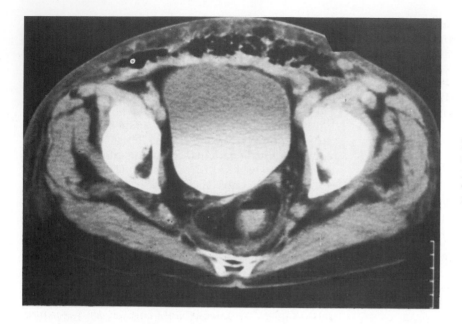

Figure 2. Computerized tomographic scan of the abdomen demonstrating the presence of gas within the rectus muscle compartments compatible with necrotizing fasciitis.

lowing which IL-1β, and then IL-6 and IL-8 are released. This process is termed the *cytokine cascade*, as it appears to be similar to other biologic processes that involve a series of effector molecules. In experimental animal models of infection and in humans, release of TNF-α occurs 1.5 to 2 hours after endotoxin injection. Administration of TNF-α itself reproduces almost all of the effects observed after endotoxin injection, and anti–TNF-α antibody administration provides protective capacity against a lethal challenge of either endotoxin or gram-negative bacteria.

Current antimicrobial therapy for the septic patient is dictated by the organisms most likely to be encountered at the site of infection. Thus, most surgical patients should receive therapy directed against gram-negative and gram-positive aerobes as well as anaerobes until culture results become available. The local site of infection should be actively sought, and local infection must be eradicated. Because neutropenic patients who develop gram-negative bacterial sepsis benefit from the use of two antimicrobial agents directed against the specific pathogen, two agents also are often used in normal individuals because of the high mortality of this disease process. Clinical trials are underway to assess the efficacy of administration of monoclonal antibodies directed against endotoxin or TNF-α during severe sepsis. The utility of IL-1 receptor antagonist that blocks the activity of IL-1β, and combination therapy using several of these new reagents together, is being examined also. It is important to note that these agents are used in conjunction with other standard forms of therapy.

FUNGAL INFECTIONS

Candida albicans and various other *Candida* species (*C. glabrata, C. parapsilosis, C. kruesii, C. tropicalis*) are capable of causing both local and disseminated infection in hospitalized surgical patients. Overgrowth of *Candida* occurs at mucocutaneous surfaces and in the intestinal tract of immunocompromised and diabetic patients and in individuals receiving broad-spectrum antibacterial agent therapy, particularly of long duration. Although the use of oral, nonabsorbable antifungal agents such as nystatin reduces such colonization, fungemic episodes can still occur. As an inhabitant of the lower small intestine and colon, *Candida* species are not infrequently isolated from samples obtained at the time of laparotomy during which a perforated viscus is discovered. Retrospective studies indicate that increased survival is associated with treatment using amphotericin B during either fungemia or peritonitis caused by *Candida*, although this hypothesis has not been strictly tested in the confines of a randomized trial. In general, patients should receive 350 to 500 mg amphotericin B for the treatment of such disease processes, and because most of these infections are polymicrobial, concurrent antibacterial therapy should be administered. Some data suggest that the addition of a second antifungal agent such as 5–fluorocytosine (5–FC) may be of benefit. The use of new triazole antifungal agents such as fluconazole or itraconazole may provide similar benefit in this setting. These agents are less potent and less nephrotoxic compared to amphotericin B, and fluconazole is not active against certain types of *Candida* such as *C. kruesii*. The surgeon may also be called upon to treat aggressive skin, pulmonary, or cerebral disease caused by other fungal pathogens such as *Aspergillus, Mucor,* or *Rhizopus* species. Extirpative therapy is warranted in virtually all patients if it is anatomically feasible, and because of the aggressive nature of these infections, a prolonged course of amphotericin B often combined with 5–FC and rifampin should be administered to prevent recurrence. In addition, solid-organ transplant patients should undergo a concurrent reduction in immunosuppressive therapy.

VIRAL INFECTIONS

Surgeons commonly encounter significant infections caused by viral pathogens in immunocompromised patients. The most common types of viral infections are those caused by viruses belonging to the *Herpesviridae* group. These include herpes simplex virus (HSV) types I and II, cytomegalovirus (CMV), Epstein-Barr virus (EBV), herpes virus type 6, and varicella-zoster virus. HSV can cause severe mucosal ulceration, and occasional cases of severe pneumonitis, hepatitis, encephalitis, or widespread dissemination have been reported. The nucleoside analog acyclovir should be used to treat HSV infection. Disease caused by CMV infection is associated with substantial morbidity and mortality after solid organ and bone marrow transplantation, and patients can develop protean manifestations. These can be grouped according to severity: (1) mild manifestations consist of fever, malaise, and leukopenia; (2) moderate manifestations include pneumonitis and hypoxemia, abdominal pain, or retinitis; and (3) severe CMV disease may consist of hypotension, severe pulmonary infection requiring ventilatory support, massive upper or lower gastrointestinal bleeding due to CMV intestinal ulceration, hepatitis, pancreatitis, MOF, and death. The occurrence of serious tissue-invasive CMV disease is increased by a CMV-seronegative recipient receiving tissue from a donor who is CMV-seropositive and the use of large amounts of immunosuppressive drugs. A reduction in the incidence of CMV disease has been accomplished by use of prophylactic, long-term administration of acyclovir or immune globulin with activity against CMV. Treatment of disease requires the use of antiviral agents with a greater degree of efficacy against CMV such as ganciclovir or foscarnet. EBV infections are of interest because they cause a spectrum of disease ranging from a self-limited mononucleosis-type syndrome, to polyclonal and aggressive monoclonal B cell lymphomas in immunocompromised patients. Treatment of acute EBV infection requires use of acyclovir, while investigational studies using α-interferon or chemotherapy to treat EBV-induced lymphomas are currently being conducted.

At least four different types of hepatitis viruses (A, B, C, and δ) have been identified, and two (B and C) are of considerable importance to the surgeon because of the occupational exposure risk that they represent. Hepatitis B virus (HBV) is a hepatotrophic pathogen that can cause disease ranging from asymptomatic mild liver dysfunction, to acute, fulminant hepatic necrosis. Parenteral transmission is most common, and immunologic and liver function tests serve to establish the diagnosis. Initially, IgM directed against surface and core antigens (HBsAg and HBcAg, respectively) is observed, during which time elevation of hepatic enzymes and liver dysfunction occurs. HBV surface antigenemia followed by identification of IgG directed against HBsAg, HBcAg, or both, then takes place. A small number of patients develop fulminant hepatic necrosis, coma, and death, often due to certain types of HBV (HBeAg), while a slightly larger number may shed HBsAg chronically and without symptoms or demonstrate evidence of chronic persistent or chronic active hepatitis. These latter groups of patients are all highly infectious and generally should not be allowed to donate blood or tissue. Prophylaxis against HBV is extremely effective and consists of three separate immunizations with a recombinant vaccine that provokes a protective IgG response directed against HBsAg. All surgeons should receive this vaccine. Nonimmune individuals who are exposed to HBV should receive HBV immune globulin and undergo vaccination.

Hepatitis C virus (HCV) was formerly termed non-A, non-B hepatitis due to the lack of a diagnostic test for this pathogen. Use of a recombinant form of viral antigens in a diagnostic test has facilitated the detection of endogenous antibody directed against this virus. HCV probably is the most common cause of transfusion-associated hepatitis, and it is likely that the impact of this disease process will be diminished by careful screening and exclusion of HCV-positive donors. Unfortunately, the available tests are imperfect, and precise determination of the presence of infection requires use of tests to detect the presence of HCV nucleic acid (e.g., recombinant immunoblot assay, polymerase chain reaction). Several different retroviruses, including human immunodeficiency virus types 1 and 2 (HIV-1, HIV-2) have been identified and appear to be causative agents of the acquired immunodeficiency syndrome (AIDS). Although treatment of patients suffering from AIDS with azidothymidine (AZT) and other agents has been studied, mortality rates remain extremely high. Transmission of these viral agents is of considerable concern, and a variety of barrier devices are being developed to reduce contact of personnel with blood and other body fluids in the operating room environment. Currently, there are no vaccines available for either HCV or HIV.

REFERENCES

Burd RS, Cody CS, Dunn DL: Immunotherapy of Gram-Negative Bacterial Sepsis. Medical Intelligence Unit. Austin, TX, RG Landes Company, 1992.

Dunn DL, Barke RA, Knight NB, Humphrey EW, Simmons RL: Role of resident macrophages, peripheral neutrophils, and trans-lymphatic absorption in bacterial clearance from the peritoneal cavity. Infect Immun 49:257–264, 1985.

Dunn DL, Mayoral JL, Gillingham KJ, Loeffler CM, Brayman KL, Kramer MA, Erice A, Balfour HH, Fletcher CV, Bolman RM III, Matas AJ, Payne WD, Sutherland DER, Najarian JS: Treatment of invasive cytomegalovirus disease in solid organ transplant patients with ganciclovir. Transplantation 51:98–106, 1991.

Dunn DL, Sawyer MD: Deep soft tissue infections. Curr Opinion Infect Dis 3:691–696, 1990.

Dunn DL, Simmons RL: The role of anaerobic bacteria in intra-abdominal infections. Rev Infect Dis 6(suppl 1):S139–146, 1984.

Sawyer MD, Dunn DL: Antimicrobial therapy of intra-abdominal sepsis. Infect Dis Clin North Am 6:545–570, 1992.

14
SURGICAL ASPECTS OF THE ACQUIRED IMMUNODEFICIENCY SYNDROME

J. MICHAEL DiMAIO, M.D.   H. KIM LYERLY, M.D.

Although the acquired immunodeficiency syndrome (AIDS) was not recognized as a clinical entity until 1981, the human immunodeficiency virus type 1 (HIV-1) has reportedly been transmitted by sexual and parental routes to more than 12 million people in the world. The end-stage manifestation of infection with a human retrovirus, HIV-1, is characterized by defects in cellular immunity leading to opportunistic infections and unusual neoplasms, and is termed AIDS. While HIV-1 infection has been treated primarily by antiretroviral therapy, the surgical therapy of specific complications is a prominent feature of the clinical management of this infection, and surgical procedures in infected patients are increasingly common.

EPIDEMIOLOGY

Patients at greatest risk for HIV-1 infection and the development of AIDS include homosexual or bisexual males, intravenous drug users, hemophiliacs with a history of significant factor XIII concentrate administration, heterosexual partners of infected individuals, recipients of contaminated blood or blood products, and children born to an infected mother. Although transmission of HIV-1 continues through sexual contact with infected partners and through perinatal transmission from infected mothers to their offspring, surgeons are particularly concerned about parenteral routes of transmission, by transfusion and direct exposure to infected cells, body fluids, or transplanted organs.

Transfusion-Associated AIDS

The transmission of HIV-1 has been documented after transfusions of whole blood, packed red cells, fresh frozen plasma, cryoprecipitate, platelets, and pooled plasma. Transmission by transfusion has decreased considerably since the exclusion of donors at risk for HIV-1 and the institution of routine testing of all donations for antibodies to HIV-1. Factor VIII and factor IX concentrates are also currently heat treated to inactivate HIV-1. Although these tactics have reduced the risk of transfusion-acquired HIV-1, transmission is still possible because persons recently infected with HIV-1 may donate blood in the period before detectable antibodies to HIV-1 have developed, rendering HIV-1 exposure undetectable by present screening methods. Therefore, individuals at high risk for infection are not good candidates for blood or organ donation.

The risk of acquiring hepatitis from a single transfusion is much higher than the estimated risk of acquiring HIV-1. Recent reports using the direct detection of HIV-1 by sensitive DNA amplification techniques (polymerase chain reaction) and by viral culture confirm the low rates of HIV-1 in donor blood that has been screened for the absence of anti–HIV-1 antibodies. Furthermore, epidemiologic studies have confirmed that the actual risk of HIV-1 infection following a single blood transfusion ranges between 1 in 30,000 to 1 in 60,000.

Parenteral Exposure

HIV-1 can be transmitted by parenteral exposure, which is of particular concern to health care workers due to the risk of occupational exposure. However, assessment of the magnitude of this risk remains difficult. Combined data from prospective studies indicate that the risk of HIV-1 transmission from single parenteral exposure is approximately 1 in 300. There is no evidence of HIV-1 transmission following a single mucous membrane exposure. Occupational exposure is minimized by implementation of universal blood and body fluid precautions, but the continued risk of parenteral exposure has led to the development of strategies to reduce this risk. Postexposure prophylaxis with antiretroviral agents such as *zidovudine* (AZT) has been advocated for health care workers exposed to HIV-1. However, no reports indicate a reduction in seroconversion rates following prophylactic antiretroviral therapy. There have been anecdotal reports of HIV-1 seroconversion despite AZT administration following parenteral exposure.

The acquisition of HIV-1 by five patients of a dentist who died of AIDS has raised the possibility that HIV-1–infected health care workers who perform invasive procedures may potentially transmit the virus to others. As there have been no other documented reports of HIV-1 seroconversion from infected health care workers to several thousand evaluable patients, firm support for such a risk has not been established.

PATHOGENESIS

While the pathogenesis of HIV-1 infection has been under intense scrutiny, the long latent period between infection and disease progression and the lack of an animal model of HIV-1 infection has delayed complete understanding of HIV-1 immunopathogenesis. HIV-1 selectively enters cells bearing the $CD4^+$ molecule that typically includes T helper/inducer cells and monocyte/macrophages. Following entry into $CD4^+$ T cells, HIV-1 is thought to exist in a latent, nonintegrated form or as an integrated form that is not productive. On activation of the immune system, productive HIV-1 infection can occur, followed by the release of infectious HIV-1 and the destruction or dysfunction of the infected cell. Recent data suggest that in secondary lymphoid organs such as lymph nodes, progeny virus production occurs continually, leading to infection

and destruction of susceptible $CD4^+$ T-lymphocytes. It is the quantitative and qualitative deficiency in the $CD4^+$ T–helper-inducer lymphocyte population that appears to produce the profound immune effects associated with AIDS. Other immune defects may also be related to abnormal cytokine release or other viral-associated factors such as soluble HIV-1 glycoprotein release. Nonetheless, $CD4^+$ T-cell deficiency ultimately causes immune impairment and secondary opportunistic infections and malignancies.

DIAGNOSIS

Standard methods for documenting HIV-1 infection rely on detection of HIV-1–specific antibodies by *enzyme-linked immunosorbent assay* (ELISA) and confirmed by Western blotting. These antibodies are generally not detectable until 6 to 8 weeks after infection. Therefore, individuals may remain seronegative, yet infectious, for a period of weeks. Confirmation of HIV-1 infection in this group relies on the direct detection of HIV-1 by viral culture or by the demonstration of HIV-1–specific proteins or nucleic acids in body fluids or cellular material. Patients who have had a recent exposure to HIV-1 but are seronegative are usually retested at 6 and 12 weeks and at 6 and 12 months to exclude occult infection and the late development of antibodies.

CLINICAL MANIFESTATIONS

Two to 12 weeks after exposure to HIV-1, a mononucleosis-like syndrome may occur. Following acute infection, a variable asymptomatic period may occur that can persist for more than 10 years. However, 80 per cent of infected adults are usually symptomatic within 10 years of infection. The period of symptomatic disease is marked by a progressive depletion of $CD4^+$ T cells and may consist of constitutional signs including weight loss, fever, and night sweats, or infections that do not meet the criteria for the complete syndrome of AIDS. Other manifestations of progressive HIV-1 infection include immune thrombocytopenia and neurologic disease.

AIDS, which represents the most severe manifestation of HIV-1 infection, develops in 50 per cent of infected adults within 10 years and is characterized by progressive $CD4^+$ T-cell lymphopenia manifested by susceptibility to life-threatening opportunistic infections and malignancies. The $CD4^+$ lymphocyte count has emerged as predictive of disease progression, and $CD4^+$ counts under $100/mm^3$ indicate a high mortality within the subsequent 12 to 18 months.

Medical Management

Although there is currently no curative therapy for HIV-1 infection, the life expectancy of infected individuals has increased with improvement in antiretroviral therapy and with improved management of opportunistic infections. Zidovudine (AZT) is a nucleoside analog that acts as a chain terminator for reverse transcriptase–driven elongation of HIV-1 DNA. The use of AZT has led to improvement in the quality and length of life in patients with AIDS and has decreased the number and severity of opportunistic infections. It has also been used for patients who have not yet developed AIDS but whose $CD4^+$ counts are less than $200/mm^3$. Asymptomatic patients with $CD4^+$ counts less than $500/mm^3$ are currently being treated with antiretroviral therapy, but this use has come into question. The emergence of AZT-resistant HIV-1 has complicated the treatment of HIV-1. Recently, other nucleoside analogs, including didanosine (DDI) and zalcitabine (DDC), used alone or in combination with AZT, have been approved for use by HIV-1–infected individuals.

Manifestations of AIDS

Most of the morbidity associated with AIDS is related to opportunistic infection. Clinical syndromes that occur frequently include fever, diarrhea, central nervous system (CNS) disorders, generalized lymphadenopathy, and esophagitis. Neoplasms also occur in a relatively large number of patients with AIDS and include Kaposi's sarcoma (KS), non-Hodgkin's lymphoma (NHL), squamous cell carcinoma of the anus, and cervical dysplasia/neoplasia in women.

Kaposi's sarcoma usually occurs in homosexual and bisexual male AIDS patients. Its incidence has fallen from 40 per cent in the early 1980s to less than 20 per cent in the early 1990s. HIV-1 is not found in the KS cells themselves, and the pathogenesis of KS is unclear. Kaposi's sarcoma is characterized by the sudden onset and often widespread appearance of lesions involving not only skin but all mucosal surfaces, lymph nodes, and visceral organs. The average survival is 18 months; however, visceral involvement often means an even worse prognosis. Small localized lesions may be treated by electrodesiccation and curettage or by surgical excision, and larger tumors are generally responsive to local radiation.

Symptomatic or rapidly progressive disease should be treated with systemic chemotherapy, which establishes remission in some patients, while some have responded to treatment with α-interferon. Recent evidence suggests that growth factors involved with KS include interleukin-6 (IL-6) and Oncostatin M (Onco M). Uncontrolled growth of KS cells may occur due to interactions with HIV-1 regulatory proteins and abnormal production or sensitivity to these cytokines, and new agents to treat KS by inhibiting growth factors are being developed.

AIDS-related NHL are usually small, noncleaved, or immunoblastic tumors. Many are present in extranodal sites, including a predominance of CNS tumors. The CNS lymphomas and many of the peripheral lymphomas often contain Epstein-Barr virus (EBV) DNA, and EBV may be implicated in the pathogenesis of lymphoma. The lymphomas initially respond to conventional chemotherapeutic regimens, but patients have a poor prognosis, with frequent relapses and death usually occurring within a year. Recent treatment strategies include the administration of various hematopoietic growth factors to improve immunologic function in patients receiving chemotherapy. Some researchers advocate the use of autologous bone marrow transplantation in conjunction with AZT and chemotherapy for AIDS-associated lymphoma.

Anal squamous cell carcinoma is increasing in incidence in patients with HIV-1 infection. Treatment is usually by excisional biopsy followed by multimodality therapy consisting of chemotherapy and radiation therapy. No large series of patients with squamous cell carcinoma of the anus and HIV-1 infection has yet been reported.

HIV-infected women who have multiple sexual partners have a five- to tenfold increase in the incidence of high-grade squamous intracellular lesions on cervicovaginal examination, especially in adolescents and young adults. Women with HIV infection should obtain Papanicolaou (Pap) smears at 6-month intervals.

SURGICAL CONSIDERATIONS OF HIV-1–INFECTED INDIVIDUALS

HIV-1–infected individuals are not only susceptible to the usual medical problems and surgical disorders occurring in all patients, but also to a variety of unique conditions that may require surgical intervention. The following represent potential conditions.

Esophagus

Diffuse esophagitis secondary to *Candida albicans*, herpes simplex virus (HSV), and cytomegalovirus (CMV) are the most common lesions observed. Patients complain of dysphagia and substernal burning. Typically, a trial of empiric antifungal therapy is given prior to invasive testing, especially in the presence of oral thrush. If empiric therapy is not successful, endoscopy and biopsy may be required to differentiate the other causes of these lesions. KS of the esophagus also occurs and may bleed or cause pharyngeal obstruction, necessitating excision.

Stomach and Duodenum

Commonly encountered lesions in the stomach and duodenum include KS, NHL, and CMV infections. Kaposi's sarcoma lesions are usually asymptomatic, but are a frequent cause of upper gastrointestinal bleeding in HIV-1–infected individuals and can occasionally cause gastric outlet obstruction. Surgical excision is required if radiotherapy, chemotherapy, or immunotherapy fail to control the tumor. Non-Hodgkin's lymphoma may cause hemorrhage, obstruction, or perforation. Whereas the normal protocol for NHL is administration of chemotherapy, intestinal perforation secondary to extensive tumor lysis after chemotherapy has been reported. Therefore, surgical excision may be preferable to chemotherapy initially. Cytomegalovirus infections of the stomach and duodenum cause ulcerations which, when perforation occurs, require surgical intervention. Despite surgical repair, the morbidity and mortality are high following perforation secondary to CMV.

Liver

Most HIV-1–related opportunistic infections and neoplastic complications, including KS and NHL, may affect the liver. Constitutional symptoms and abnormal liver function tests are indicative of liver involvement. Most patients with AIDS have serologic evidence of previous hepatitis-B infection, and other types of viral hepatitis are also common. A liver biopsy is usually indicated, and liver abscesses may occasionally require an operative procedure for drainage.

Gallbladder and Biliary Tract

Acute acalculous cholecystitis has been documented in HIV-1–infected individuals. Infecting organisms include *Cryptosporidium* species, CMV, *Campylobacter*, and *Candida* species. The diagnosis of acute cholecystitis is often made by ultrasonography or radionuclide scan, and cholecystectomy is the treatment of choice. Laparoscopic cholecystectomy is currently the most common technique used for removal of the diseased gallbladder. This operation is generally well tolerated; however, in poor operative candidates, placement of a percutaneous cholecystostomy tube with guidance by ultrasound may be considered. Papillary stenosis and sclerosing cholangitis also occur. *Cryptosporidium* and CMV infection are the likely causes of extrinsic compression of the bile ducts. Sec-

ondary compression due to KS lesions, lymphadenopathy, or lymphoma should be excluded by ultrasonography or computed tomography (CT) scan. Papillary stenosis can be relieved by endoscopic sphincterotomy. Sclerosing cholangitis may often be relieved by balloon dilatation and stenting. Surgical intervention may be required for relief of extrinsic compression or when endoscopic sphincterotomy or stenting fails.

Small Intestine

HIV-1–related neoplastic lesions affecting the small intestine include NHL and KS. Lymphomas are usually symptomatic, presenting with pain, fever, night sweats, weight loss, jaundice, ascites, obstructive signs, bleeding, or perforation. Diagnosis is usually made by CT scan, and surgical intervention is frequently indicated and is advised prior to the initiation of chemotherapy to prevent intestinal perforation secondary to postchemotherapy tumor lysis. Intestinal KS lesions are present in 40 to 50 per cent of patients with cutaneous KS lesions but are usually asymptomatic. Lesions may become symptomatic by bleeding or causing obstruction, and these may then require surgical excision.

Cytomegalovirus infection may cause intestinal perforation necessitating surgical exploration and segmental resection of bowel. Morbidity and mortality after such a procedure remain high because of the lack of appropriate systemic antiviral therapy, although recent trials suggest that intravenous ganciclovir is effective against CMV. Several other organisms, including *Campylobacter*, *Shigella*, and *Salmonella* species, and *Mycobacterium avian-intracellulare*, can cause an inflammatory response of the terminal ileum that may mimic regional enteritis or appendicitis leading to surgical exploration.

Appendix

Whereas appendicitis occurs in HIV-1–infected individuals by the same mechanisms through which it occurs in non–HIV-1–infected individuals, appendiceal infection may also follow AIDS-associated neoplasms such as KS and NHL. Appendicitis is often difficult to diagnose in patients with AIDS, as they frequently have chronic abdominal complaints. The use of laparoscopic exploration allows full evaluation of the abdominal contents, including the appendix, with minimal morbidity in those in which the physical examination is difficult or unreliable.

Colon

Lesions affecting the colon in HIV-1–infected individuals are predominantly infectious in nature. Cytomegalovirus infection may lead to perforation requiring surgical intervention. A number of bacterial and parasitic organisms can cause severe colitis, which usually presents with abdominal pain and diarrhea.

Anus and Rectum

Anorectal complaints are common in HIV-1–infected individuals, especially homosexuals and AIDS patients. Symptoms include pain, discharge, incontinence, bleeding, mass, and/or tenesmus. Such symptoms may be caused by a wide variety of viral, bacterial, fungal, protozoal, and helminthic infections; lesions such as anal fissures and fistulas and perirectal abscesses; and tumors such as KS, lymphoma, or squamous cell carcinoma. The frequency of these lesions in AIDS patients appears to increase their risk of developing anal and rectal carcinomas. Treatment of the various rectal lesions should be as conservative as possible because patients usually heal poorly after attempted surgical therapy. Inflammatory bowel disease may also occur with HIV-1 infection. Patients with refractory inflammatory bowel disease should undergo surgical exploration with resection in the presence of toxic megacolon, as do non–HIV-1–infected individuals. It is interesting that this supposed autoimmune disease may occur in the setting of HIV-1 and be refractory to treatment with immunosuppressive corticosteroids. Systemic antibiotic prophylaxis is recommended, as these patients are prone to postoperative wound infections.

Lungs

In addition to malignancies, an increase in the incidence of tuberculosis is associated with HIV-1 infection. Pulmonary manifestations of tuberculosis appear as described; however, there is a high incidence of drug-resistant tuberculosis associated with HIV-1 infection. It is unknown whether this is due to an aggressive pathogen or to the tendencies for patients with pulmonary tuberculosis and HIV-1 to intermittently cease antitubercular therapy allowing resistant strains to evolve. Tuberculosis may continue to be a major clinical problem in HIV-1–infected individuals.

EVALUATION BY CLINICAL SIGNS AND SYMPTOMS

Abdominal Pain

Abdominal pain in HIV-1–infected individuals is divided into three broad categories: abdominal pain secondary to standard surgical problems, abdominal pain secondary to AIDS-related surgical problems, and nonsurgical abdominal pain. Abdominal pain requiring surgical intervention in this population is uncommon. However, as more HIV-1 infections are reported, the probability is high that an increasing number of patients will have standard surgical problems. Abdominal pain may occur secondary to appendicitis, cholecystitis, perforated gastric or duodenal ulcer, diverticulitis, adhesions, small-bowel obstruction, or incarcerated hernias. In general, the more immunocompromised the HIV-1–infected patient (as determined by the presence of a low $CD4^+$ count), the more often an atypical presentation and a poor outcome can be expected.

AIDS-related conditions leading to abdominal pain and requiring surgical intervention include KS and NHL. Such lesions may cause gastrointestinal bleeding, obstruction, or perforation. Cytomegalovirus infection may lead to enteritis or colitis, causing abdominal pain, bleeding, and diarrhea. Surgical intervention is required for free perforation, massive hemorrhage, or if toxic megacolon occurs; however, intravenous ganciclovir therapy is often able to inhibit CMV. Evaluation of patients with abdominal pain includes standard diagnostic studies, such as endoscopy with biopsy and culture, stool examination, and CT scanning.

Gastrointestinal bleeding is an unusual occurrence in HIV-1-infections. Lesions causing this problem are directly related to HIV-1 infection and include KS and NHL. Because these lesions are frequently amenable to surgical intervention, gastrointestinal bleeding should be treated aggressively.

Lymphadenopathy

Generalized lymphadenopathy is a relatively common finding in patients with HIV-1 infection. The development of accurate serologic tests for HIV-1–specific antibodies has rendered routine diagnostic lymph node biopsy unnecessary for the diagnosis of HIV-1. However, selected use of diagnostic lymph node biopsy may be useful in the diagnosis of a specific infection, lymphoma, or other disease process and thus assists in management. Typically, incisional lymph node biopsy is advocated in patients with dominant lymph nodes. In addition to pathologic evaluation for tumor and lymphoma, routine fungal and microbacterial cultures are obtained. Cytopathologic evaluation of lymph nodes is dependent on the availability of experts in the evaluation and interpretation of specimens from the AIDS population.

Immune Thrombocytopenic Purpura

Splenectomy may have a role in the treatment of HIV-1–associated immune thrombocytopenic purpura

(ITP). These patients are usually treated with anti-retroviral therapy, but corticosteroids and intravenous immune globulin may be required. If patients have no response to medical therapy or if they are suffering from complications of steroid therapy, splenectomy may be considered as an option. Short-term results include a rise in circulating platelets, but long-term follow-up has been limited.

OTHER SURGICAL CONSIDERATIONS

Postoperative Care

Postoperative morbidity and mortality appear to be related to the patient's underlying immunocompetence and the nature of the underlying disease requiring operation. HIV-1–infected patients who are asymptomatic with relatively normal CD4$^+$ counts can undergo elective surgical procedures without problems with wound healing and postoperative infection that are significantly different from those of the general population. Surgical intervention in these patients has been reported to occasionally exacerbate the underlying HIV-1 infection, but there is no evidence to support this view. High morbidity and mortality have been reported following emergent operative procedures in AIDS patients; however, this may reflect the role of delayed diagnosis due to nonspecific symptoms or opportunistic infections associated with HIV-1 more than HIV-1 itself.

Trauma

Surgeons must consider the risk of occupational exposure to HIV-1 when managing severely injured patients, especially those who are actively bleeding and who may require multiple invasive procedures in the emergency clinic. In one study, approximately 3 per cent of all patients seen in the emergency clinic were HIV-1–seropositive at the time of presentation and did not have a previous history of HIV-1 infection. The highest prevalence was among patients undergoing operation for penetrating trauma and in populations that have a likely incidence of intravenous drug use, usually patients between the ages of 25 and 34. The policy of universal blood and body fluid precautions should be followed by all health care workers regardless of knowledge of HIV-1 infection.

REFERENCES

Carpenter CCJ, Mayer KH, Stein MD, et al: Human immunodeficiency virus infection in North American women: Experience with 200 cases and a review of the literature. Medicine 70:307–325, 1991.

Diettrich NA, Cacioppo JC, Kaplan G, Cohen SM: A growing spectrum of surgical disease in patients with human immunodeficiency virus/acquired immunodeficiency syndrome. Arch Surg 126:860–864, 1991.

Lo B, Steinbrook R: Health care workers infected with the human immunodeficiency virus. JAMA 267:1100–1105, 1992.

Mann J: AIDS-the second decade: A global perspective. J Infect Dis 165:245–250, 1992.

Simonds RJ, Holmberg SD, Hurwitz RL, et al: Transmission of human immunodeficiency virus type 1 from a seronegative organ and tissue donor. N Engl J Med 326:726–732, 1992.

Stein DS, Korvick JA, Vermund SH: CD4$^+$ lymphocyte enumeration for prediction of clinical course of human immunodeficiency virus disease. J Infect Dis 165:352–363, 1992.

15
TRAUMA

MITCHELL P. FINK, M.D.

Every year, one of every three people in the United States sustains a nonfatal injury, and patients with life-threatening injuries constitute 10 to 15 per cent of individuals hospitalized for trauma. Among children and adults less than 44 years of age, trauma is the leading cause of death. The cost of trauma care is in excess of $100 billion annually, making trauma a public health problem of epidemic proportions.

INITIAL MANAGEMENT

The initial evaluation and therapy of the trauma victim should follow a planned approach. During the primary survey, the goals are to secure a patent airway, ensure adequate ventilation, maintain or restore circulation, and assess global neurologic status. Simple diagnostic studies, such as routine bloodwork, urinalysis, lateral cervical spine and anteroposterior chest radiographs, and, in some instances, a one-shot intravenous pyelogram, are obtained during the primary survey. If hemodynamic stability can be maintained or restored, then a secondary survey is performed during which more complicated and time-consuming diagnostic studies (e.g., abdominal computed tomographic [CT] scans) are obtained.

The crucial first priority in the management of the injured patient is ensuring that there is an adequate *airway*. Indications for endotracheal intubation include: inability to secure an airway using noninvasive means, such as the chin-lift maneuver; hemoptysis; obtundation or coma due to severe head trauma, asphyxia, or intoxication; or shock. Endotracheal intubation is most often performed via the orotracheal route. In all victims of blunt trauma (and in many victims of penetrating trauma), cervical spine injury should be assumed to be present even if the lateral cervical spine radiograph (which should be obtained early in the primary survey) is normal. Therefore, during orotracheal intubation, the neck should be held in a neutral position, and not placed in the usual "sniffing" attitude. When the patient has no evidence of soft tissue or bony injury of the midface and is breathing spontaneously, the blind nasotracheal approach is an acceptable alternative to orotracheal intubation. In some patients, particularly those with laryngeal or extensive maxillofacial injuries, the airway is best secured by performing a cricothyroidotomy or tracheostomy. Assisted ventilation should be instituted if spontaneous ventilation is inadequate for any reason.

Even as efforts are being made to ensure the adequacy of ventilation, the surgeon should make an assessment of the patient's circulatory status. Inadequate tissue perfusion (i.e., shock) is suggested by the presence of some or all of these readily discernible clinical findings: cool extremities, slow capillary refill, rapid and thready pulse, altered mentation, and/or arterial hypotension. Shock in trauma victims is most often due to inadequate circulating volume secondary to hemorrhage. The neck veins in hypovolemic shock are flat. If the patient is shock-like and the neck veins are distended, then five diagnostic possibilities must be considered: tension pneumothorax, pericardial tamponade, air embolism, myocardial contusion, and myocardial infarction. Of these possibilities, the first two, which are discussed below, are by far the most common. Two large-bore intravenous lines should be placed in the upper extremities or the groin, taking care not to position them distal to extremity wounds with known or possible vascular injuries. Cut-downs are rarely necessary. Intraosseous catheters are sometimes useful in children under age 3. Subclavian and jugular lines are best used for monitoring, not for fluid administration. In adults, fluid resuscitation should start with 1 L lactated Ringer's solution. In children, the initial bolus should be 20 ml/kg body weight. Initial laboratory studies, including hematocrit, amylase, toxicologic screen, and blood typing and cross-matching, should be obtained as soon as the first intravenous line has been secured. Catheters, including a nasogastric tube, urinary (Foley) catheter, and, in some instances, a central venous pressure catheter, should be placed during this stage of the initial resuscitation. The adequacy of resuscitation is assessed by monitoring blood pressure, urine output (which should be 0.5 ml/kg of body weight per hour), capillary refill, and central venous pressure (which should be 5 to 15 cm H_2O).

A brief neurologic examination should be performed to assess level of consciousness, pupillary responses to light, and movement of extremities in response to commands or noxious stimuli. The information thereby gained can be used to calculate the Glasgow Coma Scale (Table 1), which aids in both quantitating central nervous system dysfunction over time and providing prognostic information about the likelihood of future recovery. The neurologic assessment should be performed repeatedly over time, because deterioration of central nervous system function is the most important indicator of serious injury to the brain.

If immediate life-threatening problems can be stabilized, the patient should undergo a complete, albeit brief, reexamination, looking for other injuries. Further history, including such facts as drug allergies, con-

current medical problems, and current medications, should be sought at this time either from the victim or from family or friends. Additional laboratory and radiographic studies should be obtained as indicated by the history or physical examination findings. Special diagnostic tests, such as peritoneal lavage, are performed at this time as well.

INJURIES TO THE CHEST

Rib fractures are the most common thoracic injury. Symptomatic relief of pain is usually the only treatment required. Fractures of ribs 1 to 3 are indicative of severe chest trauma, and should increase the index of suspicion for associated injuries, particularly rupture of the thoracic aorta. Severe chest wall instability can be caused by unilateral anterior and posterior fractures or bilateral anterior (or costochondral) fractures of four or more ribs. This instability leads to paradoxic respiratory motion of the involved thoracic wall segment, a condition that is referred to as *flail chest*. Although presence of a flail segment undoubtedly leads to mechanical impairment of ventilation, the main problem in this condition is the associated *pulmonary contusion*, which is almost invariably present. Treatment of pulmonary contusion and flail chest consists of providing adequate analgesia, avoiding fluid overload, and, if necessary, supporting the patient with mechanical ventilation.

Pneumothorax (i.e., air in the pleural space) results from laceration of the chest wall or lung and can be caused by either blunt or penetrating trauma to the chest. *Tension pneumothorax* develops when there is a flap valve such that air can enter the pleural space during inspiration but cannot leave during expiration. In tension pneumothorax, intrapleural pressure rises, leading to collapse of the ipsilateral lung, compression of the great veins, and embarrassment of cardiac output. The diagnosis of tension pneumothorax is suggested by shock, subcutaneous emphysema, absent breath sounds, tracheal deviation (away from the affected hemithorax), distended neck veins, and ineffective ventilation. This condition is a true emergency; diagnosis and treatment cannot wait for a chest film. If the diagnosis is suspected, a needle should be inserted in the ipsilateral second intercostal space. If the diagnosis is confirmed by a gush of air, a tube thoracostomy should be performed. The presence of a large defect in the chest wall constitutes an *open pneumothorax* or "sucking chest wound." This also is an immediate life-threatening problem, which should be treated by closing the defect with a sterile dressing and venting the pleural space with a chest tube connected to a flutter valve or a closed system drainage device. The diagnosis of *simple pneumothorax* is made by ex-

TABLE 1. THE GLASGOW COMA SCALE*

Eyes open	Never	1
	To pain	2
	To verbal stimuli	3
	Spontaneously	4
Best verbal response	No response	1
	Incomprehensible sounds	2
	Inappropriate words	3
	Disoriented and converses	4
	Oriented and converses	5
Best motor response	No response	1
	Extension (decerebrate rigidity)	2
	Flexion abnormal (decorticate rigidity)	3
	Flexion withdrawal	4
	Localizes pain	5
	Obeys	6
Total		3–15

*From Jurkovitch GJ, Carrico CJ: Trauma: Management of acute injuries. *In* Sabiston DC Jr (ed): Textbook of Surgery: The Biological Basis of Modern Surgical Practice, ed 14. Philadelphia, WB Saunders Company, 1991, p 260, with permission.

amining the chest roentgenogram. Treatment is tube thoracostomy. *Hemothorax* (i.e., bleeding into the pleural space) is adequately managed by tube thoracostomy and nothing more in 85 per cent of cases. Exploratory thoracostomy is indicated if the initial chest tube drainage exceeds 1500 ml or ongoing drainage of blood exceeds 250 ml/hr for 3 hours.

In blunt trauma, *tracheal and bronchial injuries* are caused by compressive and/or shearing forces, such as those generated by sudden deceleration of the sternum against the steering wheel in head-on motor vehicle accidents. Findings with these injuries include subcutaneous emphysema, hemoptysis, hemopneumothorax, and respiratory distress. Definitive diagnosis is usually made by fiberoptic bronchoscopy. Definitive repair of major airway injuries requires operation, which is preferably performed early to prevent stricture formation.

Myocardial contusion occurs in 20 per cent of cases of blunt chest trauma. Usually this lesion is clinically silent although, rarely, severe complications (e.g., ventricular rupture) can result. In hemodynamically unstable patients, the diagnosis is best made echocardiographically. In most instances, however, extensive studies to make the diagnosis of myocardial contusion are unwarranted. *Cardiac tamponade* results from accumulation of blood in the pericardial sac, leading to impaired filling of the cardiac chambers and, hence, cardiogenic shock. Although most often caused by penetrating injuries to heart, tamponade also can occur as a complication of blunt trauma (leading, for example, to rupture of the right ventricular free wall). The classic findings of Beck's triad (distended neck veins, muffled heart sounds, and hypotension) are present in only a third of patients with this condition. If tamponade is suspected, the diagnosis is best made by echocardiography if this study can be obtained expeditiously. For patients in extremis, diagnosis and initial treatment can be provided by percutaneous pericardiocentesis, by creation of a subxiphoid pericardial window, or by immediate thoracotomy. The latter two procedures are best performed in the operating room.

Rupture of the thoracic aorta causes 15 to 40 per cent of fatalities due to motor vehicle accidents. Most often, this injury leads to immediate exsanguination and death. In about 20 per cent of cases, however, hemorrhage is controlled by the periaortic adventitia, resulting in the formation of a traumatic aneurysm. Since the adventitial tissues containing the hematoma are tenuous, survival depends upon expeditious diagnosis. Aortic rupture should be suspected if the chest film shows widening of the mediastinum (to >10 cm), loss of aortic contour, deviation of the trachea to the right, elevation of the left mainstem bronchus, depression of the right mainstem bronchus, shift of the nasogastric tube to the left, left-side hemothorax, apical capping, or presence of a retrocardiac density. Aortography remains the diagnostic study of choice. Surgical repair, which almost always requires a Dacron interposition graft, should be performed as soon as the diagnosis is established.

Laceration or rupture of the diaphragm is usually due to penetrating trauma. Herniation of abdominal viscera through the rent may not occur immediately; thus, diagnosis is often delayed. When the diagnosis is made early (either at exploratory laparotomy for other causes, or as a result of abnormalities on the chest film or CT scan), repair should be via the abdominal approach. When diagnosis has been delayed, a thoracic approach may be preferable in some instances.

Blunt *injury to the esophagus* is rare, and perforating injuries are rarely isolated to this organ. The common presentation is extreme pain, followed by fever. All patients with gunshot wounds traversing the mediastinum or stab wounds near the posterior midline should be endoscopically or radiographically evaluated to exclude esophageal injury. If diagnosed early, esophageal injuries should be sutured and drained. If the diagnosis is delayed longer than 12 to 24 hours, conservative therapy consists of drainage, proximal diversion, and feeding gastrostomy.

ABDOMINAL TRAUMA

In awake, alert patients, history and physical examination are often sufficient to establish or exclude the presence of intra-abdominal injuries. However, in patients with an altered sensorium (due to brain injuries or intoxication), additional diagnostic modalities are typically needed. Diagnostic peritoneal lavage (DPL) is performed by infusing 1000 ml of crystalloid solution into the peritoneal cavity via a catheter inserted either percutaneously or with an open technique. The effluent is sampled and examined for the presence of erythrocytes, leukocytes, amylase, or food particles. One criterion for a positive test is the presence of greater than 100,000 red cells per microliter. Diagnostic accuracy is about 97 per cent with this technique. Abdominal CT scans are most useful in the evaluation of hemodynamically stable patients with equivocal findings on physical examination or hematuria. Gunshot wounds to the abdomen mandate operative exploration.

The *spleen* is the most commonly injured intra-abdominal organ. Splenic hemorrhage is easily controlled by splenectomy, but removal of this organ increases the risk of overwhelming infections with certain bacteria, particularly *Streptococcus pneumoniae*. The true incidence of overwhelming postsplenectomy sepsis (OPSI) is poorly defined, but mortality due to posttraumatic OPSI has been estimated to be approximately 0.8 per cent. Because of the risk of OPSI, splenectomy should be reserved for cases with massive injuries to this organ or other concurrent and immediately life-threatening problems. In children, many splenic injuries can be successfully managed nonoperatively, but results with this approach have not been as good in adults. For splenic injuries in adults, splenic repair ("splenorrhaphy") should be performed, unless contraindicated because of persistent hemodynamic instability or destruction of splenic parenchyma. Patients requiring splenectomy should receive polyvalent pneumococcal vaccine in the postoperative period.

The *liver* is the most commonly injured organ in penetrating abdominal trauma and the second most injured organ in blunt abdominal trauma. The majority of liver injuries either are not bleeding at the time of laparotomy or require only minor suturing or application of topical hemostatic agents. Severe liver injuries, although uncommon, carry a high mortality rate. Resection of hepatic parenchyma is rarely necessary; formal lobectomy is almost never indicated. Perihepatic packing and planned reexploration in 24 to 72 hours is often life saving.

Isolated injuries to the *portal vein, hepatic artery,* or *common bile duct* are rare; usually two or all three of these structures are injured simultaneously, often in combination with trauma to the liver, duodenum, or other upper abdominal organs. Injuries to these structures are difficult to manage, life-threatening bleeding being the usual immediate problem and stricture of the biliary tree being the main late one. Hemorrhage from the portal vein is best controlled by the Pringle maneuver followed by isolation and venorrhaphy or interposition grafting. Ligation of the portal vein is compatible with survival under some circumstances, but does not represent optimal management. Common bile duct injuries involving less than 50 per cent of the wall are usually best managed by repair over a stent with external drainage of bile. For more extensive injuries, the incidence of late stricture can be reduced to about 5 per cent by performing a choledochoenterostomy, rather than attempting direct repair or duct-to-duct anastomosis, approaches which are complicated by stricture formation in more than 50 per cent of cases. Injuries to the *gallbladder* are best managed by cholecystectomy.

Most full-thickness injuries to the *stomach* are due to penetrating trauma and can be treated by simple débridement and closure. In penetrating abdominal trauma, the *small intestine* is injured in about 50 per cent of cases. Injuries to the small bowel due to blunt abdominal trauma, which occur in 5 to 15 per cent of cases, are caused by three mechanisms: (1) crushing between anterior abdominal wall and the vertebral column; (2) sudden increase in intraluminal pressure; and (3) tears at the junction between mobile and fixed

segments, the latter consisting of the duodenojejunal flexure, the ileocecal junction, and sites of adhesions. Although most patients with enteric perforations manifest signs of peritoneal irritation, clinical findings are sometimes minimal for days. The DPL is more accurate than CT for detecting enteric perforations. During laparotomy for trauma, the entire small bowel should be examined thoroughly. Perforations usually can be débrided and sutured, although when damage is extensive, segmental resection is warranted.

Injuries to the *colon* and *rectum* carry mortality rates of 3 to 12 per cent and 4 to 22 per cent, respectively. The morbidity and mortality associated with these injuries can be reduced by prompt diagnosis and treatment. Because large portions of the colon are retroperitoneal, DPL can miss colonic injuries due to stab wounds in the back or flank. Patients with these injuries should undergo abdominal exploration or abdominal CT scanning using intravenous, oral, and intrarectal contrast enhancement. In an effort to minimize septic complications from rectal or colonic trauma, all patients at risk for having injury to these organs should receive appropriate broad-spectrum antibiotics in the emergency department. Colonic injuries can be managed with primary closure, provided that the following general criteria are met: (1) operation is performed within 4 to 6 hours after injury; (2) the requirement for blood transfusion is less than 6 U; (3) hemodynamic stability is maintained; (4) there is minimal soilage of the peritoneal cavity; (5) injury is limited to one part of the colon; (6) there are no injuries to the colonic vascular supply; (7) synthetic mesh is not needed to repair the abdominal wall; (8) there are no associated renal or pancreatic injuries; and (9) injuries to multiple intra-abdominal organs are not present. When these criteria are not satisfied, most colonic injuries should be managed by resection with creation of a proximal colostomy or ileostomy and a distal mucous fistula or Hartmann's pouch. Rectal injuries, except those that are distal to the dentate line, are best managed by débridement, closure if possible, proximal diverting colostomy, placement of presacral drains, and irrigation of the rectal stump with antiseptic solution.

Approximately three fourths of injuries to the *duodenum* are caused by penetrating trauma. The remainder are due to blunt trauma, often involving impact of the abdomen against the steering wheel of a motor vehicle. Whereas penetrating injuries to the duodenum are usually easily diagnosed at laparotomy, injuries resulting from blunt trauma are frequently diagnosed late, greatly increasing attendant morbidity and mortality. The diagnosis of blunt duodenal trauma is suggested by the mechanism of injury and/or the presence of hyperamylasemia; the diagnosis is confirmed or excluded by findings on a Gastrografin upper gastrointestinal series or an abdominal CT with oral and intravenous contrast enhancement. DPL is unreliable for detecting duodenal, pancreatic, and other retroperitoneal injuries. About 80 per cent of duodenal injuries can be repaired primarily; the remainder are severe injuries that require more complex procedures, including débridement or segmental resection and primary anastomosis, Roux-en-Y duodenojejunostomy, the Berne "duodenal diverticularization procedure" (Fig. 1), or very rarely, pancreatoduodenectomy.

Because of its protected retroperitoneal location, trauma to the *pancreas* is relatively uncommon. Still, pancreatic trauma leads to mortality in 10 to 25 per cent of cases and major complications (including hemorrhage, pseudocyst formation, and fistulization) in 30 to 40 per cent of patients who survive their initial injury. Because the pancreas is surrounded by other major organs and blood vessels, accompanying injuries are common. In blunt trauma, pancreatic trauma should be suspected on the basis of mechanism of injury and elevated amylase concentration in serum or DPL fluid. Further diagnostic information can be provided by abdominal CT. At operation, excluding the presence of pancreatic trauma requires full mobilization of the duodenum ("Kocher maneuver") and opening of the gastrocolic ligament to inspect the contents of the lesser sac. Mobilization of the spleen and tail of the pancreas may be necessary to inspect the posterior aspect of the gland. Most injuries are adequately treated with drainage alone; more complex injuries require more extensive procedures, such as distal pancreatectomy, duodenal diverticularization (see above) or, rarely, pancreatoduodenectomy.

The mortality from major *abdominal vascular trauma* is 30 to 60 per cent despite improvements in emergency transport and resuscitation. Mortality from aortic wounds (40 to 80 per cent) is higher than from caval injuries (10 to 40 per cent). Wounds to the suprarenal portions of these vessels carry the highest mortality rates. Other major vascular structures in the abdomen that can be wounded or disrupted include the iliac and superior mesenteric vessels. A third of patients with major abdominal vascular injuries present in shock, and immediate laparotomy (or in rare instances, left thoracotomy followed by laparotomy) is indicated to obtain rapid control of the hemorrhage. When the diagnosis is uncertain, DPL or abdominal CT (only in hemodynamically stable patients) can be helpful.

The intraoperative management of *retroperitoneal hematomas* warrants special discussion. Midline infrarenal hematomas should be opened and explored. In cases of blunt trauma, nonexpanding lateral hematomas should not be disturbed if the kidneys are well perfused on an intravenous contrast-enhanced CT or intravenous pyelogram and there is no evidence of a urinary leak. Lateral hematomas associated with penetrating trauma should be explored, but vascular control should be obtained prior to opening the Gerota's fascia. Pelvic hematomas secondary to blunt trauma should not be explored, whereas penetrating pelvic wounds require exploration of the pathway of the projectile or knife.

URINARY TRACT

If blood is present at the urethral meatus in males, or the mechanism of injury suggests a high likelihood of urethral injury, retrograde urethrography should be performed prior to urinary catheterization. Rectal examination should precede Foley catheterization; ina-

Figure 1. Illustration of the Berne "duodenal diverticulization" (*left*) and the Vaughan "pyloric exclusion" procedure (*right*) utilized as adjuncts to repair of severe duodenal or combined duodenopancreatic injury. Note that the Berne diverticulization includes vagotomy and antrectomy, whereas the Vaughan pyloroplasty is intended to be a temporary duodenal bypass. (From Jurkovich GJ, Carrico CJ: Management of pancreatic trauma. Surg Clin North Am 70:575, 1990, with permission.)

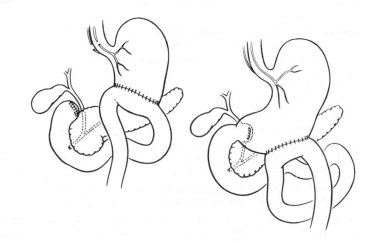

bility to palpate the prostate in males is suggestive of complete urethral transection. Evaluation of the upper urinary tract is indicated when there is hematuria or the mechanism of injury suggests a high likelihood of renal trauma. Abdominal CT with intravenous contrast provides more detailed information than intravenous pyelography (IVP). If either of these studies suggest absence of function in all or a segment of a kidney, then immediate arteriography is indicated. Evidence of urinary extravasation from the bladder on these studies is an indication for retrograde cystography. This latter test also is indicated in cases of massive pelvic trauma or when there is blood at the urinary meatus. Whereas nearly all victims of penetrating renal trauma should be explored, most cases of blunt renal trauma can be managed nonoperatively. Indications for exploration in blunt renal trauma include shattered kidney by CT or IVP, renal pedicle injury, or cortical laceration with extensive extravasation. Ureteral injuries are usually due to penetrating trauma and are repaired by primary anastomosis (upper and middle thirds) or ureteroneocystostomy (lower third). Stenting is sometimes indicated. In some instances, percutaneous nephrostomy and delayed repair of the ureteral injury is the preferred method of management. Extraperitoneal bladder injuries can be managed with simple urinary drainage unless the anterior wall of the organ has been perforated by a fragment of bone from a pelvic fracture. In these cases, the fracture should be reduced, the spicule of bone removed, the bladder débrided and closed, and urinary drainage provided. Intraperitoneal bladder ruptures mandate operative closure and urinary drainage.

TRAUMA TO THE PELVIS AND PERINEUM

The mortality from complex pelvic crush injuries and open pelvic fractures exceeds 50 per cent. The major causes of death are uncontrolled hemorrhage and complications due to injuries to associated organs. In the initial management of these injuries, the pneumatic antishock garment (PASG) often is used to stabilize the pelvic fractures and tamponade pelvic bleeding. The initial objective in these injuries is control of bleeding, which is most often venous in origin; thus, angiographic embolization is only rarely of value. Operative control of pelvic bleeding in this circumstance also is fruitless. The best results are obtained with early skeletal stabilization using external fixators, transfusion of packed cells and coagulation factors as needed to resuscitate the patient, and application of the PASG. Extensive injuries involving the *perineum* often require

temporary colostomy to divert the fecal stream away from the site of soft-tissue damage. These wounds should be débrided and irrigated, a process that often needs to be repeated many times.

CENTRAL NERVOUS SYSTEM TRAUMA

It is important to remember that *brain* injuries rarely cause hypotension. Thus, other causes of shock, such as external or internal hemorrhage, tension pneumothorax, or cardiac tamponade, must be sought. Furthermore, efforts to restore perfusion are very important in head trauma victims to limit exacerbation of central nervous system injury. Definitive diagnosis in head trauma is established by CT, and obtaining a cranial CT should have a high priority in the evaluation of patients with an altered sensorium or lateralizing neurologic signs. Focal injuries with significant mass effect require operative evacuation. Diffuse brain injuries are managed nonoperatively. Serious brain injuries, whether focal of diffuse, are best managed with continuous monitoring of intracranial pressure. Measures to control intracranial hypertension include hyperventilation, administration of mannitol, and, possibly, administration of barbiturates. Although representing only about 1 per cent of the total number of trauma cases requiring hospitalization, *spinal cord* injuries are responsible for a disproportionate share of the costs, in terms of both disability and financial outlay, associated with trauma. Motor vehicle accidents are responsible for approximately 60 per cent of spinal cord injuries, the remainder being due to falls (20 to 30 per cent) and diving accidents (5 to 10 per cent). When transporting victims with a potentially unstable spine, gentle traction should be used to stabilize the head, which should be turned to the midline and taped to a padded spine board. Sandbags and a Philadelphia-type cervical collar should be used to provide additional stability. The lower spine should be protected by strapping the patient to a long back board.

The initial neurologic examination should establish the spinal cord level of the deficit and whether the deficit is total or partial. Immediately after severe spinal cord injury there can be a transient period of disordered neurologic function; this phenomenon is termed spinal shock. During this period, no reflexive or voluntary activity is evident distal to the level of injury. The normal sacral reflexes (i.e., the bulbocavernosus reflex and anal wink reflex) are the earliest to recover after spinal shock; if neurologic impairment is incomplete, sacral reflexes typically recover within 24 hours. Recent laboratory and clinical studies suggest that prompt administration of high doses of methylprednisolone for 24 hours can improve long-term neurologic outcome in some cases of incomplete spinal cord injury. New therapeutic strategies, particularly use of a class of compounds called 21-aminosteroids or *lazeroids*, are currently undergoing evaluation.

INJURIES TO THE NECK

The neck contains multiple vital structures in a small area. Most significant neck injuries are the result of penetrating trauma. Fatality rates for penetrating neck wounds range from 2 per cent for stab injuries, to 50 per cent for rifle or shotgun blasts. Wounds that fail to penetrate the platysma are considered superficial and do not warrant extensive evaluation. Wounds that penetrate the platysma mandate hospital admission and further evaluation. All authorities agree that exploration is mandatory for patients with serious neck trauma and clinical signs of significant injury, such as shock, expanding hematomas, external hemorrhage, diminished carotid pulsations, subcutaneous emphysema, hemoptysis, dysphagia, stridor, hoarseness, dysphonia, or lateralized neurologic deficits. Controversy exists, however, regarding the proper management of neck wounds that penetrate the platysma when clinical signs of significant injury are absent. Some authorities advocate exploration routinely, whereas others favor a selective approach, using repetitive examination and nonoperative diagnostic studies (arteriography, esophagoscopy, and laryngo-bronchoscopy) to determine which patients actually require surgery. Neck CT is particularly helpful in evaluating severe blunt trauma to the neck.

EXTREMITY AND PERIPHERAL VASCULAR INJURIES

Hemorrhage from disruption of major blood vessels represents the only immediately life-threatening complication of trauma to the extremities. Nevertheless, early stabilization of long-bone fractures decreases the incidence of subsequent pulmonary complications, particularly the adult respiratory distress syndrome. In order to minimize the risk of soft-tissue infections, all lacerations and penetrating injuries of the extremities should undergo early and thorough irrigation and débridement. If the viability of remaining muscle or other soft tissue remains in question, then there should be a plan for subsequent, early reexploration. Rapidly spreading erythema, crepitus, or unexplained pain in an injured extremity is an indication for immediate exploration and débridement. Tetanus is caused by toxins released by *Clostridium tetani*, an obligately anaerobic gram-positive bacillus. Prevention of this complication depends upon adequate débridement of devitalized tissue as well as appropriate administration of tetanus and diphtheria toxoids with or without tetanus immune globulin (Table 2). Prophylactic antibiotics are of unproven benefit in the prevention of tetanus. Fractures are often associated with arterial injuries, particularly in the leg. Fracture-dislocation of the knee is often complicated by injury to both the popliteal artery and vein. Arteriography should be performed routinely in cases of posterior knee dislocation. In some instances, a plastic interposition shunt can be temporarily positioned to restore perfusion to the distal popliteal artery while orthopedic stabilization of the knee is completed. Definitive arterial repair then follows.

In order to decrease the risk of compartment syndrome, massive myonecrosis, and myoglobinuric renal damage, fasciotomies should be performed routinely in cases of combined popliteal artery and vein injury, extensive bony and muscular injury, prolonged shock in association with major extremity trauma, or whenever the extremity has been ischemic for more than a few hours. In general, major venous injuries in the extremities should be repaired. If ligation is necessary because of the complexity of the injury or because other injuries assume priority, then the extremity should be elevated and provided with elastic wrappings for a prolonged period postoperatively, in an effort to reduce edema and late morbidity.

TABLE 2. IMMUNIZATION SCHEDULE*

Verify a history of tetanus immunization from medical records so that appropriate tetanus prophylaxis can be accomplished.

Td: Tetanus and diphtheria toxoids adsorbed (for adult use)
TIG: Tetanus immune globulin (human)

History of Adsorbed Tetanus Toxoid (Doses)	Tetanus-Prone Wounds		Nontetanus-Prone Wounds	
	Td†	TIG	Td†	TIG
Unknown or fewer than 3	Yes	Yes	Yes	No
3 or more‡	No§	No	No‖	No

*From Advanced Trauma Life Support Course Manual. Chicago, American College of Surgeons, 1988, p 272, with permission.

†For children less than 7 years old: DTP (DT, if pertussis vaccine is contraindicated) is preferable to tetanus toxoid alone. For persons 7 years old and older, Td is preferable to tetanus toxoid alone.

‡If only three doses of fluid toxoid have been received, a fourth dose of toxoid, preferably an adsorbed toxoid, should be given.

§Yes, if more than 10 years since last dose.

‖Yes, if more than 5 years since last dose. (More frequent boosters are not needed and can accentuate side effects.)

REFERENCES

Burch JM, Ortiz VB, Richardson RJ, Martin RR, Mattox KL, Jordan GL Jr: Abbreviated laparotomy and planned reoperation for critically injured patients. Ann Surg 215:476, 1992.

Cogbill TH, Moore EE, Jurkovich GJ, Feliciano DV, Morris HA, Mucha P, Shackford SR: Severe hepatic trauma: A multicenter experience with 1335 liver injuries. J Trauma 28:1433, 1988.

Feliciano DV, Martin TD, Cruse PA, et al: Management of combined pancreatoduodenal injuries. Ann Surg 205:673, 1987.

Flint L, Babikian G, Anders M, Rodriguez J, Steinberg S: Definitive control of mortality from severe pelvic fracture. Ann Surg 211:703, 1990.

Trunkey D: Initial treatment of patients with extensive trauma. N Engl J Med 324:1444, 1991.

16
SURGICAL COMPLICATIONS

JAMES A. SCHULAK, M.D.

After every operation, complications may occur that, if not recognized early and acted upon, can cause morbidity or even death. The aim of this chapter is to familiarize the student with the variety of postoperative complications encountered following surgical operations. Both during and after a surgical procedure, the patient should be monitored for fever, tachycardia, tachypnea and dyspnea, hypotension, oliguria, jaundice, progressive abdominal distention, and pain out of proportion to the incisional trauma. Also of importance is the development of mental status changes such as anxiety, confusion, somnolence, stupor, and coma. Most surgical complications are manifested by one or more of these signs (Table 1).

POSTOPERATIVE FEVER

An elevation in temperature is frequently observed following operation, but is not always indicative of a serious complication. Fever may be due to atelectasis, blood transfusion reactions due to mismatch or contamination, dehydration, drug therapy (e.g., amphotericin B, penicillin, and cephalosporin antibiotics), or phlebitis at intravenous site, as well as being a natural physiologic response to stress and trauma. Fever may also signal the presence of infections such as pneumonia, cystitis, intraperitoneal abscess, central venous line sepsis, or wound infection. Rarer causes of fever include anesthesia-induced hyperthermia, deep vein thrombophlebitis, pulmonary embolism, myocardial infarction, and the underlying disease. Common causes of postoperative fever are summarized in Table 2.

Frequently, postoperative fever can be traced to the lungs, due either to atelectasis or pneumonitis. Accordingly, inspection of the patient's breathing pattern

and auscultation of the lungs are essential components of the initial evaluation of fever. Routine chest films are not advocated unless either physical signs of pneumonia are present or the fever persists despite measures taken to reexpand the lungs. Because urinary tract infection (UTI) is the most frequently encountered nosocomial infection in patients following either catheterization or instrumentation of the bladder, it too is a frequent cause of postoperative fever. Analysis of a urine sample may reveal leukocytes and bacteria or leukocyte esterase activity, all indicative of an acute UTI. Intravenous cannulation sites should be carefully examined for phlebitis. Catheter removal may resolve the fever; however, with septic thrombophlebitis, complete excision of the suppurative vein is recommended. Blood cultures should be obtained as part of the initial evaluation in many patients with a fever of greater than 38.5°C. Additional laboratory tests are indicated in immunosuppressed patients such as recipients of cancer chemotherapy or organ transplants because the variety of possible infections is greater, including those caused by fungi, parasites, and viruses. Wound infection may occur at any time following operation, and examination of the wound is mandatory in the postoperative evaluation of fever.

INFECTION

Intra-abdominal Abscess

Postoperative intraperitoneal abscesses may occur at any site in the peritoneal cavity and are best demonstrated by computed tomography (CT). While they may occur at any time, fever, chills, leukocytosis, or abdominal pain may not develop until a week or more after operation. Often rectal and/or vaginal examina-

TABLE 1. PHYSICAL SIGNS AND SYMPTOMS OF SURGICAL COMPLICATIONS AND THEIR COMMON ASSOCIATED CONDITIONS

Symptom	Associated Conditions
Fever	Atelectasis, infections, transfusion reactions, drug therapy, thrombophlebitis, pulmonary embolus
Tachycardia	Anxiety, hypovolemia, hypoxemia, fever, cardiac arrhythmia, sepsis, pain
Tachypnea and dyspnea	Anxiety, atelectasis, pneumonia, pulmonary edema, pulmonary embolus
Hypotension	Hypovolemia, sepsis, cardiac failure, anaphylaxis, hemorrhage
Oliguria	Hypovolemia, renal failure, urinary tract obstruction
Jaundice	Hemolysis, hepatitis, sepsis, central venous nutrition, biliary tract obstruction, bile fistula
Abdominal distention	Paralytic ileus, intra-abdominal hemorrhage, bowel obstruction, constipation, ascites
Wound pain	Infection, dehiscence, intra-abdominal infection
Mental status change	Hypoxemia, sepsis, drugs, alcohol withdrawal, stroke, fever, postoperative psychosis

tion suffice to make the diagnosis of pelvic abscess by revealing a tender mass. Subphrenic and subhepatic abscesses may present with upper abdominal pain and fullness, as well as back, pleuritic, or shoulder pain. Upright chest films may reveal a pleural effusion on the side of the abscess, an elevated hemidiaphragm and the presence of air bubbles, or an air-fluid level immediately under the diaphragm. Although subhepatic abscesses may occur after operations on the biliary tract or duodenum, most fluid collections following right upper quadrant procedures are sterile and do not require drainage. All intra-abdominal abscesses require drainage, which often can be accomplished by a

TABLE 2. COMMON CAUSES OF FEVER IN THE POSTOPERATIVE PATIENT

1. Pulmonary causes
   Aelectasis
   Pneumonia
   Pulmonary embolism
2. Infections
   Intravenous line inflammation and sepsis
   Urinary tract infection (UTI)
   Intra-abdominal abscess
   Peritonitis
   Empyema
   Wound infections
   Cholecystitis
   Parotitis
3. Deep vein thrombosis and phlebitis
4. Drug therapy (penicillin, cephalosporin, amphotericin)
5. Transfusion reactions

CT-guided percutaneous catheter. Surgical drainage of pelvic abscesses may be performed through the rectum or the vagina or through a small lower abdominal incision, and subphrenic abscesses may be drained through either an extraperitoneal or intraperitoneal approach. Other abscesses include those loculated by the omentum and/or visceral surfaces and those in the solid organs. Patients with interloop abscesses may present with localized pain and tenderness and bowel obstruction in addition to the usual systemic signs described above. Visceral abscesses in the liver, spleen, pancreas, kidney, and female adnexae are demonstrated best by CT. Laparotomy is often necessary to achieve complete drainage of these complex infections.

Peritonitis

Generalized peritonitis following surgery is often associated with anastomotic breakdown that usually occurs 5 to 7 days after operation, but also may be due to spontaneous perforation of the bowel, caused by either occult intraoperative injuries or fecal erosion of the colon (stercoral ulcer) in the presence of postoperative obstipation. Symptoms include unexplained tachycardia, fever, abdominal pain, and sometimes mental status changes. The diagnosis, which is suggested by free air on an abdominal film, may be confirmed by demonstration of extravasation using water-soluble contrast radiography in patients with either an upper gastrointestinal or a colonic anastomosis. Paracentesis may be helpful by demonstrating the presence of bile, leukocytes, food particles, amylase, or bacteria in the aspirated fluid. Anastomotic breakdown or visceral perforation requires urgent reoperation to either revise or exteriorize the anastomosis. Some bowel injuries and anastomotic leaks may cause enterocutaneous fistulas without generalized peritonitis or abscess formation because the leaked bowel contents track directly to the incompletely healed wound. Frequently, these fistulas can be managed successfully by placing the bowel at rest and instituting central venous nutrition. Fistulas that develop in ischemic or irradiated bowel, that are associated with the presence of a foreign body, or that occur in a loop of bowel that is either obstructed distally or involved with malignancy are unlikely to close without reoperation.

Intrathoracic Infections

Postoperative infections in the thorax include pneumonia, lung abscess, empyema, and mediastinitis. Lung abscess due to incompletely treated bacterial, tuberculous, or fungal infection often appears as cavitary lesions on either chest film or CT scan. Therapy consists of long-term administration of antibiotics, respiratory therapy to affect spontaneous drainage, and bronchoscopic evacuation of the abscess when appropriate. Operation is indicated for lung abscess when symptoms persist, when thickened walls do not resolve, when the lesion cannot be distinguished from malignancy, or following severe hemoptysis due to erosion of the abscess cavity into a blood vessel.

Empyema, a collection of pus in the pleural space, occurs most commonly following thoracic operations for esophageal resection, abscess, or exploration for penetrating chest trauma. The chest film may reveal a pleural effusion or mass, and diagnosis is confirmed by aspiration of purulent material. Empyemas are treated by systemic antibiotic therapy and chest tube drainage. Operative intervention is reserved for those with multiple loculations.

Mediastinitis is most commonly caused by esophageal anastomotic leaks, but esophageal perforation following endoscopy or dilatation also occurs. Signs of mediastinitis include fever, tachycardia, leukocytosis, chest pain, and subcutaneous emphysema. Chest films may reveal hydropneumothorax or air-fluid levels in the mediastinum, and an esophageal injury can be demonstrated by extravasation on a water-soluble contrast esophagogram. Broad-spectrum antibiotic therapy and nasogastric aspiration may be sufficient treatment for small, immediately diagnosed esophageal perforations. However, prompt operative drainage and repair of the esophageal defect is usually indicated in all other cases of mediastinitis.

WOUND COMPLICATIONS

All operations require an incision, and healing of the wound must occur before the operation can be considered a success. Complications in wound healing are in three categories: (1) simple wound hematomas and seromas; (2) wound infections; and (3) wound dehiscence. They occur because of imperfect surgical technique and alterations in wound healing due to many influences that are discussed in Chapter 10.

Hematoma and Seroma

Inadequate wound hemostasis causes the accumulation of blood in the wound after its closure. Coagulopathies due to the patient's disease or due to the perioperative administration of aspirin, heparin, warfarin, or dextran can also contribute to the development of wound hematomas. Physical findings include swelling and pain in the wound and drainage of blood from the suture line if the hematoma is superficial. If bleeding is arterial, the hematoma may dissect between tissue planes and grow to considerable size.

Rapidly expanding hematomas may compress adjacent vital structures such as the trachea causing ventilatory stridor, the carotid artery causing a neurological deficit, or the renal veins causing renal dysfunction. Wound hematomas often resolve spontaneously, but large, expanding, and painful hematomas require surgical reexploration. Wound collections of nonhematogenous fluid may be classified as seromas or lymphoceles. Their development is usually due to the creation of large subcutaneous spaces within the wound that collect serum and/or lymph. Simple seromas usually resolve either spontaneously or after aspiration, but true lymphoceles due to active secretion from a major lymphatic channel may require repeated aspirations or suction drainage to cure. With either technique, sterility must be maintained to prevent development of a secondary wound abscess.

Wound Infections

Wound infections may occur in as many as 20 per cent or more of cases in which the operative field was *contaminated* during the operation. Conversely, clean operations not involving the gastrointestinal tract should have an infection rate of 2 per cent or less. Signs of wound infection include fever, wound tenderness, and inflammation in the early stages. Swelling, purulent drainage, tissue ischemia, and wound breakdown may eventually occur if the infection is not recognized and treated expeditiously. Wound sepsis can occur within 24 hours following operation if the causative organisms are *Streptococcus* or *Clostridia* species. Infections due to the latter are extremely serious, as clostridial myonecrosis (gas gangrene) can develop rapidly. A thin serous discharge, crepitus, and wound ischemia signal its presence, and urgent surgical débridement is mandatory. More commonly, wound infections become evident between the fourth and seventh postoperative day, due to either gram-negative bacteria or *Staphylococcus* species. Antibiotic therapy may be useful in treating early wound cellulitis, but unless systemic sepsis is present, it is generally of little aid after adequate surgical débridement and drainage have been accomplished.

Wound Dehiscence

Disruption of the surgical wound may occur anytime after an operation, but is most common approximately 1 week after operation. Wound dehiscence can involve part or all of the wound layers. Skin dehiscence usually is of little consequence because the wound can be reapproximated rather easily, often without return to the operating room. Fascial dehiscence, however, is a much more serious complication because it (1) requires operative repair to prevent an incisional hernia, (2) is often due to a wound infection, and (3) may lead to evisceration. The latter occurs when the viscera (usually small intestine in an abdominal wound) protrude through the wound or onto the abdominal wall. Evisceration is a surgical emergency requiring careful replacement of the viscera into the peritoneal cavity, protection from injury and drying by use of saline-soaked gauze as a covering, and prompt return to the operating room for surgical repair. Wound dehiscence can be precipitated by many factors, including obesity, malnutrition, diabetes, renal failure, ascites, abdominal distention, persistent coughing or vomiting, wound infection (up to 50 per cent of cases), suture breakage, and wound ischemia due to improper suture techniques. Most commonly, dehiscence of an incision is due to faulty surgical technique. Dehiscence is often signaled by sudden drainage of serosanguinous fluid from the wound between 5 and 8 days after operation. When this is observed, the wound should be carefully palpated for signs of breakdown, and if necessary, several stitches or staples should be removed so that integrity of the fascial closure can be ascertained.

RESPIRATORY COMPLICATIONS

Respiratory complications are the most common problems experienced by patients undergoing an operation and include: (1) atelectasis, (2) pneumonia, (3) acute postoperative respiratory insufficiency, (4) adult respiratory distress syndrome (ARDS), and (5) pulmonary embolism. Normal ventilatory and respiratory mechanisms are often adversely affected by surgical procedures because of long-duration anesthesia, mechanical ventilation, pain due to surgical incisions, administration of certain analgesic agents that depress respiratory drive, and use of nasogastric tubes. Intrinsic factors that predispose the patient to pulmonary complications include old age, obesity, poor nutritional status, chronic obstructive or restrictive pulmonary disease, and cigarette smoking. A brief discussion of the common respiratory complications follows. The student also is referred to Chapters 46 and 48 for a more in-depth consideration of these topics.

Atelectasis

Atelectasis, or incompletely ventilated lung, occurs to some degree after all operations and is a common cause of postoperative fever. Although atelectasis can be caused by bronchial mucus plugs and extrinsic compression from hemopneumothorax, alveolar hypoventilation due to shallow breathing is most common. The treatment of atelectasis is reexpansion of the lungs, which usually causes rapid resolution of the fever. This can be accomplished by early postoperative ambulation, which allows for a fuller diaphragmatic excursion and by deep breathing and coughing exercises, as well as through the use of incentive spirometers. Of equal importance is the provision of adequate analgesia. Atelectasis that is progressive and accompanied by dyspnea or increasing fever may be due to a mucus plug blocking a segmental or lobar bronchus. The diagnosis is suggested by lobar collapse on chest film, and treatment consists of aggressive chest physiotherapy and bronchoscopy when necessary for extrication of the plug.

Pneumonia

Postoperative pneumonia is usually a nosocomial infection and, as such, has a greater potential for morbidity and mortality because of the many resistant organisms that can be contracted in a hospital environment. Risk factors include old age, presence of underlying pulmonary or cardiovascular disease, cigarette smoking, long preoperative hospitalization, thoracic or upper abdominal incisions, immnosuppressive therapy, and the necessity for prolonged ventilatory support. The most common cause of postoperative pneumonia is aspiration. Nasogastric intubation enhances the possibility of aspiration by interfering with the normal defense mechanisms of swallowing, coughing, and gagging. Inhalation of bacteria that may contaminate the ventilator itself, although rare, should be considered in all ventilated patients with pneumonia, especially those in an intensive care unit where other patients with pneumonia may have been. Lymphohematogenous spread of bacteria from infections in the bladder, the wound, or an abscess occurs, and identification of the causative organism at these sites may be helpful in selection of appropriate antibiotic therapy.

The diagnosis of postoperative pneumonia is suggested by the presence of fever, tachypnea, cough, rales or signs of consolidation on pulmonary auscultation, purulent sputum production, and pulmonary infiltrates on chest film. However, the latter may lag behind the development of clinical signs by several days. Generally, lobar consolidation is indicative of a bacterial pneumonia, and interstitial infiltrates are indicative of a viral pneumonia. Confirmatory evidence is obtained through isolation of a pathogen. Sputum samples should contain leukocytes to be considered adequate and are obtained by endotracheal lavage in the intubated patient and either nasotracheal or transtracheal aspiration in the nonintubated patient who cannot produce a suitable specimen by coughing. In immunosuppressed patients, where early and specific antibacterial therapy is of critical importance, the diagnosis may require transpleural needle aspiration, bronchoscopy, or even open lung biopsy. Treatment of postoperative bacterial pneumonia includes administration of the appropriate antibiotics and facilitation of adequate pulmonary toilet. In patients with suspected aspiration, it is important to include an agent that provides coverage for anaerobic bacteria.

Acute Respiratory Insufficiency

Acute postoperative respiratory insufficiency may present as either failure of the patient to meet acceptable criteria for extubation following operation (see below) or the urgent necessity for reintubation with resumption of ventilator support. Prolonged ventilator dependency following general endotracheal anesthesia is most frequently experienced by elderly patients with preexisting pulmonary disease, by patients who have undergone long operations, and by those who are nutritionally depleted and thereby lack adequate energy for the muscular work of ventilation. Pulmonary edema, which can develop unexpectedly during an operation, also alters pulmonary gas exchange and thereby may impede successful extubation in the early postoperative period.

The need for urgent reintubation also may have a pharmacologic etiology. Anesthetic agents such as methoxyflurane can accumulate in the adipose tissue of obese individuals and be released in a rebound manner, causing respiratory depression after extubation. Muscle relaxants administered during the operation may also accumulate and interfere with resumption of spontaneous ventilation, especially in patients with renal failure. Postoperative suppression of ventilatory drive also can be due to overdosage with narcotic analgesics, and treatment consists of pharmacologic reversal with the narcotic antagonist naloxone.

Successful endotracheal extubation can generally be predicted in the majority of patients by the following criteria: evidence that neuromuscular blockage is reversed; a PCO_2 of 40 mm Hg or lower; a breathing rate of 15 to 25 breaths per minute; a tidal volume of 5 to 7 ml/kg, and a PO_2 of at least 65 to 70 mm Hg with the patient breathing room air. Indications for urgent reintubation include respiratory distress with an increasing rate of greater than 30 to 40 breaths per minute, a low tidal volume of less than 300 ml per breath, carbon dioxide retention with PCO_2 in the greater than 50 mm Hg range, and arterial blood hypoxia with PO_2 of less than 65 mm Hg.

Adult Respiratory Distress Syndrome

Adult respiratory distress syndrome is distinctly different from acute postoperative ventilator dependence in that pathologic changes occur in the lungs. Adult respiratory distress syndrome, which has been observed in the pediatric age group as well, commonly occurs in the setting of massive trauma, shock from any cause, intracranial injury, burns, sepsis, pancreatitis, long-bone fractures, and multiple transfusions. The clinical manifestations of ARDS are usually associated with satisfactory pulmonary function in the immediate postoperative period, with later development of tachypnea, anxiety, and breathing fatigue. Increased arteriovenous shunting causes hypoxemia, and bilateral pulmonary infiltration invariably develops. Pulmonary function studies reveal a decrease in compliance and functional residual capacity. Endothelial and alveolar membrane injury causes accumulation of fluid and protein in the alveolar air space, severe pulmonary edema, and the development of hyaline membranes. Microvascular obstruction due to cytokine-mediated attraction of white blood cells and upregulation of intercellular adhesion molecules on the endothelial cells also contribute to injury. Neither reducing the amount of intravenous fluid administration nor increasing the amount of inspired oxygen is adequate to overcome this situation in most cases.

The treatment of ARDS requires mechanical ventilation with positive end-expiratory pressure (PEEP). The use of diuretics may be warranted to reduce pulmonary edema, and patients with renal failure may benefit from urgent dialysis. Positive airway pressure prevents further alveolar collapse and promotes reinflation of collapsed alveoli. This increases functional residual capacity, decreases arteriovenous shunting, and improves oxygenation. The use of PEEP permits reduction in the FIO_2, thereby decreasing the risk of pulmonary fibrosis due to oxygen toxicity. Complications of positive-pressure ventilation include alveolar rupture with development of pneumothorax, pneumomediastinum, and pneumoperitoneum. A decrease in cardiac output may also occur due to reduced venous return from the lungs. Consequently, frequent auscultation of the chest, serial chest x-rays, and monitoring of cardiac output is necessary for all patients being ventilated with positive airway pressure.

RENAL DYSFUNCTION

Postoperative oliguric renal insufficiency is defined as urine output of less than 500 ml/day or less than 0.5 ml/kg/hr and is a hallmark of impending acute renal failure (ARF). Complete anuria is rare and is seen primarily in patients with a postrenal obstruction or with irreversible cortical necrosis. Renal insufficiency also may be manifested by high-volume urine output and, as such, may not be appreciated early in its course. Renal failure has been classically subdivided into three categories depending upon the site of abnormal physiology: prerenal, renal, and postrenal. An in-depth discussion of renal failure is presented in Chapter 17.

ALIMENTARY TRACT DYSFUNCTION

Anorexia, Nausea, and Vomiting

Anorexia is mediated by the hypothalamus and is generally associated with decreases in gastrointestinal motility due to intra-abdominal inflammation, carcinoma, intestinal obstruction, hepatitis, congestive heart failure, and adrenal insufficiency, as well as many other conditions. Nausea, a sensation that encompasses anorexia, gastric bloating, and the need to vomit, may be secondary to paralytic ileus, mechanical small-bowel obstruction, intra-abdominal abscess and inflammation, and the administration of various drugs. Treatment consists of limiting oral intake to liquids and using antiemetic agents. Nausea and vomiting due to paralytic ileus or bowel obstruction may also require decompression by a nasogastric tube. Physiologic consequences of vomiting include hypovolemia, hypokalemia, alkalosis, and aspiration pneumonia.

Diarrhea and Colitis

Postoperative diarrhea is often due to mechanical, infectious, or physiologic consequences of the operation performed. Diarrhea may be the first sign of pelvic abscess, enterocolic or gastrocolic fistula, or fecal impaction. Therefore, all patients require a careful rectal examination, proctoscopy and, possibly, a contrast enema radiograph if a fistula is suspected. Diarrhea may also occur as a consequence of ingestion of large amounts of magnesium-containing antacids.

Infectious colitis is a frequent cause of postoperative diarrhea. While salmonella, shigella, staphylococci, campylobacter, and parasitic or protozoan infections are occasionally seen, development of pseudomembranous enterocolitis due to *Clostridium difficile*, a toxin-releasing anaerobic bacterium, is a more common complication. Pseudomembranous colitis, which often follows systemic antibiotic therapy, presents initially with cramping abdominal pain and distention, but fever, chills, and diarrhea may soon follow. Proctoscopic examination reveals an edematous and friable colonic mucosa that is covered with the thin yellow pseudomembranes. Diagnosis is confirmed by isolation of *C. difficile*, or its toxin, from the stool. The disease may be mild, with self-limited diarrhea; or progressive, with the development of intractable diarrhea, toxic colonic dilatation, and even perforation. Ther-

apy is supportive, with immediate cessation of unnecessary antibiotics, fluid and electrolyte resuscitation, and oral administration of vancomycin or metronidazole. Urgent total abdominal colectomy may be required in the event of toxic megacolon or perforation.

Constipation and Fecal Impaction

Constipation in the immediate postoperative period is often due to paralytic ileus and is self-limited in duration. Constipation in elderly and diabetic patients, many of whom are laxative dependent, is often due to the loss of normal muscular tone in the colon and gastrointestinal neuropathy. In both situations, early intervention with stool-softening agents and cathartics may be appropriate, since spontaneous bowel movements are rare. Pharmacologic causes of constipation include aluminum-containing antacids, some calcium channel blockers, and narcotic analgesics. When oral intake is satisfactory, a high-fiber diet and increased fluids may be helpful in establishing a regular pattern of defecation. Rectal examination should be performed on constipated patients to evaluate for fecal impaction, which may require digital extrication in addition to enemas. Lubricating agents such as mineral oil given by mouth may also be helpful. Caution should be taken, however, in prescribing osmotically active oral preparations if total or near total obstruction is present, as this may cause marked distention and further increase in discomfort. Fecal impaction that is not successfully treated may lead to development of a stercoral ulcer and subsequent colonic perforation with fecal peritonitis. Patients who have not passed either flatus or feces should also be evaluated for postoperative bowel obstruction.

Paralytic Ileus

Paralytic ileus, defined as either a lack of peristaltic activity or disorganized contraction of the gut, is most commonly associated with intraperitoneal operations, inflammatory processes (abscess, hematoma, peritonitis), and retroperitoneal injuries. Stasis of swallowed air and intraluminal fluid in the stomach and small bowel gives rise to nausea, abdominal distention, and sometimes vomiting. Visceral distention may be severe enough to cause the patient extreme discomfort, especially if it causes an acute gastric or colonic dilatation. Peristaltic bowel sounds are either absent or infrequent, helping to distinguish this entity from postoperative mechanical bowel obstruction, in which bowel sounds are hyperactive and peristalsis may be visible through the abdominal wall. Abdominal radiographs reveal gas-filled loops of bowel throughout the abdomen including both large and small intestine, whereas mechanical small-bowel obstruction is suggested by the presence of air-fluid levels and little or no colonic gas. Treatment of paralytic ileus consists of aspiration of the stomach with a nasogastric tube and provision of adequate intravenous fluids to compensate for third-space losses. Peristalsis usually returns to the small intestine and stomach within 24 hours of operation, but paralysis of the colon, particularly the sigmoid colon, may last up to 72 hours or longer. Persistent or progressive colonic dilation, especially with a cecal diameter greater than 10 to 12 cm, may require colonoscopic decompression to prevent perforation. Paralytic ileus that persists for greater than 4 days may be signaling the presence of peritonitis, hypokalemia, anastomotic leak, intraperitoneal abscess, hematoma, or incipient mechanical bowel obstruction.

Postoperative Bowel Obstruction

Postoperative bowel obstruction should be suspected in patients who do not regain bowel function in the time course described above and who demonstrate the clinical and radiographic criteria for mechanical obstruction. When in doubt, however, the diagnosis can be confirmed by use of barium contrast enteroclysis. Early mechanical small-bowel obstruction is often self-limited in duration and is treated by a slightly prolonged period of nasogastric intubation. Operative intervention should be elected whenever the patient has evidence for a complete or closed loop obstruction or intestinal gangrene manifested by tachycardia, fever, leukocytosis, rebound tenderness, and peritonitis. Failure of a postoperative obstruction to resolve spontaneously within a week of onset often warrants reexploration, as the morbidity of such an operation may be less than that of continued observation.

Acute Gastric Mucosal Hemorrhage

Hemorrhage from diffuse gastric mucosal ulceration usually occurs in severely ill patients who have experienced either a major operation or extensive trauma. Endoscopy, which is essential to exclude other causes of upper gastrointestinal hemorrhage, reveals diffuse shallow mucosal ulcers and hemorrhage throughout the stomach. Treatment primarily consists of neutralization of the gastric pH by administration of antacids, histamine receptor antagonists, or the parietal cell inhibitor, omeprazole. Rarely, total gastrectomy may be necessary to control life-threatening hemorrhage.

HEPATOBILIARY COMPLICATIONS AND JAUNDICE

The development of postoperative hyperbilirubinemia may be due to overproduction of bile pigments, decreased ability of the liver to process the pigment load due either to parenchymal disease or to cholestasis, or obstruction of the biliary ductal system. The initial step in evaluating the newly jaundiced patient is to determine to which of these broad categories the patient belongs (see Table 3).

Intravascular hemolysis and reabsorption of extravasated blood from intra-abdominal, retroperitoneal, and pelvic hematomas are the two most common sources of increased pigment load in the postoperative period, and both are manifested by indirect hyperbilirubinemia. Hemolysis may be due to transfusion of mismatched blood, hemoglobinopathy, autoimmunity, or sepsis, or may be precipitated by administration of various drugs. Diagnosis of hemolysis is confirmed by an elevated unconjugated serum bilirubin fraction, reduced serum haptoglobin concentration, and normal liver enzyme profile. Therapy of hemolytic jaundice is directed to correction of the underlying cause.

Parenchymal hepatic disorders are responsible for the development of postoperative jaundice in a large portion of patients. Hypotension, hypoxia, and septic shock may cause anoxic liver cell injury which, in turn, causes decreased cellular excretion of bilirubin, intrahepatic cholestasis, and hepatocyte necrosis. Cholestatic jaundice also may be due to drug therapy and central venous nutrition. Hepatocellular injury due to

TABLE 3. COMMON CAUSES OF JAUNDICE IN POSTOPERATIVE PATIENTS

1. Hemolysis
    Extravasated blood, hematomas
    Transfusion reactions
    Drug reactions
    Sepsis
    Hemaglobinopathies
2. Hepatic parenchymal disease
    Exacerbation of preexisting liver disease
    Viral hepatitis
    Drug (anesthesia)-induced hepatitis
    Shock-induced injury
    Intrahepatic abscess
3. Cholestasis
    Drug induced
    Sepsis
    Central venous nutrition
4. Biliary tract disease
    Choledocholithiasis
    Inadvertent bile duct ligature
    Bile fistula or leak
    Cholecystitis
    Pancreatitis with bile duct obstruction
    Bile duct stricture due to injury

chronic hepatitis or alcoholism may predate the operation. Postoperative anesthesia-induced hepatitis is an often-implicated but rarely proven event that has been associated with administration of either halothane or methoxyflurane to patients who presumably have a hypersensitivity to these agents.

Viral hepatitis due to transfusion of infected blood is not observed until several weeks or more after surgery due to the necessary incubation periods of the various viral pathogens. Because of diligent screening protocols, hepatitis B is less prevalent now than in the past, but hepatitis due to cytomegalovirus, or hepatitis C, is being diagnosed more commonly. Consequently, evaluation of postoperative jaundice should include tests for all of these viral pathogens. Postoperative biliary tract obstruction is most commonly observed in patients who have undergone a biliary tract procedure. Hyperbilirubinemia is of the conjugated variety, is associated with an absence of urinary urobilinogen, and is accompanied by a marked rise in serum alkaline phosphatase. The presence of fever, chills, and pain suggests the development of cholangitis and sepsis and requires appropriate antibiotic therapy and expedient surgical or endoscopic drainage. Diagnosis of biliary obstruction is confirmed using radiologic techniques. If a T-tube is in place, a cholangiogram should be performed. Cholescintigraphy with ^{99m}technetium-labeled iminodiacetic acid (IDA) derivatives may be useful in diagnosing the presence of obstructive jaundice in patients who do not have a common bile duct drain. Although ultrasonography of the bile ducts may be helpful by demonstrating choledochal calculi and ductal dilation, percutaneous transhepatic cholangiography (PTC) or endoscopic retrograde cholangiopancreatography (ERCP) provide the most definitive imaging of the biliary ductal system in patients who cannot undergo T-tube cholangiography. The appropriate therapeutic measures and surgical options for the patient with postoperative obstructive jaundice or biliary fistula are considered in Chapter 33.

Extrahepatic biliary obstruction may also be due to cholecystitis and/or pancreatitis. Although in most cases acute cholecystitis is associated with gallbladder stones, acalculous cholecystitis is sometimes encountered in the postoperative period. Diagnosis is made by eliciting physical signs of right upper quadrant inflammation and obtaining either ultrasound or CT evidence for gallbladder edema and dilation. Radionuclear cholescintigraphy can provide supporting data by revealing nonvisualization of the gallbladder. Laparoscopic evaluation of the upper abdomen is beginning to gain acceptance as a means of making this diagnosis in difficult cases. Because of the risk of gangrene, acute postoperative acalculous cholecystitis usually requires urgent cholecystectomy.

DEEP VENOUS THROMBOSIS AND PULMONARY EMBOLISM

Deep Venous Thrombosis

Preoperative and postoperative venous stasis in the lower extremities coupled with postoperative hypercoagulability leads to thrombosis in the deep veins. Other predisposing factors for deep venous thrombosis (DVT) include obesity, cancer, chronic venous insufficiency, and long operations. Most often, DVT occurs in the calf and thigh veins, but may also occur in the iliac veins from where subsequent progression to pulmonary embolism is more common. Signs of DVT are tenderness, swelling, pain upon movement, and sometimes fever. Diagnosis of DVT, however, requires plethysmographic, Doppler ultrasonographic, or radiographic techniques to demonstrate venous obstruction or presence of thrombus. Clinical signs alone may be false-positive indicators of DVT in up to 50 per cent of cases.

The treatment of DVT requires therapeutic anticoagulation with intravenous heparin therapy and eventual conversion to oral warfarin therapy in order to prevent pulmonary embolism. A period of up to 1 week of bed rest also may be indicated for patients in whom the thrombus does not appear to be adherent to the vein wall on either Doppler duplex scan or venography. The best treatment is prevention, which can be achieved by early postoperative ambulation, use of intermittent compression stockings both during and after operation and, in some cases, use of low-dose perioperative heparin therapy.

Pulmonary Embolism

Pulmonary embolism (PE) is the most serious complication of DVT because it can lead to respiratory compromise and sudden death. The symptoms of PE include dyspnea, coughing, and bronchospasm, but many patients may be asymptomatic. Clinical signs include tachypnea, tachycardia, and fever, and laboratory analysis should reveal a low PaO_2 of less than 70 mm Hg. Diagnosis is strongly suggested by a vascular filling defect on a pulmonary nuclear perfusion scan. Normal scans safely exclude major PE, but intermediate scans are not helpful. Definitive diagnosis can be obtained by pulmonary artery angiography. Pulmonary embolism is treated by systemic anticoagulation as described for DVT. Recurrent PE in the face of anticoagulation, septic pulmonary embolization, and a contraindication to use of anticoagulation therapy indicates the need for vena caval interruption (ligation or filter insertion) to prevent further embolization from the pelvic or lower extremity source. Recent increased use of subclavian vein venous catheters has increased the incidence of subclavian vein thrombosis and PE from that site. A more detailed discussion of pulmonary embolism can be found in Chapter 46.

MENTAL STATUS ABNORMALITIES

Mental status changes following operation include failure to awaken following operation, somnolence, coma, confusion, disorientation, agitation, and convulsions. These disturbances may be the result of physiologic abnormalities such as hypoxia, hypoglycemia, uremia, and elevated blood ammonia; or by various drugs such as narcotic analgesics, tranquilizers, and cimetidine in the elderly. Specific intracranial lesions such as strokes, brain abscess, and unrecognized injuries in victims of multiple trauma can also cause disorders of consciousness and orientation. Failure to awaken after operation is most often due to persistence of the anesthetic agents and is usually self-limited in duration. Cerebrovascular accident, however, must be considered in all patients with preoperative carotid bruits, those undergoing operations in which the carotid artery was cross-clamped, and in those with significant hypotensive periods during the operation. Although agitation and anxiety in the immediate postoperative period are usually due to pain, discomfort from indwelling endotracheal and nasogastric tubes, or inability to empty a full bladder, hypoxemia and intra-abdominal hemorrhage must also be considered. Postoperative hallucinations may be due to meperidine or pentazocine therapy and improve after the parenteral analgesic agent is switched. The somnolence of narcotic overdose can be treated with naloxone.

Mental status changes that occur several days after operation are often due to metabolic abnormalities. Hyponatremia, hypoglycemia, and hypercalcemia may cause somnolence or coma; while hypocalcemia, hypomagnesemia, and hypophosphatemia are associated with tremors and agitation. Postoperative convulsions are often due to preexisting epilepsy, but may also be secondary to metabolic abnormalities. Therapy consists of maintenance of the airway, protecting the patient from injury, and administration of the usual anticonvulsant drugs including diazepam, barbiturates, and phenytoin. Alcoholic patients may experience delirium tremens due to sudden cessation of alcohol intake. Symptoms of this serious complication include agitation, tremulousness, disorientation, hallucinations, and convulsions. Fever, dehydration, and adrenal insufficiency may also occur. Treatment consists of sedation, rehydration, mechanical restraints if necessary and, occasionally, administration of alcohol in difficult-to-control cases.

Psychiatric disturbances after surgery are frequently observed in elderly patients, patients undergoing cardiac operations, and patients experiencing prolonged stays in an intensive care unit. Elderly patients may lose their orientation at night and become confused or even combative. This syndrome, commonly referred to as "sundowning," may be explained by the loss of familiar surroundings. Treatment consists of reassurance from the medical staff and, more importantly, from the patient's family. Tranquilizing agents, however, should be used cautiously in the elderly because they may cause paradoxic agitation in some and may precipitate respiratory and hemodynamic failure in others. Hallucinations, disorientation, and delirium are also frequently encountered in patients who are in an intensive care unit setting. While metabolic factors are sometimes implicated, environmental factors such as loss of chronologic orientation and the complete dependence upon nursing personnel also play a major etiologic role.

REFERENCES

Civetta JM, Taylor RW, Kirby RR (eds): Critical Care. Philadelphia, JB Lippincott Company, 1992.

Howard RJ, Simmons RL (eds): Surgical Infectious Diseases, ed 2. Norwalk, CT, Appleton & Lange, 1988.

Moossa AR, Mayer AD, Lavelle-Jones M: Surgical complications. In Sabiston DC Jr (ed): Textbook of Surgery, ed 14. Philadelphia, WB Saunders Company, 1991.

Rossi RL (ed): Complications in general surgery. Surg Clin North Am 71, 1991.

Wilmore DW, Brennan MF, Harken AH, Holcroft JW, Meakins JL (eds): Care of the Surgical Patient. Perioperative Management and Techniques. Scientific American, Inc, 1992.

17
ACUTE RENAL FAILURE IN SURGICAL PATIENTS

SCOTT K. PRUITT, M.D.

Despite advances in medical care, acute renal failure (ARF) remains a significant cause of morbidity and mortality, accounting for almost 5 per cent of hospital admissions in the United States. In the critically ill surgical patient, the mortality associated with ARF is greater than 50 per cent. Because many causes of renal injury are preventable and prompt therapy of ARF can often lead to recovery of renal function, an understanding of the pathogenesis and treatment of this complication is of much importance.

Classification

Acute renal failure is clinically defined as an acute loss of kidney function with the accumulation of the nitrogenous wastes blood urea nitrogen (BUN) and creatinine (Cr). When the urine output is less than 400 ml/day, ARF is classified as *oliguric*. A patient with a daily urine output of less than 50 ml/day is classified as *anuric*. In *nonoliguric* renal failure, the urine output is either normal or supranormal. Because the mortality and morbidity associated with nonoliguric ARF is almost half that seen in the oliguric form of this disease and because nonoliguric ARF is easier to manage clinically, many of the therapeutic strategies discussed below are designed to convert the oliguric to the nonoliguric form.

NORMAL RENAL FUNCTION

Renal Anatomy

A thorough understanding of normal renal anatomy and physiology is necessary to understand the pathophysiologic changes associated with ARF. The anatomic arrangement of the normal nephron is depicted in Figure 1. The blood flow to the kidneys is supplied by the renal arteries which branch from the aorta at approximately the level of the first lumbar vertebra. These vessels successively branch into interlobar, arcuate, and interlobular arteries and finally into the afferent arterioles that supply each glomerulus. The glomerular capillaries exiting the glomerulus then rejoin to form the efferent arteriole. The glomerulus is surrounded by Bowman's capsule within which is Bowman's space, the beginning of the renal tubule. Glomerular filtration rate (GFR), the rate at which substances pass from the capillary lumen into the lumen of Bowman's capsule, depends on the pressure within the glomerular capillaries (and the pressure within the tubular lumen), which is controlled by the afferent and efferent arterioles. These vessels can relax or contract in response to changes in blood pressure and thus maintain glomerular filtration pressure until the systemic blood pressure falls below 60 to 80 mm Hg. Blood from the efferent arteriole flows into another capillary bed surrounding the renal tubules, where many of the filtered substances in the tubular lumen reenter the circulation. Venules leaving this bed coalesce into larger and larger veins, finally forming the renal veins, which enter the inferior vena cava. This anatomic arrangement allows the normal kidney to efficiently perform a variety of vital functions, including (1) maintenance of extracellular fluid volume and electrolyte composition, (2) excretion of nitrogenous wastes, (3) acid-base regulation, and (4) calcium and phosphate metabolism.

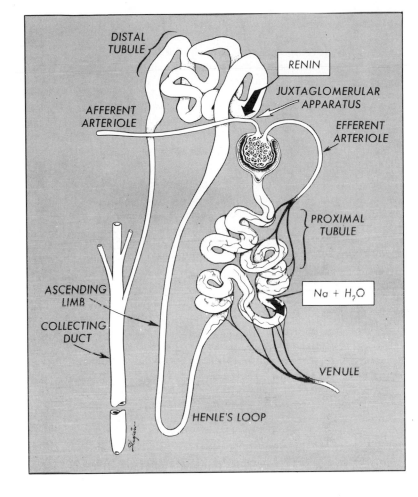

Figure 1. Principal structural features of the nephron and its blood supply. Blood enters the glomerulus through the afferent arteriole and exits through the efferent arteriole. Active dilation and constriction of these muscular vessels significantly modulate glomerular filtration. The tubule receives its blood supply primarily from the efferent arteriole. Renin is secreted by the juxtaglomerular apparatus in response to afferent blood flow and distal nephron urinary flow and composition (From Bollinger RR, Schwab SJ: Acute renal failure in surgical patients: Prevention and treatment *In* Sabiston DC Jr [ed]: Textbook of Surgery: The Biological Basis of Modern Surgical Practice, ed 14. Philadelphia, WB Saunders Company, 1991, p 319, with permission.)

Normal Renal Physiology

To regulate extracellular fluid volume, the kidney carefully controls sodium resorption from the glomerular filtrate. Sodium is resorbed by active transport in the proximal tubule, and water passively follows. Additionally, when renal blood flow is reduced, as occurs when the patient is hypovolemic, the juxtaglomerular apparatus responds by secreting renin, an enzyme which, in turn, activates plasma angiotensinogen to angiotensin I. Angiotensin I is then converted to angiotensin II by angiotensin-converting enzyme (ACE) present on vascular endothelial cells, predominantly in the lungs. Among the many systemic effects of angiotensin II is stimulation of aldosterone secretion by the adrenal glands. Aldosterone acts on the distal convoluted tubule to enhance the rate of resorption of sodium, which is passively followed by water. Osmoreceptors in the posterior pituitary gland also help control extracellular fluid volume by responding to hypertonicity of the extracellular fluid with secretion of antidiuretic hormone (ADH). The ADH then

acts at the level of the distal convoluted tubule and the collecting duct to increase permeability, allowing increased water resorption and concentration of the urine.

The thiazide diuretics (chlorothiazide, hydrochlorothiazide) block resorption of sodium in the distal convoluted tubule, which diminishes the amount of water resorbed, increases the amount of urine, and decreases the extracellular fluid volume. The loop diuretics (furosemide, ethacrynic acid) block active chloride transport in the ascending loop of Henle. Since positively charged sodium ions normally follow the negatively charged chloride ions to maintain charge neutrality, less sodium is resorbed and urine output is increased. Osmotic diuretics such as mannitol are filtered in the glomerulus, but are not reabsorbed from the tubular lumen. This raises the intraluminal oncotic pressure and inhibits passive resorption of water, increasing urine flow.

The other major electrolyte controlled by the kidney is potassium, which is secreted in the distal convoluted tubule. Because potassium secretion is directly proportional to the flow of urine through this portion of the nephron, it is easily understood why hyperkalemia can quickly develop during ARF, especially in the oliguric form of this disease. Excretion of the nitrogenous wastes, BUN and uric acid, by the kidney also depends on urine flow rate. Creatinine is filtered from the blood in the glomerulus; thus, its removal depends on GFR, which is dependent upon renal blood flow as well as tubular integrity.

The kidneys serve to regulate acid-base balance through excretion of acids and through resorption of bicarbonate (HCO_3^-) in both the proximal tubule and distal nephron. Resorbed bicarbonate combines with protons in the tubular cells to form carbonic acid (H_2CO_3). The enzyme carbonic anhydrase then catalyzes the conversion of carbonic acid to water and carbon dioxide, which is delivered to the lungs by the circulation where it is removed from the body by ventilation. When the negatively charged bicarbonate anion is resorbed, the cation which follows to maintain charge neutrality is sodium. By blocking proximal tubule bicarbonate resorption, the carbonic anhydrase inhibitor diuretic, acetazolamide, increases the sodium concentration in the tubular lumen, thus increasing urine flow.

Calcium resorption occurs in several portions of the nephron and is enhanced by parathyroid hormone. In addition, vitamin D_3, which facilitates calcium absorption from the intestines, is converted from the 25-hydroxy form to the active 1,25-dihydroxyvitamin D_3 form by the kidney. The normal kidney also excretes phosphates.

CAUSES OF ARF

The causes of ARF can be classified as prerenal, intrarenal, or postrenal (Table 1). In many patients, especially critically ill surgical patients, however, a variety of insults may combine to cause renal injury.

Prerenal Causes

Prerenal causes of ARF are those that cause hypoperfusion of the kidneys. Hypovolemia, whether occurring because of blood loss, dehydration, or "third-spacing," is a common cause of prerenal ARF and should be the first cause considered in the surgical patient with impaired renal function. Acute renal failure in this situation responds to volume infusion, but if prompt correction of the fluid deficit is not achieved, intrarenal damage occurs, with the development of acute tubular necrosis (ATN). Prerenal azotemia can also occur during cardiogenic or septic shock, conditions in which renal perfusion is diminished. Treat-

TABLE 1.   COMMON CAUSES OF SURGICAL ACUTE RENAL FAILURE*

Prerenal
  Hypotension
  Hypovolemia
  Arterial occlusion or stenosis
  Cardiac failure

Intrarenal
  Toxins (radiographic contrast, endotoxin)
  Drugs (aminoglycosides, cyclosporine, amphotericin B, nonsteroidal anti-inflammatory drugs)
  Pigment nephropathy (myoglobin, hemoglobin)

Postrenal
  Ureteral obstruction or tear (stones, trauma, surgical injury)
  Bladder dysfunction (anesthetic, nerve injury, drugs)
  Urethral obstruction (trauma, BPH, malignancy)

*From Bollinger RR, Schwab SJ: Acute renal failure in surgical patients: Prevention and treatment. *In* Sabiston DC Jr (ed): Textbook of Surgery: The Biological Basis of Modern Surgical Practice, ed 14. Philadelphia, WB Saunders Company, 1991, p 318, with permission.

ment is directed toward the underlying cardiac or infectious disease. Renal vascular occlusion, caused by stenosis, emboli, thrombosis, or operative damage to the renal artery during prolonged cross-clamping, can also lead to prerenal ARF.

Intrarenal Causes

Intrarenal causes of ARF are those that directly damage the kidney. Acute tubular necrosis, the most common intrarenal cause of ARF, is usually caused by prolonged renal hypoperfusion and is, therefore, usually a "prerenal-induced" intrarenal injury. The causes of prerenal ARF previously mentioned as well as preservation-induced injury in the transplanted kidney can all lead to ATN. In addition, any prolonged postrenal damage to the kidney can lead to ATN. Thus, rapid correction of prerenal and postrenal insults can reduce the chance of developing ATN.

Pigment nephropathy is another cause of intrarenal ARF. Large amounts of myoglobin can be released into the circulation following crush injury, burns, or major operative procedures. Free hemoglobin can be released during intravascular hemolysis, such as occurs following a mismatched blood transfusion. Metabolites of both hemoglobin and myoglobin, generated within the tubule lumen in an acidic environment, are toxic to the tubular cells.

The third major cause of intrarenal azotemia is nephrotoxic drugs, and among the many agents with renal toxicity, several are commonly encountered in the surgical patient. Aminoglycoside antibiotics (e.g., gentamicin, tobramycin), the antifungal agent amphotericin, and the immunosuppressant cyclosporine can all cause nephrotoxicity. Nonsteroidal anti-inflammatory drugs cause direct renal damage and also can produce renal vasoconstriction. Finally, radiographic contrast agents are toxic to tubular cells and cause renal vasoconstriction. The newer and much more expensive nonionic contrast agents may be less nephrotoxic.

Postrenal Causes

The third major category of causes of ARF is postrenal. Urinary obstruction is the most common cause of postrenal ARF and can be due to blood clots, calculi, catheter obstruction, prostatic hypertrophy, or traumatic injury. Extravasation of urine into the peritoneal cavity can also lead to ARF and is often the result of trauma. Iatrogenic ureteral injury can also lead to postrenal azotemia and should be considered when ARF develops following pelvic or retroperitoneal surgical procedures.

EVALUATION OF THE PATIENT WITH ARF

Diagnosing the cause of ARF can be difficult because in many critically ill patients, a variety of factors may contribute to renal injury. However, routine clinical and laboratory tests, many of them simple and inexpensive, can often be extremely helpful in establishing the cause of ARF in critically ill and less complicated patients.

History and Physical Examination

As with all patients, a detailed history should be obtained, with emphasis on preexisting renal disease, nephrotoxic drug exposure, cardiac dysfunction, and sepsis. During the physical examination, the volume status should be assessed by measuring heart rate, blood pressure, and orthostatic changes in blood pressure. Invasive monitoring of central venous pressure or Swan-Ganz catheterization may be necessary to adequately assess the patient's volume status and cardiac function. Daily weights and fluid intake and output records should also be reviewed. Rectal examination may reveal an enlarged prostate as a possible cause of obstruction, while abdominal examination may reveal a distended bladder. In male patients experiencing pelvic trauma, a displaced prostate on rectal examination suggests urethral damage and obstruction as the cause of ARF. Although obstruction can cause distention of the renal capsule and flank pain, this physical sign is nonspecific and can be caused by both renal infarction and pyelonephritis.

Laboratory Evaluation

A variety of routine laboratory tests are particularly helpful in determining the cause of ARF. Routine urinalysis with microscopic examination of the urine can provide a great deal of information and should be performed for all patients. The presence of casts in the urine usually implies ATN, but is sometimes seen with prerenal ARF. Elevated protein levels suggest renal disease, while more than 2 to 3 red blood cells per high-power field (RBC/HPF) is also consistent with underlying intrinsic renal disease. If the urine dipstick test is positive for blood but no RBC are present on microscopic examination of the urine, free hemoglobin or myoglobin are present in the urine, and pigment nephropathy is likely. Urate crystals indicate uric acid nephropathy. Urine osmolality should also be evaluated, with a value of greater than 500 mOsm suggesting prerenal ARF.

Spot measurements of urine sodium and creatinine should also be performed. In prerenal ARF, the kidney attempts to conserve sodium and the urine sodium concentration is usually less than 20 mEq/L. Comparisons between these urine levels and those from simultaneously drawn plasma are even more helpful in making a diagnosis. A urine/plasma osmolality ratio of more than 1.25 suggests prerenal ARF. A urine/plasma creatinine ratio of less than 20 is consistent with ATN, while a value greater than 40 suggests a prerenal cause of ARF. Most importantly, these laboratory values can be used to calculate the fractional excretion of sodium (FE_{Na}) using the formula:

$$FE_{Na} = (U_{Na} \times P_{creat})/(P_{Na} \times U_{creat})$$

Where U_{Na} and P_{Na}, and U_{creat} and P_{creat}, are the urinary and plasma concentrations of sodium and creatinine, respectively. A value of less than 1 strongly suggests prerenal ARF, while a value of greater than 1 suggests intrarenal or postrenal causes. A summary of useful laboratory tests in the diagnosis of the cause of ARF is found in Table 2.

Radiologic Examination

In determining the cause of ARF, ultrasound is a valuable and noninvasive method to evaluate obstruc-

TABLE 2. DIAGNOSTIC INDICES IN ARF

	Cause of ARF		
	Prerenal	*Intrarenal*	*Postrenal*
Urine osmolality (mOsm)	>500	<350	Variable
U/P osmolality	>1.25	<1.1	Variable
U/P creatinine	>40	<20	<20
Urine sodium (mEq/L)	<20	>40	>40
FE sodium	<1	>3	>3

Abbreviations: ARF = acute renal failure, U/P = urine/plasma ratio, FE = fractional excretion.

tion. Other radiologic tests that are occasionally useful in the evaluation of ARF include plain film of the abdomen (KUB), which may show enlarged kidneys or radiopaque stone, abdominal CT scan; and more invasive tests such as cystography, urethrography, and cystoscopy, for evaluation of obstruction. The intravenous pyelogram (IVP) may be useful in evaluating ureteral obstruction, intrarenal pathology, and diminished renal perfusion, but the risk of nephrotoxicity due to the intravenous contrast agent should be considered.

TREATMENT OF ARF

General Considerations

The most effective treatment of ARF is prevention, with prompt response to any conditions that might lead to further renal injury. First, adequate renal perfusion and oxygen delivery should be maintained. In the critically ill patient, "renal dose" dopamine (1 to 3 μg/kg/min intravenously) can be administered to increase GFR, renal blood flow, and urine output and, thus, may help convert oliguric to the more easily managed nonoliguric form of ARF. Diuretic therapy (usually with a loop or osmotic diuretic) is also commonly used to help convert oliguric to nonoliguric ARF, but should only be instituted after adequate intravascular volume has been achieved. Second, pigment-induced nephropathy can be lessened by expanding the extracellular volume with intravenous fluids to increase urine flow and "flush out" the myoglobin or hemoglobin from the kidney. The osmotic diuretic, mannitol, should also be administered to help increase urine flow. Alkalization of the urine to a pH of more than 7.0 by sodium bicarbonate should be given to prevent the generation of toxic metabolites of hemoglobin and myoglobin in the tubular lumen, which occurs at acidic pH. Third, drugs with nephrotoxic potential should be administered with caution and with careful attention to dosage and levels. It is particularly important to monitor serum levels of aminoglycosides and adjust dosage accordingly. If possible, nephrotoxic drugs should be discontinued if ARF develops. When radiologic studies utilizing contrast agents are necessary, the potential for renal injury can be minimized by adequate hydration prior to the diagnostic procedure.

Finally, sources of mechanical obstruction should always be considered when oliguria develops and should be strongly suspected if anuria develops suddenly. Any obstruction should be relieved immediately to minimize renal damage. Thus, when ARF develops, reversible causes of renal impairment should be sought and treated immediately. Otherwise, treatment is aimed at correcting the host of systemic alterations encountered when the kidneys are no longer able to function normally.

SYSTEMIC ALTERATIONS IN ARF

Uremia

Uremia is caused by the accumulation of nitrogenous wastes. Elevated levels of BUN and serum creatinine are useful as markers for uremia, but symptoms are more likely to develop when levels are rising rapidly rather than when a certain level is reached. Uremia can lead to altered mental status, and uremic pericarditis may develop, although this latter condition is more common in chronic renal failure. Dialysis should be instituted when BUN levels reach 80 to 100 mg/dl, or when creatinine levels reach 8 to 10 mg/dl, but should be utilized earlier if symptoms develop.

Hypervolemia

Volume overload is a common complication of ARF. Daily weights and accurate input and output records are critical in managing the patient with ARF. All possible sources of fluid input should be considered including "KVO" fluids, fluids used to flush intravenous lines, intravenous medications, and water in humidified respirators. More invasive hemodynamic monitoring with central venous pressure measurements, or even Swan-Ganz catheterization, may be necessary to accurately assess the patient's volume status. Signs and symptoms of fluid overload include peripheral edema, pulmonary edema, and congestive heart failure. Treatment usually begins with diuretic therapy, but these agents are only administered if adequate intravascular volume is present. Otherwise, the administration of diuretics worsens ARF. When diuretics and fluid restriction fail to control volume overload, dialysis should be instituted. In those patients with ARF requiring total parenteral nutrition (which necessitates large volumes of intravenous fluids) or multiple blood transfusions, dialysis should also be utilized.

Hyperkalemia

Hyperkalemia occurs in half of patients with ARF and is the most common reason for dialysis in these patients. Because damaged tissues release large amounts of potassium, patients with traumatic injury are more prone to develop this complication. Also, serum potassium levels rise in any patient with acidemia, because cells exchange extracellular protons for intracellular potassium ions. The major complication associated with hyperkalemia is cardiac irritability, which usually occurs when the serum potassium level is more than 6.0 mEq/L. The earliest electrocardiographic (ECG) changes associated with elevated serum potassium levels are peaked T waves. As potassium rises and the myocardium becomes more irritable, ECG changes progress to prolonged P-R interval, loss of P waves, widening of the QRS complex, AV block, and finally ventricular fibrillation and cardiac arrest. If the serum potassium is greater than 6.0 mEq/L and any of these conduction abnormalities develop, a potentially life threatening condition exists, and immediate therapy should be instituted with intravenous administration of 10 per cent calcium gluconate (10 ml over 5 to 10 minutes). Hypertonic glucose (50 per cent dextrose) and insulin (10 U with the glucose bolus) followed by a continuous infusion of glucose and insulin as well as the administration of intravenous sodium bicarbonate also decrease serum potassium levels. All of these therapies transiently lower the serum potassium and help avert cardiac arrest; however, none alter the amount of total body potassium. In those patients with functioning gastrointestinal tracts, the oral administration of cation exchange resins (Kayexalate) binds potassium and lowers body stores of this cation. Rectal administration of these resins is less effective. Intake of potassium, both dietary and intravenous, should also be limited to less than 40 mEq/day. If these measures fail to control serum potassium levels, dialysis should be instituted.

Hyponatremia

Hyponatremia may also develop in the patient with ARF and is usually secondary to excess free-water intake. Symptoms include altered mental status that can progress to convulsions and cerebral edema. Free-water intake should be restricted in these patients, and dialysis should be utilized if any symptoms develop.

Acid-Base Disturbances

Metabolic acidosis is another manifestation of ARF and is more likely to develop in the hypercatabolic patient in whom acid production is increased. Acidosis can also worsen the hyperkalemia seen in ARF. When the serum pH is less than 7.2, therapy should be initiated. While intravenous or oral administration of sodium bicarbonate corrects the base deficit, this sodium load can lead to volume overload in these patients. Dialysis is very effective in correcting this abnormality.

Coagulopathy

Coagulopathy often develops in the patient with ARF, due to platelet dysfunction secondary to the bio-

chemical alterations associated with this state. The platelet count is normal in these patients. This platelet defect, the anticoagulant therapy used during hemodialysis, combined with stress gastritis in these critically ill patients all combine to make acute gastrointestinal hemorrhage the second highest cause of death (after infection) in patients with ARF. As with any critically ill patient, antacids and/or H$_2$ blockers should be administered prophylactically to decrease the incidence of gastrointestinal ulceration and hemorrhage.

Altered Calcium and Phosphate Regulation

Hypocalcemia and hyperphosphatemia are two biochemical alterations seen in patients with ARF, especially those with tissue injury, which releases phosphates. Elevated phosphate levels in plasma inhibit the conversion of 25-hydroxyvitamin D$_3$ to its active form (1,25-dihydroxyvitamin D$_3$), which leads to decreased absorption of calcium from the intestine. Also, when serum phosphate levels rise, calcium and phosphate precipitate in tissues if the product of their serum concentrations (mg/dl) is greater than 55, and this further contributes to hypocalcemia. Therefore, phosphate levels should be controlled by using aluminum-containing (nonmagnesium) antacids to bind phosphates, limiting dietary intake of phosphates, and débriding necrotic tissue. If not treated, hypocalcemia may develop, with clinical tetany. The intravenous administration of calcium should be used to correct the hypocalcemia in symptomatic patients, but may lead to increased precipitation of calcium and phosphates in the soft tissues. Dialysis is effective in correcting these abnormalities.

RENAL REPLACEMENT

If any of the biochemical abnormalities of ARF cannot be controlled with more conservative therapy, dialysis should be instituted immediately. Dialysis should always be instituted early to avoid the complications associated with uremia. The indications for dialysis in ARF are listed in Table 3. Contraindications to dialysis include terminal disease, hypotension, and cardiovascular instability. Currently, dialysis can be achieved using one of three modalities: hemodialysis, peritoneal dialysis, and hemofiltration.

Hemodialysis

Hemodialysis is the most efficient and rapid method for dialysis. It requires vascular access with an in-

TABLE 3.   INDICATIONS FOR DIALYSIS*

Absolute indications (when unresponsive to conservative management)
1. Volume overload
2. Electrolyte abnormalities
3. Acidosis
4. Uremic signs and symptoms

Relative indications (when needed for improved patient management)
1. BUN > 100 mg/dl in patient with ARF
2. Need for enteral or hyperalimentation in patient with ARF
3. Need for multiple transfusions in patient with ARF
4. Hemorrhagic complications in patient with ARF
5. Drug intoxication with hemodialyzable substance

*From Bollinger RR, Schwab SJ: Acute renal failure in surgical patients: Prevention and treatment. *In* Sabiston DC Jr (ed): Textbook of Surgery: The Biological Basis of Modern Surgical Practice, ed 14. Philadelphia, WB Saunders Company, 1991, p 331, with permission.
Abbreviations: BUN = blood urea nitrogen, ARF = acute renal failure.

dwelling central line, and although systemic heparinization is usually not necessary, regional citrate anticoagulation is required. Because this method is so efficient, one of the complications may be hypotension. Other complications include a reduction in arterial oxygen saturation upon initiation of dialysis, bleeding due to anticoagulation, and cardiac arrhythmias.

Peritoneal Dialysis

Peritoneal dialysis requires the insertion of an intraperitoneal dialysis catheter, but offers the advantages that no vascular access and no anticoagulation are required. Also, while this form of dialysis is much slower and is a continuous process (24 hours a day), it does not produce the hemodynamic instability associated with hemodialysis. Therefore, peritoneal dialysis is the method of choice for dialysis of cardiac patients with ARF. The use of peritoneal dialysis is contraindicated in patients following abdominal surgery, especially those with vascular grafts. Complications of peritoneal dialysis include catheter infection and peritonitis, hyperglycemia due to the hypertonic glucose in the dialysate, diaphragmatic compromise from the fluid-filled abdomen leading to respiratory complications, and protein loss in the dialysate.

Hemofiltration

The newest form of dialysis for patients with ARF is hemofiltration, which utilizes continuous arteriovenous hemodialysis through indwelling arterial and venous catheters, usually in the femoral vessels. It is the treatment of choice for ARF in surgical patients, especially following abdominal surgery. This form of dialysis is slower than standard hemodialysis and, as such, is not ideal for the highly catabolic or hyperkalemic patient, but the slower rate minimizes hemodynamic instability. In addition, hemofiltration does not require systemic heparinization, but the hemofiltration device must be heparinized.

REFERENCES

Bollinger RR, Schwab SJ: Acute renal failure in surgical patients. *In* Sabiston DC Jr (ed): Textbook of Surgery, ed 14. Philadelphia, WB Saunders Company, 1991.
Gamelli RL, Silver GM: Acute renal failure. *In* Deitch EA (ed): Multiple Organ Failure. New York, Thieme Medical Publishers, Inc, 1990.
Mault JR, Currin SM: The renal system. *In* Lyerly HK, Gaynor JW (eds): The Handbook of Surgical Intensive Care: Practices of the Surgery Residents at the Duke University Medical Center, ed 3. Chicago, Year Book Medical Publishers, Inc, 1992.

18
TRANSPLANTATION

ROBERT C. HARLAND, M.D.

HISTORY

The concept of transplantation of body parts has long been a source of fascination and interest. In Greek mythology one finds descriptions of *chimaira*, a creature created from transplanted animal parts. Artists have portrayed the legend of Cosmos and Damian, patron saints of medicine, who transplanted the black leg of a dead Moor to a patient whose leg had been amputated. The Scottish surgeon John Hunter, widely regarded as the father of experimental surgery, performed several experiments in transplantation, such as transplanting a cock's spur to its own comb. The technique of skin grafting was developed in the 19th century and was used experimentally and clinically.

It was the pioneering work of Carrell and Guthrie in the first decade of the 20th century that provided the techniques necessary to successfully perform vascularized organ transplants. This work, which led to a Nobel Prize for Carrel in 1912, included autografts, allografts, and xenografts of a number of organs (Table 1). He utilized fine continuous suture to create vascular anastomoses without thrombosis. With this technical barrier overcome, it became apparent that there existed a separate process, later labeled rejection, that occurred in allografts and xenografts. This recognition of the immune system and its effect on foreign tissues led to declining interest in the prospects for organ transplantation. Further advances had to await a more complete understanding of rejection and its treatment. This was provided by a number of investigators who described the important role of leukocytes and antibodies, as well as the importance of tissue antigens, in the rejection of foreign tissues and organs.

The successful performance of kidney transplantation between identical twins by Murray and others in Boston in the 1950s proved that clinical transplantation was technically feasible. Newly available immunosuppressive agents such as corticosteroids and 6-mercaptopurine were utilized for cadaveric and living-related renal transplants and led to a new era of excitement in transplantation. In the 1960s, advances were made in the techniques for transplantation of the heart, liver, and other organs, but widespread clinical application of such nonrenal allografts only came after improvements in immunosuppression, mostly with the introduction of cyclosporine in the early 1980s.

IMMUNOBIOLOGY OF TRANSPLANT ANTIGENS

Cell Surface Antigens

Rejection of a transplanted organ depends on recognition by the host that the transplanted tissue is foreign or "nonself." This recognition is dependent on the presence on donor cells of distinctive cell surface proteins called *histocompatibility antigens*. In humans, these proteins are called human leukocyte antigens (HLA) and are an inherited trait coded for by the *major histocompatibility complex* (MHC) located on the short arm of human chromosome 6.

Two general types of HLA cell surface antigens are coded for by the genes of the MHC. Class I antigens (HLA-A, B, and C) contain a unique 44,000-dalton glycoprotein and a constant 12,000-dalton subunit called β_2-microglobulin, which is involved in intracellular transport and cell surface expression. Class I antigens are expressed to varying degrees on virtually all nucleated cells and are recognized by the T-cell receptor of recipient CD8$^+$ T lymphocytes (cytolytic T cells).

TABLE 1.   TRANSPLANTATION TERMINOLOGY

Recent Nomenclature	Older Nomenclature	Relationship of Donor and Recipient of Graft
Syngeneic graft	Autograft	Same individual
(Isogeneic graft)	Isograft	Same species and genetically identical
Allogeneic graft (allograft)	Homograft	Same species but not genetically identical
Xenogeneic graft (xenograft)	Heterograft	Different species

Class II molecules (HLA-DR, DP, and DQ) consist of an α (34,000-dalton) and a β (28,000-dalton) subunit. Class II antigens are present on B cells, antigen-presenting cells like macrophages, and capillary endothelial cells in humans. Class II antigens are recognized by the T-cell receptor of recipient CD4$^+$ T lymphocytes (helper T cells). The number of molecules on the surface of cells is increased by the presence of a number of cytokines such as tumor necrosis factor and interferon-γ.

In the recipient, the "self" HLA molecules present on the surface of leukocytes have an important role in the generation of the immune response. Foreign antigens, including donor HLA molecules, are *processed* and *presented* to recipient T cells with the aid of recipient HLA molecules. They provide an antigen-binding site for the foreign antigens and facilitate the interaction with the recipient T cells, aiding in the generation of the immune response. Recipient Class I molecules act as antigen-binding sites for foreign *intracellular* peptides, which are presented to Class I T cells bearing CD8 antigens. Recipient Class II molecules participate in the processing and have an antigen-presenting site for *exogenous* peptide antigens, which are presented to T cells bearing CD4 antigens. This recognition of foreign antigens in the context of self HLA molecules also provides for *MHC restriction* whereby stimulation of the immune system by this method can only be performed with the aid of antigen-presenting cells that have self HLA molecules on their cell surface.

Many Class I and Class II antigens have been identified using sera from individuals exposed to nonself antigens by blood transfusions, pregnancy, or transplantation, making it possible to "type" a potential recipient of a graft. It is well documented that limiting the number of foreign antigens on a renal allograft by matching the donor and recipient improves the chances of avoiding rejection and having long-term graft survival. This has led to a system of trying to transplant kidneys into the best matched recipient available.

GENERATION OF AN IMMUNE RESPONSE

Exposure to foreign antigens initiates a complex array of events that leads to the generation of an im-

mune response. In transplanted tissue, donor HLA molecules are recognized by a T-cell receptor on recipient lymphocytes, either on a donor-antigen–presenting cell that was transplanted with the graft or after processing by a recipient antigen-presenting cell. The activation of lymphocytes to generate an immune response is thought to require two signals. The binding of foreign antigen to a lymphocyte is the first signal. The second, or costimulatory signal, is provided by cytokines released by the antigen-presenting cell and later released by T cells. Interleukin-1 (IL-1) activates T helper cells. IL-2 is required for the activation of T cytotoxic cells, and the activation of B cells to make antibody requires the release of IL-4. The secretion of these and other cytokines leads to recruitment of other inflammatory cells, increased blood flow, and increased vascular permeability. The relative involvement of antibody and cellular elements dictates the pathologic findings of rejection. The patterns of graft rejection usually described are presented below.

Acute Cellular Rejection

Acute cellular rejection is probably the most common type of allograft rejection and is characterized by a lymphocytic infiltrate with associated macrophages, polymorphonuclear leukocytes, eosinophils, and plasma cells. Edema and, occasionally, hemorrhage are associated. Lymphocyte subset staining with antibodies usually demonstrates many CD4$^+$ or CD8$^+$ T cells. Clinically, acute cellular rejection is seen most commonly between 1 week and 6 months following transplantation, and it is manifest by graft dysfunction and often by a low-grade fever. The clinical setting and results of imaging tests may strongly suggest rejection, but a definitive diagnosis requires a transplant biopsy. Acute cellular rejection is usually treated effectively by bolus corticosteroids and/or antilymphocyte agents such as OKT3, ATG, or ALG.

Accelerated Cellular Rejection

If a patient has been remotely sensitized by blood transfusions, pregnancy, or previous transplantation, previous exposure to HLA molecules of the type found on the donor organ is possible. In this case, the cellular immune response represents a reactivation of a previous stimulus. Therefore, this anamnestic rejection response is characterized by an accelerated tempo, often beginning 4 to 6 days following transplantation. The histology is similar to that in acute cellular rejection, with a tendency toward a more dense lymphocytic infiltrate in the graft. Treatment measures are similar to those utilized in acute cellular rejection.

Hyperacute Rejection

The transplantation of a donor organ into a recipient with circulating antibody against the donor can lead to a dramatic rejection response mediated by binding of anti–donor antibody, complement activation, and severe vascular injury, leading to loss of the organ, often within minutes. Once the process begins, graft loss is difficult to avoid. Renal and cardiac allografts experience the most dramatic hyperacute rejection, but preformed antibody also adversely affects pancreas, liver, and lung allografts.

This reaction is mediated by anti-A or anti-B antibodies when transplantation is performed across the ABO barrier. For this reason, ABO incompatible transplantation is generally not performed. If the recipient has preformed antibodies against donor MHC antigens, hyperacute rejection can also occur. Screening for preformed antibody is routinely performed on all potential transplant recipients, and the specificity of the antibody or antibodies present in sensitized individuals is determined. A *crossmatch* can be performed to test for antibody in the serum against a specific donor by mixing donor lymphocytes with the serum of the potential recipient. Evidence of antibody binding to the cells, or cell lysis following the addition of complement, indicates preformed anti–donor antibody. A pretransplant crossmatch is performed before kidney transplantation and prior to transplantation of other organs when the recipient has known anti-HLA antibodies. In an unsensitized recipient of a heart or liver, the crossmatch is not required prior to transplantation because the desirability of short cold ischemic times for hearts and livers makes routine pretransplant testing difficult.

Accelerated Acute Humoral Rejection

Antibody can be produced after transplantation and cause rejection. Usually a component of rejection that includes a cellular element, it often occurs 4 to 7 days following transplantation and may represent an anamnestic response. Humoral rejection is difficult to reverse, although removing antibody by plasmapheresis has been utilized as has treatment with cyclophosphamide to diminish antibody production.

Chronic Rejection

Chronic rejection is an increasingly important cause of graft loss, accounting for much of the late (> 1 year) attrition of allografts. Common features are present in most organs. There is a predominance of injury to the antigenic targets of rejection, including arterioles, bile ducts, pancreatic acini, bronchiolar epithelium, and renal tubules. Fibrosis is prominent, as is a chronic mononuclear infiltrate. The manifestations are somewhat organ specific. Cardiac allografts demonstrate accelerated atherosclerosis, lung allografts have obliterative bronchiolitis, and livers develop "vanishing bile duct syndrome." Renal allografts usually demonstrate a progressive loss of function over several months. Grafts with a very good HLA match may be less susceptible to chronic rejection. The exact etiology (or etiologies) of chronic rejection are unclear. Some have postulated that it represents the end result of multiple episodes of acute rejection, many of which may not have been clinically apparent. There is some evidence that low levels of antibody directed against the graft may have a role. Cytomegalovirus infection has also been suggested as a factor in the development of chronic rejection, since it upregulates the expression of HLA class II molecules on graft cells. Finally, the initial damage from harvest, preservation, and reperfusion may play a role in the development of chronic rejection. Unfortunately, reliable interventions to treat chronic rejection are not available, although studies are underway with some new immunosuppressive agents.

PRINCIPLES OF IMMUNOSUPPRESSION

The successful transplantation of a kidney between identical twins in 1954 demonstrated that transplantation could be performed with technical success and that control of rejection presented the greatest obstacle to overcome. Attempts to perform successful transplantation between nonidentical twin siblings or from unrelated donors were pursued at a few centers. Immunosuppression in the 1950s was limited to total body irradiation and relatively low-potency corticosteroids. Irradiation was largely abandoned due to problems with bone marrow suppression. In the early 1960s, corticosteroids were combined with 6-mercaptopurine and, later, its derivative, azathioprine. This combination proved to be successful and served as the mainstay of immunosuppression for allotransplantation for over 20 years. It was also demonstrated at that time that acute rejection could be reversed with large doses of corticosteroids.

In the late 1970s a soil fungal metabolite, *cyclosporine*, was discovered that improved success rates of all transplants and made nonrenal transplantation a much more viable treatment option. Antilymphocyte agents such as antithymocyte globulin (ATG) and antilymphocyte serum or globulin (ALS, ALG) have been developed and are useful in the treatment of acute rejection and as induction agents in the immediate post-transplant period. Monoclonal antilymphocyte agents such as OKT3 have also found a place in the treatment of transplant recipients. New agents are being developed constantly and are added to the armamentarium of transplant clinicians when they become available. A brief description of the most widely used immunosuppressive agents follows.

Corticosteroids

These compounds are the mainstay of most immunosuppressive regimens. The precise mechanism of action is not known, although it is known that steroids block the production of IL-1 by macrophages and IL-2 by T cells. They also have anti-inflammatory properties. Side effects include glucose intolerance, weight gain, fluid retention, inhibition of wound healing, osteonecrosis, and susceptibility to infection, and they are associated with significant gastrointestinal side effects such as gastric ulcers and perforation. Many of the serious adverse effects are dose related. Fortunately, the introduction of cyclosporine has allowed a reduction in the steroid doses necessary in most protocols.

Azathioprine

Azathioprine is a purine analogue that is converted to the active metabolite 6-thioinosinic acid in the liver. This agent blocks cell proliferation by limiting DNA and RNA synthesis, thereby inhibiting replication of rapidly dividing cells, such as lymphocytes responding to the presence of a foreign graft. Its main toxicity is bone marrow suppression, and the dose is titrated according to the white blood cell count. It is also known to cause hepatitis and pancreatitis, and long-term use may increase susceptibility to skin cancer. Care must be exercised in the use with xanthine oxidase inhibitors such as allopurinol, as these affect the metabolism of azathioprine and toxic side effects may be enhanced.

Polyclonal Antiserum Against T Cells

Several preparations have been made by immunization of horses or rabbits with human thymocytes or lymphocytes to create antisera directed against human cells: ALS, ALG, and ATG. T cells are lysed when these agents are administered, rendering them quite effective for the treatment of allograft rejection. The main disadvantage of these agents is that they are foreign proteins themselves and can elicit an immune response, which can cause serum sickness and similar reactions if used repeatedly. Its potent anti–T-cell activity also causes susceptibility to infections, particularly viral infections such as cytomegalovirus.

Monoclonal Antibodies

Relatively pure and homogeneous preparations of antibodies against human lymphocytes can be made by monoclonal methodology. Currently, the most widely used monoclonal antibody is OKT3, a mouse monoclonal antibody that binds to the CD3 T-cell receptor, which is present on all mature T lymphocytes. This T-cell receptor is necessary for the recognition of Class I and Class II antigens by the lymphocyte and is necessary for the generation of effector T cells. When administered to a patient, OKT3 rapidly depletes circulating $CD3^+$ T cells. Continued therapy binds to remaining targets, blocking binding of other cells to the CD3 receptor or modulating the CD3 molecule off the surface of T cells, inhibiting their ability to respond to alloantigen.

The major side effects include a fairly profound first-dose effect manifest by fever, chills, dyspnea, and pulmonary edema, which are caused by the release of lymphokines (TNF, IFN-γ, and IL-1) from the target T cells. Pretreatment with acetaminophen, steroids, and antihistamines can limit these symptoms. Because the antibody is a mouse protein, an antimurine response may be elicited, which occasionally limits the effectiveness of subsequent courses of OKT3 therapy.

Monoclonal antibodies have been developed against other T-cell surface molecules such as CD4, as well as to receptors such as the IL-2 receptor. These hold the promise of even more specific therapy to treat rejection or possibly even induce long-term tolerance.

Cyclosporine

The introduction of this fungal metabolite into widespread clinical use in about 1980 changed transplantation in a number of ways. Because it is a potent inhibitor of the cellular response, it allows less reliance on high-dose corticosteroids and their associated complications, improving patient and graft survival. It also significantly improves the results with transplantation of extrarenal organs, opening the door for advances in the transplantation of liver, heart, pancreas, and lungs.

Cyclosporine acts on T cells by interrupting the calcium-dependent signal transduction necessary for the transcription of several early T-cell activation genes, including IL-2, IL-3, IL-4, and IFN-γ. With inhibition of synthesis and release of these cytokines, activation of helper and cytotoxic T cells is blocked. Cyclosporine also has other activities, including the inhibition of IL-1 production by macrophages.

Cyclosporine is usually used in combination with corticosteroids and azathioprine. OKT3, ALG, or ATG may also be added to the regimen in the immediate posttransplant phase. Adverse effects of cyclosporine include nephrotoxicity, especially during the recovery phase of acute tubular necrosis in renal transplants. Many centers delay initiation of cyclosporine therapy until good renal function is achieved. Chronic cyclosporine nephrotoxicity can occur, appearing as interstitial fibrosis with tubular atrophy. Cyclosporine can also cause hypertension, hyperkalemia, hypercholesterolemia, hirsutism, and neurologic abnormalities including tremors, seizures, confusion, depression, and somnolence.

FK506

FK506 is another derivative of a soil fungus with immunosuppressant effects 10 to 100 times more potent than cyclosporine. FK506 blocks T-cell activation by inhibiting cytokine transcription in T cells, as does cyclosporine. FK506 also blocks expression of IL-2 receptors on allostimulated T cells. FK506 has been shown to reverse rejection in liver transplant recipients that is resistant to conventional therapy, and it has been used in combination with low-dose corticosteroids for primary immunosuppression for hepatic allografting with favorable results. It also appears to be useful in pediatric transplantation, making it possible to wean many patients completely off corticosteroids, allowing more normal growth and development. The application of FK506 to other types of organ transplants awaits the results of ongoing trials. The toxicities of FK506 include nephrotoxicity, neurotoxicity, and glucose intolerance.

COMPLICATIONS OF IMMUNOSUPPRESSION

Infection

The development of more potent immunosuppression has been paralleled by the development of infectious complications in transplant recipients. Most patients experience at least one infection following transplantation. Initially, patients are susceptible to the common infections that occur following surgical procedures, including bacterial wound infections, pneumonia, and urinary tract infections. From 1 to 6 months following transplantation, the heavily immunosuppressed recipient is susceptible to a number of life-threatening infections, including viral and fungal infections, some of which may have been transmitted with the transplanted organ. *Cytomegalovirus* (CMV) deserves special mention because it is a relatively common infection and is the cause of significant morbidity and mortality. Cytomegalovirus is most common in patients who are heavily immunosuppressed, particularly with antilymphocyte agents. It may be transmitted with the transplanted organ or with blood products to a naive recipient, leading to a severe primary infection. The latent virus may also be reactivated in a recipient previously exposed to CMV, causing a symptomatic secondary infection. Fever and leukopenia are the most common findings. Pneumonitis, hepatitis, gastrointestinal ulcers, and encephalitis can occur. Prophylactic protocols that utilize hyperimmune globulin, ganciclovir (DHPG), and/or acyclovir are part of recipient management at most transplant centers. Treatment of symptomatic episodes relies primarily on intravenous ganciclovir.

Other significant viral infections include Epstein-Barr virus (EBV), herpes simplex virus, and herpes varicella-zoster virus. Fungal infections often occur, with *Candida* species being the most common, and are treated with antifungal agents and by minimizing broad-spectrum antibiotics. Fortunately, serious fungal infections such as those caused by *Aspergillus*, *Cryptococcus neoformans*, and *Nocardia* species, and mucormycosis are rare and usually require therapy with amphotericin B plus appropriate surgical intervention. Finally, *Pneumocystis carinii* is an important cause of pneumonia in immunocompromised patients. Prophylaxis is often administered in the form of trimethoprim sulfamethoxazole.

Malignancy

The incidence of neoplasms in immunosuppressed transplant recipients increases with time, and it is unclear whether this is due to impaired immune surveillance mechanisms, activation of latent oncogenic viruses, or a direct oncogenic effect of immunosuppressive agents. The most common malignancies in this population are nonmelanoma skin cancers. As in the general population, the incidence is related to the type of complexion and exposure to ultraviolet light. Conventional surgical and medical therapy is indicated for treatment. Squamous cell carcinoma appears to be more virulent than in nonimmunosuppressed patients, with a 25- to 100-fold increase in the incidence of lymph node metastases.

Malignant lymphomas and lymphoproliferative diseases are the second most common malignancy in transplant recipients, accounting for 15 to 20 per cent of cancers in this population. Many of these are patients with B-cell lymphoproliferative disease that is thought to represent a response to activation of EBV, which over time progresses to a monoclonal lymphoma. Reduction of immunosuppression or administration of antiviral agents may be useful, at least in patients with an EBV-associated lymphoproliferative process.

Cervical carcinoma is also more common in transplant recipients, which emphasizes the importance of routine health care maintenance in such patients. Conventional treatment is indicated, as dictated by stage of disease.

CADAVERIC DONOR SELECTION AND MANAGEMENT

The greatest obstacle to transplantation for many patients is the lack of a suitable donor organ. In 1992, over 28,000 patients were on waiting lists for transplantation, and just over 16,000 transplants were performed. Many potential transplant recipients on waiting lists expire before a suitable donor is available. The use of a living donor, usually a relative, is possible for some of those in need of a kidney, but otherwise patients must rely on brain-dead, heart-beating donors. Such cadaveric donors are most often seen following trauma or intracerebral hemorrhage. Once an unequivocal diagnosis of brain death has been established by an independent examiner, usually a neurologist, consent for donation is obtained from the next of kin. Ideally, donors should be free of chronic disease and demonstrate hemodynamic stability since the event precipitating brain death. The scarcity of suitable donors has eliminated absolute age limits for donors, and consideration is given to transplantation of organs from donors older than 65 years. Successful transplantation of kidneys and livers from donors older than 80 years has been reported. Donors less than 5 years of age are best utilized as donors for pediatric recipients because this allows optimal size matching. There is some controversy about the success of kidney transplantation from donors less than 5 years into adult recipients, but many centers do this routinely if no pediatric recipients are available.

A detailed history is obtained from the medical staff and family, with attention to any history of hepatitis or substance abuse. Contraindications to donation include active systemic infection and serologic evidence of viral hepatitis or human immunodeficiency virus (HIV). A history of malignancy is also a contraindication to donation, due to the risk of tumor cells being transplanted with the organs. Rapid tumor growth has been observed in the heavily immunosuppressed recipient. One exception to this is a donor with a primary brain tumor where the risk of systemic spread is extremely low.

Evaluation of specific donor organ function is performed with routine laboratory determinations and parameters such as the urine output. Most events leading to brain death cause progressive intracranial hy-

pertension, which is associated with increased sympathetic activity and the release of catecholamines, which can promote cardiac arrhythmias. Once brain herniation occurs, hypotension can ensue due to a decrease in catecholamines and loss of sympathetic tone. Furthermore, failure of the central hormonal axis occurs with brain death, and loss of antidiuretic hormone leads to diabetes insipidus with massive urine output and hypernatremia. There is also evidence that thyroid hormone, cortisol, and insulin levels decrease in brain death.

Restoration of tissue perfusion is performed by volume administration to a central venous pressure of 10 to 12 cm H_2O and transfusion of red blood cells if necessary. The arterial oxygen saturation is maintained at greater than 95 per cent and donor temperature is maintained at greater than 35°C. Inotropic support, if necessary, is provided by dopamine, preferably at a dose less than 10 to 15 μg/kg/min. Vasopressin is sometimes given to treat diabetes insipidus, and electrolyte abnormalities are corrected with intravenous replacement. Thyroid hormone is often given to improve hemodynamic stability.

Organ Harvest Procedure

The thoracic and abdominal organ procurement teams perform a coordinated procedure in the operating room. A long midline incision is made from the sternal notch to the pubis. A thorough exploration is performed to identify tumor, infection, or unexpected organ injury. The thoracic team mobilizes the aorta, pulmonary artery, and lungs, and the abdominal aorta and inferior vena cava are exposed from the superior mesenteric artery to their bifurcations. The aorta at the crus of the diaphragm is isolated for later cross-clamping. Dissection as necessary is performed around the liver, pancreas, and kidneys. The identification of aberrant arterial anatomy is important, especially with regard to the hepatic arteries.

After systemic heparinization, cannulas are inserted in the aortic root, pulmonary artery (if lungs are to be procured), distal abdominal aorta, and a portal vein tributary (if liver is to be procured). Simultaneously, the aorta is cross-clamped in the chest at the innominate artery and in the abdomen at the crus of the diaphragm while cold preservative solutions are administered into the aorta and portal vein. Topical hypothermia is achieved with iced saline slush. Once flushing and cooling are complete, the organs are carefully removed along with lymph nodes for tissue typing and are sterilely packaged for transport.

Organ Preservation

Successful organ transplantation depends on the ability to transport organs without sustaining injury from which the organ cannot recover. Hypothermia is an important aspect of organ preservation. At 5°C, cellular metabolism is reduced to 5 per cent of the rate seen at 37°C, which slows consumption of cellular energy stores. The most commonly used preservative solution, at least for abdominal organs, is one developed at the University of Wisconsin (UW). UW solution (ViaSpan) consists of intracellular concentrations of electrolytes and large molecules to serve as osmotic agents that limit cell swelling. It also contains some compounds designed to limit free radical–induced reperfusion injury and substrate for adenosine triphosphate (ATP). Kidneys are safely stored at 4°C in this solution for 36 to 48 hours, while the liver and pancreas can reliably be preserved as long as 18 to 24 hours. Preservation of hearts is usually accomplished with hyperkalemic, crystalloid cardioplegia identical to that used for intraoperative cardioplegia; UW solution has also been utilized for cardiac preservation with good results.

Some institutions utilize pulsatile pump preservation of kidneys rather than simple cold storage. Kidneys on a perfusion pump may be maintained for as long as 72 hours and generally display less early graft dysfunction. This method, however, is more expensive and requires continuous monitoring of the kidney and perfusion apparatus during transport.

KIDNEY TRANSPLANTATION

Nearly 10,000 kidney transplants were performed in 1992, 22 per cent of them from living donors. The transplantation of a kidney is recognized as an excellent method of treatment for many patients with end-stage renal disease. Even diabetic patients, who once were thought to be poor candidates for transplantation, can enjoy longer and better lives following renal transplantation. Contraindications to transplantation include the presence of infection (including HIV), malignancy, and inability to comply with long-term medications or follow-up. The pretransplant evaluation includes a thorough medical evaluation, including an assessment for significant cardiac disease and an examination of the lower urinary tract.

Living Donor Selection

Living donor kidney transplantation permits the elective transplantation of a well-matched kidney with minimal cold ischemic time. Most living donor transplants have been between relatives, offering the opportunity for haplo-identical or HLA-identical transplants, which have a 1-year survival of approximately 90 per cent, with the potential for many years

of excellent renal function. Transplantation can be performed prior to the need for dialysis, once it is established that the need for renal replacement therapy is imminent.

Donors should be in excellent health with no evidence of disease processes such as diabetes or hypertension that might lead to later renal insufficiency in the donor. Donor anatomy is evaluated with arteriography. Above all, donors must be true volunteers and willing to undergo the risks of anesthesia and a surgical procedure.

Once a donor organ is identified and a crossmatch between donor cells and potential recipient serum is negative, the patient is brought to the operating room and placed under general anesthesia. A lower quadrant incision is utilized to expose the iliac vessels. While maintaining hypothermia, the renal vein and artery of the donor kidney are anastomosed to the iliac vessels of the recipient. The kidney is reperfused, hemostasis is achieved, and the ureter is implanted in the bladder. A Foley catheter and sometimes a ureteral stent remain in the bladder.

Postoperatively, attention is directed at maintenance of a euvolemic to slightly hypervolemic state. Immunosuppression is initiated before transplantation and is continued. A period of acute tubular necrosis (ATN) may prevent immediate function, but supportive care, including dialysis if necessary, usually allows the transplanted kidney to recover.

Graft Function and Complications

Function of the transplanted kidney is assessed by urine output and creatinine clearance. A period of acute tubular necrosis may be observed, especially after a long cold ischemic time (> 24 hours). Many centers avoid the use of cyclosporine during a period of posttransplant ATN because it may delay the recovery of kidney function. If cyclosporine is withheld, an antilymphocyte agent is usually given to prevent rejection in the immediate postoperative period.

Renal function can be assessed by radionuclide scan, confirming adequate blood flow to the kidney and quantitating function. Ultrasound easily documents patency of the vessels and evaluates for ureteral obstruction. Rejection can be seen at any time but is most common in the weeks immediately following transplantation. It is manifest by a rise in the serum creatinine and, often, a low-grade fever and graft tenderness. Percutaneous needle biopsy confirms the presence of rejection, which is treated with bolus steroids and/or an antilymphocyte agent.

Technical complications include acute thrombosis, ureteral leak, and obstruction. Divided lymphatics in the iliac fossa may lead to the accumulation of fluid, creating a lymphocele, which can cause ureteral obstruction. Maintenance of gastrointestinal function is important to avoid colonic distention, and prophylaxis for gastroduodenal ulcers is usually given. Expected graft survival rates at 1 and 5 years for cadaveric transplants are 80 to 85 per cent and 65 to 70 per cent, respectively, with even better rates following living-related transplantation. An excellent HLA match confers the best long-term survival. Late graft losses are most often due to chronic rejection or death of a recipient with a functioning graft from an unrelated illness.

LIVER TRANSPLANTATION

Liver transplantation is a technically demanding procedure requiring the involvement of a multidisciplinary team of surgeons and support staff. Improvements in immunosuppression and technique have allowed this form of therapy to become routine for many acute and chronic diseases of the liver. More than 4000 liver transplants were performed in the United States in 1992.

Indications

Orthotopic liver transplantation has been performed for nearly all causes of hepatic insufficiency (Table 2). This includes viral hepatitis, cirrhosis from a number of causes, and cholestatic diseases. Inborn errors of metabolism and primary tumors of the liver and bile ducts that are not amenable to partial hepatic resection may also be treated in this manner. A thorough pretransplant evaluation is performed, with at-

TABLE 2. DISEASES TREATED BY ORTHOTOPIC LIVER TRANSPLANTATION

Autoimmune hepatitis
Fulminant hepatic failure
  Toxin induced
  Viral
Hepatitis B
  Chronic hepatitis B
  Chronic active hepatitis B
Hepatitis C
Cirrhosis
  Cryptogenic
  Alcoholic
  Primary biliary
  Posthepatic
Budd-Chiari syndrome
Biliary atresia
Sclerosing cholangitis
Caroli's disease
Hepatic adenomatosis
Primary hepatocellular carcinoma
Cholangiocarcinoma
Inborn errors of metabolism

tention to determination of the urgency of transplantation, underlying medical problems, and specific technical problems that might be encountered. The liver size and blood supply are evaluated by radiographic methods. Patients with primary malignancies are evaluated to exclude metastatic disease, and hepatic encephalopathy, coagulopathy, and nutritional deficiencies are documented and corrected as much as is possible. Any active infection is sought and treated. Baseline viral and fungal serologies are obtained. The goal during the evaluation is to maintain the patient in as stable a condition as possible in order to minimize complications in the peritransplant period and hasten recovery. Variceal bleeding from portal hypertension should be treated with endoscopic sclerotherapy. Portal decompression is best accomplished with a transvenous portosystemic shunt through the hepatic parenchyma (TIPS). This is superior to a surgically placed shunt because it does not create adhesions that make subsequent transplantation more difficult.

Some patients present with fulminant hepatic failure, most often from viral hepatitis or exposure to a hepatotoxin. Transplantation, if performed prior to the onset of significant cerebral edema, can allow recovery. In such patients, the evaluation may need to be expedited and abbreviated to permit transplantation as soon as an appropriate liver is available.

Recipients are placed on a waiting list according to their degree of medical urgency. A higher priority is given to patients who are hospitalized, and the highest priority given to those patients in an intensive care unit with a life expectancy of less than 7 days.

Donor Selection

The selection of the specific organ for a recipient depends on a number of factors. Ideally, transplantation is performed with a liver from an ABO-compatible donor. Size matching is necessary, although a portion of the liver is often transplanted into a pediatric recipient because the supply of pediatric donor organs is much less than the number of patients needing them. In addition, certain anatomic considerations in the recipient may affect selection of the donor organ.

The ideal donor organ is from a donor with no hemodynamic instability. There should be no history of hepatitis, HIV exposure, significant ethanol use, or intravenous drug use. The serum transaminases, coagulation studies, and bilirubin should be normal. The liver is examined in the operating room and biopsied if necessary. The gallbladder is usually removed prior to implantation.

Recipient Operation

Transplantation of the liver is a major operation with three distinct phases. The *hepatectomy phase* involves isolation of the blood supply to and from the liver as well as division of the bile duct in preparation for removal of the diseased native liver.

The *anhepatic phase* begins when the vena cava superior and inferior to the liver is clamped, the portal structures are divided, and the liver is removed. In adults, venous return to the heart is usually maintained using a venovenous pump that carries blood from the femoral and portal veins to the axillary vein. During this phase the patient is dependent on exogenously administered clotting factors. The suprahepatic vena caval anastomosis is performed initially, followed by the infrahepatic vena caval anastomosis. The portal vein is joined to the recipient portal vein and the hepatic artery is anastomosed to the donor artery.

The *reperfusion phase* begins with release of clamps and restoration of blood flow to the new liver. Hyperkalemia and acidosis can occur as the preservative solution is flushed from the liver. During this phase, the patient is warmed and control of bleeding is achieved. The biliary reconstruction is performed either with a choledochocholedochostomy or with a choledochojejunostomy, usually over a T tube or other type of stent (Fig. 1).

Pediatric Liver Transplantation

Biliary atresia and other causes of hepatic dysfunction in children can successfully be treated with transplantation. For patients with biliary atresia, a Kasai procedure (hepaticojejunostomy) may still be of benefit as a temporizing procedure to allow an infant to grow. The availability of donor livers is less limiting, and the procedure is technically easier in a larger child compared to an infant. Reduced size organ allografts have been utilized to transplant small recipients. A lobe of the liver, or even the left lateral segment, can be used from a donor up to ten times the size of the recipient. These techniques have been used to split the same liver into transplantable segments for two recipients. However, technical complications are greater in such "split-liver" procedures; therefore, they are currently utilized only in limited situations.

Another approach for providing donor liver tissue for infants and children is from a living donor. The left lateral segment or an entire lobe, usually from a parent or grandparent, is transplanted. As in living kidney donation, this permits transplantation to be an elective procedure. The donor should be carefully selected after an evaluation to identify any contraindications. Partial hepatectomy is performed at most centers with minimal mortality and morbidity, but donors should be made aware of the risks of donation during the initial stages of the evaluation process.

Complications and Long-Term Results

Five to 10 per cent of livers demonstrate minimal function following transplantation, probably from preservation injury or from an undetected process in the donor. If this does not reverse rapidly, retransplantation is indicated to permit patient survival. Rejection, as with other organs, usually presents after the first week and before 6 months. It is heralded by an increase in the serum transaminases, can be confirmed by liver biopsy, and is treated in the same manner as rejection in other organs.

Infection remains the single most frequent complication following liver transplantation. Early infections are most often bacterial. Later infections reflect those in immunocompromised patients, including fungal and viral infection. Cytomegalovirus is a frequent viral infection, especially after the use of lymphocyte-depleting agents such as OKT3 or ATG. Biliary complications continue to affect 15 to 20 per cent of recipients. Early complications are most commonly bile leaks and often require operative repair. Late complications are more likely to be biliary strictures that can often be managed with percutaneous transhepatic dilatation and stenting or with endoscopic techniques. Most centers report patient survival rates of 70 per cent at 1 year and about 60 per cent at 5 years.

INTESTINAL TRANSPLANTATION

The replacement of intestine lost from tumor, congenital anomalies, or vascular catastrophe is emerging as a new arena for transplantation. Initial series of small bowel, small bowel plus colon, and liver plus intestine are being reported. It appears that potent immunosuppression, most often in the form of FK506, is useful. Graft-versus-host disease has not been a problem with this regimen, despite the large volume of donor lymphoid tissue transplanted with the intestine. Arterial inflow to the intestinal graft is via the superior mesenteric artery, which is attached to the recipient aorta, and venous drainage is preferably through the liver. At least one graft stoma is created that permits frequent biopsies of the intestine to monitor for rejection.

Complications include bacterial infection, perhaps in part due to translocation of bacteria from the lumen of the graft. Currently, it appears that survival is better in recipients of a liver and intestine, which is thought to be a reflection of the liver's capacity to modulate rejection of the intestine.

PANCREAS TRANSPLANTATION

The normalization of glucose homeostasis in diabetes has long been a goal of diabetologists and trans-

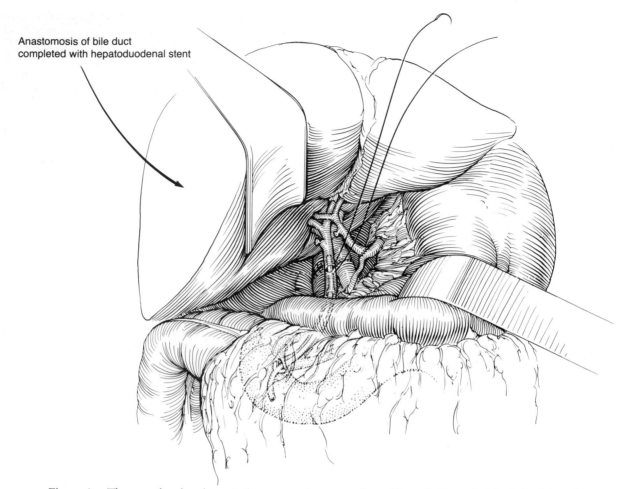

Anastomosis of bile duct
completed with hepatoduodenal stent

Figure 1. The completed orthotopic liver transplant procedure. (From Sabiston DC Jr [ed]: Atlas of General Surgery. Philadelphia, WB Saunders Company, in press, with permission.)

plant surgeons. In the last several years, this has become a reality with the development of safe methods to transplant the whole pancreas.

Indications

Patients with type I diabetes (insulin-dependent, juvenile-onset) are the population that might benefit from pancreas transplantation. Currently, three major settings are considered. *Pancreas transplantation alone* (PTA) can be performed in patients without significant diabetic nephropathy and with the hope of preventing the end-organ complications of diabetes. For patients who have already developed diabetic nephropathy and the need for dialysis or kidney transplantation, transplantation of the pancreas can be accomplished either after kidney transplantation (PAK) or simultaneously with kidney transplantation (SPK). In the last two groups, the beneficial effects of kidney transplantation to treat renal failure is already well established, as is the need for chronic immunosuppression for the kid-

ney transplant. The addition of a pancreas transplant, therefore, adds a small amount of risk to the procedure itself, but does not significantly add to long-term risk from chronic immunosuppression. The proven benefits of pancreas transplantation include avoidance of diabetic nephropathy in the transplanted kidney, improvement in peripheral neuropathy, and an improved quality of life without the need for glucose monitoring and insulin administration.

Potential recipients undergo an evaluation similar to that performed in potential kidney transplant recipients, in which the degree of neuropathy is evaluated as well as any retinopathy. The incidence of occult coronary disease in diabetics is significant. Therefore, either cardiac catheterization or a functional cardiac test is performed prior to transplantation.

Donor Selection

Because many patients with head injuries have elevated glucose and amylase levels, the best assessment of the quality of the pancreas is made in the operating room. The absence of injury and edema is important to assure graft function, and the pancreas is harvested with the other organs. The frequency of arterial anomalies supplying the liver and pancreas requires careful examination and discussions between the liver and pancreas teams to decide where vessels are to be divided to facilitate transplantation of each organ.

Recipient Operation

The whole pancreas is usually transplanted to the iliac fossa with arterial inflow through the splenic artery and superior mesenteric artery. If a patch of aorta is not obtained with the graft, a Y-graft of donor iliac artery is used to join these two vessels prior to implantation. The portal vein provides venous outflow and is usually anastomosed to the iliac vein. In the past, the handling of the exocrine output from the pancreas was a major problem in pancreas transplantation. The pancreatic duct was injected or ligated, but problems with pancreatitis and graft thrombosis were common. Drainage into a loop of intestine avoids these problems but is associated with an increased incidence of intra-abdominal infection. Currently, the preferred technique is to anastomose a segment of donor duodenum containing the ampulla of Vater to the bladder, draining the exocrine secretions from the bladder with a Foley catheter. This has several advantages. The risk of infection is much less without an enterotomy in the recipient, and graft function can easily be determined by measuring the urinary pH and amylase excretion. If a kidney is also transplanted, it is placed in the opposite iliac fossa, using standard technique.

Posttransplant Care

Control of glucose is initially achieved with intravenous insulin, which is usually discontinued within a few hours of transplantation. Immunosuppression consists of corticosteroids, cyclosporine, and azathioprine, with an initial induction course of OKT3 or ATG/ALG. Rejection is more common than in kidney transplantation alone, occurring in about 75 per cent. If simultaneous kidney transplantation has been performed, rejection is usually detected in the kidney first by a rise in the serum creatinine, and biopsy of the kidney can be performed. The urinary amylase excretion can decrease, but the blood glucose is usually not elevated until rejection is advanced. Antirejection therapy with corticosteroids and/or antilymphocyte agents usually reverses the rejection episode.

Complications and Results

Infectious complications are similar to those of other transplant recipients. Thrombosis of the pancreas transplant can occur, leading to graft loss. Anticoagulation, either with heparin or antiplatelet agents, is usually given. The loss of fluid and bicarbonate from the pancreas makes replacement of these losses important. Adequate fluid intake is encouraged and sodium bicarbonate supplementation is given. In 10 to 20 per cent of recipients, bicarbonate losses or bladder/urethral irritation requires conversion of the pancreas transplant from bladder to enteric drainage. The best results are seen with SPK transplants, at least in part due to the ability to monitor for rejection of both organs by observing renal function. Pancreatic endocrine function at 1 year is 85 to 90 per cent in these patients.

PANCREATIC ISLET CELL TRANSPLANTATION

The transplantation of pancreatic islet cells to treat Type I diabetes mellitus has been attempted for many years. Largely due to the immunogenicity of islets and difficulty monitoring for rejection, these attempts have not been successful in rendering patients permanently free from the need for insulin. Current attempts involve transplanting islet tissue by the portal vein to the liver under fairly heavy immunosuppression around the time of kidney transplantation. Encapsulating the islet tissue in chambers that exclude recipient leukocytes is also under study. The long-term results of these studies have yet to be reported.

HEART TRANSPLANTATION

Experimental cardiac transplantation was performed by Carrel and Guthrie in the early part of this century and experimental heterotopic cardiac transplants were performed in the Soviet Union by Demikhov, but cardiac transplantation became a clinical reality in the 1960s. Activity at many centers produced over 100 cardiac transplants in the year after clinical introduction of the technique in 1967. Unfortunately, although the technical barriers had been overcome, there remained significant obstacles to patient survival, including control of rejection. Persistent efforts at a few centers through the 1970s demonstrated the importance of repeated sampling of the myocardium with endomyocardial biopsies to diagnose rejection. Antilymphocyte agents were added as immunosuppression for rejection and, with the introduction of cyclosporine, results improved, ushering in a new growth in cardiac transplant programs and procedures.

Indications

Patients accepted for cardiac transplantation have end-stage heart disease, with an expected survival of less than 1 year, and other medical or surgical treatment options have already been exhausted. Most of the potential recipients are patients with ischemic or idiopathic cardiomyopathies. Congenital cardiac defects may also be treated with cardiac transplantation, even in neonates. Patients over age 65 are generally not accepted for transplantation. The existence of diabetes mellitus, significant pulmonary disease, and renal or hepatic insufficiency may preclude consideration for transplantation. Elevated pulmonary artery pressures are a contraindication due to the problem of right heart failure when a nonhypertrophied, normal right ventricle is transplanted into such a patient. Treatment for congestive heart failure in the recipient is optimized, which may require inotropic support with agents such as dobutamine. Some patients deteriorate and require support with intra-aortic balloon pump, a ventricular assist device, or a total artificial heart. However, the outcome following transplantation in this group of patients is significantly poorer than that achieved in more stable patients.

Donor Selection and Operation

The ideal donor is less than 45 years old with no history of cardiac trauma or previous cardiac disease. Echocardiography is a routine part of the evaluation, and coronary arteriography may be performed, particularly in older donors. A median sternotomy is used to expose the heart. The great vessels and vena cavae are isolated. In concert with harvesting other organs, the vena cavae are ligated and divided, following which an aortic crossclamp is applied and cardioplegic solution is administered into the aortic root. Once the heart is fully flushed, the aorta, pulmonary artery, and atria are divided and the heart is removed. In general, standard hyperkalemic cardioplegic solution has been utilized, although preliminary studies with the UW solution demonstrate the ability to prolong the cold ischemic time beyond 4 to 5 hours.

Recipient Operation

In most cases, the recipient is anesthetized while the donor harvest is being performed. The native heart, however, is not excised until the donor heart has arrived in the operating room. Standard cardiopulmonary bypass is utilized. The new heart is anastomosed to the cuffs of the left and right atrium, followed by the pulmonary artery and aorta. After removing air from the chambers of the heart, cardiopulmonary bypass is weaned. Inotropic support may be required.

Most patients are extubated within 48 hours of transplantation. Inotropic support is weaned as tolerated. The chest tubes are usually removed on the second or third postoperative day, and an oral diet is resumed at that time. Frequent endomyocardial biopsies are performed in the weeks and months following transplant, beginning 7 days following transplant. A grading system for the histology of rejection has been described and is used to guide therapy. Maintenance immunosuppression usually consists of cyclosporine, azathioprine, and corticosteroids. An initial induction course of an antilymphocyte agent is sometimes administered, and therapy for rejection consists of bolus corticosteroids and an antilymphocyte agent if necessary.

An important part of improved clinical results has been the development of prophylactic regimens to prevent infectious complications. Prophylaxis is administered for both CMV and herpes viruses. In addition, most patients receive trimethoprim sulfamethoxazole as prophylaxis against *Pneumocystis carinii* pneumonia.

Long-Term Results

Utilizing modern surgical techniques and immunosuppression, 1-year graft and patient survival is close to 90 per cent in most series. Long-term graft loss is primarily a result of chronic rejection, which presents as progressive graft atherosclerosis. It is unclear whether this represents a manifestation of vascular rejection, CMV infection, or preservation injury in the donor heart. Retransplantation has been performed in some cases.

Heterotopic Cardiac Transplantation

Heterotopic heart transplantation is occasionally performed in patients with elevated pulmonary artery pressures. In addition, it might also be indicated if the donor heart is small compared to the size of the recipient. The donor heart is placed next to the native heart and is utilized as a pumping chamber to provide additional left ventricular support. Although there are many cases of survival following such a procedure, the success rate is much lower than that for orthotopic heart transplantation. Therefore, many agree that it is preferable to lower pulmonary artery pressures pharmacologically, allowing subsequent orthotopic transplantation. Alternatively, combined heart and lung transplantation can be pursued in patients with persistently elevated pulmonary pressures.

LUNG TRANSPLANTATION

Lung transplantation represents one of the most recent advances in clinical transplantation, becoming a reality with improvements in the treatment of rejection and infection. One of the initial obstacles in lung transplantation was difficulty with the healing of the airway anastomosis. The bronchial arteries are small and have a variable anatomy, making direct anastomosis between the graft and recipient not feasible. As a result, the bronchial anastomosis is relatively ischemic for a period of time and susceptible to breakdown. The recognition that steroids were deleterious to airway healing and introduction of the technique of wrapping the anastomosis with a portion of omentum have permitted the conquest of this technical obstacle.

Indications and Pretransplant Evaluation

Pulmonary transplantation is generally offered to patients less than 60 years of age who have irreversible lung disease with a life expectancy of less than 1 year. End-stage lung disease due to a number of causes has been successfully treated with this method of therapy. *Restrictive lung disease* as well as *obstructive lung disease* may be treated with transplantation. Even patients with cystic fibrosis have undergone bilateral lung transplantation as treatment for their chronic lung disease caused by recurrent infection. In addition, patients with primary or secondary pulmonary hypertension have been treated with lung transplantation.

Contraindications to lung transplantation include the presence of significant other diseases such as coronary artery disease. Patients also require adequate psychosocial support, as both the preoperative and postoperative regimens are quite involved. In the preoperative period, the focus is placed on maintaining freedom from infection and optimizing skeletal muscle strength to improve respiratory effort.

Donor Selection

Appropriate donors are screened by plain radiographic films as well as bronchoscopy. The presence of significant pneumonia or purulent sputum is a contraindication to lung donation. Fluid overload and the resulting lung edema is avoided. Lung harvesting is performed in conjunction with other transplant teams. The pulmonary vasodilator *prostaglandin E_1* is injected into the pulmonary artery prior to flushing it with crystalloid solution (Euro-Collins solution). This provides a more uniform distribution of the flush solution. A portion of the left atrium remains with the pulmonary veins as a cuff for anastomosis to the recipient. Optimal cold ischemic times are generally less than 6 hours, although successful lung function has been documented with cold ischemic times as long as 10 hours.

Recipient Operation

The decision to perform single lung or bilateral lung transplantation depends on recipient factors, primarily the cause of the end-stage lung disease as well as donor lung availability. It is now apparent that patients with chronic infections such as cystic fibrosis require replacement of both lungs. Single-lung transplantation is well suited to those patients with restrictive lung disease, such as pulmonary fibrosis, and appears to be adequate for many patients with emphysema. Patients with pulmonary hypertension have been successfully treated with both single-lung and bilateral lung transplantation. The preferred technique has yet to be established.

The recipient is anesthetized and the operation begun while the donor harvest is underway. Single-lung transplantation is performed through a posterolateral thoracotomy with anastomoses of the bronchus, pulmonary artery, and cuff of the left atrium to the corresponding structures of the recipient. Bilateral lung transplantation is performed through bilateral thoracotomies with division of the sternum. Most often, the operation can be performed without cardiopulmonary bypass by performing replacement of each lung in sequence. The gastrocolic omentum is sometimes utilized to reinforce the bronchial anastomosis and is brought up through a small defect created in the diaphragm.

Patients are maintained on cyclosporine, azathioprine, and an antilymphocyte agent. Corticosteroids are withheld until 1 week after transplant to aid bronchial healing. Early extubation is encouraged. Patients are followed by blood gas determination as well as the chest radiograph. Infection remains the most significant cause of morbidity and mortality. Prophylactic antibiotics are directed at the prevailing bacterial flora. Cytomegalovirus infection is a frequent complication, and control of this pathogen starts with selection of the donor based on the CMV status of the recipient. Patients who have not previously been exposed to CMV are generally not transplanted with lungs from donors who have been exposed to CMV. In addition, prophylactic regimens of hyperimmune globulin, ganciclovir, and/or acyclovir are used to prevent significant CMV episodes.

In addition to the chest film, frequent determinations of the forced expiratory volume in 1 second (FEV$_1$) are performed. Any evidence of decline in function suggests the possibility of infection or rejection, and bronchoscopy with transbronchial biopsy can be performed to ascertain the presence of these complications.

Acute rejection is treated by pulse steroids and, if necessary, an antilymphocyte preparation. Chronic rejection is manifest in lung transplants as obliterative bronchiolitis, which can cause gradual deterioration of pulmonary function and eventual loss of the graft. Most patients improve shortly after transplantation and show markedly improved exercise tolerance. Expected survival is in the range of 60 to 70 per cent at 1 year. Long-term results await further experience.

Heart and Lung Transplantation

The advent of single-lung or bilateral lung transplantation for pulmonary hypertension has largely replaced combined heart and lung transplantation as a method of treatment for these patients, permitting utilization of scarce thoracic donor organs for up to three patients instead of only one patient. Patients who might require combined heart and lung transplantation are those patients with congenital cardiac anomalies and resulting pulmonary hypertension in whom replacement of anything less than heart and lungs would not be sufficient. The techniques and immunosuppressive protocols are similar to those used for transplantation of the individual organs.

XENOTRANSPLANTATION

The transplantation of organs between members of different species has long been a goal of transplant scientists. Successful xenotransplantation would eliminate the current limits on transplantation imposed by donor scarcity, would make transplantation an elective operation, and would allow selection of the donors based on size. Manipulation of donors by genetic engineering could conceivably allow creation of organs with enhanced function and reduced antigenicity.

A number of attempts have been made at transplantation between closely related species (*concordant* xenografts) that have included kidney, heart, and liver transplants from baboons and chimpanzees. To date, the longest survival has been with a chimpanzee kidney transplanted into a human who survived 9 months after a course that was quite similar to that seen after renal allotransplantation. Several problems may limit the use of nonhuman primates as organ donors, including limited availability, small size, and the possibility of transmission of infectious diseases.

Attempts to transplant organs between more distantly related species such as pigs to humans (*discordant* xenografts) have been fewer in number and have had limited success. The rejection reaction observed following discordant transplantation is a vigorous one, with features similar to hyperacute rejection. The antibody involved seems to be a naturally occurring, preformed antibody that activates complement and readily causes endothelial injury. An understanding of this naturally occurring antibody and its target(s) as well as the potential cellular response to a discordant xenograft will be necessary before transplantation between widely disparate species is possible.

AUTOTRANSPLANTATION

Autotransplantation was documented as early as 700 BC in the *Sushruta Samhita*, a Sanskrit text of India that described pedicle grafts for reconstruction of various facial features. In recent years, autografts of various tissues and organs have developed into techniques important in every surgical discipline.

Autografts may be transferred without an attempt to preserve blood supply, such as in skin grafting. A pedicle graft maintains its blood supply through the base of the pedicle until the graft is revascularized from ingrowth of vessels in the new location. Finally, whole segments of tissue may be transferred as a *free graft* with reanastomosis of the blood supply in the new location.

Skin Grafts

Skin grafts are both the oldest and most widely used type of autograft. They are useful to cover cutaneous defects created by burn or injury as well as to reconstruct various body parts. The split-thickness skin graft is a thin layer removed with a dermatome and is best transferred to a well-vascularized, relatively clean graft site. It survives for the first few days on nutrients exchanged from the serum and interstitial fluid before capillary ingrowth occurs. The donor site reepithelializes cells that remain on the dermis. Split-thickness skin grafts are usually meshed, permitting coverage of a larger area. Full-thickness skin grafts are used when resistance to contraction and pigment matching are important. They require a better blood supply for survival than split-thickness grafts and a cleaner graft site. They are usually used for small areas at cosmetically important sites.

Pedicled grafts, or flaps, are rotated to an adjacent area to be covered. The grafts depend on dermal and subdermal vessels for blood supply until ingrowth of vessels in the new location occurs. A myocutaneous flap, on the other hand, is supplied by perforating vessels from the muscle bed and can, therefore, be longer or contain a skin island as long as the major vessel supplying the flap is preserved. Examples of this flap include the pectoralis major flap and the latissimus dorsi flap.

Free graft tissues can now be transferred to provide tissue coverage in remote sites. An example is the latissimus flap transferred to the leg to cover an area resected for a soft-tissue tumor, accomplished by isolating the vascular pedicle supplying the tissue graft and anastomosing the artery and vein to appropriate vessels in the new location with the use of microvascular techniques. Free bone grafts have also been transferred with their vascular supply. For instance, a free vascularized fibula graft may be inserted into the femur of a patient with early avascular necrosis of the femoral head.

Other Autografts

The transfer of veins from one area of the body to another is one of the most widely used autotransplant techniques. The greater saphenous vein is the preferred conduit. It is usually reversed so that the one-way valves do not impede the flow of blood. In general, it easily withstands the arterial pressure when utilized for arterial bypass. Vein grafting into the venous circulation is less successful, with thrombosis a common problem.

Nerve autografts are used to bridge defects in motor nerves caused by trauma or surgical excision, and serve as conduits for nerve regeneration, a slow process, as regrowth of axons proceeds at a rate of 1 mm/day.

Bone grafts are frequently used for improving healing of fractures and to supplement arthrodesis of joints. The graft serves as a matrix for ingrowth of new cells and bone. The most commonly employed donor sites include iliac crest, ribs, and the fibula. Cartilage is also used for reconstructing the nose, the ear, and the orbit. Fascia lata is often used for hernia repair and as a substitute for damaged ligaments in joint repairs.

Endocrine Autografts

Parathyroid autotransplantation is the most commonly employed endocrine autograft. After removal of the parathyroid tissue from the neck of a patient with severe secondary hyperparathyroidism or generalized parathyroid hyperplasia, small slices are placed in muscle pockets in the forearm. Tissue may also be cryopreserved in the event that an inadequate volume of parathyroid tissue is transplanted initially. Continued hypercalcemia can be treated by removal of a portion of the transplanted pieces.

Autotransplantation of a portion of the pancreas to a heterotopic location has been attempted for benign diseases such as chronic pancreatitis in an effort to preserve endocrine function. Continued problems with the exocrine portion of the pancreas and compromise of the islets has limited application of this technique. Fortunately, synthetic hormone replacement for endocrine function exists, making endocrine autotransplants rarely necessary.

VASCULAR ACCESS PROCEDURES FOR RENAL REPLACEMENT THERAPY

Hemodialysis Access

The development of an effective means of access to the systemic circulation was necessary to allow successful *chronic hemodialysis* (HD). The initial development was the Scribner shunt, a Silastic tube with Teflon ends, which was usually inserted into the radial artery and cephalic vein. The tubing of the shunt could be connected to the dialysis circuit and provided arterial and venous access. Although rarely used today, it provided the 150- to 250-ml/min flow rate necessary for hemodialysis, at least on a short-term basis.

Temporary access for HD today is most often achieved by placement of a dual-lumen catheter in the jugular, subclavian, or femoral vein. Depending on type of catheter and location, it can remain in place for weeks or months. Infection is the major complication, occurring in approximately 5 per cent, and is usually treated by removal of the catheter.

Chronic access for HD is obtained by the creation of an arteriovenous (AV) fistula, either with autogenous vein or bioprosthetic material. The optimal method remains the subcutaneous primary AV fistula described by Brescia and Cimano. With this technique, the radial artery is anastomosed to the cephalic vein at the level of the wrist, which can produce a durable fistula that provides adequate venous access for many years without further intervention. The success of this procedure depends on the presence of adequate vessels, and in particular, the presence of an adequate vein.

The absence of suitable vein as a conduit requires the use of a bridge graft to connect an artery and vein. Originally, materials such as bovine artery, allogeneic vein grafts, and human umbilical vein grafts were utilized, but expense, sizing difficulty, aneurysm formation, and degradation by infecting bacteria have led to their abandonment by nearly all surgeons. In recent years, polytetrafluoroethylene (PTFE) has emerged as the most satisfactory and widely used prosthetic material for vascular grafts. Six- or 8-mm grafts are tunneled in a subdermal plane and anastomosed to the radial or brachial artery and to an appropriate outflow vein in the forearm or upper arm. Grafts are usually allowed to mature in place for 2 to 6 weeks prior to use to avoid bleeding and hematoma formation. Multiple revisions may be required to maintain patency. In some patients who have had many access procedures, bridge grafts may need to be placed in the leg or across the chest (axillary artery to axillary vein or jugular vein) to provide access for HD.

The major complications of angioaccess fistulae are thrombosis, infection, and arterial steal. Thrombosis may occur from external pressure or from intimal hyperplasia, which most often occurs at the venous anastomosis. Thrombectomy is usually a simple procedure, performed with a Fogarty balloon catheter under local anesthesia. Intimal hyperplasia may require anastomotic revision in some. Graft infection may be associated with a needle site infection and is unusual in grafts utilizing autogenous vein. Infections associated with prosthetic graft material are treated with intravenous antibiotics (which often may be dosed at prolonged intervals due to renal failure). Fever, tenderness, or abscess formation may require incision and drainage in the operating room. Ligation of the graft is indicated if hemorrhage is a possibility, particularly for infections in the area of an anastomosis.

Arterial steal is caused by limited distal blood flow due to easy runoff to the low pressure venous circulation through the fistula. It is more common in diabetics and with larger, more proximal fistulae. Narrowing the arterial anastomosis may help, but often urgent ligation of the fistula is required.

Peritoneal Dialysis

The utilization of the peritoneum as a dialysis membrane has several advantages. Direct exposure to blood is avoided, dialysis is continuous, and dialysate changes can be performed at various times during the day, conforming to the patients schedule. This often causes less interference and a more productive lifestyle.

Dialysate consists of glucose-containing sterile solutions. The glucose concentration is varied to remove volume as needed. Dialysate is introduced by a cuffed Silastic catheter that is surgically placed in the peritoneal cavity and tunneled to an exit site lateral to the umbilicus. Relative contraindications to peritoneal dialysis include intra-abdominal infection and prior operations with adhesion formation.

Disadvantages of peritoneal dialysis include relatively inefficient dialysis by the peritoneum and the risk of peritonitis. Peritonitis may be treated by the addition of antibiotics to the dialysate, and removal of the catheter is required for persistent infection.

REFERENCES

Brodsky FM, Guagliardi LE: The cell biology of antigen processing and presentation. Ann Rev Immunol 9:707–744, 1991.

Kaiser LR, Cooper JD: The current status of lung transplantation. Adv Surg 25:259–307, 1992.

Marx AB, Landmann J, Harder FH: Surgery for vascular access. Curr Probl Surg 27:5–48, 1990.

Robertson RP, Sutherland DE: Pancreas transplantation as therapy for diabetes mellitus. Ann Rev Med 43:395–415, 1992.

Starzl TE, Demetris AJ: Liver transplantation: A 31-year perspective. Curr Probl Surg 27:49–240, 1990.

19
NEOPLASTIC DISEASE

I
Principles of Surgical Oncology

H. KIM LYERLY, M.D.

Cancer continues to be the second leading cause of death in the United States and causes over 450,000 deaths annually. Approximately 30 per cent of Americans develop cancer at some point during life, and two thirds die of the disease. Carcinoma of the skin is the most common cancer and, fortunately, usually has a good prognosis. The leading sites of invasive cancer include the lung, prostate, and colorectum in males; and the breast, colorectum, uterus, and lung in females. Tumors in these locations comprise over half of all malignancies, with leukemias and lymphomas being only 7 to 8 per cent of malignancies. Definitive surgical resection is the treatment of choice for most solid tumors.

The treatment of solid tumors has changed as the understanding of the biology of tumors has evolved. It has become apparent that many malignant tumors may have already metastasized microscopically at the time of diagnosis, thus precluding surgical extirpation of all malignant cells. Surgical therapy is therefore being integrated with other therapeutic modalities to achieve local, regional, and systemic control. Recently, an interest in the role of the immune system in the management of cancer has been renewed, adding yet another modality to consider in the treatment of cancer. Modern surgical practice encompasses more than the diagnosis and excision of solid tumors in the management of the patient with cancer. For example, reconstruction to restore cosmetic and functional deficiencies has an important role in the treatment of patients with cancer. Staging of tumors is often accomplished by operation, as in axillary lymph node dissection for breast cancer, or splenectomy and staging laparotomy for Hodgkin's disease, to provide prognostic information about the primary tumor and serve as a guide to the administration of primary or adjuvant therapy. Surgical intervention also has a role in the *prevention* of cancer, clearly exemplified by the surgical management of familial polyposis of the colon, in which prophylactic proctocolectomy may eliminate the patient's risk of developing cancer of the colon. While total proctocolectomy formerly meant a permanent ileostomy, now, fecal continence can be maintained in many patients with reconstruction of the alimentary tract by an ileoanal pull-through procedure. Operation can also be considered for metastatic lesions. In situations in which extirpation of primary tumors is not warranted, palliative surgical intervention can be utilized to relieve symptoms from complications of cancer, such as intestinal or biliary obstruction, hemorrhage, perforation, or compression of vital structures.

The expansion of knowledge regarding the biology of cancer has clearly altered oncologic management, and advances in imaging and surgical techniques have significantly influenced care and outcome of the patient with cancer as well. A role for *minimally* invasive operative therapy in the diagnosis and management of these patients has emerged, but long-term results have not been evaluated. The advantages of decreased perioperative morbidity must be weighed against the goals of surgical intervention in local and regional cancer control. A fundamental understanding of the biology of cancer and the advantages and limitations of evolving technologies is necessary prior to clinical decision making in oncologic management. For this reason, an overview of the fundamental principles of the biology of cancer with an emphasis on immunobiologic aspects is provided.

CARCINOGENESIS, ONCOGENES, AND TUMOR SUPPRESSOR GENES

Recently, much attention has been focused on the genetic events leading to the development of cancer. The occurrence of cancer in an individual is postulated to represent the accumulation of multiple genetic events in a normal cell producing the necessary changes for full development of the features of a malignant cell. The fundamental concept that underscores this paradigm is the accumulation of genetic events, which fit the observations of cancer occurrence seen in many patients. For example, some of the requisite genetic changes may be inherited through the germ line. Individually, these inherited genetic changes may not be sufficient for a cell to become malignant, but they may lead to the development of large numbers of premalignant cells susceptible to the secondary genetic changes required for malignant transformation. These secondary genetic changes may be due to exposure to environmental irradiation, carcinogens, viruses, or other agents, or may represent random mutations that increase as the cells age. The consequence of these germ-line mutations is not the development of cancer or precancerous lesions at birth, but rather an increase in susceptibility and in incidence of cancer at an early age.

The accumulated genetic events leading to malignant transformation usually include activation of oncogenes or deactivation or loss of tumor suppressor genes. Proto-oncogenes (cellular oncogenes) are normal constituents of cells and usually regulate normal cell growth and differentiation. An oncogene is a tumor-promoting gene that is activated by disruption of the proto-oncogene by amplification, mutation, or translocation. Examples of proto-oncogenes and tumor suppressor genes and their associated tumors are shown in Table 1. Amplification of proto-oncogene sequences has been detected in some tumors, including N-*myc*, which is amplified in neuroblastoma, and *neu*/erb-B2, which is amplified in breast cancer. In these cancers, proto-oncogene amplification is associated with a poorer prognosis, suggesting that enhanced expression of these genes may be critically related to disease progression. An example of proto-oncogene activation occurring via mutation is the *ras* oncogene; *ras* genes normally encode *guanosine triphosphate* (GTP)-binding proteins. Mutated *ras* proteins usually contain single amino acid substitutions. The mutated *ras* proteins are capable of neoplastic

TABLE 1. PROTO-ONCOGENES AND TUMOR SUPPRESSOR GENES

FAMILY	EXAMPLES	ASSOCIATED TUMORS
Tyrosine-specific protein kinase	c-*fms* c-*abl* c-*src*	Sarcoma Chronic myelogenous leukemia Sarcoma
Serine-threonine protein kinase	c-*mos* c-*raf*	
Steroid type growth factor receptor	c-*erb*-A (Thyroid hormone receptor)	
Guanosine triphosphate (GTP) binding protein	c-Ha-*ras* c-K-*ras*	Sarcoma Pancreatic, colon carcinoma
Growth factor	c-*sis* (PDGF)	Sarcoma
Growth factor receptor acting via tyrosine specific protein kinase	PDGF receptor c-*erb*-B (EGF receptor)	
Nuclear transcripton factor	c-*myc* c-*fos* c-*jun*	Carinomas, sarcomas, leukemias
Tumor suppressor genes	Retinoblastoma gene p53 APC DCC NF-1 WT-1	Retinoblastoma Li-Fraumeni syndrome, etc. Colon carcinoma Colon carcinoma Wilms' tumor Von Recklinghausen

transformation and are associated with several human malignancies including colon and pancreatic cancer.

A tumor suppressor gene is a normal constituent of the cell and usually regulates normal cell growth and differentiation. Progression toward the malignant phenotype is achieved through the loss of function of a tumor suppressor gene, usually by mutation or deletion. Tumor suppressor genes were first described for the rare childhood tumor, *retinoblastoma*. The gene-encoding susceptibility to retinoblastoma was identified, cloned, and characterized, and it was found that introduction of the retinoblastoma gene (RB) into normal cells did not transform them. In contrast, introduction of the RB gene into tumor cells caused phenotypic alterations suggestive of a decrease in malignant potential. A single, intact copy of the RB gene is sufficient to prevent tumorigenesis; hence, both copies of the RB gene on chromosome 13 must be deleted or disrupted for retinoblastoma tumors to ensue. Various genetic lesions have been found to involve RB in tumorigenesis, all acting to delete or disrupt gene function. This information helps in understanding the peculiarities of retinoblastoma. A child can acquire a defective RB allele at conception and develop normally because of the activity of the normal allele. Only when the surviving intact allele is lost in one or another of the retinal cell genomes does that cell begin neoplastic growth. Hence, an inherited susceptibility to retinoblastoma is seen (Fig. 1). Another syndrome associated with the loss of a tumor suppressor gene is familial polyposis. This syndrome is clinically manifested by inheritance of a disorder predisposing to cancer of the colon.

Proto-oncogenes and tumor suppressor genes in cellular DNA are targets for various carcinogens. Although any one carcinogen is unlikely to act upon a single site to produce cancer, the underlying paradigm is that accumulation of multiple genetic events allow neoplasia to occur over long periods. The consequence of these accumulated mutations is either cell death or an internal milieu that disturbs the cellular balance between promotion and inhibition of growth, causing malignant transformation. These accumulated mutations may also serve as targets that can be recognized by the human immune system, and this recognition is the framework for modern immune-based antitumor strategies.

IMMUNOBIOLOGY OF SOLID TUMORS

The immune system is thought to have an important role in the control of solid tumors. This view is supported by a number of animal and human experiments in which immunodeficient animals or patients were found to be more susceptible to the development of solid tumors than were immunocompetent animals or patients. Profound immunodeficiency, however, is most often associated with fatal infections; thus, an increased incidence in the development of solid tumors in the immunodeficient may be obscured due to the high death rate secondary to infectious organisms. Improvement in the management of the infectious complications prolongs the life of individuals with immunodeficiency syndromes and, therefore, has led to an increase in the incidence of unusual malignancies. In addition, iatrogenically immunosuppressed patients, including those receiving immunosuppressive agents following solid-organ transplant or lymphocytotoxic chemotherapy for the treatment of malignancies, appear to have an increase in the development of solid tumors. Although most malignant tumors associated with immunosuppression are of the lymphoid system, other forms, including Kaposi's sarcoma, squamous cell carcinoma of the anus, dysplasia/neoplasia of the cervix, and squamous cell carcinoma of the skin, are seen with increased frequency.

From a historic perspective, the detection of a putative antitumor response such as a lymphocytic infiltrate in a tumor has not uniformly correlated with an improved prognosis in patients with cancer. However, in a study of 293 patients with cancer of the stomach, breast, or rectum who received only surgical treatment, it was concluded that the "uniform consistency of increased length of postoperative life (in the presence of lymphocytic infiltration, fibrosis, hyalinization, and cellular differentiation) suggests that these factors play a significant role as part of the natural defensive mechanism against cancer after it has been developed."

The hypothesis that immune reactivity against malignant cells leads to an improved survival directed early efforts toward stimulation of host immunity against growing tumors involving either nonspecific or specific attempts at active immunization. These attempts utilized substances such as *bacille Calmette-Guérin* (BCG), *methanol-extracted residue* (MER), *Corynebacterium parvum*, or *Nocardia rubia* administered in the hope that they would nonspecifically increase immune reactivity and, thus, concomitantly increase the putative immune response against a growing malignancy. Alternatively, attempts have been made to utilize specific active immunization against cancer using cancer vaccines composed of inactivated cancer cells or cancer cell extracts administered alone or in conjunction with immune adjuvants. Although there was initial enthusiasm for these approaches in active immunotherapy, early reports of success could not be confirmed.

More recent efforts to enhance the immune response have included specific active immunotherapy using in-

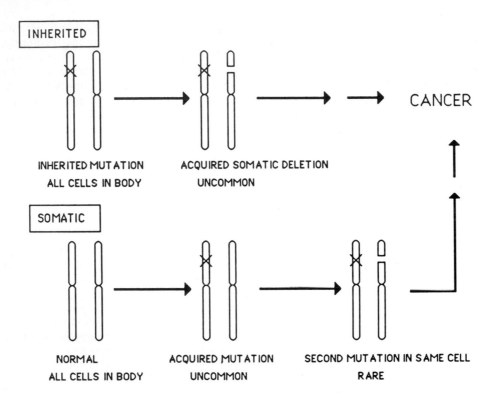

Figure 1. Tumor suppressor genes in the pathogenesis of cancer. Two mechanisms are shown for the inactivation of both copies of a tumor suppressor gene. *Top*, Individuals who have an inherited mutation or deletion of the suppressor gene carry only a single functional allele in every cell in their bodies. In the uncommon event of a somatic mutation occurring in the remaining allele, cancer may result. (This usually occurs in 1 in 10^6 cells, or several per individual on average.) *Bottom*, Individuals who inherit two normal copies of the tumor suppressor gene are much less susceptible to the development of cancer. In order for these cells to become malignant, both cells must undergo somatic mutation. The acquired somatic mutations have a frequency of only 1 in 10^{12} cells, or once in many thousands of individuals.

tact tumor cells as an immunizing antigen or purified tumor-associated antigen preparations that may elicit tumor-specific immune response and delay subsequent tumor growth. Specific active immunotherapy trials have been performed in patients with both melanoma and colorectal carcinoma. Patients with melanoma have been immunized with intact autologous or allogeneic cells or with a viral lysate prepared from such cells. The results of these studies suggest that a statistically significant therapeutic benefit is realized in some high-risk patients. Human subjects with colorectal carcinoma have been immunized with irradiated autologous tumor cells, but this approach has limited clinical use.

ADOPTIVE IMMUNOTHERAPY FOR SOLID TUMORS

An alternative to active immunotherapy involves the passive administration of immune reagents to react against cancer. It has been shown that the cellular arm of the immune system, rather than the humoral arm, is involved in tissue and organ allograft rejection and in the rejection of experimental tumors. Animal studies have demonstrated that immunity to tissue present in highly immunized mice could be transferred to naive mice by the adoptive transfer of lymphocytes, whereas the transfer of serum containing large amounts of antibody was relatively ineffective in transferring immunity. These studies led to the use of lymphocytes from highly immunized mice to treat established tumors in other animals, and the encouraging results motivated efforts to transfer lymphocytes among cross-immunized cancer patients. These studies were unsuccessful due to the limited ability to immunize patients against allogeneic cancer-associated antigens in vivo and the limited survival of allogeneic lymphocytes in the host. Recently, several approaches have been developed to generate immune cells from cancer-bearing patients with specific immune reactivity against cancer and to expand the cells in large numbers. This approach represents the first successful cellular therapy for advanced cancer in humans and includes generation of *lymphokine-activated killer* (LAK) cells, *in vitro–stimulated* (IVS) cells, and *tumor-infiltrating lymphocytes* (TILs).

Clinical trials of adoptive immunotherapy have demonstrated both complete and partial responses in patients with a number of solid tumors. Clinical trials in patients with metastatic melanoma and renal cell carcinoma receiving TILs and interleukin-2 (IL-2) have shown partial or complete regression of the cancers in approximately 15 to 20 per cent. Responses have not been as significant with other tumor types. Genetic modification of lymphocytes for adoptive immunotherapy has also been developed as a therapeutic modality. Initially, lymphokine-activated TILs were genetically modified to carry a marker gene (neomycin phosphotransferase) by transduction with retroviral vectors. These gene-modified TILs were then reinfused into patients and were shown to circulate to the tumor sites and retain their transduced marker gene. In vitro studies demonstrated that these retroviral transduced TILs maintained their specificity and function for lysis of autologous tumor.

Recent studies have utilized genetically modified TILs to secrete tumor necrosis factor (TNF). The hypothesis of this strategy is that the TILs that reach the tumor secrete TNF within the microenvironment of the tumor. High levels of TNF produced in this microenvironment should be cytotoxic to the tumor cells and should not be present in the systemic circulation, thus avoiding the profound systemic effects of TNF that make high systemic dosing of TNF unwarranted in patients.

GENE-MODIFIED TUMOR IMMUNOTHERAPY

Although the effector cells adoptively transferred to patients with advanced cancer had objective responses in only a few patients, these experiments did demonstrate an effector phenotype that clearly had an antitumor effect. This evidence for an effective antitumor immune response, combined with advances in the understanding of the immune response to human tumors, has renewed interest in active immunotherapy. The immune response to tumors is dependent on the existence of antigens within tumors that can be recognized as foreign by the host. Virally induced tumors and some tumors induced by mutagens have foreign or mutated proteins thought to serve as tumor antigens recognized by *cytotoxic T lymphocytes* (CTLs). Spontaneously arising tumors are also thought to express tumor-specific antigens that can elicit an immune

response. However, they are felt not to present these antigens properly for immune recognition.

CTLs are now known to recognize peptides derived from endogenously synthesized proteins and presented on the cell surface together with *major histocompatibility* (MHC) class I molecules. Consequently, antigens include any primary amino acid sequence in any cellular proteins, either membrane bound or intracellular. It has been shown that, for tumors rendered immunogenetic by mutagen treatment, CTLs recognize peptides derived from point-mutated intracellular proteins. Because spontaneously arising cancers are thought to have multiple mutational events within the same cell, peptides from the mutated proteins may bind to the MHC class I molecules and could be recognized by CTLs. These peptides, unique to the tumor cells, may serve as target antigens for a specific CTL response and may also serve as targets for other cytotoxic cell types such as *natural killer* (NK) and *lymphokine-activated killer* (LAK) cells, which appear to demonstrate specificity for tumor cells, although the nature of their ligand binding remains undefined.

As the details of CTL recognition of peptide antigens emerge, the failure of an immune response to spontaneously arising tumors is hypothesized to be due not entirely to the absence of tumor antigens, but rather, in part, to a failure of T-cell help or a failure of antigen processing. Most CTL responses require *T helper* (Th) cells, and a prime component of Th function is the local secretion of cytokines such as IL-2. The local secretion by tumor cells of a helper lymphokine critical for CTL activation might bypass a deficient Th arm of the immune system. In fact, in experimental animal models in which IL-2 was provided locally by the tumor cell target in vivo, potent antitumor immune responses were generated. Recent studies have shown that animal tumors that are poorly immunogeneic can be recognized by MHC class I–restricted, CD^{8+} cytotoxic T cells if the tumor cells are engineered by gene transfection to secrete IL-2 or IL-4.

The prospect of active immunotherapy for human cancers has improved with these recent advances. In animal models, increasing the immunogenicity of tumors to secrete lymphokines by use of gene transfection has led to the use of *gene-modified tumor* (GMT) vaccines that appear to provide protective immunity against tumor challenge. The GMT vaccines are not only protective against non–gene transduced tumors, but also elicit immune responses that cause regression of established tumors in animal models. The effector arm of the immune system that mediates the antitumor effect is thought to be the MHC class I–restricted, CD^{8+} cytotoxic T-cell arm. Clinical trials are underway to demonstrate the efficacy of GMT vaccines with solid tumors.

REFERENCES

Broder S (ed): Molecular Foundations of Oncology. Baltimore, Williams & Wilkins, 1991.

Fearon ER, Pardoll DM, Itaya T, et al: Interleukin-2 production by tumor cells bypasses T-helper function in the generation of an antitumor response. Cell *60*(3):397–403, 1990.

Golumbek PT, Lazenby AJ, Levitsky HI, et al: Treatment of estab-

lished renal cancer by tumor cells engineered to secrete interleukin-4. Science *254* (5032):713–716, 1991.

Moore MW, Carbone FR, Bevan MJ: Introduction of soluble protein into the class I pathway of antigen processing and presentation. Cell *54*:777–785, 1988.

Townsend ARM, Rothbard J, Gotch FM, et al: The epitopes of influenza nucleoprotein recognized by cytotoxic T lymphocytes can be defined with short synthetic peptides. Cell *44*:959–968, 1986.

II
Malignant Melanoma

CRAIG L. SLINGLUFF, Jr., M.D.

Melanoma is a malignant neoplasm arising from melanocytes, and approximately 90 per cent of primary melanomas arise from the skin, originating at the dermal/epidermal junction. A small percentage arise from unknown primary sites and present with metastatic disease, and the remainder arise from rarer sites including the eye, the mucous membranes, and the viscera. The distribution of cutaneous primary sites is presented in Table 1. Since early in this century, the incidence of melanoma has increased substantially in the United States, and it is now estimated that the lifetime risk of melanoma is approximately 1 in 100. In

1990, 32,000 new cases were reported in the United States, with an estimated 6500 deaths. Although over 80 per cent of patients are diagnosed during their productive years, between the ages of 25 and 65, melanoma ranks second behind leukemia as a cause of cancer deaths in males 15 to 34 years of age in the United States. The management of malignant melanoma involves prevention, early diagnosis, surgical extirpation, and management of metastatic disease. Recent trends in therapy have included aggressive surgical treatment of isolated distant metastases, hyperthermic limb perfusion, and application of experimental immunotherapeutic methods. Debate continues regarding the role of elective lymph node dissection (ELND) and about the optimal margin of excision.

CAUSATIVE FACTORS

The population at risk for melanoma is all-inclusive, but most melanomas occur in patients with a Celtic complexion (fair and freckled skin that burns easily, blond or red hair, blue eyes). Approximately 99 per cent of melanomas in the United States arise in Caucasians. In addition to skin pigmentation, other risk

TABLE 1. DISTRIBUTION OF CUTANEOUS PRIMARY SITES FOR MELANOMA*

Primary Site	Incidence
Trunk	38%
Upper extremity	13%
Lower extremity	19%
Head and neck	16%
Volar (palms, soles)	2%
Subungal	1%

*Data derived from Slingluff CL, Seigler HF: Duke Melanoma Database, 8-18-91, 8075 patients.

factors include sun exposure, dysplastic nevus syndrome, xeroderma pigmentosum, a history of nonmelanoma skin cancer, higher socioeconomic status, and family history of melanoma. Chromosomal abnormalities have been implicated in melanoma patients, but the specific genetic basis of melanoma is unknown. The environmental factor most associated with melanoma is sun exposure; in particular, exposure to ultraviolet (UV) radiation. Although prospective randomized data on sun exposure in humans do not exist, the epidemiologic evidence implicating sun exposure as an etiologic factor for melanoma in sun-sensitive individuals is significant. It is thought that severe burns early in life are of greater risk than chronic sun exposure, and sun block is recommended, especially in children and in individuals with fair skin, for prevention of severe burns.

CLINICAL PRESENTATION

The usual presentation of melanoma is a pigmented skin lesion that has recently changed. Melanomas typically have irregular borders, variegated pigmentation ranging from pink to blue to black, and a raised irregular surface. Although melanomas arise de novo in the majority of patients, they may arise from preexisting nevi in 10 to 50 per cent. Advanced lesions present with itching and bleeding, presumably signs that the lesion has invaded the cutaneous nerve plexus or superficial capillary bed. Advanced lesions also may be ulcerated, and any change in a nevus such as change in color, a papule arising in the center of an existing nevus, bleeding, and ulceration are important signs that suggest the possibility of malignancy. Melanoma may also elude prompt diagnosis because of atypical presentation such as amelanotic (unpigmented) melanoma, unknown primary melanoma, and melanomas arising from noncutaneous sites (ocular sites, mucous membranes, meninges, and viscera). Visceral melanomas (esophagus, lung, adrenal gland) are very rare, and ocular melanomas are the most common of the noncutaneous melanomas.

DIAGNOSIS OF CUTANEOUS MELANOMA

Careful examination of the skin is a beginning in diagnosis. Any lesion that has irregular borders, variations in pigmentation, black color, or an irregular surface—especially if it has undergone recent change, is raised, or has begun to itch or to bleed—should arouse suspicion. The lymph node basins draining the region of the lesion also must be examined carefully.

Whenever melanoma is suspected in a skin lesion, a full-thickness biopsy of the skin is advised. Prognosis depends on the measured thickness, and shave biopsies and partial thickness excisions prevent assessment of Breslow thickness. Complete excisional biopsy, with narrow margins, is the ideal diagnostic procedure. On the extremity, it is critical to orient the incision longitudinally so that reexcision, if needed, may be performed without skin grafting. In some cases, such as with large facial lesions when complete excision of a pigmented lesion would be unreasonably deforming, partial excision is recommended for diagnosis, with a full-thickness portion of the most suspicious region included in the specimen. Diagnosis is determined by histologic examination of the biopsy specimen.

HISTOLOGIC ASPECTS AND PROGNOSTIC FACTORS

There are four major histologic types of cutaneous melanoma (Table 2). *Superficial spreading melanoma* (SSM) is most common and may occur on any cutaneous site. It grows radially for months to years, with little or no surface elevation (radial growth phase). Eventually it enters a vertical growth phase, at which time a nodular component is evident. *Nodular melanoma* (NM) has a vertical growth phase but lacks a radial growth phase, is usually diagnosed when it is thick, and has a correspondingly less favorable prognosis. *Lentigo maligna melanoma* (LMM) arises on sun-exposed surfaces, especially the face, typically arises from a macular brown lesion, often large in diameter that has been present for decades (Hutchinson's freckle), and has a more favorable diagnosis. *Acral lentiginous melanoma* (ALM) has a prolonged radial growth phase and characteristically arises on the glabrous skin of the palms and soles or in a subungual position (acral sites). This lesion is more common among blacks than are any of the other histologic types, and it tends to have a poor prognosis.

PROGNOSTIC FACTORS

Histologic evaluation of the primary melanoma is the first step toward assessing prognosis. Clark classified melanomas based on the level of invasion into and through the layers of the skin. These levels are defined in Table 3. The more invasive lesions have a less favorable prognosis. In 1970, Breslow reported that the thickness of the lesion, as measured by the pathologist with an ocular micrometer, also predicts prognosis. It is now generally accepted that Breslow thickness has greater prognostic value than Clark

TABLE 2. CLINICAL AND HISTOLOGIC CHARACTERISTICS OF THE FOUR PREDOMINANT GROWTH PATTERNS OF CUTANEOUS MELANOMA*

Growth Pattern	Relative Incidence	Mean Thickness	Mean Age (years)	Percentage Male	Percentage Black	Mortality (%)/Median Follow-Up (years)
LMM	5%	1.9 mm	60.1	63%	0.6%	29%/3.8 years
SSM	67%	1.7 mm	46.0	52%	0.3%	25%/4.3 years
Nodular	19%	3.6 mm	49.2	57%	0.3%	41%/3.8 years
ALM	5%	2.8 mm	56.3	47%	12.1%	50%/4.5 years

*Data derived from Slingluff CL, Seigler HF: Duke Melanoma Database, 8-18-91, 8075 patients.
Abbreviations: LMM = lentigo maligna melanoma, SSM = superficial spreading melanoma, ALM = acral lentiginous melanoma.

level. Mortality rates associated with a 1-mm lesion, a 3-mm lesion, and a 6-mm lesion are approximately 20, 45, and 70 per cent, respectively.

Other characteristics of primary melanomas also have prognostic significance. A better prognosis has been associated with the following: absence of ulceration, extremity primary site, lentigo maligna histology, absence of a vertical growth phase, and the presence of lymphocytes infiltrating the tumor. Among the clinical prognostic factors are gender and race. Females have an increased risk of melanoma but have an improved outcome, as they are more likely than males to develop melanoma on an extremity, which partially explains the improved prognosis. Caucasians are far more likely to develop melanoma than blacks, but blacks who develop melanoma have a poorer prognosis. Blacks are more likely to present with thick primaries and with acral and mucocutaneous primaries, which have a poorer prognosis.

STAGING

There are two principal staging systems for melanoma. The system defined by the American Joint Committee on Cancer (AJCC) is a tumor node metastasis (TNM) system and is summarized in Table 4. The older system, still in use by many cancer centers and prevalent in the literature, is a three-stage system that benefits from simplicity. Stage I indicates localized disease, including local recurrences less than 5 cm from the primary; stage II involves lymph node metastasis; and stage III involves distant metastatic disease. The advantage of the AJCC classification is that it takes into account the microstaging information available from Breslow thickness and/or Clark level. Neither system includes all relevant prognostic factors. Because many relevant prognostic factors have been defined for melanoma, it is inappropriate when comparing or describing patient groups to limit information to stage alone, regardless of the staging system used.

The history and physical examination are the most valuable staging procedures. Eighty per cent of first recurrences are to local or distant skin or to regional nodes and are best identified by physical examination of the primary site, skin, and the draining nodal basins. Palpable nodes larger than 1 cm should arouse suspicion of metastatic disease and can be evaluated by fine-needle aspirate cytology or by biopsy. Because the most common first visceral site of metastatic disease is the lung (Table 5), a chest radiograph is a useful screening procedure to detect hematogenous metastases. The most common abdominal visceral site of first metastases is the liver. A serum lactate dehydrogenase (LDH) level is obtained by some clinics as a screening test for liver metastases, but its value for asymptomatic patients is not documented. Because of the biologic tendency of melanoma to metastasize widely, it is not surprising that clinicians often believe

TABLE 3. CLARK LEVELS OF MELANOMA INVASION

	Description	Mortality (Clark)
Level I	In situ melanoma, confined to the epidermis (i.e., above the basement membrane)	—
Level II	Invasion into the papillary dermis	8%
Level III	Invasion through the papillary dermis, without invasion into the reticular dermis	35%
Level IV	Distinct invasion into the reticular dermis	47%
Level V	Invasion through all layers of the dermis and into the subcutaneous tissue	52%

TABLE 4. AJCC STAGING FOR MELANOMA

Stage*	Description
I	Localized <1.5 mm thick
II	Localized >1.5 mm thick
III	Nodal metastases involving only one regional nodal basin or 1 to 4 in-transit nodes
IV	Advanced regional metastases or any distant metastases

*Stage I is further subdivided into IA (<0.76 mm thick) and IB (0.76 to 1.5 mm thick), and stage II is further subdivided into IIA (1.5 to 4 mm thick) and IIB (>4 mm thick). When Breslow thickness is not available, stages IA, IB, IIA, and IIB can be defined by Clark levels, II, II, IV, and V, respectively.
Abbreviation: AJCC = American Joint Committee on Cancer.

TABLE 5. INCIDENCE OF FIRST AND SECOND
METASTASES IN EACH SITE*

Site	Percentage of First Metastases	Percentage of Second Metastases
Local skin	15.9	19.6
Nodes	60.0	24.4
Distant skin	4.4	12.2
Lung	8.4	15.2
Liver	2.5	6.8
Bone	1.4	4.1
CNS	3.1	9.5
GI	1.1	2.7
Other	3.1	5.1

*Data derived from Slingluff CL, Seigler HF: Duke Melanoma Database,
8-18-91, 8075 patients.
Abbreviations: CNS = central nervous system, GI = gastrointestinal.

they are compelled to perform an extensive work-up by ordering screening computed tomography (CT) scans of the brain, chest, and abdomen, at the time of diagnosis, for staging purposes. The cost of these screening tests is high, and in asymptomatic patients without clinical evidence of metastases, the yield of false-positives exceeds the yield of true-positives. Many visceral, central nervous system, and bone metastases are evident by history, and evidence of gastrointestinal symptoms, neurologic changes, or bone pain should be sought. When there is evidence of more advanced disease by history or physical examination, a more exhaustive radiologic examination is warranted.

TREATMENT OF THE PRIMARY LESION AND INITIAL MANAGEMENT OF REGIONAL NODES

Once the diagnosis of melanoma has been made by biopsy, a wide reexcision, also referred to as wide local excision (WLE), should be performed to reduce the risk of local recurrence. There is some variation among institutions about the margins obtained. A reasonable scheme, based on available data, is 0.5 cm for melanoma in situ, 1 cm for 1-mm invasive melanoma, and 2 to 3 cm for thicker lesions. Elective lymph node dissection has long been in the armamentarium of surgeons managing melanoma, but its role continues to be debated. The theoretical purpose of ELND is to remove occult nodal metastases before metastases occur. In patients with thin melanomas, the risk of recurrence and mortality is quite low (approximately 5 per cent recurrence rate for lesions <0.76 mm thick), and the potential benefit from ELND, if any, would be very small. On the other hand, thick melanomas (>4 mm) metastasize so frequently to distant sites that resection of clinically negative nodes would not be expected to alter the risk of mortality, and data support

this contention. Several retrospective reviews from the major melanoma clinics worldwide have reported an improved survival among patients with intermediate thickness melanoma who receive ELND. Prospective randomized trials have failed to show any survival benefit for ELND in similar patients, and recent major retrospective reviews have failed to support the earlier findings of a survival benefit.

Currently, it is within the standard of care to perform ELND in patients with intermediate thickness lesions (1.5 to 4 mm) and single draining nodal basins and who do not have medical contraindications to operation. Lymphoscintigraphy (using ^{99m} technetium antimony sulfur colloid) has been suggested as a means of mapping the lymphatic drainage from a primary site and, therefore, to determine the nodal basin for ELND. Because the putative value of ELND is modest at best, it is also reasonable (and not outside the standard of care) to follow all nodal basins clinically and to perform node dissections only for palpable nodes. The incidence of positive nodes at ELND depends on thickness of the primary tumor and is approximately 5 per cent for 0.76 to 1.5 mm thickness, 16 per cent for 2 to 3 mm thickness, and 35 to 40 per cent for thicknesses greater than 3 mm.

METASTATIC PATTERNS AND PATTERNS OF FAILURE

The natural history of a melanoma is to enlarge locally and to metastasize by lymphatic and hematogenous dissemination. After excision of the primary lesion, the patient may experience recurrence of disease locally, regionally, or systemically. Among those patients who develop recurrent or metastatic disease, the metastases are local in 16 per cent of cases, nodal (lymphatic metastases) in 60 per cent, and distant (hematogenous metastases) in 24 per cent. After the first recurrence, subsequent recurrences are more likely to be distant rather than local or regional, and the second recurrence is distant in 56 per cent of cases (Table 5). Once melanoma has metastasized to distant sites, it usually becomes so widely disseminated that, at autopsy, it can be found in virtually any organ. The typical clinical course after the development of recurrent diseases is progressive nodal disease with extension to visceral and distant skin sites. Central nervous system metastasis is commonly the terminal event. Prognosis in distant metastatic disease depends primarily on the extent and resectability of metastatic disease. A patient with an isolated metastasis may have a good outcome if resection is complete. Rarely, patients may also show benefit from systemic therapy or radiation therapy, as discussed below. Overall survival after the appearance of a distant metastasis is less than 5 per cent.

MANAGEMENT OF DISTANT METASTATIC DISEASE

When a patient presents with advanced disease (distant metastases or extensive regional nodal disease) for which resection is being considered, it is appropriate to perform CT scans to exclude occult metastases that diminish the chance of long-term survival after resection of the known metastatic disease. Resection of apparent solitary metastases does, in selected cases, provide palliation and extension of the disease-free interval, or even long-term survival. Resection of isolated nodal metastases is associated with up to 40 per cent 10-year survival. Although pulmonary metastases are associated with 70 per cent mortality within 1 year and a 4 per cent 5-year survival, it has been reported that resection of solitary pulmonary metastases was associated with a 20 per cent 5-year survival rate. Patients with isolated pulmonary metastases should be considered seriously for resection with curative intent. Similarly, complete resection of isolated metastases from the adrenal gland is associated with a 2-year median survival, and complete resection of gastrointestinal metastases is associated with a mean survival of 5 years. It is suggested that the diagnosis and resection of isolated metastases may improve patient prognosis. When complete resection of metastatic disease is not possible, radiation therapy or systemic therapy should be considered. Malignant melanoma is generally considered relatively radioresistant, but there have been reports of significant reductions in tumor mass with radiation therapy given in large fractions (>400 to 500 rads). In clinical practice, radiation therapy is not a major therapeutic arm but does have a place in several clinical situations. Treatment of unresectable brain metastases with radiation stabilizes or diminishes tumor size. Because the brain is relatively radioresistant, a therapeutic dose can be administered with minimal toxicity. Any unresectable bulk tumor may be considered for radiation therapy as palliation, alone or in combination with chemotherapy. The decision for each patient is based on multiple factors including tumor location and available alternatives. The patient who presents with massive regional disease may undergo resection (e.g., therapeutic node dissection) with removal of all gross tumor but with near certainty that microscopic or other nondetected tumor remains regionally. Radiation may be performed in an attempt to delay regional recurrence.

Chemotherapy has not been effective in the adjuvant mode, and its use is reserved for treatment of unresectable advanced disease. The most active single agent is dacarbazine (DTIC), with overall response rates of 20 per cent and uncommon complete responses. Other agents, each with lower response rates, include the nitrosureas (e.g., BCNU, CCNU, methyl-CCNU), the vinca alkaloids (vindesine), cisplatin, and dibromodulcitol. These and several others have been used in clinical trials alone or in combination. The most successful regimen is DTIC, BCNU, cisplatin, and tamoxifen. The response rates have been approximately 50 per cent, with 15 to 20 per cent complete responses. Tamoxifen appears to be a critical component of this regimen, for unknown reasons, and it is recommended as the first-line treatment for unresectable advanced disease. The role of immunotherapy for melanoma is controversial, but evidence suggests that melanoma-specific T-cell responses can be generated from patient lymphocytes and are therapeutically useful.

RECOMMENDATIONS FOR FOLLOW-UP

The patterns of metastasis and recurrence suggest that careful examination of the skin surrounding the primary lesion, the draining nodal basins, and the chest film will identify approximately 90 per cent of recurrent or metastatic lesions and are appropriate for follow-up visits. These patients have a risk of recurrence for decades, and once recurrence is clinically evident, it may progress rapidly. Therapeutic resection of nodes or of isolated distant metastases is associated with a reasonable chance of long-term survival. Based on these observations, it is appropriate to follow melanoma patients closely and probably for life. In the early years after diagnosis, this is best done by the original physician seeing the patient frequently. It can later be done by a family practitioner.

SUMMARY

Malignant melanoma is a neoplasm arising from melanocytes at the dermal/epidermal junction that usually begin by growing radially, and when they enter a vertical growth phase, there is greater likelihood of metastasis. Early diagnosis depends on a high level of suspicion. The typical characteristics of melanoma include irregular borders, dark and variegated color, and recent or progressive change or growth. Curative treatment for a primary melanoma is surgical excision with wide margins. Approximately one third of patients with melanoma who undergo appropriate surgical management of the primary lesion eventually develop recurrent disease. Usually, the first site of recurrent or metastatic disease is a regional lymph node, and the most common site of first hematogenous metastasis is the lung. Because most melanomas arise during patients' productive years, the impact of the disease is significant. Future progress in diminishing mortality and morbidity due to melanoma depends on (1) educational programs aimed at developing a national awareness of melanoma with the goal of earlier diagnosis, and (2) new approaches to the prevention and treatment of metastatic disease.

REFERENCES

Balch CM, et al (eds): Cutaneous Melanoma, ed 2. Philadelphia, JB Lippincott Company, 1992.

Breslow A: Thickness, cross-sectional areas and depth of invasion in the prognosis of cutaneous melanoma. Ann Surg 172:902–908, 1970.

Clark WH Jr, From L, Bernardino EA, Mihm MC: The histogenesis and biologic behavior of primary human malignant melanoma of the skin. Cancer Res 29:705–726, 1969.

Evans RD, Kopf AW, Lew RA, Rigel DS, Bart RS, Friedman RJ, Rivers JK: Risk factors for the development of malignant melanoma— I: Review of case-control studies. Dermatol Surg Oncol 14:393–408, 1988.

Ferrone S (ed): Human Melanoma. Berlin, Springer-Verlag, 1990.

III
Soft Tissue Sarcomas

H. KIM LYERLY, M.D.

PATHOGENESIS

Soft tissue sarcomas are malignant tumors arising in the extraskeletal connective tissue of the body. They are relatively uncommon neoplasms, constituting less than 0.5 per cent of malignant tumors, yet their estimated annual death rate is over 3000. The etiology of soft tissue sarcomas is poorly understood. An area known to be at high risk for the development of sarcoma is the field of radiation following therapy for breast cancer and Hodgkin's disease. Lymphangiosarcomas may occur in a lymphedematous arm after axillary node dissection for breast cancer (Stewart-Treves syndrome). Certain inherited conditions also predispose to the development of sarcomas. Fibrosarcomas occur in 15 per cent of patients with neurofibromatosis, and patients with Gardner's syndrome are known to be at risk for desmoid tumors. Finally, agents such as Thorotrast, a radiologic contrast agent

no longer in use, and polyvinyl chloride have been associated with angiosarcomas of the liver.

PATHOLOGY

Soft tissue sarcomas occur throughout the body. Approximately half are found in the lower extremities, 13 per cent in the upper extremities, and 33 per cent on the trunk and the retroperitoneum. The pathologic classification of soft tissue sarcomas is based on the putative cell of origin of the tumor. Light microscopy, electron microscopy, immunohistochemical studies, and genetic studies have recently been utilized in combination for the precise identification and histopathologic classification of these tumors. The myogenic, neurogenic, or epithelial origin of tumors can often be demonstrated using specific antibodies in immunohistochemical analysis. In addition, cytogenetic abnormalities can facilitate a diagnosis. For example, chromosomal translocations are seen in synovial sarcomas (x;18), alveolar rhabdomyosarcoma (2;13), and myxoid liposarcoma (12;16). Malignant fibrous histiocytomas, malignant peripheral nerve sheath tumors, and some leiomyosarcomas are distinguished by the absence of translocation. The most important components of pathologic classification are the *tissue type*, whether benign or malignant, and the *histopathologic grade* of malignant tumors. Consequently, a number of soft tissue sarcomas have been described, each with distinguishing histologic features and biologic behaviors and varying tendencies for local infiltration and distant metastases.

Histologic types of soft tissue sarcomas include liposarcomas, malignant fibrohistiosarcomas, leiomyosarcomas, fibrosarcomas, and rhabdomyosarcomas. There are soft tissue tumors that appear histologically malignant with the capacity for aggressive local invasion but which rarely metastasize, including desmoid tumors, dermatofibrosarcoma protuberants, and well-differentiated liposarcomas. Metastases of other soft tissue sarcomas occur most frequently to the lungs by the hematologic route. Some of these tumors, especially synovial sarcomas, embryonal rhabdomyosarcomas, epithelioid sarcomas, and malignant fibrohistiocytomas, may metastasize to regional lymph nodes in 10 to 20 per cent of patients, with the malignant fibrohistiocytomas having the highest incidence of lymphatic spread in adults.

The histologic grade of a soft tissue sarcoma is widely accepted as the most important indicator of the biologic behavior. Estimation of nuclear DNA content and altered gene expression also has prognostic significance. Approximately one third of soft tissue sarcomas are low grade, and low-grade sarcomas tend to grow locally and invade aggressively but metastasize in only 14 per cent of patients. High-grade tumors are more likely to metastasize to distant sites. The most commonly used system of classification ranks sarcomas as *low*, *intermediate*, or *high* grade depending on certain criteria, including mitotic rate, nuclear morphology, degree of cellularity, cellular anaplasia or pleomorphism, presence of necrosis, amount of surrounding stroma, and vascularity.

CLINICAL PRESENTATION

A sarcoma typically occurs as a painless mass or may gradually enlarge until it becomes painful or interferes with function. Pain may be caused by either hemorrhage or necrosis within the tumor or compression of peripheral nerves and is present in about one third of patients. Superficially located sarcomas are usually small when discovered, whereas in fleshy areas or in the retroperitoneal region they may be quite large before detection.

DIAGNOSIS

Because no reliable physical signs or historic data distinguish benign from malignant soft tissue lesions, all soft tissue masses that persist should be biopsied. Small soft tissue masses that have been present and unchanged for many years may be followed, but lesions larger than 3 cm, as well as any enlarging tumors, should be biopsied or removed. Aspiration cytology has a less useful role in the diagnosis of soft tissue sarcomas because of limited sampling and difficulty in differentiating between the cellular elements of reactive and benign neoplasms and those of malignant neoplastic lesions. Core needle biopsy is simple and may be performed to establish a diagnosis of a primary soft tissue sarcoma, but is more often used to confirm residual or recurrent disease following treatment. Contamination of surrounding tissue planes is minimal if only one pass is made into the tumor. A disadvantage of core needle biopsy to confirm a diagnosis of a primary sarcoma is that a small, potentially unrepresentative sample may be obtained. Multiple needle passes are to be avoided due to the risk of local recurrence in the needle tracks. The skin puncture site on the needle track must be placed so as to be readily included in the excision if the mass proves to be sarcoma.

The most reliable method of confirming a diagnosis of soft tissue sarcoma is open biopsy. Small lesions can be sampled by excisional biopsy, but an incisional biopsy is preferred for most lesions. Biopsy incisions should be made along a longitudinal axis of the extremity so that the site of biopsy may be included in subsequent wide excisions, if indicated, without sacrificing unnecessary overlying skin. Biopsy and histologic grading is mandatory before proper therapy can be initiated.

Clinical evaluation is directed at determining the site, size, and depth of the tumor and possible bone and neurovascular involvement. Regional lymph node metastases are rare, and the most common site of first metastasis is the lung. Routine radiographs of soft tissue sarcomas are of little clinical value. However, chest films and computed tomographic (CT) scans are useful to exclude pulmonary metastases. Computed tomography and magnetic resonance imaging (MRI) are the most useful modalities for evaluation of soft tissue sarcomas, as they allow visualization of major vascular, gastrointestinal, and genitourinary structures. Magnetic resonance imaging appears to offer better delineation of the tumor and surrounding muscles and permits visualization of the tumor from the coronal and diagonal aspects.

MANAGEMENT

Several staging systems based on prognostic factors have been proposed, and they are based primarily on histologic grade, which is the most important prognostic indicator. The staging system from the American Joint Committee on Cancer is based on three histologic grades: tumor size, status of regional nodes, and the presence of distant metastases. Survival decreases with increasing stage, and the inclusion of lymph node status may be unnecessary, as nodal metastases from sarcomas are uncommon.

An increased knowledge about the natural history of sarcomas, their biology, and their response to adjuvant therapy has facilitated advances in the surgical management of soft tissue sarcomas. In the past, local excision with little or no margin was commonly advocated. Soft tissue sarcomas tend not to be encapsulated; rather, they possess a pseudocapsule, which is composed of malignant cells compressed against normal cells. Local excision often "shells out" the tumor, leaving a perimeter of malignant cells. This residual tumor was associated with a high local recurrence rate, predictably followed by distant metastases and death. Therefore, more radical surgical excisions of wide local excision with a margin of normal tissue were advocated with improved local control rates. Currently, the primary objective of the surgeon is to resect the tumor, with a wide margin (2 to 3 cm) of local tissue spanning the limb.

Despite improved local control, survival rates at 5 and 10 years following radical resections remained poor. Hence, combined-modality therapy was introduced for the management of soft tissue sarcoma. Interest in multimodality therapy was stimulated by experience with rhabdomyosarcoma in children, in which adjuvant chemotherapy and radiation therapy improved survival from less than 10 per cent to 60 to 70 per cent.

Adjuvant radiation therapy minimizes the need for amputation. In randomized prospective trials, with the use of adjuvant chemotherapy, wide en bloc resection with adjuvant external beam radiation therapy to 6000 rad was equivalent to amputation. Brennan showed that local recurrence is significantly decreased by adjuvant radiation therapy, but it had no impact on long-term survival. The local recurrence rate was reduced by radiation therapy due to its affect on high-grade tumors (i.e., those tumors most likely to develop subsequent metastatic disease). Therefore, further studies are needed to document the impact on survival of radiation therapy for low-grade tumors, which have a low risk of metastases. Other questions regarding radiotherapy include its method of use.

A number of other modalities have been used for the treatment of soft tissues sarcoma, including both intra-arterial chemotherapy, preoperative radiation therapy, isolated lymph profusion, and hyperthermia in various combinations. Each of these has shown some efficacy, but their precise role in the management of patients with sarcoma is not clearly defined. The value of chemotherapy has not been clearly defined in the adult population. Although some reports have suggested a long-term survival benefit, others have been contradictory. High-risk patients should consider combined-modality therapy with chemotherapy.

Although metastatic disease from extremity lesions is predominantly to the lung, other sites can be involved. Pulmonary resection has been advocated for metastatic sarcoma, as 5-year survival rate of 30 per cent can be expected in patients who have had complete resection. Unfortunately, most patients develop metastatic disease at other sites and, of those patients who have pulmonary metastases, only half are suitable for operation. Retroperitoneal sarcomas represent another common site for soft tissue sarcoma. They are unusual tumors, comprising 0.1 to 0.2 per cent of all malignant tumors, and because of their location, symptoms are usually subtle and many are quite large at the time of initial diagnosis. Most patients present with a palpable abdominal mass that may or may not be painful due to compression of peripheral nerves or nerve routes. It is very uncommon for patients to experience intestinal obstruction. Myosarcomas and liposarcomas are common histologic types in this location. As with the extremity sarcomas, CT is the most common investigative modality, but this is being replaced by MRI. The primary treatment modality remains complete surgical excision. It is significant that a large percentage of patients with retroperitoneal sarcomas require resection of other retroperitoneal organs, commonly the kidney. Operability rates have increased and operative morbidity and mortality have decreased, survival being related primarily to the completeness of resection. In those patients with a complete resection, the most important factor in survival is the histologic grade of the tumor. At this time adjuvant radiation and chemotherapy do not appear to have significant survival benefit, but their use should be considered with patients with high-grade tumors.

REFERENCES

Brennan MF, Casper ES, Harrison LB, Shiu MH, Gaynor J, Hajdu SI: The role of multimodality therapy in soft tissue sarcoma. Ann Surg 214:328–338, 1991.

Geer RJ, Woodruff J, Caspar ES, Brennan MF: Management of adult primary small (5 cm or less) soft tissue sarcomas at the extremity. Arch Surg 127:1285–1289, 1992.

Lawrence W, Donegan WL, Natarajan N, et al: Adult soft tissue sarcomas. A pattern of care. Survey of the American College of Surgeons. Ann Surg 205:349– 359, 1987.

Lawrence W, Neifeld JP: Soft tissue sarcomas. Curr Probl Surg 26: 759–827, 1989.

Řosenberg SA, Tepper J, Glatstein E, Costa J, Baker A, et al: The treatment of soft tissue sarcoma of the extremities: Prospective randomized evaluations of (1) lymph-sparing surgery plus radiation therapy compared with amputation and (2) the role of adjuvant chemotherapy. Ann Surg 196:305–315, 1982.

IV
Tumor Markers

H. KIM LYERLY, M.D.

Physical examination and radiographs rarely detect tumor masses of less than 1 cm^3, a size that reflects approximately 1×10^9 tumor cells. Because the optimal management of patients with cancer continues to be dependent on early detection and treatment of minimal tumor burden, tumor markers or alternative methods to detect tumor or tumor-specific products are continually sought. The potential uses for tests to detect minimal tumor burden include screening of asymptomatic populations, diagnosis, prognosis, assessment of therapeutic efficacy, and detection of residual recurrent disease. A number of tumor markers are useful in screening high-risk populations and as index of response to treatment and recurrence of disease. A list of tumor markers with their corresponding malignant and nonmalignant conditions is presented in Table 1.

A tumor marker used for screening should possess a high sensitivity for the detection of early, curable lesions in asymptomatic patients. An excellent example of such a marker is *calcitonin*, which is detected in the plasma of individuals following provocative testing and can be used to detect surgically curable C-cell carcinoma or medullary thyroid carcinoma in situ in patients with familial multiple endocrine neoplasia type IIA (MEN-IIA). A more widely applicable but less specific test is *prostatic specific antigen* (PSA), used for the detection of prostatic carcinoma.

The most widespread current application for the measurement of circulating tumor markers is the assessment of treatment efficacy and follow-up for recurrent disease. For example, detection of rising serum levels of *carcinoembryonic antigen* (CEA) suggests recurrence of malignant tumors or a poor response to therapy. In these settings, measurement of marker levels may influence management decisions, such as continuing or discontinuing therapy or performing imaging studies or surgical therapy at the site of recurrent disease. Tumor markers may also be used to confirm the diagnosis of a particular tumor, especially by detection of circulating tumor-specific products or secretions such as hormone markers of endocrine tumors. More frequently, the measurement of tumor markers may yield prognostic rather than diagnostic information. For example, detection of CEA in the serum of patients is not diagnostic of colorectal carcinoma, but patients with colorectal cancer and those with high serum levels of CEA at the time of diagnosis have a worse prognosis than those with low levels of CEA.

CATEGORIES OF TUMOR MARKERS

Tumor markers are classified into *tumor-specific antigens*, *tumor-specific enzymes*, and *tumor-specific hormones*, but it is clear that few, if any, of the cur-

TABLE 1. TUMOR MARKERS ASSOCIATED WITH MALIGNANCIES

Tumor Marker	Normal Limit	Associated Malignancies	Associated Nonmalignant Conditions	Sensitivity (%)	Specificity (%)
Carcinoembryonic antigen (CEA)	3–5 μg/ml	Colon, pancreas, stomach, lung, breast, thyroid, and ovarian cancers	Smokers, peptic ulcer disease, gastritis, pancreatitis, cirrhosis, inflammatory bowel disease, hepatitis, jaundice, bronchitis, emphysema, benign prostatic hypertrophy, and renal failure	42–96	10–90
Alpha-fetoprotein (AFP)	15 μg/ml	Hepatocellular, gastric, pancreatic, colon, and lung cancers Nonseminomatous germ cell tumors	Pregnancy, alcoholic and viral hepatitis, cirrhosis, inflammatory bowel disease, ataxia telangiectasia	60–90	60 100
Prostatic-specific antigen (PSA)	2.5 μg/ml	Prostatic cancer, myeloma, bony metastases from nonprostatic cancers	Benign prostatic hypertrophy, osteoporosis, hyperthyroidism, hyperparathyroidism	33–99	82–97
β-Human chorionic gonadotropin (BHCG)	3 IU/ml	Trophoblastic tumors; germ cell neoplasms; adenocarcinomas of ovary; pancreatic, gastric, and hepatocellular cancers	Pregnancy	60–100	40 90
CA 125	35 μg/ml	80% of ovarian cancer, 20% of nongynecologic cancers	1% healthy controls, 5% benign disease	40–86	86–99

rently detected markers are *tumor specific*. Rather, evolving technologies have provided increasingly sophisticated measures to differentiate between normal and malignant cells, and these approaches have been applied to the detection of tumor-associated products in the serum or body fluids of patients. For example, the earliest and best characterized tumor markers include the enzyme *acid phosphatase* for the detection of prostate cancer and the antigen *CEA* for the detection of gastrointestinal malignancies. However, even the biologic tests for enzyme activity can be replaced by immunoassays for specific proteins, replacing the usually cumbersome bioassays and blurring the distinctions between tumor-specific enzymes and antigens. Tumor antigens have also been subcategorized as *oncofetal antigens*, and *polyclonal* or *monoclonal antibody-defined antigens*. Oncofetal antigens are produced during normal development by the placental complex and are also produced by neoplastic tissue and include CEA, *alpha-fetoprotein* (AFP), and *β-human chorionic gonadotropin* (BHCG). As polyclonal and monoclonal antibody technology advances, an evolving category of tumor markers is being defined by antibodies directed against tumor extracts or cell lines, or products elicited from the tumors. Some of these carcinoma antigens are CA125, CA99, and CA15.3.

Finally, the directly measured activated oncogenes or mutated tumor suppressor genes may be evaluated for their ability to serve as tumor markers. For example, detection of mutated *ras* genes in the intestinal tract of patients with colorectal carcinoma has been reported. The detection via DNA amplification of other genes in body fluids or plasma may produce the most sensitive and specific tumor markers to date.

Carcinoembryonic Antigen

Carcinoembryonic antigen is a classic example of a tumor marker that is widely used, but is not an ideal marker because of low specificity and sensitivity. Serum levels are usually less than 2.5 ng/ml in normals, and concentrations greater than 5 ng/ml are considered elevated. Elevations in CEA are primarily associated with cancer of the colon, but serum levels may also be elevated in patients with cancer of the pancreas, stomach, lung, breast, thyroid, and ovary. In addition, CEA may be elevated in patients with nonmalignant conditions including peptic ulcer disease, gastritis, pancreatitis, inflammatory bowel disease, cirrhosis, hepatitis and jaundice, bronchitis and emphysema, as well as benign prostatic hypertrophy and renal failure. Although CEA is not specific for colorectal tumors, the highest concentrations in tissue and serum have been found in patients with colorectal carcinomas. In addition to being nonspecific, serum CEA levels are insensitive, as elevated CEA levels occur in only 5 per cent of patients with localized, surgically curable colon cancer and 65 to 90 per cent of patients with either distant or locally advanced disease. Carcinoembryonic antigen cannot be used to screen normal populations for colon cancer, in which small tumors would be expected. Screening of patients with conditions such as ulcerative colitis or polyposis coli, that predispose to colorectal cancer, has also been unsuccessful because these diseases themselves may produce elevated serum levels of CEA. Some reports indicate that preoperative serum CEA concentrations before definitive resection of primary colorectal cancer are an independent prognostic parameter of subsequent survival. Thus, the higher the preoperative serum CEA level, the poorer the prognosis of a patient with colon cancer.

Detection of CEA is most often used to follow patients after resection of a tumor. Elevated serum levels of CEA indicate recurrent colorectal cancer, usually 4 to 6 months before it is clinically evident. In general, serum CEA levels are elevated in approximately two of three patients before any other evidence of recurrent colon or rectal cancer is present. These levels need not have been elevated preoperatively to be elevated postoperatively as a marker of tumor recurrence following resection. When a rise in CEA is noted, a careful physical examination should be performed and radiographic and endoscopic examinations for recurrent or metastatic disease should be done. Following detection of recurrent disease, a second-look exploratory procedure with resection of recurrent disease is often appropriate. The results of CEA-initiated second-look procedures vary, with some reporting complete resection in 70 per cent of patients and others finding this approach of little, if any, benefit. The strategy of reoperation can provide a cure for a small percentage of patients and may be used to document definite recurrence of colorectal carcinoma in most patients. Potential improvement in the selection of patients and results for CEA-initiated second-look operative procedures may be achieved through better preoperative localization of the extent of disease. Some advocate a method using radiolabeled antibody to CEA and scintigraphy for the detection of the exact location and extent of recurrent tumor. Patients with resectable recurrent disease or liver disease can then be selected for second-look operation. Serum levels of CEA appear to correlate with distant disease extent in patients with colorectal cancer. Serum levels usually rise with disease progression and fall with regression, but once markedly elevated, the levels do not always correlate directly with tumor burden. Serum CEA levels have been used to monitor the response to chemotherapy in patients with metastatic colorectal cancer. For those with metastatic colorectal cancer who had elevated serum CEA levels and responded to chemotherapy, 89 per cent showed a decrease in serum CEA levels. In patients who had progressive disease despite therapy, 90 per cent had an increase in serum CEA levels compared to pretreatment levels.

Alpha-Fetoprotein

Alpha-fetoprotein was the first oncofetal antigen discovered to be a useful tumor marker for primary hepatocellular carcinoma and nonseminomatous cell tumors of the testes. Abnormal serum levels of AFP usually occur with malignant neoplasms but can also occur in nonmalignant diseases of endodermal-derived organs, such as hepatitis, inflammatory bowel disease, ataxia-telangiectasia, and hereditary tyrosinemia. However, highly elevated serum levels of AFP are present exclusively in primary hepatocellular and nonseminomatous testicular tumors. Eighty per cent of patients with hepatocellular carcinoma have elevated serum levels of AFP. Approximately 20 per cent of patients with gastric or pancreatic cancer and 5 per cent of patients with colorectal or lung cancer also have significant elevations in serum AFP. Investigators have assessed AFP levels in detection of hepatocellular carcinoma in at-risk populations, but the results have been disappointing. Serum AFP levels may be normal in 30 to 50 per cent of patients with hepatocellular carcinoma. In a few patients with hepatocellular carcinoma, serum levels of AFP fall despite continued tumor growth. In the presence of cirrhosis, a serum level of AFP greater than 500 ng/ml is diagnostic of hepatocellular carcinoma.

Serum levels of AFP may also be of prognostic value for the subgroup of patients with normal serum levels and a relatively good prognosis. In these patients the primary factor predicting better prognosis may be the absence of cirrhosis. Normal serum AFP levels are more common in patients without underlying cirrhosis. Serum measurement of AFP levels can be helpful before and after presumed curative surgical resection in patients with hepatocellular carcinoma. However, serum levels of this tumor do not always show the presence of recurrent hepatocellular carcinoma, as it may recur without elevation due to variation in AFP synthesis in different parts of the same tumor. Thus, the ability of the tumor to secrete AFP may change with growth. If specific chemotherapy is effective, serum AFP levels usually fall continuously, indicating tumor regression and effective treatment. If serum AFP levels show a continued rise despite antitumor treatment, the tumor is probably resistant to the treatment, and an alternative regimen should be used. Monitoring of serum AFP levels in hepatocellular carcinoma can help abort prolonged ineffective use of toxic chemotherapy.

Prostatic-Specific Antigen

Prostatic-specific antigen is a glycoprotein specific for prostatic tissue with utility as a very sensitive tumor marker for prostatic cancer. Approximately 90 per cent of normal males have detectable serum levels of PSA, with normal being defined as less than 2.5 ng/ml. Some 96 per cent of patients with early carcinoma of the prostate and 100 per cent of patients with more advanced disease have elevated serum levels of PSA. However, 86 per cent of patients with benign prostatic hypertrophy have *moderate* elevations of serum PSA levels, thus limiting its utility as a screening test for prostatic cancer. The level of the serum marker may also increase following prostatic massage, prostatic biopsy, and transurethral resection.

Despite the nonspecific nature of the PSA, it is currently being used for screening for prostatic carcinoma. If the level of PSA is from 0 to 4 μg/ml, the patient is considered to be at low risk for prostatic carcinoma. If, however, the value is greater than 4, prostatic ultrasound should be considered. Core needle biopsies are obtained of any nodules that are palpable or evident by prostatic ultrasound, and blind biopsies of either lobe may be obtained for persistently elevated PSA. Values that appear to be greater than 12 are unlikely to be due to benign causes.

REFERENCES

National Institutes of Health Consensus Development Conference. Carcinoembryonic antigen: Its role as a marker in the management of cancer. Ann Intern Med 94:407–409, 1981.

Norton JA, Fraker DL: Tumor markers. *In* Sabiston DC Jr (ed): Textbook of Surgery: The Biological Basis for Modern Surgical Practice, ed 14. Philadelphia, WB Saunders Company, 1991, pp 491–509.

Sell S (ed): Serological Cancer Markers. Totowa, NJ, Humana Press, 1992.

Sell S: Cancer markers of the 1990s. Clin Lab Med 10:1–37, 1990.

20
THE BREAST

I
The Breast

CHRISTINA WELTZ, M.D.   H. KIM LYERLY, M.D.

Common breast diseases include disorders of normal physiologic function, inflammatory disorders, and benign or malignant neoplasms. Disorders of normal physiologic function include fibrocystic changes that may cause pain (mastodynia), fullness, nipple discharge, galactorrhea, or cyst formation. Although these disorders are common, therapy is currently directed toward excluding breast neoplasms as a cause of these symptoms, as well as providing symptomatic relief. In addition to disorders of function, inflammatory disorders may occur and may require surgical evaluation and intervention. Benign breast tumors are common and, although not life threatening, may be the cause of much concern while the possibility of a malignant process is excluded. Benign tumors commonly include breast cysts and fibroadenomas.

Disorders of the breast that are most concerning are malignant neoplasms. Breast cancer is the most common cancer in women in the United States, diagnosed in over 180,000 women in 1993. The lifetime risk for developing breast cancer for a woman in the United States is greater than 10 per cent (Table 1). Risk of breast cancer varies with a woman's age, and the greater than 10 per cent risk is based on a theoretical lifetime of 110 years. Thus, the evaluation of a patient presenting with a breast disorder requires not only an accurate history, physical examination, and interpretation of diagnostic tests, but also a high index of suspicion for carcinoma, detailed knowledge of breast physiology, and indications for more invasive diagnostic tests.

In addition to the skills necessary for early detection and diagnosis, expertise in the treatment of breast cancer is required for managing patients with breast lesions. The management of breast cancer has dramatically changed over the past several decades, and current knowledge concerning the multimodality therapy of breast carcinoma is required to make rational therapeutic decisions. This requires knowledge of the evaluation of breast disorders as well as familiarity with the natural history of precancerous breast disorders and the histologic subtypes of breast carcinoma.

TABLE 1. PROBABILITY OF DEVELOPING BREAST CANCER DURING VARIOUS AGE INTERVALS*

Age Interval	Risk of Developing Breast Cancer (in situ or invasive)
20–30	0.04%
35–45	0.88%
50–60	1.95%
65–75	3.17%
Cumulative Birth to 110	10.2%

*From Seidman H, Mushinski MH, Gelb SK, Silverberg E: Probabilities of eventually developing or dying of cancer—United States, 1985. CA 35(1):36–56, 1985, with permission.

In addition, keen interpretation is required when assessing additional information about breast tumors, such as DNA content, hormone receptor expression, percentage of cells in the S phase of the cell cycle, oncogene expression, and other measures of biologic behavior. The indications for adjuvant treatment has continued to evolve, and knowledge of the current indications and options for adjuvant therapy is required to make rational decisions regarding its use.

ANATOMY

During the first trimester of fetal life, bilateral milk lines develop in the fetus and extend from the axilla to the pubis. By the ninth week, only the milk bud, or the pectoral portion of the milk line, remains. Hence, in the normal adult, breast tissue is usually located only in the pectoral region, but variations in anatomy may occur that reflect the embryologic development of the breast. Commonly, breast tissue extends into the fold of the axillary space.

The breast is composed of epithelium, fibrous stroma and supporting structures, and fat, in various relative amounts. Throughout the fat of the breast, strands of dense connective tissue provide shape and support to the breast by connecting the underlying deep fascia to the skin. These are termed *Cooper's ligaments* which, due to their attachments to the skin, may reflect deep changes in the breast by dimpling. The glandular structure of the breast is organized as an array of successfully branching ducts connecting the milk-producing lobules to the nipple via the large subareolar lactiferous sinus, which opens onto the surface of the nipple through 15 to 20 orifices. At the terminal end of the ductal system, the ducts end blindly in the terminal ductules or acini to form lobules.

Important clinical features of the gross anatomy of the breast are elucidated by considering the surgical principles of mastectomy, the goal of which is removal of all perceptible breast tissue. The anatomic relations of the breast on the chest wall define the extent of dissection and excision. The breast is bordered anteriorly by the superficial layer of the superficial pectoral fascia, which lies deep to the dermis (Fig. 1). Skin flaps are created by dissecting in the plane between the dermis and this superficial layer of fascia. The width of this plane, and hence the potential thickness of the flap, varies with the patient's body fat content.

The medial border of breast tissue and skin-flap creation is the sternal edge, and the lateral border is the midaxillary line, defined operatively by the latissimus dorsi muscle. Inferiorly, the breast extends to the inframammary fold, which corresponds to the sixth and seventh ribs. The superior border of the breast overlies the second and third ribs, and dissection is normally performed to the lower level of the clavicle. The breast is excised from the chest wall by dissecting immediately above the pectoralis muscle. The excised specimen thus includes the retromammary space, consisting of the loose areolar tissue that enables mobility of the breast relative to the chest wall.

Most breast lymphatic drainage is through the axilla. Excision and pathologic analysis of axillary lymph nodes determines staging and treatment of breast cancer and is thus a standard component of modified radical mastectomy. The five major axillary node groups are depicted in Figure 2. Three levels of axillary nodes relative to the pectoralis minor muscle have been described (Fig. 3). Level I nodes are lateral to the muscle and include the external mammary, subscapular, and axillary vein groups. Level II lies deep to the muscle and consists of the central axillary group. Level III contains the subclavicular group, is medial to the pectoralis minor, and usually requires division of that muscle near its insertion at the coracoid process for adequate exposure and excision. Lymph tissue also flows through the interpectoral (or Rotter's) nodes, and through the medially located internal mammary nodes. These groups are not dissected in the conventional modified radical mastectomy.

Axillary dissection requires knowledge of two nerves. The long thoracic nerve to the serratus anterior muscle courses medially through the axilla. During axillary dissection, it should be identified and maintained against the chest wall while the axillary contents are freed and excised. Injury to the nerve can cause a winged scapula deformity. The thoracodorsal nerve courses more laterally in the axilla and enters the medial aspect of the latissimus dorsi muscle at the level of the second and third ribs. This nerve enables medial rotation and adduction of the arm. The arterial supply to the breast is from branches of the internal mammary, lateral thoracic, and axillary artery. Venous drainage follows the course of arterial supply. The axillary vein is the principal drainage.

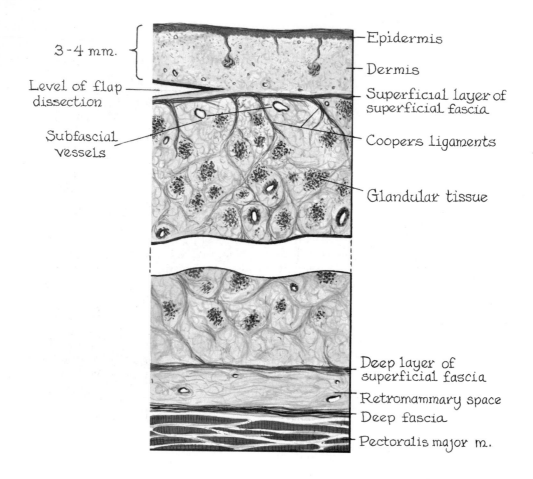

3-4 mm.

Level of flap dissection

Subfascial vessels

Epidermis

Dermis

Superficial layer of superficial fascia

Coopers ligaments

Glandular tissue

Deep layer of superficial fascia

Retromammary space

Deep fascia

Pectoralis major m.

Figure 1. Cross-sectional depiction of breast tissue revealing anatomic relations to skin, fascia, and muscle. The breast is bordered anteriorly and posteriorly by the superficial and deep layers of the superficial pectoral fascia. During mastectomy, skin flaps are created in the plane between the dermis and superficial layer of superficial fascia. The breast is excised by creating a plane immediately overlying the pectoralis muscle. The excised specimen includes the retromammary space. (From Haagensen CD: Diseases of the Breast, ed 3. Philadelphia, WB Saunders Company, 1986, p 15, with permission.)

PHYSIOLOGY

Development and function of the breast are under hormonal control, primarily estrogen and progesterone, and the physiology of the breast reflects changing levels of these hormones (Fig. 4). During infancy and childhood, estrogen levels are low and the breast is quiescent, consisting of fat and stroma, with few ducts and no lobules. At puberty, ovarian secretion of estrogen stimulates development of the ductal epithelium and stroma, while progesterone initiates differentiation of the lobules. Ongoing cyclical changes in hormone levels following menarche promote increased breast adipose content, darkening of the nipple/areolar complex, further proliferation of ductules and lobules, and attainment of the mature, hemispherically shaped breast. Each menstrual cycle is marked by late luteal or premenstrual glandular hypertrophy and dilatation and stromal edema. These changes are effected by the premenstrual surge of estrogen and progesterone levels and are clinically manifest as breast pain, tenderness, and nodularity on physical examination.

During pregnancy, high estrogen and progesterone levels are maintained by the corpus luteum during the first trimester and by the placenta thereafter. This leads to marked hyperplasia of ducts and lobules and development of lobuloalveolar units, with replacement of surrounding stroma and fat. Lactation begins in the third trimester. Secretion of prolactin by the anterior pituitary initiates differentiation of alveolar cells destined to secrete milk products. Immediately postpartum, estrogen and progesterone levels fall, enabling an

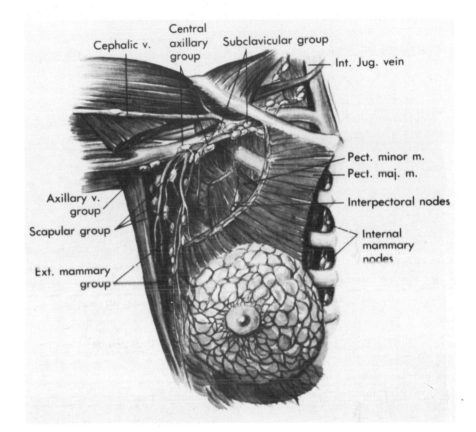

Figure 2. Depiction of the lymphatic drainage of the breast. The five axillary groups are external mammary, scapular, axillary vein, central axillary, and subclavicular. The breast lymph also drains via the interpectoral, or Rotter's nodes and internal mammary nodes. These two groups are not excised during the standard modified radical mastectomy. (From Donegan WL, Spratt JS: Cancer of the Breast, ed 3. Philadelphia, WB Saunders Company, 1988, p 325, with permission.)

enhanced prolactin effect and, hence, milk synthesis within the lobule. Suckling stimulates immediate release of oxytocin from the posterior pituitary causing contraction of ductular myoepithelial cells and milk expulsion. Prolactin is also maintained by suckling, and this explains the cessation of lactation with weaning. Ovarian and estrogenic decline during menopause results in atrophy of the breast ducts, lobules, and stroma with replacement by adipose tissue.

EVALUATION OF BREAST ABNORMALITIES

History

The presence of a breast mass detected by self-examination should lead to an evaluation by a physician. A complete history is critical to the evaluation of breast masses (Table 2). Determining the time of onset and duration of the mass is important, as is determining the patient's menstrual and reproductive history, the use of exogenous hormones, and obtaining a relevant history of previous breast disorders and any surgical procedures. A history of nipple discharge should also be sought. A pertinent family history is very important in defining possible risk factors for breast cancer.

Physical Examination

Physical examination of the breast requires careful palpation and inspection. Inspection may reveal dimpling that could indicate the presence of a cicatrizing breast mass, suspicious for carcinoma. Edema and erythema may be present, consistent with inflammation. Although these findings are consistent with infection, inflammatory breast carcinoma may also be associated with these findings (termed *peau d'orange*) and a biopsy is required to exclude carcinoma in suspicious lesions. The erythema and edema present in inflammatory breast carcinoma are due to invasion of the dermal lymphatics by cancer.

Skin changes involving the nipple and areola may be a sign of Paget's disease (intraepithelial carcinoma). In this condition, the intraductal carcinoma within the subareolar ducts invades across the epidermal/epithelial junction and enters the epidermal layer of the skin on the nipple, producing a dermatitis that originates on the nipple and secondarily encompasses the areola.

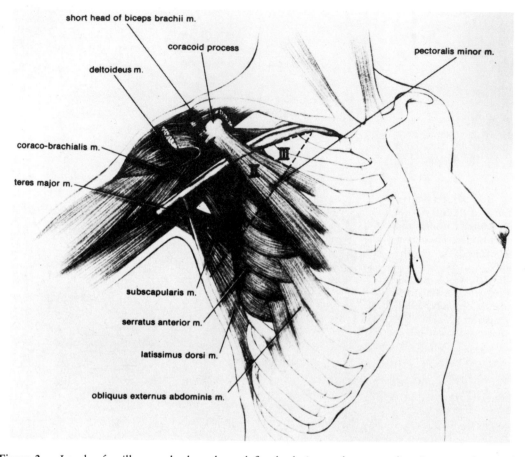

short head of biceps brachii m.

coracoid process

deltoideus m.

pectoralis minor m.

coraco-brachialis m.

teres major m.

subscapularis m.

serratus anterior m.

latissimus dorsi m.

obliquus externus abdominis m.

Figure 3. Levels of axillary nodes have been defined relative to the pectoralis minor muscle in order to standardize description of surgical dissection and pathologic analysis. Level I nodes lie lateral to the pectoralis minor. Level II lies deep to the pectoralis minor. Level III lies medial to the pectoralis minor and can normally only be excised by dividing that muscle. (From Donegan WL, Spratt JS: Cancer of the Breast, ed 3. Philadelphia, WB Saunders, 1988, p 425, with permission.)

Other signs of breast cancer include nipple retraction and ulceration.

By palpation, breast masses are characterized by their size, shape, consistency, location, and fixation to the surrounding breast tissue, skin, or chest wall. A breast mass should be definitively evaluated to exclude a carcinoma by a pathologic examination in all women at risk for carcinoma. Three quarters of early breast cancers are palpable, and it is important that physicians instruct all adult women to perform a careful monthly breast self-examination, as the smallest mass that can be palpated is usually only 1 cm in diameter. In addition, a breast examination should also be performed annually by a physician.

Breast Imaging

Screening mammography is most likely to be beneficial if studies are obtained annually after the age of 50 years. The benefit of an annual or biannual screening mammogram may extend to those between the ages of 40 and 50 years, but increased survival has been difficult to demonstrate for women in this age group. Women with a personal family history or other risks of breast cancer may benefit from early screening mammography beginning at age 35. The radiation dose is approximately one tenth of that delivered 20 years ago, and the potential benefits of screening outweigh the risks of radiation.

Mammography is the most sensitive and specific test that can be used in conjunction with the physical examination for evaluation of the breast and is considered complementary to the history and physical examination in the evaluation of a specific breast lesion. Mammographic features of malignancy include abnormalities of density, such as masses, asymmetries, and architectural distortions and microcalcifications. Densities with indistinct margins, or signifi-

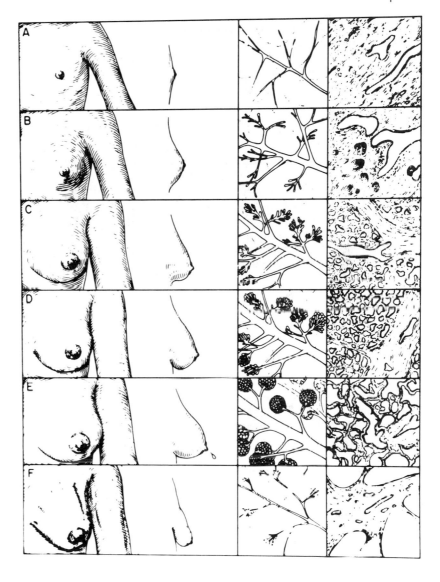

Figure 4. Physiology of the breast reflects changing levels of hormones, most importantly estrogen and progesterone. Breast physiology, as manifest by gross (left column) and histologic (right columns) appearance, is depicted during (*A*) childhood, (*B*) puberty, (*C*) maturity, (*D*) pregnancy, (*E*) lactation, and (*F*) postmenopausal state. (From Bland KI, Copeland EM [eds]: The Breast: Comprehensive Management of Benign and Malignant Diseases. Philadelphia, WB Saunders Company, 1991, p 20, with permission.)

cant architectural distortion surrounding the parenchyma, are most likely to be malignant. Microcalcifications may be very small (detected by magnification) and are not compressible unless associated with an abnormal density palpable on physical examination.

Diagnostic mammography is a valuable test in the evaluation of the breast, as it detects carcinomas less than 0.5 cm in diameter. Unfortunately, 10 per cent of breast cancers may not be detected by mammography, regardless of size; therefore, the presence of a carcinoma cannot be definitively excluded by mammography alone. Routine use of mammography in women under the age of 25 is generally not appropriate, as dense hormonally active breast tissue may make interpretation difficult.

Other Diagnostic Tests

Although an accurate history, physical examination, and mammography are essential components of the evaluation of a breast abnormality, it is often difficult to distinguish clinically benign breast lesions such as fibroadenomas, lipomas, inflammatory masses, and cysts from malignant ones, especially in premenopausal women. Unfortunately, mammography may not only be nonsensitive, but may also be nonspecific. Mammographically defined lesions may be considered highly suspicious for carcinoma, abnormal, or normal. Further evaluation of a breast lesion following a history, physical exam, and mammogram is directed, in large part, by the probability of the lesion representing a malignancy.

Mammographically detected abnormalities suspicious for a malignancy are usually evaluated by open biopsy if palpable, or needle localization and open biopsy if not palpable. A large number of lesions detected by mammogram may be simply abnormal. To avoid many unnecessary biopsies, thoughtful consideration should be given to a variety of complementary procedures that may be utilized to evaluate abnormal mammographic findings. These include ultrasonography, fine-needle aspiration, stereotactic needle biopsy, and interval reevaluation. Although these procedures can be utilized to avoid more invasive testing, the current standard to exclude a diagnosis of breast carcinoma includes the histologic examination of dominant breast masses detected by palpation or by mammography. An algorithm demonstrating the possible uses of the tests discussed below is shown in Figure 5.

Ultrasonography

Ultrasonography is indicated as a complement to mammography or physical examination but has no proven benefit in screening. The principal utility of ultrasonography is to distinguish solid from cystic masses. Cystic masses are more likely to be benign functional cysts and may be clinically followed by interval reevaluation. If the cyst is palpable, direct needle aspiration is possible, otherwise ultrasound-guided aspiration is required. If a nonpalpable abnormality is present on mammogram and ultrasound examination reveals a solid or indeterminate abnormality, cytologic or histologic evaluation is indicated. Currently, a variety of modalities are useful in acquiring tissue for the cytologic and histologic evaluation of breast lesions. These include fine-needle aspiration (FNA), stereotactic breast biopsy, or needle localization followed by excisional biopsy.

Fine-Needle Aspiration

Fine-needle aspiration of a palpable breast mass determines whether it is solid or cystic, as aspiration of

TABLE 2.   RISK FACTORS FOR CARCINOMA OF THE BREAST

Increasing age
Familial history of breast cancer
First- and second-degree relatives with breast cancer
Premalignant breast lesions
Previous carcinoma in one breast
Early menstruation
Late menopause
Nulliparity
Radiation therapy to the chest
Family history of carcinoma of the ovary, uterus, or colon
Obesity

a cyst causes resolution of the mass. Cystic fluid is commonly green or amber, and if the mass disappears after the aspiration and the fluid is nonbloody, a diagnosis of a functional cyst is made. If the mass is solid, cytologic evaluation of cells obtained by FNA by an experienced cytopathologist may be diagnostic. Because FNA has a false-negative rate of approximately 5 per cent, a negative or nondiagnostic FNA of the solid mass should be followed by a breast biopsy to exclude a carcinoma. An FNA that is diagnostic of carcinoma allows the surgeon to make a diagnosis and discuss management options with the patient. Usually, histologic confirmation of the carcinoma is made prior to definitive treatment.

Stereotactic Needle Biopsy

A recently developed modality used for biopsy and histologic examination of a nonpalpable breast abnormality is stereotactic needle biopsy, which uses a coring biopsy needle (true-cut needle biopsy). Typically, following stereotactic localization of the mammographic abnormality, local anesthesia is infiltrated into the skin and a true-cut needle is inserted into the breast allowing core biopsies (usually five) to be obtained. A postbiopsy mammogram is obtained to ensure that the mammographic abnormality of interest has indeed been biopsied and removed. Histologic examination of each of the core biopsies is performed. Recent studies have demonstrated that the accuracy of this test may be 90 to 95 per cent. Histologic confirmation of a breast malignancy allows the surgeon to discuss management options with the patient. A negative or nondiagnostic biopsy is usually managed based on the probability that the mammographically defined lesion is malignant. A negative stereotactic needle biopsy of a lesion that is suspicious for malignancy may be followed by a needle localization and excisional breast biopsy. A negative stereotactic needle biopsy of a lesion that is abnormal, but not suspicious for malignancy, may be followed by observation and interval reevaluation. The current utility of stereotactic needle biopsy in the management of breast lesions is evolving, and long-term studies of outcome following biopsy are needed.

Needle Localization Followed by Excisional Biopsy

For nonpalpable masses that are not adequately biopsied using FNA or stereotactic needle biopsy, histologic diagnosis is determined by mammographic needle localization followed by excisional breast biopsy. Mammographically detected abnormalities are

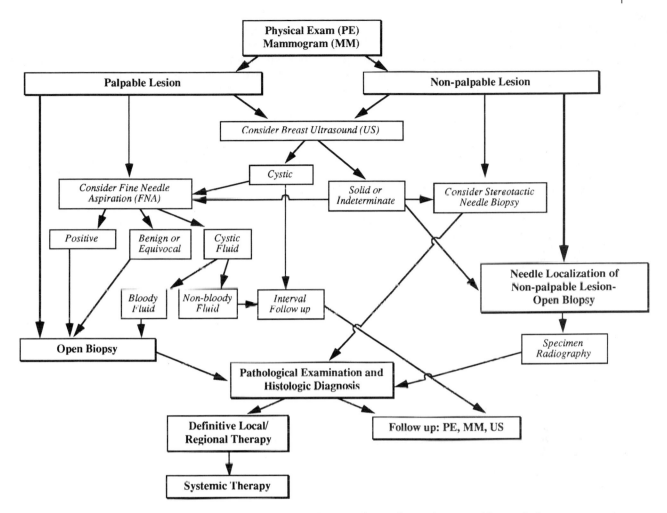

Figure 5. Algorithm demonstrating the possible uses of tests for evaluation of breast lesions.

localized by stereotactic implantation of fine wire with an embedding hook that allows the tip of the wire to be fixed in the region of the mammographic abnormality. Following placement of this needle under local anesthesia, an excisional breast biopsy is performed in the operating room. Instead of excising a palpable mass, the surgeon performs an excisional biopsy that incorporates the tip of the guidewire as the localizing focal point with excision of breast tissue surrounding this localizing wire.

Following removal of the specimen, a radiograph is obtained of it to confirm the presence of the mammographic abnormality of interest within the specimen. A histologic diagnosis is then made, and treatment is planned based on the findings. The management of patients with benign lesions includes an interval baseline mammogram obtained after changes from the operation have resolved. Patients are counseled regarding the diagnosis, including the management of premalignant and malignant lesions. It is

important to emphasize that a breast biopsy does not eliminate the risk of breast cancer, and patients must continue breast self-examination as well as annual mammograms and physical examinations as indicated.

Interval Reevaluation

Some breast abnormalities detected by mammography are associated with a low rate of breast carcinoma. In these patients, an interval evaluation, usually performed 4 to 6 months following the initial evaluation, permits determination of the stability of the abnormality. Stable abnormalities are usually followed at 4- to 6-month intervals, for a period of 18 months, at which time annual mammography and physical examination are resumed. Any evidence of progression warrants histologic evaluation as described above.

CLINICAL SYNDROMES

Although malignant lesions of the breast are the most concerning, a variety of benign clinical syndromes have significant clinical impact on a woman's health.

Mastodynia

Breast pain is a common clinical problem in young women, occurring in 30 to 40 per cent of premenopausal women. Pain may be continuous or cyclical, may be associated with breast swelling and tenderness, and may occur primarily in the luteal phase of the menstrual cycle. Breast pain is often the cause of much concern and is evaluated to exclude breast carcinoma as the cause of the pain. Treatment of mastodynia follows an evaluation of the breast for any abnormality. If a dominant mass or mammographic abnormality is detected, complete evaluation is indicated, even if distant from the painful area of the breast.

Management of breast pain usually follows a progressive interventional approach. Avoidance of caffeine, dietary fat, and cigarettes is advocated by some; however, careful studies documenting the usefulness of this approach have been limited. Mild nonnarcotic analgesics may be used to provide symptomatic relief. Hormonal manipulation with tamoxifen, danazol, and bromocriptine have been utilized, but many women experience resolution of the pain without specific intervention. Surgical excision has had limited clinical utility in the management of breast pain.

Nipple Discharge

Nipple discharge is a common cause of concern in younger women, but is usually associated with a benign disorder. It is important to determine if blood is present in the nipple discharge, which can be determined by visual inspection or testing for occult blood. It is also important to determine if the nipple discharge is from one or both breasts and if it is from one or multiple nipple orifices. This can be determined by careful palpation around the nipple in a clockwise manner. If nipple discharge is present from a single duct when a discreet location is palpated, a pathologic disorder is likely. If nipple discharge is present from bilateral or multiple ducts, it is more likely to be a functional disorder. Certain hormones, tranquilizers, and antihypertensives may lead to watery or milky nipple discharge, and a history of such use should be investigated.

The presence of a palpable mass or radiographic abnormality under the involved nipple and areolar complex should be sought. In these patients, surgical bi-opsy is recommended. Biopsy may also be indicated with discharge from a discreet, dilated duct. This usually involves ductal cannulation and a circumareolar incision with excision of the dilated duct. Wider excision of subareolar tissue is indicated if the involved duct cannot be identified. Usually an intraductal papilloma is found. This is a polyp-like epithelial lesion with papillary architecture projecting from the wall of a dilated duct. Single papillomas are usually located beneath the nipple/areolar complex and commonly present with bloody nipple discharge. *Papillomatosis* is a commonly used term that means an epithelial hyperplasia, not the true polyp formation as in solitary and multiple papilloma.

Galactorrhea or milky discharge associated with regular menses is usually a benign disorder. If it is associated with *amenorrhea*, it may indicate a serious condition such as a pituitary tumor. The measurement of a serum prolactin level is helpful, because the prolactin level is normal in 85 per cent of patients with idiopathic galactorrhea. *Hyperprolactinemia* is present in 70 per cent of patients with galactorrhea associated with amenorrhea. Hyperprolactinemia may be associated with a prolactinoma if levels are greater than 300 ng/ml, or a variety of conditions if levels are less than 300 ng/ml, including postpartum or postpill states, endocrine disease, or drug therapy.

Nipple discharge is rarely purulent and indicates a breast abscess. Abscesses of the breast usually occur around the nipple and areola, presumably originating in the large subareolar lactiferous sinuses but may be in any location. Treatment is usually conservative and consists of administration of antibiotics. Incision and drainage is reserved for the unusual case that cannot be controlled with antibiotics and is usually directed by fluctuance or tenderness. Chronic recurrent subareolar mastitis may respond to excision of the subareolar ductal tissue when the process is quiescent.

Gynecomastia

Hypertrophy of the male breast is a common condition that occurs in adolescent males and in older men and is frequently unilateral. It may be associated with systemic disease such as hepatic and renal disorders. On physical examination, the breast hypertrophy is smooth, firm, sometimes tender, and symmetrically distributed under the areola. Surgical therapy is rarely needed in the treatment of gynecomastia except to establish a diagnosis or for cosmetic reasons.

Breast Masses

All palpable breast masses in women at risk for breast cancer should be evaluated by cytologic or histologic examination. Often, a mass represents fibrocystic changes in the breast, which refers to firm, fibrous breast tissue with cyst formation. On histologic examination, the fibrocystic complex contains cysts, fibrosis, and a variable amount of epithelium, hyperplasia, and adenosis. Fibrocystic changes are a health risk in only a small group of patients. Of great concern is the connection between benign breast lesions and invasive breast cancer. There is a strong relationship between lobular carcinoma in situ and ductal carcinoma in situ and invasive breast cancer in that both of these lesions are premalignant. Although benign lesions are not thought to be as strongly associated with invasive carcinoma as these premalignant lesions, there are conditions that are associated with an increased risk of invasive breast cancer. Hyperplasia and papilloma with a fibrovascular core are associated with a slight increase in risk for invasive carcinoma, while hyperplasia *with atypia* is associated with a moderate increase in risk for invasive carcinoma, generally estimated to be five times the baseline risk.

Breast Cysts

Breast cysts are fluid-filled epithelial cavities varying in size from microscopic to large and palpable masses. Formation, enlargement, and regression of cysts are influenced by varying hormone levels. The incidence of large cysts peaks after the age of 35 and is rare in women before the age of 25. Breast cysts are also uncommon after menopause without exogenous hormone replacement. The diagnosis of a cyst is made by needle aspiration or by ultrasonography. Simple cysts may be observed, and biopsy is reserved for complex lesions that do not resolve or recur after aspiration, or those that contain bloody fluid.

Fibroadenoma

This is the most common breast neoplasm in patients younger than age 30. Physical examination is often suggestive of the diagnosis, as a fibroadenoma is usually a solitary, rubbery, firm, mobile, round mass. Patients may experience variation in size with menstrual cycles and an overall increase in size with time. The sharply circumscribed nature is apparent during surgical excision, and the excised gross specimen has a smooth, white appearance. The histologic appearance reveals epithelial and particularly fibrous stromal proliferation without cellular atypia. Although breast masses in young women under the age of 20 might be presumed to be benign on physical examination, FNA and/or excisional biopsy should be performed if there is any doubt. In older women, those with risk factors for breast cancer, or for breast masses that enlarge or

fail to regress, FNA and/or excisional biopsy is often performed.

Phyllodes Tumor and Phyllodes Sarcoma

The traditional term *cystosarcoma phyllodes* has been rejected by some authors, both because the lesion is typically solid and because the term *sarcoma* inappropriately implies malignancy in all cases. The term phyllodes (*phyllon*—leaf; *eidos*—form) describes the gross leaf-like appearance of these lesions' borders. *Phyllodes tumor* describes the more common benign lesion, while *phyllodes sarcoma* is reserved for the rare malignant form. Phyllodes sarcomas are large, usually unilateral, nontender lesions presenting in patients ranging in age from 35 to 55. They can grow rapidly, dominate the entire breast, and progress to skin fixation and ulceration, but without fixation to the chest wall.

Phyllodes lesions are histologically characterized by dense proliferation of stromal spindle cells. The epithelial component is unremarkable. Prediction of malignant behavior is not exact, but is based on degree of stromal cellular density, cytologic atypia, and mitotic figures. Surprisingly, malignancy does not correlate with size, breast domination, or skin changes. When metastases are detected, their histology recapitulates the stromal, not epithelial, component of the primary tumor. Treatment is largely determined by tumor size and presumption of malignant potential is based on histology. Local excision is appropriate for smaller, probably benign lesions, with the realization that recurrence may follow incomplete excision but does not imply malignancy. Large, dominant, or presumably malignant lesions require mastectomy, sometimes requiring skin grafting if the skin is extensively involved. Management of metastatic phyllodes sarcoma includes chemotherapy and hormonal manipulation, but has not been well defined.

Fat Necrosis and Sclerosing Adenosis

Fat necrosis is a rare lesion, the significance of which is in its mimicry of breast cancer. It presents as a firm, sometimes fixed breast mass and is manifest mammographically as a dominant lesion that can contain calcifications. Frequently, the patient does not recall a history of breast trauma. Fine-needle aspiration of a lesion may reveal fat globules, foamy macrophages, and occasionally an inflammatory reaction. Despite the clinical resemblance to breast cancer, fat necrosis is not premalignant. Like fat necrosis, sclerosing adenosis may mimic breast cancer on physical examination and mammograms may show calcifications. This lesion is a proliferation of terminal ducts, lobules, and surrounding stroma without histologic epithelial distortion suggesting malignancy.

Malignant Tumors of the Breast

Adherence to an anatomic hypothesis of tumor dissemination has historically determined the approach to the treatment of carcinoma of the breast. The spread of breast cancer was thought to occur in an orderly manner, with enlargement of the primary tumor, followed by spread to the axillary nodes by the lymphatics, followed by systemic dissemination to the bone, lungs, and intra-abdominal organs. Although this hypothesis is attractive, it appears to be inconsistent with clinical data regarding the natural history of breast cancer. Over 60 per cent of women with breast cancer that has spread to the axillary lymph nodes at the time of diagnosis later present with systemic disease, despite complete removal of the breast and the associated lymph nodes and lack of detectable distant metastasis at the time of diagnosis and initial treatment. In fact, as many as one in four women without lymph node metastasis treated by mastectomy and axillary node dissection develop systemic recurrence. The historic trend toward increasingly radical operations, designed to extirpate all possible tumor, has not led to increased survival in these patients. It is now thought that variations in local treatment may not influence long-term survival in patients with occult micrometastatic disease.

Breast cancer, however, is clearly a heterogeneous disease, manifesting a wide spectrum of biologic behavior. For example, one third of women with lymph node metastases at the time of diagnosis are long-term survivors following radical mastectomy, suggesting that systemic micrometastases were not present. Variations in the local treatment of breast cancer may be critical for patients without micrometastatic systemic disease, whereas local therapy has a minimal impact on survival in those with micrometastatic systemic disease. This hypothesis has led to trends toward less radical operations in combination with radiotherapy for the treatment of certain subsets of patients with operable breast cancer. As predicted, this approach has not led to diminished survival among these patients. A fundamental understanding of the biology of breast cancer, as well as the natural history of histologic subtypes, must be achieved to design rational treatment strategies for patients with operable disease.

ONCOGENES AND BREAST CANCER

As attempts to understand the etiology and pathogenesis of breast cancer have progressed, new knowledge about specific genetic mutations present in primary breast tumors has gradually emerged. Such mutations can be thought of in two broad categories: either cellular proto-oncogenes or tumor suppressor genes. To date, a number of mutations have been found to occur frequently in primary human breast cancers. Three of these, c-myc, int-2/hst and c-erb-B2, are genetic alterations that can be classified as amplifications of cellular proto-oncogenes. The remaining eight mutations are categorized as loss of heterozygosity; that is, losses of the normal expression of specific genes (chromosomes 1p, 1q, 3p, 11p, 13q, 17p, 17q, and 18q).

Studies in mammary carcinogenesis in transgenic mice and other murine studies in the mouse mammary tumor virus (MMTV) have provided information on the potential ways in which these mutations contribute to the development and progression of breast cancer. Insertion of MMTV into murine DNA causes the activation by insertional mutagenesis of five previously silent genes. The mammary glands of transgenic mice containing one of these genes (int-1) developed preneoplastic hyperplasia and later focal cancers. Two other of these genes (int-2 and hst) show homology with the basic fibroblast growth factor gene family and have been shown to encode for products that may act as profound growth factors.

Other oncogenes that may be important in the development of breast cancer are c-myc, v-H-ras, and neu (erb-B2). Transgenic mice containing c-myc or v-H-ras transgenes undergo normal mammary development but develop mammary cancers later. In contrast, male and female transgenic mice containing the neu (erb-B2) oncogene develop bilateral polyclonal tumors early in development. Such studies suggest that the effect of an oncogene may depend on the developmental stage of the mammary gland. It is also consistent with the paradigm of tumorigenesis, in that multiple mutations are probably needed for frankly invasive cancer to arise. Mutations in breast cancer that lead to loss of heterozygosity (LOH) are believed to inactivate tumor suppressor genes that function to inhibit cell proliferation. Approximately 20 to 70 per cent of primary breast cancers have been shown to contain loss of heterozygosity in one of eight chromosomal locations; however, little is known about which specific genes are being activated in breast cancers with LOH. One target gene in several human cancers, including breast cancer, appears to be the tumor suppressor gene, RB (retinoblastoma gene), on chromosome 13. Approximately 19 per cent of primary human breast cancers have altered DNA at the RB locus and 29 per cent of breast cancers do not express the RB gene product. Frequent loss of heterozygosity has been reported in 61 per cent of human breast cancers on chromosome 17. A target for this deletion is the

P53 gene, which encodes for the transformation-associated suppressor protein, P53, and primary human breast cancers show point mutations within remaining P53 alleles, usually manifest by overexpression of the mutant P53 gene product. Thirty per cent of primary human breast cancers examined in other studies show loss of heterozygosity on 3p. It is of interest that other proto-oncogenes are located within this frequently deleted region.

Investigators have hypothesized that some subsets of breast cancers can be classified on the basis of the particular group of mutations they contain. As discussed, this is believed to follow the hypothesis that multiple accumulated mutations are needed for tumor development and progression. Therefore, certain specific sets of mutations sufficient for neoplastic transformation should be definable for certain tumors. An interesting corollary to this hypothesis is that the presence of any of these specific mutations or accumulate mutations may predict biologic behavior and, therefore, be useful as surrogate markers of prognosis. Several intriguing series have been reported in this regard, especially pertaining to overexpression of erb-B2, but no single mutation has definitively been shown to be a consistent predictor of outcome. Recent studies have demonstrated that not only may prognosis be predictable based on the presence of genetic markers, but there may be other biologic behaviors that may be predicted, such as the response to chemotherapy.

Another interesting area of research in the next decade concerns the specific genetic abnormalities present in familial patterns of breast cancer and in the germ lines of cancer-free individuals and high-risk families. Linkage analysis of several large families with hereditary breast carcinoma have identified a putative gene of the long arm of chromosome 17 that may be associated with familial breast cancer (BRCA1). This genetic region is quite interesting, as it also contains the loci for a number of other genes including erb-B2, thyroid hormone receptor (THR), retinoic acid receptor-α (RARA), topoisomerase 2 (TOP2), and estradiol dehydrogenase (EDH17B).

As the ability to detect patients at risk for developing breast cancer becomes possible through the use of genetic analysis, there will be an enormous need for effective interventions to prevent the development of further mutations and the consequent invasive disease. Concomitant with the development of predictive and prognostic genetic markers for breast cancer, there must be development of effective preventive strategies and more effective methods to prevent tumor progression in patients with early disease. The biologic behavior of breast cancer and its relationship to other factors, such as growth factors, outside of the cancer cell may provide a key to possible interventions.

Growth Factors

The control of breast cancer growth is believed to be mediated by the complex relationship between growth stimulatory and growth inhibitory factors and the breast cancer cells themselves, as well as in the breast stroma. It is clear that one growth factor in particular, estrogen, is critical to the genesis of breast cancer. The frequency of occurrence of breast cancer in women who have never had functional ovaries is only 1 per cent of the frequency in women with active ovarian function.

Estrogen, in combination with its receptor, interacts with genetically determined elements to induce or alter specific gene expression. It has been shown that estrogen-dependent tumors secrete a number of growth factors that act to modulate tumor growth. The production of these growth factors is controlled by the presence of estrogen in these tumors. Growth inhibitors, such as antiestrogens, appear to act by turning off the production of growth stimulatory factors and introducing the production of specific growth inhibitory factors. Estrogen-independent breast cancer cells have been shown to produce the same growth stimulatory factors constitutively, thereby bypassing the need for estrogen stimulation.

Evidence is mounting that breast cancer growth is controlled not only by growth factors produced by the tumor itself, but also by the mesenchymal stromal elements, fibroblasts, mononuclear cells, and endothelial cells that comprise normal breast tissue. Malignant breast cells secrete peptides such as transforming growth factor β (TGF-β) and platelet-derived growth factor (PDGF), which stimulate the growth of stromal cells. Likewise, stromal elements secrete proteins that may stimulate the growth of breast cancer cells. These complex interactions offer potential targets for novel therapeutic strategies.

Retinoids, which include vitamin A and synthetic derivatives of vitamin A, also exhibit important growth inhibiting effects in both epithelial and mesenchymal cells. Both TFG-β and the retinoids inhibit the growth of breast cancer cells in vitro and in vivo, and recent studies have demonstrated that the combination potentiates the antiproliferative effects of either molecule alone on human breast cancer cell lines. One possible mechanism for this potentiation is the induction of TGF-β by retinoic acid. Retinoic acid has been shown to induce the expression of TGF-β receptors on breast cancer cells (HL60 cells), which do not constitutively express these receptors. Retinoic acid also has been shown to upregulate the expression of TGF-β_2 itself in cultured keratinocytes. Retinoic acid has synergistic antiproliferative effects against breast cancer cell lines when combined with α- or γ interferon.

Strategies aimed at inducing the production of antiproliferative growth regulator factors of breast cancer cells represent very significant and innovative approaches to therapy for future research. It has been emphasized that the antiestrogen tamoxifen stimulates the production of TGF-β by breast cancer cells. Tamoxifen thus may work by interfering with the autocrine loop that stimulates cell growth. There may be a basis for combining tamoxifen, which stimulates the production of a type-2 form of TGF-β, with retinoic acid, which stimulates the more common type-1 form of TGF-β. Clinical trials addressing the effectiveness of these combined agents in treating metastatic and possibly localized breast cancer are of considerable interest.

Other methods of interrupting the growth factor cascades that control proliferation of breast cancer include the use of anti–growth factor compounds that are functionally related to heparan sulfate. Heparan sulfate is an important component of the extracellular matrix found in all animal cells. Heparan, an analog of heparin sulfate, binds the growth factors and other components of the extracellular matrix including fibronectin, thrombospondin, fibroblast growth factor, and laminin. It is believed that heparan sulfate has an important role in the regulation of cell growth, perhaps by its ability to bind to critical molecules that stimulate cellular proliferation.

Recent studies of breast cancer cells in vitro have shown that surinamine, functionally related to heparan sulfate, can inhibit the growth of several breast cancer cell lines and that this inhibition is partially overcome by the addition of estrogen to the culture medium. It is believed that surinamine's antiproliferative effects may be caused by interference with growth factor receptor interactions and inhibition of cells in the cell cycle. Other novel approaches to the treatment of growth factor–dependent human tumors, such as breast cancer, will undoubtedly arise from further studies of the interactions between growth factors.

The locations of several growth factor receptors on the plasma membrane constitute potential targets for monoclonal antibody therapy, and several investigators have successfully controlled tumor growth in experimental systems utilizing anti–growth factor and antireceptor antibodies. It is believed that this inhibition is due to monoclonal antibody–mediated interference with the autocrine growth factor stimulation loops driving these cells. Other approaches include the production of small polypeptide analogs that block receptor function.

Risk Factors

The greatest risk factors for breast cancer are sex and age, as cancer is quite uncommon in males and in females under the age of 30. A family history of breast cancer is most important when primary relatives had cancer when they were young or if the breast cancer was bilateral. Epithelial hyperplasia with atypia is associated with a fivefold increase in the risk of breast cancer. Fibrocystic changes do not predispose to breast cancer unless associated with atypical hyperplasia. The presence of *lobular carcinoma in situ* (LCIS) and *ductal carcinoma in situ* (DCIS) both increase the likelihood of development of mammary carcinoma. LCIS and DCIS are both noninvasive lesions, distinguished by a lack of invasion of the basement of the membrane of the lobule or the duct seen by light microscopy. However, these lesions may coexist with invasive disease in the same malignant tumor.

LOBULAR CARCINOMA IN SITU

The characteristic feature of LCIS is replacement of the regular two-cell layered lobular epithelium with a disorderly, amorphous proliferation of relatively benign-appearing cells. The cells are larger than those of the normal epithelium, nuclei are proportionately sized, and mitotic figures are absent. The cytoplasm is pink, pale, and contains vacuolated areas. The cells ultimately obliterate the lumen, causing lobular distention. Despite its name, this process is not limited to the lobule, but can extend to the terminal ducts. The cells do not undergo necrosis as in DCIS, though it has been suggested that obliteration of a terminal duct obstructs the distal lobule, causing necrosis and calcification. Whether this is related to reported findings of LCIS in association with microcalcifications is speculative.

The average age of patients diagnosed with LCIS is 45, and 90 per cent are premenopausal, suggesting an etiologic role of estrogen. The diagnosis of LCIS is usually made as an incidental finding. LCIS cannot be detected clinically, as it causes no perceptible changes on examination of the breast and has no mammographic findings beyond an unsubstantiated, nonspecific association with microcalcifications. Rather, it presents as an unanticipated, incidental finding on microscopic examination of between 1 and 4 per cent of breast specimens obtained following biopsy of breast lesions. LCIS is typically found in association with, but is not related to, benign breast disease, most commonly gross cystic disease and fibroadenomas.

LCIS has a high rate of multicentricity, and attempts at local excision result in residual LCIS in the remaining breast tissue. Complete excision of LCIS from an involved breast requires a simple mastectomy. This disorder also has a high rate of bilaterality, as two thirds of patients are found to have disease in both breasts. Therefore, complete eradication of LCIS usually involves bilateral simple mastectomy. The controversial and clinically significant feature of LCIS is the risk of subsequent invasive cancer. A series of clinical studies published in the 1970s found that patients with LCIS have an incidence as high as 29 per cent of developing a subsequent invasive breast cancer, which represents a ninefold higher risk of cancer over age-matched women in the general population.

Two theories have been proposed to explain the increased risk of invasive breast carcinoma in women with LCIS. The *transformation theory* states that the in situ process evolves into an infiltrating cancer by penetration of the basement membrane. Evidence supporting this includes the 36 per cent incidence of the relatively uncommon infiltrating lobular cancer in patients with a prior diagnosis of LCIS. In addition, electron microscopy has revealed protrusion of the cytoplasm of in situ cells into the breast stroma through disrupted areas of the basal lamina, suggesting the origins of invasive behavior. A second theory, known as the *risk theory*, purports that LCIS represents a marker of conditions in the breast that predispose the patient to the subsequent development of invasive cancer. Proponents of this theory emphasize that the majority of infiltrating cancers developing in LCIS patients are ductal, not lobular. Infiltrating cancers do not necessarily occur at the site of previously diagnosed LCIS but can occur anywhere, including the contralateral breast, with equal frequency.

Estrogen may have an etiologic role both in LCIS and in the invasive cancers that subsequently develop, and may therefore be the mechanism behind the risk theory. The young age and premenopausal status of patients diagnosed with LCIS supports this concept. More than 50 per cent of patients with LCIS are also premenopausal when invasive cancer is diagnosed, and, on average, they are younger than patients diagnosed with infiltrating cancer with no prior diagnosis of LCIS.

Treatment options for LCIS are radically divergent, and are based on the known tissue distribution and natural history of the disease. One option includes close surveillance for early detection of an invasive breast cancer, which involves frequent breast examinations and mammography, typically performed every 6 months. This program must be continued indefinitely, as the risk of breast cancer is ongoing and has been estimated to approach 20 to 25 per cent over 20 years. The second option advocated by some includes prophylactic bilateral mastectomy with the option of reconstruction. The rationale for the latter includes the multicentricity and bilaterality of LCIS and the proven concept that, in LCIS, both breasts should be conceived of as a single organ at risk of development of invasive cancer. Advocates of bilateral mastectomy site the alarmingly high rate of invasive cancer development and mortality. Compliance with lifetime close surveillance may be impractical. However, no proven benefit to prophylactic mastectomy has been demonstrated as yet by a clinical trial. The ultimate decision on management of LCIS lies with the patient, who must be fully informed of the risk of future invasive cancer and the expectations and limitations of surveillance.

DUCTAL CARCINOMA IN SITU

Ductal carcinoma in situ, or intraductal carcinoma, is characterized histologically by proliferation of malignant-appearing cells, which by definition, are contained by the basement membrane. The cells form one of a number of distinct architectural patterns: *cribriform, solid, papillary, micropapillary,* or *comedo*. The last of these is characterized by filling of the duct followed by central necrosis, which produces a mammographic finding of microcalcifications.

Prior to the widespread use of mammography, DCIS was a relatively rare form of breast cancer (1 to 2 per cent of all detected). It typically presented as a palpable breast mass and was routinely treated by mastectomy, as were most breast cancers before and during the 1970s. The advent of mammography has markedly changed the presenting clinical features of DCIS, and it now represents 15 to 20 per cent of breast cancers detected in patients undergoing routine mammography. It is typically detected as a focus of microcalcifications, and the average size of the lesion is 6 mm, hence it is not detectable on physical examination.

A knowledge of the natural history of mammographically detected DCIS is limited by the past practice of routinely treating DCIS with mastectomy. While the process is contained by the basement membrane, three aspects of the natural history are worrisome: (1) multicentricity, (2) the risk of development of invasive cancer, and (3) the coexistence of invasive disease. Multicentric DCIS has been reported to be as high as 30 to 40 per cent, as determined by pathologic examination of breast specimens of patients treated by mastectomy. The risk of subsequent invasive cancer in patients with DCIS has been studied by following the course of patients with a retrospective, and hence untreated, finding of DCIS on biopsy. These studies describe a 28 to 53 per cent incidence of subsequent invasive cancer. Typically, the cancer occurs within 10 years of the original biopsy revealing DCIS and develops in the ipsilateral breast, at or near the site of the biopsy, suggesting that DCIS is directly involved in the pathogenesis of the infiltrating cancer. Finally, the incidence of coexisting invasive carcinoma has been reported to be as high as 46 per cent. However, the incidence of simultaneous axillary metastasis, an indicator of invasive disease, is low (1 to 2 per cent), and current studies of patients with microscopic foci of DCIS clearly show a low incidence of nonde-tected coexisting invasive carcinoma.

Mastectomy has been viewed as the standard ther-apy against which all other treatments for DCIS must be compared. Ipsilateral mastectomy is generally con-sidered appropriate because the overall risk of contra-lateral occult disease is about the same as invasive dis-ease. The value of axillary dissection is limited and, in most instances, is not performed if invasive disease is not documented by pathologic review. Collective re-views reveal a 3 per cent recurrence and a 2.3 per cent mortality in patients with DCIS treated with mastec-tomy. Nonetheless, the proven efficacy of breast-con-serving procedures for invasive cancer has prompted the investigation of the role of less invasive procedures for DCIS. While preservation of the breast should be a goal of treatment, in the evaluation of breast con-servation therapy for DCIS, one must consider that recurrent disease is equally divided between recurrent DCIS and recurrent invasive carcinoma. Therefore, lo-cal failure rates are of considerable importance in de-fining the optimal therapy.

One study compared patients with DCIS treated with mastectomy, segmental resection, and segmental resection and radiation, all with axillary dissection. Recurrence rates were 0, 23, and 7 per cent, respec-tively. Residual DCIS at the biopsy site has been re-ported to be as high as 66 per cent, which may ac-count for this pattern of recurrence. While advocates of mastectomy hold that these results demonstrate that DCIS must be treated by mastectomy, others have per-sisted in attempts to establish the appropriateness of breast-conserving procedures. Lagios stratified DCIS based on size and found that small (<2.5 cm), mam-mographically detected DCIS is associated with a de-creased incidence of multicentricity and occult invasive cancer. A prospective analysis of such lesions treated by segmental mastectomy revealed a 12.6 per cent re-currence and no mortality. Radiation following seg-mental resection decreases local recurrence, although follow-up has been limited and the question remains whether radiation prevents, or simply delays, recurrent disease.

The current management of DCIS includes total mastectomy with axillary node sampling, usually without formal axillary lymph node dissection. This strategy is usually applied to large and histologically or radiologically extensive manifestations of DCIS. Al-ternatives to total mastectomy may still be considered when lesions present as a small focus of disease or focal microcalcifications. These may be appropriately treated by segmental mastectomy. Such lesions must be excised with clear surgical margins. Radiation fol-lowing segmental resection has been shown to de-crease the rate of local recurrence, and the patient must be willing to undergo close observation. Treat-ment of DCIS with chemotherapy and/or hormonal therapy remains inadequately studied, and it is hoped that ongoing prospective trials will clarify the role of mastectomy, segmental resection, radiation, hormonal therapy, and chemotherapy.

Paget's Disease

Paget's disease is a chronic eczematoid eruption of the nipple that arises as an intraductal carcinoma and involves the epidermis of the nipple and areola by ep-ithelial spread. Patients complain of burning, itching, tenderness, and occasionally bleeding, and the surface of the nipple areola complex is encrusted, scaly, hy-peremic, and enlarged. The nipple is always involved, while the areola may have varying degrees of involve-ment. A definable, palpable, subareolar mass is com-mon. Biopsy of the nipple and the associated subar-eolar mass is diagnostic, as intraductal carcinoma is usually found associated with an invasive carcinoma; however, Paget's disease may be associated with an intraductal carcinoma in situ alone.

Invasive Carcinoma

Infiltrating ductal carcinoma is the most common malignant breast disease diagnosed by biopsy. The term *infiltrating* means that it has invaded beyond the basement membrane of the breast and is found in the surrounding stroma, and *ductal* refers to its origin in the ductal epithelium. Neoplastic cells are typically ar-ranged in small clusters or in single rows occupying the irregular spaces between collagen bundles. A spec-trum of well-differentiated–to–anaplastic variants may be observed within the same tumor mass, and invasive ductal carcinoma is commonly found coexist-ing with intraductal carcinoma. This tumor represents at least 75 per cent of invasive carcinoma of the breast.

Medullary carcinoma is characterized by the pres-ence of anaplastic tumor cells that appear to be infil-trated by lymphocytes. Medullary carcinoma is rec-ognized by its soft hemorrhagic gross appearance with a zone of encircling fibrosis and lymphatic infiltration on histologic examination, which is often confused with a lymph node filled with tumor. It represents ap-proximately 3 to 5 per cent of breast cancers and has a better 5–year survival than invasive ductal or lobu-lar carcinoma. The significance of the infiltrating lymph nodes in this histologic subtype is unknown, and axillary lymph node metastases remain a common route of dissemination.

Comedocarcinoma comprises 5 to 10 per cent of invasive breast carcinomas and has characteristic plugs of pasty material that can be expressed from the sur-face of the neoplasm. These tumors may be of appreciable size at the time of presentation, but they tend to grow slowly and the 5–year survival for invasive comedocarcinoma averages 73 per cent. The tumor is usually well circumscribed. Histologically, cores of highly cellular epithelial tissue with focal calcification occlude the ducts. Of interest, the intraductal counterpart of comedocarcinoma tends to behave aggressively, in comparison to other intraductal carcinomas.

An adenocarcinoma of ductal origin, *colloid* or *mucinous carcinoma* is a relatively rare tumor with a slow growth rate and limited potential for metastasis. The tumor is usually well demarcated but not encapsulated. Histologically, many multilocular cysts containing amorphous material are surrounded by islands of tumor cells. Colloid carcinomas have a similarly favorable prognosis as comedocarcinoma.

Papillary and tubular carcinomas are unusual but have favorable features. Papillary carcinomas are usually bulky and centrally located lesions occurring in young women, with lowest frequency of axillary lymph node metastasis and the best 5- and 10-year survival of any truly invasive adenocarcinomas of ductal origin. Histologically, large sheets of viable tumor cells form a papillary pattern. Tubular carcinomas represent only 1 per cent of all breast carcinomas but also have an excellent long-term prognosis. Histologically, the tumor is characterized by small, well-formed ductal structures, may mimic sclerosing adenosis, and must be differentiated from focal atypical hyperplasia. Survival is over 90 per cent when the carcinoma contains over 90 per cent of a tubular component.

Invasive lobular carcinoma probably originates from the epithelial lining of the breast lobules and is distinguishable from lesions arising in the larger lactiferous ducts. It constitutes between 3 and 15 per cent of all invasive breast tumors. Clinically, lobular carcinomas behave very similarly to their ductal counterpart.

SURGICAL THERAPY FOR OPERABLE BREAST CANCER

The goals of treatment for breast cancer include control of local disease, staging, a satisfactory cosmetic result, rehabilitation, and cure. Each of these goals must be discussed with the patient to achieve an acceptable treatment plan. As discussed above, the treatment of invasive carcinoma is distinct from the management of premalignant conditions or carcinoma in situ, where the goal is the prevention of invasive cancer. Three surgical options are available to treat patients with early stage invasive breast carcinoma: modified radical mastectomy, breast conservation procedures with radiation, and breast reconstruction either at the time of mastectomy (immediate) or some

time later (delayed). For most patients the goals of therapy include the preservation or creation of a normal appearing breast. Details of the surgical options are described in Table 3.

Currently, patients who are candidates for modified radical mastectomy should be considered for conservative breast procedures, and this alternative should be carefully discussed. Exactly which groups of patients should be offered radiation and which are better treated by mastectomy is important. Generally, all patients should be considered candidates for conservative therapy, and then specific contraindications to breast conservation therapy should be reviewed. Following this, general discussion regarding the advantages and disadvantages of each of the surgical options available to the patient should be presented. Following operation, pathologic review of the tumor and the draining axillary lymph nodes is performed. The most commonly used method for staging breast carcinoma is the tumor node metastasis (TNM) system proposed by the American Joint Committee on Cancer and the International Union Against Cancer, which is depicted in Table 4. At times, the optimal method of treatment may not be apparent until operation and the pathologic staging has been performed.

Modified Radical Mastectomy

Standard modified radical mastectomy consists of removal of the entire breast and an axillary node dissection. At present, the histologic status of the axillary nodes (positive or negative) and the extent of nodal involvement (number of positive nodes) are the best indicators of prognosis. Although there is no evidence that removal of axillary nodes improves survival rates, an axillary node dissection provides more reliable staging than clinical assessment of the axilla and reduces the risk of a subsequent regional recurrence. A formal level I and II axillary node dissection (removal of axillary lymph nodes lateral to and behind the pectoralis minor muscle) accurately defines prognostic subsets of patients (i.e., those with one to three positive nodes versus those with four or more). In addition to preserving the thoracodorsal neurovascular structures and long thoracic nerve, care should be taken to avoid injury to the pectoralis nerves innervating the pectoralis major muscle. However, the intercostal brachial nerve may be sacrificed because its branches course anatomically through the lower axillary lymph nodes. The patient should be made aware preoperatively that this sacrifice causes anesthesia of the skin in the axilla and posteromedial aspect of the upper arm. The patient is usually instructed on active range-of-motion exercises to use in the postoperative period.

TABLE 3.   TREATMENT OPTIONS FOR OPERABLE BREAST CANCER

	Breast Conservation Surgery with Radiation	Modified Radical Mastectomy	Breast Reconstruction
Description of Breast Procedure	Excision of the breast lesion with a margin of normal tissue	Removal of the entire breast	Removal of the entire breast and breast reconstruction
Description of Axillary Procedure	Axillary node dissection	Axillary node dissection	Axillary node dissection
Advantages	Preservation of the breast including the nipple	Lowest local recurrence rate	Reconstruction of the breast to recreate a normal-appearing breast
Disadvantages	Local recurrence rate higher than modified radical mastectomy	Removal of breast tissue	Multiple procedures required
Risks and Side Effects	Radiation risks include edema and altered sensation of the skin, fibrosis of the breast parenchyma, contraction of the breast, rib fractures, brachial pexopathy, damage to the underlying heart and lung, and rarely development of sarcoma in the treatment field		Prosthetic material may be required
Survival	Equivalent to other alternatives	Equivalent to other alternatives	Equivalent to other alternatives

BREAST CONSERVATION PROCEDURES AND RADIATION

Breast conservation refers to conservation of breast tissue without compromising treatment of the tumor. The goal of combined surgery and irradiation is to achieve cancer treatment and an acceptable cosmetic outcome while minimizing the risk of local recurrence. A multimodality approach is best employed when discussing breast conservation therapy, as radiation is a necessary component of optimal treatment. This is achieved by including the radiation therapist in pretreatment discussions before breast conservation procedures are pursued to ensure that the patient is a candidate for this approach. Even more important is the information acquired by the patient that allows a rational decision about the best treatment option. In addition, the patient should be adequately informed about the specific plan for delivery of the radiation, including the duration of treatment, as well as about the potential short- and long-term side effects.

Surgical risks of breast conservation therapy include an unacceptable cosmetic result following excision of a relatively large portion of the breast and the risk of a subsequent breast recurrence that may require mastectomy or lead to decreased survival. Of importance is the realization that the axillary node dissection, with its inherent complications, is also a requisite part of breast conservation therapy. The number of complications following axillary lymph node dissection should be equivalent following modified radical mas-

tectomy and following breast conservation therapy. Specific risks of radiation include edema and altered sensation of the skin, fibrosis of the breast parenchyma, contraction of the breast, brachial plexopathy, damage to the underlying heart and lung, and, rarely, rib fractures and development of sarcoma in the field of treatment.

Numerous prospective randomized studies have shown that survival is not significantly different for selected patients who undergo breast conservation procedure plus irradiation than for those who receive a modified radical mastectomy for early stage breast cancer. However, patterns of failure, including locoregional recurrence, are significantly different between these two groups and should be distinguished. Patients failing therapy following a standard mastectomy usually develop a recurrence within 2 years of operation and have a poor prognosis. Local and regional recurrence in the chest wall is difficult to manage and is often associated with distant metastases. These patients have 5-year survival of only 15 per cent.

Patients treated with breast conservation therapy and irradiation have a higher local and regional failure rate than patients treated with standard modified radical mastectomy. However, in contrast to the poor prognosis of patients with local failure after mastectomy, most have a relatively good prognosis, with recurrence following breast conservation therapy. Recurrent disease following breast conservation therapy and radiation is usually not on the chest wall, but develops at the site of the primary lesion. With careful

TABLE 4. TNM BREAST CANCER CLASSIFICATION SYSTEM

Primary Tumor (T)
TX	Primary tumor cannot be assessed
T0	No evidence of primary tumor
Tis	Carcinoma in situ or Paget's disease of the nipple with no associated tumor
T1	Tumor 2 cm or less in greatest dimension
T2	Tumor more than 2 cm but not more than 5 cm in greatest dimension
T3	Tumor more than 5 cm in greatest dimension
T4	Tumor of any size with direct extension to chest wall or skin

Regional Lymph Node (N)
NX	Regional lymph nodes cannot be assessed
N0	No regional lymph node metastasis
N1	Metastasis to ipsilateral axillary lymph nodes
N2	Metastasis to ipsilateral axillary lymph node(s) fixed to one another or other structures
N3	Metastasis to ipsilateral internal mammary lymph node(s)

Distant Metastases (M)
MX	Presence of distant metastasis cannot be assessed
M0	No distant metastasis
M1	Distant metastasis (includes metastasis to supraclavicular lymph nodes)

interval examination and early detection, these patients can usually be salvaged by further surgery and achieve a 5-year survival of 60 to 70 per cent. Nonetheless, careful attention must be given those factors associated with a higher local failure rate following breast conservation therapy and radiation as depicted in Table 5.

Patients must have a strong desire to preserve the breast, as they must be willing to have daily outpatient irradiation for a 5- to 6-week period. A fear of or aversion to irradiation must also be addressed, as local failure is more common if radiation therapy is not completed. Patients must be able to return indefinitely for interval evaluation to exclude treatment failure. Advanced age is not considered a contraindication to breast conservation, and younger women may actually have a higher rate of failure of therapy in the treated breast. However, the disease-free and overall survival rates are not significantly different.

A solitary lesion smaller than 3 to 4 cm in diameter is preferable, depending on the size of the breast and the location of the tumor, as tumor margins should be negative. Patients with multiple primary tumors are not candidates for breast conservation procedures.

TABLE 5. RISK FACTORS ASSOCIATED WITH LOCAL RECURRENCES FOLLOWING BREAST CONSERVATION SURGERY

Risk Factor	Recurrence Rate (%)
No breast irradiation	25–43
Surgical margin positive or near tumor	20–35
Extensive DCIS (especially in younger patients)	20–25
Young age (<40 years)	20–25
Multiple tumors	16–35
High nuclear grade of tumor	10–20

Abbreviation: DCIS = ductal carcinoma in situ.

When there are two small lesions or microcalcifications that can be completely excised by the removal of a 3- to 4-cm diameter region of the breast with negative margins, breast conservation procedures can be considered. Conservative procedures for larger tumors are considered investigational. Biopsy sites should be reexcised if inadequate or unknown margins are reported by the pathologist or if physical examination or mammography suggests residual cancer. Patients with stage III disease, consisting of fixed or matted axillary nodes, should undergo induction chemotherapy and be reassessed for breast conservation surgery if a response is achieved.

No significant difference in local recurrence has been detected among histologic subtypes of invasive breast cancer. Among the risk factors associated with local failure, the presence of *extensive intraductal carcinoma* (EIC) deserves special mention. As noted above, intraductal carcinoma is often multicentric and extensive disease may need to be treated by mastectomy. A report from the Joint Center for Radiation Therapy in Boston showed that the presence of EIC occupying 25 per cent or more of the tumor lesion with extension outside the invasive component was associated with 10-year local failure of 35 per cent, as compared with 8 per cent when EIC was absent. The relapse rate is reportedly higher when EIC occurs in younger women. Therefore, if an invasive carcinoma coexists with extensive intraductal carcinoma, both tumor types must be considered when planning therapeutic strategies. Alternatively, if a focus of intraductal carcinoma that is completely excised is found with an invasive carcinoma, breast conservation therapy with radiation can be considered.

Because the goal is to avoid local recurrence and preserve the breast with acceptable cosmetic results, other factors that may impact on these goals should be discussed with the patient. Breast size appears to have more of an impact on the cosmetic result than on local failure or survival. Because a negative surgical margin should be achieved for breast conservation therapy, the breast should be of adequate size to allow appropriate tumor excision with an acceptable cosmetic result. A superficial, centrally located or subareolar tumor may require removal of the nipple/areolar complex to excise the tumor with negative margins. However, the resulting breast mound may be cosmetically satisfactory to the patient. An increased incidence of fibrosis and contraction may be seen with large, pendulous breasts due to technical difficulties in delivering a uniform dose of radiation. Irradiation of a small breast with a subcutaneous implant also may cause severe capsular contraction. The acute and chronic side effects of radiation may be exaggerated in patients with discoid or systemic lupus crythematosus or with scleroderma.

In performing a segmental mastectomy (wide local excision), an elliptical incision is placed directly over the breast mass and includes the needle track or scar from any previous biopsy. To achieve the best cosmetic result, a curvilinear transverse incision that conforms to the contour of the breast is used, although a radial (vertical) incision may be preferred for large tumors in the lower quadrants of the breast to diminish downward retraction of the nipple/areolar complex. The incision for the segmental mastectomy should be separate from the incision for the axillary node dissection. This diminishes subsequent retraction of the breast toward the axilla and also enables the radiation therapist to give a radiation boost to the primary tumor site if necessary.

After the incision is made, flaps are raised in all directions to free the skin from the underlying breast tissue. These flaps are relatively thick unless the tumor is superficially located. An en bloc excision around the tumor or biopsy cavity is performed with a 1-cm or greater margin of normal breast tissue obtained in all three dimensions. Excising the entire quadrant of the breast is unnecessary and may cause greater distortion of the contour of the breast. The pectoralis major fascia may be included for deep-seated tumors. When the specimen is removed, the surgeon should orient and mark it for the pathologist and request that any close margin be checked by frozen section examination. A portion of the tumor should also be sent for hormone receptor assays and flow cytometry analysis. Radiopaque hemoclips may be used to mark the bed of tumor resection for the radiation therapist. Meticulous homeostasis should be obtained. The defect in the breast is not closed with sutures, and drains are not necessary. The skin is closed with a continuous subcuticular suture for cosmesis. A level I and II axillary node dissection is performed as in the standard modified radical mastectomy.

Radiation therapy is begun 2 to 3 weeks after operation when the wounds have healed and the patient is able to abduct the arm out of the treatment field. If adjuvant chemotherapy is given, radiation therapy can be deferred until the chemotherapy has been completed. If the patient had stage I disease, only the breast is irradiated, with a dose of 50 Gy given through tangential ports to include the breast and underlying chest wall. Computerized dosimetry is used to ensure a uniform dose throughout the breast. It remains controversial whether a boost dose of 1000 cGy is necessary to achieve local disease control. Axillary irradiation should not be performed in a patient who has had a level I and II axillary dissection. Axillary irradiation may be considered when there is extensive extranodal tumor or multiple positive axillary nodes. The combination of complete axillary dissection and radiation therapy is likely to significantly increase the risk of breast and arm edema, and there is no additive benefit gained by using the combination of treatments when either alone is sufficient for local disease control. A potential risk factor for young women who have undergone breast radiation is an increase in incidence of contralateral breast carcinoma.

In most studies, satisfactory cosmetic results have been achieved if extensive axillary node dissection combined with axillary irradiation is avoided and if the radiation dose to large volumes is restricted to 50 Gy. Excessively wide resection of normal breast tissue surrounding the tumor also produces a less satisfactory appearance. In addition, the use of concomitant adjuvant chemotherapy may increase the radiation-induced fibrosis of the breast and thus augment breast retraction. The psychologic effects of preserving the breast as compared with the effects of mastectomy are most significant in terms of positive body image. However, there are no major differences between treatment groups with respect to general psychologic adjustment, anxiety, and marital satisfaction.

THE ROLE OF ESTROGEN AND THE ESTROGEN RECEPTOR

It has been demonstrated that the presence of estrogen receptors provides a molecular basis for the distinction between those human breast carcinomas that are responsive to hormonal therapy or organ ablation and those that are not. Investigators have suggested that the ability of a breast cancer to bind estrogen may be predictive of a patient's response to endocrine therapy. Numerous studies have shown that approximately half of all biopsy samples of malignant breast tumors contain estrogen receptors. The results from the National Institutes of Health (NIH) Consensus Development Conference suggest that a 50 to 60 per cent response rate may be expected from a breast cancer given hormonal manipulation when only the status of the estrogen receptor is considered (Table 6).

Analysis of estrogen receptors in primary lesions indicates that patients with estrogen receptor–positive tumors have a favorable prognosis with an increased disease-free survival when compared to patients with tumors that did not contain estrogen receptors. This appears to be independent of the patients' menopausal status and the presence of metastases in the axillary lymph nodes. These data clearly indicate that the estrogen receptor status is a useful predictive index of a response to endocrine manipulation and is a prognostic indicator for the course of the disease.

Unfortunately, not all women with breast cancer containing estrogen receptors respond to hormonal therapy. It is possible that the estrogen receptor binding may be insufficient due to defects in the intercellular cascade of events that normally control biologic responsiveness. Therefore, the determination of progesterone receptor status has been advocated to increase the accuracy for selected breast cancer patients most likely to respond to hormone therapy. This is based on animal work in which progesterone receptor formation is regulated by estrogen receptors, thereby acting as a surrogate marker for the presence of estrogen receptor. Table 6 provides a summary of results presented at the NIH Consensus Development Conference showing the relationship between steroid receptor status of the breast and patients' objective response to endocrine therapy. Of note is the poor response to tumors that are estrogen receptor– and progesterone receptor–negative. However, it is noted that 45 per cent of estrogen receptor–negative tumors respond to endocrine therapy if progesterone receptor–positive. These data suggest that the progesterone receptor may be useful in the selection of patients for endocrine manipulation in conjunction with the status of the estrogen receptor.

ADJUVANT THERAPY FOR OPERABLE BREAST CANCER

A summary of pathologic stage, options for therapy, and 5-year survival for breast carcinoma is shown in Table 7. After operation for breast cancer, an important decision must be made about the use of adjuvant systemic therapy, either chemotherapy or hormonal therapy. This decision will depend on information from the pathologic examination of the excised specimen and axillary lymph nodes, including assays for tumor markers and hormone receptors. The decision-making process for adjuvant systemic therapy involves

TABLE 6. RELATIONSHIP BETWEEN HORMONE RECEPTOR STATUS OF BREAST TUMOR AND PATIENT RESPONSE TO ENDOCRINE THERAPY

Estrogen Receptor	Progesterone Receptor	Response
+	+	78%
+	−	34%
−	+	45%
−	−	10%

two basic steps: estimating the risk of systemic micrometastases based on prognostic factors, and assessing the known benefits, risks, and complications of each systemic drug regimen. Patients can be categorized into one of three groups using currently available prognostic factors: low risk (10 to 20 per cent) for systemic metastases, intermediate risk (20 to 50 per cent), and high risk (>50 per cent). Tumor size and nodal status are the primary factors used to delineate risk groups for metastatic disease, but a number of factors are currently being evaluated to determine their role in assigning risk of metastasis (Fig. 6). Numerous other prognostic factors correlate with survival, such as estrogen receptor status, presence or absence of the oncogene *erb*-B2, levels of protease cathepsin D and angiogenesis factor VIII, nuclear grade, flow cytometry DNA index, and the percentage of cells in the S phase of the cell cycle.

In general, patients with tumors at low risk for recurrence or metastasis following operation and/or radiation therapy should not be considered for adjuvant systemic therapy, except in prospective protocols, because there is no proven benefit for any of the currently available agents that are associated with risks and additional costs. Alternatively, patients at high risk for recurrence or metastasis should be considered for adjuvant systemic therapy as standard treatment, because the benefits outweigh the risks, as documented in prospective randomized clinical trials. Patients with tumors that are at an intermediate risk for recurrence or metastasis might also be considered for adjuvant therapy. Early results from clinical trials suggest that women in this subgroup with node-negative cancer may benefit from systemic therapy in terms of disease-free survival. However, an increased overall survival rate has been demonstrated for patients with node-negative tumors larger than 3 cm in diameter.

As specific forms of chemotherapy are being intensely investigated, a number of clinical trials are available for entry. Generally, recommendations by the 1990 NIH Consensus Development Conference are being accepted as standard care. Adjuvant chemotherapy and/or hormone therapy is usually recommended for women with positive axillary nodes. Postmenopausal women with metastatic disease who

TABLE 7. STAGE, THERAPY, AND SURVIVAL FOR BREAST CARCINOMA

Stage	T	N	M	Local/Regional Therapy	Systemic Therapy Premenopausal	Postmenopausal	5-Year Survival
Stage 0 (in situ carcinoma)							
a. Intraductal carcinoma in situ	Tis	N0	M0	Wide local excision with or without postoperative radiation therapy, or total mastectomy (with or without axillary node dissection)			over 95%
b. Lobular carcinoma in situ (commonly occurs bilaterally)				No further treatment, unilateral or bilateral total mastectomy			
Stage I: Primary tumor less than 2 cm, negative axillary lymph nodes and no distant metastases	T1	N0	M0	Wide excision or quadrantectomy with axillary lymph node dissection and postoperative radiation therapy, or modified radical mastectomy			85%
Stage IIA: Primary tumor less than 2 cm, and positive axillary lymph nodes or primary lesion between 2 and 5 cm in diameter with negative nodes	T0 / T1 / T2	N1 / N1 / N0	M0 / M0 / M0	Wide excision or quadrantectomy with axillary lymph node dissection and postoperative radiation therapy, or modified radical mastectomy	Chemotherapy	Hormone therapy for ER+ tumors, possible chemotherapy	75%
Stage IIB: Primary tumor between 2 and 5 cm in diameter with positive axillary lymph nodes or primary lesion greater than 5 cm in diameter with negative nodes	T2 / T3	N1 / N0	M0 / M0	Wide excision or quadrantectomy with axillary lymph node dissection and postoperative radiation therapy, or modified radical mastectomy	Chemotherapy	Hormone therapy for ER+ tumors, possible chemotherapy	65%
Stage IIIA: Primary tumor greater than 5 cm in diameter with ipsilateral axillary node involvement or fixed axillary lymph nodes	T0 / T1 / T2 / T3	N2 / N2 / N2 / N1,N2	M0 / M0 / M0 / M0	Surgery, radiation	Chemotherapy, hormone therapy in varying sequences		50%
Stage IIIB: Internal mammary nodes are involved; tumor extends to the chest wall and ulcerates the skin	T4 / Any T	Any N / N3	M0 / M0	Surgery, radiation	Chemotherapy, hormone therapy		41%
Stage IV: Distant metastases	Any T	Any N	M1	Surgery, radiation	Chemotherapy, hormone therapy		10%

Abbreviation: ER+ = estrogen receptor–positive.

are hormone receptor–positive are treated with various combinations or sequences of tamoxifen, progestin, and occasionally, oophorectomy, adrenalectomy, and androgens. For postmenopausal patients who have a hormone receptor–positive tumor and nodal metastasis, tamoxifen alone has been proven to have a survival benefit almost equivalent to that of cytoxan, methotrexate, and 5-fluorouracil type chemotherapy regimens. For those with hormone receptor–negative tumors or who no longer respond to hormonal manipulation, combination chemotherapy is commonly given.

Premenopausal women with positive axillary nodes are also treated with adjuvant combination therapy. A number of different chemotherapeutic agents are used in varying dosages and combinations, including cyclophosphamide, doxorubicin, methotrexate, and 5-fluorouracil. Experimental high-dose chemotherapy with granulocyte colony stimulating factor or granulocyte macrophage colony stimulating factor or with bone marrow transplantation is currently being studied. The antiestrogen drug tamoxifen causes an objective response in one third of initially treated patients. This response correlates closely with the presence of hormone receptors for estrogen and progesterone on the primary tumor. Antiestrogens block the uptake of estrogen by the target tissue following cytosol binding to the estrogen receptor. A poor response at a low dose may be improved by a higher dose. The optimal duration of therapy with tamoxi-

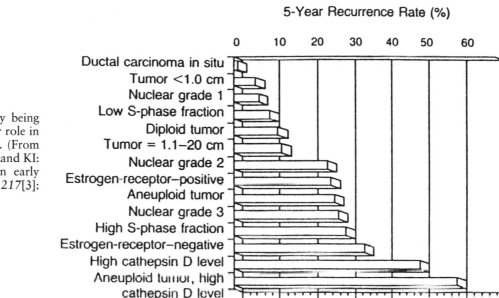

5-Year Recurrence Rate (%)

Figure 6. Factors currently being evaluated to determine their role in assigning risk of metastasis. (From Balch CM, Singletary SE, Bland KI: Clinical decision making in early breast cancer. Ann Surg 217[3]: 207–208, 1993.)

fen is unknown, but a minimum of 2 to 5 years has been recommended. Tamoxifen may cause hypercalcemia and bone pain when initiated, but usually has few side effects. It may cause hot flashes, and a few experience serious complications such as phlebitis and pulmonary embolism.

LOCALLY ADVANCED BREAST CANCER

The diagnosis of inflammatory breast cancer is based on the clinical findings of erythema, edema or *peau d'orange*, and wheals or ridging of the skin and is confirmed by the dermal lymphatics filled with tumor cells. A delay in the diagnosis of inflammatory breast cancer is usually due to confusion with bacterial infections of the breast. The differential diagnosis of erythema of the nonlactating breast must include inflammatory breast cancer, and a tissue biopsy should be performed to confirm the clinical impression.

Prior to the advent of current forms of combination chemotherapy, inflammatory breast cancer had a 5-year survival of only 3 to 5 per cent. With the use of any one of the combination chemotherapeutic programs, approximately 60 to 75 per cent of individuals have a dramatic regression of the breast lesion. Following two to three drug cycles, an extended simple mastectomy may be done to remove the remaining malignant disease from the chest wall. The skin flaps, peripheral lymphatics, and apical axilla are then treated with radiation therapy. Using multimodality

treatment, 5-year survival of inflammatory breast cancer has improved to 30 per cent.

Combination chemotherapy has also been valuable in the treatment of stage III disease. Often, axillary nodes are large and matted; thus, completion of a mastectomy may not be feasible. Preoperative chemotherapy may cause the malignant deposits to regress, allowing a mastectomy with the use of skin grafts. The use of radiation therapy to the chest wall and the peripheral lymphatics ensures better control of disease remaining on the chest wall. Chest wall recurrence has been limited to 4 to 6 per cent, and 5- and 10-year survival has been 45 and 28 per cent, respectively.

BREAST CANCER IN PREGNANCY

Although breast cancer is the most common malignancy in pregnancy, it is rare, occurring in only 3 of 10,000 pregnancies. Despite hormonal and immunologic changes of pregnancy, there is no certain evidence that pregnancy increases the risk of developing breast cancer, advances disease stage, or worsens prognosis. The only known differences inherent to pregnancy are delayed diagnosis and treatment limitations.

Relative to age-matched patients, pregnant women present with more advanced disease and, hence, have an overall worse prognosis. Most authors attribute this to the difficulty of examining enlarged, firm, often nodular breasts, and a tendency to dismiss masses as physiologic and, hence, delay diagnosis (Fig. 5). Mammography is not contraindicated, provided the abdomen and pelvis are shielded, and breast biopsy has been proven safe if anesthetic considerations are appropriately managed. The treatment of stage I and stage II breast cancer is oriented toward mastectomy instead of breast-conserving procedures because of the risk to the fetus of radiation therapy. A decision must also be made as to whether adjuvant chemotherapy should be delayed until delivery, although little is known about the teratogenic properties of these agents during the second and third trimesters. Consideration of aborting a pregnancy becomes relevant only in stage III and stage IV breast cancer. The risks of radiation and chemotherapy, which are standard treatments for advanced breast cancer, and realization of the mother's limited life expectancy influence these decisions.

MALE BREAST CANCER

Male breast cancer is rare. Less than 1000 cases per year are reported in the United States. This represents less than 1 per cent of all breast cancers and less than 1 per cent of all cancers in men. Unlike female breast cancer, the incidence has remained unchanged in recent years. Klinefelter's syndrome, gynecomastia, trauma, and radiation exposure have all been reported to increase risk.

Patients present with a nontender, firm mass, usually centrally located, and sometimes with nipple inversion, bloody discharge, or skin ulceration. Largely because of rarity and decreased awareness of this disease, males have traditionally presented at a later stage relative to female patients, although this trend is improving with public awareness of breast cancer. The male breast is physiologically atrophic. Lobules are absent and male breast cancers are ductal in origin. Because of delayed presentation and prevalence of pectoralis muscle invasion, radical mastectomy was historically the common treatment for male breast cancer. Surgical therapy has adapted to earlier presentation, and modified radical mastectomy, simple mastectomy, and even local excision are currently employed. Some cancers are steroid receptor–positive, and hormonally based treatment, including tamoxifen, additive hormonal therapy, orchiectomy, and adrenalectomy, decrease recurrence rate and slow progression of metastatic disease. Effectiveness of chemotherapy has yet to be proven, although a presumption of effectiveness is based on the concept that male breast cancer is similar to female. For comparable stage, survival data between males and females is the same. As in female breast cancer, lymph node involvement is the best indicator of survival.

TABLE 8. COMMONLY USED COMBINATIONS OF CHEMOTHERAPY TO TREAT ADVANCED AND METASTATIC BREAST CANCER*

Cyclophosphamide-Based Regimens

CMFVP

C = cyclophosphamide	2 mg/kg/day orally
M = Methotrexate	0.7 mg/kg/wk intravenously × 8 wk
F = 5-fluorouracil	12 mg/kg/day × 4, then 500 mg/wk intravenously
V = vincristine	0.035 mg/kg/wk intravenously
P = prednisone	0.75 mg/kg/day orally

CMF

C = cyclophosphamide	100 mg/m^2/day orally on days 1–14
M = methotrexate	30–40 mg/m^2 intravenously on days 1 and 8 every 28 days
F = 5-fluorouracil	400–600 mg/m^2 intravenously on days 1 and 8 every 28 days

CFP

C = cyclophosphamide	150 mg/m^2/day orally × 5
F = 5-fluorouracil	300 mg/m^2/day intravenously × 5 q 6 wk
P = prednisone	30 mg/day × 7

Doxorubicin-Based Regimens

FAC

F = 5-fluorouracil	500 mg/m^2 intravenously on days 1 and 8
A = doxorubicin hydrochloride (adriamycin)	50 mg/m^2 intravenously on day 1 every 28 days
C = cyclophosphamide	500 mg/m^2 intravenously on day 1

ACMF

A = adriamycin	40 mg/m^2 on day 21
C = cyclophosphamide	1000 mg/m^2 on day 1
M = methotrexate	30 mg/m^2 on days 21, 28, and 35
F = 5-fluorouracil	400–600 mg/m^2 on days 21, 28, and 35; repeat cycle q 6 wk

AC

A = adriamycin	40 mg/m^2
C = cyclophosphamide	200 mg/m^2 on days 3 to 6; repeat cycle q 21 days

*From Iglehart JD: The Breast. *In* Sabiston DC Jr [ed]: Textbook of Surgery: The Biological Basis of Modern Surgical Practice, ed 14. Philadelphia, WB Saunders Company, 1991, p 543, with permission.

METASTATIC BREAST CANCER

Patients with metastatic breast cancer, including supraclavicular lymph node metastasis, are treated primarily with chemotherapy, but control of the local chest wall disease is often achieved by a limited surgical procedure possibly combined with radiation therapy. The choice of these procedures is individualized to each patient and the timing is dictated by the need to control metastatic disease.

Responses to combination chemotherapy have been observed for metastasis to bone, liver, soft tissue, lung, and occasionally, brain. Table 8 summarizes commonly used combinations of chemotherapy to treat advanced and metastatic breast cancer. Clinical trials have demonstrated a response rate of 25 per cent with single agents, which increases to 50 and 60 per cent with combination therapy. Dose intensification has led to the use of high-dose chemotherapy with autologous bone marrow transplantation after marrow purging in selected patients with stage IV carcinoma of the breast.

Patients who fail combination chemotherapy may still be eligible for hormonal manipulation, particularly if the tumor is hormone receptor–positive. For hormonal therapy to be of value, approximately 2 to 3 months of therapy are required before an objective response can be obtained.

REFERENCES

Balch CM, Singletary SE, Bland KI: Clinical decision making in early breast cancer. Ann Surg 217(3):207–225, 1993.

Bland KI, Copeland EM (eds): The Breast: Comprehensive Management of Benign and Malignant Diseases. Philadelphia, WB Saunders Company, 1991.

Haagensen CD: Diseases of the Breast, ed 3. Philadelphia, WB Saunders Company, 1986.

Harris JR, Hellman S, Henderson IC, Kinne DW: Breast Disease. Philadelphia, JB Lippincott Company, 1987.

Lagios MD, Westdahl PR, Margolin FR, et al: Duct carcinoma in situ: Relationship of extent of noninvasive disease to the frequency of occult invasion, multicentricity, lymph node metastases, and short-term treatment failure. Cancer 50:1309, 1982.

Rosen PP, Lieberman PH, Braum DW Jr, et al: Lobular carcinoma in situ of the breast: Detailed analysis of 99 patients with average follow-up of 24 years. Am J Surg Pathol 2:225, 1978.

II
Reconstructive and Aesthetic Breast Surgery

GREGORY S. GEORGIADE, M.D.

The role of reconstructive and aesthetic breast surgical reconstruction is important to many female patients who undergo ablative breast procedures. Congenital and developmental breast abnormalities, including hypermastia, hypomastia, breast asymmetry, and ptosis of the breast, as well as ablative operations following malignant lesions of the breast, affect the patient's self-image and confidence, and create an ever-present desire for aesthetic and breast reconstruction to correct these deformities. The psychologic effects associated with ablative breast operations for breast cancer should not be underestimated, and the aesthetic improvements achieved with reconstruction of the breast have a very positive affect on the patient's self-image and mental health.

BREAST RECONSTRUCTION FOLLOWING ABLATIVE SURGERY

The desire for reconstruction of the breast mound following ablative operations has greatly increased, particularly as surgical techniques and mammary implants have improved. The timing of breast reconstruction can vary from the time of the initial ablative procedure to months or years later. Whether immediate or delayed, there are three options for reconstruction. The most common reconstructive procedure is a permanent or temporary expander type of saline implant placed beneath the pectoralis major and serratus anterior muscles, and the superior rectus fascial area. After submuscular placement, the inflatable prosthesis is gradually expanded in increments of up to 100 ml every few weeks until the desired breast mound is obtained. It is then overexpanded to reduce the incidence of dense scarring or capsular contractures surrounding the permanent implant. This overexpansion is maintained for a period of approximately 2 months. The temporary expander can then be replaced with a permanent prosthesis, or the permanent type of expander prosthesis can be adjusted in volume and remain in place.

The second option requires approximately 5 hours of additional operative time and considerably more technical skill with more hazard and involves the elevation of a suitably sized rectus abdominis musculo-cutaneous flap based on one or both superior epigastric vessels. This is the composite autologous tissue flap of choice, and usually composite abdominal tissue can be transferred to obviate the necessity for a prosthesis (Figs. 1 and 2). Latissimus dorsi myocutaneous flaps can also be transferred, although this is usually a second choice because this flap is limited in reference to the defect that remains at the donor site. Postoperative scarring and the size of the breast mound that can be reconstructed by this approach may also be negative factors. The third option involves the use of a free rectus abdominis musculocutaneous flap. The inferior epigastric vessels can usually be anastomosed to the thoracodorsal artery and vein, and the abdominal tissue can be transferred as a free flap.

In patients with unilateral breast cancer, the contralateral breast should be carefully evaluated from an aesthetic and oncologic standpoint. Surgical procedures such as mastopexy may be required to produce symmetry, and reconstruction of the nipple on the breast mound can be performed following attainment of symmetric breasts. The nipple is usually recon-

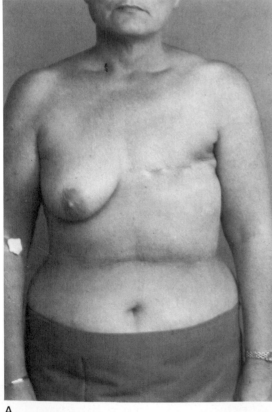
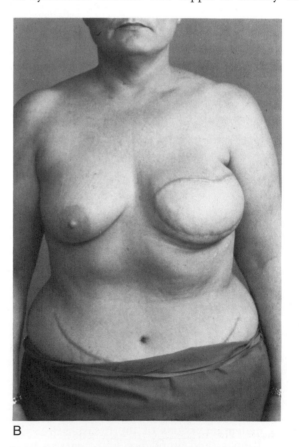

A   B

Figure 1. *A*, Preoperative view of a 47-year-old patient who had a left modified radical mastectomy for extensive intraductal carcinoma 6 months previously. *B*, Three-month postoperative view of the same patient following the elevation and transfer of a contralateral rectus abdominis flap to reconstruct the breast mound (the patient refused nipple-areola reconstruction).

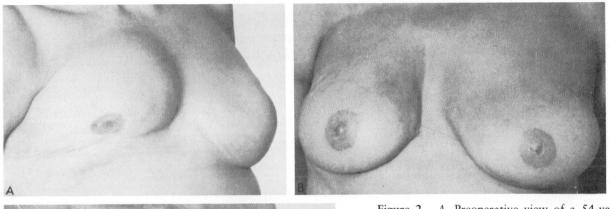

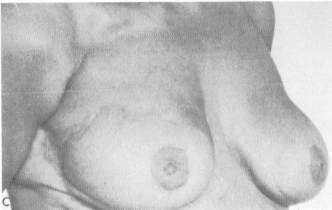

Figure 2. *A*, Preoperative view of a 54-year-old patient who had a long complicated history of attempted breast reconstruction elsewhere, which resulted in loss of tissue in the left and right breasts with attempted transfer of a latissimus dorsi musculocutaneous flap into the right chest area. *B*, and *C*, One-year postoperative views of the same patient following the elevation and transfer of two rectus abdominis flaps, each based on separate rectus abdominis muscle, into the right and left breast mound area recreating two satisfactory breast mounds. (From Sabiston DC Jr [ed]: Davis-Christopher Textbook of Surgery. ed 13. Philadelphia, WB Saunders Company, 1986, p 575, with permission.)

structed using a local breast flap or by sharing a portion of the contralateral nipple as a composite graft positioned appropriately on the reconstructed breast mound. The areola is reconstructed utilizing a full-thickness skin graft from the groin area that usually has sufficient pigment to simulate the appearance of a normal areola. Alternatively, tattooing may be used to pigment the areola.

REDUCTION MAMMOPLASTY

Mammary hyperplasia can create a serious functional disability for women; limit physical activity; and produce neck, back, and shoulder pain. There may be associated inframammary skin excoriations and discomfort. The correction of the ptosis and reduction in breast size can be accomplished by several techniques usually involving the use of nipple areola and dermal pedicle flaps. The procedure utilized most often involves maintenance of a pyramidal central core of breast tissue with the associated nipple areola complex. Resection of the excess breast tissue in the medial, superior, and lateral positions around this inferior

pedicle of breast tissue appears to be the safest technique, which permits the patient to lactate and yields the most normal sensation to the nipple areola area. The use of a pyramidal-based inferior pedicle allows the surgeon to carry reductions of up to 3000 gm of tissue from each breast, minimizing the inferior and vertical incisions and resultant scars (Fig. 3). Alternate techniques for massive breast hypertrophy usually necessitate utilization of an amputative technique with immediate grafting of a free nipple areola.

AUGMENTATION MAMMOPLASTY

Hypomastia can be improved by utilizing a suitable saline-filled prosthesis constructed of a microtextured Silastic shell. The microtexturing process of the shell has the advantage of disrupting the linear scar formation that occurs around the entire prosthesis and produces a lower incidence of capsular contracture or firmness of the breast mound than with a smooth-walled prosthesis. Inflatable saline prostheses are available in various sizes and shapes. The breast can be augmented by an intramammary incision or

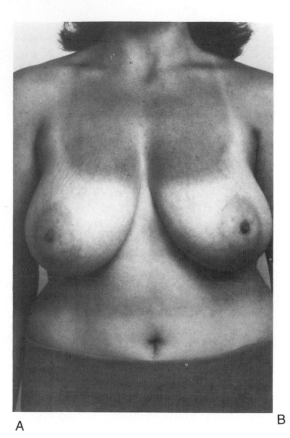

A

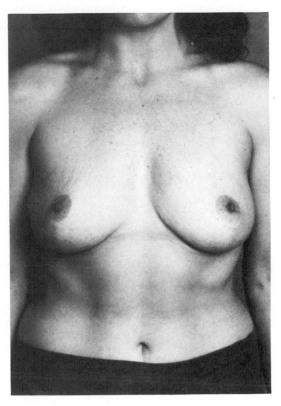

B

Figure 3. *A,* Preoperative view of a 21-year-old patient who complained of back problems related to the weight of her massively enlarged pendulous breasts. *B,* Five-year postoperative view of the same patient; 550 gm of tissue had been removed from each breast utilizing an inferior pyramidal flap technique.

through a circumareolar incision, transareolar incision, or an axillary approach. The prosthesis can be placed beneath the breast or in the subpectoral position. Generally, a normal appearance of the breasts is obtained when the prosthesis is placed in the submammary position.

Capsular contracture or firmness of the prosthesis may occur after an augmentation mammoplasty, noticeably in as many as 10 per cent, and is of considerable concern. The development of the microtextured, silicone-walled prosthesis has decreased the incidence of capsular contracture. Fortunately, infection occurs seldom, but if present, necessitates removal of the prosthesis. Nipple anesthesia occurs in approximately 2 per cent and is due to injury to the fourth intercostal nerve. The placement of any prosthesis, particularly a large one, should be viewed as a potential hazard because the intercostal nerves can be injured. Therefore, care should be taken in the dissection to isolate or identify these nerves and protect them during the creation of the pocket.

BREAST PTOSIS

Breast ptosis is an aesthetic problem that varies in severity depending on the relationship of the nipple and areola to the inframammary fold. Usually, breast ptosis can be corrected, if there is an associated atrophy of the breast or lack of breast tissue, by insertion of a breast prosthesis with simultaneous elevation of the nipple areola complex. This procedure, with augmentation, can be performed under local anesthesia and intravenous sedation on an outpatient basis. If there is adequate breast tissue, a redraping and elevation of the skin envelope may be used to correct the ptotic breast.

SUMMARY

Developmental, aesthetic, and mastectomy-related deformities of the breast can be corrected by specially designed surgical procedures. Over the last 20 years, dramatic improvements in the techniques available in the area of breast reconstruction have allowed reconstruction to start in selective patients at the time of the mastectomy, as well as on a delayed basis. The techniques available vary from the use of breast tissue expanders and permanent implants, to the use of composite autogenous tissue such as rectus abdominis flap reconstruction. Aesthetic breast procedures involve the correction of both cosmetic and functional deformities including breast reduction, augmentation mammoplasty, and ptosis of the breast. The techniques have continued to improve as have the prostheses. Aesthetic breast procedures produce major psychologic and physiologic benefits.

REFERENCES

Bostwick J (ed): Plastic & Reconstructive Breast Surgery. St. Louis, Quality Medical Publishing, Inc, 1990.

Georgiade GS: Reconstructive and aesthetic breast surgery. *In* Sabiston DC Jr (ed): Textbook of Surgery: The Biological Basis of Modern Surgical Practice, ed 14. Philadelphia, WB Saunders Company, 1991.

Georgiade GS, Georgiade N, Riefkohl R, Barwick W: Textbook of Plastic, Maxillofacial and Reconstructive Surgery, ed 2. Baltimore, Williams & Wilkins, 1992.

Georgiade N, Georgiade GS, Riefkohl R: Aesthetic Surgery of the Breast. Philadelphia, WB Saunders Company, 1990.

21

SURGICAL DISORDERS OF THE THYROID

H. KIM LYERLY, M.D.

ANATOMY

The thyroid gland develops from the entoderm of the floor of the pharynx, descending to emerge as a bilobed diverticulum, maintaining its connection to the pharynx by a narrow stalk known as the thyroglossal duct, which is usually obliterated, but can be identified in the normal adult at its two ends: in the tongue as the foramen cecum and, in 75 per cent of cases, at the thyroid end as a pyramidal lobe that arises from the isthmus. The normal adult thyroid weighs approximately 15 to 20 gm and has two lobes along the lower half of the lateral margins of the thyroid cartilage. The isthmus joins the two lobes just below the cricoid cartilage.

Thyroglossal duct cysts and fistulas are conditions associated with a persistent thyroglossal duct. Thyroglossal duct cysts are most common in children and usually present at around age 5 as painless, cystic swellings in the midline in the region of the hyoid bone. Cysts frequently present with infection and are treated by incision and drainage followed by excision of the fistula. The middle of the hyoid bone must be excised with the fistula because the duct usually courses through it. Other abnormalities include thyroid tissue in the thyroglossal duct between the tongue and the root of the neck and a lingual thyroid gland, a very rare abnormality in which the thyroid gland develops at the base of the tongue and may represent the only thyroid tissue.

The developing thyroid meets and accommodates tissue from the ultimobranchial bodies, which develop from brachial pouches at the fifth to sixth week to form C cells. Histologically, the thyroid has numerous follicles (acini) arranged in subunits of 20 to 40 and demarcated by connective tissue to form lobules, each supplied by an individual artery. The height of the epithelial cells lining the follicles varies with the state of functional activity. The follicular lumen is filled with a proteinaceous colloid that appears homogeneous and moderately dense.

Directly anterior to the thyroid gland are the sternothyroid and sternohyoid muscles, and the investing fascia of the neck, encasing the sternocleidomastoid muscles and the anterior jugular veins (Fig. 1). The sternothyroid muscles lie on the thyroid capsule, and are innervated at their cranial ends by the descendens hypoglossi nerves and at the caudal end by the ansa hypoglossi. The carotid artery, the internal jugular vein, the cervical sympathetic trunk, and the inferior thyroid artery are lateral and posterior to the thyroid. Posterior and medial are the parathyroid glands, the esophagus, and the recurrent laryngeal nerve, which ascends in the tracheoesophageal sulcus.

The blood supply to the thyroid is by the paired inferior thyroid arteries and the paired superior thyroid arteries. The superior arteries, usually arising as the first branches from the external carotid arteries, are closely related to the superior laryngeal nerves; they enter the superior poles of the thyroid to divide into anterior and posterior branches. The thyroidea ima artery, a vestige of the embryonic aortic sac, varies from a minute vessel to one the size of the inferior thyroid artery and may originate from the innominate artery, the internal mammary artery, or the aortic arch and may be present in up to 12 per cent of cases. The superior thyroid veins drain into the internal jugular or common facial veins, the middle thyroid veins into

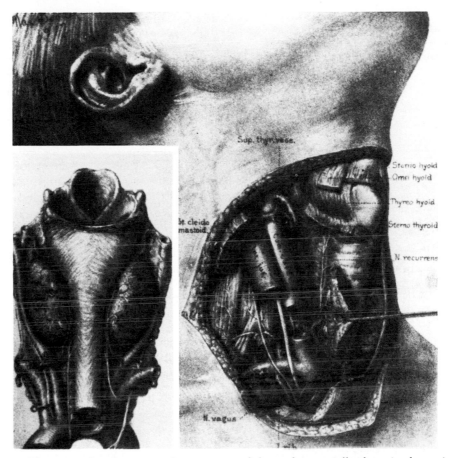

Figure 1. Dissection showing anatomic structures of the neck, especially those in the region of the thyroid gland. The nerve to the left of the vagus is the phrenic. Note location of parathyroid glands and recurrent laryngeal nerve. The amount of thyroid gland on the right side of the trachea is twice the amount that is left after subtotal thyroidectomy. (Drawing from dissections made by Mr. Max Brödel for Professor W.S. Halsted; original drawing in the Max Brödel Archives, The Department of Art as Applied to Medicine. The Johns Hopkins School of Medicine.)

the internal jugular veins, and the inferior thyroid veins into the brachiocephalic veins. The thyroid has a lymphatic capillary network that drains into lymph nodes on the larynx above the isthmus (Delphian node), paratracheal nodes near the recurrent laryngeal nerve, and nodes on the anterior surface of the trachea. From these nodes, lymph drains into the cervical lymph node chains.

PHYSIOLOGY

The thyroid gland functions primarily to produce thyroid hormone for development and regulation of metabolism. Production of thyroid hormone is regulated by the anterior pituitary hormone thyrotropin, or thyroid-stimulating hormone (TSH), and by a system of autoregulation within the thyroid gland. Iodine is necessary for the synthesis of thyroid hormones, which is reduced to iodide ion in the intestine and absorbed. The thyroid, which receives 4 to 6 ml/gm/min of blood flow, actively transports and concentrates iodide in the thyroid follicular cell where it is rapidly oxidized and bound to tyrosine residues in thyroglobulin. After its synthesis and intracellular transport, thyroglobulin accumulates as colloid in the follicle lumen. The thyroid gland has a storage reserve of approximately 3 weeks. After being bound to thyroglobulin, iodide is incorporated in thyroxin (T_4) and triiodothyronine (T_3) via monoiodotyrosine (MIT) and diiodotyrosine (DIT) (Fig. 2). By a complex coupling mechanism, two molecules of DIT combine to form T_4, and a molecule of DIT and a molecule of MIT form T_3. Thyroglobulin breakdown and thyroid hormone release occur when colloid is engulfed and forms endocytotic vesicles that fuse with lysosomes, where

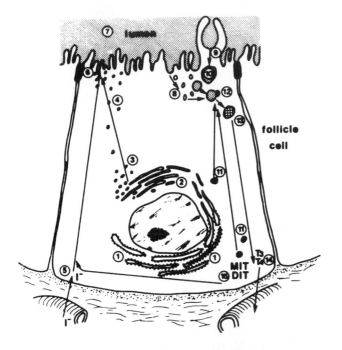

follicle
cell

Figure 2. Diagrammatic schema of thyroid hormone formation and secretion. *1*, Thyroglobulin (Tg) and protein synthesis in the rough endoplasmic reticulum. *2*, Coupling of the Tg carbohydrate units in the smooth endoplasmic reticulum and Golgi apparatus. *3*, Formation of exocytotic vesicles. *4*, Transport of exocytotic vesicles with noniodinated Tg to the apical surface of the follicle cell and into the follicular lumen. *5*, Iodide transport at the basal cell membrane. *6*, Iodide oxidation, Tg iodination, and coupling of iodotyrosyl to iodothryronyl residues. *7*, Storage of iodinated Tg in the follicular lumen. *8*, Endocytosis by micropinocytosis. *9*, Endocytosis by macropinocytosis (pseudopods). *10*, Colloid droplets. *11*, Lysosomes migrating to the apical pole. *12*, Fusion of lysosomes with colloid droplets. *13*, Phagolysosomes with Tg hydrolysis. *14*, T_3 and T_4 secretion. *15*, MIT and DIT deiodination. (From Sabiston DC Jr [ed]: Textbook of Surgery: The Biological Basis of Modern Surgical Practice, ed 14. Philadelphia, WB Saunders Company, 1991, p 561, with permission.)

the thyroglobulin is hydrolyzed to iodothyronines and secreted. Although T_4 is the principal secretory product of the thyroid gland, T_3 is produced by peripheral conversion of T_4 in the liver, heart, and kidneys.

Hormone-binding proteins are the principal intravascular factors influencing total hormone concentration. The major serum thyroid hormone-binding proteins are *thyroxin-binding globulin* (TBG), thyroxin-binding prealbumin, and albumin. Because alterations in TBG may alter the total hormone concentration independently of the metabolic status of the body, free hormone, rather than the total hormone, is a more accurate indicator of the thyroid hormone-dependent metabolic state. The concentration of total thyroxin is

30 to 50 times the concentration of T_3. However, only 0.03 per cent of the total serum T_4 and 0.3 per cent of the total serum T_3 is present in the unbound or biologically active form, making T_3 the principal active hormone.

Thyroid hormones produce numerous metabolic effects. Enhancement of the basal metabolic rate as reflected by increased oxygen consumption is one of the classic actions of thyroid hormone. An optimal amount is also necessary for balanced growth and maturation. Many of the effects of thyroid hormones on carbohydrate metabolism appear permissive with respect to the effects of other hormones. They characteristically lower the level of serum cholesterol by enhancing excretion in the feces and conversion of cholesterol to bile acids. The generalized metabolic response increases the demand for vitamins and cofactors, and a magnified catecholamine effect is produced by excess thyroid hormone. The manifestations of acute hyperthyroidism or thyroid storm include hyperthermia, tachycardia, intense irritability, profuse sweating, hypertension, extreme anxiety, eventual prostration, hypotension, and death. Sympatholytic treatment has been the most effective, and reserpine and guanethidine have been used to dissipate the thyroid crisis gently and effectively. β-Adrenergic blockade is used to control the tachycardia, tremor, and anxiety. Oxygen is delivered, as well as liberal amounts of intravenous glucose. Large doses of adrenal steroids have been advised because cortisol breakdown is accentuated by excess thyroid hormone. Intravenous sodium or potassium iodide (1 to 2.5 gm) is also recommended to reduce thyroid iodide uptake. This effect of iodide on thyroid hormone regulation is discussed further.

REGULATION OF THYROID HORMONE

The principal regulatory mechanisms of the thyroid gland are the hypothalamic-pituitary-thyroid control system and the intrathyroidal autoregulatory system (Fig. 3). *Thyroid-stimulating hormone* is a glycoprotein hormone with α- and β-subunits. The β-subunit is responsible for its biologic and immunologic specificities. Thyroid-stimulating hormone is required for the normal production and secretion of thyroid hormone and has a major role in thyroid growth. Iodide deficiency and blockers of iodide binding to thyroglobulin cause increased TSH secretion and thyroid enlargement.

Thyrotropin-releasing hormone (TRH) is a tripeptide (pyroglutamyl-histidylprolineamide) produced by the supraoptic and paraventricular nuclei of the hypothalamus that courses down their axons to the

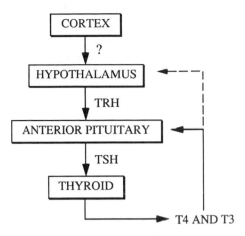

Figure 3. The normal hypothalamic pituitary thyroid axis. Both T₄ and T₃ feed back negatively on the pituitary and inhibit the secretion of thyroid-stimulating hormone (TSH). A similar process may regulate the hypothalamic secretion of thyrotropin-releasing hormone (TRH).

median eminence, where it is stored. Secretion into the pituicytes stimulates TSH secretion and synthesis, as well as prolactin release and synthesis. The primary role of TRH appears to be tonic stimulation of TSH-producing cells within the pituitary because the normal secretion of TSH and thyroid hormone is dependent on hypothalamic stimulation.

In addition to hypothalamic-pituitary control, the thyroid gland has the intrinsic ability to alter the production and release of thyroid hormone. As iodide levels in plasma increase, there is an increase in the amount absorbed and bound by the thyroid gland. After a critical amount of iodide accumulates, there is a progressive inhibition of iodide binding. The Wolff-Chaikoff block (acute block of iodide binding) is induced by an elevation of the plasma iodide concentration to approximately 25 mg/dl. Monovalent anions, including thiocyanate, perchlorate, and nitrate, inhibit iodide uptake. Thiocyanate and perchlorate both stimulate discharge of free iodide from the thyroid gland, and thiocyanate also inhibits iodide binding and iodotyrosine coupling.

Thyroid Function Tests

The fundamental issues in the evaluation of thyroid disease are the metabolic status of the patient, the etiology of the disease process responsible for the hormonal imbalance, and the etiology of the thyroid gland abnormality in the euthyroid patient. Tests of thyroid disease can be classified in the evaluation of thyroid function or anatomic abnormalities of the thyroid gland and are listed in Table 1.

HYPERTHYROIDISM

Hyperthyroidism is caused by increased levels of thyroid hormone and loss of the normal feedback mechanism controlling the secretion of thyroid hormone. Common types of hyperthyroidism include diffuse toxic goiter (Graves' disease), toxic adenoma, and toxic multinodular goiter. Graves' disease is a systemic autoimmune syndrome with variable expression that includes goiter with hyperthyroidism, exophthalmos, and pretibial myxedema. A thyroid adenoma is benign and is associated with excess secretion of thyroid hormone and is thus a localized disease. Uncommon causes of hyperthyroidism include thyrotoxicosis factitia, functioning metastatic thyroid carcinoma, trophoblastic tumors that secrete human chorionic gonadotropin that possess thyroid-stimulating properties, inappropriate secretion of thyrotropin by pituitary tumors, struma ovarii, iodide-induced hyperfunction, and thyroiditis.

Graves' Disease

The incidence of Graves' disease is 36 females and 8 males per 100,000 of the general population. The relative incidence of Graves' disease compared with adenomatous hyperthyroidism varies geographically, but Graves' disease is usually three to ten times more common. A hereditary component of Graves' disease has been suggested, and susceptibility to the development of thyrotoxicosis in response to an emotional problem has been reported. Consumption of excess iodide and use of thyroid hormone have also been implicated as activators of hyperthyroidism.

Although the origin of Graves' disease remains obscure, current evidence suggests that it is an autoimmune disorder caused by thyroid-stimulating immunoglobulins produced against an antigen in the thyroid. These polyclonal immunoglobulins appear to be directed to TSH receptors and can be detected by radioreceptor assays. Substantial levels of thyroid-stimulating immunoglobulins are present in over 90 per cent of patients with active Graves' disease, and the levels are sensitive and specific and correlate with the activity of hyperthyroidism. Thyroid-stimulating immunoglobulin levels have been reported to decrease to normal in approximately 50 per cent of patients treated with antithyroid medications or radioactive iodine and in 83 per cent after successful subtotal thyroidectomy.

Clinical Features

The symptoms and signs of hyperthyroidism are well known and include heat intolerance, increased

TABLE 1. THYROID FUNCTION TESTS

Test	Description
Thyroidal radioiodide uptake (RAIU)	After oral ingestion of ^{123}I (which has a short half-life and is associated with minimal radiation, compared with ^{131}I), the thyroid uptake as counted with a gamma counter is near its peak at 24 hours. Normal values for 24-hour RAIU in most parts of North America are approximately 15 to 30%.
Total thyroxin and total triiodothyronine (T_4 And T_3)	Measurement of T_4 and T_3 in serum and the estimation of their free concentration have become the most commonly used tests for the evaluation of thyroid hormone-dependent metabolic status. The usual concentration of T_4 in adults ranges from 5 to 11.5 μg/dl. Normal serum T_3 concentration in the adult is 80 to 190 μg/dl. Although total levels do not reflect the metabolic state of the patient, the free T_4 index remains a popular indirect measure of free T_4. Free T_3 and T_4 can be measured most specifically and easily by radioimmunoassay.
Resin triiodothyronine uptake (RT_3U)	RT_3U measures the unoccupied thyroid hormone binding sites on TBG by measuring the competitive binding for radioactive T_3 between TBG and a resin and provides an indirect measure of T_4. The radioactive T_3 added to the system is bound preferentially by the resin if the thyroid hormone binding sites on TBG are occupied by T_4. The resin uptake of T_3 is directly proportional to the fraction of free T_4 in the serum and inversely related to the TBG binding sites. RT_3U is high in thyrotoxicosis. Normal values of RT_3U are 25 to 35%. The test serves as an indirect measurement of the unbound fraction of T_4 and is valuable because it is simpler to perform than are other measurements of T_4. The free T_4 index is total T_4 multiplied by the ratio of the patient's RT_3U to the normal RT_3U: $$FT_4I = TT_4 \times \frac{RT_3U \text{ (Patient)}}{RT_3U \text{ (Normal)}}$$
Serum thyroglobulin	Elevated serum levels are present in patients with goiter, hyperthyroidism, thyroiditis, and thyroid tumors. Serum thyroglobulin is suppressed in factitious thyrotoxicosis, a feature that helps differentiate this condition from subacute thyroiditis. The major clinical application of serum thyroglobulin levels is in the management of thyroid carcinoma, in which elevation may suggest recurrent disease.
Serum calcitonin	Serum calcitonin is elevated in association with a number of conditions. Clinically, the most important is medullary thyroid carcinoma.
Thyrotropin (TSH)	Concentrations of TSH become elevated before there is any measurable reduction in serum T_4 and T_3, so the elevated TSH levels observed in primary hypothyroidism help confirm this diagnosis. Since reliable detection of low levels of TSH is difficult, a true absence of the hormone is difficult to distinguish from a nondetectable level that may be observed in some normal individuals. However, a low or undetected TSH level in association with a low thyroxin concentration is indicative of pituitary or hypothalamic disease.
Thyrotropin stimulation test	This test is employed to differentiate primary thyroid failure from thyroid hypofunction caused by inadequate TSH stimulation. If an increase in radioactive iodine uptake of 10% or more or a rise in T_4 of at least 2 μg/dl can be demonstrated, it is likely that the thyroid can respond to exogenous TSH stimulation.
Thyroid-releasing hormone (TRH) stimulation test	The TRH stimulation test measures the increase of pituitary TSH in serum in response to the administration of synthetic TRH. The magnitude of the TSH response to TRH is modulated by the thyrotrope response to active thyroid hormone and is thus inversely proportional to the concentration of free thyroid hormone in serum. The test provides a unique method of distinguishing between secondary and tertiary hypothyroidism. A TSH response is indicative of a hypothalamic disorder, and a failure to respond is compatible with intrinsic pituitary dysfunction.
Thyroid suppression test	This test is based on the principle that the administration of thyroid hormone suppresses the patient's thyroid function unless normal homeostatic mechanisms are disrupted. RAIU is performed after administration of thyroid hormone. Autonomously functioning thyroid tissue will continue to take up ^{123}I.

sweating, weight loss, hyperkinetic movements, insomnia, proximal muscle weakness, tremor, scant menses, tachycardia, and atrial fibrillation. The optic effects of Graves' disease include a continuum from mere stare and lid lag to complete visual loss from corneal or optic nerve involvement. The pathogenesis of the eye changes is not well understood, and the possibilities include pituitary exophthalmos–producing substances, circulating antibodies that bind specifically to eye muscle antigens, circulating lymphocytes sensitized to an antigen in the extraocular tissue, and a complex of thyroglobulin and antithyroglobulin antibody formed in the blood that is bound by the external orbital muscles.

Hyperthyroidism is usually confirmed by measuring circulating T_4, but other tests may be useful. Elevated radioactive iodine uptake is also diagnostic of hyperthyroidism. Thyroid suppression tests can confirm the diagnosis of hyperthyroidism because autonomously functioning thyroid should not be suppressible. Patients with Graves' disease also have a flat response to the TRH stimulation test.

Treatment

Thyroid hypersecretion, or thyrotoxicosis, can be controlled by reducing the functional mass of thyroid tissue with operative removal of a large part of the gland or by destruction of most of the gland with radioiodine. It can also be controlled with antithyroid drugs for reduction of the secretion of thyroid hormone and by drugs that block β-adrenergic receptors.

Antithyroid Drugs

Thionamides such as methimazole and propylthiouracil are commonly used and impair the covalent binding of iodine to thyroglobulin and iodide peroxidase. Unfortunately, these agents may succeed in inducing a permanent remission in only a minority of adults and in approximately 20 per cent of children. Prolonged use is limited because of toxic side effects such as rash, liver dysfunction, neuritis, arthralgia, myalgia, lymphadenopathy, psychosis, and the occasional development of irreversible agranulocytosis. β-receptor blockade effectively controls some of the major effects of thyrotoxicosis, but has not been effective as monotherapy.

Radioiodine

Radioiodine therapy is useful for many patients with thyrotoxicosis except in newborns, in pregnant females, or when precluded by a low iodine uptake. This treatment is highly effective, although progressive hypothyroidism requiring thyroid replacement is common. Radioactive iodine is absolutely contraindicated in pregnant women because destruction of the fetal thyroid follows. Antithyroid drugs in conventional doses may lead to the development of fetal goiter that may obstruct the fetal airway at birth. Minimal-dose antithyroid drug therapy reduces this risk. In the middle trimester of pregnancy, subtotal thyroidectomy after a short course of antithyroid drugs and propranolol has been an effective treatment.

Subtotal Thyroidectomy

Indications for subtotal thyroidectomy for Graves' disease include (1) intolerance or noncompliance with antithyroid drug therapy, and (2) contraindications to radioiodine therapy. Subtotal thyroidectomy is indicated for Graves' disease in children and adolescents, for women who are potential mothers, for patients under the age of 20 years who are unlikely to undergo remission because of a large goiter, and in those who do not experience a remission as indicated by persistent thyromegaly or the need to continue antithyroid medication beyond 1 or 2 years. Surgical management of hyperthyroidism is directed toward removal of sufficient thyroid tissue to render the patient euthyroid. Surgical risks are minimal but include recurrent laryngeal nerve injury, hypoparathyroidism, and permanent hypothyroidism. Patients with Graves' disease with antithyroid antibodies are particularly susceptible to hypothyroidism after subtotal thyroidectomy. Subtotal thyroidectomy should be performed after thyrotoxicosis is controlled medically, accomplished by the use of propylthiouracil to inhibit thyroid hormone synthesis and limit peripheral conversion of T_4 to T_3. Thyroidectomy performed immediately after control of thyrotoxicosis is associated with a risk of thyroid crisis; thus, it is preferable to wait approximately 2 months after a patient is euthyroid.

Thyrotoxic patients are usually treated with iodide and iodine (Lugol's solution) 10 days before operation to decrease the vascularity of the gland. Thyroid hormone, rather than iodine, can also be used to reduce the vascularity of the gland treated with propylthiouracil, because adequate doses of thyroid hormone suppress the TSH increase associated with propylthiouracil and decrease the thyroid vascularity stimulated by that mechanism. β-Adrenergic blockade alone has been prescribed for preoperative preparation but is more commonly used as an adjunct to thionamides. Propranolol may be used alone or in conjunction with Lugol's solution in the preparation of the patient intolerant of antithyroid drugs or who is noncompliant. Subtotal thyroidectomy effectively and immediately controls thyrotoxicosis. The incidence of recurrent disease is 1 to 5 per cent and is inversely related to the incidence of hypothyroidism. Within 1 to 2 years, hypothyroidism may develop in 5 to 50 per cent of patients, with a slight additional increase in subsequent years. The associated morbidity, related primarily to damage to the recurrent laryngeal nerves and parathyroid glands, is estimated to be 0.5 to 3 per cent. Although exophthalmos frequently occurs in hyperthyroidism, most patients require specific measures for a condition that is self-limiting and that to a variable degree regresses. Treatment is directed toward reducing periorbital swelling and safeguarding against infection.

TOXIC ADENOMA

Hyperfunctioning adenomas are often first recognized on a thyroid scan, on which they appear as hot nodules. Often the patient is euthyroid because, even though the adenoma is hypersecreting independently of the pituitary feedback system, suppression of thyroid secretion from the normal gland maintains a physiologic net secretion rate of thyroid hormone. Only when the normal gland can no longer be suppressed does hyperthyroidism ensue.

In adenomatous disease, the recognition of symptoms is delayed because an older age group is involved, especially in multinodular disease, and there is more commonly a predominance of cardiac symptoms. However, the presence of ophthalmopathy and pretibial myxedema differentiates patients with Graves' disease. The diagnosis of toxic adenoma may rest with the character of the goiter, since paranodular tissue and the contralateral lobe are functionally suppressed and are usually minimally palpable. The diagnosis is suggested by thyroid scanning after administration of radioiodine. When the diagnosis is in doubt, a suppression test can be useful. The autonomous nodule has persistently elevated radioactive iodine uptake, whereas normal thyroid tissue is suppressed. For purposes of control of hyperthyroidism, surgical excision of the thyroid lobe containing the hyperfunctioning adenoma is simple, safe, and effective. Radioactive iodine therapy for a hyperfunctioning nodule is also effective, although there is a high risk of permanent hypothyroidism.

THYROIDITIS

Thyroiditis is the infiltration of the thyroid gland by inflammatory cells caused by a diverse group of infectious and inflammatory disorders. Inflammation of the thyroid may be organ specific or part of a multisystem process that may be acute and self-limiting or chronic and progressive. *Autoimmune thyroid disease* encompasses a group of conditions characterized by the presence of circulating thyroid antibodies and immunologically competent cells capable of reacting with certain thyroid constituents. These autoimmune thyroid diseases include Hashimoto's disease (lymphocytic thyroiditis); primary myxedema; and juvenile, fibrous, focal, and painless varieties of thyroiditis.

Hashimoto's Disease (Lymphocytic Thyroiditis)

Hashimoto's disease is the most common cause of goitrous *hypothyroidism* in adults and sporadic goiter in children. The incidence is 0.3 to 1.5/1000/year and is 10 to 15 times more common in women than in men, with the highest incidence in the age group of 30 to 50 years. In Hashimoto's disease thyroid tissue is damaged by immunologic factors and is replaced by lymphocytes, plasma cells, and fibrosis. Antithyroid antibodies in the serum of patients with Hashimoto's disease have been demonstrated to be directed against elements in the thyroid cell or colloid and are usually detectable at some time in the course of the disease. In contradistinction to Graves' disease, no antibodies to the TSH receptor of the cell surface have been associated with Hashimoto's disease. The enlarged thyroid is pale and firm, with a finely nodular surface and a pale yellow color. On histologic examination, there is diffuse infiltration of the gland by lymphocytes and plasma cells, with formation of lymphoid follicles and germinal centers.

Symptoms of hypothyroidism in association with a painless, firm goiter are frequent presenting complaints, but patients may be euthyroid. The diagnosis of Hashimoto's disease begins by documenting hypothyroidism with thyroid function tests. Transient (2 to 8 weeks) hyperthyroidism may be present when inflammatory changes cause disruption of follicles with leakage of thyroid hormone into the circulation. Tests for thyroglobulin and microsomal antibodies should be performed because the presence and the titer of these antibodies correlate with the severity and extent of the autoimmune process. Hypothyroidism associated with a goiter but negative thyroid antibodies suggests use of goitrogen, a dyshormonogenetic goiter, or an endemic goiter. If thyroid neoplasia is suspected, due to asymmetry of the goiter, cervical lymphadenopathy, pressure symptoms, hoarseness, or enlargement of the goiter despite adequate thyroid replacement, fine-needle aspiration or open biopsy of the suspicious area should be performed. There is a strong relationship between thyroiditis and malignant thyroid lymphoma. These patients are usually followed medically, and replacement therapy with T_4 is begun in patients with hypothyroidism that is symptomatic or associated with a goiter that is causing pressure symptoms. Surgical resection of goiter should be performed if severe pressure symptoms are present that have not responded to corticosteroid therapy, and usually consists of subtotal thyroidectomy. Biopsy is performed for exclusion of malignancy in nodules suspicious for thyroid carcinoma (usually papillary) or lymphoma as indicated.

De Quervain's (Subacute or Giant Cell) Thyroiditis

Subacute thyroiditis represents approximately 1 per cent of all thyroid disease and is much less common than Hashimoto's thyroiditis, with only an eighth the incidence of Graves' disease. It often follows upper respiratory tract infections, which suggests that it is due to a viral infection. There is generally moderate thyroid enlargement, which may be asymmetric. The inflammatory reaction involving the thyroid may cause adherence of the gland to the capsule and immediate extrathyroid tissues. Histologic features include desquamation of the follicular cells and disturbance and loss of colloid material.

Pain in the thyroid gland often develops relatively suddenly, often following radiation to the jaw and ears, and may be associated with marked tenderness and dysphagia. The gland is generally moderately enlarged. Laboratory findings include an increased erythrocyte sedimentation rate, a generalized increase in immunoglobulins, and a neutrophil leukocytosis or lymphocytosis in some patients. The changes in thyroid function are quite characteristic, with an early thyrotoxic stage followed by hypothyroidism and usually euthyroidism. This condition remits spontaneously after a variable period from a few days to a few months and relapses occasionally before the disease remits permanently. The treatment consists of analgesics such as aspirin or ibuprofen in mild cases. Steroids are effective in controlling symptoms in the more severe cases. However, spontaneous recovery occurs in over 90 per cent of patients, and therefore subtotal thyroidectomy is not indicated.

Acute Suppurative Thyroiditis

This is a rare condition of the thyroid gland that is usually due to bacterial infection from *Streptococcus*, *Staphylococcus*, *Pneumococcus*, and rarely *Salmonella* or *Bacteroides* species. Histologic examination of the gland reveals a marked polymorphonuclear leukocytic and lymphocytic infiltrate in the acute phase, which may be associated with frank thyroid necrosis and abscess formation followed by fibrosis. Symptoms occur acutely and include tenderness, enlargement, warmth, erythema, and neck pain exacerbated by neck extension and swallowing. Septicemia or direct extension to the neck or chest may occur. Although the clinical characteristics of acute suppurative thyroiditis are usually straightforward, differentiation from de Quervain's thyroiditis is important. Primary treatment of suppurative thyroiditis consists of appropriate antibiotics against the causative organism. Thyroid abscesses should be drained, and cysts communicating with the pyriform sinus or trachea require exclusion.

Riedel's Thyroiditis

Riedel's thyroiditis is a rare inflammatory condition of unknown etiology. It appears likely that the invasive fibrous thyroiditis represents one aspect of a generalized process that is not specifically related to the thyroid gland. The gland is involved wholly or in part by dense, invasive fibrosis that extends to include the surrounding tissues so that the capsule and anatomic margins of the gland cannot be precisely defined. There is no lymphocytic infiltrate in the tissue, but a lymphocytic perivasculitis is observed in most patients. Patients generally present with a history of rapid increase in thyroid size, which is frequently associated with symptoms of tracheal or esophageal compression. The gland is often described as "woody" in texture; is generally uniformly enlarged, nontender, and strikingly hard on palpation; and is often mistaken for thyroid carcinoma. There are no characteristic laboratory findings except absent to low titers of antithyroid antibodies. In late stages of disease, hypothyroidism may be present, but the diagnosis can be confirmed only by biopsy. Medical therapy includes thyroid replacement if hypothyroidism is present. Surgical treatment is indicated if pressure symptoms in the neck require relief, and partial thyroidectomy is required in most patients. The operation requires meticulous dissection because fibrosis may involve surrounding structures, including the trachea, the carotid sheath, and the recurrent laryngeal nerve.

Multinodular Goiter

Goiter may be caused by a deficiency of dietary iodine, dietary substances or medications that impair hormone synthesis, absence of an enzyme essential for hormone synthesis, or thyroiditis, which damages follicular cells and impairs hormone production. It reflects the compensatory effects of TSH and its ability to promote thyroid growth for inadequate thyroid hormone production. Multinodular goiters rarely cause symptoms; however, an enlarging goiter can compress neck structures, causing dysphagia, cough, or a feeling of fullness in the neck. Although airway obstruction is unusual, it should be viewed with concern. Plain radiographs may show deviation or compression of the trachea. Further airway compromise due to a foreign body or tracheitis with edema may eliminate an adequate airway, causing respiratory insufficiency.

The treatment of goiter is based on suppression of TSH by administration of exogenous thyroid hormone. Although most multinodular goiters regress very little, patients may be comfortable for many years on thyroid hormone replacement if the goiter remains stable. Indications for surgical therapy include the presence of obstructive symptoms or cosmetic problems related to the size of the goiter. Once obstructive symptoms occur, replacement of thyroid hormone is unlikely to produce improvement. The goal of surgical therapy is removal of all abnormal, nodular thyroid tissue, correction of the current problem, and prevention of recurrence of the goiter.

Thyroid tissue may be present in the anterior mediastinum, and substernal goiter may develop in this location in continuity with the thyroid in the neck. The thyroid remains within its capsule, and the arterial supply and venous drainage of such a gland are by the normal routes. Rarely, posterior mediastinal thyroid tissue is found, and from it may arise large goiters that may or may not be continuous with the cervical thyroid gland. Because the goiter is growing in a confined space with many critical structures, the potential for complications is significant. Substernal goiter rarely regresses with suppression of thyroid hormone and is usually managed by surgical removal. Most substernal goiters can be removed through a standard cervical incision.

MANAGEMENT OF THYROID NODULES

Thyroid nodules are common in adults but must be evaluated to determine if benign or malignant. Because most thyroid nodules are benign, the management strategies must incorporate noninvasive diagnostic tests to identify patients who require surgical intervention (Table 2). Findings on the physical examination that suggest malignancy include firm texture, irregularity, fixation to surrounding structures, and enlarged ipsilateral cervical lymph nodes. Thyroid function tests are of little value in establishing the benign or malignant nature of a thyroid nodule.

Ultrasound Scanning

Although there are no specific ultrasonographic criteria for malignancy, ultrasonography is a noninvasive test that can be used to distinguish between solid and cystic lesions.

Radioactive Scanning

Radioactive scanning using radioiodine or technetium is very useful in distinguishing a solitary nodule from a multinodular goiter. Malignant thyroid nodules usually do not concentrate iodine; thus hypofunctional nodules are more likely to be malignant than are functioning nodules. Those that are hypofunctioning by scan usually require surgical resection, because approximately 20 per cent are thyroid carcinomas. Hyperfunctioning nodules are rarely malignant; however, radionuclide scanning does not clearly differentiate benign from malignant lesions. Radionuclide scanning is also helpful in localizing aberrant thyroid tissue in the tongue and in the line of the thyroid's descent down the midline of the neck.

Fine-Needle Aspiration

Fine-needle aspiration (FNA) is often used as the initial diagnostic technique in management of thyroid nodules because it is the most precise screening method for differentiating benign from malignant thyroid nodules. A satisfactory FNA requires a representative specimen from the nodule and examination by an experienced cytologist. While sampling errors may occur with lesions larger than 4 cm, and while lesions smaller than 1 cm may be difficult to aspirate, a correct diagnosis is nonetheless achieved in over 90 per cent of papillary, medullary, and undifferentiated carcinomas. Follicular carcinoma is difficult to diagnose accurately by FNA because malignancy is often determined by the histologic presence of invasion. Therefore, when a hypercellular aspirate is obtained, these lesions are classified as follicular tumors or suspicious for malignancy and should be excised unless they are hyperfunctioning on radionuclide scanning. Nodules that are benign by needle-aspiration biopsy must be followed with repeat aspirations periodically, as there is a 10 per cent false-negative diagnosis rate. Despite these limitations, needle biopsy has reduced the number of patients requiring operation, while increasing the relative incidence of malignancy in resected nodules.

Thyroid Carcinoma

Thyroid carcinoma is relatively uncommon in the United States, occurring at a rate of 36 to $60/10^6$/year, with an annual mortality rate of only $6/10^6$. Although the cause of thyroid carcinoma is unknown, exposure of the gland to external radiation is directly related to the subsequent development of benign and malignant thyroid nodules. Postirradiation thyroid malignancies usually develop within 3 to 5 years, with a peak incidence at 15 to 25 years following exposure. Although the types of thyroid cancer seen following irradiation are similar to those that develop in nonirradiated individuals of comparable age, multi-

TABLE 2. ETIOLOGY OF THYROID NODULES

Lesions	Prevalence
Benign thyroid nodule	40%
Multinodular goiter	20%
Cyst	12%
Thyroiditis	10%
Follicular adenoma	12%
Carcinoma	6%

centric tumors are found in up to 55 per cent of the irradiated patients. Nonetheless, the prognosis of patients with radiation-associated thyroid carcinoma is identical to nonirradiated patients in the same age group. Other significant prognostic variables include age at the time of diagnosis. Although a high percentage of children and young adults have nodal metastases at the time of diagnosis, patients under 40 years of age have a better prognosis than those older. The influence of nodal metastases on prognosis is controversial but generally represents a more extensive thyroid tumor and is associated with an increased recurrence rate and a poorer prognosis. Patients whose cancers have invaded into the adjacent structures of the neck have a poorer prognosis, and the presence of distant metastases is associated with the poorest prognosis.

Most experienced surgeons agree that thyroid lobectomy and isthmusectomy is the appropriate initial procedure for a thyroid nodule suspected of being cancer. Small anterior nodules or nodules at the isthmus may be locally resected with the anterior third of each lobe. The histologic subtype of thyroid cancer has a significant influence on the prognosis. Follicular carcinoma is slightly less favorable than papillary carcinoma, and the prognosis is generally poorer in patients with medullary carcinoma and is least favorable in those with undifferentiated cancer.

Papillary Carcinoma

The surgical management of papillary carcinoma is determined by the extent of tumor and may consist of lobectomy, near-total thyroidectomy, or total thyroidectomy. In a number of patients, papillary carcinoma is bilateral. Because the risk of complications (such as injury to the recurrent nerve and hypoparathyroidism) increases with the extent of the thyroidectomy, total thyroidectomy is appropriate in patients with gross evidence of bilateral carcinoma and is thought by many surgeons to be appropriate in all patients with tumors larger than 1.5 cm. Others recommend that thyroid lobectomy or near-total thyroidectomy for papillary carcinoma confined to one lobe is more appropriate, because more extensive total thyroidectomy does not improve survival but substantially increases the complication rate. Because papillary carcinoma has an excellent prognosis, the more extensive operations should be performed only if they can be done with very low morbidity. Routine prophylactic neck dissection is not indicated, although there is frequently metastatic involvement of regional lymph nodes. However, when total thyroidectomy is performed for papillary carcinoma, the central neck nodes, including nodes in the ipsilateral tracheoesophageal groove, in the pretracheal area, along the recurrent laryngeal nerve and inferior thyroid veins, and in the anterior mediastinum, are removed with the operative specimen. In addition, in patients with clinically enlarged lateral cervical nodes, a modified neck dissection is indicated.

Follicular Carcinoma

Follicular carcinomas typically occur in older patients, with a peak incidence in the fifth decade of life and constitute 15 to 20 per cent of thyroid cancers. Lymph node metastases are much less common than in papillary carcinoma, as follicular carcinoma does not invade lymphatic channels but frequently disseminates hematogenously to bone, lung, brain, and liver. The minimally invasive follicular carcinoma can be managed by total lobectomy when it is confined to one lobe, as it is well differentiated, rarely multicentric, rarely metastasizes, and is generally associated with an excellent prognosis. In contrast, widely invasive follicular carcinoma usually presents with locally aggressive tumors, frequently showing extension through the thyroid capsule into surrounding structures, or proven metastatic disease. This is best treated with near-total or total thyroidectomy, which optimizes the effectiveness of ^{131}I treatment for residual or distant disease.

Undifferentiated Carcinoma

Undifferentiated or anaplastic carcinoma, which constitutes 5 to 10 per cent of thyroid cancers, is the most aggressive, predominantly seen in patients over age 50 years, with a peak incidence at approximately 65 years of age. Most undifferentiated carcinomas present after invasion to vital structures in the neck, precluding surgical resection. Therapy with external radiotherapy and chemotherapy may provide limited palliation.

Medullary Carcinoma

Medullary carcinoma arises in the parafollicular C cells and is a distinct and separate carcinoma with a high propensity for lymph node metastasis. Approximately 20 per cent of these tumors occur in genetically predisposed families, either with other endocrine abnormalities or with medullary carcinoma alone. Standard operative therapy includes total thyroidectomy with consideration of ipsilateral lymph node dissection.

Lymphoma

Rarely, primary lymphoma of the thyroid may present as a rapidly enlarging, firm, painless mass in older females. The diagnosis may require surgical exploration and should be followed by staging. Survival is not affected if only a biopsy is performed at the time of exploration, as patients with disease confined to the neck are treated with radiation therapy. Patients with more extensive disease or those who relapse are treated with chemotherapy.

ADJUVANT THERAPY

The role of radioiodine in the postoperative management of patients with well-differentiated thyroid carcinoma remains controversial. However, convincing studies have demonstrated that the lowest recurrence and death rates are found in patients who have received both radioiodine and thyroid hormone suppression. This survival advantage is seen primarily in patients with follicular and mixed papillary/follicular tumors. For the radioiodine to be most effective, the normal thyroid tissue must first be removed, as it accumulates the isotope more avidly than does thyroid cancer. Postoperative ^{131}I scans are usually performed 2 to 3 months following operation for well-differentiated thyroid carcinoma. Patients with significant residual functioning tissue and evidence of metastatic disease are candidates for radioiodine ablation. Ablation of residual thyroid tissue can usually be accomplished with one dose of 30 μCi of ^{131}I. Patients with metastatic deposits in the neck are given 75 to 100 μCi, and those with distant metastases are given 150 to 200 μCi. Radioiodine scan and treatment are then repeated at 6- to 9-month intervals until tumor uptake of the isotope is abolished or adverse effects of radioiodine are encountered.

Nearly all patients who undergo operation for well-differentiated thyroid carcinoma should receive exogenous thyroid hormone to prevent hypothyroidism but also to inhibit TSH-stimulated growth of differentiated thyroid carcinoma. Serum thyroglobulin measurements are helpful in determining the presence of recurrent disease in patients who have undergone ablative therapy of all thyroid tissue, as increasing levels of thyroglobulin are suggestive of disease recurrence.

REFERENCES

Cady B, Rossi RL: Surgery of the Thyroid and Parathyroid Glands, ed 3. Philadelphia, WB Saunders Company, 1991.

Foster RS Jr: Morbidity and mortality after thryoidectomy. Surg Gynecol Obstet 146:423–430, 1978.

Goldstein R, Hart IR: Follow-up of solitary, autonomous thyroid nodules treated with ^{131}I. N Engl J Med 309:1473–1475, 1983.

Rosen I, Provias J, Walfish P: The pathological nature of cystic thyroid nodules selected for surgery by needle-aspiration biopsy. Surgery 100:606–612, 1986.

Sridama V, McCormick M, Kaplan EL, et al: Long-term follow-up of compensated low-dose ^{131}I therapy for Graves' disease. N Engl J Med 311:426–431, 1984.

22

THE MULTIPLE ENDOCRINE NEOPLASIAS

JEFFREY A. NORTON, M.D.   SAMUEL A. WELLS, Jr., M.D.

Tumors of the endocrine system most often develop within a single gland. Some genetic disorders, however, are characterized by a predisposition to the development of neoplasms in multiple endocrine glands. In these diseases, which are usually familial, the endocrine tumors may be benign or malignant and develop either synchronously or metachronously. The pathologic change in affected glands is characteristically multicentric and may be expressed as hyperplasia, adenoma, or carcinoma. The multiple endocrine neoplasia (MEN) syndromes are classified according to the pattern of involvement. In its full expression, MEN-I is characterized by the concurrence of parathyroid hyperplasia, pancreatic islet cell neoplasms, and adenomas of the anterior pituitary gland. It is also associated with thyroid adenoma, adrenal adenoma, lipomas, and carcinoid tumors. MEN-IIa is characterized by the concurrence of medullary thyroid carcinoma (MTC), adrenal pheochromocytoma, and parathyroid hyperplasia; whereas MEN-IIb consists of MTC, pheochromocytoma, mucosal neuromas, a distinctive "marfanoid" habitus, but not parathyroid disease. All of these syndromes are transmitted as mendelian autosomal dominant traits (Table 1).

MULTIPLE ENDOCRINE NEOPLASIA TYPE I

Historical Background

In 1954, Wermer described the familial occurrence of tumors involving the pituitary gland, parathyroids, and pancreatic islets. The disease was subsequently termed multiple endocrine adenomatosis and more recently has been designated multiple endocrine neoplasia type I. In the family studied by Wermer, the father and four of nine children were affected. Four of the five had pituitary tumors and peptic ulcer disease, while three had hypercalcemia and pancreatic adenomas. Wermer proposed that the syndrome in this family was caused by an autosomal dominant gene with a high degree of penetrance.

Genetic Studies and Pathogenesis

The mendelian autosomal dominant inheritance pattern of the trait for MEN-I has been clearly established. Recent studies using DNA probes to detect linkage between restriction fragment length polymorphisms (RFLPs) and the disease locus have mapped the MEN-I gene to the long arm of chromosome 11. It appears likely that the parathyroid, pancreatic islet, and pituitary derangements all result from a single mutated locus. Oncogenesis in the MEN syndromes may require two separate mutational events. According to this model, the first mutation is inherited in the germ line and confers susceptibility to neoplastic change in the involved endocrine tissues. Elimination of the remaining normal allele through a second somatic mutational event, or "second hit" (such as a gene deletion), unmasks the inherited recessive mutation, and results in the development of adenoma or carcinoma. The occurrence of multiple second hits would then result in multiple clones of neoplastic cells and the multicentric involvement characteristically seen in affected endocrine tissues. In fact, the use of DNA probes that detect RFLPs to compare constitutional and tumor tis-

TABLE 1. MULTIPLE ENDOCRINE NEOPLASIA (MEN)
SYNDROMES

	MEN-I	MEN-IIa	MEN-IIb
Chromosome with genetic defect	11	10	10
MTC	No	Bilateral	Bilateral
Pheochromocytoma	No	70% Bilateral	70% Bilateral
Parathyroid disease	Hyperplasia	Hyperplasia	No
Specific phenotype	No	No	Yes
Familial, autosomal dominant trait	Yes	Yes	Yes
Course of MTC	None	Variable, frequently indolent	Generally more virulent
Pancreatic endocrine tumors	Yes	No	No
Duodenal endocrine tumors	Yes	No	No

Abbreviation: MTC = medullary thyroid carcinoma.

sue genotypes from patients with MEN-I has demonstrated allelic deletions on chromosome 11 (11q 12-13) (Table 1).

Clinical Features and Management

The clinical expression of MEN-I most often develops in the third or fourth decade, and the onset of symptoms is rare before age 10. Males and females are affected equally, as predicted by the autosomal dominant inheritance pattern. The gene for MEN-I is transmitted with nearly 100 per cent penetrance, but with variable expressivity, such that each affected individual exhibits some but not necessarily all of the components of the syndrome. The distribution of endocrine involvement varies according to the method of study and the patient population. However, approximately 90 to 97 per cent of patients have biochemical evidence of hyperparathyroidism, while pancreatic islet cell neoplasms are manifested in 30 to 80 per cent, and pituitary tumors occur in 15 to 50 per cent. If followed long enough, most affected individuals eventually develop pathologic involvement in all three endocrine tissues. The clinical manifestations of patients with MEN-I depend on the endocrine tissue involved and the overproduction of a specific hormone. Symptoms may also arise as a result of the tumor mass itself. In a classic review of 85 patients by Ballard and associates in 1964, the most frequent mode of clinical presentation was peptic ulcer disease or its complications. Manifestations of hypoglycemia represented the second most common presenting feature, while symptoms of primary hyperparathyroidism (kidney stones) or complaints referable to pituitary dysfunction (headaches, visual field defects, and secondary amenorrhea) least often led to the diagnosis.

Parathyroids

The most common endocrine abnormality in patients with MEN-I is primary hyperparathyroidism (HPT), occurring in greater than 90 per cent of patients. Most affected individuals exhibit generalized parathyroid hyperplasia with involvement of all four glands. Although there has been some debate among pathologists with respect to the occurrence of multiple adenoma versus asymmetric or nodular hyperplasia in MEN-I, most agree that generalized chief cell hyperplasia is the characteristic pathologic lesion. The symptoms of primary hyperparathyroidism in the setting of MEN-I are similar to those of patients with sporadic disease. Asymptomatic hypercalcemia may be present in many patients over a long period of observation. Symptomatic patients usually develop renal or ureteral lithiasis and/or nephrocalcinosis, as urinary levels of calcium are more elevated than serum levels. Skeletal manifestations of hyperparathyroidism occur but are uncommon. The diagnosis is made by measurement of serum levels of calcium and parathormone.

Patients with MEN-I and parathyroid hyperplasia have most often been managed by subtotal (3.5-gland) parathyroidectomy. Unfortunately, the incidence of recurrent hyperparathyroidism postoperatively has been as high as 40 per cent, while the incidence of permanent hypoparathyroidism has been in the range of 25 per cent. For these reasons, in patients with multiglandular hyperplasia, total parathyroidectomy with autotransplantation of parathyroid tissue into an ectopic site such as the nondominant forearm muscle has been advocated. The potential advantages of this technique include a lower incidence of hypocalcemia and the feasibility of managing recurrent hyperparathyroidism, should it develop, by excision of a portion of the grafted parathyroid tissue under local anesthesia (obviating the morbidity of repeat neck exploration).

Pancreas

The second most frequent expression of MEN-I is neoplasia of the pancreatic islet cells. The pathologic change is typically multicentric, and diffuse hyperplasia and microadenoma formation may be present in areas of the gland distant from grossly evident tumor. Either single or multiple islet cell tumors may be within the wall of the duodenum. The most common clinical pancreatic islet cell lesion in patients with MEN-I is gastrinoma. Clinically, patients present with a severe peptic ulcer disease. Gastrinomas associated with MEN-I account for 20 per cent of all cases of Zollinger-Ellison syndrome (ZES). The diagnosis of gastrinoma is made by the documentation of hyperacidity (gastric acid hypersecretion) and elevated fasting serum levels of gastrin (>100 pg/ml). The diagnosis can be confirmed by an abnormal secretin test. Secretin, 2 U/kg, administered intravenously causes an increment of serum levels of gastrin greater than 200 pg/ml.

Islet cell tumors that develop in patients with MEN-I are usually multicentric and may be malignant as indicated by the presence of regional or distant metastases. Because of the multicentricity, the true gastrinoma may not be localized by computed tomographic (CT) scanning, angiography, or portal venous sampling and measurement of plasma gastrin levels. Previously, the accepted surgical therapy for this disease was total gastrectomy. However, H_2-receptor antagonists and proton pump inhibitors like omeprazole are effective in controlling acid hypersecretion and its attendant complications. In MEN-I patients with ZES and HPT, surgical correction of HPT greatly facilitates medical control of gastric acid hypersecretion. Resection of the islet cell tumors may be attempted if the tumor is identifiable on CT or angiogram and measures 2 to 3 cm in size. Operation is recommended to control the tumoral process, as 50 per cent of tumors this size are malignant with lymph node or liver metastases. Although the gastrinomas in patients with the MEN-I syndrome can be malignant, the disease progression is indolent in many patients. With aggressive medical management and surgery to limit tumor progression, affected individuals may tolerate the malignancy well and enjoy long survival.

The second most common pancreatic islet cell neoplasm in patients with MEN-I is insulinoma. The insulinomas are usually distinct (>2 cm), but may be multiple in contrast to those that occur sporadically where nearly all are solitary. Patients commonly present with recurrent symptoms of neuroglycopenia: sweating, dizziness, confusion, or syncope. The diagnosis of insulinoma is made by documenting symptomatic hypoglycemia concomitant with inappropriately elevated plasma levels of insulin and C peptide. There is no ideal medical therapy for insulinoma; therefore, these lesions are most often treated by surgical resection (subtotal pancreatectomy). Often, surgically treated patients become asymptomatic with normoglycemia. Approximately 10 per cent of insulinomas occurring in patients with MEN-I are malignant. Patients with disseminated or diffuse carcinomas may respond to treatment with streptozotocin, and some control of hypoglycemia may be achieved by the administration of either diazoxide or octreotide. Other pancreatic islet cell neoplasms, such as glucagonoma, somatostatinoma, and tumors secreting vasoactive intestinal peptide or pancreatic polypeptide, occur rarely in association with MEN-I.

Pituitary

Pituitary neoplasms occur in 15 to 50 per cent of patients. The majority of these tumors are prolactin-secreting adenomas. Pituitary tumors cause symptoms either by hypersecretion of hormones or compression of adjacent structures. Large adenomas may cause visual field defects by pressure on the optic chiasm or manifestations of hypopituitarism through compression of the adjacent normal gland. Prolactin-secreting tumors result in amenorrhea/galactorrhea in females or hypogonadism in males. Approximately 30 per cent of patients exhibit acromegaly resulting from growth hormone overproduction. Much less commonly, patients present with Cushing's disease. Pituitary tumors, either functioning or nonfunctioning, may require ablation by surgery or irradiation. Bromocriptine, a dopamine agonist and an inhibitor of prolactin secretion, has been used to treat prolactinomas medically.

Other Tumors

Forty per cent of patients with MEN-I develop adrenocortical lesions including adenomas, but adrenocortical hyperfunction is rare. Thyroid carcinomas or adenomas can occur in up to 15 per cent of patients. Rarely, multiple lipomas and carcinoid tumors may also occur.

MULTIPLE ENDOCRINE NEOPLASIA TYPES IIa AND IIb

Historical Background

Medullary thyroid carcinoma (MTC), first described in 1959 by Hazard and associates, was distinguished by material in the stroma with the staining properties of amyloid. Sipple noted an association of thyroid carcinoma with pheochromocytoma, and Williams later observed that this thyroid neoplasm was MTC and was derived from the parafollicular calcitonin-secreting "C" cells. The term MEN-II was originally introduced by Steiner and associates in 1968 to describe the familial occurrence of MTC, pheochromocytoma, and parathyroid hyperplasia. This is now known as MEN-IIa. Williams and Pollack described patients with MTC, pheochromocytoma, and multiple mucosal neuromas. Chong and associates suggested that this syndrome be termed MEN-IIb to distinguish it from MEN-IIa. It has also been called MEN-III.

Genetic Studies and Pathogenesis

Both MEN-IIa and MEN-IIb are inherited in an autosomal-dominant pattern. Recent genetic linkage studies have mapped the locus for MEN-IIa to the pericentromeric region of chromosome 10 (Table 1). Linkage for MEN-IIb has also been to the same region (Table 1). Importantly, identification of more tightly linked markers to the MEN loci allows presymptomatic genetic diagnosis of the trait with a high level of confidence. A possible unifying explanation for the pathogenesis of the MEN syndromes, particularly MEN-IIa and MEN-IIb, is provided by embryologic and cytochemical studies. Thyroid C cells derive embryologically from the neural crest. These cells are members of a class of polypeptide-producing cells termed *amine precursor uptake and decarboxylation* (APUD) cells. These cytochemical attributes are shared by a dispersed family of endocrine cells. The chromaffin cells of the adrenal medulla are also derived from the neural crest and have APUD cell characteristics. The inheritance of simultaneous MTC and pheochromocytoma may result from a single defect or combination of defects in the development of neural crest tissue.

This explanation is particularly attractive in the case of MEN-IIb, which consists of MTC and pheochromocytoma developing in cells of neural crest origin and widespread involvement of peripheral nerves. However, the occurrence of HPT in MEN-IIa is inconsistent with this hypothesis. Parathyroid cells are not derived from the neural crest and do not have the biochemical properties of APUD cells. It appears that parathyroid hyperplasia is a primary feature of MEN-IIa, and its relationship to the other tumors is not well understood.

Clinical and Pathologic Features

The MEN-IIa and MEN-IIb syndromes are inherited in an autosomal dominant pattern. As is the case for MEN-I, the traits for MEN-IIa and MEN-IIb are transmitted with near 100 per cent penetrance, but with variable expressivity. Bilateral MTC occurs in virtually every affected individual with MEN-IIa and MEN-IIb. In addition, patients with MEN-IIa may have associated pheochromocytoma (50 per cent) or parathyroid hyperplasia (50 per cent).

Medullary thyroid carcinoma occurs in MEN-IIb syndrome in association with pheochromocytoma, mucosal neuromas, intestinal ganglioneuromas, skeletal abnormalities, and a "marfanoid" habitus. Affected individuals are often recognizable at birth or in early infancy. Significantly, the MTC in MEN-IIb occurs earlier (sometimes before 2 years of age) and is much more aggressive than in patients with MEN-IIa. Patients with MEN-IIb may die from widespread metastatic MTC at an early age. Owing to the aggressive nature of the disease, kindreds with MEN-IIb are characteristically small, encompassing only two or three generations.

Medullary Thyroid Carcinoma

Medullary thyroid carcinoma accounts for 5 to 10 per cent of all thyroid malignancies. Approximately 80 per cent of these represent sporadic cases of MTC. Twenty per cent of MTC cases occur in a familial setting, either in association with MEN-IIa, MEN-IIb, or less commonly as familial MTC not associated with other endocrinopathies (FMTC). Medullary thyroid carcinoma is usually the first abnormality expressed in both MEN-IIa and MEN-IIb. The peak incidence of MTC in the setting of MEN-IIa or MEN-IIb is in the second or third decade, compared with a peak incidence in the fifth or sixth decade for patients with sporadic MTC. Medullary thyroid carcinoma usually appears grossly as a circumscribed, gritty, whitish tan nodule. Microscopically, it consists of nests or sheets of uniform round or polygonal cells separated by variable amounts of fibrovascular stroma. Medullary thyroid carcinoma can be diagnosed immunohistochemically by demonstrating calcitonin within the MTC cells.

Sporadic MTC is almost always unilateral. In patients with MEN-IIa or MEN-IIb, MTC virtually always occurs as bilateral, multicentric foci of tumor in the middle and upper portions of each thyroid lobe. A diffuse premalignant proliferation of C cells in the thyroid gland of patients with familial MTC has been described and termed C-cell hyperplasia (CCH). Parafollicular clusters of C cells represent the early manifestation of hyperplasia or microinvasive carcinoma that progress to multifocal MTC. The presence of bilateral MTC strongly suggests the presence of familial disease.

Medullary thyroid carcinoma cells secrete calcitonin, which serves as a sensitive plasma marker for the presence of tumor. Medullary thyroid carcinoma may be detected when it is clinically occult. Asymptomatic members of kindreds with MEN-IIa or FMTC may be diagnosed as having MTC by detecting an elevated plasma calcitonin level either basally or following the administration of calcium and/or pentagastrin. These patients are likely to have their MTC confined to the thyroid gland, and almost all of them are cured by total thyroidectomy (Table 2). Patients with clinically evident MTC present with a palpable thyroid nodule

TABLE 2. OUTCOME OF PATIENTS WITH MEN-IIa AND MEDULLARY THYROID CARCINOMA (MTC) ACCORDING TO METHOD OF DIAGNOSIS

Method of Diagnosis of MTC	Number	Follow-Up (years)	Cured Patients (%)	Dead From Disease (%)
Screening	41	12	38 (93)	0
Mass	17	19	5 (29)	2 (12)

* From Gagel RF, et al: N Engl J Med *318*:478–484, 1988; and Alexander HR, Norton JA: Ann Intern Med *115*:133–147, 1991, with permission.

or a multinodular thyroid gland and often have lymph node metastases. These patients are less often curable.

Pheochromocytoma

Pheochromocytomas in patients with MEN-IIa and MEN-IIb are characterized by their tendency to appear in the second or third decade of life. These tumors are seldom malignant. They occur within the adrenal, and approximately 60 to 80 per cent are bilateral. The majority of these tumors are diagnosed concurrent with, or a few years subsequent to, the detection of MTC. The histologic appearance of the tumor cells is similar to that seen in pheochromocytomas that occur in a nonfamilial setting. Pheochromocytomas in patients with MEN-IIa or MEN-IIb may either be clinically silent or associated with dramatic clinical symptoms such as severe pounding frontal headaches, episodic diaphoresis, palpitations, and vague feelings of anxiety. Hypertension, if present, may be sustained or episodic.

Parathyroids

Hyperfunction of the parathyroid glands in patients with MEN-IIa is the most variable component of the syndrome. The parathyroid lesions consist primarily of generalized chief cell hyperplasia, and typically there is multiple gland enlargement. Many patients are asymptomatic, and recognition stems from the finding of hypercalcemia during routine laboratory studies. The most common symptom of altered calcium homeostasis in patients with MEN-IIa is the presence of asymptomatic or symptomatic renal stones. More advanced signs of hyperparathyroidism, such as osteitis fibrosa cystica or nephrocalcinosis, are unusual. Primary hyperparathyroidism does not occur in patients with MEN-IIb.

Nonendocrine Manifestations of MEN-IIb

In addition to MTC and pheochromocytoma, patients with MEN-IIb develop abnormalities of the musculoskeletal and nervous systems. Unlike patients with MEN-I or MEN-IIa, patients with MEN-IIb have a characteristic phenotype, including a tall, thin "marfanoid" body habitus. Multiple neuromas develop on the lips, tongue, and oral mucosa and result in the appearance of thick, "bumpy" lips. Slit lamp examination of the eyes often reveals hypertrophied corneal nerves. Patients may develop diffuse ganglioneuromatosis of the gastrointestinal tract that can cause crampy abdominal pain, constipation, and even megacolon. There is also a high incidence of skeletal anomalies, including pes planus or cavus, pectus excavatum, kyphosis, and scoliosis (Fig. 1).

Diagnosis

Because MTC occurs in virtually 100 per cent of patients with MEN-IIa and MEN-IIb and is usually the first abnormality expressed, diagnosis of the disease in kindred members at risk is accomplished by screening for the presence of elevated basal or stimulated plasma levels of calcitonin (CT), which are diagnostic for MTC. In 1970, Tashjian and associates first described the measurement of human calcitonin by radioimmunoassay and documented that virtually all patients with clinically detectable MTC have elevated plasma CT levels. In normal individuals, basal plasma CT levels are either very low or less than 200 pg/ml. Patients with clinically palpable MTC generally have plasma CT levels greater than 1000 pg/ml. With extensive disease, basal plasma values may exceed several thousand picograms per milliliter.

Initially, either calcium infusion or pentagastrin injection was used as a provocative agent for the early diagnosis of MTC in individuals at risk. Subsequently, it has been shown that the sequential intravenous administration of calcium gluconate (2 mg/kg over 1 minute) followed by a bolus injection of pentagastrin (0.5 µg/kg over 5 seconds) stimulated higher peak levels of plasma CT than either agent alone. Kindred members with clinically occult MEN-IIa whose MTC was diagnosed by provocative testing were younger, had smaller primary tumors, had a lower incidence of positive lymph nodes, and were more often cured following total thyroidectomy (Table 2).

We recommend that members of kindreds at risk for developing MTC undergo annual calcium pentagastrin stimulation testing beginning as early as age 5 years and continuing until the age of 40 to 45 years. In families with MEN-IIa or FMTC, stimulated plasma CT levels greater than 300 pg/ml are highly suggestive of MTC. The diagnosis is virtually assured in patients with plasma CT levels exceeding 1000 pg/ml. Occasionally, kindred members are found whose basal plasma CT levels are undetectable but increase modestly (250 to 1000 pg/ml) following provocative testing. In these patients, selective thyroid venous catheterization and measurement of CT levels in blood collected after provocative testing have identified patients with early MTC and clearly separated them from subjects with non–C-cell disorders.

The diagnosis of pheochromocytoma in patients with MEN-IIa and MEN-IIb can be made biochemically by measurement of the urinary excretion of catecholamines and catecholamine metabolites. Patients with symptoms characteristic of pheochromocytoma should have a 24-hour urine collection for measurement of total urinary catecholamines, epinephrine, norepinephrine, metanephrines, and vanillylmandelic acid (VMA). It is imperative that patients with MEN-

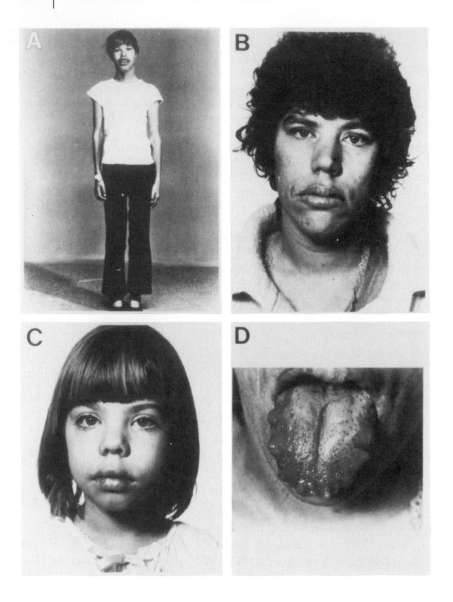

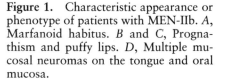

Figure 1. Characteristic appearance or phenotype of patients with MEN-IIb. *A*, Marfanoid habitus. *B* and *C*, Prognathism and puffy lips. *D*, Multiple mucosal neuromas on the tongue and oral mucosa.

IIa and MEN-IIb have a pheochromocytoma excluded prior to undergoing a thyroidectomy. This is particularly important because the pheochromocytoma may be unsuspected clinically. If a patient with MTC is found to have a pheochromocytoma, adrenalectomy should be performed first, followed by a thyroidectomy in 1 to 2 weeks.

If the 24-hour urinary excretion rates of catecholamines and metabolites are equivocal and there is concern about the presence of a pheochromocytoma, magnetic resonance imaging (MRI) of the abdomen should be performed to exclude an adrenal tumor. Pheochromocytomas appear bright on the T2-weighted image, and tumors as small as 1 cm can be detected. ^{131}I-metaiodobenzylguanidine (^{131}I-MIBG) scintigraphy is another study that may be useful to

diagnose pheochromocytoma. It is very specific for pheochromocytomas, and positive identification has been possible in 90 per cent of patients. There have been less than 5 per cent false-positive tests. The diagnosis of hyperparathyroidism in patients with MEN-IIa depends largely on serial measurements of the plasma calcium concentration. If an individual is hypercalcemic, elevated peripheral plasma levels of parathyroid hormone confirm the diagnosis.

Genetic Screening by DNA Polymorphism Analysis

Screening members of families with MEN-IIa by provocative testing to detect the presence of MTC in its earliest stages has been the most sensitive way to identify affected individuals. A significant contribution to the presymptomatic diagnosis of families with the MEN syndromes will undoubtedly be provided by the identification of chromosomal markers closely linked to the disease loci. Tight genetic linkage exists when two loci are closely situated on the same chromosome such that the probability of crossover between them is very low. In families with parents who are informative (heterozygous) for the marker used, inheritance of the disease can be predicted with a high level of confidence by demonstrating coinheritance with the marker. Preclinical diagnosis using DNA polymorphism analysis may eventually allow early identification of affected patients, who should then be followed closely for the development of MTC. The availability of this technology may lead to the performance of prophylactic thyroidectomy in patients identified as carrying the gene for the disease. It almost certainly will obviate endocrine testing in patients with a minimal likelihood of possessing the trait.

SURGICAL MANAGEMENT

Pheochromocytoma

If pheochromocytoma is detected, the patient should have a bilateral subcostal incision and exploration of both adrenal glands, the sympathetic chain, and the organ of Zuckerkandl. Bilateral pheochromocytomas require bilateral adrenalectomy. Although a matter of some controversy, in MEN-IIa or MEN-IIb patients with unilateral pheochromocytoma and a palpably normal contralateral gland, it is acceptable policy to perform a unilateral adrenalectomy. Such patients should be followed carefully at 6-month to yearly intervals for recurrence in the contralateral gland. It is recognized that approximately 30 per cent of patients initially managed by unilateral adrenalectomy may develop pheochromocytoma in the remaining gland. Preoperatively, patients with pheochromocytomas receive α-adrenergic blockade with phenoxybenzamine. β-Adrenergic blockade may be necessary if tachycardia or arrhythmias develop with phenoxybenzamine. β-Blockade without prior α-blockade is dangerous because without it patients are subjected to unopposed vasoconstriction. Intraoperative control of hypertension, which frequently occurs with manipulation of the tumor, is most effectively achieved with sodium nitroprusside or phentolamine.

Medullary Thyroid Carcinoma

The surgical treatment of familial or sporadic MTC is total thyroidectomy. Meticulous removal of all thyroid tissue should be undertaken at the initial opera-

tion, because MTC in the setting of MEN-IIa or MEN-IIb is virtually always multicentric and bilateral and may metastasize early to cervical lymph nodes. Dissection of the nodes in the central compartment of the neck (between the jugular veins and from the hyoid bone to the sternal notch) should be performed in all patients with either clinically evident or occult MTC. Patients with macroscopic regional lymph node metastases should undergo ipsilateral neck dissection in addition to total thyroidectomy. Postoperatively, residual or recurrent MTC can be readily detected by repeat calcium-pentagastrin stimulation and measurement of plasma CT levels. Until recently, repeat neck exploration in an attempt to resect residual disease has infrequently resulted in normalization of elevated plasma CT levels. However, one group has reported 4 of 11 patients with residual MTC who normalized elevated plasma CT levels by undergoing meticulous superior mediastinal and bilateral lymph node dissection.

Hyperparathyroidism

The characteristic parathyroid lesion in patients with MEN-IIa and primary hyperparathyroidism is hyperplasia with involvement of all four glands. Although some surgeons prefer a subtotal (3.5-gland) parathyroidectomy in patients with parathyroid hyperplasia and MEN-IIa, we perform total parathyroidectomy with autograft of parathyroid tissue into the nondominant forearm musculature.

Prognosis

The course of patients with MEN-IIa and MEN-IIb is essentially that of MTC. Medullary thyroid carcinoma is an intermediate grade of thyroid malignancy, as compared with the more malignant anaplastic or less malignant papillary or follicular carcinoma. Medullary thyroid carcinoma can exhibit variable biologic aggressiveness within different MEN syndromes and different kindreds. Medullary thyroid carcinoma in the setting of MEN-IIb is very aggressive, and patients may die at a young age. Medullary thyroid carcinoma in patients with MEN-IIa or familial MTC is usually indolent and progresses very slowly. In some patients, the disease may have a more aggressive course. Not surprisingly, it has been demonstrated that patients whose MTC is diagnosed biochemically have a more favorable pathologic stage than do patients whose tumor is diagnosed clinically (Table 2). The ideal treatment of patients with nonresectable metastatic MTC is unclear. Medullary thyroid carcinoma is relatively resistant to radiation therapy, and various chemotherapeutic agents have infrequently demonstrated significant responsiveness. It is imperative that families with hereditary MTC be identified and managed by an aggressive screening program, because early diagnosis and thyroidectomy cures MTC in a large percentage of patients.

REFERENCES

Ballard HS, Frame B, Hartsock RJ: Familial multiple endocrine adenomapeptic ulcer complex. Medicine 43:481–516, 1964.

Larsson C, Skogseid B, Oberg K, Nakamura Y, Nordenskjold M: Multiple endocrine neoplasia type 1 gene maps to chromosome 11 and is lost in insulinoma. Nature 332:85–87, 1988.

Mathew CGP, Chin KS, Easton DF, Thorpe K, Carter C, Liou GL, Fong, SL, Bridges CDB, Haak H, Meuwenhuijzen Kruseman AC, Schifter S, Hansen HH, Telenius H, Telenius-Berg M, Ponder BAJ: A linked genetic marker for multiple endocrine neoplasia type 2a on chromosome 10. Nature 328:527–528, 1987.

Norum RA, Lafreniere R, O'Neal LW, et al: Linkage of multiple endocrine neoplasia type 2b gene (MEN-IIb) to chromosome 10 markers linked to MEN-IIa. Genomics 8:313–320, 1990.

Pipeleers-Marichal M, Somers G, Willems G, Foulis A, Imrie C, Bishop AE, et al: Gastrinomas in the duodenums of patients with multiple endocrine neoplasia type 1 and the Zollinger-Ellison syndrome. N Engl J Med 322:723–727, 1990.

Simpson NE, Kidd KK, Goodfellow PJ, McDermid H, Myers S, Kidd JR, Jackson CE, Duncan AMV, Farrer LA, Brasch K, Castiglione C, Genel M, Gertner J, Greenberg CR, Gusella JF, Holden JJA, White BN: Assignment of multiple endocrine neoplasia type 2a to chromosome 10 by Linkage. Nature 328:528–530, 1987.

23
THE PARATHYROID GLANDS

JEFFREY A. NORTON, M.D.   SAMUEL A. WELLS, Jr., M.D.

HISTORICAL ASPECTS

In 1880, Ivar Sandstrom first described the parathyroid glands, and in 1891, Gley demonstrated that excision of these glands caused tetany. Others found that the tetany could be corrected by infusion of calcium salts. Von Recklinghausen described a disease of bone in 1891 that later was found to be caused by hyperparathyroidism. The first to describe the association of bone disease and parathyroid neoplasia was Askanazy in 1904. In 1907, Erdheim studied several patients who had died of osteomalacia and incorrectly concluded that the marked parathyroid hyperplasia observed was secondary to the bone disease. However, Schlagenhaufer subsequently held that it was unlikely for compensatory hypertrophy to involve only a single gland and suggested that some parathyroid tumors were primary and caused secondary changes in the skeleton. Mandl confirmed this hypothesis 10 years later when he excised an enlarged parathyroid gland and, following operation, the calcium in the blood and urine decreased, and the bones became more dense and pain free. The first successful parathyroidectomy was performed at Barnes Hospital in St. Louis in 1929. In 1934, Albright and others noted an association of osteitis fibrosa cystica with renal stones and subsequently identified a group of patients with hyperparathyroidism who had calculi or nephrocalcinosis but no bone disease. Biologically active parathyroid extracts were first prepared by Collip in 1925. Parathyroid hormone was isolated and purified by Aurbach and others in 1959, and Berson and associates developed a radioimmunoassay for parathyroid hormone in 1963.

EMBRYOLOGY

The superior parathyroid glands arise from the fourth pharyngeal pouch, and the inferior from the third. During the branchial complex stage, the glands are intimately associated with the derivatives of their respective pouches, the inferior parathyroids with the thymus and the superior parathyroids with the lateral thyroid complex. As the embryo matures and the thymus descends, the inferior parathyroids migrate caudally. Typically, the separation of these glands from the thymus becomes complete when they lie posterior to the lower pole of the thyroid lobe. This migration is extremely variable and, as a result, the inferior glands are more likely to be found in an ectopic location than the superior glands.

ANATOMY

Typically, there are four parathyroid glands. However, more than four glands have been detected in some series (5 per cent). Most often, the supernumerary gland is located in the thymus. The anatomic location of the parathyroid glands demonstrates considerable constancy and is shown in Figure 1. The vascular supply to the parathyroid glands is usually from the inferior thyroid artery, but it can arise from the superior thyroid artery; the thyroid ima artery; and arteries in the larynx, trachea, esophagus, or mediastinum or from anastomoses between these vessels. The inferior, middle, and superior thyroid veins

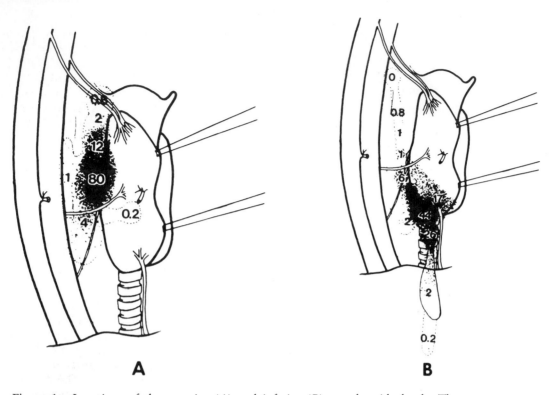

Figure 1. Locations of the superior (*A*) and inferior (*B*) parathyroid glands. The more common locations are indicated by the darker shading. The numbers represent the percentages of glands found at the different locations. (From Akerstrom G, Malmaers J, Bergstrom R: Surgical anatomy of human parathyroid glands. Surgery 95:17, 1984, with permission.)

drain the parathyroid glands. Approximately 50 per cent of all parathyroids are found adjacent to the area where the inferior thyroid artery enters the thyroid parenchyma. The normal glands tend to be flat and ovoid, but on enlargement, they become globular. Normally, they measure 5 to 7 mm by 3 to 4 mm by 0.5 to 2 mm. The combined weight of the parathyroid glands ranges from 90 to 200 mg, and the upper glands generally are smaller than the lower. In adults, the parathyroids are usually red-brown to yellow, whereas in the newborn, they are gray and semitransparent. The superior parathyroid glands are usually embedded in fat and located on the posterior surface of the middle or upper portion of the thyroid lobe close to the point where the recurrent laryngeal nerve enters the larynx. The superior parathyroid glands are superior to the inferior thyroid artery and posterolateral to the recurrent laryngeal nerve. The lower parathyroid glands reside more ventrally close to the lower pole of the thyroid gland and the "thyrothymic ligament." In approximately 1 to 5 per cent of patients, an inferior parathyroid gland is located in the deep mediastinum. The inferior glands are inferior to the inferior thyroid artery and anteromedial to the recurrent laryngeal nerve.

PHYSIOLOGY

Mineral Metabolism

Calcium is a constituent of all animal fluids and is involved in a variety of physiologic processes ranging from blood coagulation and bone formation, to milk production. It represents a major cellular messenger and is critical in both muscle contraction and membrane repolarization. It constitutes about 2 per cent of the adult body weight, and almost all is contained in the skeleton. Plasma calcium measures 9.0 to 10.5 mg/dl (4.5 to 5.2 mEq/L) and is about equally divided between an ionized and a protein-bound phase. Five per cent is bound to organic anions. Approximately 80 per cent of the bound calcium is complexed to albumin. The amount of protein and the body fluid pH are the two most important factors regulating the distribution of calcium in plasma. Hydrogen ion competes with calcium for the same binding sites for all the calcium-binding proteins in plasma. In general, for each gram of alteration of the total protein there is a similar 0.8 mg/dl change in the total serum calcium. Of greatest importance is the ionized calcium that is the form most immediately related to the activity of the parathyroid glands.

Calcium, in the inorganic form, is absorbed in the upper small intestine. On a regular diet, approximately 1 gm is ingested daily. The calcium in the extracellular fluid is constantly being exchanged with that in the exchangeable bone, the intracellular fluid, and the glomerular filtrate, 99 per cent of which is reabsorbed by the normal kidney. The adult body contains about 700 gm of phosphate, most being located in the bones and teeth. On a regular diet, approximately 1500 mg of phosphate is ingested daily. Plasma phosphate measures 2.5 to 4.3 mg/dl. The plasma levels of calcium and phosphate vary inversely with one another. Normally, the relationship is such that the product of plasma calcium and phosphate (measured in milligrams per deciliter) is constant and ranges between 30 and 40. Magnesium, the fourth most abundant metal in mammals and the second most prevalent intracellular cation, is located primarily in the mineral phase of bone. Approximately 300 mg is ingested daily. Magnesium is important in the activation of enzymes necessary for intermediary metabolism and phosphorylation, in protein and nucleic acid synthesis, and in mitochondrial regulation.

Regulation of Calcium Metabolism

The primary agents responsible for regulation of calcium metabolism are parathyroid hormone, vitamin D, and calcitonin.

PARATHYROID HORMONE. Parathyroid hormone (PTH) is synthesized within the parathyroid as a larger precursor, preproparathyroid hormone, which is cleaved to proparathyroid hormone, and then to the final 84–amino acid PTH. The hormone is secreted and then metabolized in the liver into hormonally active N-terminal and inactive C-terminal fragments. Parathyroid hormone secretion is inversely related to the serum level of calcium and also to the levels of 1,25-dihydroxyvitamin D_3. It has direct effects on the kidney and skeleton and indirect effects on the gastrointestinal tract through vitamin D. Parathyroid hormone promotes a release of calcium from the skeleton. It inhibits osteoblasts and stimulates osteoclasts. It causes a decrease in calcium clearance by the kidney. It also causes an increased excretion of renal phosphate and bicarbonate. Finally it stimulates hydroxylation of 25-hydroxy to 1,25-dihydroxyvitamin D_3 in the kidney, and this latter metabolite causes enhanced absorption of calcium from the intestine.

VITAMIN D. The major D vitamins are vitamin D_2 and vitamin D_3. The most important physiologically is vitamin D_3, which is derived from ultraviolet activation of 7-dehydrocholesterol in the skin. The bulk of commercially prepared vitamin D is vitamin D_2. It is derived from ergosterol and is the major form of vitamin D used clinically in the treatment of certain skeletal diseases. Vitamin D increases the intestinal absorption of calcium, and secondarily phosphate, and increases the mobilization of calcium and phosphate from bone to blood. Vitamin D appears to exert a growth-promoting effect that is not explained by mineral retention.

CALCITONIN. Calcitonin inhibits bone resorption and produces hypocalcemia when administered to experimental animals. The hormone also induces urinary excretion of calcium and phosphate. Calcitonin has not been demonstrated to be important in the control of serum levels of calcium in humans.

In summary, serum calcium is closely regulated by the action of parathyroid hormone. A reduction in serum ionized calcium increases secretion of parathyroid hormone that secondarily stimulates production of 1,25-dihydroxyvitamin D_3. Conversely, a rise in serum calcium inhibits both PTH secretion and the formation of active calciferol.

DISORDERS OF THE PARATHYROID GLANDS

Hyperparathyroidism

The cause of spontaneous hyperfunction of the parathyroid glands is unknown, and overactivity is recognized because of the peripheral effects of excess hormone. Primary hyperparathyroidism occurs when the normal feedback control by serum level of calcium is disturbed and there is increased production of parathyroid hormone. Secondary hyperparathyroidism occurs most commonly in patients with renal disease. There is a defect in mineral homeostasis leading to a compensatory increase in parathyroid gland function and size. Occasionally, with prolonged compensatory stimulation, a hyperplastic gland develops autonomous function. This state is called tertiary hyperparathyroidism.

PRIMARY HYPERPARATHYROIDISM. The incidence of hyperparathyroidism is approximately 25 per 100,000 in the general population, and approximately 50,000 new cases occur annually. The incidence of the disease increases markedly with age, and it is especially common in postmenopausal women; in females over age 65 years the incidence is between 2.5 and 5 per 1000.

Etiology

The etiology of hyperparathyroidism is unknown and probably varies with the underlying pathology.

Single-gland or adenomatous disease is more consistent with a mechanism involving spontaneous hyperfunction, whereas multiglandular disease suggests the presence of some exogenous stimulus. Several investigators have reported an increased incidence of hyperparathyroidism in patients exposed to low-dose ionizing irradiation, usually in childhood. In one study, 8 (14 per cent) of 58 persons found to have hyperparathyroidism had received ionizing irradiation to the neck at a young age. Nine of 58 normal subjects matched for age and sex had not been previously irradiated. Several other investigators have confirmed an association of radiation exposure to the neck and hyperparathyroidism. Recent data on the etiology of hyperparathyroidism in multiple endocrine neoplasia type I (MEN-I), may have significance for sporadic disease as well. Friedman and associates have identified chromosome 11 deletions, including a gene locus previously associated with MEN-I, in 10 of 16 parathyroid tumors from patients with known MEN-I. Similar losses were demonstrated in 11 of 34 sporadic adenomas. Another less common (3 per cent) mechanism of parathyroid adenoma initiation is DNA rearrangement involving the PTH gene. One of these DNA rearrangements forms an oncogene, PRAD-1, which is a protein like the cyclins. Thus, the initiation of parathyroid tumor growth is heterogeneous, from deletion of a tumor suppressor gene to induction of an oncogene.

Clinical Presentation (Signs and Symptoms)

Since the advent of routine screening by measuring serum levels of calcium and phosphate, primary hyperparathyroidism has been detected with increasing frequency. While in the past most patients presented with severe bone or renal disease, an increasing percentage of patients today are apparently asymptomatic. On the other hand, when carefully questioned, many of these patients describe symptoms or associated conditions that can be related to hyperparathyroidism, and these symptoms may improve after successful parathyroidectomy. The most frequent symptoms in 100 sequential patients evaluated are shown in Table 1. The usual symptomatic patient with hyperparathyroidism is in the chronic phase of disease, with signs and symptoms from secondary changes in the genitourinary system and skeleton. The earliest complaints, such as muscle weakness, anorexia, nausea, constipation, polyuria, and polydipsia, occasionally cause the patient to seek medical advice.

RENAL COMPLICATIONS. Renal complications are generally the most severe clinical manifestations of primary hyperparathyroidism. The presenting symptoms are usually related to nephrolithiasis, which occurs in about 30 per cent of patients; conversely, about 5 to

TABLE 1. PRESENTING SYMPTOMS IN 100 PATIENTS WITH PRIMARY HYPERPARATHYROIDISM

Symptoms	Percentage Population
Nephrolithiasis	30
Bone disease	2
Peptic ulcer disease	12
Psychiatric disorders	15
Muscle weakness	70
Constipation	32
Polyuria	28
Pancreatitis	1
Myalgia	54
Arthralgia	54

10 per cent of previously unscreened patients presenting with nephrolithiasis have hyperparathyroidism. Patients complain of back pain, hematuria, and the passing of renal calculi. Nephrocalcinosis represents calcification within the parenchyma of the kidneys. It occurs in only 5 to 10 per cent of patients with primary hyperparathyroidism. Although renal stones can be treated surgically or with lithotripsy, little can be done for nephrocalcinosis. Renal damage is much more common in patients with nephrocalcinosis, but it can occur in the absence of renal calcification. If renal impairment is severe preoperatively, it tends to remain unchanged or to become progressively worse postoperatively; mild degrees of renal damage are usually functional and reversible. Careful evaluation of renal function reveals some degree of abnormality in 80 to 90 per cent of patients with hyperparathyroidism.

BONE DISEASE. Many of the first descriptions of hyperparathyroidism were of patients who had severe bone disease characterized by osteitis fibrosa cystica generalisata, a condition with a unique radiographic picture that is pathognomonic of hyperparathyroidism. Although the incidence of bone disease in patients with primary hyperparathyroidism reported in earlier studies was as high as 50 to 90 per cent, the reported incidence in more current series has ranged from 5 to 15 per cent. Skeletal involvement is most readily demonstrated by radiographic films of the hands. Subperiosteal resorption is usually evident on the radial aspect of the middle phalanx of the second or third fingers. In more advanced cases, cysts are present and there is tufting of the distal phalanges. The skull is the second most commonly affected skeletal site and presents a mottled appearance often associated with diffuse granularity and cystic lesions. Also, with advanced disease, osteoclastomas or "brown tumors" may be present. With the use of more sophisticated and sensitive technology, such as x-ray spectrophotometry and phosphate absorptiometric analysis, subtle derangements in bone density can be detected and the incidence of "bone disease" in patients with hyperparathyroidism has been shown to be relatively common. Although the significance of subtle bone loss has been questioned, recent studies demonstrate an increased prevalence of vertebral fractures in patients undergoing parathyroidectomy.

GASTROINTESTINAL MANIFESTATIONS. An increased incidence of peptic ulcer disease in patients with primary hyperparathyroidism was first reported in 1946. Most, but not all, subsequent studies have confirmed this association. The association of pancreatitis and hyperparathyroidism was first reported in 1940. Even though an increased incidence of pancreatitis was reported from various clinics in the subsequent two decades, there were no carefully controlled studies evaluating the relationship. In a more recent study, postoperative hyperamylasemia (>300 IU) occurred in 35 per cent of patients following parathyroidectomy, and clinically significant pancreatitis (serum amylase of >1000 IU associated with abdominal pain) occurred in 10 per cent. Finally, there may be an increased incidence (25 to 35 per cent) of cholelithiasis in patients with primary hyperparathyroidism, but gall stones are common and an increased incidence is difficult to demonstrate unequivocally.

EMOTIONAL DISTURBANCE. Patients with hypercalcemia of any cause may develop neurologic or psychiatric disturbances ranging from depression or anxiety, to psychosis or coma. Most of the mental derangements associated with hyperparathyroidism are subtle. Some individuals experience personality change, inability to concentrate, or recent memory loss. Many patients after successful parathyroidectomy experience a sense of well-being and relief of fatigue and dullness that often was not fully appreciated preoperatively.

OTHER MANIFESTATIONS. There is an increased prevalence of chondrocalcinosis and pseudogout in patients with primary hyperparathyroidism, the incidence being 3 to 7 per cent. Characteristically, one can see radiographic evidence of calcium pyrophosphate deposition in the articular cartilages and menisci. Vascular and cardiac calcification, skin necrosis, and band keratopathy of the cornea have all been reported. Muscular weakness and fatigue may occur. Most commonly, the weakness is in the proximal muscle groups. Most patients with primary hyperparathyroidism demonstrate some signs or symptoms of weakness, easy fatigability, and muscle atrophy.

Physical Findings

The diseased parathyroid glands are rarely palpable in patients with primary hyperparathyroidism. A palpable mass in the neck should suggest either the presence of a thyroid nodule or parathyroid carcinoma in a patient with severe hypercalcemia.

Laboratory Diagnosis

The diagnosis of hyperparathyroidism is dependent upon the documentation of an elevated serum calcium concentration, usually in conjunction with an elevated serum level of parathyroid hormone. Normal serum calcium values usually are between 8.5 and 10.5 mg/dl. Theoretically, one should be concerned with the ionized or free fraction of serum calcium rather than that portion which is bound to protein or inorganic anions. The measurement of ionized calcium is possible using a calcium-sensitive flow-through electrode. Studies have demonstrated that the serum level of ionized calcium is a more sensitive index of primary hyperparathyroidism than the total calcium. Following successful operation for primary hyperparathyroidism, the values of total and ionized calcium return to normal. It may seem that the most efficient method of diagnosing primary hyperparathyroidism is to document an increased concentration of parathyroid hormone in plasma. It is important to remember that the finding of an elevated plasma level of parathyroid hormone does not by itself establish the diagnosis of hyperparathyroidism. One must determine the parathyroid hormone level as a function of the serum calcium concentration. Subjects with increased serum concentrations of both calcium and parathyroid hormone almost certainly have hyperparathyroidism (Fig. 2).

Following secretion, parathyroid hormone is very rapidly cleaved into an N-terminal fragment and a C-terminal fragment. The intact molecule and the biologically active N-terminal fragment have half-lives of minutes, whereas the inactive C-terminal fragment has a half-life of hours. Generally, antibodies directed against the C-terminal fragment have been more useful in radioimmunoassay to establish the diagnosis of hyperparathyroidism. The concentration of serum phosphate varies between 2.5 and 4.5 mg/dl. Approximately half the patients with primary hyperparathyroidism have hypophosphatemia. However, in the presence of significant renal impairment, levels may be considerably elevated. The serum concentration of alkaline phosphatase is normally below 110 IU/dl. Between 10 and 40 per cent of patients with hyperparathyroidism have increased levels. In such patients, there is almost always some degree of bone disease, and following operation, the serum calcium concentration may fall more rapidly to lower levels compared with patients whose serum alkaline phosphatase levels are normal. Alkaline phosphatase level is not helpful in diagnosing hyperparathyroidism because it is also very often elevated with other causes of hypercalcemia.

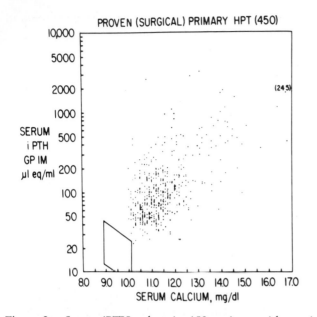

Figure 2. Serum iPTH values in 450 patients with surgically proven primary hyperparathyroidism as a function of serum calcium concentration. Serum iPTH was measured with a radioimmunoassay using GP Im antiserum. The area enclosed by the solid lines represents the normal range + 2 SD for serum iPTH and serum calcium. Note that there is a 10 per cent overlap of serum iPTH with the normal range, but that greater than 95 per cent of normal sera and all hyperparathyroid sera have measurable iPTH. Formal discriminative analysis of serum iPTH and serum calcium separates 100 per cent of hyperparathyroid patients from normal subjects. (From Arnaud CD, et al: Excerpta Medica International Congress Series. No. 270, 1973, p 281, with permission.)

Because of the effect of PTH on bicarbonate excretion in the kidney, patients with hyperparathyroidism often have a hyperchloremic metabolic acidosis at the time of diagnosis. The serum concentration of chloride as a function of the serum concentration of phosphate has been used as a diagnostic test for patients with hyperparathyroidism. The Cl/PO_4 ratio was above 33 in 96 per cent of the patients. Conversely, in 27 patients with hypercalcemia of other causes, the ratio was less than 30 in 92 per cent. The Cl/PO_4 ratio may have value in patients in whom the differential diagnosis of hypercalcemia is difficult. The serum concentration of magnesium is below normal in only 5 to 10 per cent of patients with hyperparathyroidism. If there is concomitant hypocalcemia and hypomagnesemia following parathyroidectomy, it is difficult to correct the hypocalcemia until the serum magnesium concentration has been returned to normal. The serum concentrations of calcium, phosphate, alkaline phosphatase, and chloride, as well as the Cl/PO_4 ratio, in 100 consecutive patients with primary hyperparathyroidism are depicted in Figure 3.

Special Diagnostic Tests

NEPHROGENOUS CYCLIC ADENOSINE MONOPHOSPHATE. The interaction of parathyroid hormone with specific receptors in the renal tubule causes the activation of adenylate cyclase and an increase in cyclic adenosine monophosphate (cAMP) inside the cell. Because the cAMP leaks into the tubular fluid, increased concentrations of cAMP are present in the urine of patients with hyperparathyroidism. When measured as a function of creatinine clearance (nephrogenous cAMP), it has been demonstrated that approximately 90 per cent of patients with hyperparathyroidism have increased urinary levels. The measurement of nephrogenous cAMP has been useful in the differential diagnosis of hyperparathyroidism, although it may be elevated in certain patients with malignancy-associated hypercalcemia.

URINARY CALCIUM. In hyperparathyroidism, urinary calcium excretion is almost always elevated, which has assumed increasing importance in differentiating hyperparathyroidism from the recently recognized syndrome of familial hypercalcemic hypocalciuria, a condition that is not treated by operation.

BONE BIOPSY AND DENSITOMETRY. Iliac crest bone biopsy and photon beam bone scanning can detect subtle changes when conventional radiographs are negative. These findings may help to establish the diagnosis and document the degree of bone demineralization.

Less Common Manifestations

FAMILIAL HYPERPARATHYROIDISM. The familial incidence of hyperparathyroidism is well established. In its simplest form, it occurs as a single disease with no associated abnormalities; whereas in its more complex form, it presents as a part of one of the multiple endocrinopathy syndromes. MEN-I is characterized by the association of parathyroid hyperplasia, pituitary adenomas, pancreatic islet cell neoplasia, and, occasionally, tumors of the thyroid or adrenal cortex. MEN-IIa consists of medullary thyroid carcinoma, pheochromocytoma, and parathyroid hyperplasia. Each of the MEN syndromes is inherited as an autosomal-dominant trait.

Familial hypercalcemic hypocalciuria (FHH) is a syndrome characterized by the familial occurrence of hypercalcemia, hypocalciuria, and generalized mild parathyroid gland enlargement. These patients have no apparent morbidity from the hypercalcemia, and the hypercalcemia is difficult to correct by surgical resection. Despite resection of 3.5 glands, incidence of

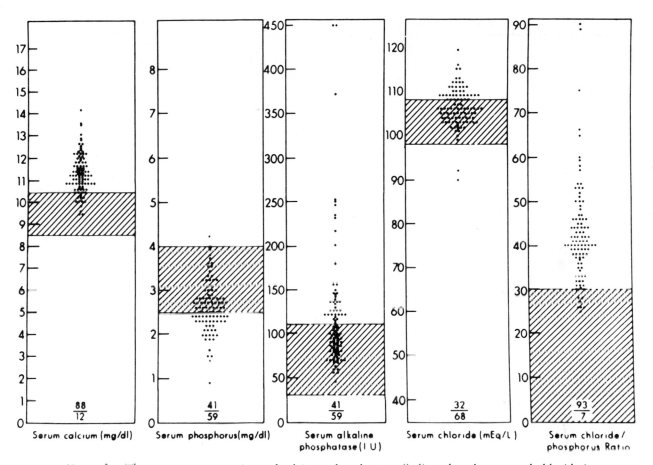

Figure 3. The serum concentrations of calcium, phosphorus, alkaline phosphatase, and chloride in 100 consecutive patients with surgically proven hyperparathyroidism. The ratio of serum chloride to phosphorus is also shown (*extreme right*). The fractions at the bottom of each bar represent the number of abnormal values over the number of normal values. The laboratory values shown represent the determinations made at the time of hospital admission for parathyroidectomy. Even though 12 patients had serum calcium concentrations in the normal range, all had been demonstrated to be hypercalcemic on several preoperative determinations. (From Wells SA Jr, Leight GS, Ross AJ: Primary hyperparathyroidism. Curr Probl Surg 17:400, 1980, with permission.)

persistent or recurrent hypercalcemia postoperatively is high. Most experts think that surgical resection is not indicated for patients with FHH.

HYPERPARATHYROIDISM IN PREGNANCY. Primary hyperparathyroidism in pregnancy is rare and is associated with neonatal tetany, stillbirth, and abortion. The risk of fetal complications seems to be higher if the hyperparathyroidism is left untreated. When the diagnosis is made, the mother should undergo operation, if possible during the second trimester.

PARATHYROID CARCINOMA. Parathyroid carcinoma is rare and represents the cause of the primary hyperparathyroidism in less than 1 per cent of patients. Parathyroid carcinoma usually presents with more severe disease than parathyroid adenoma (Table 2). The diagnosis is most securely based on the pres-

ence of local invasion of surrounding tissues or metastases to regional lymph nodes or distant sites. However, some pathologists suggest that the diagnosis can be made when there is histologic evidence of fibrous bands, vascular invasion, frequent mitotic figures, and capsular invasion. Characteristically, the serum concentrations of calcium, PTH, and alkaline phosphatase are markedly increased compared with concentrations in patients with adenoma or hyperplasia (Table 2). In approximately 50 per cent of patients with parathyroid carcinoma, the involved parathyroid gland is palpable clinically, a finding rarely seen in patients with adenoma. The majority of patients with parathyroid carcinoma are symptomatic at the time of diagnosis and complain of nausea, vomiting, polyuria, generalized weakness, and weight loss. Furthermore, both the

TABLE 2. BENIGN PRIMARY HYPERPARATHYROIDISM VERSUS PARATHYROID CARCINOMA

Author	Benign		Malignant		
	Mallette et al.*	Heath et al.†	Holmes et al.‡	Shane and Bilezikan§	Fraker et al.‖
Period of review	1965–1972	1974–1976	1933–1968	1968–1981	1982–1989
Number of cases	57	51	46	62	4
Female/male ratio	1.4:1	3.6:1	0.8:1	1.2:1	3:1
Average age (years)	51	62	44	48	52
Serum calcium (mg/dl)	11.7	10.8¶	15.9	15.5	14.4
Renal involvement	21 (37%)	2 (4%)	15 (32%)	37 (60%)	2 (50%)
Skeletal involvement	8 (14%)	10 (209%)#	34 (73%)	34 (55%)	3 (75%)
No symptoms	13 (23%)	26 (51%)		1 (2%)	0

*Mallette et al: Medicine 53:127, 1954.
†Heath et al: N Engl J Med 302:189, 1980.
‡Holmes et al: Ann Surg 169:631, 1989.
§Shane and Bilezikan: Endocr Rev 3:218, 1982.
‖Fraker et al: Ann Surg 213:58, 1991.
¶The normal range for serum calcium in this study was 8.9 to 10.1 mg/dl, lower than the range reported for the others (approximately 8.8 to 10.7).
#This number included patients with osteoporosis.

kidneys and the skeleton are commonly affected. It is important to recognize the presence of cancer at the initial neck exploration because radical resection of the malignant parathyroid gland, the ipsilateral thyroid lobe, and involved adjacent soft tissue and lymph nodes offers the only possibility for cure. If the disease recurs, a repeat surgical procedure may be indicated (including resection of pulmonary or liver metastases), but usually involves resection of ipsilateral local recurrences in soft tissues or lymph nodes. Management of the severe hypercalcemia in patients with unresectable disease poses a significant challenge, as radiation and chemotherapy are generally ineffective.

Hyperparathyroid Crisis

Rarely, patients with primary hyperparathyroidism may become acutely ill with urgent symptoms that sometimes prove fatal. The term hyperparathyroid crisis has been used to describe this presentation. The onset is usually characterized by rapidly developing muscular weakness, nausea and vomiting, weight loss, fatigue, drowsiness, and confusion. Males and females are affected equally. The serum calcium concentration is extremely elevated, usually 15 mg/dl, and mild azotemia is present. This clinical picture may also be seen in patients with acute hypercalcemia accompanying other diseases. The offending parathyroid gland(s) is usually large, which is explained by the fact that larger parathyroid glands are associated with higher serum levels of calcium than smaller ones. The pathophysiology of the condition involves uncontrolled PTH secretion, followed by hypercalcemia, polyuria, dehydration, decreased renal function, and worsening hypercalcemia.

Although the definitive therapy is resection of the hyperfunctioning parathyroid tissue, operation must be postponed until the calcium concentration is lowered. The cornerstone of therapy is rehydration and diuresis. Normal saline is infused at rates between 250 and 500 ml/hr until urinary output is approximately 100 ml/hr. When urinary output becomes satisfactory, potassium chloride should be administered. The diuretic furosemide should then be used to increase urinary calcium excretion (20 to 40 mg every 8 to 12 hours). This aggressive therapy reduces serum levels of calcium to less than 12 mg/dl in the majority of patients, and then operation can be performed safely. In general, patients with primary hyperparathyroidism as the cause of severe hypercalcemia respond to saline hydration and furosemide. If a patient doesn't respond, the hypercalcemia is more likely to be due to a malignant process including parathyroid cancer and metastatic cancer from other sites. Other agents that are known to lower the serum calcium concentration should then be administered (Table 3). If primary hyperparathyroidism is the etiology of the hyperparathyroid crisis, surgical resection of the abnormal gland or glands provides dramatic reversal of the hypercalcemia. However, parathyroid surgery should not be attempted until the serum level of calcium is less than 12 to 13 mg/dl and the serum level of parathyroid hormone is determined to be elevated.

Secondary Hyperparathyroidism (Renal Osteodystrophy)

Since the initiation of maintenance dialysis and renal transplantation, the lives of patients with chronic renal failure (CRF) have been prolonged. Secondary hyperparathyroidism develops as a result of the metabolic alterations occurring in CRF. Phosphate retention and hyperphosphatemia in conjunction with a decrease in the renal production of 1,25-dihydroxy-

TABLE 3.   AGENTS USED IN THE TREATMENT OF HYPERCALCEMIA*

Agent	Dosage	Administration	Comment
Calcitonin	2–6 MRC U/kg 10–20 MRC U	Subcutaneous every 6–8 hr Intravenous, hourly	Nausea and vomiting are side effects; allergy is the only contraindication; onset of calcium-lowering effect is rapid
Mithramycin	25 µg/kg	Intravenously over 1 hr in 100 ml 0.9% saline or 5% dextrose	Contraindications are renal or hepatic dysfunction; calcium-lowering effect occurs within 24 hr; drug is useful when diuretic and intravenous saline are contraindicated; nausea and vomiting are side effects
Glucocorticoids	Prednisone 40–50 mg/day Prednisolone phosphate 40 mg	Oral Intramuscularly or intravenously every 8 hr	Lag period may be used 7–10 days; glucocorticoids are safe for short-term use; alternate-day oral program may be used for long-term use
Orthophosphate	1–2 gm/day	Oral	Dosage must be adjusted for renal impairment; soft tissue calcification may occur; intravenous phosphate is not recommended
Prostaglandin synthetase inhibitors	Indomethacin, 25–50 mg 3 times a day	Oral	Unless increased prostaglandin secretion is measured, this drug should not be used alone
Diphosphonates Etidronate	7.5 mg/kg/day	Intravenously in 250 ml saline over several hours	Effective for severe hypercalcemia caused by hyperparathyroidism or cancer; takes 2–10 days to lower calcium to normal

*From Purnell DC, van Heerden JA: Management of symptomatic hypercalcemia and hypocalcemia. World J Surg 6:702, 1982, with permission.

vitamin D_3 reduce the serum level of calcium, producing secondary hyperparathyroidism. Also, aluminum present in the dialysate water and in oral phosphate binder medications accumulates in bone and contributes substantially to the osteomalacia component of the disease. Therapy should be directed toward controlling the serum phosphate by dietary restriction and phosphate gels, maintaining adequate calcium intake, administering vitamin D sterols, and reducing aluminum in the dialysate bath and the diet.

Differential Diagnosis

Many other diseases are associated with hypercalcemia (Table 4). They must be excluded before subjecting a patient with suspected hyperparathyroidism to operation. However, the most likely cause of hypercalcemia is primary hyperparathyroidism. If the patient has hypercalcemia and elevated serum levels of parathormone on a reputable immunoassay, the diagnosis is certain. In patients with sarcoidosis or multiple myeloma, the serum globulin levels are usually elevated and there are characteristic radiographic findings. If patients with hypercalcemia are on thiazide diuretics, the drug should be discontinued and, if this is responsible, the calcium returns to normal within a few weeks. The presence of cancer is another common cause of hypercalcemia, and, generally, patients can be divided into three groups: (1) hematologic malignan-

cies (30 per cent), (2) solid tumors and lytic bone metastases (50 per cent), and (3) solid tumors without bone metastases (20 per cent). Hematologic malignancies that cause hypercalcemia include multiple myeloma, lymphosarcoma, or lymphoma. Bone lesions are lytic secondary to increased bone resorption. Bone resorption and hypercalcemia is caused by osteoclast-activating factor (OAF), a lymphokine secreted by the neoplastic lymphoid cells. Prostaglandin synthesis by monocytes can regulate OAF production. Patients with carcinoma of the breast, lung, kidney, or pancreas may have hypercalcemia from lytic bone metas-

TABLE 4.   DISEASES CAUSING HYPERCALCEMIA

Hyperparathyroidism
Malignancy
   With skeletal metastases
   Without skeletal metastases (pseudohyperparathyroidism)
Hyperthyroidism
Multiple myeloma
Sarcoidosis and other granulomatous disease
Milk-alkali syndrome
Vitamin D intoxication
Vitamin A intoxication
Paget's disease
Immobilization
Thiazide diuretics
Addisonian crisis
Familial hypocalciuric hypercalcemia
Idiopathic hypercalcemia of infancy

tases. The exact mechanism of bone resorption is unclear. It involves either the tumor cell, or OAF and prostaglandin secreted by lymphoid cells in response to tumor. Some tumors secrete a PTH-like peptide that causes hypercalcemia. This peptide is immunologically distinct from PTH so it doesn't cause false-positive results in most assays. The skeleton from these patients shows increased osteoclast bone resorption and decreased bone formation.

Localization

In the hands of an experienced surgeon, approximately 95 per cent of patients with primary hyperparathyroidism are cured at initial neck exploration. One must keep this in mind when evaluating the need for methods that can localize the site of hyperfunctioning parathyroid tissue. No study has yet demonstrated that preoperative localization reduces either the duration of the operation or the incidence of complications. Generally, localization techniques are not indicated before the first operation for hyperparathyroidism. Most surgeons feel that these techniques should be reserved for the patient undergoing reexploration after a failed initial procedure. In this situation, the normal tissue planes are obscured and dissection is tedious. High-resolution, real-time ultrasonography differs from conventional ultrasound scanning in that the emitted sound waves are of higher frequency (5 to 10 MHz), permitting better resolution of structures and limiting focal depth of visualization to shorter distances from the transducer. It is observer dependent, and in the best hands has an accuracy rate of 76 per cent. This technique may be useful in patients with hypercalcemic crisis in whom rapid diagnosis of a parathyroid mass lesion is advantageous. It images abnormal glands that are near or within the thyroid because parathyroid glands appear sonolucent compared to the more echodense thyroid. Sonographically guided fine-needle aspiration with either cytology or determination of parathyroid hormone concentration may also be helpful.

Computed tomographic (CT) scanning appears to be about equally as effective as ultrasound. It is more expensive, but is less operator dependent than sonography. Unlike ultrasound, CT images abnormal glands that are either within the anterior mediastinum or along the esophagus in the posterior neck and mediastinum. Magnetic resonance imaging (MRI) provides similar images to CT, except the abnormal gland appears bright on the T2-weighted images, which enhances tumor detection. Technetium-thallium scintigraphy depends on the uptake of ^{201}thallium by both the thyroid and parathyroid, while ^{99m}technetium is taken up only by the thyroid. The technetium image is subtracted from the thallium image by computer,

leaving only the abnormal parathyroid gland as a hot spot. This is theoretically appealing, but has a sensitivity that is less than ultrasound and CT.

Invasive localization including either selective angiography or digital subtraction angiography and selective venous sampling for PTH must be reserved for only patients who have failed prior operations. Each study is expensive and has associated complications. Arteriogram provides a blush that identifies the abnormal gland. Venous sampling provides a PTH gradient in either one side of the neck or the mediastinum that localizes the tumor. These studies have the best sensitivity of any localizing study, but their sensitivity is less than the success rate of an initial operation by an experienced surgeon. Therefore, these studies are reserved for patients who are candidates for parathyroid reoperations who have failed noninvasive imaging techniques.

Treatment

With the use of automated technology for determining the serum concentration of calcium, the diagnosis of hyperparathyroidism is made increasingly more often in asymptomatic patients. Whether all patients with hyperparathyroidism should undergo operation has been questioned, and some physicians have proposed that asymptomatic patients be followed intermittently without operative intervention. Selby and Peacock have demonstrated that postmenopausal women with primary hyperparathyroidism can be treated with estrogen to reduce bone turnover rates and serum levels of calcium. Others state that all patients with clear biochemical evidence of primary hyperparathyroidism should undergo operation. The National Institutes of Health held a recent consensus conference to address this controversy. The panel stated that there is a population of patients with primary hyperparathyroidism who can be safely followed and managed medically. Patients with only mildly elevated serum levels of calcium, no prior episodes of severe hypercalcemia, and normal renal and bone status are eligible for nonoperative management. This remains a controversial point and requires further contemplation. Before making a decision about nonoperative management, four facts should be considered. First, the ability of meticulous operation by an experienced parathyroid surgeon to cure patients is greater than 95 per cent. Second, the typical patient with no family history of endocrine disease diagnosed by screening most likely has a solitary adenoma as a cause for primary hyperparathyroidism. Third, it has been demonstrated that many of the asymptomatic patients with primary hyperparathyroidism are not without symptoms. These patients have subtle symptoms like memory loss, personality change, inability to concentrate, exercise fatigue, back pain, and others that are not uncommon in daily living that may totally disappear following successful operation. Finally, this operation can be performed with minimal complications (<1 per cent recurrent laryngeal nerve injury rate, no transfusion requirement, and essentially no mortality risk). It is due to these four facts that we contend that healthy "asymptomatic" patients with primary hyperparathyroidism should undergo operation.

Before subjecting a patient to operation, the surgeon should be confident of the diagnosis and have adequate experience to systematically explore the neck, recognizing in the process the normal and abnormal parathyroid glands. The patient should be made fully aware of the complications associated with the neck exploration, including potential damage to the superior and recurrent laryngeal nerves and the development of hypocalcemia with associated symptoms of tetany. In the asymptomatic patient, the alternative of nonoperative or medical management should be presented. Lastly, the possibility of an unsuccessful parathyroid search should be mentioned, and the patient should be made aware that repeat operation, including a mediastinal exploration, may be required if the planned operation is unsuccessful. Although the likelihood of these complications is small, it is best to discuss them prior to the initial neck exploration.

A second exploration of the neck because of failure to find the lesion at the initial procedure is very difficult and should be avoided by an assiduous primary operation. If reoperation is required, not only is parathyroid tissue more difficult to identify, but damage to the recurrent laryngeal nerve is more likely. General anesthesia is used, and the neck is opened through a transverse cervical incision. After the strap muscles are separated in the midline, a chosen lobe of the thyroid gland is elevated and rotated medially. The tissues inferior to the thyroid lobe are cleaned down to the trachea to expose the recurrent laryngeal nerve and the inferior thyroid artery. In the majority of patients, the nerve lies in the tracheoesophageal groove, less commonly lateral to the trachea, and rarely anterolateral to the trachea, where it is especially vulnerable to injury. A direct laryngeal nerve may branch off in the neck without looping around the right subclavian artery. The external branch of the superior laryngeal nerve is the most important tensor of the vocal cords, and it usually lies immediately adjacent and medial to the vascular pedicle of the superior thyroid lobe. With mobilization of the lobe, care must be taken not to injure this nerve. Four or more parathyroid glands may be present and abnormal, and the reconnaissance of the neck area requires great patience. One also needs the help of an experienced pathologist, because frozen-section identification of the parathyroid glands is helpful. It should be remembered that although the pathologist can distinguish parathyroid tissue from nonparathyroid tissue by frozen section, it is difficult to determine histologically whether parathyroid tissue is normal or abnormal. The upper parathyroid glands are more easily found and are usually located far dorsally on the surface of the thyroid lobe at the level of the upper two thirds of the gland. The lower glands are larger than the upper and less constant in location, being normally distributed from well above the upper half of the thyroid to well within the mediastinum. The lower glands are usually more anterior than the upper glands. If the upper glands are identified and normal, but either of the lower glands cannot be found, the thymus pedicle on the side of the unfound gland should be carefully examined and removed. It is possible to totally remove the thymus through the neck incision. The majority of parathyroid adenomas located in the mediastinum can be removed through the cervical incision.

If no parathyroid tissue is found after the thymus pedicle is removed, the surgeon should mobilize, examine, and palpate both lobes of the thyroid gland, because occasionally a parathyroid is completely encapsulated within the thyroid parenchyma. Removal of a thyroid lobe on the side where a parathyroid gland is not found is occasionally indicated as a last resort, but should by no means substitute for a meticulous search for parathyroid tissue. It is also helpful to follow the branches of the inferior thyroid artery, especially if one is enlarged, because these often lead to an abnormal parathyroid gland or adenoma. Because of the possibility of multiple gland involvement, every effort must be made to identify all four parathyroids. To ensure that one has actually identified parathyroid tissue, small biopsies of the suspected glands should be taken. The organs must be handled with extreme care, however, because they are delicate structures and their blood supply is easily damaged.

PARATHYROID ADENOMA. The operative management depends upon the number of enlarged parathyroid glands. The most common cause of primary hyperparathyroidism is an adenoma, a single abnormal parathyroid gland (86 per cent). Parathyroid hyperplasia or multiple gland involvement is the second most common cause (14 per cent) and generally occurs in inherited syndromes, but may also occur in the sporadic setting. Parathyroid carcinoma is a rare cause of primary hyperparathyroidism (<1 per cent) (Table 5). It may be unclear in some patients whether the diagnosis is multiple adenomas or hyperplasia. If one gland is large and the remaining three are of normal size, the diagnosis is adenoma and resection of

TABLE 5. PRIMARY HYPERPARATHYROIDISM: ETIOLOGY, INCIDENCE, PATHOLOGY, SURGERY, AND OUTCOME

Diagnosis	Etiology	Incidence	Pathology	Surgical Procedure	Recurrence Rate
Adenoma	Associated with irradiation	86%	Single enlarged gland, brownish red	Resection of abnormal gland, biopsy normal glands	<1%
Hyperplasia	Familial pattern	14%	Multiple abnormal glands, brownish red	Either 3.5-gland resection or 4-gland resection with autograft	10–30%
Carcinoma	Some families reported	<1%	Massively enlarged gland, locally invasive, whitish grey, firm to palpation	Resection of abnormal gland with ipsilateral thyroid and medial lymph nodes	50%

the enlarged gland is curative in virtually all patients. In the event that two or three parathyroid glands are enlarged, most surgeons resect them, leaving the normal-sized glands undisturbed except for a biopsy. The question of whether these represent multiple adenomas or primary hyperplasia has not been resolved.

PARATHYROID HYPERPLASIA (GENERALIZED [FOUR-GLAND] PARATHYROID ENLARGEMENT). This phenomenon occurs in two forms: water-clear cell hyperplasia and chief cell hyperplasia. Water-clear cell hyperplasia is indistinguishable from the hyperparathyroidism associated with single-gland disease, but the gross appearance at operation is characteristic. All four glands are diffusely enlarged and dark brown with uneven surfaces. Microscopically, the glands are composed almost entirely of water-clear cells. In primary chief cell hyperplasia, the glands are often nodular and red-brown and grossly are characterized by the presence of fibrous septa within the parenchyma. Histologically, chief cells predominate, but there are also nests of water-clear and oxyphil cells. It is now known that chief cell hyperplasia is the pathologic entity most commonly associated with familial hyperparathyroidism, particularly MEN-I and MEN-IIa. The standard therapy for patients with hyperparathyroidism and generalized parathyroid enlargement has been radical subtotal (3.5-gland) parathyroidectomy. However, this procedure has been associated with a high incidence of persistent and recurrent hyperparathyroidism (7 to 13 per cent) and a similar incidence of hypoparathyroidism (5 to 20 per cent). Because of the relatively increased incidence of postoperative hypoparathyroidism and hyperparathyroidism in patients with "parathyroid hyperplasia," we have elected to manage them by total parathyroidectomy and heterotopic autotransplantation.

MEDIASTINAL EXPLORATION. If after diligent search in the neck, including exploration of the upper mediastinum, retroesophageal area, carotid sheaths, thyroid gland, and undescended location near the carotid bifurcation, no enlarged parathyroid gland has been found, a decision must be made regarding median sternotomy. Most surgeons favor delay of this procedure, reasoning that the blood supply to the hyperfunctional gland might have been damaged during manipulation or that the pathologist may find the abnormal gland on further sectioning of the submitted tissues. Median sternotomy is indicated in only about 1 to 2 per cent of patients with primary hyperparathyroidism. In mediastinal exploration, a vertical incision is made from the center of the cervical incision to the xiphoid. The sternum is completely divided in the midline, and a retractor is inserted. Any remaining thymus tissue is first isolated and examined, because an adenoma is most likely found associated with this structure located anterior to the great vessels. In parathyroid adenomas that are true mediastinal organs, the blood supply is often from the mediastinal vessels and not the inferior thyroid artery. If the anterior mediastinal exploration is negative, the posterior mediastinum is next examined, especially posterior and lateral to the trachea. Mediastinal parathyroid glands are usually located within the thymus, posterior to the thymus along the aortic arch, or rarely within the aortopulmonary window.

SURGERY FOR PERSISTENT OR RECURRENT HYPERPARATHYROIDISM. Persistent hyperthyroidism is defined as no change in serum level of calcium following the initial operative procedure. Recurrent hyperparathyroidism means that the serum level of calcium dropped into the normal range for at least 6 months, then the patient developed recurrent hypercalcemia. Persistent disease generally implies missed adenoma or unrecognized parathyroid hyperplasia. Recurrent disease implies parathyroid cancer, incompletely resected adenoma or hyperplasia. Evaluation should begin with reconfirmation of the diagnosis of primary hyperparathyroidism. Familial hypercalcemic hypocalciuria should be excluded by urinary calcium excretion. The patient should have symptoms related to the disease, including kidney stones or nephrocalcinosis, bone disease, and/or serum level of calcium greater than 12 mg/dl. Noninvasive and invasive localization procedures are necessary to guide the operation. Reoperations for primary hyperparathyroidism are associated with lower success rates than initial operations (80 versus 95 per cent) and greater complication rates (6 versus 1 per cent recurrent laryngeal nerve injury, 20 versus 1 per cent hypoparathyroidism). However, with experience, proper selection of patients, and use of localization studies, most of these patients have successful reoperations without complication.

MANAGEMENT OF SECONDARY HYPERPARATHYROIDISM. There are four indications for parathyroidectomy in patients with secondary hypoparathyroidism: (1) persistent and symptomatic hypercalcemia in prospective renal transplant patients, (2) bone pain or pathologic fractures, (3) ectopic calcification, and (4) intractable itching. These patients can be managed by subtotal (3.5-gland) parathyroidectomy or total parathyroidectomy with heterotopic (forearm) autotransplantation. Andress and associates have demonstrated that parathyroidectomy can actually enhance aluminum deposition in the bone so that all aluminum excess should be corrected by chelation before operation.

PARATHYROID TRANSPLANTATION. There are certain conditions in patients with hyperparathyroidism in which it is preferable to reduce the total parathyroid mass and yet still have a portion of functional parathyroid tissue. As previously mentioned, parathyroid hyperplasia, either primary or secondary, has been most frequently treated by subtotal 3.5-gland parathyroidectomy. If patients develop hypercalcemia after this operation, a second neck exploration with all its attendant risks is usually required. It has been demonstrated in animals that parathyroid glands can be transplanted. The success of the transplantation depends upon the freshly removed parathyroid tissue being sliced into very small pieces for subsequent implantation into a muscle bed. This technique has been used in patients with both primary and secondary parathyroid hyperplasia. A total 4-gland parathyroidectomy is performed, and approximately twenty 1- by 2-mm fragments of parathyroid tissue are autografted to the nondominant forearm musculature. If the patient subsequently develops hypercalcemia from the grafted parathyroid tissue, a few of the pieces can be removed. The fact that the transplanted parathyroid tissue functions is documented by the patient's maintaining normocalcemia with the grafted tissue as the only source of parathyroid hormone. Furthermore, large concentrations of parathyroid hormone are detectable in the antecubital vein draining the graft bed compared with normal parathyroid hormone levels in the contralateral antecubital vein. It has also been demonstrated that parathyroid glands can be viably stored

frozen in dimethyl sulfoxide and autologous serum. This capability offers the surgeon great versatility. When one is uncertain about the amount of parathyroid tissue remaining in the neck following resection of hyperplastic parathyroid tissue, a portion can be frozen viably to be grafted at a subsequent time. If the patient remains hypoparathyroid, part of the frozen autologous parathyroid tissue can be grafted months later into the forearm under local anesthesia.

Hypoparathyroidism

The most common cause of hypoparathyroidism is damage to the parathyroid glands during operation involving the thyroid, and it occurs more commonly with total thyroidectomy. It is not at all unusual for patients undergoing operative procedures on the thyroid gland to experience a drop in serum level of calcium after operation. This probably represents bruising or compromise of the blood supply to the parathyroids, and the hypocalcemia is transient. Following successful surgical correction of hyperparathyroidism in patients with significant bone disease, there may be excessive calcium demands for skeletal deposition, termed "bone hunger." Serum calcium reaches its lowest level in about 48 to 72 hours and returns to normal 2 to 3 days thereafter. The major signs and symptoms of hypocalcemia are directly attributable to the reduction of plasma level of ionized calcium, which leads to increased neuromuscular excitability. Clinically, the earliest manifestations are numbness and tingling in the circumoral area, the fingers, and the toes. Mental symptoms are common, and patients are anxious, depressed or, occasionally, confused. Tetany may develop, characterized by carpopedal spasms, tonic clonic convulsions, and laryngeal stridor, which may prove fatal. On physical examination, contraction of the facial muscles is elicited by tapping on the facial nerve anterior to the ear (Chvostek's sign). This sign is present in a small number of normal persons. Trousseau's sign is elicited by occluding blood flow to the forearm for 3 minutes. The development of carpal spasm indicates hypocalcemia. The treatment of acute hypocalcemia is the intravenous administration of calcium gluconate or calcium chloride. Vitamin D and oral calcium are used for long-term management.

REFERENCES

Andress DL, Oh SM, Maloney NA, Sherard DJ: Effect of parathyroidectomy on bone aluminum deposition in chronic renal failure. N Engl J Med 312:468, 1985.
Christensson T: Hyperparathyroidism and radiation therapy. Ann Intern Med 89:216, 1978.

Friedman E, Sakaguchi K, Bale AE, Falchetti A, Streeter E, Zimering MB, Weinstein LS, McBride WO, Nakamura Y, Brandi M, Norton JA, Aurbach GD, Spiegel AM, Marx SJ: Clonality of parathyroid tumors in familial multiple endocrine neoplasia type 1. N Engl J Med *321*:1057, 1989.

Motokura T, Bloom T, Kim HG, et al: A novel cyclin encoded by a bc11-linked candidate oncogene. Nature *350*:512, 1991.

Potts JT Jr, Ackerman IP, Barker CF, et al: Diagnosis and management of asymptomatic primary hyperparathyroidism: Consensus development conference statement. Ann Intern Med *114*:593, 1991.

Selby PL, Peacock M: Ethinyl estradiol and norethindrone in the treatment of primary hyperparathyroidism in postmenopausal women. N Engl J Med *314*:1481, 1986.

24

THE PITUITARY AND ADRENAL GLANDS

RICHARD F. GROSSMAN, M.D.   STEFANIE S. JEFFREY, M.D.
ORLO H. CLARK, M.D.

THE PITUITARY AND HYPOTHALAMUS

Anatomy

The pituitary gland normally measures 13 mm by 10 mm by 6 mm and weighs about 0.5 gm. It lies within the bony confines of the sella turcica in the sphenoid bone at the base of the skull. Superiorly, the pituitary is bounded by the diaphragma sellae, which is a fibrous reflection of the dura (Fig. 1). Although in 50 per cent of individuals the diaphragma sellae tightly adheres to the pituitary stalk, in 40 per cent there is an opening around the pituitary stalk greater than 5 mm, and in 10 per cent of patients the diaphragma is very thin. In patients with an incomplete diaphragma sellae, pituitary tumors may preferentially extend superiorly into the region of the optic chiasm and suprasellar cistern. If the diaphragma sellae tightly adheres to the pituitary stalk, pituitary tumors tend to extend inferiorly into the sphenoid sinus. The lateral boundary of the sella turcica is formed by the cavernous sinus, which contains the intracavernous portion of the internal carotid arteries and cranial nerves III, IV, and VI.

The pituitary gland is divided anatomically and physiologically into anterior (adenohypophysis) and posterior (neurohypophysis) lobes. The superior hypophyseal artery, a branch of the internal carotid, supplies the anterior lobe of the pituitary, the stalk, and the median eminence. The anterior lobe also receives blood from a portal system from the hypothalamus. The inferior hypophyseal artery, also a branch of the

internal carotid artery, supplies the posterior lobe (Fig. 2). Venous blood drains into the cavernous sinus.

The neuronal connections between the hypothalamus and the pituitary differ for the adenohypophysis versus the neurohypophysis. Axons of the parvicellular neurons of the hypothalamus terminate in the median eminence and regulate the adenohypophysis through their secretion of specific releasing and inhibiting factors into the portal venous system. In general, one specific cell type in the anterior pituitary is thought to interact with one group of releasing and inhibiting factors and to secrete one polypeptide hormone; however, the gonadotroph cell is known to secrete both luteinizing hormone (LH) and follicle-stimulating hormone (FSH). The axons that connect the hypothalamus to the neurohypophysis originate from cells in the supraoptic and paraventricular nuclei and are referred to as magnocellular neurons owing to the relatively large size of their cell bodies (Fig. 3). In contrast to the parvicellular neurons, which produce and release factors that act on the pituitary to influence its production of hormones in situ, within the magnocellular neurons of the supraoptic and paraventricular nuclei are produced the very hormones (antidiuretic hormone [ADH] and oxytocin, respectively), albeit in immature form, that the posterior pituitary secretes after cleaving them from their carrier molecules.

Physiology

Anterior Pituitary

The following hormones are secreted by the anterior pituitary gland: growth hormone (GH), adrenocorti-

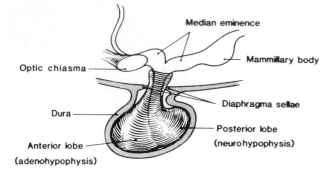

Figure 1. Anatomic relationships of hypothalamus, diaphragma sellae, and pituitary.

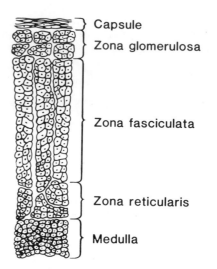

Figure 3. Neuronal connections between the hypothalamus and neurohypophysis.

cotropic hormone (ACTH), prolactin (PRL), thyroid-stimulating hormone (TSH), luteinizing hormone (LH), follicle stimulating hormone (FSH), endorphins, and enkephalins.

GROWTH HORMONE. Growth hormone is a large polypeptide comprised of 191 amino acids (molecular weight, 21,500) that is secreted by somatotroph cells. The secretion of GH is stimulated by growth hormone–releasing hormone (GH-RH), synthesized in the parvicellular hypothalamic neurons. Somatostatin, another hypothalamic factor, directly inhibits the secretion of GH. Growth hormone secretion increases during periods of physical exercise, stress, hypoglycemia, or protein depletion. Hypothalamic secretion of GH occurs periodically throughout the day, with a prominent surge during the early morning hours. The major metabolic effects of growth hormone include stimulation of the growth of the musculoskeletal system and solid viscera. It antagonizes the effects of insulin peripherally but, within the pancreas, stimulates insulin secretion.

ADRENOCORTICOTROPIC HORMONE. Adrenocorticotropic hormone is synthesized by corticotroph cells and is a peptide made up of 39 amino acids (mo-

lecular weight, 4500). The secretion of ACTH is negatively regulated by feedback from adrenocortical hormones (primarily cortisol) and stimulated by the release of corticotropin-releasing factor (CRF) by the hypothalamus. The secretion of ACTH follows a diurnal rhythm, with peak secretion during the early morning and a nadir in the late afternoon and evening. In addition to direct stimulation by the hypothalamus, a variety of other factors may increase ACTH secretion, including stress, trauma, fever, hypoglycemia, and exposure to extreme cold. Adrenocorticotropic hormone is initially synthesized as part of a larger precursor molecule (prohormone) known as proopiomelanocortin (POMC). Proopiomelanocortin contains a number of active polypeptides including ACTH, melanocyte-stimulating hormone (MSH), and β-endorphin, which are later cleaved from this molecule. The primary metabolic effects of ACTH are to stimulate

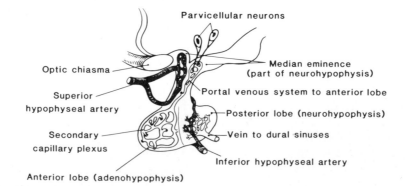

Figure 2. Vascular system of the pituitary.

the growth of the adrenal cortex and the production and secretion of adrenocorticosteroid hormones.

PROLACTIN. Prolactin is a large, 198–amino acid polypeptide hormone (molecular weight, 23,000) secreted by the lactotroph cells. A prolactin-releasing factor (PRF) has recently been identified in the posterior pituitary, but is not yet well characterized. Suckling also stimulates PRL release, whereupon PRL induces the female breast to lactate.

THYROID-STIMULATING HORMONE. Thyroid-stimulating hormone, or thyrotropin, is a glycoprotein (molecular weight, 28,000) synthesized by the thyrotroph cells in response to stimulation by the hypothalamic tripeptide thyrotropin-releasing hormone (TRH). Thyroid-stimulating hormone stimulates thyroid growth and the synthesis of thyroid hormones, and circulating thyroid hormones directly inhibit TSH release. Peak release of TSH occurs in the early morning.

FOLLICLE-STIMULATING AND LUTEINIZING HORMONE. Follicle-stimulating hormone and LH are glycoproteins (molecular weight, 29,000 for each) secreted by the gonadotroph cells. Structurally, FSH and LH have identical alpha subunits and different beta subunits. Hypothalamic regulation of both FSH and LH is under the control of a single factor known as gonadotropin-releasing hormone (GRH), which is secreted in a pulsatile manner. In the female, FSH and LH undergo cyclical secretion in response to a complex interaction of estradiol, progesterone, and GRH pulsations during the follicular and luteal phases of the menstrual cycle. A major surge in LH (and to a much lesser extent, FSH) occurs just prior to ovulation. Follicle-stimulating hormone aids in the development of ovarian follicles and stimulates them to produce estrogen. Luteinizing hormone maintains the corpus luteum and stimulates its production of progesterone. In males, FSH promotes spermatogenesis, while LH stimulates production of testosterone.

ENDORPHINS AND ENKEPHALINS. Endorphins and enkephalins are peptides that bind to opiate receptors in the central nervous system and gut. They arise through the cleavage of POMC secreted by the corticotroph cells. Their physiologic role appears to be as mediators of stress and pain, and they also influence the secretion of several of the other pituitary hormones.

Posterior Pituitary

ANTIDIURETIC HORMONE. The magnocellular neurons of the supraoptic nuclei synthesize a large prohormone that migrates to the posterior pituitary. The prohormone is then cleaved, with separation of ADH from its carrier protein, neurophysin II. Antidiuretic hormone acts on the kidney to promote the reabsorption of filtered water, thereby regulating plasma volume and osmolarity. Antidiuretic hormone secretion rises when plasma volume decreases by 5 per cent or more and when plasma osmolarity rises above 285 mOsm. Conversely, reduced serum osmolarity inhibits the secretion of ADH. Antidiuretic hormone is also known as vasopressin.

OXYTOCIN. Oxytocin is structurally similar to ADH, is also synthesized as a large prohormone within the magnocellular neurons, and is cleaved from its carrier, neurophysin I, in the posterior pituitary. Uterine distention and suckling are stimuli for the release of oxytocin. Oxytocin stimulates uterine contraction during labor and promotes milk secretion in the lactating breast.

Pituitary Tumors

RADIOLOGIC EVALUATION. Although plain films of the skull may demonstrate bony abnormality of the sella, contrast-enhanced computed tomography (CT) or magnetic resonance imaging (MRI) are the imaging methods of choice for diagnosing pituitary tumors. Following injection of intravenous iodinated contrast, the normal pituitary stalk and body demonstrate significant enhancement on CT scan. The excellent density discrimination of CT affords ready detection of abnormal pituitary enlargement and extension of pituitary tumors either inferiorly into the sphenoid sinus or superiorly through the diaphragma sellae. Magnetic resonance imaging has the advantage of using neither iodinated contrast nor ionizing radiation and, with gadolinium injections, is a more sensitive technique than CT scanning.

CLASSIFICATION OF PITUITARY TUMORS. Historically, pituitary tumors were classified according to the appearance of different cell types under light microscopy and were divided into chromophobic, eosinophilic, and basophilic types. With the development of immunohistochemistry, it is now possible to classify pituitary tumors according to the type of hormone secreted (endocrine-active tumors). Immunohistochemistry also identifies tumors that are nonsecretory (endocrine-inactive).

Endocrine-Inactive Tumors

Patients with endocrine-inactive tumors ("chromophobe adenomas" under the old nomenclature) may present with visual disturbances, such as bitemporal hemianopsia, owing to compression of the optic chiasm. Hormonal symptoms, if present, result from tumoral compression of the adenohypophysis with loss of secretion of GH, LH/FSH, TSH, and, ultimately, ACTH. Rarely, diabetes insipidus occurs through decreased secretion of ADH. In a small percentage of patients, tumor necrosis occurs with subarachnoid bleeding, which may be associated with acute loss of vision. It may also cause panhypopituitarism, a dramatic clinical event termed "pituitary apoplexy." Pituitary glands in pregnant women may also infarct postpartum, causing a form of pituitary apoplexy called Sheehan's syndrome.

The differential diagnosis of endocrine-inactive mass lesions in the vicinity of the pituitary includes juxtacellular meningiomas, aneurysms, hypothalamic gliomas, chordomas, teratoid tumors, gliomas of the optic chiasma, metastatic tumors, and granulomas. Craniopharyngiomas, however, are the most important nonpituitary tumors that arise in the vicinity of the sella turcica. They originate from embryologic rest cells of Rathke's pouch and, though they may be cystic or solid, contain calcifications in 75 per cent of cases, a feature helpful in making the diagnosis. They may arise above or below the diaphragma sellae. Compression of the pituitary may cause pituitary deficiency with absent or arrested puberty, diabetes insipidus, and dwarfism (in children), while compression of the optic chiasm or surrounding cerebrum may cause visual field defects and headache. Treatment is by surgical excision, when possible, versus cyst drainage and radiation therapy.

Endocrine-Active Tumors

PROLACTIN-SECRETING TUMORS (PROLACTINOMA). Prolactinomas are the most common endocrine-active pituitary tumors, comprising 30 to 60 per cent of pituitary neoplasms. In females, hypersecretion of PRL may produce amenorrhea and galactorrhea. In males, symptoms usually do not occur until the tumor is large enough to cause mass effects, with hormonal symptoms such as impotence and decreased libido occurring in only 15 per cent . Thus, the diagnosis is usually established earlier in women. Contrast-enhanced CT or MRI is used to exclude a PRL-secreting adenoma, but may not demonstrate microadenomas (< 1 cm). Elevated levels of prolactin must be documented to establish the diagnosis. The normal level of prolactin is less than 20 ng/ml, and in patients with levels exceeding 150 ng/ml, prolactinoma is almost invariably present. However, mild elevations of prolactin may be produced by renal failure, hypothyroidism, cirrhosis, drugs, stress, nipple stimulation, spinal cord lesions, hypothalamic lesions, or estrogen therapy. Transsphenoidal resection is recommended for larger or growing lesions (macroadenomas) and for women with small lesions who wish to become pregnant. Medical therapy with bromocriptine, which antagonizes PRL (and GH) release by elevating dopamine levels within the pituitary portal circulation, is used to treat relapses after operation and is recommended by

some authorities as the initial therapy in a variety of instances, such as very large, invasive prolactinomas. Patients with prolactinomas over 2 cm in diameter or with basal prolactin levels over 200 ng/ml may require combined therapy with surgery, radiation, and bromocriptine.

GROWTH HORMONE-SECRETING TUMORS. The syndrome that results from excess secretion of GH by an endocrine-active pituitary tumor is termed "acromegaly" in adults and "giantism" in children. The most prevalent sign of acromegaly is acral enlargement; that is, enlargement of the hands and feet. However, growth hormone promotes the growth of many tissues. Therefore an overall coarsening of facial features, frontal bossing, and jaw protrusion; along with enlargement of the heart, liver, spleen, and kidney; and kyphosis, hypertension, atherosclerosis, and osteoarthropathy also occur. Cardiovascular disease is the most common cause of death in untreated patients. While the classic clinical features may take years to develop, assays for serum GH permit early diagnosis. Growth hormone–secreting tumors are often associated with menstrual abnormalities in women because the tumor compresses the pituitary gland or pituitary stalk or because the tumor secretes PRL along with GH. Treatment is by surgical resection often followed by radiation therapy and is directed at decreasing GH levels below 5 ng/ml. If extirpation and radiation fail, high doses of bromocriptine may be used in an attempt to suppress GH secretion. Bromocriptine reduces GH levels in 60 to 80 per cent of patients, but in only about 40 per cent do the levels become normal (< 10 ng/ml).

CORTICOTROPIN-SECRETING TUMORS (CUSHING'S DISEASE). Excess pituitary secretion of ACTH causing hypercortisolism and bilateral adrenal cortical hyperplasia is known as Cushing's disease. Cushing's disease is distinguished from Cushing's syndrome, which refers to any state of glucocorticoid excess, including excess glucocorticoid production by adrenal tumors, glucocorticoid administration, and ectopic (i.e., nonpituitary) production of ACTH. Adults with longstanding hypercortisolism have a typical body habitus of truncal obesity, thin extremities, and fat accumulation on the posterior neck ("buffalo hump") and face ("moon facies"). Cushing's disease is the cause of 80 per cent of cases of Cushing's syndrome, and approximately 80 per cent of these are due to pituitary microadenomas. The remainder of cases of Cushing's disease are caused by diffuse hyperplasia or macroadenomas. If CT scan or MRI of a patient with hypercortisolism fails to reveal a pituitary lesion, as occurs frequently with microadenomas because 50 per cent are less than 5 mm in diameter, bilateral selective venous catheterization of the petrosal sinuses during CRF administration may be performed. Pituitary microadenomas have an exaggerated ACTH response to CRF. If these tests are equivocal, an exhaustive search must be made for an adrenal cause of cortisol excess and for ectopic sources of ACTH, such as oat cell carcinoma of the lung. (The evaluation of the patient with Cushing's syndrome is discussed in greater detail in the section "The Adrenal Gland," later in this chapter.)

Patients with Cushing's disease are treated with exploration of the sella and resection of the pituitary gland. Pituitary procedures can be performed through either a transsphenoidal or transcranial approach. The former is less traumatic and preferred for tumors 1 cm or less in diameter. Surgical excision produces remission in 60 to 90 per cent of patients with microadenomas, although the recurrence rate is 10 to 15 per cent. Adrenocorticotropic hormone secretion often ceases for 6 to 12 months after surgery, so postoperative replacement with cortisone must be administered. The outcome of surgical treatment in patients with macroadenomas and in those with suprasellar extension is poorer (25 to 50 per cent success rate). If no adenoma is found, a total hypophysectomy may be performed, which effectuates panhypopituitarism and necessitates permanent endocrine replacement.

Radiation or heavy particle therapy may be required for patients with unresectable or recurrent pituitary tumors. Up to 90 per cent of patients so treated may experience remission and restoration of the normal circadian rhythm of ACTH secretion, but the response time is slow, often taking 6 to 18 months. Until the effects of radiation are realized, chemotherapy with cyproheptadine, a serotonin antagonist, may be used to suppress ACTH secretion.

THE EMPTY SELLA SYNDROME. This syndrome refers to the enlargement of the sella turcica, and its name belies the persistence of normal pituitary function in most patients. The sella is enlarged usually as the result of asymptomatic extension of the subarachnoid space through a defect in the diaphragma sellae, and often, there is associated cerebrospinal fluid (CSF) hypertension. Computed tomographic scan or MRI in such cases reveals a CSF-containing space within the sella. Other causes of the empty sella syndrome include loss of pituitary mass and, often, pituitary function, degenerating and necrosing tumors, gummas, or other inflammatory lesions. If enlargement is due to a pituitary adenoma, a syndrome of hormonal excess may exist.

THE ADRENAL GLAND

Anatomy

The adrenals are a pair of pyramid-shaped glands located one each on the superior medial aspect of the upper pole of the kidneys, each weighing approximately 4 gm. There are usually three main adrenal arteries, arising from the inferior phrenic artery superiorly, the aorta medially, and the renal artery inferiorly. A single vein generally drains each adrenal. On the right, the adrenal vein is short and drains directly into the inferior vena cava. On the left, the adrenal vein drains into the left renal vein or, rarely, the vena cava directly.

Adrenal Histology

The adrenal cortex is physiologically and histologically different from the adrenal medulla. The cortex is derived from mesoderm and demonstrates three separate functional zones: the zona glomerulosa, the zona fasciculata, and the inner zona reticularis (Fig. 4). Aldosterone is synthesized in the zona glomerulosa. Synthesis of cortisol and other glucocorticoids as well as production of adrenal androgens and small amounts of estrogens occur in both the zona fasciculata and zona reticularis. The adrenal medulla is derived from ectodermal cells of the neural crest and is a site of production of the class of neurotransmitters called catecholamines.

Physiology of the Adrenal Cortex

The adrenal cortex is the primary site of synthesis of the glucocorticoids (cortisol and corticosterone) and mineralocorticoids (aldosterone). Each of the adrenocortical hormones derives from a common precursor: cholesterol. The precursor to all the sex hormones (androstenedione), a weak androgen (dehydroepiandrosterone [DHEA]), and progesterone are intermediates in the pathway, and the former two can accumulate

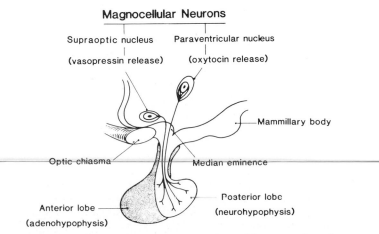

Figure 4. Diagrammatic representation of human adrenal cortical histology.

in a variety of enzyme-deficiency states (the adreno-genital syndromes). As noted earlier, the hypothalamus releases CRF, stimulating the anterior pituitary to release ACTH, which in turn directly acts on the zona fasciculata and zona reticularis to promote glucocorticoid production and secretion. A negative feedback system regulates glucocorticoid secretion: increasing serum levels of cortisol inhibit ACTH release, even in the face of constant CRF levels, causing decreased cortisol production. Secretion of cortisol follows a remarkably constant diurnal rhythm. Peak periods of cortisol secretion occur between approximately 6:00 and 8:00 a.m. The lowest level of cortisol secretion is generally between 10:00 p.m. and 2:00 a.m. In patients with Cushing's syndrome, this pattern of diurnal variation in cortisol levels is lost.

Cortisol, like all steroid hormones, enters the target cell by diffusion and acts directly in the nucleus to influence RNA synthesis. Cortisol is metabolized in the liver, and the inactive metabolites conjugated with glucuronate are excreted in the urine. The amount of cortisol excreted into the urine is small, but it may be measured and reflects the overall level of cortisol synthesis. The metabolic effects of glucocorticoids oppose those of insulin and are mainly catabolic, except in the liver. Glucocorticoids increase lipolysis, protein breakdown, and nitrogen excretion, and inhibit protein synthesis. This increases substrate delivery to the liver where glucocorticoids promote gluconeogenesis. In addition, glucocorticoids possess immunosuppressive and anti-inflammatory properties mediated by several mechanisms, including T-cell cytolysis, reduced lymphocyte adherence to vascular endothelium, antagonism of the effects of migration inhibitory factor (MIF), and impaired histamine release. They retard wound healing by impairing collagen formation and fibroblast function. Prolonged exposure to supraphysiologic levels of glucocorticoids causes a chronic catabolic state, with muscle wasting, insulin-resistant diabetes mellitus and, in adults, redistribution of body fat characterized by truncal or centripetal obesity. Both cellular and humoral immunity may be suppressed, predisposing the patient to life-threatening infection.

Androgens and estrogens are synthesized in far greater amounts by the gonads than by the adrenals, and gonadal steroidogenesis is primarily controlled by LH and FSH. However, abnormally high levels of adrenal androgen accumulate in the pathologic conditions of adrenogenital syndrome, congenital adrenal hyperplasia, and some adrenocortical tumors. Androgens directly stimulate growth of body hair and development of muscle mass as well as growth of the genitalia. Androgen excess in developing girls causes masculinization with clitoral hypertrophy and labial

fusion. In young males, it produces mild enlargement of the genitalia and atrophy of the suppressed testicles.

The primary mineralocorticoid is aldosterone, and its major metabolic function is to conserve sodium and excrete potassium. The renin-angiotensin system is the primary regulatory mechanism governing aldosterone secretion. Renin is an enzyme produced by the kidney in response to a decrease in serum sodium concentration or a decrease in mean renal arterial pressure. Renin catalyzes the conversion of angiotensinogen to angiotensin I, which is then converted in the lung to angiotensin II by the angiotensin-converting enzyme (ACE). Angiotensin II is an extremely potent vasoconstrictor that acts directly upon the glomerulosa cells of the adrenal cortex to stimulate aldosterone synthesis. An elevated serum potassium level also stimulates aldosterone secretion. Aldosterone stimulates the renal tubule to excrete potassium and hydrogen ion in exchange for sodium. Excess aldosterone causes hypokalemia, metabolic alkalosis, and hypertension.

Physiology of the Adrenal Medulla

The primary secretions of the adrenal medulla are the catecholamines dopamine, norepinephrine, and epinephrine. Epinephrine comprises 80 per cent of the catecholamine content of the adrenal medulla and is usually not produced elsewhere in the body (except the organ of Zuckerkandl), while the other catecholamines are synthesized in the brain and sympathetic neurons, as well as in the adrenal. Epinephrine affects a wide variety of tissues, producing a response that is dependent on the tissue type and its expression of β versus α receptors. Representative β responses include stimulation of heart rate and contractility; enhanced lipolysis and intestinal relaxation (β_1 receptor); and bronchodilatation, vasodilatation, and uterine relaxation (β_2 receptor). Certain α responses are contrary to the β responses (e.g., vasoconstriction and uterine contraction), and these predominate in response to stimulation with norepinephrine, or epinephrine at higher levels. Catecholamines are rendered inactive by the enzymatic action of catechol-O-methyl transferase (COMT) or monoamine oxidase (MAO). Their metabolites (normetanephrine, metanephrine, and vanillylmandelic acid) can be measured in the urine and are useful in diagnosing pheochromocytoma, a tumor of neural crest origin.

Adrenal Imaging and Diagnosis of Adrenal Masses

Computed tomography and MRI are noninvasive imaging techniques that can identify adrenal lesions as small as 1 cm. Incidental adrenal masses are noted in about 1.5 per cent of abdominal CT scans performed for other clinical indications. When such a lesion is without endocrine activity (i.e., nonfunctioning), less than 3.5 cm in size, homogeneous, with a smooth capsule and without adjacent adenopathy, the patient may be followed with a repeat CT scan in 3 to 6 months. All adrenal masses that increase in size or have endocrine function should be resected. Lesions larger than 3.5 cm, whether functioning or not, should be resected, as the risk of adrenal carcinoma is higher.

Bilateral adrenal masses are seen with pheochromocytomas, adrenal metastases, adrenal hyperplasia, and bilateral adrenal hemorrhage. Diagnosis of pheochromocytoma may also be aided by radionuclide scanning using the agent ^{131}I-metaiodobenzylguanidine (^{131}I-MIBG). Scintiscanning with NP-59 ([6β-^{131}I]iodomethyl-19-norcholesterol) for primary hyperaldosteronism may differentiate between adenoma and bilateral hyperplasia and is helpful in the evaluation of patients with aldosterone excess. When suspected, small (< 1 cm) functioning lesions in patients with primary hyperaldosteronism are not detected by CT, adrenal venous catheterization and sampling to document elevated levels of hormone secretion may be necessary for tumor localization. A simultaneous serum cortisol level is obtained to be certain the sample has been obtained directly from the adrenal vein.

Cushing's Syndrome

Cushing's syndrome is the clinical state that follows hypercortisolism of any etiology. There are three categories of lesion that produce Cushing's syndrome: (1) Cushing's disease, the overproduction of ACTH by the pituitary, is the cause of hypercortisolism in 80 per cent of cases of Cushing's syndrome; (2) excess corticosteroid secretion stimulated by an ectopic source of ACTH production accounts for about 10 per cent of cases; and (3) primary overproduction of cortisol by an adrenal adenoma, carcinoma, or bilateral nodular hyperplasia accounts for the remaining 10 per cent of cases. (The aforementioned form of nodular hyperplasia is primary and of adrenal origin, differing from the secondary hyperplasia induced by Cushing's disease.) Exogenously administered steroids may also produce the syndrome.

Clinical Features

Cushing's syndrome is more common in women than men and has a peak incidence at between 20 and 30 years of age. Most cases of nonpituitary Cushing's syndrome, as noted above, are caused by adrenal adenoma or ectopic sources of ACTH secretion, and the former is more common in females than in males. A

rare cause is adrenocortical carcinoma, which occurs most often in patients between 30 and 50 years of age. It is a highly aggressive malignancy rarely cured by current therapies. Approximately two thirds of these tumors have endocrine function and may produce Cushing's syndrome, virilization or feminization, or hyperaldosteronism. An abdominal mass may be palpated in approximately half these patients and the tumor may be identified by CT scan or MRI. Bilateral nodular hyperplasia is the most common cause of Cushing's syndrome in children, accounting for some 2 per cent of all patients with Cushing's syndrome. The most common source of ectopically produced ACTH is oat cell carcinoma of the lung, other sources including carcinoma of the pancreas, medullary thyroid carcinoma, thymoma, bronchial adenomas, and carcinoid tumors. Many of these tumors are highly malignant, and often the metabolic effects of the tumor are more prominent than the effects of cortisol excess, so the patient appears cachectic rather than cushingoid.

Many of the symptoms and signs of Cushing's syndrome follow the excess secretion of cortisol. The most specific are muscle wasting, truncal obesity, hirsutism, fungal infections (tinea versicola), purple striae, easy bruisability, and hyperpigmentation (Table 1). If left untreated, the disease is usually fatal due to the effects of muscle wasting, atherosclerosis, and hypertension, or as a result of infection.

Diagnosis

The diagnosis of Cushing's syndrome is made by the demonstration of hypercortisolism. Cortisol levels may be assayed in a 24-hour urine collection or measured in plasma. Plasma levels may be normal or high, but remain relatively constant without the normal di-

TABLE 1. CLINICAL MANIFESTATIONS OF CUSHING'S SYNDROME*

Manifestation	Incidence (%)
Obesity	95
Hypertension	85
Glucosuria and decreased glucose tolerance	80
Menstrual and sexual dysfunction	76
Hirsutism and acne	72
Striae	67
Weakness	65
Osteoporosis	55
Easy bruisability	55
Psychiatric disturbances	50
Edema	46
Polyuria	16
Ocular changes	8

* From Frohlich ED: Pathophysiology: Altered Regulatory Mechnaisms in Diseases. Philadelphia, JB Lippincott Company, 1984, with permission.

urnal variation, the absence of which may be detected by measuring plasma cortisol at 8:00 a.m. and midnight. Patients with Cushing's disease, or Cushing's syndrome due to ectopic ACTH production, have mild to markedly elevated plasma ACTH levels, respectively, whereas in adrenal Cushing's, ACTH levels are suppressed by the intact feedback mechanism of cortisol on the pituitary. A variety of tests is used to differentiate between a pituitary, ectopic ACTH, or adrenal etiology of Cushing's syndrome (Table 2).

DEXAMETHASONE SUPPRESSION TEST. The dexamethasone suppression test is useful in distinguishing pituitary from adrenal causes of hypercortisolism. Dexamethasone is a synthetic corticosteroid that suppresses ACTH release from the pituitary more potently than does cortisol. A 1-mg dose at night blocks ACTH release in normal individuals, and the resultant overnight fall in cortisol production is detected on plasma cortisol measurement the next morning (overnight dexamethasone suppression test). Patients with Cushing's syndrome, on the other hand, have abnormal secretion either of ACTH or cortisol and, on the morning after a 1-mg dose of dexamethasone, continue to have high cortisol levels. The pituitary in Cushing's disease is not truly autonomous, but reset, and higher doses of dexamethasone suppresses ACTH secretion. Therefore, when challenged with high doses of dexamethasone (8 mg/day), most patients with Cushing's disease suppress cortisol secretion to 50 per cent of baseline levels, whereas most patients with high levels of cortisol production from ectopic ACTH secretion or from autonomous cortisol secretion by an adrenal tumor do not.

METYRAPONE TEST. Metyrapone is a compound that also aids in the discrimination of pituitary versus nonpituitary Cushing's through its partial inhibition of the cortical enzyme 11-hydroxylase. Instead of producing cortisol, the adrenal gland produces 11-deoxycortisol, which does not negatively feedback on the pituitary gland. The pituitary, in turn, increases ACTH secretion, and more 11-deoxycortisol is produced. The 11-deoxycortisol is detected directly in serum, or in the urine as increased 17-hydroxycortico-steroid (17-OHCS). Patients with Cushing's disease respond to metyrapone challenge with a greater than normal increase in urinary 17-OHCS. In patients with autonomous adrenal tumors or ectopic production of ACTH, the pituitary is suppressed, and 11-deoxycortisol and 17-OHCS levels do not change after metyrapone challenge.

RADIOGRAPHIC STUDIES AND SCANS. When a pituitary source of excess ACTH production is suspected, the patient should have a CT scan or MRI of the sella. As noted previously, approximately 50 per cent of microadenomas are 5 mm or less in diameter and may not be detected. If an adrenal etiology is postulated, CT scan or MRI of the abdomen should be performed. In patients with adrenal adenoma or carcinoma, an ipsilateral mass may be seen, while the contralateral adrenal is often suppressed and atrophic. In bilateral nodular hyperplasia, both adrenals are enlarged.

A scintigraphic localization technique uses [131]I-19-iodocholesterol, which is taken up by the adrenals, as cholesterol is the precursor of all the cortical hormones. Cushing's disease causing bilateral adrenal hyperplasia shows bilaterally increased uptake of the isotope, adrenal adenoma usually shows unilateral uptake of the isotope, and adrenal carcinoma evidences either a low isotope uptake in the malignancy or no uptake on either side.

Treatment

The treatment of Cushing's disease has been discussed previously. Treatment of Cushing's syndrome is directed toward removal of the source of cortisol excess and is, therefore, principally surgical. Adrenalectomy is the treatment of choice for adrenal adenoma or adrenal carcinoma. Patients undergoing unilateral adrenalectomy for adrenal adenoma tend to do very well postoperatively, although steroid replacement therapy is necessary for at least several months until the suppressed pituitary and contralateral adrenal recover. Surgical resection of adrenocortical carcinoma frequently includes the kidney, and adjuvant

TABLE 2. TYPICAL LABORATORY VALUES IN NORMAL SUBJECTS AND PATIENTS WITH CUSHING'S SYNDROME*

	Normal	Adrenal Tumor	Cushing's Disease	Ectopic ACTH Syndrome
Plasma cortisol	10–25 μg%	High	High	Very high
	Rhythmic	No rhythm	No rhythm	No rhythm
Plasma ACTH	0.1–0.4 mU%	Low	High	High
17-OHCS response to ACTH	3- to 5-fold	+ ,0	+ ,0	+ ,0
Response to metyrapone	2- to 4-fold	0	+	+ ,0
Response to dexamethasone	0–3 mg/day	No fall	Partial fall	No fall

* Adapted from Liddle GW: Am J Med 53:638, 1972, with permission.
Abbreviations: 17-OHCS = 17-hydroxycorticosteroid, ACTH = adrenocorticotropic hormone.

chemotherapy with mitotane may also be used (see below). Unfortunately, there are few long-term survivors. Bilateral nodular hyperplasia in children is treated either by total adrenalectomy or total removal of one gland and subtotal removal of the other. Total adrenalectomy has been used in the past for bilateral adrenal hyperplasia secondary to Cushing's disease, but is presently reserved for the severest cases in which there is an inadequate response to hypophysectomy.

Complications of adrenalectomy include infection and wound dehiscence with impaired wound healing. Deaths have been reported from pulmonary embolism. The use of preoperative metyrapone, low-dose heparin, prophylactic antibiotics, and preoperative vitamin A (to counteract corticosteroid effects by stabilizing lysosomal membranes) has reduced postoperative morbidity. An important late complication of bilateral total adrenalectomy is Nelson's syndrome, the development of a pituitary tumor after cortisol inhibition has been removed. It occurs in approximately 10 per cent of patients following total adrenalectomy. Some centers have, therefore, used preoperative pituitary irradiation prior to total adrenalectomy to prevent Nelson's syndrome.

Chemotherapy of Cushing's syndrome is directed toward the blockade of cortisol synthesis, generally to bring levels under control prior to surgery, or after surgery if the reduction in cortisol levels is inadequate. Metyrapone, as noted earlier, lowers cortisol production by blocking 11 hydroxylation in the adrenal cortex. Aminoglutethimide blocks the conversion of cholesterol to pregnenolone and thus lowers levels of all the adrenocortical hormones. Metyrapone and aminoglutethimide are often used in combination. Mitotane is an insecticide that causes necrosis of adrenocortical cells and inhibits cortisol synthesis in the zona fasciculata and zona reticularis without affecting aldosterone production.

When Cushing's syndrome is caused by a paraendocrine source of ACTH production, therapy is focused on the eradication of that tumor. If treatment of the primary lesion is unsuccessful or no lesion can be found, bilateral adrenalectomy may be palliative. Metyrapone or mitotane may also be helpful. Hypophysectomy is contraindicated.

Primary Aldosteronism (Conn's Syndrome)

Conn's syndrome, or primary aldosteronism, is the clinical syndrome that results from excessive secretion of aldosterone due to the presence of an adrenal adenoma (75 per cent), bilateral adrenal hyperplasia (25 per cent) or, rarely, adrenal carcinoma. An idiopathic variant is suppressible by dexamethasone and is frequently familial. Hypertension and hypokalemia are the major presenting features. Primary aldosteronism

is a curable form of hypertension found in 1 per cent of all hypertensive patients. Secondary aldosteronism results when decreased renal artery perfusion pressure causes a rise in renin secretion from the renal juxtaglomerular apparatus, an increase in angiotensin, and therefore increased release of aldosterone from the zona glomerulosa. Primary aldosteronism is associated with low renin levels, whereas secondary aldosteronism has high renin levels. Causes of secondary aldosteronism are renal artery stenosis, cirrhosis, congestive heart failure, and nephrotic syndrome. Bartter's syndrome is a unique cause of hyperaldosteronism associated with hyperplasia of the juxtaglomerular cells, increased renin levels, hypokalemic alkalosis, and normotension. These patients frequently present as children with growth failure, polyuria, and weakness.

Clinical Features

Primary aldosteronism is more common in females than in males and occurs in the fourth to sixth decade of life. Children and young adults occasionally are affected. Although cases of normotensive primary aldosteronism have been described, hypertension and hypokalemia are present in most patients. The hypertension is usually moderate, with diastolic blood pressure in the 100- to 130-mm Hg range. Sodium retention and potassium wasting by the renal tubule is a direct effect of aldosterone. Low potassium levels cause proximal muscle weakness and cramps. Hypokalemia has toxic effects on the kidney, producing a nephrogenic form of diabetes insipidus. Laboratory tests show a decreased serum potassium level associated with an increased serum bicarbonate level and a high-normal or mildly increased serum sodium level. The urine potassium level is inappropriately high compared to the serum potassium level.

Diagnosis

The diagnosis of primary hyperaldosteronism is based on finding high aldosterone levels in combination with low plasma renin levels. Aldosterone is assayed under conditions that normally would cause low levels: with the patient supine, following sodium loading with normal saline infusion or high-sodium diet. Renin levels are measured under conditions that normally would cause increased secretion, such as the upright position, a low-sodium diet, or following two doses of the diuretic furosemide. Computed tomographic scans of the adrenals are used to identify adenomas, but bilateral hyperplasia usually cannot be differentiated from normal adrenal glands. Scintiscanning with NP-59 identifies hyperfunctioning lesions, and uptake is unilateral in the case of an adenoma and bilateral in the case of hyperplasia. Selective adrenal vein catheterization for aldosterone sampling is also useful when it is difficult to distinguish unilateral from bilateral disease. Samples from an adrenal vein draining an adenoma have a higher aldosterone/cortisol ratio than samples obtained from the normal contralateral gland. Samples from hyperplastic glands both show higher than normal aldosterone/cortisol ratios, with less disparity between the two glands.

Therapy

The treatment of primary aldosteronism due to an adrenal adenoma is unilateral adrenalectomy. The aldosterone antagonist spironolactone is given preoperatively with potassium replacement. Postoperatively, as renin levels normalize, hypertension improves and is cured in 70 per cent of patients. Potassium wasting ceases. Transient hypoaldosteronism with hypotension and hyperkalemia may be seen rarely and resolves within a few days. Surgery is not performed on patients with hyperaldosteronism due to bilateral adrenal hyperplasia, as it would benefit only 20 to 30 per cent of them. Instead they are treated with spironolactone, or the potassium-sparing diuretic, amiloride. Side effects of spironolactone therapy include gynecomastia and impotence in men. Dexamethasone is used to treat the glucocorticoid-suppressible form.

Adrenogenital Syndrome

The adrenogenital syndromes are a group of disorders resulting from a deficiency, partial or complete, of one or more of the enzymes that convert cholesterol to the various adrenocortical hormones (Fig. 5). In the most common type, 21-hydroxylase deficiency (94 per cent of all cases), cortisol synthesis is diminished, ACTH secretion by the pituitary rises, and the adrenal cortex becomes hyperplastic. In patients with a partial enzyme deficiency, increased ACTH produces normal levels of cortisol. However, cortisol precursors produced in great excess are shunted to synthesis of androstenedione which, in turn, is metabolized to testosterone. In females this causes virilization and, in males, premature acquisition of adult secondary sexual characteristics. If there is complete absence of the 21-hydroxylase enzyme, there is neither cortisol nor aldosterone production at all, and infants with this condition are born with adrenal insufficiency as well as androgen excess. Diagnosis is confirmed by demonstrating markedly elevated levels of 17-hydroxyprogesterone in plasma and urine. Prenatal diagnosis of the enzyme deficiency is now possible with amniocentesis and human leukocyte antigen (HLA) typing. Treatment of 21-hydroxylase deficiency involves administration of glucocorticoid and, if necessary, min-

eralocorticoid. Virilized females should undergo genital reconstruction during the first years of life.

The second most common deficiency (5 per cent) is of 11-β-hydroxylase, which also causes low cortisol levels and elevated androgens. A deficiency of 17-hydroxylase decreases cortisol and androgen production, with resultant excess mineralocorticoid, hypertension, and hypokalemia. Adults who develop adrenogenital syndrome generally harbor a malignant adrenal neoplasm.

Adrenocortical Insufficiency (Addison's Disease)

Addison's disease refers to the hormonal sequelae of destruction of the adrenal cortices bilaterally. Related terms, "addisonian crisis" or acute adrenocortical insufficiency, refer to the metabolic effects of a sudden deficit of adrenocortical hormones. The deficiency may be caused by sudden adrenal destruction, such as bilateral adrenal hemorrhage, or may occur without adrenal destruction, such as when chronic glucocorticoid therapy is abruptly ceased and the suppressed adrenals cannot produce adequate quantities of hormone. Although Addison's disease was formerly most often due to bilateral adrenal tuberculosis, the most prevalent form of adrenocortical insufficiency today is autoimmune destruction of the adrenal cortex. Bilateral adrenal hemorrhage is another common cause and may occur spontaneously, most often in anticoagulated, hypertensive, or poorly nourished persons. It may also occur in the setting of meningococcal septicemia (Waterhouse-Friderichsen syndrome), during pregnancy, in burn patients, and in patients with sepsis or intra-abdominal infection. The clinical presentation of adrenal insufficiency is variable, ranging from chronic, low-grade illness, to fulminant addisonian crisis presenting with shock and coma. In patients with chronic adrenal insufficiency, clinical signs and symptoms are secondary to both glucocorticoid and mineralocorticoid deficiency. Major symptoms of chronic glucocorticoid deficiency include lethargy, weakness, weight loss, hypotension, nausea and vomiting, and abdominal pain. Mineralocorticoid deficiency causes salt craving and electrolyte disturbances including hyponatremia, hyperkalemia, and mild acidosis. Hyponatremia causes a decreased extracellular fluid volume with cardiovascular effects including hypotension, decreased cardiac output, and decreased renal blood flow with prerenal azotemia. Increased MSH causes hyperpigmentation of the extensor surfaces, buccal mucosa, and palmar surfaces. Chronic replacement therapy with cortisone acetate is given orally (20 mg hydrocortisone in the morning and 10 mg in the evening). Treatment with mineralocorticoid is usually not necessary.

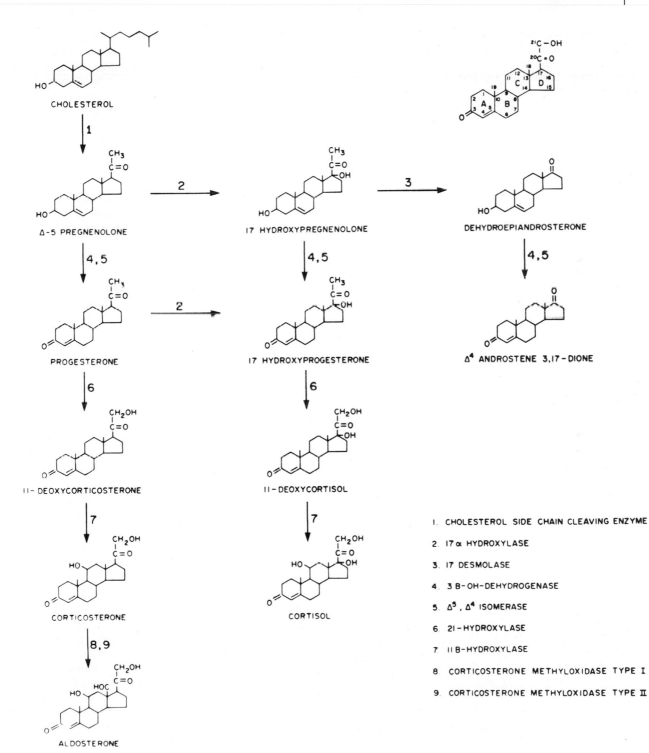

Figure 5. The biosynthetic pathways of adrenal corticosteroids.

Patient mortality follows the failure to recognize and treat acute adrenal insufficiency. The signs and symptoms are nonspecific: fever, nausea and vomiting, abdominal pain, hypotension, and often a change in mental status. When addisonian crisis is suspected, serum cortisol and ACTH levels should be obtained. Laboratory tests may show hyponatremia, hyperkalemia, low cortisol levels, and increased ACTH levels. However, treatment must be initiated before these laboratory tests are available. This requires large amounts of intravenous fluids and corticosteroids (initially, hydrocortisone 100 mg intravenously every 6 hours, or its equivalent).

Pheochromocytoma

Pheochromocytoma is a chromaffin cell tumor arising from cells of neural crest origin in the adrenal medulla or in extra-adrenal sympathetic nervous tissue. The organ of Zuckerkandl is para-aortic nervous tissue located in the region of the inferior mesenteric artery and aortic bifurcation. It is a common site for extra-adrenal pheochromocytoma. The adrenal medulla and the organ of Zuckerkandl are unique among nervous tissues in that they contain the enzyme that converts norepinephrine to epinephrine. Thus, pheochromocytomas arising in the adrenal medulla or organ of Zuckerkandl may produce both epinephrine and norepinephrine, while other extra-adrenal pheochromocytomas produce only norepinephrine. Most pheochromocytomas (85 to 90 per cent) are located in the adrenal medulla and about 10 per cent are bilateral. Approximately 10 per cent of pheochromocytomas are malignant, more frequently in females, while 20 per cent of familial tumors are malignant. When pheochromocytomas are extra-adrenal in location, 30 to 40 per cent are malignant. Approximately 10 per cent of pheochromocytomas occur in children, usually males. There is an association with the autosomal dominant multiple endocrine neoplasia type IIa (MEN-IIa) (Sipple's syndrome); that is, pheochromocytoma, medullary cancer of the thyroid, and parathyroid hyperplasia as well as an association with the rarer MEN-IIb, consisting of pheochromocytoma, medullary cancer of the thyroid, multiple mucosal neuromas, ganglioneuromatosis, and marfanoid habitus. There is also an association of pheochromocytoma with von Recklinghausen's disease (neurofibromatosis) and von Hippel-Lindau disease (retinal angiomatosis and hemangioblastoma of the cerebellum or spinal cord).

Clinical Features

Signs and symptoms of pheochromocytoma are related to the circulating excess catecholamines and include hypertension, tachycardia, perspiration, palpitations, tremor, anxiety, abdominal pain, constipation, fever, weight loss, and glucose intolerance. Hypertension may be sustained (50 per cent) or paroxysmal (50 per cent). However, children with pheochromocytomas usually show persistent hypertension as do patients with malignant pheochromocytomas. Untreated tumors may cause myocarditis, congestive heart failure, ventricular fibrillation, stroke, and gastrointestinal infarction. Paroxysmal catecholamine release may occur in response to tumor palpation, stress, exercise, or even micturition (especially in the case of pheochromocytomas present in nervous tissue adjacent to the bladder wall).

Diagnosis

Pheochromocytoma produces elevations in norepinephrine and epinephrine, and their metabolites normetanephrine, metanephrine, and vanillylmandelic acid (VMA), which may be measured in the urine. If pheochromocytoma is diagnosed, the patient is placed on the α-adrenergic antagonist phenoxybenzamine at least 10 days before tumor localization is attempted. This blocks many of the cardiovascular effects of catecholamine excess, but the diminished vascular tone causes hypovolemia. Patients should be vigorously hydrated during treatment. Side effects of phenoxybenzamine include postural hypotension, nasal congestion, weakness, nausea, and inability to ejaculate. If tachycardia or arrhythmias are present, a β-adrenergic blocker such as propranolol may be added. β-Blockade should never be initiated before α-blockade, as unopposed α-stimulation may precipitate cardiac failure or a hypertensive crisis, nor should it be administered to a patient with asthma, chronic obstructive pulmonary disease, or congestive heart failure. Computed tomography or MRI scanning may demonstrate lesions with a diameter as small as 1 cm within the adrenal gland. The scanning agent ^{131}I-MIBG is taken up by adrenergic tissues and is the most sensitive means of localizing ectopically situated pheochromocytomas. ^{131}I-MIBG scanning also determines whether a mass seen by other diagnostic techniques has adrenergic function. Selective arteriography is rarely used, but can demonstrate pheochromocytomas, owing to their highly vascular nature. All patients must be prepared with α-blockers, however, because arteriography may precipitate a hypertensive crisis.

Treatment

Patients with pheochromocytoma are treated by surgical excision of the adrenal tumor(s) after preoperative adrenergic blockade and vigorous hydration. Careful monitoring is essential for managing intraoperative hypertension, tachyarrhythmias, and postremoval hypotension. Intraoperative hypertension is most often treated with intravenous sodium nitroprusside, a smooth muscle relaxant, because it acts rapidly. The tumor should be manipulated as little as possible during the operative procedure to avoid a surge of catecholamine release into the circulation. In spite of localizing techniques, most authors still recommend an anterior surgical approach to examine both adrenals and the para-aortic sympathetic chain. In patients with familial pheochromocytoma, some surgeons perform bilateral adrenalectomies because of the high incidence of developing another pheochromocytoma (sometimes malignant) in the contralateral gland. Operative mortality is less than 2 per cent. Approximately 90 per cent of patients with episodic hypertension become normotensive, and approximately 5 per cent of patients develop recurrent disease. The

5-year survival for patients with malignant pheochromocytoma is 30 to 40 per cent. Metastases are most commonly found in bone, lymph nodes, liver, and lung. Metastatic disease is treated by surgical debulking procedures, chemotherapy, or radiation, and high dose ^{131}I-MIBG is used for palliative and adjunctive treatment of patients who have significant uptake in the metastatic deposits.

REFERENCES

Besser G, Rees L (eds): The Pituitary-Adrenocortical Axis. Philadelphia, WB Saunders Company, 1985.
Goodrich I, Lee KJ: The Pituitary. Amsterdam, Elsevier, 1988.
Nelson D (ed): New Aspects of Adrenal Cortical Disease. Philadelphia, WB Saunders Company, 1991.
Scott HW (ed): Surgery of the Adrenal Glands. Philadelphia, JB Lippincott Company, 1990.
Thompson NW, Vinik AI: Endocrine Surgery Update. New York, Grune & Stratton, 1983.

25

THE ESOPHAGUS

ANDRÉ DURANCEAU, M.D.

ANATOMY

The esophagus is the narrowest segment of the digestive tract and joins the hypopharynx and the stomach. It is a collapsed muscular tube that measures 22 to 28 cm in length and is closed proximally by the upper esophageal sphincter (UES) and distally by the lower esophageal sphincter (LES) (Fig. 1). There is an external fibrous layer, the adventitia, and the muscularis is a longitudinal layer that parallels the axis of the esophagus with an inner circular layer that thickens over 3 cm immediately above the gastroesophageal junction. The submucosa is composed of elastic and collagenous fibers with a meshwork of abundant blood vessels and lymph vessels. The esophageal mucosa is a stratified squamous epithelium supported by the muscularis mucosa. Functional innervation of the esophagus is provided primarily by the vagus nerves. Sympathetic nerves have an influence on glands and blood vessels. The vascular supply to the upper, middle, and lower esophagus arises from the inferior thyroid arteries, the tracheobronchial arteries, and the esophageal branches of the left gastric arteries. Lymphatic drainage is abundant along the submucosa and is of importance in patients with esophageal malignancies. The topographic relationship of the esophagus to adjacent structures is important in the assessment of patients with esophageal neoplasms. In the neck, chest, and abdomen, the esophagus lies on the spine. At the thoracic inlet and within the thoracic cavity, it lies behind the trachea and pericardium adjacent to the azygos vein and the thoracic duct on the right and to the descending aorta on the left.

PHYSIOLOGY

Esophageal function is assessed through manometric recordings. These studies document the finely reg-ulated mechanisms of action that allow comfortable swallowing. Voluntary swallowing begins with an upward and posterior thrust of the tongue with closure of the soft palate by contraction of the velopharyngeal muscles, and the pharynx then becomes a closed cavity. Upon motor stimulation from the deglutition centers, a peristaltic wave passes down the pharynx causing intraluminal pressures of 200 to 600 mm Hg. The single contraction peak occurs during 0.2 to 0.5 seconds and progresses through the pharynx at a speed of 9 to 25 cm/sec.

Upper Esophageal Sphincter

The body of the esophagus is closed proximally by the UES. This is a high-pressure zone created by the sling action of the cricopharyngeus muscle that is attached to both posterior ends of the cricoid cartilage. Through vagal and glossopharyngeal stimulation, the cricopharyngeus is maintained in a tonic state at rest, with a resulting pressure of 20 to 80 mm Hg. During deglutition, inhibition of the tonic innervation to the sphincter occurs with relaxation of the high-pressure zone to ambient cervical esophageal resting pressure. This relaxation occurs simultaneously with the pharyngeal contraction, a coordination which allows the normal accommodation of the bolus propulsed by the pharynx. A postdeglutitive contraction closes the sphincter, generating pressures that are often twice the pressure of the resting sphincter. The normal resting pressure is then resumed in the UES (Fig. 2A). With the closure of the UES, the peristaltic contraction proceeds to sweep the cervical esophagus. Both UES contraction and peristalsis prevent the regurgitation of the swallowed bolus from the cervical esophagus back into the pharynx.

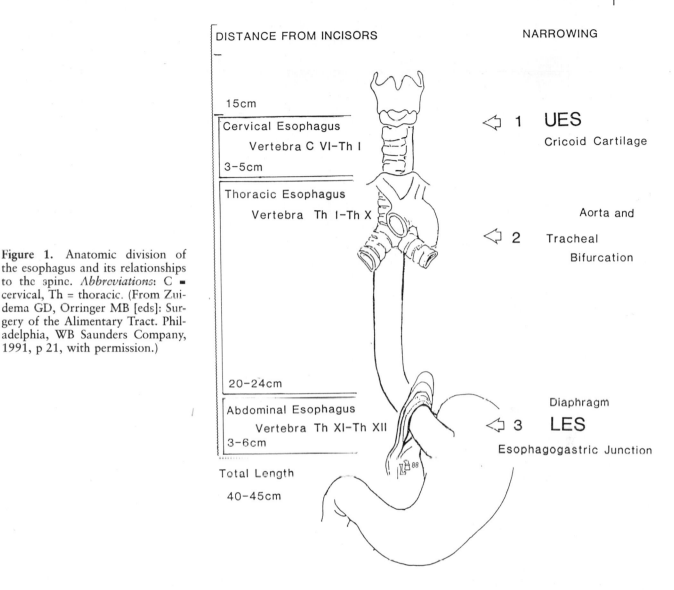

DISTANCE FROM INCISORS

NARROWING

15cm

Cervical Esophagus

Vertebra C VI–Th I

3–5cm

Thoracic Esophagus

Vertebra Th I–Th X

20–24cm

Abdominal Esophagus

Vertebra Th XI–Th XII

3–6cm

Total Length

40–45cm

1 **UES**
Cricoid Cartilage

Aorta and

2 Tracheal
Bifurcation

Diaphragm

3 **LES**
Esophagogastric Junction

Figure 1. Anatomic division of the esophagus and its relationships to the spine. *Abbreviations:* C = cervical, Th = thoracic. (From Zuidema GD, Orringer MB [eds]: Surgery of the Alimentary Tract. Philadelphia, WB Saunders Company, 1991, p 21, with permission.)

Esophageal Body

In response to cholinergic stimulation, the esophageal contraction moves with a velocity of 2 to 5 cm/sec. The contraction accelerates in the smooth muscle part and slows again in the distal esophagus, just before the lower sphincter. The resting pressure in the esophagus reflects the negative intrathoracic pressure. In the proximal half of the esophagus, contraction pressures may vary between 20 and 70 mm Hg, while the contractions generate pressures of 50 to 100 mm Hg in the distal half of the esophagus. Contraction duration is from 4 to 6 seconds (Fig. 2B).

Swallowing induces a peristaltic wave that progresses down the esophagus, termed a *primary contraction*. In the absence of deglutition, esophageal distention or irritation may initiate a normal propulsive wave. This is secondary peristalsis, a response to local stimuli of the normal esophageal wall. Tertiary contractions are nonpropulsive and are characterized on the manometric recording by a simultaneous pressure rise at different recording levels. These contractions occur spontaneously or in response to a deglutition (Fig. 2D). Tertiary contractions in response to deglutition are usually considered abnormal and can be occasionally observed in healthy individuals. Spontaneous tertiary activity is also seen in healthy individuals and can be influenced by psychogenic factors.

Lower Esophageal Sphincter

The esophagus is separated from the stomach by a physiologic sphincter that creates a high-pressure zone of 2 to 4 cm in length. Myogenic and neurogenic

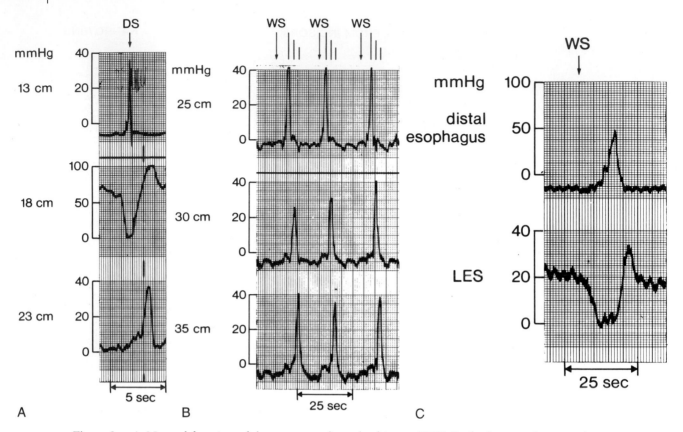

Figure 2. *A*, Normal function of the upper esophageal sphincter (UES). Peak pharyngeal contraction occurs simultaneously with the nadir of UES relaxation. Sphincter opening accommodates the duration of pharyngeal contraction. Contraction of the UES continues into the cervical esophagus as primary peristalsis. *B*, Normal peristalsis in esophageal body. Following a wet swallow (WS), separation of the three wave peaks is shown by the three vertical lines. *C*, Normal lower esophageal sphincter (LES). Relaxation of the sphincter anticipates the oncoming peristaltic wave. Closure of the LES occurs with the passing contraction. *Illustration continued on following page*

mechanisms help maintain the resting tone of the distal sphincter with probable hormonal influences. Just as in the remainder of the esophagus, the resting tone observed varies with the recording technique. In the LES, it usually ranges between 15 and 25 mm Hg, and causes a positive-pressure barrier against gastroesophageal reflux. Upon swallowing and while esophageal peristaltic wave progresses in the esophageal body, relaxation to resting intragastric pressure occurs allowing proper transit of the alimentary bolus from esophagus to stomach. This relaxation is essential for normal sphincter function, and the opening period of the sphincter must accommodate the duration of esophageal body contraction (Fig. 2C). The peristaltic wave, as it crosses the sphincter area, creates a closing contraction, and the lower esophageal sphincter and then returns to normal resting pressure.

Distal sphincter pressures may vary from moment to moment in any individual. Neurologic, myogenic, and hormonal influences have been mentioned. Mechanical influences are important, and emotions, although poorly quantifiable, may have an effect on LES function as well as on the remainder of the esophagus. Theophylline, alcohol, nicotine, nitroglycerin, and diazepam, as well as fats and chocolate are known to cause distal sphincter hypotension. Conversely, urecholine and metoclopramide as well as ingestion of protein increase the LES resting pressure.

EVALUATION OF THE PATIENT WITH ESOPHAGEAL DISORDERS

Symptoms

The assessment of symptoms is usually responsible for further investigation of potential esophageal problems.

Dysphagia has different etiologies depending on the level of presentation. Oropharyngeal dysphagia is clas-

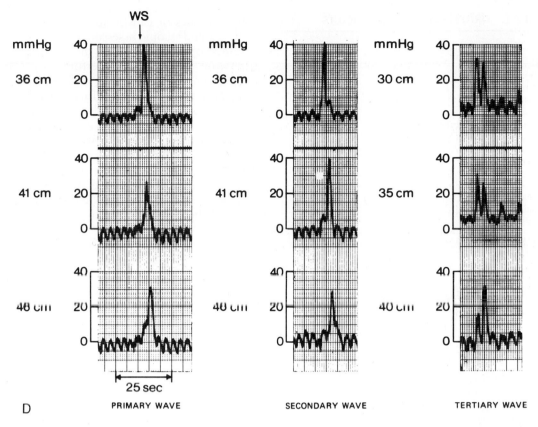

Figure 2. *Continued. D,* Primary, secondary, and tertiary contractions. (From Hurwitz AL, Duranceau A, Haddad J: Disorders of Esophageal Motility in Major Problems in Internal Medicine, vol 16, Philadelphia, WB Saunders Company, 1979, with permission.)

sically described at the level of the sternal notch or above (Table 1). Substernal dysphagia, either as a sticking sensation or as complete blockage of the bolus, suggests esophageal disease (Table 2). *Odynophagia* refers to pain on swallowing. A constricting pain irradiating to the back or to the neck may present with functional or mechanical obstruction. *Regurgitation* of freshly ingested food is likely to be a motor disorder. *Regurgitation* associated with *heartburn* suggests reflux of gastric content toward the esophagus and is typically increased when lying down, particularly at night, or when bending. These symptoms must be documented by objective methods prior to confirming their etiology.

Radiology

Dynamic radiology is necessary to document anatomic abnormalities of the esophagus at rest and following swallowing. Motor dysfunction, mucosal lesions, strictures, and distortions or compressions are documented through barium studies. The type of hiatal hernia is classified accurately by radiology, but reflux disease cannot be documented precisely through radiographic assessment alone.

Emptying Scintiscan

Radionuclide pharyngoesophageal transit studies add quantitative information on the esophageal emptying capacity. Since rapid emptying of both liquid and solid boluses occurs in the normal, abnormal retention is usually seen with pathologic conditions.

Motility Studies

Manometric recordings of the esophagus and both its sphincters are essential for an accurate diagnosis of motor disorders. Clinical and radiologic suspicion of such disorders, especially with normal endoscopic findings, indicate the need for a motility study.

pH Recording

Twenty-four–hour pH recording in the esophagus with a single electrode placed 5 cm above the lower

TABLE 1. OROPHARYNGEAL DYSPHAGIA

Neurogenic
  Central
  Peripheral
Myogenic
  Motor end-plate disease
  Skeletal muscle disease
Idiopathic dysfunction of UES
  Without pharyngoesophageal diverticulum
  With pharyngoesophageal diverticulum (Zenker's)
Iatrogenic
  Neck surgery
  Irradiation
Gastroesophageal reflux and distal esophageal dysfunction
Mechanical causes
  Endoluminal
  Extraluminal

Abbreviation: UES = upper esophageal sphincter.

esophageal sphincter or with multilevel pH probes is now recognized as the most accurate method of documenting abnormal acid reflux from the stomach.

Endoscopy

Esophagoscopy and esophageal biopsies provide the most objective assessment of esophageal mucosal damage. Gastroesophageal reflux disease and malignant lesions of the esophageal mucosa and of the esophagogastric junction are the conditions for which endoscopy confirms clinical and radiologic abnormalities. Esophageal symptoms, esophageal compression, established motor disorders, and esophageal injury by foreign bodies or caustic substances are other indications for endoscopic assessment.

Endoscopic evaluation of the esophagus may cause significant morbidity. Perforation, hemorrhage, cardiopulmonary problems, and sepsis are the most frequent complications. Perforation is the most dangerous and occurs in less than 1 per cent of all examinations. Persistent pain and fever after an endoscopic procedure should always be considered as a perforation. The proper diagnostic procedures to confirm or exclude this problem should be performed immediately. A recent myocardial infarct, hemodynamic instability, agitation, and large thoracic aneurysms are some of the contraindications to the performance of esophagoscopy.

MOTOR DISORDERS OF THE ESOPHAGUS

Oropharyngeal Dysphagia

Oropharyngeal dysphagia is a symptom complex at the oropharyngeal level and includes difficulties in swallowing or in initiating swallows, hesitation, and poor handling of the bolus from mouth to pharynx. When present with oropharyngeal dysphagia, misdirection of the bolus causes pharyngo-oral and pharyngonasal regurgitation and/or tracheobronchial aspiration.

TABLE 2. ESOPHAGEAL DYSPHAGIA

Motor		Mechanical	
		Esophageal Wall	*Periesophageal*
1. Oropharyngeal dysphagia	1. Congenital	Embryonic rest	Vascular
2. Hypomotility disorders	2. Traumatic	Foreign body—	Trauma
Achalasia		induced injury	Surgical; previous
		Medication	esophageal surgery
		Caustic	
		Endoscopic	Lung and mediastinal
			operations
3. Hypermotility disorders	3. Inflammatory	Complications of reflux	Mediastinal nodes
Diffuse esophageal spasm		disease	Fibrosing mediastinitis
Nutcracker esophagus		Rings and webs	
(hyperperistalsis-		Infections	
supersqueeze)			
Hypertensive LES			
Nonspecific motor disorders (NEMD)			
4. Motor dysfunction and reflux disease	4. Neoplastic	Benign	Mediastinal tumors
Idiopathic		Malignant	Lung tumors
Secondary			Metastatic disease
Scleroderma			
Diabetes			
Alcoholism			

Abbreviations: LES = lower esophageal sphincter, NEMD = nonspecific motor disorders.

Etiology and Pathogenesis

The various causes of oropharyngeal dysphagia are summarized in Table 1. The etiology of these symptoms is quite different from that seen with substernal dysphagia (Table 2). In patients with neurologic damage, poor pharyngeal propulsion is frequently associated with incomplete, absent, or delayed opening of the upper esophageal sphincter. When muscular disease is responsible for the symptoms, it is mostly the weakness of pharyngeal contraction against the normal tone and resistance of the upper sphincter that causes dysphagia. When there is no obvious neurogenic or myogenic disease to explain the symptoms, it is termed *idiopathic dysfunction* of the upper sphincter. In this situation, the presence of a pharyngoesophageal diverticulum on radiologic studies is a complication of the upper sphincter dysfunction with hypopharyngeal mucosa herniating through the muscularis just above the abnormally functioning cricopharyngeus. Disease or dysfunction in the distal esophagus must be excluded even if the manifestation of symptoms is at the oropharyngeal level.

Diagnosis

A careful clinical assessment of symptoms remains the most appropriate method of classifying dysphagia at the oropharyngeal level. A video esophagogram provides objective evidence of pharyngeal, laryngeal, and upper sphincter behavior. The remaining esophagus and proximal digestive tract must be assessed as well. Manometric studies should clarify the dysfunction at upper sphincter level (Fig. 3A). However, difficulties with recording at that level may lead to an underestimation of the existing dysfunction. Pharyngeal emptying scintiscans may assist in documenting and quantitating abnormal retention, with either liquids or solids, above the upper esophageal sphincter. Endoscopic examination is made with extreme care and is usually avoided when a diverticulum is present.

Treatment and Prognosis

Medical treatment aims at controlling symptoms whenever the dysphagia is secondary to a medical condition. The dysphagia of myasthenia gravis or the muscular dysfunction of metabolic myopathy are examples of such management. In neurogenic disease, selection of patients for surgical treatment by cervical esophagomyotomy is important. When neurologically damaged patients show intact voluntary deglutition with good lingual muscle movement and proper phonation, significant improvement in swallowing can be obtained in approximately 80 per cent of patients. Cricopharyngeal myotomy also improves dystrophy pa-

tients in the same proportion by decreasing resistance to pharyngoesophageal transit. In these patients, the progress of the underlying disease is unaltered.

Cricopharyngeal myotomy for idiopathic dysfunction of the upper sphincter causes significant improvement of symptoms when a good correlation is found between clinical and radiologic abnormalities. If a pharyngoesophageal diverticulum is present, surgical treatment is the only effective therapy. Uniformly excellent results are obtained by sectioning the abnormally functioning muscle with either resection or suspension of the diverticulum.

Idiopathic Motor Disorders

Idiopathic dysfunctions of the esophagus are classified as hypomotility disorders and hypermotility disorders (Table 2).

Hypomotility: Achalasia

DEFINITION AND PATHOGENESIS. Achalasia is a lack of relaxation of the LES accompanied by loss of peristalsis affecting the entire body of the esophagus. This loss of function is caused by denervation and loss of ganglion cells in Auerbach's plexus. Inhibitory nerves at the postganglionic level, by losing their control, are then responsible for increased tone in the lower sphincter, impaired relaxation, and loss of peristalsis.

CLINICAL PRESENTATION. Early achalasia is suggested by dysphagia and pain on swallowing (odynophagia). Chest pain may appear spontaneously between meals and during the night. Regurgitation of fresh undigested food is common. Symptoms are increased by stress. Progression of the disease results in less pain but persistent dysphagia and regurgitation. Late achalasia may be accompanied by pulmonary aspiration and secondary septic complications.

DIAGNOSIS. If symptoms are present, they are highly suggestive. Dynamic radiologic studies of the esophagus confirm the poor contraction of the esophagus and the poorly relaxing LES that gives a "bird's beak" appearance. Dilatation of the esophageal body is frequently seen. Motility studies are diagnostic and the only way to classify this motor disorder properly (Fig. 3B,C). Endoscopy is essential to exclude other causes of esophageal obstruction at the cardia, especially carcinoma.

TREATMENT AND PROGNOSIS. Management of achalasia whether invasive or noninvasive provides only palliation, since the motor abnormalities remain unchanged. Pneumatic or hydrostatic dilatation of the LES area is considered less invasive. It stretches and ruptures the muscle fibers of the abnormally function-

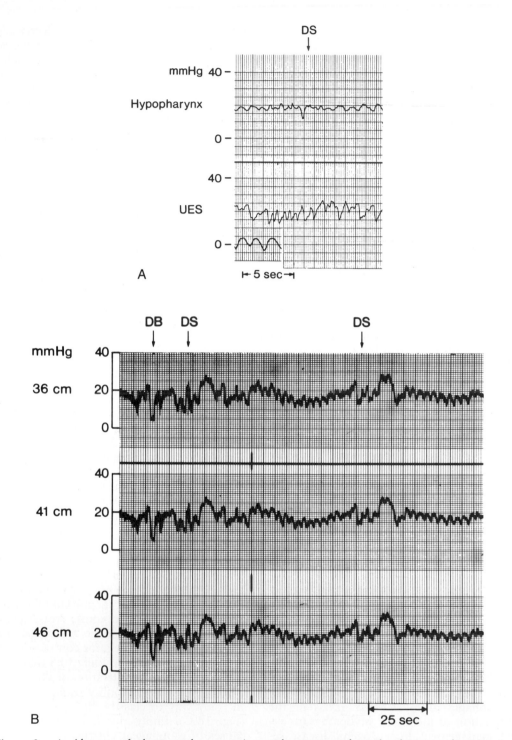

Figure 3. *A,* Absence of pharyngeal contraction and upper esophageal sphincter relaxation in a patient with neurologic dysphagia. *B,* Motor dysfunction of achalasia: elevated esophageal body resting pressures and flat, nonperistaltic contractions are seen in response to all deglutitions. *Illustration continued on opposite page*

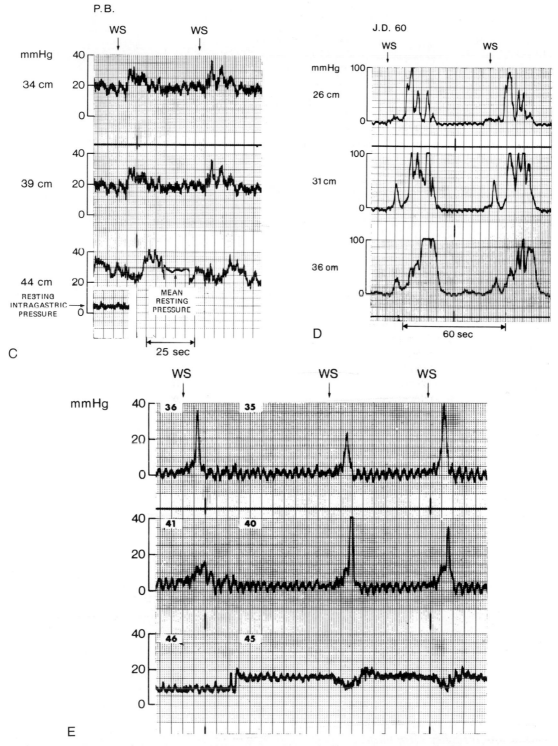

Figure 3. *Continued. C,* Lower esophageal sphincter (LES) function in achalasia. The resting pressure is at the upper limits of normal, and relaxation to resting intragastric pressure is incomplete. *D,* Repetitive, nonpropulsive, and prolonged duration activity as seen in hypermotility disorders. *E,* The idiopathic dysfunction of reflux disease: the lower esophageal sphincter in the lower recording panel is virtually absent while normal peristaltic activity is retained in the esophageal body. *Illustration continued on following page*

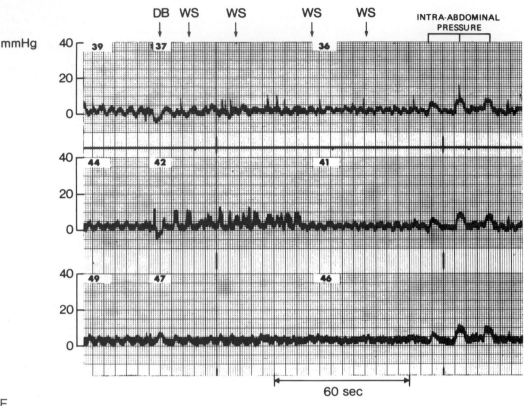

F

Figure 3. *Continued. F*, Absent LES and absent motor activity seen in severe reflux disease secondary to scleroderma. As shown on the right, pressure elevations in the esophagus in response to increased intra-abdominal pressures suggests that esophagus and stomach have become a single communicating cavity.

ing sphincter. Symptoms and esophageal emptying are improved in approximately 60 per cent of patients. The main risk of pneumatic dilatation is perforation, which is about 4 per cent in most series.

Surgical treatment consists of an extramucous myotomy under direct vision at laparotomy or thoracotomy. Thoracoscopic myotomy may well provide a significant alternative approach. Good to excellent relief of obstructive symptoms is obtained in more than 90 per cent of patients, with improvement in esophageal emptying. Gastroesophageal reflux is the main problem that may follow operation and is prevented by the addition of a partial fundoplication of the stomach at the time of the operation.

Hypermotility: Diffuse Esophageal Spasm, Supersqueeze or Nutcracker Esophagus, Hypertensive Lower Esophageal Sphincter

DEFINITION AND PATHOGENESIS. Although typically described as hyperdynamic motor abnormalities in patients with dysphagia and chest pain, the pattern of contraction abnormalities varies with the type of disorder. The etiology of these problems remains unclear, but strong psychological influence is likely.

CLINICAL PRESENTATION. This disorder is seen in hyperactive patients who present with chest pain of undetermined origin. The pain is typically substernal and radiates toward the interscapular area or toward the neck and mandible. Dysphagia and odynophagia are frequent.

DIAGNOSIS. If angina is suspected, it must be excluded first because lethal complications may follow. Radiographs show curling or segmentation of the esophagus, mostly in its smooth muscle portion. An associated diverticulum in the distal third of the esophagus is related to the motor dysfunction. Motility studies are essential to classify the motility disorder, using precise manometric criteria (Fig. 3D; Table 2). Endoscopy must be performed to exclude mucosal disease or lesions in the distal esophagus.

TREATMENT AND PROGNOSIS. Management of hyperdynamic esophageal disorders is not surgical initially. Reported results are not as favorable as for achalasia patients. This is possibly related to selection and diagnosis. Psychological assessment is important with these problems because those with hypochondriacal personalities tend to seek medical care early for symptoms. Reassurance, removal of triggering stimuli, and medication (nitroglycerin, calcium channel blocking agents) often reduce the effects of abnormal contractions. Medication to control anxiety is often helpful. Benefit from pneumatic dilatation is less evident than in achalasia except for some 30 per cent of patients who show LES relaxation abnormalities. Long esophageal myotomy covering the abnormally functioning muscle as documented by manometry is offered only following a prolonged conservative follow-up with appropriate medication. Approximately 60 per cent of treated patients are improved.

Motor Disorders and Reflux Disease

Definition and Pathogenesis

Lower esophageal sphincter hypotension is caused by an idiopathic dysfunction. When constantly hypotensive, the LES allows more frequent gastroesophageal reflux episodes to occur. Damage from reflux leads to more reflux, and further progression of damage leads to weaker defense mechanisms (Fig. 3E). Secondary reflux disorders are seen in scleroderma. Smooth muscle atrophy with collagen infiltration leads to loss of peristalsis and weaker contractions. Reduction or absence of LES pressures removes all defense mechanisms to the esophagus. Diabetes and alcohol abuse can lead to similar dysfunction (Fig. 3F).

Clinical Manifestations

Patients with these functional abnormalities present with regurgitations and heartburn. Dysphagia may be caused by poor contractions or stricture formation of the esophageal body as seen in complication of severe reflux disease.

HIATAL HERNIA AND GASTROESOPHAGEAL REFLUX

Definition

Herniation of the stomach through the esophageal hiatus can be classified into four types. Type I is the smallest sliding type and is a condition in which a few centimeters of the proximal stomach may ascend into the chest with intact supporting structures in the hiatus (Fig. 4A). Type II hernia is paraesophageal and the esophagogastric junction is in normal position (Fig. 4B). Through a defect in the phrenoesophageal membrane, the entire stomach may roll into the chest in a paraesophageal position. Type III hernia results

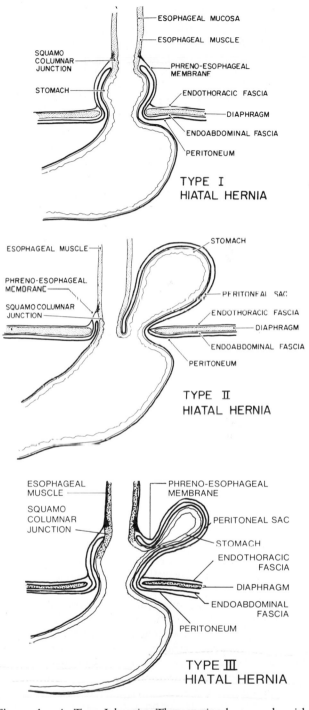

Figure 4. *A*, Type I hernia. The proximal stomach with supporting structures slides into the mediastinum across the hiatus. *B*, Type II hernia. The esophagogastric junction remains in proper position. Part or all of the stomach may roll into the chest to adopt a paraesophageal position. *C*, Type III hernia. Components of both type I and II hernias are identified. When accompanying organs are in the hernia sac, a type IV hernia is created. *Illustration continued on following page*

STAGING OF SEVERITY IN GASTROESOPHAGEAL REFLUX

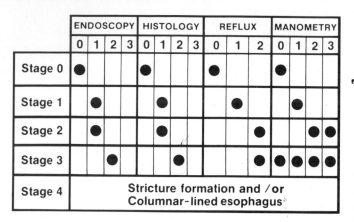

	ENDOSCOPY				HISTOLOGY				REFLUX			MANOMETRY			
	0	1	2	3	0	1	2	3	0	1	2	0	1	2	3
Stage 0	●				●				●			●			
Stage 1		●				●				●			●		
Stage 2		●				●					●			●	●
Stage 3			●				●				●	●	●	●	●
Stage 4	Stricture formation and /or Columnar-lined esophagus														

Figure 4. *Continued. D,* The four areas of investigation that help to document reflux disease objectively. Each method of investigation has a severity index. The more severe the disease, the higher the staging level. (From Jamieson GG, Duranceau A [eds]: Gastroesophageal Reflux. Philadelphia, WB Saunders Company, 1988, p 110, with permission.)

from a progressive enlargement of a sliding hernia through the hiatus (Fig. 4C). A hernia is formed with components of both the sliding and paraesophageal types. Type IV hernias show a large paraesophageal stomach with other organs such as the colon or small bowel in the hernia sac.

Etiology and Symptoms

Types II, III, and IV hernias cause mostly mechanical problems, and postprandial fullness and dyspnea may occur. Epigastric, left subcostal, and chest pain may follow meals. Dysphagia suggests acute angulation of the esophagus entering into a rolled stomach. Type I hernia alone causes no clinical problems if not associated with significant reflux disease. The typical symptoms of gastroesophageal reflux disease are regurgitations and heartburn. Symptoms related to complicated reflux disease are dysphagia and odynophagia, suggesting motor abnormalities or stricture and spoliation manifest as unexplained anemia, melena, or hematemesis. Asthma, oropharyngeal dysphagia, and chest pain of undetermined origin must be carefully considered prior to associating them with reflux disease.

Pathophysiology

Transient relaxation of the lower esophageal sphincter occurs normally during meals. With these relaxa-

tions, regurgitations of gastric content may occur into the distal esophagus. If these episodes increase in frequency and duration, mucosal damage in the esophagus follows. Over time, very low resting pressures in the lower esophageal sphincter lead to more frequent episodes of reflux. The potential for reflux is linearly related to LES pressures. Tobacco, alcohol, chocolate, mint, and medication affecting smooth muscle may lead to increased reflux episodes.

Diagnosis

Radiologic procedures have a role in classifying the type of hernia as well as the presence or absence of related esophageal complications, but are not sufficiently accurate to document the presence or absence of pathologic reflux. Four important features should be quantified as objectively as possible to assess the severity of gastroesophageal reflux disease: (1) endoscopic visualization of the mucosa, (2) documentation of mucosal and submucosal pathology by histology, (3) proof of esophageal exposure to acid by long-term pH testing, and (4) documentation of the physiologic abnormalities leading to pathologic reflux disease by manometry (Fig. 4D).

Treatment and Prognosis

Medical management should control reflux symptoms in a large majority of patients. Treatment objectives are: (1) to remove the abnormal stimuli potentially involved in increasing reflux episodes (medication, alcohol, tobacco); (2) to remove mechanical factors influencing reflux, to reduce weight to normal weight/height ratio, and to improve gravity drainage of esophagus with elevation of the head of the bed at night; (3) to reduce the irritation by modifying the reflux (antacids, alginic acid, ranitidine, omeprazole); (4) to improve LES tone (bethanechol, domperidone, cisapride); and (5) to improve gastric emptying (bethanechol, domperidone, cisapride). These attempts in medical management must be tried for a period of 6 months to 1 year prior to any other therapy.

Surgical treatment of gastroesophageal reflux if proposed solely to patients with well-staged and documented complications of reflux disease (erosive and ulcerative esophagitis with or without stricture, circumferential columnar lined esophagus). Weight reduction is essential to prevent intra-abdominal pressure from inducing abnormal tension on the repair. Most antireflux operations are directed toward restoration of competence to the esophagogastric junction by some form of fundoplication around an intra-abdominal esophagus.

BENIGN TUMORS OF THE ESOPHAGUS

Definition

In order of frequency, benign tumors of the esophagus are a leiomyoma, an intramural lesion developing in the muscularis, or an esophageal cyst considered to be an embryologic remnant within the wall. All components of the esophageal wall may participate in the formation of a benign lesion.

Clinical Presentation

Often asymptomatic, these lesions may cause intermittent dysphagia if sufficiently large to cause obstruction of the lumen. Rarely, bleeding can occur from an ulcerated leiomyoma.

Diagnosis

Radiologic examination suggests a semilunar compression in the wall with intact mucosa. Esophagoscopy confirms the absence of mucosal lesions with an endoluminal tumor bulge covered by normal mucosa. Biopsies of these lesions are unnecessary because of the expected subsequent operation which needs to be planned. Computed tomographic scan of the chest may clarify the location and consistency of the lesion in the esophagus.

Treatment

Once documented, these tumors should be removed to establish a definite histologic diagnosis and to prevent eventual complications from the tumor. Extramucosal resection of these lesions can be completed through a standard thoracotomy or through video-assisted thoracoscopy.

MALIGNANT TUMORS OF THE ESOPHAGUS

Definition

Malignant lesions of the esophagus are usually epithelial in origin. Squamous cell carcinoma remains the most frequent esophageal mucosal cancer, while adenocarcinomas involving the cardia and arising in columnar lined mucosa are increasing in North America.

Etiology

In industrialized countries, the association of alcohol intake with tobacco use is known as a potentiating factor leading to the development of esophageal malignancies. In nonindustrialized societies, dietary factors with known carcinogens favor the development of such tumors. Patients with achalasia, lye strictures, and Barrett's esophagus are at risk of developing esophageal tumors.

Symptoms

Dysphagia (Table 2) is present in over 80 per cent of patients due to gradual closure of the esophageal lumen when a significant proportion of its circumference is involved. The dysphagia is usually progressive in nature, initially with solids and later with soft foods and liquids as the degree of obstruction becomes more severe. Weight loss is almost uniformly present and is responsible for the catabolic status of the patient. Pain, when present, is an ominous symptom suggesting extraesophageal invasion or metastasis of the tumor. Coughing on swallowing suggests a communication between the esophagus and the tracheobronchial tree.

Diagnosis

An esophagogram should localize the lesion, usually in the middle esophagus for squamous cell carcinomas and in the distal esophagus or cardia for adenocarcinomas. Deviation of the esophageal axis suggests infiltration of the tumor to the periesophageal tissues.

Esophagoscopy is the method of choice to diagnose these lesions and demonstrate their upper and lower limits. Submucosal extension of the tumor at a distance from the primary site must be sought. Biopsies and brush cytologies should provide accurate histologic documentation of the tumor. Endoscopic ultrasound is useful in evaluating the depth of penetration and in identifying involved nodes or invasion of major vessels. Bronchoscopy is essential to exclude invasion of the trachea or major bronchi. Computed tomography often demonstrates periesophageal extension if present, and an abdominal echography shows hepatic spread of the disease and clarifies the status of periceliac nodes. Radionuclide scanning of the bones and brain is indicated only when patients have symptoms suggestive of metastatic spread.

Staging Esophageal Cancer

The TNM classification helps to assess the extent of disease and prognosis. T refers to depth of invasion independent of size and length of the lesion, N1 to periesophageal nodes and N2 to regional nodes, and M to the presence or absence of metastasis. Accurate staging is obtained only after surgery.

Treatment

Preparation for operation requires the patient's motivation to stop smoking and to participate in active pulmonary physiotherapy to optimize lung function. Patients with significant weight loss benefit from intravenous or enteral alimentation to counteract debilitation and to decrease postoperative morbidity and mortality.

Resectable Carcinoma

When no clinical contraindications to treatment are found on preoperative assessment, over 90 per cent of esophageal carcinomas are resectable. However, more than 75 per cent of patients who are resected have stage III or IV tumors (transmural extension of metastasis beyond regional nodes). Thus, for the majority of these patients palliation of dysphagia is the first aim

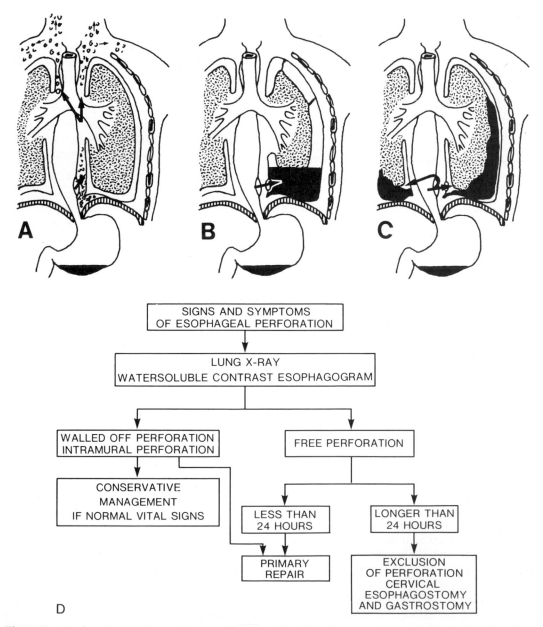

Figure 5. Perforation of the esophagus. Clinical and radiologic presentation. *A*, Mediastinal emphysema with spread along the fascial planes. *B*, Left hydropneumothorax. *C*, Bilateral hydrothorax. *D*, Diagnosis and management of esophageal perforation.

of therapy, as long-term survival cannot be expected. The overall 5-year survival is 5 per cent. When a "curative" resection is done, there is a 30 per cent 5-year survival, and the main prognostic factors are wall penetration and node status. Current protocols using adjuvant chemotherapy and radiotherapy usually show increased benefit for those patients in whom the tumor disappears. Reconstruction following esophagectomy is usually completed using the stomach or colon. Surgical resection and reconstruction has a hospital mortality of between 5 and 10 per cent.

Unresectable Tumors

Irradiation administered as palliation initially succeeds in controlling dysphagia in a large number of patients. However, recurrent dysphagia within a year is observed in 80 per cent of these patients. In patients in whom the tumor invades the tracheobronchial tree, irradiation and chemotherapy may lead to the formation of a tracheoesophageal fistula. Palliation offered through a surgical bypass procedure without esophageal resection causes a disproportionate morbidity and mortality for the benefit afforded. Where feasible, the simplest form of comfortable palliation is dilatation and transtumoral intubation using reinforced tubing. This is installed endoscopically by placing the prosthesis in position, or by laparotomy and gastrotomy with the tube being pulled into position by traction. The prosthesis is then sutured to the lesser curvature of the stomach to prevent migration. Complications of prosthetic installation for unresectable carcinomas are perforation, hemorrhage, and migration of the prosthesis.

CAUSTIC BURNS OF THE ESOPHAGUS

Definition and Presentation

Caustic burns of the esophagus are caused by chemical injury from the ingestion of alkaline or acid substances (mostly household cleaning agents). Medication tablets such as potassium chloride, ascorbic acid, and doxycycline are also known to produce esophageal burns. These lesions are seen mostly following accidental ingestion in children or following a suicide attempt in adults.

Pathophysiology

The extent of injury depends on the nature, concentration, and amount of the substance, as well as how long the esophagus was exposed to the damaging agent. Alkaline caustic agents cause immediate cell destruction with liquefaction necrosis, allowing diffusion of the substance through the esophageal wall. The damage is present within 30 seconds of exposure to a concentrated alkaline agent. In contrast, strong acids (sulfuric, hydrochloric) cause coagulation necrosis on the exposed mucosa. In the esophagus, this causes superficial burns, but in the stomach, long exposure causes severe burns with gastric destruction.

Symptoms

Burns in the mouth and oropharynx may cause local pain. Respiratory difficulties are seen with laryngeal injury. Esophageal damage usually causes neck and chest pain. Bacterial invasion causes fever and tachycardia. Dysphagia is secondary to esophageal obstruction by edema in the acute phase or by granulation and stricture formation in the more chronic phase. Symptoms and signs of mediastinitis and peritonitis suggest perforation of the esophagus or stomach or both.

Evaluation

Evaluation is made by a barium swallow that should clarify the initial damage and exclude perforation. Control evaluation at 1 month and 1 year after injury rules out late-appearing complications. Damage at the level of the three natural esophageal narrowings (pharyngoesophageal junction, aortic arch, lower sphincter) must be sought. Early endoscopic evaluation is important to determine the extent of injury. It is not performed distally if lesions are present. Superficial injury shows mostly hyperemia and edema. Deeper injury is more difficult to assess and ranges from exudates and ulcers with granulation tissue, to sloughing, obliteration, or full thickness necrosis and perforation.

Treatment

During the acute phase, respiratory and hemodynamic stability are ensured. Antibiotics are administered to prevent bacterial invasion through damaged tissues. The use of steroids is proposed to decrease inflammation and scar formation during the chronic phase, and periodic dilatation of established strictures is performed initially using rigid bougies passed on a guidewire. Eventually, mercury-weighted Maloney bougies should help maintain a proper diameter for comfortable swallowing.

Indications for Operation

In the acute phase, total esophageal destruction with or without gastric damage may require emergency esophagectomy with possible resection of adjacent damaged organs. During the chronic phase, long tight strictures, marked irregularities and pocketing of the esophagus, fistulas, or the impossibility of maintaining an adequate esophageal lumen favor esophageal resection and reconstruction.

DIVERTICULA OF THE ESOPHAGUS

Definition

Diverticula are pouches found at all levels of the esophagus from the pharyngoesophageal junction to the gastric inlet. When histologic examination of these pouches shows all layers of the esophageal wall, it is a true diverticulum. If the diverticulum shows only mucosa, submucosa, and thinned out muscular fibers, a *false* diverticulum is diagnosed.

Pathogenesis

The true diverticulum is usually formed by traction on the esophageal wall by periesophageal inflammation, while a false diverticulum is a herniation of mucosa and submucosa through the muscular layers and is secondary to abnormal pressures within the esophagus, as seen with established motor disorders.

Clinical Presentation

The pharyngoesophageal diverticulum (or Zenker's) is a pulsion diverticulum that is diagnosed in patients with oropharyngeal symptoms. Proximal and midthoracic diverticula are small, show a wide mouth, are usually asymptomatic, and represent deformation of the esophageal wall by inflammation. Diverticula of the distal half of the esophagus may be asymptomatic or they may be associated with dysphagia, odynophagia, fresh food regurgitations, and chest pain. This suggests the presence of a motor disorder.

Diagnosis

Radiologic studies are essential to locate the diverticulum. Symptomatic patients should undergo motility studies to exclude a primary motor disorder. Endoscopy is not attempted when the diverticulum is located at the pharyngoesophageal junction unless an accompanying lesion is suspected. Endoscopy is completed for diverticula located in the esophageal body.

Treatment

Surgical therapy is the only successful approach for a pharyngoesophageal diverticulum. Therapy for dis-

tal diverticulum, which is asymptomatic, is unnecessary. When symptoms are present, management is directed toward treatment of the motor disorder. Esophageal myotomy with either resection or suspension of the diverticulum is successful in controlling symptoms in most of these patients.

PERFORATION OF THE ESOPHAGUS

Definition and Pathogenesis

Perforation of the esophagus and disruption of the esophageal wall with contamination and infection of the mediastinum is a serious problem. The most frequent cause of esophageal perforation is instrumentation by endoscopy and dilatation. Spontaneous or postemetic perforation are caused by tremendous increases in intra-abdominal pressure that cause sudden overdistention of the proximal stomach and distal esophagus, usually after severe vomiting. Foreign bodies impacted at natural narrowings of the esophagus may cause erosion and perforation. Esophageal disease, mostly ulcers in a columnar lined esophagus, or carcinoma may cause perforation.

Clinical Presentation

Intense chest pain relating to neck, back, or shoulder is the first symptom, with tachypnea, dyspnea, and pleuritic pain following. Abdominal tenderness warrants the diagnosis of acute abdomen in some patients with involvement of the distal esophagus. Tachycardia and hypotension caused by massive liquid sequestration in the mediastinum usually follow. Fever and sepsis occur and are caused by progression of the contamination along the cellular planes of the posterior mediastinum. Subcutaneous emphysema is observed in some 50 per cent of the patients. A left pleural effusion occurs rapidly with hypoventilation and, occasionally, hydropneumothorax on the left. Mediastinal infection may progress and involve both pleural cavities.

Diagnosis

The morbidity and mortality of an esophageal perforation are directly related to the time between the occurrence of the injury and its diagnosis and treatment. The chest film may show mediastinal emphysema and a left pleural effusion. An esophagogram with water-soluble contrast medium is essential to locate precisely the site of the perforation. Liquid barium is used if the perforation is not evident. Examination of neck soft tissues may reveal retropharyngeal space thickening and air trapping. Endoscopy is not indicated for fear of diffusing the mediastinal contamination and creating a tension pneumothorax by the endoscope's air feed (Fig. 5).

Management

The principles of management include: (1) immediate administration of fluids and antibiotics covering aerobic and anaerobic bacteria; (2) immediate surgical exploration; (3) complete débridement of all devitalized tissue around the esophagus and within the esophageal wall; (4) appropriate repair of the laceration; and (5) drainage. Perforation at the pharyngoesophageal junction or in the neck usually requires drainage and antibiotic therapy. Lacerations with thoracic contamination have a mortality of 10 to 20 per cent when the repair is performed within the first 24 hours, but mortality increases to 60 per cent or more when diagnosis is late and treatment is more than 24 hours after injury. Late perforations with sepsis may require esophagectomy, esophagostomy, gastrostomy, and jejunostomy. Control of sepsis with adequate nutritional repletion should permit delayed reconstruction with gastric or colon interposition.

REFERENCES

Bonavina L, Khan NA, DeMeester TR: Pharyngoesophageal dysfunctions: The role of cricopharyngeal myotomy. Arch Surg 120: 541–549, 1985.

Castell DO, Richter JE, Dalton CB: Esophageal Motility Testing. New York, Elsevier, 1987.

Clouse RE, Lustman PJ: Psychiatric illnesses and contraction abnormalities of the esophagus. N Engl J Med 309:1337–1342, 1982.

Csendes A, Velasco N, Braghetto I, Henriquez A: A prospective randomized study comparing forceful dilatation and esophagomyotomy in patients with achalasia of the esophagus. Gastroenterology 80:789–795, 1981.

Delarue NC, Wilkins EW, Wong J: Esophageal Cancer. Volume 4 of International Trends in General Thoracic Surgery. St Louis, CV Mosby, 1988.

Dodds WJ: The pathogenesis of gastroesophageal reflux disease. AJR 151:49–56, 1988.

Duranceau A, Lafontaine ER, Taillefer R, Jamieson GG: Oropharyngeal dysphagia and operations on the upper esophageal sphincter. Surg Ann 19:317–362, 1987.

Ferguson MK, et al: Early evaluation and therapy for caustic esophageal injury. Am J Surg 157:116–120, 1989.

Jamieson GG, Duranceau A: Gastroesophageal Reflux. Philadelphia, WB Saunders Company, 1988.

Michel L, Grillo HC, Malt RA: Operative and non-operative management of esophageal perforation. Ann Surg 194:57–63, 1981.

Okike N, Payne WS, Neufeld DM, Bernatz PE, Pairolero PC, Sanderson DR: Esophagomyotomy versus forceful dilatation for achalasia of the esophagus: Results in 899 patients. Ann Thorac Surg 28:119–125, 1979.

Postlethwait RW: Benign tumors and cysts of the esophagus. Surg Clin North Am 63:925–931, 1983.

Richter JE, Castell DO: Diffuse esophageal spasm: A reappraisal. Ann Intern Med 100:242–245, 1984.

Skinner DB, Little AG, DeMeester TR: Management of esophageal perforation. Am J Surg 139:760–764, 1980.

Spechler SJ, Goyal RK: Barrett's Esophagus: Pathophysiology, Diagnosis, and Management. New York, Elsevier, 1985.

26
THE ACUTE ABDOMEN

STEPHEN J. FERZOCO, M.D.   JAMES M. BECKER, M.D.

The *acute abdomen* presents one of the most difficult challenges in clinical medicine and implies severe abdominal pain arising rather suddenly and often less than 24 hours in duration. Its causes are often conditions that require immediate operation, and the decision of whether to operate is dependent on an ability to diagnose the problem accurately as based on a complete medical history, thorough physical examination, and pertinent diagnostic tests. The primary goal is to establish whether the acute abdominal condition requires operative intervention and when it must be performed. Further decisions must also be made regarding additional diagnostic evaluation and the role of medical therapy.

The age has considerable influence on the differential diagnosis of the acute abdomen, and the causes of an acute abdomen in the adult and the child may be quite different (Table 1). A common cause of abdominal pain in children is appendicitis. Less common causes include bowel obstruction, bowel perforation, intussusception, ovarian cysts, cholecystitis, and primary peritonitis. In adults, biliary tract disease, intestinal obstruction, peptic ulcer disease, diverticulitis, appendicitis, pancreatitis, and incarcerated hernia are often causes, with less common conditions including rupture of abdominal aortic aneurysms, mesenteric ischemia, and perforation of a viscus due to a malignant tumor.

An understanding of the neurophysiology of pain in the abdominal organs is important in establishing a diagnosis of an acute abdomen. The embryologic derivation of the structures of the abdomen provides a basis for the location and distribution of pain. Pain arising in structures originating from the foregut, including the stomach, pancreas, duodenum, and biliary tree, localizes in the epigastric region. Pain from the small bowel and right and transverse colon, which are derivatives of the midgut, localize in the periumbilical region, while pain from the hindgut derivatives, such as the left colon, sigmoid, and rectum, have pain fibers that localize lower in the hypogastric region.

The nerve supply to the parietal peritoneum is derived from the somatic nerves that also supply the adjacent abdominal wall and skin. Sensory pathways for visceral pain are present in the lower thoracic and lumbar splanchnic nerves and in the parasympathetic nerves of the vagus and sacral plexus. In general, two types of abdominal pain occur with an acute abdomen. The first is steady, well-localized abdominal pain, that usually occurs following ischemia, perforation, inflammation, or hemorrhage. The second is intermittent colicky, poorly localized abdominal pain, found with obstruction of the gastrointestinal tract.

HISTORY

An accurate clinical diagnosis depends on obtaining a careful and complete history. The time of onset of pain, its location, and change in character and location are all very important.

Location and onset of the pain helps to determine the organ system involved. Pain characterized as vague, diffuse, and nonlocalizing tends to be visceral in nature. Pain that is of sudden onset or rapid in progression suggests perforation, rupture, or ischemia of a visceral organ. Pain with a gradual onset suggests a subacute process such as peptic ulcer disease, gastritis, inflammatory bowel disease, and diverticulitis. Pain from appendicitis, pancreatitis, cholecystitis, and pelvic inflammatory disease also tends to begin gradually with a gradual increase in intensity and, within 24 hours, often becomes an acute abdomen.

TABLE 1. DIFFERENTIAL DIAGNOSES OF ACUTE ABDOMINAL PAIN BY AGE

Childhood
Common
  Appendicitis
  Nonspecific abdominal pain
Less common
  Bowel obstruction
  Bowel perforation
  Intussusception
  Ovarian cyst
  Cholecystitis
  Spontaneous peritonitis
Elderly
Common
  Biliary tract disease
  Intestinal obstruction (colonic, small-bowel)
  Ulcer disease
  Diverticulitis
  Appendicitis
  Pancreatitis
  Hernia (incarcerated)
Less common
  Ruptured aneurysm
  Mesenteric ischemia
  Perforated cancer

The *course and characteristics* of the symptoms provide useful information in establishing the correct diagnosis. Pain that is episodic or fluctuates suggests obstruction, while pain that is steady and increasing over time suggests ischemia or peritoneal inflammation. Sudden, sharp pain indicates an acute vascular lesion, infarction, or rupture of a viscus. Dull or vague pain that is poorly localized indicates an inflammatory process. Crampy or colicky pain can be characteristic of gastroenteritis, mechanical small bowel obstruction, and cholecystitis. The more common causes of an acute abdomen are depicted in Figure 1.

It is critically important to accurately record the patient's history because associated diseases of the cardiac, pulmonary, or renal systems determine the safety of surgical intervention and because acute abdominal symptoms may arise as a consequence of chronic illness. A careful gynecologic history is imperative in women because gynecologic disease is a major differential factor in establishing an accurate diagnosis of acute abdominal pain. A history of pelvic inflammatory disease, vaginal discharge, previous abortion, abnormal masses, and timing of symptoms within the menstrual cycle is important. A careful family history is sought to detect patients harboring heritable diseases that may cause or mimic an acute abdomen.

While obtaining the history, it is important to observe additional modifying factors that may mask or accentuate the characterization of the pain, such as the dietary history. Ingestion of certain foods or drugs can precipitate abdominal discomfort, and it is important

to record the patient's most recent bowel movement. If there is absence of flatus and no bowel movement over 24 hours, intestinal obstruction should be suspected. It is also useful to know if there are certain activities or positions that lessen or worsen the pain; for example, pain exacerbated by breathing, coughing, or moving suggests peritonitis.

Associated signs and symptoms of abdominal pain can be helpful in determining the origin of the pain, especially the localization of the pain (Fig. 2). Referral pain is also important, and a knowledge of the sites of referral is essential (Fig. 3). Nausea and vomiting in the early stages of an illness suggest autonomic activation. With intestinal obstruction, continued vomiting can lead to hypochloremic, hypokalemic metabolic alkalosis. Fever suggests an inflammatory process, but in the elderly, it may occur late in the disease and is not often impressive in the setting of an acute abdomen, while in children fever occurs in most illnesses. Diarrhea and constipation are additional factors, as profuse, watery diarrhea suggests an infectious process or inflammatory bowel disease.

PHYSICAL EXAMINATION

The physical examination begins with a general assessment of the patient's condition (Table 2). The ability to answer questions, degree of discomfort, and position in bed provide important diagnostic aids in determining the status of the patient. A patient who appears relaxed, able to answer questions, and breaths normally must be distinguished from the patient who is anxious, pale, restless, or lying motionless in bed and obviously is in pain.

The initial and most important part of the physical examination is *inspection of the abdomen*. Evidence of previous scars, hernia, or any obvious masses are important. Patients with significant peritonitis may have flexed hips and knees to lessen the pain. A distended abdomen is evidence of intestinal obstruction.

The abdomen is then *auscultated* in all four quadrants for several minutes to be certain of the character of the bowel sounds. The frequency and pitch of bowel sounds are noted, and absence of bowel sounds after several minutes is consistent with ileus. High-pitched tones with splashes, tinkles, and rushes, especially with abdominal distention, suggest small-bowel obstruction, although proximal intestinal obstruction may be present without these findings.

The abdomen is then palpated beginning in a quadrant free of pain and progressing slowly toward the point of maximal tenderness. It should also be performed gently to avoid causing pain early in the examination. It is important to reconfirm the point of maximal tenderness in context with the patient's his-

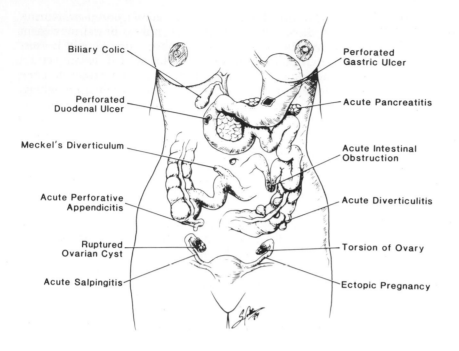

Biliary Colic

Perforated Duodenal Ulcer

Meckel's Diverticulum

Acute Perforative Appendicitis

Ruptured Ovarian Cyst

Acute Salpingitis

Perforated Gastric Ulcer

Acute Pancreatitis

Acute Intestinal Obstruction

Acute Diverticulitis

Torsion of Ovary

Ectopic Pregnancy

Figure 1. Common causes of abdominal pain. (From Sabiston DC Jr [ed]: Textbook of Surgery: The Biological Basis of Modern Surgical Practice, ed 14. Philadelphia, WB Saunders Company, 1991, p 738, with permission.)

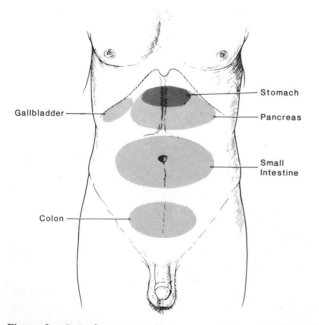

Gallbladder

Colon

Stomach

Pancreas

Small Intestine

Figure 2. Pain from intra-abdominal viscera. (From Sabiston DC Jr [ed]: Textbook of Surgery: The Biological Basis of Modern Surgical Practice, ed 14. Philadelphia, WB Saunders Company, 1991, p 737, with permission.)

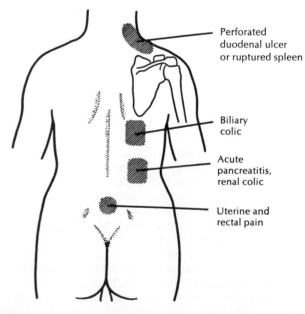

Perforated duodenal ulcer or ruptured spleen

Biliary colic

Acute pancreatitis, renal colic

Uterine and rectal pain

Figure 3. Sites of referred pain for specific problems in the differential diagnosis of the acute abdomen. (From Silen W: Cope's Early Diagnosis of the Acute Abdomen, ed 17. New York, Oxford University Press, 1987, p 11, with permission.)

TABLE 2. PRINCIPLES OF EXAMINATION

Assessment
Inspection
Auscultation
Palpation
Percussion
Rectal/pelvic examination

tory, and evidence of guarding or spasm should be noted. *Percussion* of the abdomen is useful in determining the amount of distention in the bowel. Costovertebral tenderness may be associated with urinary tract disease. The presence of rebound tenderness suggests peritoneal irritation and can be elicited by palpation with quick but not exaggerated release of the pressure by the hand.

Other important parts of the physical are the *rectal and pelvic examinations*, during which the lower pelvis is fully evaluated and any masses or tenderness are noted. In addition, the stool should be inspected and tested for occult blood. The presence of cervical discharge or vaginal bleeding is important, and a bimanual examination can elicit uterine or adnexal tenderness or masses.

LABORATORY TESTS

In addition to the physical findings, important information leading to a clear understanding of the clinical manifestations is provided by specific laboratory tests (Table 3). A *complete blood count* (CBC) is important, and an elevated leukocyte count and shift in the differential indicate an inflammatory process. A normal leukocyte is often found in elderly patients or in those who are immunosuppressed. The hematocrit is obtained, and if low, may reflect anemia or chronic bleeding, while an elevated hematocrit suggests dehydration.

A *urinalysis* is routinely performed to determine if a urinary infection may be the cause of the abdominal pain. The presence of blood, protein, or glucose may

TABLE 3. DIAGNOSTIC ASSESSMENT

CBC, electrolytes
Urinalysis, amylase, liver function tests
Additional blood tests
Radiographic Imaging
  Plain films
  Ultrasound
  Computed tomography
  Angiography
  Barium studies
Laparoscopy or laparotomy

Abbreviation: CBC = complete blood count.

offer additional data to the etiology, while the urine-specific gravity reflects the status of the patient's blood volume. A pregnancy test may also be useful when applicable to the diagnosis of pelvic disease.

Patients suspected of having acute pancreatitis frequently have an elevated *serum or urine amylase*. Amylase levels can also be elevated in patients with mesenteric thrombosis, intestinal obstruction, or a perforated duodenal ulcer. Liver function tests are useful in the diagnosis of disorders of the biliary tract. It is important to obtain serum electrolytes to identify and correct any underlying abnormalities prior to admission to the hospital or in preparation for an operative procedure.

The role of diagnostic peritoneal lavage to evaluate blunt abdominal trauma is well established, and it may also be useful in evaluating peritonitis. Evidence of blood, purulent material, or bacteria suggests the need for surgical intervention and exploration.

RADIOGRAPHIC IMAGING

Plain Supine and Erect Radiographs

Radiographic imaging can also provide much useful information in the diagnosis of an acute abdomen. The initial evaluation consists of a plain film of the abdomen with the patient in the supine and erect positions. A standard chest film is usually appropriate, as basilar pneumonia can mimic the symptoms of an acute abdomen, and the presence of free air under the diaphragm due to a perforated viscus usually indicates the need for surgical intervention. Plain films of the abdomen are especially useful in the evaluation of obstruction of the gastrointestinal tract and allow visualization of air-fluid levels in distended loops of small bowel or colon due to an ileus or obstruction.

Ultrasound

Ultrasound provides a safe and painless method of evaluating an acute abdomen and can provide a quick assessment of many organs including the liver, spleen, biliary tract, pancreas, appendix, kidneys, and ovaries. In addition, pulsed Doppler ultrasound provides assessment of many vascular abnormalities including aortic and visceral arterial aneurysms, arteriovenous fistulas, and venous thrombi.

Computed Tomography

Computed tomography (CT) is another safe, noninvasive, rapid, and efficient method of investigating the acute abdomen. It provides detailed information on a variety of structures with views of the bowel wall, mesentery, and the retroperitoneum. In particular, the kidneys, pancreas, duodenum, and aorta are better seen and with more detail than with other diagnostic modalities. In addition, CT provides sensitive detection of free air, abscesses, calcifications, and collections of intraperitoneal fluid. Magnetic resonance imaging (MRI) requires more time and is generally less useful than CT scanning.

Angiography

Although of limited use in the early stages, angiography is useful in confirming diagnoses and in therapeutic embolization of many vascular lesions with bleeding causing abdominal pain. After initial ultrasound or CT studies have led to suspicion of a vascular abnormality, angiography is apt to further delineate the diagnosis.

Barium Studies

The role of barium studies has diminished with the increased use of other imaging modalities such as CT. Although not useful in the setting of a questionable perforation, barium enemas can delineate an obstructing lesion such as a carcinoma or volvulus as well as provide evidence for mucosal disease in various forms of colitis.

Endoscopy

Visual examination of the alimentary tract by direct endoscopy is often successful in establishing a diagnosis. Upper gastrointestinal lesions, including peptic ulcers, obstructing strictures, neoplasms, and sources of acute bleeding, can be identified. Colonoscopy is useful in the diagnosis of inflammatory bowel disease, obstructing neoplasms, intussusception, and volvulus.

LAPAROSCOPY AND LAPAROTOMY

Laparoscopy has been employed by gynecologists for decades in evaluating women with acute lower abdominal pain. As general surgeons have become more familiar with this technique, it has an increasingly greater role in the diagnosis and treatment of many patients with acute abdominal pain. It is especially useful in differentiating appendicitis from other causes of lower abdominal pain, including pelvic disease, when the diagnosis of acute appendicitis is unclear. In addition, laparoscopy can be therapeutic for cholecystitis, appendicitis, and intestinal obstruction. In some patients, exploratory laparotomy is ultimately required for a final diagnosis. When the patient contin-

ues to show serious signs of an acute abdomen and the diagnosis remains unclear despite a thorough preoperative assessment, abdominal exploration may be the only option.

PRESENTATION OF COMMON CONDITIONS LEADING TO AN ACUTE ABDOMEN

Peritonitis (Gastrointestinal Tract Perforation)

Patients with a perforated viscus or peritonitis often present with diffuse, severe abdominal tenderness. Guarding or rigidity is often present. On physical examination, there is an absence of bowel sounds and often evidence of systemic sepsis. The upright chest film may show free intraperitoneal air under the diaphragm.

Appendicitis

The classic signs and symptoms of appendicitis are mild fever and focal right lower quadrant (McBurney point) pain with rebound tenderness. Anorexia, nausea, and vomiting are common, and while not usually necessary, ultrasound and CT may be helpful in confirming the diagnosis. These imaging modalities have largely replaced the barium enema in situations of diagnostic uncertainty. A pelvic examination in women and rectal examination in all patients are essential. A moderate leukocytosis is usually present.

Pancreatitis (Acute)

Pancreatitis often presents with a relatively rapid onset of severe epigastric pain radiating to the back that is frequently accompanied by anorexia, nausea, and vomiting. Tenderness is localized to the midepigastric region, and patients often have mild rebound tenderness. The bowel sounds may be hypoactive or absent, and tests that should be obtained include CBC, to discern an elevated white count or a depressed hematocrit, as well as serum amylase, an ultrasound, and/or CT scan.

Cholecystitis (Acute)

Acute cholecystitis commonly occurs in women between the ages of 40 and 60 years who are overweight and have a previous history of pregnancy. Cholecystitis may be difficult to differentiate from self-limited biliary colic. Patients present with right upper quadrant tenderness that is accentuated by inspiration and accompanied by nausea and vomiting. These patients are febrile, and the abdomen may be slightly distended with guarding. Bowel sounds are often hypoactive, and tenderness is localized to the right upper quadrant. Ultrasound remains the most effective method of evaluating the gallbladder and biliary tree in an emergency situation and often demonstrates gallstones and permits assessment of the presence or absence of edema and thickening of the gallbladder wall or dilatation of the bile ducts. Acute cholecystitis is suggested if, on radionuclide hepatobiliary scanning, the cystic duct is occluded and the gallbladder fails to take up the HIDA-labeled bile.

Diverticulitis

Diverticulosis and diverticulitis increase in incidence with age. Although diverticulitis can involve the entire colon, the disease is most frequently limited to the left and sigmoid colon. Patients present with left lower quadrant tenderness, chills, and fever. On examination, the tenderness is usually localized to the left lower quadrant with rebound and guarding and absent bowel sounds. Computed tomography and interval barium enema may be helpful to confirm the diagnosis, with the barium enema performed only after resolution of the acute inflammatory process.

Small-Bowel Obstruction

Patients with small-bowel obstruction present with nausea, bilious vomiting and, not infrequently, sudden, sharp, colicky abdominal pain. In the advanced stages of small-bowel obstruction, tachycardia, hypotension, and fever may be present. On examination, abdominal distention is frequently present with distal small-bowel obstruction. Typically, hyperactive and high-pitched bowel sounds are auscultated. Supine and erect plain films of the abdomen are most useful in the diagnosis. Dilated loops of bowel can often localize the general site of obstruction. Other diagnostic tests that may be performed include an upper gastrointestinal radiographic contrast study and endoscopy for a proximal small bowel obstruction and barium enema in a distal bowel obstruction.

Large-Bowel Obstruction

Patients with large-bowel obstruction present with constipation and abdominal distention, and pain is gradual in onset. The most common causes of large-bowel obstruction include carcinoma of the colon, acute diverticulitis, and volvulus. On physical examination, abdominal tenderness is often present, but the degree of tenderness to palpation is minimal. Radio-

graphic tests that aid in the diagnosis include plain films of the abdomen and retrograde contrast studies that localize the area of obstruction. An upper gastrointestinal contrast series is contraindicated in a patient with suspected colonic obstruction.

Meckel's Diverticulitis

A diagnosis of Meckel's diverticulitis is often difficult to establish preoperatively. The signs and symptoms are often mistaken for those of acute appendicitis. Most laboratory data and radiographic studies are often unremarkable, and small-bowel contrast studies, including small-bowel enteroclysis, may occasionally be useful. If the Meckel's diverticulum contains heterotopic gastric mucosa, a technetium radionuclide scan (Meckel's scan) may be useful in identifying the anomaly. The presence of a Meckel's diverticulum is often recognized only during surgical exploration.

Mesenteric Ischemia

The most common complaint of patients with mesenteric ischemia is sudden onset of very severe abdominal pain. Additional symptoms include nausea, vomiting, diarrhea, and gastrointestinal bleeding. The classic finding of acute mesenteric ischemia is pain out of proportion to the amount of tenderness elicited by abdominal palpation. Hypotension, tachycardia, fever, and hypovolemia are also apt to rapidly appear. The plain abdominal films are nonspecific, and an accurate diagnosis is confirmed by angiography.

Ruptured Aortic Aneurysm

Expanding or ruptured abdominal aortic aneurysms often present with abdominal pain. Patients complain of upper abdominal tenderness and back pain and are often hypovolemic and in shock. On physical examination, a pulsatile supraumbilical mass is present. It is important to recognize the urgency of such a situation and the need for rapid surgical intervention. Although ultrasound, CT, and angiography can confirm the diagnosis, time frequently does not permit obtaining these studies.

Gynecologic Causes

Although a variety of gynecologic disorders present with abdominal pain, the most life-threatening is a ruptured ectopic pregnancy. A detailed gynecologic history including menstrual irregularities, vaginal bleeding, and crampy abdominal pain should be elicited. Pregnancy tests should be performed on any female with abdominal pain with the suspicion of a possible ectopic pregnancy. *Pelvic inflammatory disease* is a common cause of acute abdominal pain in females between 15 and 35 years of age. Patients manifest lower or diffuse abdominal pain combined with high fever. Most present either during or just after the most recent menstrual period and often have a past history of pelvic inflammatory disease. Pelvic examination reveals a hyperemic, extremely tender cervix with vaginal discharge. A positive diagnosis can be established with a cervical smear and culture, and a pelvic ultrasound may identify a tubo-ovarian abscess. *Ovarian cysts* often present acutely in either the right or left lower quadrants. Accurate diagnosis is based on a thorough pelvic examination. If rupture occurs, generalized peritonitis occurs following intraperitoneal bleeding. Other gynecologic causes of abdominal pain include endometriosis, gonorrhea, ovarian cysts, ruptured tubo-ovarian abscess, ruptured uterus, and ovarian torsion.

Nonsurgical Causes

It is important to emphasize that patients with an acute abdomen require surgical intervention. The list of nonsurgical causes of the abdominal pain is extensive and must be considered prior to any surgical intervention. *Myocardial infarction* as well as *acute pericarditis* may mimic the symptoms of acute pancreatitis or perforated duodenal ulcer. The pain is localized to the midepigastric region and is sudden in onset. An electrocardiogram demonstrates the underlying cardiac abnormality. The most common pulmonary cause of an acute abdomen is a *pneumonia* involving the diaphragmatic pleura. Patients present with either right or left upper quadrant abdominal pain. Other pulmonary processes such as pleuritis or a pleural effusion require radiographic studies to distinguish them from other surgical causes.

A common gastrointestinal cause of acute abdominal pain is *gastroenteritis.* In addition to severe abdominal pain, this disorder is often accompanied by nausea, vomiting, and diarrhea. On history, patients often note a specific food intake or additional family members who are affected. Treatment is supportive, and symptoms usually resolve within 12 hours. Sickle cell anemia is a common hematologic cause of acute

abdominal pain, and the diagnosis depends on a careful history, as most patients have had previous episodes. Of note is the common occurrence of cholelithiasis in this group, which may lead to acute cholecystitis. Several urologic conditions can be associated with abdominal pain, including *pyelonephritis,* which presents with dysuria, frequency, or urgency with flank pain and tenderness. Urinalysis is crucial in the diagnosis. Organisms such as *Escherichia coli, Proteus mirabilis,* and *Klebsiella* species are the common organisms responsible for infection. Proteinuria and hematuria are often seen in addition to bacteria. Patients with *urolithiasis* initially present with flank pain. As the stone passes distally, the location of the pain also migrates lower in the abdomen and, in males, may be referred to the testes. Urinalysis and microscopic examination of the urine help to establish the diagnosis. In addition, the plain film of the abdomen sometimes reveals renal calculi, as about 90 per cent are radiopaque. An intravenous pyelogram may also reveal the calculi and the point of obstruction or a delayed visualization on the obstructed side.

Of increasing importance are the acute abdominal conditions being observed in patients with acquired immunodeficiency syndrome (AIDS). Acute abdominal pain in AIDS may be secondary to a number of causes, including cytomegalovirus enterocolitis, opportunistic infection, lymphoma, or Kaposi's sarcoma of the gastrointestinal tract. Patients may present with peritonitis from perforation or infection, distention, obstipation, or gastrointestinal bleeding. Evaluation should include clinical assessment, serum testing for AIDS, and diagnostic testing with CT scanning, endoscopy, and barium contrast studies.

REFERENCES

Barone JE, Gingold BS, Arvanitis ML, Nealon JF: Abdominal pain in patients with acquired immune deficiency syndrome. Ann Surg 204:619, 1986.

Davies AH, Mastorakou I, Cobb R, et al: Ultrasonography in the acute abdomen. Br J Surg 78(1):1178–1180, 1991.

Diethelm AG, Stanley RJ: The acute abdomen. *In* Sabiston DC Jr (ed): Textbook of Surgery: The Biological Basis of Modern Surgical Practice, ed 14. Philadelphia, WB Saunders Company, 1992, pp 736–755.

Paterson-Brown S, Vipond MN: Modern aids to clinical decision-making in the acute abdomen. Br J Surg 77:13, 1990.

Silen W: Cope's Early Diagnosis of the Acute Abdomen, ed 18. New York, Oxford University Press, 1991.

27

THE STOMACH AND DUODENUM

WALLACE P. RITCHIE, Jr., M.D., Ph.D.

The stomach, duodenum, and pancreas act together as an elegantly integrated unit to initiate the digestion of swallowed foodstuffs, each having a specific role. The stomach secretes a highly caustic acid and a powerful proteolytic enzyme that begins the digestion of protein. It also mixes and grinds the food and delivers it as small particles in an orderly manner into the duodenum. The duodenum acts in association with the pancreas and hepatobiliary system to adjust intraluminal pH and osmolarity, to promote further hydrolysis of protein and carbohydrate, and to alter dietary fat into an absorbable form. On occasion, the process can become faulty, leading to autodigestion of the gastric or duodenal mucosa, and the result is a *peptic* ulcer. In addition, a variety of neoplasms can develop in the stomach that may require the attention of a surgeon. In this chapter, the normal anatomy and physiology of the stomach and duodenum are reviewed, the operative treatment of peptic ulcers of these organs is outlined, and the surgical therapy of the more common benign and malignant conditions of the stomach is discussed.

SURGICAL ANATOMY OF THE STOMACH AND DUODENUM

The stomach is the first organ of the alimentary canal in the abdominal cavity. Its external surface is divided into anatomic regions based approximately on the cell types found in the subjacent mucosa (Fig. 1). The proximal stomach (body) contains the vast majority of the stomach's complement of *parietal* cells, the source of hydrochloric acid (HCl) and intrinsic factor, and of *chief* cells, the major source of pepsinogen. The body is bounded superiorly by the cardia (that portion of the stomach immediately below the gastroesophageal junction) and the fundus (the portion of the stomach lying to the left and superior to the gastroesophageal junction). The most distal portion of the stomach is the antrum, which contains mucus-secreting glands as well as G cells, the source of the hormone *gastrin*.

The duodenum curves around the head of the pancreas in a C-shaped manner, beginning at the pylorus and ending at the ligament of Treitz. It is divided, by convention, into four parts: superior (first part), descending (second part), horizontal (third part), and ascending (fourth part). In its course, it receives the common bile duct and both the major and minor pancreatic ducts.

The stomach and duodenum are organs that are extremely well vascularized, deriving their blood supply from a rich network of anastomotic interconnections (Fig. 2). Both the celiac axis and the superior mesenteric artery are involved. After arising from the abdominal aorta, the celiac axis divides into the left gastric, the hepatic, and the splenic arteries. The left gastric artery supplies the lesser curvature and the lower esophagus, and it anastomoses with the right gastric artery, which is one of the branches of the hepatic artery. The greater curvature receives its blood supply from the right gastroepiploic artery, a branch of the gastroduodenal artery (itself a branch of the hepatic), from the left gastroepiploic artery, and from the short gastric arteries, both of which are derived from the splenic artery. The gastroduodenal artery also supplies the duodenum. Its proximity to the pos-

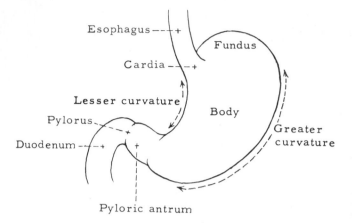

Figure 1. Divisions of the stomach. (From Shackelford RT, Zuidema GD [eds]: Surgery of the Alimentary Tract, ed 3, vol 2. Philadelphia, WB Saunders Company, 1991, p 3, with permission.)

terior duodenal wall distal to the pylorus renders it susceptible to acid peptic digestion with consequent upper gastrointestinal hemorrhage. The terminal branch of the gastroduodenal artery is the superior pancreaticoduodenal, which anastomoses with the inferior pancreaticoduodenal artery, the first branch of the superior mesenteric artery.

The parasympathetic nerve supply to the stomach (the vagus nerves) traverses the thoracic cavity as two branches in close proximity to the esophagus (Fig. 3). After forming a plexus in the region of the esophageal hiatus, the anterior and posterior vagus nerves (also known as the nerves of Latarjet) emerge. The left anterior trunk innervates not only the entire stomach including the antrum, but also, via its hepatic branch, the duodenum, pancreas, liver, gallbladder, and bile ducts. The right posterior trunk also supplies the stomach and antrum and, via its celiac branch, joins the celiac plexus to innervate the remainder of the small bowel and the colon up to the level of the splenic flexure.

SURGICAL PHYSIOLOGY OF THE STOMACH AND DUODENUM

Gastric Acid Secretion

Hydrochloric acid is secreted in the proximal stomach by parietal cells, which contain three distinct receptors on their basolateral membranes: an H_2-receptor, responsive to histamine; a gastrin receptor, responsive to the peptide hormone gastrin; and a muscarinic receptor, responsive to acetylcholine released during vagal stimulation. Stimulation of one or all of these receptors activates a variety of intracellular events that culminate in the excitation of an H^+, K^+-ATPase located in the apical cell membrane, which promotes secretion of H^+ in exchange for absorption of luminal K^+. A variety of inhibitors interact in this system: H_2-receptor antagonists competitively inhibit the H_2-receptor locus; atropine blocks the muscarinic receptor; the prostaglandins inhibit intracellular events; and omeprazole destroys membrane-bound H^+, K^+-ATPase.

In the gastric lumen, the concentration of HCl far exceeds that of the subjacent tissue. In any other semipermeable membrane of the body, this would promote massive diffusion of H^+ into the mucosa. Under ordinary circumstances, however, this does not occur in the stomach because of the *gastric mucosal barrier*. Factors thought to promote this barrier include the existence of a viscid mucus gel at the apices of the cells at greatest risk, the surface epithelial cells; the capacity of surface cells to secrete bicarbonate into the mucus; the ability of the gastric mucosa to increase its nutrient blood flow in response to topical injury; the peculiar capacity of the gastric mucosa to be nonwettable; and the ability of mucosa to restore itself rapidly once surface cells are damaged.

The physiologic stimulus to HCl secretion is the ingestion of a meal. By convention, three distinct yet interrelated phases of secretion have been described. The first is properly called the *vagal* or *cephalic phase*. The sight, smell, or thought of food excites neural centers in the cortex and hypothalamus, which transmit signals through the vagus nerves to the stomach. Acid production during the cephalic phase results primarily from direct vagal stimulation of the perietal cells, although the vagus also has the capacity to simulate the release of gastrin from antral G cells. Additionally, vagal excitation causes the release of mucus from surface epithelial cells and of the preenzyme pepsinogen from chief cells. Pepsinogen becomes fully active as the pH of intragastric content falls to less than 3. Although the magnitude of the acid response seen during the cephalic phase surpasses that produced during the other phases of secretion, its duration is short, and therefore, it accounts for only 20 to 30 per cent of the total volume of gastric acid produced in response to a meal.

The gastric phase of secretion is mediated by the hormone gastrin. This peptide is released from G cells in response to vagal excitation, antral distention, and the presence of partially digested protein in contact with antral mucosa. The gastric phase of secretion persists for the several hours required for gastric emptying to occur; therefore, it accounts for approximately 60 to 70 per cent of the total acid output seen in response to a meal. The final phase of gastric acid production is the intestinal phase, which is the least well under-

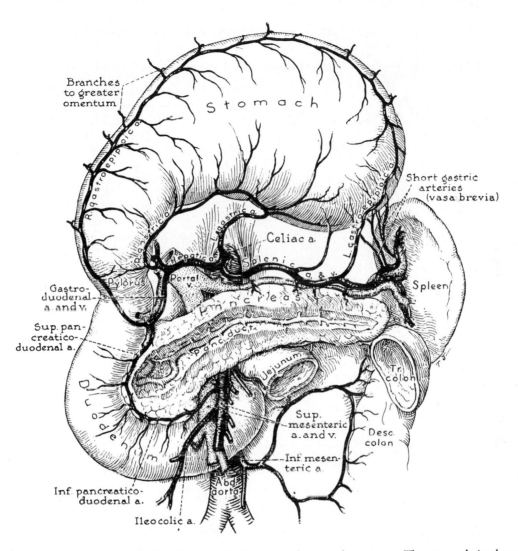

Figure 2. Blood supply of the stomach, duodenum, spleen, and pancreas. The stomach is shown reflected upward, and the pancreatic duct is exposed. (From Shackelford RT, Zuidema GD [eds]: Surgery of the Alimentary Tract, ed 3, vol 2. Philadelphia, WB Saunders Company, 1991, p 5, with permission.)

stood and the least important of the three. It occurs after complete gastric emptying and continues for as long as chyme remains in the proximal small intestine. The mediator of this phase has not been identified and accounts for only 5 to 10 per cent of total acid output after eating.

Once initiated, gastric acid production does not proceed indefinitely. The stimulus (the meal) is transient, and several important mechanisms capable of inhibiting further acid production are also activated. The first is referred to as the *acid brake* on antral gastrin release. When the pH of intraluminal content in contact with the antrum falls below 2.5, gastrin output is

almost completely arrested in normal individuals. In addition, it is now clear that vagal excitation can stimulate somatostatin release from specialized cells in the antrum, which further modulates antral gastrin output. Finally, transfer of an acid load into the proximal duodenum also serves to inhibit gastric acid production. Secretin, a hormone released from the proximal duodenum as the pH of duodenal chyme falls, inhibits gastrin release and stimulates pancreatic bicarbonate secretion. A second hormone, cholecystokinin (CCK), is released by intraluminal fat and protein and acts as a competitive inhibitor of gastrin at the parietal cell level. It seems likely that other intestinal peptides

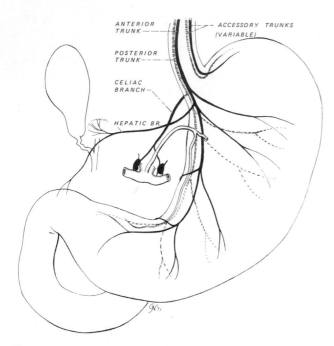

ANTERIOR TRUNK

POSTERIOR TRUNK

CELIAC BRANCH

HEPATIC BR.

ACCESSORY TRUNKS (VARIABLE)

Figure 3. Anatomy of the vagus nerves in relation to the stomach. (From Sabiston DC Jr [ed]: Textbook of Surgery, ed 14. Philadelphia, WB Saunders Company, 1991, p 776, with permission.)

probably play an equally important role in the inhibition of gastric acid production under physiologic circumstances.

Gastric Motility

The stomach serves as a commodious reservoir for large volumes of ingested solids and liquids. At the same time, it ensures that this material is delivered to the duodenum as small particles in isosmotic solution at physiologic pH. Gastric emptying of liquids is modulated primarily by the proximal stomach, which is capable of increasing its intraluminal volume more than 15 times relative to its resting volume without an appreciable rise in intragastric pressure. This phenomenon is known as *receptive relaxation* and is mediated in large part by the vagus nerves. Thus, following denervation of the proximal stomach, receptive relaxation is impaired, the proximal stomach cannot accommodate as well, intragastric pressure rises, and gastric emptying of liquids is accelerated as a result.

Gastric emptying of solids is more complex. As solid food reaches the antrum, antral muscular contractions increase in both frequency and amplitude. This response is also mediated, at least in part, by the vagus. Initially, the pylorus remains closed so that forward propulsion of ingested foodstuffs is followed by their retropulsion into the proximal stomach, resulting in a

mixing and grinding action. Once solid food is of an appropriate particle size (~1 mm), the pylorus opens in response to an integrated peristaltic wave, permitting solid food to empty into the duodenum. Vagotomy of the antrum ablates this mechanism, causing delayed gastric emptying of solids. In contrast, resection of the antrum causes rapid gastric emptying of solids into the duodenum. Once food has entered the duodenum, gastric motility is inhibited. Both physical and physiologic factors are involved in this response, which is most profound when the duodenum is exposed to fat.

Physiology of Gastric and Duodenal Digestion

The stomach and duodenum are responsible primarily for initiating digestion of ingested carbohydrates, fats, and proteins. Absorption takes place in the more distal small intestine. Digestion of dietary proteins (long-chain polypeptides) begins in the stomach. In the presence of gastric acid, the zygomen *pepsinogen* is secreted and converted to pepsin, an exopeptidase. In the duodenum, partially digested protein and fat cause the release of CCK which, in concert with vagal stimulation, stimulates secretion of pancreatic trypsin, chymotrypsin, and carboxypeptidase. Each is elaborated as an inactive precursor that is subsequently activated intraluminally by the duodenal hormone, enterokinase. In their active forms, these enzymes promote further digestion of proteins that are ultimately absorbed in the distal small intestine as individual amino acids.

The principal form of ingested dietary fat is triglyceride, three fatty acids linked to glycerol. The pancreatic enzyme that hydrolyzes triglycerides, *lipase*, is insoluble in fat, so that initially the large fat globules entering the duodenum are fragmented into smaller units, a process known as *emulsification*. Once emulsified, triglycerides are hydrolyzed to fatty acids and monoglycerides. Hydrolysis alone is insufficient to ensure absorption, however, so that these moieties must be rendered water soluble by bile acids, which form them into *micelles*. Digestion of carbohydrates is somewhat less complex. The process is initiated by salivary amylase, which hydrolyzes ingested sugars into maltose and isomaltose. The reaction continues in the stomach until sufficient acid is secreted to inactivate the enzyme. The greater part of dietary carbohydrate is hydrolyzed in the duodenum by pancreatic amylase, reducing polysaccharides to the disaccharides, lactose and sucrose. These sugars in turn are reduced to monosaccharides by enzymes located in the brush borders of the intestinal mucosal cell and are subsequently absorbed as such.

PEPTIC ULCER DISEASE

An ulcer is a disruption in the integrity of what is normally a contiguous sheet of cells. A *peptic* ulcer is one that requires for its development the presence of acid and pepsin. In this sense, all ulcerative lesions of the upper gastrointestinal tract are peptic in origin. By convention, an ulcer involves the full thickness of the mucosa, whereas less than full-thickness lesions are termed erosions. Two major variants of peptic ulcers are commonly encountered in clinical practice: *duodenal ulcers* and *gastric ulcers*.

Duodenal Ulcer

Although the number of hospitalizations and operations for duodenal ulcer disease has fallen precipitously in the United States over the past 30 years, approximately 1 in 15 Americans can still expect to suffer from duodenal ulcer disease during his or her lifetime. Duodenal ulcers are found most frequently in middle-aged males and are characterized by frequent episodes of exacerbation and remission. In general, duodenal ulcer is a benign condition: 80 to 90 per cent of patients can be treated successfully by nonoperative means. Anatomically, duodenal ulcers are found in three major locations:

1. Most commonly, distal to the pylorus on the posterior duodenal wall. As noted previously, the proximity of these ulcers to the gastroduodenal artery can precipitate massive hemorrhage.

2. Less commonly, distal to the pylorus on the anterior duodenal wall. Free perforation into the peritoneal cavity can result.

3. Least commonly, in the pyloric channel. This location can predispose to obstruction.

Pathogenesis

It is important to recognize that duodenal ulcer disease is heterogeneous in origin and that not all identified pathophysiologic abnormalities are present in every patient. In general, however, patients with duodenal ulcer have approximately twice the number of parietal cells as do normal individuals. Thus, they secrete increased amounts of acid, both in response to exogenous stimulants such as histamine and in response to a meal. Meal-stimulated acid secretion persists for a longer period of time in patients with ulcer than in normal individuals. Current evidence also suggests that the individual parietal cells in patients with duodenal ulcer are more sensitive to any given stimulant. Hydrogen ion delivery to the duodenum is greater in afflicted patients, and in some, this is a con-

sequence of a rapid rate of gastric emptying. The gastrin response to feeding is also significantly exaggerated in duodenal ulcer disease.

Defects in resistance factors have also been identified. Gastrin release in response to a meal is incompletely inhibited to low pH in duodenal ulcer subjects, suggesting a defective *acid brake* on antral gastrin release. Duodenal ulcer patients also demonstrate an impaired ability to synthesize prostaglandins in duodenal mucosa. This is of some importance because the prostaglandins, which are ubiquitous in the stomach and duodenum, have the peculiar capacity to protect the gastric and duodenal mucosa from the injurious effects of a variety of topically damaging agents. In addition, patients with duodenal ulcer secrete less duodenal bicarbonate in response to instilled acid than do normals. As additional information accumulates, it is likely that other defects in resistance will be identified.

Considerable recent interest has been directed to the possibility that duodenal ulcer may have an infectious origin, at least in part. The spiral organism *Helicobacter pylori* has been identified in the mucus layer of the upper portion of the gastric pits of the antrum in large numbers of patients with duodenal ulcer, particularly those that are refractory to conventional treatment. The fact that gastric metaplasia is common in the region of a duodenal ulcer may be germane in this regard. Importantly, complete eradication of *Helicobacter pylori* from the stomach causes very high rates of ulcer healing and extraordinarily lower rates of ulcer relapse. The case is not definitively proved, however. *Helicobacter pylori* infection is extremely common worldwide, yet the vast majority of afflicted patients have no ulcer. Obviously, further data are required to clarify the precise role of this organism in the pathogenesis of duodenal ulcer disease.

Diagnosis

In the majority of patients, the diagnosis of duodenal ulcer disease is not difficult because the history is quite typical: intermittent episodes of epigastric pain aggravated by fasting and temporarily relieved by eating or by the ingestion of antacids. Occasionally, the pain will radiate through to the back, raising the suspicion that the ulcer has penetrated into the pancreas. Definitive diagnosis is established most cost-effectively by upper gastrointestinal barium studies. In the usual case, endoscopic confirmation of the presence of the ulcer and analysis of gastric acid output are not required.

Indications for Operation

Longitudinal studies of large numbers of patients with duodenal ulcers indicate that the vast majority live in harmony with their disease, often requiring no medication whatsoever. In approximately 10 per cent, however, surgical intervention will be required. The classic indications for operative therapy include hemorrhage, perforation, obstruction, and failure of nonoperative management (*intractability*).

Approximately 10 per cent of patients with duodenal ulcer can expect to experience ulcer-related bleeding. In most, the magnitude of the hemorrhage is mild and will stop spontaneously. In some patients, however, bleeding is massive—at least 1000 ml of replacement volume is required to resuscitate the patient, and at least 500 ml every 6 to 8 hours is needed to maintain hemodynamic stability. Patients at risk for massive hemorrhage or early rebleeding in hospital are those with visible vessels in the ulcer crater and those who are actively bleeding at the time of admission. The mortality of hemorrhage from duodenal ulcer is increased as the magnitude of the bleed and the age of the patient increase. In the hands of a skilled endoscopist, correct diagnosis can be accomplished in 95 to 100 per cent of instances. Although controversy exists as to whether or not endoscopy should be employed routinely in all patients with upper gastrointestinal bleeding, it is clear that those with massive hemorrhage should undergo this procedure. The likelihood that surgical intervention is required in this group is great, and operative mortality is significantly reduced if the correct bleeding site has been identified preoperatively. Furthermore, a variety of endoscopic hemostatic techniques are available (injection of the ulcer with sclerosant, heater probe coagulation, multipolar electrocautery) which, in experienced hands, may be efficacious in arresting hemorrhage.

Ulcers located on the anterior duodenal wall may perforate into the free peritoneal cavity, resulting in the sudden onset of severe generalized abdominal pain associated with a rigid abdomen on examination. In approximately one half of instances, patients with perforation have a long history compatible with chronic ulcer disease; conversely, perforation may be the index symptom in as many as one third of patients. An erect abdominal film demonstrates free air under the diaphragm in approximately 85 per cent. Laboratory studies usually reveal a leukocytosis with increased immature forms. Occasionally, an elevated serum amylase is noted as duodenal content spills into the peritoneal cavity and is absorbed systemically.

Gastric outlet obstruction may be the consequence of cicatricial scarring in the region of an ulcer that has undergone repeated cycles of activation and healing. Alternatively, obstruction may be due to edema secondary to ulcer reactivation. Differentiation is important, since the former almost always mandates surgical intervention, while the latter may not. Clinical features include nausea, fullness, vomiting, and weight loss. In severe cases, marked dehydration and electrolyte imbalance may ensue. The finding of a dilated stomach that fails to empty on upper gastrointestinal barium studies establishes the diagnosis, which must be confirmed endoscopically. Initial treatment should be directed toward decompressing the stomach, correcting electrolyte and volume deficits, and providing maximum nonoperative antiulcer therapy. If the obstruction persists on this regimen, surgical management is warranted.

The final indication for operative therapy is *intractability* (i.e., the inability of maximal nonoperative treatment to provide symptomatic relief). Simple in concept, the fact remains that there are as many intractable patients (those who cannot comply with such a regimen) as there are intractable ulcers. In the precimetidine era, intractability was the most common indication for operation. The introduction of H_2-receptor antagonists has dramatically reduced the relative numbers of patients coming to operation on this basis.

Operations for Duodenal Ulcer

The aim of operative therapy for duodenal ulcer is to cure the disease (something most nonoperative approaches rarely, if ever, achieve) without producing excessive immediate or long-term morbidity. Based on an understanding of the pathophysiology of duodenal ulcer, several options are available: interruption of the cephalic phase of secretion (vagotomy), interruption of the cephalic phase and ablation of the gastric phase (vagotomy and antrectomy), or ablation of the gastric phase in combination with removing a generous portion of the end organ, the parietal cell mass (subtotal gastrectomy, currently an operation of historic interest only). It is unfortunate that those procedures with the highest potential for cure are also those most likely to produce untoward postoperative sequelae.

The most popular resective procedure used today is a distal gastrectomy (antrectomy) (Fig. 4) combined with resection of the truncal vagus nerves at the esophageal hiatus. Gastrointestinal continuity can be restored either by constructing a gastroduodenostomy (Billroth I) or a gastrojejunostomy (Billroth II, also illustrated in Fig. 4). Vagotomy with antrectomy is associated with the lowest recurrence rate of any ulcer operation (<2 per cent at 15 years) and is relatively safe in accomplished hands. Unfortunately, the incidence of unpleasant postoperative symptoms is relatively high (10 to 20 per cent).

Truncal vagotomy associated with a drainage procedure is also a popular operation in the United States today. Its efficacy depends solely on its capacity to interrupt the cephalic phase of secretion. The drainage procedure is necessitated by the fact, already discussed, that denervation of the antrum impairs the capacity of the distal stomach to empty solids. A variety of techniques are available to accomplish drainage.

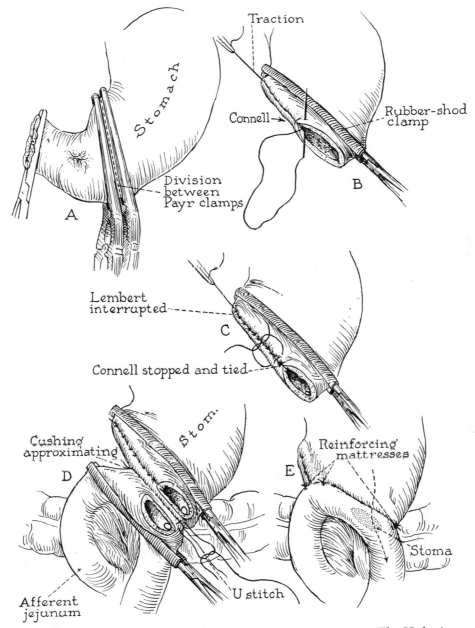

Figure 4. Distal gastrectomy with reconstruction as a gastrojejunostomy. (The Hofmeister modification of the Billroth II operation is shown.) The operation is completed by performing a truncal vagotomy. (From Shackelford RT, Zuidema GD [eds]: Surgery of the Alimentary Tract, ed 3, vol 2. Philadelphia, WB Saunders Company, 1991, p 158, with permission.)

The most popular is to perform one of the several available types of pyloroplasty such as the Heineke-Mikulicz (Fig. 5), Finney, or Jaboulay. All aim to enlarge the gastric outlet. An alternative approach is to create a gastrojejunal anastomosis at the most dependent portion of the stomach. Both types of drainage are efficacious and neither is superior in terms of reducing the risk of recurrent ulcer. Truncal vagotomy and drainage is a safe procedure with a mortality rate of less than 1 per cent. Its main disadvantage is that the risk of recurrent ulcer disease is relatively high (10 per cent recurrence in 10 years, 25 per cent in 15 years). In addition, even though gastric reservoir function is to a degree preserved, unpleasant late sequelae can occur in 10 to 15 per cent of instances.

Selective vagotomy is a variant of truncal vagotomy that was very popular for a brief period. In this procedure, the entire stomach is denervated, but the vagal

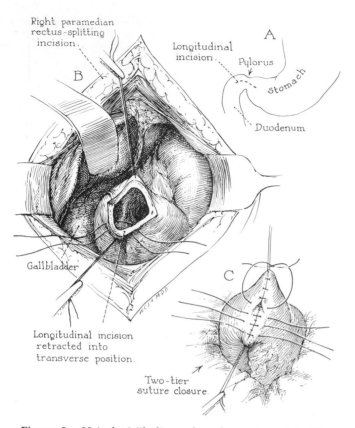

Figure 5. Heineke-Mikulicz pyloroplasty. *A* and *B*, The longitudinal incision is converted into one continuing transversely by traction on the marginal traction sutures. *C*, Two-layer closure is shown. (From Shackelford RT, Zuidema GD [eds]: Surgery of the Alimentary Tract, ed 3, vol 2. Philadelphia, WB Saunders Company, 1991, p 143, with permission.)

branches to the hepatobiliary tree and to the celiac plexus are preserved. It was thought that an intact visceral vagal innervation would reduce the incidence of late postoperative side effects. Unfortunately this has not been the case in most studies because the presence of the necessary drainage procedure promotes rapid gastric emptying.

The most recent innovation in the operative therapy of duodenal ulcer is parietal cell vagotomy, a procedure that attempts to denervate the parietal cell mass only (Fig. 6). Thus, the motor function of the antrum and pylorus is maintained intact with the result that gastric emptying of solids is normal. For this reason, a drainage procedure is *unnecessary*, and as a result, postoperative side effects are almost completely eliminated. Morbidity and mortality are low, and recurrence rates at 5 years approximate those of truncal vagotomy and drainage. Long-term (15 to 25 years) recurrence rates may be considerably higher, however. The procedure is a difficult one to master and should

be performed only by surgeons experienced in the technique. Significantly, the operation is contraindicated in patients with prepyloric or pyloric ulcers because of excessively high recurrence rates early after operation.

The operative approach to patients with bleeding or perforation requires special comment. In the patient with massive hemorrhage, it is mandatory to resuscitate the patient adequately prior to operation. As mentioned, endoscopy is a highly useful adjunct to confirm the diagnosis and may be therapeutic as well. It is generally agreed that, in addition to controlling hemorrhage, an acid-reducing procedure is appropriate if operation is required. Truncal vagotomy associated with oversewing of the bleeding ulcer through a pyloroplasty accomplishes both of these objectives admirably. Although no consensus exists as to the best procedure for the perforated duodenal ulcer, current evidence suggests that simple closure of the ulcer with an omental patch is appropriate if the patient is unstable perioperatively, if the perforation is of long duration, or if the patient has severe intercurrent disease. On the other hand, if the patient is stable and rela-

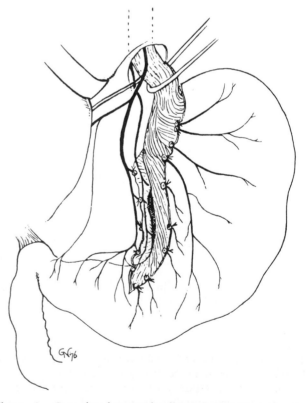

Figure 6. Completed parietal cell vagotomy. Note the absence of a drainage procedure. (From Sabiston DC Jr [ed]: Textbook of Surgery, ed 14. Philadelphia, WB Saunders Company, 1991, p 777, with permission.)

tively healthy and if the amount of contamination is minimal, an acid-reducing procedure can be performed safely with excellent long-term results.

Some surgeons prefer a truncal vagotomy with pyloroplasty to include the ulcer. Many others feel that a parietal cell vagotomy combined with patch closure is most appropriate under these circumstances.

Benign Gastric Ulcer

Ulcerations of the stomach proper are encountered less commonly than are duodenal ulcers. They occur in older patients and are slightly more common in females than in males. The most prevalent type (type I) heals readily with nonoperative therapy, but has a marked tendency to recur. An additional clinical challenge is to differentiate such ulcers from gastric carcinomas.

Pathogenesis

Not all gastric ulcers are etiologically similar. Three types have been distinguished. Type III benign gastric ulcers (15 per cent of the total) are prepyloric in that they are found within 2 cm of the pylorus. The etiology of these ulcers is probably similar to that of duodenal ulcer. Type II benign gastric ulcers (20 per cent) occur in association with an active or healed duodenal ulcer that has partially obstructed the gastric outlet. For both type III and type II ulcers, an operation appropriate for duodenal ulcer gives excellent results when operative therapy is required. The most common of the benign gastric ulcers (65 per cent) is type I. These occur on the lesser curvature, usually at the incisura but occasionally more proximally. Not infrequently, they may be found on the greater curvature, where distinction from gastric carcinoma can be difficult. Current evidence suggests that these ulcers are a consequence of excessive reflux of upper intestinal content into the stomach. Of all peptic ulcers of the upper gastrointestinal tract, this type is most clearly related to defects in mucosal resistance. Excessive ingestion of nonsteroidal anti-inflammatory drugs (NSAIDs) has been clearly implicated in their development in certain patients.

Diagnosis

The clinical manifestations of gastric ulcer are quite variable. As with duodenal ulcer, pain is the most common presenting complaint. However, the sequence of pain relieved by food is not nearly as clear in gastric ulcers; in fact, food may exacerbate the symptoms. Thus, weight loss is a frequent accompaniment of the disease. In addition, it is not uncommon to encounter completely asymptomatic gastric ulcers, particularly in users of NSAIDs. Under these conditions, bleeding or perforation may be the index clue as to their presence.

The definitive diagnosis of gastric ulcer is made endoscopically. Gastroscopy is extremely important in this situation because it is mandatory to distinguish a benign ulcer from a malignant one. Besides allowing direct visualization of the ulcer, multiple biopsies and brushings can be obtained for histologic and cytologic examination.

When benign status is ensured, a trial of nonoperative therapy is indicated. This approach is usually successful with a benign ulcer. Failure to heal on an adequate regimen suggests malignancy and is an indication for operation. Even in those patients who do heal, relapse may occur in as many as two thirds. In the opinion of most surgeons, this circumstance is also an indication for operation. Finally, 10 to 16 per cent of benign gastric ulcers can either bleed or perforate, necessitating urgent surgical therapy.

Operations for Benign Gastric Ulcer

As indicated previously, patients with type II and type III benign gastric ulcers should undergo operations appropriate for duodenal ulcer. In type I benign gastric ulcer, the performance of a distal gastrectomy to include the ulcer without concomitant vagus resection is associated with a 96 per cent cure rate. Most surgeons prefer reconstruction as a Billroth I gastroduodenostomy. Some feel that a truncal vagotomy should be added if the ulcer is a consequence of NSAID abuse. Truncal vagotomy with drainage procedure may also be appropriate if the ulcer is concomitantly excised. Early results with parietal cell vagotomy and ulcerectomy have also been salutory.

The morbidity and mortality associated with bleeding and perforated gastric ulcer are considerably greater than that seen under similar circumstances with duodenal ulcer, because delay in diagnosis is common and because afflicted patients tend to be elderly. The aims of operation under these conditions are to excise the ulcer, to perform an acid-reducing procedure, either distal gastrectomy or truncal vagotomy, and to allow for drainage. Parietal cell vagotomy is probably inappropriate under these emergent circumstances.

STRESS EROSIONS: ACUTE HEMORRHAGIC GASTRITIS

Stress erosions are multiple punctate hemorrhagic lesions of the proximal stomach that develop in the setting of severe and unremitting physiologic stress.

They rarely penetrate deeply and are unassociated with chronic inflammation. In the absence of effective prophylaxis, stress erosions coalesce in up to 20 per cent of instances to form multiple ulcerations resulting in upper gastrointestinal hemorrhage of life-threatening severity. This condition is known as *acute hemorrhagic gastritis*. Patients hospitalized in intensive care units, those sustaining severe trauma, and those with major body burns are at particular risk.

Pathogenesis

Stress erosions are acute in onset and multiple in number. Because they are located primarily in the proximal stomach, acid and pepsin are undoubtedly important in their evolution even though they are not usually associated with hypersecretion of gastric acid. Stress erosions and their clinical endpoint, acute hemorrhagic gastritis, are the ultimate expression of failed *cytoprotection*, the capacity of the gastric mucosa to prevent autodigestion. Although all of the barriers that normally contribute to cytoprotection could, in theory, be defective in the setting in which stress ulcer disease develops, current evidence suggests that both intraluminal acid and mucosal ischemia are indispensable to their development.

Diagnosis and Clinical Course

If patients at risk are subjected to endoscopy within 24 to 48 hours following the precipitating insult, more than 60 per cent demonstrate stress erosions. However, the clinical onset of hemorrhage is often delayed for 5 to 10 days. The diagnosis should be suspected whenever a critically ill patient develops upper gastrointestinal tract hemorrhage. Upper endoscopy is the diagnostic modality of choice and produces a correct identification of the bleeding source in more than 90 per cent of instances.

A variety of nonoperative regimens have been advocated as treatment for acute hemorrhagic gastritis. Regrettably, they are either demonstrably ineffective (antacid titration, systemic H_2-receptor blockade) or effective only temporarily and associated with high morbidity and mortality (selective or systemic vasopressin infusion). Surgical therapy is only slightly more efficacious. All operative approaches are associated with poor initial control and high rates of rebleeding. This is especially true following nonresective procedures. For these reasons, the best treatment of acute hemorrhagic gastritis is its prevention.

The most effective proven prophylactic measures are those designed to control intraluminal pH, either intravenous H_2-receptor blocking agents or intragastric antacid titration to maintain intraluminal pH above 5.

Although the most effective form of prophylaxis has been the matter of some debate, it is probable that they are, for all intents and purposes, equivalent. Other forms of prevention have also been developed. Two classes of compounds in particular have been studied in this regard. The first, sucralfate, is a basic sulphated aluminum salt of sucrose that forms a viscid and impermeable gel over the lesion because its negative charge binds to positively charged exposed protein. This, in turn, promotes healing of the subjacent gastric erosion. Some feel that sucralfate prophylaxis is associated with a lower incidence of nosocomial pneumonia because intragastric pH remains low. The second class of compounds, the prostaglandins, are normally present in abundance in the gastric mucosa. In experimental animals, they are cytoprotective against a variety of noxious insults. In humans, there is good evidence to suggest that prostaglandins are as efficacious as prophylactic agents as is antacid titration, albeit, at considerably greater cost.

ZOLLINGER-ELLISON SYNDROME

In 1955, Zollinger and Ellison described a triad of findings in a small group of patients with intractable ulcer disease: massive hypersecretion of acid, leading to a virulent duodenal and jejunal ulcer diathesis, associated with a nonbeta islet cell tumor of the pancreas. Shortly thereafter, it was demonstrated that such pancreatic tumors elaborated large amounts of gastrin. With accumulated experience, it is now clear that the majority (80 per cent) of Zollinger-Ellison syndrome (ZES) tumors arise in the so-called *gastrinoma triangle* (a triangle bounded by the junction of the cystic and common ducts, the junction of the second and third portions of the duodenum, and the junction of the head and body of the pancreas), that they are microscopic in 50 per cent of patients, multiple in two thirds, and clinically malignant in more than 60 per cent. Although malignant gastrinoma may be indolent and compatible with long survival, it may prove fatal to the patient because of extensive metastatic disease. On the other hand, several large current series suggest that between 40 and 80 per cent of appropriately selected patients can be resected in anticipation of rendering them eugastrinemic, at least for a period of time.

The presence of a Zollinger-Ellison tumor should be suspected in any patient with difficult-to-control ulcer disease. Radiographic signs include giant rugal folds, an indication of an increase in perietal cell mass, increased gastric and intestinal secretion, and a rapid intestinal transit time. In fact, diarrhea is a frequent presenting complaint (occasionally, the only presenting complaint). The diagnosis is established by the finding of massive hypersecretion of gastric acid associated with basal hypergastrinemia, which increases paradoxically by greater than 150 pg/ml when the patient is given purified secretion. A combination of these studies serves to differentiate the syndrome from all other causes of elevated serum gastrin.

Occasionally ZES is found in association with the multiple endocrine neoplasia type I syndrome (MEN-I). This syndrome consists of hyperfunctioning tumors of the parathyroid, pituitary, and pancreatic islet cells. It is distinctly unusual to find resectable gastrinoma in these patients.

For many years, the standard approach to the treatment of patients with isolated ZES was to remove the target organ completely (i.e., to perform a total gastrectomy). With the demonstration that H$_2$-receptor blockage markedly decreased acid output (without affecting serum gastrin levels) and provided symptomatic control in most patients with ZES, *pharmacologic gastrectomy* using these agents became the rule. The advantage of this approach is that the risks associated with operation are avoided and control of the hypersecretory state with resolution of symptoms is accomplished, at least initially, in 80 per cent of patients. With experience, disadvantages of the regimen have also become apparent. Patients must be totally compliant with a lifelong medication schedule; tachyphylaxis develops with time; when complications do occur, they are catastrophic; and, most importantly, the potential opportunity to cure the disease is lost. Currently most surgeons believe that a third approach is preferable—patients without evidence of unresectable metastatic disease are subjected to exploratory laparotomy. Careful exploration of the gastrinoma triangle (the duodenum in particular) is followed by potentially curative resection of solitary gastrinomas in 40 to 80 per cent of patients.

COMPLICATIONS OF GASTRIC SURGERY

All operative procedures designed to ameliorate the peptic ulcer diathesis have a common and rational basis; that is, reduction in the capacity of the stomach to secrete acid. On occasion, this goal may not be achieved, resulting in recurrent ulcer. Even if the goal is realized, the patient may experience untoward sequelae, which are known collectively as the *postgastrectomy syndromes*. These result from loss of gastric reservoir function, from ablation or bypass of the pylorus, or from parasympathetic denervation, either alone or in combination.

Recurrent Ulcer

Failure to accomplish adequate reduction in gastric acid production may cause recurrent ulceration following operation, a circumstance seen more often after operations for duodenal ulcer disease than for gastric ulcer disease. Patients who undergo nonresective procedures are at greater risk than those in whom a portion of the stomach has been removed. Most recurrences are evident within the first 2 years after resection, but tend to accumulate with time after nonresective operations. Recurrent ulcers usually are located on the enteric side of the anastomosis following resection, but they may occur with equal frequency in the intestine and stomach following nonresective procedures. Diagnosis is not difficult; most patients experience the renewed onset of typical peptic ulcer pain. Confirmation of the diagnosis is made endoscopically. Incomplete division of the vagus nerve is the most common cause of recurrent ulcer, accounting for more than 80 per cent of cases. Other causes of recurrent ulcer include the existence of a previously unrecognized gastrinoma, an inadequate resection, retention of antral tissue at the duodenal stump (which causes hypergastrinemia), and an excessively long afferent limb following gastroenterostomy. Most recurrent ulcers are readily treated using H$_2$-receptor blocking agents.

Should these fail, repeat vagotomy with resection or repeat resection is indicated. The approach to the patient with a gastrinoma was discussed earlier.

Early Postprandial Dumping

Early postprandial dumping is the most common of the postgastrectomy syndromes, occurring most often after partial gastrectomy, less frequently after vagotomy combined with drainage, and almost not at all after parietal cell vagotomy. This syndrome consists of a constellation of gastrointestinal and vasomotor signs and symptoms that occur early (within the first half hour) after the ingestion of a meal. Gastrointestinal complaints include epigastric fullness, nausea, crampy abdominal pain, and explosive diarrhea. Vasomotor complaints include perspiration, weakness, dizziness, pallor followed by flushing, and palpitations. In general, the gastrointestinal components of the syndrome are more common than the vasomotor ones.

The syndrome occurs as a consequence of rapid gastric emptying of hyperosmolar chyme from the residual stomach into the small intestine. This in turn causes movement of extracellular fluid into the intestinal lumen in an attempt to achieve isotonicity which, unfortunately, also decreases the circulating plasma volume. This circumstance is thought to be responsible, at least in part, for the vasomotor components of the syndrome. In addition, distention of the proximal small intestine liberates a variety of humoral substances, which may account for the facial flushing, the increased small-bowel motility, and the explosive diarrhea encountered in severe cases.

The diagnosis of early postprandial dumping is usually made on clinical grounds alone, and characteristic postprandial symptomatology is relieved in many instances by assuming a supine position. In most cases, sophisticated diagnostic evaluation is unnecessary. In more than 90 per cent of instances, symptomatic patients can be successfully treated without operative therapy. The specific measures include frequent feeding of small meals rich in protein and fat and low in carbohydrate and the avoidance of liquids with meals. In more severe cases, the long-acting analog of the somatostatin, octreotide, may be of benefit. When operative therapy is required, the interposition of an antiperistaltic loop of jejunum between the gastric remnant in the small intestine has been reported to be quite successful. Alternatively, creation of a Roux-en-Y limb may also be effective (Fig. 7).

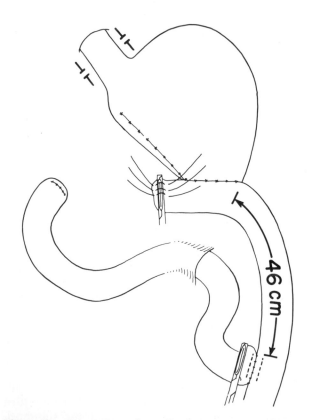

Figure 7. Conversion of a Billroth II reconstruction to a Roux-en-Y drainage. (From Fromm D: Ulceration of the stomach and duodenum. *In* Fromm D [ed]: Gastrointestinal Surgery. New York, Churchill Livingstone, 1983, with permission.)

Late Postprandial Dumping Syndrome

The *late postprandial dumping syndrome* is less common than its early counterpart and its symptoms occur much later, usually 1.5 to 3 hours following the ingestion of a carbohydrate-rich meal.

Typically, patients complain of diaphoresis, tremulousness, tachycardia, and light-headedness. The symptoms are characteristically relieved by the ingestion of carbohydrates. The basic defect responsible for late postprandial dumping is rapid gastric emptying of carbohydrates into the small intestine, where they are rapidly absorbed and produce a marked increase in blood glucose levels. Hyperglycemia triggers the release of large amounts of insulin (and perhaps enteroglucagon), which over the course of the next 2 hours not only normalizes blood sugar but also, in symptomatic patients, *overshoots* the endpoint, resulting in profound hypoglycemia. The end result is that symptoms indistinguishable from insulin shock are produced.

Nonoperative therapy is aimed toward normalizing the glucose tolerance curve, a goal that can be achieved by adding pectin to the diet. Additional measures include the use of frequent small feedings of carbohydrate-poor meals and the ingestion of carbohydrate when symptoms begin.

Afferent Loop Syndrome

The *afferent loop syndrome* is a consequence of obstruction of an afferent limb (i.e., the limb of a gastroenteric anastomosis leading to the stomach). Thus, it can only occur following gastrectomy with reconstruction as a Billroth II gastrojejunostomy.

The basic defect in the afferent loop syndrome is intermittent obstruction of the limb after eating. Typically, patients complain of epigastric fullness and crampy abdominal pain shortly after the ingestion of a meal. The symptoms are relieved by vomiting. The vomitus is usually projectile and almost invariably contains bile but no food. This clinical picture is a consequence of meal-stimulated hepatobiliary and pancreatic secretion that arrives in large volumes in the duodenum. In the presence of partial obstruction of the afferent limb, the loop rapidly distends, resulting in epigastric discomfort and cramping. Once the pressure in the loop is sufficiently great to overcome the obstruction, it decompresses itself into the stomach, causing projectile vomiting and the immediate relief of symptoms. The vomitus lacks food because the ingested meal has already passed into the efferent limb.

The treatment of the syndrome is operative correction, and the most expeditious and successful method of correcting the problem is to eliminate the loop. The creation of a long-limb Roux-en-Y with implantation of the afferent limb distal to the gastroenteric anastomosis is usually associated with an excellent outcome (Fig. 7).

Early Satiety

Early satiety, also known as the *small stomach syndrome*, is the consequence of excessive loss of gastric reservoir function. Characteristically, patients complain of an extremely unpleasant sensation of fullness after ingesting only small amounts of food. Vomiting usually ensues if the patient attempts to increase oral intake. In severe cases, only small liquid meals are tolerable and anemia and malnutrition frequently develop as a consequence. Although a variety of nonoperative measures have been advocated, none has achieved conspicuous success. Unfortunately, operative procedures also do not completely ameliorate the symptoms of early satiety. Therefore, the best treatment of the small stomach syndrome is to avoid it in the first place.

Postvagotomy Diarrhea

Increase in stool frequency may be experienced by as many as one third of patients following transection of the vagus nerves. In most instances, the condition is self-limiting. The etiology of postvagotomy diarrhea remains obscure. It is believed, however, that alterations in bile acid metabolism may play a role. This postulation is supported by the fact that the ingestion of bile acid–binding resin, cholestyramine, is effective in more than 80 per cent of instances in which it has been tried. Operative therapy is rarely necessary.

Alkaline Reflux Gastritis

Excessive reflux of upper intestinal content into the stomach following gastrectomy, gastroenterostomy, or pylorus ablating procedures has been implicated as a cause of a specific set of postoperative signs and symptoms, including burning midepigastric pain, bilious vomiting, erythema of the entire mucous membrane of the stomach, weight loss, and anemia. In the majority of patients the index procedure performed has been a gastric resection with gastrojejunostomy. The exact incidence of the syndrome is unknown, but is probably less than 3 per cent of all patients undergoing gastric surgery. Although the diagnosis can be suspected on historic grounds, it is important that excessive reflux be established in an objective manner because a poor outcome can be anticipated in up to 75 per cent of patients when remedial operation is based on symptoms alone. Several methods are available to accom-

plish this. The efficacy of nonoperative therapies in afflicted patients is questionable. When an operation is undertaken, conversion of the previous operative procedure to a long-limb (45-cm) Roux-en-Y has brought salutary results in two thirds of patients.

OTHER BENIGN CONDITIONS

Mallory-Weiss Tears

In 1929, Mallory and Weiss detailed the case histories of 15 patients in whom massive hematemesis developed following severe bouts of vomiting during an alcoholic debauch. Four patients died and, at autopsy, demonstrated fissure-like tears in the mucosa of the gastric cardia, one of which extended across the gastroesophageal junction. They attributed these lacerations to increased intragastric pressure produced as a consequence of vomiting. Initially, the Mallory-Weiss "syndrome" was considered to be rare but usually lethal. Since the advent of the widespread use of fiberoptic endoscopy, however, it is now apparent that the Mallory-Weiss tear may be responsible for 5 to 15 per cent of all upper gastrointestinal bleeds and that it is almost always a self-limiting and innocuous condition.

The diagnosis of Mallory-Weiss tears can often be established on historic grounds alone. Vomiting and retching precedes hematemesis in over 60 per cent of patients. Alcohol use is a common accompaniment. The tears are usually longitudinal and located on the lesser curvature of the stomach just distal to the gastroesophageal junction. In approximately one third of instances, the tear extends into the esophageal mucosa. The resultant bleeding is almost always arterial and is unassociated with pain.

With the recognition that the syndrome is far more common than previously appreciated, its treatment has become much less of a surgical exercise. Nonoperative management of afflicted patients is associated with cessation of hemorrhage in more than 90 per cent of patients, usually within a matter of hours. Rebleeding is uncommon. In approximately 10 per cent of instances, however, bleeding continues, necessitating active therapeutic interventions, including the use of systemic vasopressin, topical application of norepinephrine, endoscopic electrocautery, and angiographic embolization with Gelfoam or autologous clot. Should these alternative approaches fail, operative therapy to oversew the tear is warranted. Rebleeding following operation is uncommon, and the prognosis especially for nonalcoholic patients, is excellent.

Boerhaave's Syndrome

Occasionally, the forces transmitted to the distal esophageal wall are so great that an emetogenic rupture occurs (Boerhaave's syndrome). In the vast majority of patients, the rupture is located in the left lateral aspect of the distal esophagus. Characteristically, the patient complains of severe epigastric pain shortly after vomiting. Dyspnea is common. Mediastinal air may present as palpable crepitus in the suprasternal notch.

Because the syndrome is relatively rare, delay in diagnosis is common. This is unfortunate, because survival rates are excellent when patients are operated on within the first 12 hours of rupture and mortality approaches 100 per cent if operation is delayed more than 24 hours. Erect chest films yield the most information, as they may demonstrate a pleural effusion, a left pneumothorax, and/or mediastinal air. Treatment of Boerhaave's syndrome is entirely surgical.

Definitive operative therapy consists of débridement and repair of the perforation through a left thoracotomy incision with drainage of the mediastinum and pleural space.

NEOPLASMS OF THE STOMACH

Benign Tumors

Epithelial Polyp

Polyps of the gastric mucosa, although unusual, are the most common of benign gastric tumor. Two histologic types are distinguished. Hyperplastic polyps are the more frequent and consist of gastric epithelium, which is identical histologically to the morphology of the adjacent normal gastric mucosa. They are invariably small (<2 cm in diameter) and have minimal malignant potential. In contrast, the adenomatous polyp tends to be larger, is predominantly antral in location, and develops in gastric mucosa that has undergone intestinal metaplasia. It is likely that such polyps undergo malignant transformation and, indeed, malignancy has been observed in between 25 and 80 per cent of patients, either within the polyp itself or in the adjacent gastric mucosa. Adenomatous polyps that are large, sessile, and symptomatic are cause for considerable concern.

Most benign epithelial polyps are completely asymptomatic or associated with extremely vague and nonspecific complaints. On occasion, however, polyps may bleed. If appropriately situated, they may also obstruct the gastric outlet by a ball-valve–type mechanism. The diagnosis is established by endoscopy, which also permits the physician to visualize the polyp directly, to remove it, if possible, and to perform a biopsy. As with colonic polyps, complete removal for careful histologic examination is desirable. Should this be unfeasible, operative therapy should be undertaken.

Mesenchymal Tumors

Although the stomach can be the site of a variety of benign mesenchymal tumors, the most common by far is the leiomyoma. These are invariably located submucosally and are usually well circumscribed. They are frequently discovered because of upper gastrointestinal tract hemorrhage resulting from ulceration of the mucosa overlying the tumor. The diagnosis is made by the characteristic finding on upper endoscopy of a circumferential extramucosal defect often in association with an ulcer in the overlying mucosa. Definitive treatment consists of local resection of the involved portion of the stomach if at all possible. The pathologic discovery of five or more mitoses per high-power field strongly suggests malignancy (leiomyosarcoma). Occasionally, however, it is difficult to distinguish benign from malignant lesions histologically, so that not infrequently this differentiation is made by the patient's subsequent clinical course.

Malignant Tumors

Adenocarcinoma

Although the incidence of gastric adenocarcinoma has been steadily decreasing in the United States over the past several decades, it remains a lethal malignancy. Approximately 23,000 new cases are diagnosed annually. Eighty per cent of patients with this tumor come to operation, but only 40 per cent are resectable for cure and fewer than one third of resected patients are alive 5 years later.

This unpleasant fact is a consequence of the advanced stage of the disease in most patients at the time of diagnosis. The experience of the Japanese stands in marked contrast to these dismal statistics. Because of massive screening efforts to detect the disease in an early stage, fully 70 per cent of all gastric cancers in Japan are confined to the mucosa and submucosa. Surgical resection under these circumstances is followed by an 80 to 90 per cent 5-year cure rate.

Microscopically, there are two types of adenocarcinoma, an *intestinal* type and a *diffuse* type. Because the diffuse type is less well differentiated than the intestinal type, it has a worse prognosis. Grossly, three variants of adenocarcinoma are encountered. The most common is the *polypoid* type, usually seen in the distal stomach. Adenocarcinoma may also present as an *ulcerative* type that on occasion can be difficult to distinguish from benign gastric ulcer. Finally, the least common but most virulent pathologic variety is the scirrhous type, *linitis plastica*. The tumor frequently involves the entire stomach, giving it a "leather bottle" appearance because of its impliability.

Early symptoms of gastric adenocarcinoma are vague and nonspecific, including unexplained weight loss, anorexia, early satiety and, on occasion, mild epigastric discomfort. As the disease progresses, pain becomes a more prominent symptom and may be associated with vomiting and melena. Massive hematemesis is unusual. Rarely, the presenting symptoms may be related to metastatic disease and include malignant ascites, hepatomegaly, jaundice, mechanical small-bowel obstruction from peritoneal implants, and difficulty in defecation because of metastatic disease in the pouch of Douglas, the so-called *Blumer's shelf*.

A diagnosis of gastric adenocarcinoma can be made in more than 95 per cent on upper gastrointestinal endoscopy, particularly if both biopsy and cytologic evaluation are employed simultaneously. Computed tomography (CT) may be helpful in staging the disease preoperatively. Even if the CT scan suggests incurability, patients with potentially resectable disease should undergo a surgical procedure to debulk, resect, or bypass the tumor if technically feasible.

Surgery is the only therapeutic modality with potential to cure the disease. The aim of operation is to remove the primary tumor with its first tier of lymphatic drainage sites. Some surgeons advocate en bloc removal of the second and even the third tier of lymph nodes as well because of data, primarily from Japan, that suggest that this approach is associated with higher rates of long-term survival. The appropriate procedure depends upon the location and extent of the tumor. In general, adenocarcinomas of the distal stomach are best treated by extensive distal gastrectomy. Reconstruction is best accomplished as a gastrojejunostomy. Adenocarcinomas arising in the body of the stomach are best treated by total extirpation of the

organ to include the spleen. Reconstruction is usually accomplished using a Roux-en-Y esophagojejunostomy. Adenocarcinomas of the cardia and fundus present a major technical challenge because of their propensity to spread submucosally into the esophagus. In general, proximal gastrectomy with distal esophagectomy is a time-honored approach (the *Ivor-Lewis technique*). Reconstruction is accomplished by transthoracic esophagoantrostomy to which a pyloroplasty is added because the distal stomach has been vagally denervated by the dissection.

The prognosis of gastric adenocarcinoma is related primarily to the histologic type, to the depth of penetration of the tumor into the gastric wall, and to the presence or absence of lymph node metastases. Early gastric cancers are associated with an excellent prognosis—a 90 per cent 5-year survivorship. As tumors invade the muscularis propria and metastasize to lymph node, the prognosis becomes progressively worse so that, as noted, the overall 5 year survivorship of patients undergoing curative resection is 30 per cent or less. The use of adjuvant radiotherapy and chemotherapy has been advocated to improve this dismal record. Unfortunately, current data do not indicate that these modalities provide substantive benefit in terms of prolonged survival.

REFERENCES

Adam YG, Efron G: Trends and controversies in the management of carcinoma of the stomach. Surg Gynecol Obstet 169:371, 1989.

Mulholland MW, Debas HT: Chronic duodenal and gastric ulcer. Surg Clin North Am 67:489, 1987.

Norton JA, Jensen RT: Unresolved surgical issues in the management of patients with Zollinger-Ellison syndrome. World J Surg 15:151, 1991.

Ritchie WP Jr, Dempsey DT: Post-gastrectomy syndromes. *In* Moody FG (ed): Surgical Treatment of Digestive Disease. Chicago, Year Book Medical Publishers, 1990.

Wolfe MM, Soll AH: The physiology of gastric acid secretion. N Engl J Med 319:1707, 1988.

28

THE SMALL INTESTINE

MAGGIE C. LEE, B.S.   THEODORE N. PAPPAS, M.D., F.A.C.S.

The small intestine is the site of a number of disorders of the gastrointestinal tract. Quite important in this connection is the normal small-intestinal physiology, including digestion and absorption, motility, and endocrine and immunologic function. The more significant pathologic conditions are reviewed in this chapter, including intestinal obstruction, Crohn's disease, Meckel's diverticulum, benign and malignant tumors, malabsorption syndromes, and radiation injury to the small intestine. The etiology, clinical signs and symptoms, diagnosis, treatment, and prognosis of these disorders are presented.

PHYSIOLOGY

Digestion and Absorption

Protein

The digestion of protein begins in the stomach, where the acidic environment promotes denaturation of proteins and where pepsin activates proteolysis. Most of protein digestion occurs in the duodenum and proximal jejunum under the influence of pancreatic enzymes secreted into the duodenum via the duct of Wirsung. Endopeptidases (trypsin, chymotrypsin, elastase) hydrolyze the internal bonds of the protein molecule, whereas exopeptidases (carboxypeptidases) target for removal of the amino acids at the C-terminal of the peptide. The total activity of the pancreatic enzymes yields a pool of approximately 30 per cent free amino acids and 70 per cent oligopeptides. The shorter peptides are further degraded at their N-terminal positions by intestinal aminopeptidases. The amino acids and dipeptides are then absorbed into the epithelial cells by a carrier-mediated active transport process. Approximately 90 per cent of the intact peptides undergo further hydrolysis to free amino acids by intracellular peptidases before entering the portal venous system.

Carbohydrates

Carbohydrates are ingested in the form of starch, sucrose, and lactose. Dietary starch consists of the glucose polymers amylopectin and amylose. Amylopectin is more abundant, comprising 80 per cent of dietary starch, and differs from amylose in that it contains, in addition to the straight chain of 1-4 linked glucose molecules, 1-6 linked branching side chains. Salivary and pancreatic amylase hydrolyze amylose to maltose and maltotriose, whereas digestion of amylopectin produces maltose, maltotriose, and the shorter dextrins. These digestive products, as well as ingested sucrose and lactose, are hydrolyzed to monosaccharides by enzymes concentrated in the brush border of the intestinal microvilli. As final digestive products, glucose and galactose are absorbed into the cell by an active transport mechanism, requiring energy, oxygen, and sodium. Fructose, on the other hand, enters the cell via facilitated diffusion.

Fat

The digestion and absorption of lipids, ingested primarily in the form of triglycerides, occurs almost entirely in the small intestine and is contingent on two events: lipolysis and the formation of micelles. The hydrolysis of triglyceride by pancreatic lipase is aided by bicarbonate, which creates the alkaline environment necessary for optimal lipase activity. The resulting fatty acids and monoglycerides combine with bile salts to form micelles. Micelles are aggregates that coalesce to increase solubility of the digestive products by containing them in a hydrophobic interior within a hydrophilic environment. When micelles reach the brush border of the epithelial cell, they disassemble, allowing the digestive products to diffuse into the cell while the bile salts remain in the intestinal lumen for absorption later from the distal ileum and recirculation to the liver. The monoglycerides and fatty acids, once inside the cell, are resynthesized in the endoplasmic reticulum to triglycerides and transported as chylomicrons into the venous system.

Water and Electrolytes

As much as 10 L of water enters the small intestine daily, of which only a small fraction continues past the ileocecal valve. The large quantity of water resorbed in the small intestine is the net result of the water movement that occurs in the direction of lumen to plasma (absorption) and plasma to lumen (secretion). Water moves by either diffusing through pores or flowing down osmotic and hydrostatic pressure gradients created by the active transport of solutes such as sodium, glucose, and amino acids. Sodium absorption is 99 per cent efficient and occurs primarily in the jejunum by passive diffusion following bulk flow of water. Sodium is absorbed in the ileum, as well as a small fraction in the jejunum, by active transport against a concentration gradient that induces concomitant hydrogen ion extrusion. Bicarbonate secretion occurs in conjunction with this exchange, facilitating chloride absorption as well, which maintains electrical neutrality in the face of electrogenic Na^+ transport. The absorption of calcium occurs primarily in the duodenum and jejunum by active transport and is favored by a more acidic environment. Vitamin D and parathormone enhance absorption of this cation. Absorption of iron, although fairly inefficient, is an important function of the small intestine in regulating the body's iron stores.

Motility

The motility of the small intestine differs in the fed and fasting states. After feeding, a basic electrical rhythm (BER) is set by the longitudinal smooth muscle layer of the small intestine and is propagated distally at decreasing rates. The BER initiates the action potentials in the circular layer, which triggers the muscular contractions constituting small-intestinal motility. Two types of contractions are observed: *segmental* and *peristaltic*. Segmental contractions function to mix chyme with digestive enzymes and to expose the in-

testinal contents repeatedly to the absorptive surfaces. Peristaltic contractions, which occur less frequently, function to propel food through the intestine.

In the fasting state, the migrating myoelectric complex (MMC) initiates the muscular contractions of the small intestine. The MMC originates from the stomach and duodenum at regular 1- to 2-hour intervals during the interdigestive period to propel the remnants of the fed state. Motilin is known to have a significant role in the regulation of the MMC; and increased levels are associated with activation of this complex. In addition to motilin, other gastrointestinal hormones have a role in small-intestinal motility. Gastrin, cholecystokinin, and substance P stimulate muscular contractions; whereas secretin, somatostatin, vasoactive intestinal peptide (VIP), and glucagon inhibit contractile activity. Neurogenic factors regulate intestinal motility as well, with sympathetic activity generally inhibiting motility and parasympathetic influences stimulating it. Of clinical significance, the intestinointestinal inhibitory reflex responds to abnormal distention distally by decreasing motility in regions proximal to the distention.

Endocrine Function

The mucosa of the small intestine provides a rich supply of peptides that regulate the gastrointestinal tract. Secretin, the first gastrointestinal hormone described, stimulates water and pancreatic bicarbonate secretion in response to luminal acid, which alkalinizes the luminal environment for optimal digestion of lipids. In addition, secretin stimulates bile flow and inhibits gastric acid secretion and gastrointestinal motility. The functions of several other gut peptides are also known: cholecystokinin (CCK) stimulates gallbladder contractions, relaxes the sphincter of Oddi, stimulates pancreatic enzyme secretion, and increases gastric emptying; enteroglucagon inhibits intestinal motility and stimulates mucosal growth; VIP stimulates pancreatic secretion; gastric inhibitory peptide (GIP) stimulates insulin secretion; motilin activates the MMC in the fasting state; somatostatin counteracts the action of motilin on the MMC, and exerts an inhibitory influence on the release of both gastrin and gastric acid; bombesin stimulates gastrin release; and peptide YY (PYY) inhibits gastric and pancreatic secretion and gastric motility (Fig. 1).

Immunologic Function

The small bowel is an important source of immunoglobulin A (IgA), the secretory immunoglobulin. Plasma cells located in the lamina propria synthesize IgA antibodies directed at offending antigens. The IgA

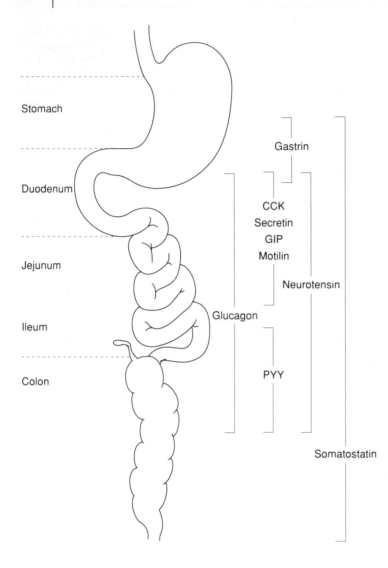

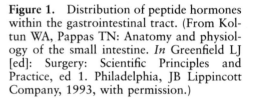

Figure 1. Distribution of peptide hormones within the gastrointestinal tract. (From Koltun WA, Pappas TN: Anatomy and physiology of the small intestine. *In* Greenfield LJ [ed]: Surgery: Scientific Principles and Practice, ed 1. Philadelphia, JB Lippincott Company, 1993, with permission.)

is subsequently secreted into the intestinal lumen. By binding directly to antigens, IgA effectively alters the uptake of these substances. IgA-antigen binding triggers mucus secretion, which can act as a protective layer to prevent bacterial and viral uptake. IgA binding can also incapacitate bacteria directly, disrupting cellular division and increasing enzymatic degradation. Secretory IgA may bind to toxins as well, impairing their biologic activity and preventing their entry across the mucosa.

SMALL-INTESTINAL OBSTRUCTION

Etiology

Intestinal obstruction, defined as a pathologic inability of luminal contents to pass distally, may result from mechanical obstruction or paralytic ileus.

Mechanical Obstruction

Mechanical obstruction is characterized by a physical occlusion of the intestinal lumen that may be partial or complete. Three types of abnormalities may lead to such obstruction: (1) extrinsic lesions, (2) intrinsic lesions, and (3) luminal compromise. The most common causes of mechanical obstruction extrinsic to the small bowel include adhesions (60 per cent), hernias (15 per cent), and masses (15 per cent). In the pediatric population, the adhesions may be congenital in origin, and in adults, adhesions usually occur following surgical procedures or from inflammation. Obstruction from adhesive bands is caused typically by kinking of the bowel or direct compression of the lumen. Incarcerated hernias may also cause obstruction, and therefore the elective repair of hernias (inguinal, femoral, umbilical, or incisional) has become accepted practice to avoid obstruction. Extrinsic masses (abscesses, neoplasms, hematomas) also produce obstruction by compression. Intestinal volvulus, usually involving the colon, may be an etiologic factor in small-intestinal obstruction as well. A volvulus is caused by the twisting of a portion of intestine about itself, often leading to compromise of the blood supply to the obstructed intestine. The intrinsic lesions that cause mechanical obstruction are mostly congenital and include atresia, stenosis, and bowel duplication. In adults, strictures from neoplasms, inflammation, and endometriosis, as well as iatrogenic causes from radiation therapy and anastomoses, may also lead to obstruction. Obstruction may also occur secondary to luminal compromise. Polypoid tumors and gallstones may cause obstruction in adults, whereas intussusception and meconium ileus are more common in children. Intussusception when observed in an adult usually signifies an underlying anatomic abnormality such as a Meckel's diverticulum or tumor.

Paralytic Ileus

Paralytic ileus is caused by paralysis of the intestinal muscle. This is a rather common event occurring in many patients following abdominal operations and usually lasts only a few days. Bowel distention, propagated by the intestino-intestinal reflex, may also lead to ileus, as well as dilatation of surrounding structures such as the ureter. Additional causes of ileus include peritonitis, trauma, electrolyte imbalances, bowel ischemia, and drugs.

Idiopathic Intestinal Pseudo-obstruction

Intestinal pseudo-obstruction is characterized by chronic symptoms of recurrent obstruction of unknown etiology. Patients with this problem lack contractile responses to intestinal distention. Whether the origin is muscular or neural is undefined, and no particular radiologic signs are notable. Treatment is nasogastric suctioning, correction of electrolyte abnormalities, discontinuation of the use of narcotics, and avoidance of surgical intervention.

Pathophysiology

Simple Mechanical Obstruction

The pathophysiology of simple mechanical obstruction involves the abnormal accumulation of gases and fluids in the portion of the small bowel proximal to the site of obstruction. With obstruction, intestinal gas is unable to pass through the bowel and collects proximally. Most of the gas causing distention is swallowed air, which is mostly nitrogen that is not readily absorbed by intestinal mucosa and can be aspirated by a nasogastric tube. Carbon dioxide, also produced in the intestinal tract, is easily absorbed and, therefore, contributes very little to pathologic distention. The absorption of fluids is impaired proximally as well, and secretion is increased, causing a net loss of fluids and electrolytes into the lumen. The loss of Na^+, Cl^-, K^+, and H^+ causes hyponatremia, hypochloremia, hypokalemia, and metabolic alkalosis, respectively. Reflex vomiting may accentuate the dehydration, with progressive fluid loss leading to oliguria, azotemia, and hemoconcentration. Without treatment, a decrease in cardiac output with hypotension and shock can ensue. Bacterial proliferation typically follows intestinal stasis, but is of little significance in simple obstruction, as intact intestinal mucosa is resistant to bacterial absorption.

Strangulated Obstruction

If the blood supply to a portion of obstructed intestine is compromised, strangulation results. A volvulus or intussusception may trap mesenteric vessels, thereby causing strangulation. Adhesive bands and hernial rings can also obstruct vascular supply. When a segment of bowel is obstructed at two sites, closed-loop obstruction follows and progresses to strangulation more rapidly than simple obstruction. Strangulation is associated with the leakage of blood and plasma into the lumen in addition to the fluid and electrolytes lost in simple obstruction. The intestinal content of a strangulated segment of bowel (i.e., bacteria, toxins, necrotic tissue, and blood) is extremely toxic, and if passed into the peritoneal cavity through a perforation in the injured bowel, septic shock can result.

Diagnosis

Signs and Symptoms

The typical symptoms of small-bowel obstruction include abdominal pain, vomiting, obstipation, abdominal distention, and failure to pass flatus. The pain is crampy and episodic, reflecting peristaltic activity against the obstruction. The crampy pain subsides after a prolonged period, with suppression of intestinal motility by the inhibitory intestino-intestinal reflex. Strangulation should be considered if the pain becomes well localized, constant, and unremitting. Biliary emesis occurs early with proximal bowel obstruction, and a thick, feculent vomitus occurs later in the course with distal obstruction. Obstipation is observed after the segment of bowel distal to the obstruction is emptied of its contents; therefore, the inability to defecate presents sooner with distal obstruction.

Physical Examination

Physical examination should include a general assessment of the patient's status, focusing on signs of dehydration. Fever, tachycardia, and hypotension reflect severe dehydration. On abdominal examination, the presence of distention, surgical scars (suggesting the possibility of adhesions), hernias, and peristaltic waves (on thin patients) should be noted. The absence of bowel sounds signifies intestinal inactivity, which may be reflective of an underlying obstruction. The abdomen should be auscultated for at least 15 minutes before the absence of bowel sounds can be accurately affirmed. The auscultatory pattern characteristic of obstruction includes rushes of high-pitched tinkles interspersed episodically with periods of quiet. An attempt should also be made to elicit peritoneal signs such as rebound tenderness and guarding. A rectal examination should also be performed to detect the presence of masses, feces, or occult blood. Blood in the feces suggests a mucosal lesion of the alimentary tract, which may result from neoplasm, infarction, or intussusception.

Radiologic Studies

Flat and upright films of the abdomen may be very helpful in supporting a diagnosis of obstruction and in identifying the site. Distended loops of bowel with air-fluid levels are highly suggestive of obstruction (Fig. 2). Involvement of the small bowel can be distinguished from the large bowel by patterns of distention and bowel markings. The small bowel typically occupies the central abdomen and is characterized by the presence of valvulae conniventes, which appear as lines traversing the entire width of the intestine. The large bowel, however, occupies more of the periphery of the abdomen and can be differentiated by its haustral markings that extend only partially across the luminal diameter. In addition, colonic obstruction with a competent ileocecal valve shows distention of the large bowel alone, whereas an incompetent valve allows distention of both the small and large bowel. Paralytic ileus appears as gaseous distention scattered uniformly throughout the stomach, small intestine, and colon.

Occasionally, when plain films are not sufficient for diagnosis, contrast studies may be necessary. Barium enemas may be useful for identifying the site and etiology of colonic obstruction. In addition, reflux of contrast into the terminal ileum may at times demonstrate the transition in the more distal segments of small bowel. Ingested barium or contrast infused by

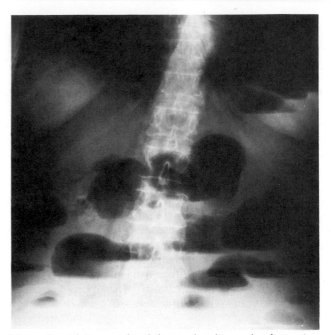

Figure 2. Plain upright abdominal radiograph of a patient with small-bowel obstruction. Note the characteristic air-fluid levels in the stomach and in the multiple, distended loops of bowel.

enteroclysis can help to differentiate paralytic ileus from partial mechanical obstruction of the small bowel. Simple upper gastrointestinal radiographs taken serially may confirm a suspected diagnosis of paralytic ileus but are not sufficient for distinguishing ileus from mechanical obstruction.

Laboratory Studies

Certain studies are helpful in monitoring dehydration and in assessing the adequacy of therapy. A patient suspected of being dehydrated should be followed with determinations of sodium, chloride, potassium, bicarbonate, and creatinine levels. Decreased levels of Na^+, Cl^-, and K^+ and elevated levels of bicarbonate and creatinine are consistent with dehydration. The hematocrit and white blood cell count (WBC) should also be obtained. A rise in the hematocrit suggests dehydration, and WBCs elevated to levels over 15,000 are consistent with strangulation. Slight elevations in WBC not exceeding 10,000, however, may be normal.

Treatment

Treatment of mechanical small-bowel obstruction often involves both nonoperative and operative management. Since dehydration is the primary concern, replacement of depleted fluids and electrolytes should be instituted immediately. Isotonic sodium chloride should be given initially, with the addition of potassium chloride when adequate urine output has been confirmed. In addition to fluid therapy, gastrointestinal decompression is helpful and is performed with a nasogastric or a longer intestinal tube used to reduce the risk of aspiration and to limit the amount of swallowed air that enters the gastrointestinal tract. Decompression may lead to resolution of the obstruction and thereby obviate the need for a surgical procedure. Failure to demonstrate progressive resolution, however, necessitates operative intervention.

The critical factor constituting an operative emergency is the suspicion of strangulated obstruction, which is associated with a higher mortality than simple obstruction. The ability to distinguish preoperatively whether bowel perfusion has been compromised is particularly difficult. Classic signs indicating the presence of gangrenous bowel include tachycardia, fever, leukocytosis, abdominal tenderness, distention, and a palpable mass. Unfortunately, these signs are not always completely reliable. When uncertainty exists, the aphorism to "never let the sun set or rise on a bowel obstruction" should be taken seriously. Operative management is indicated for all patients in whom involvement of gangrenous bowel cannot be excluded with certainty, and this means that every patient with a complete obstruction should at least be considered for abdominal exploration.

The appropriate operative procedure performed depends upon the etiologic agent causing the obstruction and includes the following: (1) lysis of adhesions, (2) reduction of hernias, (3) intestinal bypass for tumors, (4) resection of dead bowel with anastomosis, and (5) diversion by creation of a stoma, a procedure infrequently performed for small-intestinal obstruction.

In only a few instances can operation be delayed: (1) early postoperative obstruction, (2) obstruction secondary to the effects of chronic radiation, and (3) obstruction associated with chronic inflammatory disease. In the latter case, treatment of the inflammatory disease generally yields resolution of the obstruction. In patients with partial obstruction from adhesions, operative urgency is debatable; some studies have documented complete resolution with nasogastric suctioning. Determination of *partial* versus *complete* obstruction can best be accomplished radiographically, as serial plain radiographs may demonstrate eventual progression of gas distally past the obstructive site. Likewise, contrast studies may be useful for identifying an incomplete obstruction.

Treatment of Ileus

The treatment of paralytic ileus is nonoperative and involves nasogastric suctioning and intravenous fluids.

Correction of electrolytes is also important, as hypokalemia commonly causes ileus. Narcotics, chronic laxative abuse, and intra-abdominal sepsis also cause ileus, and treatment of these primary causes should also be undertaken.

CROHN'S DISEASE

Crohn's disease is a chronic granulomatous inflammatory disease of the gastrointestinal tract that was first described in detail by Crohn and his colleagues in 1932. Although any part of the alimentary tract may be involved, the small bowel and colon are the regions most commonly affected. Crohn's disease, also referred to as regional enteritis, is the most common surgical disease and the second most common pathologic entity involving the small intestine following peptic ulcer disease.

Incidence

The incidence of Crohn's disease is highest in the United States and Europe, with approximately 2 to 9 cases per 100,000 detected annually. Some studies report that the incidence is rising, but it remains less prevalent in blacks and Asians. It has a tendency to manifest primarily between the second and fourth decades; no predilection for gender has been identified.

Etiology

The etiology of regional enteritis remains unknown, although evidence for environmental, genetic, infectious, and immunologic bases exists. Recent epidemiologic studies suggest that environmental factors such as cigarette smoking and nutritional status may have a role in the pathogenesis of Crohn's disease. Interestingly, spouses of patients with Crohn's have a higher incidence of this disease than the general population. A genetic predisposition has been noted as well, with a family history of inflammatory bowel disease present in 15 to 20 per cent of patients. No clear pattern of inheritance has been identified. An infectious etiology has also been suggested. Recent investigations report the isolation of mycobacteria from several patients with this granulomatous disease, although no definitive cause-and-effect relationship has been demonstrated. An immunologic basis for Crohn's disease has also been proposed and offers perhaps the most promising evidence. The presence of antibodies directed against the gut epithelium and the clinical responsiveness to steroids support immunologic involvement. It is hypothesized that the disease is secondary to an inappropriate hyperresponsiveness of the gastrointestinal immune system to antigen stimulation.

Pathology

The inflammatory nature of Crohn's disease may involve any portion of the gastrointestinal tract from the mouth to the anus, but the terminal ileum and colon are most often affected. Disease is confined to the small intestine in approximately 30 per cent, whereas the colon is exclusively involved in 15 to 25 per cent. The majority of patients (55 per cent) with Crohn's show involvement of both the small and large intestine. The earliest gross pathologic manifestations of regional enteritis are aphthous ulcers, which are essentially shallow mucosal ulcers with white bases and raised edges. With progression of disease, the ulcers become more pronounced and confluent, and fissures tend to develop. The orientation of the fissures and ulcers around areas of intact mucosa give the luminal surface a characteristic "cobblestone" appearance. Inflammation extends *transmurally*, consuming all layers of the bowel wall, causing a progressive thickening and subsequent narrowing of the lumen. The mesentery may also become thickened and shortened from the inflammation, and extensive fat-wrapping may be observed, a phenomenon in which mesenteric fat extends circumferentially around the diseased bowel. The inflammatory process in Crohn's disease, in addition to being transmural, is also discontinuous. Skip areas, portions of normal bowel separated by diseased regions, are commonly encountered. Granuloma formation occurs later in the bowel wall in 50 to 70 per cent and in the mesenteric lymph nodes in 25 per cent of patients. Adhesions are rather common complications of inflammatory bowel disease, and at times lead to fistula formation and obstruction.

Clinical Presentation

The onset of Crohn's disease in most patients is slow, nonspecific, and insidious, and this contributes to a delayed diagnosis. Acute exacerbations and remissions characterize the initial course of the disease. As the disease progresses, however, the symptoms tend to persist and become increasingly severe. The primary symptoms are abdominal pain, diarrhea, and weight loss. Abdominal pain is the most common symptom and is described as either crampy and episodic in nature, or aching and constant. The more constant pain is suggestive of advanced disease. Diarrhea is the second most common symptom and is typically intermittent, following meals. Unlike the diarrhea associated with ulcerative colitis, the diarrhea of Crohn's disease often does not contain blood, mucus, or pus (Table 1). Weight loss tends to occur later in the course of the disease and results both from decreased food intake, which may alleviate abdominal discomfort and

TABLE 1. DISTINGUISHING FEATURES OF CROHN'S DISEASE AND ULCERATIVE COLITIS

Crohn's Disease	Ulcerative Colitis
Transmural inflammation	Disease confined to mucosa and submucosa
Discontinuous involvement with skip areas	Continuous involvement
Thickened bowel wall with "fat-wrapping"	Normal wall thickness
"Cobblestoning," fissures, deep ulcers	Shallow, wide "collar button" ulcers
Granuloma formation common	Granuloma formation rare
Perianal disease common	Perianal disease uncommon
Rectal bleeding less common	Rectal bleeding prominent
Small-bowel involvement likely	Small-bowel involvement rare
Rectum uncommonly involved	Rectum always involved

diarrhea, and from faulty digestion and absorption of food secondary to diseased portions of bowel.

Additional symptoms associated with Crohn's disease include perianal disease, fever, and anemia. Anal complications occur rather frequently in patients with regional enteritis, compared to those with ulcerative colitis. The anal fissure is the most common lesion, although fistulas and abscesses are not rare. Anal pathology is more frequently observed in patients with colonic involvement, but has been noted in patients with exclusive small-bowel disease as well. A patient may present solely with perianal disease years before the onset of intestinal disease. Therefore, any individual with a history of multiple, intermittent perianal fistulas should be examined for Crohn's disease. Fevers occur in greater than 50 per cent of patients with regional enteritis and may be the sole presenting symptom. Undetected abscesses in the bowel wall or development of a fistula may be the source of the fever. The anemia associated with inflammatory bowel disease is most often an iron deficiency or megaloblastic anemia caused by vitamin B_{12} or folate deficiency. Crohn's disease is also associated with a spectrum of extraintestinal manifestations (Table 2). Approximately 25 to 30 per cent of patients experience these manifestations, which tend to be more constant in their course and typically unresponsive to treatment. Although patients with Crohn's have been known to develop pyoderma gangrenosum, ankylosing spondylitis, sclerosing cholangitis, and active hepatitis, these disorders are more commonly seen in patients with ulcerative colitis.

Diagnosis

Crohn's disease should be suspected in any patient presenting with a chronic history of recurrent abdominal pain, diarrhea, and weight loss. The physical examination may be helpful in revealing abdominal ten-

TABLE 2. EXTRAINTESTINAL MANIFESTATIONS OF CROHN'S DISEASE

Skin
  Erythema nodosum
  Aphthous stomatitis
  Pyoderma gangrenosum
Eyes
  Iritis
  Uveitis
  Episcleritis
Joints
  Arthritis
  Hypertrophic osteoarthropathy
  Ankylosing spondylitis
Liver
  Pericholangitis
  Sclerosing cholangitis
  Hepatitis

derness, an abdominal mass, perianal involvement, or extraintestinal manifestations. However, imaging studies contribute more definitively to the diagnosis of this disease. Barium enemas have proven very useful for examining the colon and terminal ileum, whereas radiographic enteroclysis (infusion of barium contrast into the small bowel) is the most accurate technique for visualizing the upper gastrointestinal tract and small intestine. On the radiographs, ulcers, fissures, and a cobblestone appearance to the mucosa may be apparent as earlier findings. Distention of bowel proximal to areas of stricturing may also be seen. Later in the course of disease, Kantor's "string sign" may be observed, which represents the pathologic narrowing of intestinal lumen, most often of the terminal ileum, and resembles a string on the radiograph. Endoscopic examination, particularly of the terminal ileum and colon, may reveal segmental involvement of the bowel, a typical finding in Crohn's disease. Endoscopy also allows for biopsy of the diseased areas, which may show chronic inflammation and granuloma formation. While detection of a granuloma is nearly pathognomonic of Crohn's disease, only 15 per cent of patients show this finding on biopsy. The characteristic aphthous ulcers, internal fistulization, and mucosal cobblestoning may be demonstrated as well.

The list of principal differential diagnoses for regional enteritis includes ulcerative colitis, acute appendicitis, and intestinal tuberculosis. Crohn's disease may actually be very difficult to distinguish from ulcerative colitis. Acute ileitis, which may or may not be an early manifestation of Crohn's disease, may masquerade preoperatively as acute appendicitis. The diagnosis of ileitis is made during operation, upon identification of an acutely inflamed segment of terminal ileum and a normal appendix. Surgical treatment is usually unnecessary because acute regional enteritis usually resolves spontaneously. However, recommen-

dations have been made to remove the appendix to avoid confusion with appendicitis in the future, provided the cecum is *not* involved in the disease process. Tuberculosis may affect any portion of the gastrointestinal tract, although involvement distal to the cecum is uncommon.

Treatment

The initial treatment of uncomplicated Crohn's disease is essentially nonoperative. The primary principle behind treatment is the alleviation of symptoms and supportive care. Only if complications arise should the patient receive surgical therapy. Nutritional support is essential because most patients with Crohn's disease are malnourished even in the presence of inactive disease. An adjustment in diet has no beneficial effect on the progress of the disease, but an elemental diet and total parenteral nutrition can provide sufficient calories while affording the bowel rest, and this may ease symptoms. Medical therapy for Crohn's disease is palliative, not curative, and no drug therapy is known to influence the natural course of the disease. Sulfasalazine is the most commonly prescribed agent for reducing symptoms, and corticosteroids are thought to suppress inflammation. Both have shown marked effectiveness compared with placebo in treating acute disease, but combination therapy has not demonstrated additional benefit. Immunosuppressive agents have also proven more effective than placebos and, unlike sulfasalazine and prednisone, azathioprine and 6-mercaptopurine have been shown to effectively maintain patients in remission. Studies comparing cyclosporine to placebo have also shown beneficial effects in treating active disease and in maintaining remission. Additional studies are necessary to better characterize the role of cyclosporine in treating this disease.

Approximately 75 per cent of patients with regional enteritis for greater than 20 years eventually require surgical intervention. The most frequently encountered complications necessitating operation are obstructions, fistulas, and abscesses; intractable disease causing chronic debilitation is also an indication for operation. Although effective for relieving complications, surgical therapy does little to alter the progress of disease. For that reason, recurrences after operation are rather common, reaching an incidence of about 50 per cent at 10 years. The overriding principle in patients with Crohn's disease is to limit the operation to correction of the current complication. With obstruction, only the segment of bowel causing the obstructive symptoms should be removed, even if neighboring portions of bowel are involved in *chronic* disease. Likewise, for complications of bleeding, only the segment involved should be resected. Studies have indicated that increasing the margins bordering the resected segment of bowel does not improve the outcome, and conservative resection with preservation of as much bowel as possible is the recommended surgical approach. Intestinal resection with anastomosis is associated with a mortality rate of approximately 5 per cent. Bypass procedures in general should be avoided in patients with Crohn's disease because this approach leaves diseased bowel, which may develop complications in the future, including malignancy. As an alternative to resection, *stricturoplasty* has been utilized for correcting obstruction caused by strictures and has also been utilized in selected patients with duodenal disease. The more common surgical procedure for duodenal Crohn's disease, however, is *gastrojejunostomy*. Stricturoplasty is performed by making a longitudinal incision over the site of the stricture and closing it transversely. This effectively widens the lumen and avoids removal of any bowel, with few postoperative complications.

Prognosis

Currently, there is no effective treatment to cure patients with Crohn's disease. Eventually, most undergo surgery for associated complications, with a substantial number requiring a second or third procedure for recurrence. There is about a 50 per cent recurrence rate at 10 years, most frequently involving the segment of bowel proximal to the site of anastomosis. No specific factors appear to affect the rate of recurrence. The mortality for patients with Crohn's is twice that of normal individuals at any age. This observed increase in mortality is directly attributable to the disease itself and to complications. Cancer reportedly occurs more frequently in these patients (60 to 300 times more often), the most common site being the ileum, and they tend to have a worse prognosis. Although it is currently impossible to cure Crohn's disease, most patients can be maintained at a comfortable state of health with a combination of medical therapy and surgical excision and can lead relatively normal lives.

MECKEL'S DIVERTICULUM

In 1808, Meckel described the embryology and pathology of the small-intestinal diverticulum that bears his name. Meckel's diverticulum, the most frequently encountered congenital anomaly of the gastrointestinal tract, occurs in approximately 1 per cent of the population, yet remains asymptomatic in most of these patients. It is known as a *true* diverticulum, because it contains all the layers of the intestinal wall. The diverticulum almost always arises from the antimesenteric border of the ileum approximately 45 to 90 cm proximal to the ileocecal valve, and ranges in length and diameter from 1 to 12 cm. It receives its own blood supply and in many instances contains heterotopic tissue, most often gastric mucosa, with pancreatic, duodenal, and colonic tissue also being described (Fig. 3).

Embryologically, Meckel's diverticulum is an abnormal remnant following incomplete obliteration of the omphalomesenteric or vitelline duct. The omphalomesenteric duct, which connects the yolk sac with the primitive gut, typically atrophies and disappears by the seventh gestational week. Failure of the duct to obliterate appropriately may lead to the formation of an umbilical-ileal fistula, umbilical sinus, or fibrous bands joining the umbilicus to the ileum, in addition to a Meckel's diverticulum. Most patients with Meckel's diverticula are found incidentally, during either autopsy (0.3 to 3 per cent) or laparotomy. A smaller percentage of patients (approximately 6 per cent), however, become symptomatic, which is associated with greater morbidity and mortality. The most commonly observed complication is bleeding, which occurs in approximately 50 per cent of symptomatic patients. The bleeding typically follows ulceration of the surrounding ileal mucosa secondary to acid secretion from the heterotopic gastric tissue within the diverticulum and is most prevalent in the pediatric population. Intestinal obstruction, which may follow volvulus, intussusception, or diverticular incarceration within a hernia, may also be a presenting symptom. Obstruction from intussusception produces the classic "currant jelly" stool. Another complication associated with Meckel's diverticulum is inflammation that mimics acute appendicitis in presentation and leads eventually to perforation. The association of neoplasms with Meckel's diverticulum, although a rare occurrence, has been recently recorded. Carcinoid tumors are the most commonly reported tumor found coexisting within a Meckel's diverticulum, and the majority of these tumors are found at the diverticular tip. Leiomyosarcomas and adenocarcinomas have also been found in association with Meckel's, in addition to several benign neoplasms. Most of these tumors are found incidentally at autopsy or during an unrelated laparotomy, although the lesion itself may produce symptoms requiring operation.

Detection of a Meckel's diverticulum can be made preoperatively by radiographic studies. Occasionally, a barium enema or small-bowel series may show the diverticulum. Technetium scanning has also proven to be successful in identifying Meckel's diverticulum. Approximately 50 per cent of patients have heterotopic tissue within the diverticulum. In technetium scanning, ^{99m}Tc pertechnetate is absorbed by gastric mucosa, ef-

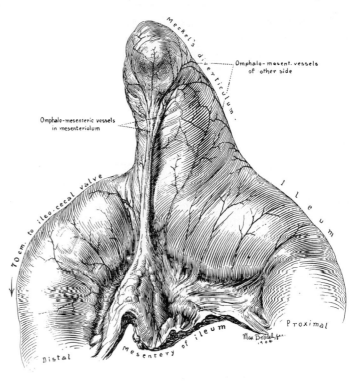

Figure 3. A large Meckel's diverticulum. Note the separate blood supply. (From Kelly HA, Hurdon E: The Vermiform Appendix and Its Diseases. Philadelphia, WB Saunders Company, 1905.)

fectively demonstrating Meckel's diverticulum with ectopic gastric tissue.

The issue of greatest controversy concerning appropriate treatment of a Meckel's is whether the diverticulum should be removed when found incidentally. Proponents hold that an incidental diverticulectomy is relatively safe, whereas the morbidity and mortality associated with surgical intervention for a complicated diverticulum is significantly higher. Opponents quote the low lifetime risk of developing symptoms and contend that the number of incidental diverticulectomies necessary to offset one death from a symptomatic Meckel's is unreasonably high. In 1983, Mackey reported 402 cases of Meckel's diverticulum over a 50-year period, which suggested that the risk of a patient developing symptoms should determine whether an incidental diverticulectomy should be performed. Patients considered to be at high risk were males under 40 years of age who had a diverticulum 2 cm in length or greater, with heterotopic tissue within the diverticulum. Other factors were considered to have negligible influence on risk status. However, the incidental removal of a Meckel's diverticulum still remains controversial. Surgical treatment of a complicated Meckel's diverticulum should involve an intestinal resection rather than a simple diverticulectomy. The most common clinical complication of a Meckel's is bleeding, and the most common source of bleeding is ulceration of the *adjacent* ileal mucosa from acid secreted by ec-

topic gastric tissue within the diverticulum. Segmental resection, including the ulcerated portion of ileum, is recommended for bleeding ulcers.

NEOPLASMS

Incidence

Primary neoplasms of the small intestine are extremely rare, and the reasons are unclear. The incidence of tumor development in the colon is approximately 40 times higher, despite the greater cell turnover and mucosal surface area of the small bowel. The majority of small-intestinal tumors occur in the ileum, with 40 to 45 per cent occurring equally in the duodenum and jejunum. The lesions may originate from any layer of the bowel, with tumors of epithelial origin being by far the most common. Reports of patients undergoing removal of the tumors show the frequency of benign tumors to be comparable to the frequency of malignant tumors. However, in autopsy, there is a marked predominance of benign neoplasms, which emphasizes that many are probably asymptomatic.

BENIGN TUMORS

The most common *benign* neoplasms of the small intestine are leiomyomas (18 per cent), lipomas (16 per cent), and adenomas (14 per cent). Tumors that occur less commonly include hamartomas, hemangiomas, fibromas, neurofibromas, fibromyomas, myxomas, and lymphangiomas (Table 3).

Leiomyomas

Leiomyomas, benign tumors of smooth muscle, are distributed rather evenly throughout the small intestine. They can penetrate intramurally and cause symptoms of intestinal obstruction, or extend both intramurally and extramurally, reaching considerable size. Bleeding may follow tumor necrosis as the mass overgrows its blood supply. Bleeding is most often caused by leiomyomas.

Lipomas

Greater than half of all gastrointestinal lipomas are found in the small intestine. They are submucosal tumors of adipose tissue, occur most commonly in the ileum, may be single or multiple, and are benign. Lipomas are most often asymptomatic and may function as lead points and cause intestinal obstruction from intussusception.

Adenomas

Half of the adenomas in the small intestine occur in the ileum, with approximately 20 per cent occurring in the duodenum and 30 per cent in the jejunum. These tumors commonly arise from the superficial mucous membrane or intestinal glands and are the most frequently encountered benign tumor of the duodenum. They tend to be asymptomatic and are most often identified at autopsy. True adenomas, villous, and

TABLE 3. SMALL-INTESTINAL NEOPLASMS

Type	Incidence
Benign	
Leiomyomas	18%
Lipomas	16%
Adenomas	14%
Polyps	14%
Hemangiomas	10%
Fibromas	10%
Neurogenic tumors	7%
Fibromyomas	5%
Myxomas	2%
Lymphangiomas	2%
Others	2%
Malignant	
Adenocarcinomas	45%
Carcinoid tumors	25%
Lymphomas	20%
Sarcomas	10%

Brunner's gland adenomas comprise the three primary types. Villous adenomas, unlike Brunner's gland adenomas, have a 35 to 55 per cent potential of malignancy and can be identified by their characteristic "soap bubble" appearance on radiograph. Often confused clinically with peptic ulcer disease, Brunner's gland adenomas are found primarily in the area of the duodenum proximal to the ampulla of Vater, where the concentration of Brunner's glands is greatest.

Peutz-Jeghers Syndrome

The Peutz-Jeghers syndrome is a dominantly inherited disorder characterized by multiple intestinal polyps and pigmented lesions on the buccal mucosa, lips, nose, palms, and soles. The intestinal polyps are thought to be hamartomas, occur most often in the jejunum and ileum, and are themselves benign, with very little malignant potential. The most frequently noted symptoms are colicky abdominal pain caused by intermittent obstruction from intussusception and anemia from occult blood loss.

Clinical Symptoms

Benign tumors of the small intestine are most often asymptomatic, and of the 10 per cent of small bowel tumors that produce symptoms, only 25 per cent are benign. The most frequently encountered symptoms are bleeding and obstruction. Bleeding, presenting in 20 to 53 per cent of symptomatic cases, tends to be occult and episodic, often leading to iron-deficiency anemia. Although all small-bowel tumors may cause bleeding, leiomyomas and hemangiomas are the most common. Obstruction, partial or complete, causes 42 to 70 per cent of the symptomatic cases and is due to narrowing of the lumen by the inwardly growing tumor mass or by intermittent intussusception. Benign tumors are the most common cause of intussusception in the adult.

Diagnosis

Since small-bowel tumors occur so infrequently and present with such nonspecific symptoms, the appropriate diagnosis is often difficult to establish. Often, a suspicion of small-bowel neoplasm is necessary to make the correct diagnosis. However, radiographic studies have proven useful as diagnostic aids. Barium studies enable visualization of a greater portion of the small bowel than does endoscopy. Endoscopy is useful for examining the proximal small bowel and allows for biopsy. Most recently, however, enteroclysis has become the technique of choice for radiographically examining the small bowel. Greater detection of small defects and mucosal changes can be achieved, and this technique is reportedly associated with a diagnostic accuracy of approximately 90 per cent.

Management

A benign tumor in the small intestine is nearly always an indication for surgical removal, to avoid further complications and to effectively exclude malignancy. Small lesions may be excised by enterotomy, while larger lesions typically require segmental resection. When a lesion is found in the bowel, the entire length of small intestine should be searched for additional lesions, as they are often multiple.

MALIGNANT TUMORS

Malignancies of the small intestine are rare and account for only 1 to 2 per cent of all gastrointestinal tract malignancies. Adenocarcinomas, occurring in 45 per cent of cases, are the most common type, with carcinoids accounting for approximately 25 per cent, lymphomas for 20 per cent, and sarcomas for 10 per cent.

ADENOCARCINOMAS

Adenocarcinomas are most often found in the duodenum (40 per cent) and proximal jejunum (38 per cent), with half of the lesions in the duodenum involving the ampulla of Vater. Adenocarcinomas associated with longstanding Crohn's disease, however, tend to occur in the ileum. The symptoms vary with the location of the tumor. Thus, duodenal involvement causes primarily jaundice and bleeding. Less specific symptoms of crampy abdominal pain, weight loss, and anemia accompany tumors located in the jejunum and ileum. Symptoms of obstruction may also follow intraluminal extension of the tumor mass or luminal constriction by an annular lesion. In general, the symptoms associated with adenocarcinoma are rather vague, which often delays the diagnosis. At the time of operation, as many as 80 per cent of patients demonstrate metastatic spread, contributing to the poor prognosis of this tumor type.

LYMPHOMAS

Gastrointestinal lymphomas are very rare, constituting only 1 per cent of all gastrointestinal neoplasms. Lymphomas generally arise from nodal tissue. The small intestine is, however, the most common site of origin for extranodal lymphomas, with the ileum most often involved because of its high concentration of gut lymphoid tissue. Often, a lymphoma that is primary to the small bowel is difficult to distinguish from a lymphoma that is a component of a more generalized disease. Dawson and his colleagues have proposed the following criteria for identifying lymphomas as primary to the small bowel: (1) absence of peripheral lymphadenopathy, (2) normal leukocyte count and differential, (3) absence of mediastinal lymph node enlargement on chest film, (4) no evidence of involvement beyond the bowel lesion and regional nodes during operation, and (5) absence of tumor involvement of the liver and spleen. Three syndromes are associated with small-intestinal lymphoma. *Western lymphoma* is seen predominantly in the adult population and may lead to severe malabsorption in 5 to 10 per cent of patients. *Mediterranean lymphoma*, recently renamed *immunoproliferative small intestinal disease*, is associated in one third of cases with abnormal IgA heavy-chain fragments. The third group is associated with childhood abdominal lymphomas (e.g., Burkitt's) and represents the most common gastrointestinal tumor seen in children.

Sarcomas

Sarcomas arise primarily from intestinal and vascular smooth muscle. The most frequently encountered type of sarcoma is *leiomyosarcoma*, which may involve any portion of the small intestine but demonstrates a preponderance for the jejunum. The lesions are typically large and ulcerative, manifesting clinically with gastrointestinal blood loss. Whereas adenocarcinomas are most apt to present with obstruction, sarcomas are apt to present with bleeding, usually in the form of melena.

Clinical Symptoms

Unlike benign tumors, which tend to be asymptomatic, approximately 75 to 80 per cent of malignant tumors produce symptoms. The most common symptoms are obstruction (with nausea, vomiting, and colicky abdominal pain) and bleeding (with anemia, weakness, and guaiac-positive stools). In addition, and unlike benign neoplasms, significant weight loss often accompanies malignancy, with lymphoma patients losing as much as 20 lbs. The obstruction observed with malignant lesions tends to follow luminal infiltration of the tumor, whereas with benign lesions, the obstruction is most often secondary to intussusception. Again, the symptoms are rather nonspecific and tend to follow an insidious course, which in most instances leads to a delayed diagnosis.

Treatment

The standard treatment for small-intestinal malignancy is wide resection with the removal of regional lymph nodes and preservation of the superior mesenteric vessels. The more radical *Whipple* procedure (pancreaticoduodenectomy) may be indicated for an attempt to cure duodenal cancers. If metastases are present at laparotomy, treatment for cure is no longer the primary goal; rather, measures for palliation should be performed. Bypass procedures may be indicated in situations where resection is not the most advantageous approach for the relief of symptoms. Chemotherapy and radiation therapy have been effective in extending the survival of patients with lymphomas, and some patients with sarcomas have shown slight improvement as well. Adjuvant therapy, however, has not proven beneficial for the treatment of adenocarcinomas.

Prognosis

Overall, patients with small-intestinal malignancies have rather poor prognoses, owing to the difficulty and delay in establishing correct diagnoses. The average 5-year survival rate for patients with adenocarcinomas is 25 per cent; for sarcomas, 30 to 40 per cent; and lymphomas, 30 to 50 per cent.

Carcinoid Tumors

Site of Origin

Carcinoid tumors may originate in the lungs, thymus, larynx, ovaries, testes, and uterine cervix. They may arise from neuroendocrine cells along the gastrointestinal tract as well. The most common gastrointestinal site is the appendix, with 50 per cent of the total arising from this site. The small intestine is involved in approximately 25 per cent, with a preference demonstrated for the ileum. The enterochromaffin or Kulchitsky cells located in the crypts of Lieberkühn are the cells of origin. The rectum is involved in 17 per cent of patients, and several reports describe carcinoid tumors arising in a Meckel's diverticulum. Carcinoid tumors originating in the ileum demonstrate the highest propensity to metastasize (35 per cent), while those in the appendix and rectum rarely metastasize (3 per cent). From 17 to 53 per cent of patients with carcinoid tumors, especially of the ileum, also demonstrate the coexistence of a second primary tumor of a different histologic type.

Clinical Symptoms

Carcinoid tumors belong to the group of neoplasms otherwise known as *apudomas*. Their distinguishing feature is an ability to secrete amines, tachykinins, and other peptides. Clinically, however, patients with carcinoid tumors demonstrate symptoms similar to those observed with other small bowel malignancies to the exclusion of those associated with the carcinoid syndrome. The most frequently encountered symptom is intestinal obstruction, which is caused more by the local fibroblastic reaction attributed to the release of serotonin by the tumor than by luminal compromise by the tumor itself. The mesentery and bowel become shortened and kinked from the reactive scarring process, causing a sclerosed mass that may be palpable on abdominal examination. Other related symptoms include diarrhea, gastrointestinal bleeding, pain, and weight loss.

Diagnosis

Evidence of carcinoid tumors may be detected radiographically. Barium studies of the small intestine may be useful in identifying kinked or fixed loops of bowel, extrinsic masses, or intraluminal masses. Intestinal enteroclysis, however, is more likely to yield positive findings. Demonstration of carcinoid malignancies of the colon and rectum may be achieved by barium enema or colonoscopy. Biopsies should be obtained whenever possible; argentaffin and argyrophil stains are helpful for identifying the carcinoid nature of tumors. Carcinoid tumors synthesize and secrete serotonin (5-hydroxytryptamine [5-HT]). Serotonin is converted by the liver to its metabolite 5-hydroxyindoleacetic acid (5-HIAA), which is secreted into the urine in large amounts. Approximately 50 per cent of patients with carcinoid tumors of the gastrointestinal tract demonstrate elevated levels of urinary 5-HIAA regardless of whether the carcinoid syndrome is present. A level of greater than 20 mg of urinary 5-HIAA collected over a 24-hour period confirms the diagnosis of carcinoid tumor.

Treatment

The appropriate treatment of carcinoid tumors depends on the size and location of the tumor. All carcinoid tumors should be removed because of their potential for metastatic spread. If the tumor is found to have already metastasized, the primary tumor should be resected to reduce future complications of obstruction and intussusception. Gastroduodenal or rectal carcinoids measuring less than 1 cm may be excised endoscopically. Certain cases of duodenal carcinoids may necessitate a Whipple procedure. En bloc resection of tumor and associated mesentery should be performed for lesions greater than 1 cm, for multiple tumors, and when widespread metastases are present. Removal of as much tumor bulk as possible has demonstrated beneficial effects on both survival and reduction of symptoms. For appendiceal carcinoids less than 1 cm in diameter, a simple appendectomy is curative. For tumors greater than 2 cm that demonstrate a greater propensity to metastasize, a right hemicolectomy should be performed.

Prognosis

Primary tumors larger than 2 cm and the presence of metastatic spread indicate a worse prognosis for patients with carcinoid tumor. The overall survival rate 5 years following resection of a small intestinal carcinoid tumor approaches 75 per cent. The presence of hepatic metastases reduces 5-year survival to 20 per cent, and the 5-year survival rate for patients with rectal or appendiceal tumors less than 1 cm (which rarely metastasize) is nearly 100 per cent.

Carcinoid Syndrome

Causes

When carcinoid tumors of the small intestine metastasize to the liver, the malignant carcinoid syndrome may follow. In the absence of metastases, carcinoid tumors of the ovaries, testes, and bronchi may induce the clinical manifestations of carcinoid syndrome by secreting their products directly into the systemic circulation. The liver functions under normal conditions to metabolize free serotonin to 5-HIAA. When liver metastases are present, the vasoactive substances secreted by the tumor escape hepatic degradation and enter directly into the systemic circulation. Approximately 10 per cent of patients with carcinoid tumors develop carcinoid syndrome.

Clinical Symptoms

The principal features of carcinoid syndrome include cutaneous flushing (80 per cent), diarrhea (83 per cent), bronchospasm (25 per cent), and right-sided cardiac valvular lesions (50 per cent). The flushing is thought to be mediated primarily by the kinin peptides secreted by the tumor. This may occur as a spontaneous manifestation or be induced by excitement, physical activity, alcohol, or certain food products. The gastrointestinal symptoms follow elevated levels of serotonin, which increases small-intestinal fluid and electrolyte secretion and intestinal motility. The diarrhea is typically episodic, watery, nonbloody, and accompanied by severe abdominal cramping. The cardiopulmonary manifestations are also attributed to the substances elaborated by the tumor. Histamine, bradykinin, and serotonin can cause bronchoconstriction,

and serotonin appears to be the primary agent involved in the valvular manifestations that occur later in the disease. Serotonin precipitates endocardial scarring, which leads to valvular stenosis and insufficiency, and the elevated levels cause fibrosis, predominantly of the tricuspid and pulmonic valves. The valves on the left side of the heart are usually spared because serotonin is inactivated by pulmonary enzymes in the lungs.

Diagnosis

A patient who presents with hepatomegaly, flushing, and diarrhea should be suspected of having the carcinoid syndrome. Confirmation of the diagnosis can be made by the repeated demonstration of elevated levels of 5-HIAA in the urine. Before collecting the urine specimen, the patient must refrain from ingesting foods rich in serotonin such as bananas, tomatoes, walnuts, and pineapples, as well as certain drugs such as phenothiazines and salicylates. Provocative tests to reproduce symptoms using epinephrine and pentagastrin have also been employed as diagnostic aids. The pentagastrin test is by far the safest and most reliable, and administration of small doses of pentagastrin in patients with carcinoid syndrome induces facial flushing, gastrointestinal symptoms, elevations in circulating 5-HT levels, and release of certain peptides. Hepatic metastases can best be detected by angiography.

Treatment

Treatment of carcinoid syndrome is both surgical and pharmacologic. In addition to surgical resection of the involved bowel and mesentery, patients with carcinoid syndrome should have resection of hepatic metastases as well for effective palliation of symptoms. Hepatic arterial embolization or ligation may provide an alternative for symptomatic relief in patients in whom resection is not possible. Valve replacements also have been reportedly performed for patients with cardiac manifestations of the carcinoid syndrome. Orthotopic liver transplants have been performed in a select few who have demonstrated unresectable metastatic involvement of the liver. Pharmacologic agents have also effectively ameliorated symptoms of the carcinoid syndrome. Serotonin antagonists, such as methysergide, cyproheptadine, and methotrimeprazine, target the diarrheal symptoms. Interferon therapy offers promising results in controlling flushing. In addition, α-adrenergic blocking agents (phenoxybenzamine and phenothiazine) block the stimulation of kallikrein, thereby reducing symptoms of flushing. Studies have also shown effective reduction in the symptoms of diarrhea and flushing with somatostatin and its analog, octreotide. To date, octreotide is the most effective pharmacologic agent for the treatment of carcinoid syndrome. Patient survival has also been shown to increase by an average of 3 years with this agent. Also, octreotide is effective as prophylaxis for patients with the carcinoid syndrome who are exposed to stressful situations, such as surgical procedures or chemotherapy. With nonresectable hepatic metastases, administration of chemotherapeutic agents in conjunction with hepatic artery occlusion has been attempted with encouraging results, using streptozocin and cyclophosphamide or 5-fluorouracil (5-FU). Radiation therapy has no beneficial role in the treatment of carcinoid syndrome.

MALABSORPTION SYNDROMES

Malabsorption may arise in several disorders involving the gastrointestinal tract including any state in which absorption is impaired. The possible etiologies are numerous, and the conditions arising from surgical procedures make up a significant proportion.

Clinical Symptoms

The primary clinical manifestations associated with malabsorption are unexplained weight loss, diarrhea, and steatorrhea. Absorption of the major constituents (fat, protein, and carbohydrate) may all be impaired, although malabsorption of fat tends to predominate. Carbohydrate malabsorption produces watery diarrhea, and fat malabsorption causes steatorrhea, which leads to altered absorption of the fat-soluble vitamins A, D, E, and K. Tetany, osteomalacia, bone pain, and pathologic fractures may be caused by the deficiency in vitamin D and calcium, and bleeding may be caused by hypoprothrombinemia, which follows loss of vitamin K. Neuropathies and glossitis are potential manifestations of vitamin B_{12} deficiency, and malabsorption of either B_{12} or iron can cause chronic anemia. Malabsorption of protein, when severe enough to produce hypoalbuminemia, leads to peripheral edema and ascites.

Diagnosis

Several tests detect malabsorption. The stool should be examined grossly for evidence of steatorrhea, appearing as bulky, malodorous, and floating stools. On microscopic examination, an increase in fat content can be visualized with Sudan III fecal B fat stain, signifying impaired absorption of fat. A more quantitative approach can be taken, in which the patient is placed on a diet fixed in fat content for a number of days. The patient's stools are then analyzed for fat: greater than 25 gm/day signifies an abnormality. Likewise, the same test can be performed for quantifying protein content, with greater than 3 gm/day being abnormal. Protein-losing enteropathies can be detected by measuring the amount of radioactivity in the stool after injection of intravenous radiolabeled albumin. The general absorptive capacity of the jejunal mucosa can be assessed by orally administering D-xylose and subsequently measuring the amount of xylose appearing in the urine. Absorption of carbohydrate can be assessed by using the standard oral glucose tolerance test. For vitamin B_{12} absorption, the Schilling test is most specific and useful and involves four stages. In the initial stage, radioactive cobalamin (vitamin B_{12}) is administered orally and the amount excreted in the urine over 24 hours is measured. Abnormally low levels indicate a defect in vitamin B_{12} absorption. The second stage involves administration of intrinsic factor along with vitamin B_{12}. Intrinsic factor (IF) is necessary for the absorption of vitamin B_{12}. Intrinsic factor is secreted in the stomach and binds to B_{12} in the intestine to enable its absorption. If cobalamin levels in the urine are normal with the addition of IF, then conclusively the B_{12} deficiency is due to a deficiency in intrinsic factor. Likewise, stage three involves administration of B_{12} but with the addition of pancreatic enzymes. Normalization in this stage suggests pancreatic insufficiency. In stage four, antibiotics are administered along with B_{12}. Normalization in this stage implicates bacterial overgrowth as the etiology for B_{12} malabsorption.

Specific Disorders

Postgastrectomy Syndrome

Malabsorption of fat, protein, calcium, iron, fat-soluble vitamins, and vitamin B_{12} have all been documented after gastric resection, both partial and complete, although the abnormalities are more pronounced following total gastrectomy. The primary clinical symptom signifying a malabsorptive complication is weight loss. Both a voluntary decrease in food intake relieving reflux esophagitis symptoms and an actual reduction in gastric storage and mixing capacities contribute to the observed weight loss. In addition to loss in weight, patients generally develop anemia following gastrectomy procedures. Iron-deficiency anemia is the most common form encountered. Pernicious anemia is observed after total gastric resection, in which the primary source of intrinsic factor is removed. The anemia does not appear clinically, however, until 3 or 4 years after surgery, after the hepatic store of intrinsic factor has been depleted. In the instances of resection for malignancy, the patients tend not to manifest with anemia at all because they generally do not survive long enough for the anemia to appear.

Patients undergoing Billroth procedures following subtotal gastrectomies manifest variable degrees of malabsorption depending upon the type of anastomosis performed. The Billroth I procedure involves anastomosis of the stomach to the duodenum, and the Billroth II, the stomach to the jejunum. In general, Billroth II reconstructions appear to be associated with more malabsorptive abnormalities than the Billroth I operation. In particular, fat malabsorption tends to be more pronounced with the former procedure, occurring in approximately 50 per cent of patients as compared to 25 per cent of patients with the Billroth I. Several reasons account for the discrepancy: (1) the primary areas of fat absorption (i.e., the duodenal and proximal jejunal mucosa) are bypassed in the Billroth II anastomosis, (2) the mixing capacity is reduced secondary to the decrease in biliary and pancreatic juice secretion, and (3) the bypassed loop of duodenum has the capacity to develop into a blind loop, in which bacteria proliferate and inactivate the bile salts necessary for appropriate fat absorption. In addition to the fat malabsorption, bacteria may interfere with the absorption of vitamin B_{12} as well, leading to megaloblastic anemia. The absorption of fat-soluble vitamins and calcium is also impaired. Since the duodenum is the primary site of iron absorption, iron-deficiency anemia tends to be more pronounced in patients with the Billroth II anastomosis as well.

Most patients who undergo total gastrectomies experience postoperative complications, including weight loss, anemia, and nutritional abnormalities. A fraction (approximately one third) of patients with partial gastrectomies manifest these symptoms as well. The treatment for these patients is generally a diet high in calories, and fat and protein if necessary. Oral pancreatic enzyme preparations may be of benefit in some patients. Supplementing the diet with iron, calcium, and vitamins, including vitamin B_{12} may also be necessary. Surgical interventions, such as conversion of a Billroth II into a Billroth I, should be left as a last resort.

Vagotomy

Vagotomies are usually performed in combination with either a partial gastric resection or a drainage procedure and rarely as an isolated operation. For this reason, it is difficult to determine the direct effects of vagotomy alone on the development of malabsorption. Experimental studies have shown that vagal denervation alters gastric mixing and storage capacity, small-bowel motility, and pancreaticobiliary secretions, all of which may lead to malabsorptive abnormalities. Clinically, postoperative diarrhea is common after vagotomy, but less than 5 per cent of patients develop complications such as secondary weight loss. The diarrhea is treatable with antispasmodics such as codeine or diphenoxylate hydrochloride. Steatorrhea is also a common finding, caused by deficient bile salt absorption.

Pancreatic Insufficiency

Because the pancreas has a large functional reserve, malabsorptive abnormalities are only evident in cases of advanced disease. Chronic pancreatitis is the main cause of pancreatic malabsorption, although cystic fibrosis of the pancreas, tumors, fistulas, and stones have all been implicated as etiologic agents. Pancreatic dysfunction causes primarily the malabsorption of fat with steatorrhea. Weight loss and abdominal pain are additional clinical findings. Because the jejunal mucosa is not altered, the D-xylose absorption test is normal in these patients. However, an altered glucose tolerance test, glucosuria, and hypocalcemia are findings consistent with pancreatic insufficiency. The secretin test, although not commonly utilized, bears mentioning: duodenal contents are examined for secretin-stimulated pancreatic enzyme secretion after an intravenous injection of secretin. Failure of the pancreas to respond to the secretin with secretion of enzymes indicates pancreatic disease.

The treatment of pancreatic dysfunction depends upon the underlying cause. Oral pancreatic enzyme extracts benefit patients with chronic pancreatitis. Ductal obstruction is best treated by pancreaticoenteric anastomoses and restoration of intestinal flow of pancreatic enzymes. Resection is the appropriate treatment for tumors. Two specific non–beta-cell tumors, elaborating gastrin and VIP, are associated with malabsorption. Gastrinomas, also known as Zollinger-Ellison tumors, hypersecrete gastrin, which hyperstimulates the parietal cells resulting in excess acid production. The treatment of this particular tumor has previously been total gastrectomy, which has often been complicated by malabsorption. Omeprazole, a hydrogen pump blocker, is currently the drug of choice for the Zollinger-Ellison syndrome. Omeprazole effectively inhibits gastric acid secretion at the level of the H^+ pump and has demonstrated relatively few adverse effects. Vasoactive intestinal peptide directly stimulates the small-intestinal mucosa to secrete water and electrolytes. Tumors elaborating VIP, therefore, result in excessive secretions, which manifest as intractable diarrhea. Removal of the tumor is the surgical treatment of choice. The use of octreotide for VIP tumors is currently under investigation and has shown promising results.

Hepatobiliary Disorders

Malabsorption from hepatobiliary disorders is caused by inadequate bile flow into the duodenum. Bile salts are necessary for the emulsification and, therefore, absorption of fats. Steatorrhea is a common finding in patients with disorders of the hepatobiliary tree. Bile flow can be impeded when the liver itself is diseased such as with acute hepatitis or cirrhosis. The flow of bile into the intestine can be obstructed, which may occur secondary to intrahepatic cholestasis or to biliary stone formation. The malabsorption of fats is accompanied by malabsorption of the fat-soluble vitamins, as well as calcium, which may lead to bone diseases such as osteomalacia and osteoporosis. The malabsorption associated with hepatobiliary disorders can be treated by correcting the cause contributing to the inadequate bile flow. Treatment of hepatitis and cirrhosis involves abstinence from agents that exacerbate the disease, such as alcohol. Administration of fat-soluble vitamins and calcium may help alleviate malabsorption secondary to obstructive etiology. Decreasing oral fat intake may also reduce steatorrhea and diarrhea. Surgical intervention is reserved for patients with extrahepatic biliary obstruction and fistulas, to restore bile flow into the intestinal tract.

Blind Loop Syndrome

This syndrome, also known as *bacterial overgrowth syndrome*, is associated with processes that cause intestinal stasis and bacterial proliferation. In addition to the well-recognized surgical causes for the blind loop syndrome, intestinal strictures, Crohn's disease, intestinal pseudo-obstruction, fistulas, and scleroderma may all lead to stasis with subsequent infection. The overgrowth of bacteria causes malabsorption by (1) rendering the bile salts inactive and, therefore, impairing fat digestion and absorption; and (2) reducing absorption of the bile salts themselves in the terminal ileum. Absorption of vitamins A, D, E, and K and calcium are also impaired. In addition, the bacteria interferes with vitamin B_{12} absorption. The mechanism causing the megaloblastic anemia is unknown, although hypotheses suggest either a competitive utilization of vitamin B_{12} by bacteria or elaboration of an inhibitory agent that hinders B_{12} absorption. The clinical hallmarks of the blind loop syndrome are vitamin deficiencies, diarrhea, steatorrhea, weight loss, and megaloblastic anemia. The test of diagnosis is the Schilling test. If, with the addition of antibiotics, B_{12} appears in appropriate amounts in the urine, the blind loop syndrome can be diagnosed. Continued use of tetracycline for approximately 3 weeks usually improves symptoms. Other beneficial drugs include clindamycin and Flagyl. Curative treatment involves surgical correction of the underlying disorder causing the intestinal stasis.

Short-Bowel Syndrome

The short-bowel syndrome results when a significant portion of the small intestine loses its absorptive capacity, either from disease or following surgical resection. Multiple resections for chronic Crohn's disease, vascular insufficiency compromising significant lengths of the intestine, and fistulas redirecting intestinal contents past absorptive surface areas may all lead to the short-bowel syndrome.

Clinical findings include malnutrition, unexplained weight loss, diarrhea, steatorrhea, and dehydration. With the loss of distal small bowel, including the ileocecal valve, the intestinal transit time is markedly reduced, leading to decreased absorption. Resection of segments of terminal ileum may lead specifically to impaired absorption of vitamin B_{12} and bile salts. Loss of proximal small-bowel interferes with calcium and iron uptake. Malabsorption is also attributable to postoperative gastric acid hypersecretion, which prevents the alkalinization necessary for optimal pancreatic enzyme activity. The initial treatment of short-bowel syndrome includes bowel rest and total parenteral nutrition therapy. When an oral diet can be adequately tolerated, fats and proteins should be administered in the partially digested form, and vitamins, electrolytes, and minerals should be administered to restore nutritional status. Histamine-receptor antagonists such as cimetidine and ranitidine are helpful for reducing gastric acid secretion. The role of surgical intervention in the treatment of short-bowel syndrome is not clearly demonstrated. Procedures to slow intestinal transit time and to control gastric hyperacidity have all been investigated without proven benefits thus far.

RADIATION INJURY OF THE SMALL INTESTINE

Radiation therapy is the treatment of choice for squamous cell carcinoma of the cervix and testicular seminoma. It has also been used significantly in combination with surgical therapy and chemotherapy for effective cure and palliation of other types of tumors. Curative or palliative radiation is administered to greater than 50 per cent of patients with cancer, and greater numbers of cancer patients are now living longer. However, the number of patients with *radiation-associated* injury to normal tissue also has risen notably. Although the goal is to limit the damage inflicted on normal tissue while effectively targeting the tumor mass, it is almost impossible to avoid exposing normal tissue to radiation of some degree, particularly since different tissue types have different sensitivities to radiation. In general, cells that rapidly divide are the most prone to damage by radiation, which include both the abnormal tumor cells as well as the normal hematopoietic, reproductive, and intestinal stem cells. The small intestine is particularly susceptible to radiation injury. Cells that rarely divide, such as neurons, are relatively resistant to injury. The features that make radiation effective in controlling tumor are actually those that cause damage to the normal tissue. Radiation may cause cellular mitotic arrest, leading primarily to cell death of rapidly dividing cells. Free radicals and abnormal macromolecules that target the cellular DNA are produced, causing radiation-induced cell death. Radiation can also produce point mutations and chromosomal rearrangements. Cellular damage may be accompanied by vascular and interstitial changes as well, which occur with chronic radiation injury. The blood supply to irradiated tissue areas may be compromised by fibrotic thickening of the blood vessel walls and surrounding connective tissue. Tissue hypoxia followed by eventual necrosis may ensue.

Acute Intestinal Injury

The acute effects of radiation injury to the small bowel occur within days to weeks of the radiation, are localized, and tend to spontaneously resolve. The cells of the crypts of Lieberkühn are the proliferative cells affected. Under normal conditions, these cells are constantly regenerating and replacing the cells exfoliated at the villous tips. With radiation, this cellular supply is actively depleted. The intestinal villi become markedly flattened, and the barrier is disturbed, causing leakage of fluid into the lumen. Symptoms of acute intestinal injury including dehydration, nausea, vomiting, crampy pain, and diarrhea then occur. Typically, these symptoms subside in several days, and supportive therapy to correct the dehydration and promote temporary symptomatic relief is all that is necessary. In cases where bacteria gain entrance to the systemic bloodstream through the incompetent intestinal barrier, the toxemia that follows should be treated accordingly.

Chronic Intestinal Injury

Unlike acute injury that primarily affects the intestinal mucosa, chronic radiation injury follows progressive vasculitis and excessive collagen deposition and fibrosis of the bowel wall. The vasculitis causes hypoxia, which may result in tissue necrosis with accompanying perforation, abscess formation, or fistu-

lization. Mucosal ulceration may occur instead, manifesting as gastrointestinal blood loss. Malabsorption may also result with compromise of a large mucosal area. The deposition of collagen, which is the other primary pathologic process contributing to chronic radiation injury, may cause severe scarring of the bowel wall and lead to intestinal obstruction. These symptoms may appear clinically as late as several months to several years after the initial course of radiation. States of low blood flow, however, such as vascular disease or congestive heart failure, may increase the hypoxic state from the radiation vasculitis and lead to earlier manifestation of clinical symptoms.

Diagnosis

The diagnosis of radiation injury should be suspected in patients who give a history of receiving radiation therapy in the past and who present with any of the symptoms involved. Physical examination may be helpful in revealing an abdominal mass, which may signal abscess formation, particularly if accompanied by a fever. In addition, peritoneal signs suggest peritonitis. Intestinal obstruction should be suspected with complaints of crampy abdominal pain and with auscultatory detection of intermittent, high-pitched bowel sounds. Obstruction, fistulization, and abscess formation may be demonstrated by radiography. Flat and upright abdominal films best reveal intestinal obstruction, with the presence of distended loops of bowel and air-fluid levels. Small-intestinal contrast studies are helpful for locating fistulas, and the abdominal computed tomography (CT) scan is preferred for identifying abscesses.

Treatment

Operative treatment is indicated for patients presenting with the complications of chronic radiation injury. Partial obstruction, however, may be managed nonoperatively with intestinal decompression and fluid replacement. At laparotomy, damaged bowel appears thickened, firm, and stenotic and has a grayish-white appearance on the serosal surface. The treatment of choice for radiation injury involves resection of the diseased bowel (containing the fistula, perforation, or ulceration) with restoration of intestinal continuity via anastomosis of unaffected bowel. To avoid creating the short-bowel syndrome by resecting too much intestine, or avoid making multiple fistulas by attempting to disengage several areas of adherent bowel, intestinal bypass may serve as a reasonable alternative to resection and anastomosis. The appropriate treatment for abscesses is drainage and irrigation.

REFERENCES

Ashley SW, Wells SA Jr: Tumors of the small intestine. Semin Oncol *15*(2):116–128, 1988.

Churnratanakul S, Wirzba B, Lam T, et al: Radiation and the small intestine. Future perspectives for preventive therapy. Dig Dis *8*(1): 45–60, 1990.

Farmer RG, Whelan G, Fazio VW: Long-term follow-up of patients with Crohn's disease: Relationship between the clinical pattern and prognosis. Gastroenterology *88*:1818–1825, 1985.

Fisher RL (ed): Malabsorption and nutritional status and support. Gastroenterol Clin North Am *18*(3):467–589, 1989.

Holder WD Jr: Intestinal obstruction. Gastroenterol Clin North Am *17*(2):317–340, 1988.

29

THE SURGICAL APPROACH TO MORBID OBESITY

WALTER J. PORIES, M.D.

Morbid obesity is a serious disease associated with a high incidence of medical complications and a significantly shortened life span. Obesity is "morbid" when the body mass index (BMI) kg/M^2, exceeds 40, equivalent to an excess weight of at least 100 lb. A direct relationship exists between the amount of excess weight and the incidence of diabetes, hypertension, biliary disease, congestive heart failure, pickwickian syndrome, arthritis, endocrine disorders, infertility, and cancers of the breast, uterus, and prostate. Sudden unexplained deaths, presumably due to arrhythmias, are common.

Of greater immediate concern to the patients, however, and the major reason for seeking surgical therapy, are the psychologic and socioeconomic consequences of morbid obesity. Fat individuals are frequently objects of public scorn and malicious ridicule. Because they have difficulty performing the activities of daily living, they frequently have difficulty finding employment, meeting family responsibilities, and maintaining social relationships. In short, morbid obesity is a serious handicap. Because treatment by diets, anorectic drugs, behavior modification, and the wiring of teeth fail almost universally, a surgical approach has become the treatment of choice for many patients. Two operations, the *vertical banded gastroplasty* and the *divided gastric bypass*, are the two most commonly performed procedures (Fig. 1). Both operations limit intake by reducing the gastric segment to a small pouch, 15 to 30 cc, and both procedures delay emptying of the gastric pouch with a small outlet, about 1 cm in diameter. However, they differ in that the gastroplasty maintains the normal pathway for food while the gastric bypass excludes the stomach, the duodenum, and the proximal jejunum.

Patients are candidates for *bariatric surgery* (i.e., surgery for the treatment of morbid obesity) when the BMI is 40 or greater if they are otherwise healthy or 35 or greater if they have comorbidities such as cardiac failure, pickwickian syndrome, diabetes, or severe arthritis. Surgery should generally be withheld if the patient is considered a prohibitive surgical risk even after intensive medical management. Other contraindications include a history of substance abuse within the previous 5 years, a failure to understand the limits in food intake that are imposed by the procedures, a likelihood of poor compliance with follow-up or the required intake of vitamins, marked resistance by other family members, significant emotional disease (especially a history of serious depression and attempts at suicide), and unrealistic expectations from the operation.

The *preoperative evaluation* for bariatric surgery generally includes a meticulous history and physical examination, complete blood count, urinalysis, an SMA-12 blood chemistry panel, chest radiograph, electrocardiogram, and upper gastrointestinal series or upper endoscopy. Thyroid panels; tests for levels of vitamins, iron, and ferritin; and skin tests for anergy have not proven to be useful. Psychiatric evaluation is useful not only for preoperative assessment, but also as a reference when, as is true in half of patients, emotional support is needed after surgery.

Although some patients are admitted several days prior to operation for medical preparation in the intensive care unit, most enter the hospital on the morning of surgery. The *preoperative orders* usually include the insertion of a nasogastric tube, catheterization of the bladder, and a prophylactic cephalosporin antibiotic. Both operations are difficult because of the mas-

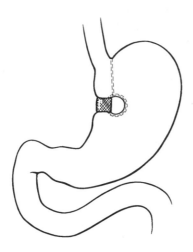 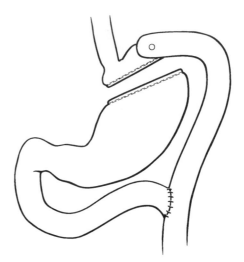

Vertical Banded Gastroplasty   Divided Gastric Bypass

Figure 1.

sive obesity, but can generally be performed in less than 2 hours. Blood transfusion is rarely needed. Patients are generally maintained on nothing by mouth for 4 days and begun on liquids by the fifth day if an upper gastrointestinal radiocontrast study reveals no leak. Patients are generally discharged on the sixth or seventh postoperative day. Progression is rapid to a full liquid diet and more slowly, over about 2 months, to soft diet with the gradual addition of fish, then chicken, then, finally, beef. Vitamin supplementation is essential to prevent neuropathies, especially after the gastric bypass, and should be monitored. Follow-up visits are scheduled for 1, 2, and 4 weeks, 3 months, and every 6 months thereafter.

The gastric bypass procedure can be performed with an operative mortality of about 1 per cent. The most common acute *complications* include wound infections, anastomotic leaks, strictures of the gastric outlet, peptic ulcer disease, pulmonary emboli, and emotional disorders. The most feared complication is infection in the right upper quadrant, usually associated with an anastomotic leak or intraoperative contamination. Postoperative infections are a major threat to the morbidly obese: a pulse rate greater than 120, an unexplained fever, or a failure to recover promptly after operation should be considered urgent indicators to consider prompt reexploration. Long-term complications include outlet obstruction (usually manageable

TABLE 1.   WEIGHT LOSS HISTORY WITH GASTRIC BYPASS OUT TO 11 YEARS

Time	N*	Mean Weight (lbs)	Mean Percentage of Excess Weight Lost	Mean Percentage of Ideal Body Weight
Preoperatively	519	297 (198–615)	0	216 (151–449)
3 months	481	240 (153–508)	37 (6– 66)	175 (120–371)
6 months	480	212 (124–449)	54 (14– 95)	156 (104–329)
12 months	453	189 (104–466)	70 (13–124)	137 (85–268)
24 months	346	182 (105–367)	72 (9–118)	134 (86–249)
36 months	269	197 (118–407)	64 (−10–108)	144 (93–263)
48 months	254	201 (114–413)	59 (−21–110)	148 (89–257)
60 months	245	202 (107–428)	59 (−14–116)	148 (86–261)
72 months	214	203 (121–399)	57 (5–104)	150 (95–271)
84 months	197	203 (113–378)	58 (−10–107)	150 (95–273)
96 months	150	202 (130–357)	56 (11–100)	152 (100–259)
108 months	122	205 (125–392)	56 (6–100)	153 (99–280)
120 months	86	209 (130–388)	53 (12–103)	156 (98–277)
132 months	31	201 (146–346)	54 (10–103)	149 (96–214)

* Number of patients with recorded weight within each time interval ranging from ±15 days at 3 months postoperatively to ±5 months at 11 years postoperatively.

with dilatation), depression (often requiring psychiatric intervention due to risk of suicide), and malnutrition, especially in patients who undergo the gastric bypass (primarily the B vitamins; specifically, vitamin B_{12}).

Bariatric surgery produces effective *weight control.* The weight loss experience of 519 morbidly obese patients undergoing the gastric bypass (GB) is presented in Table 1. Follow-up in 502 of the 519 (96.2 per cent) revealed that maximal mean weight loss (297 lb to 182 lb) is achieved at 2 years with a small increase (182 lb to 201 lb or 11 per cent) over the ensuing 9 years, reflecting those 61 (11.8 per cent) patients who had staple line breakdowns and a few others who learned to increase caloric intake into their pouches with high-calorie liquids or repeated snacks. The high number of staple line breakdowns led to division of the stomach rather than relying on staples; hence the new name, divided gastric bypass. It is believed that this modification maintains long-term weight loss within 3 to 5 per cent of the level achieved at 2 years. The gastric bypass produces about a 10 per cent greater weight loss than the gastroplasty. Whether gastroplasty provides equally good long-term weight control has not been determined.

Bariatric surgery effectively controls the *comorbidities* of morbid obesity. Gastric bypass controls non–insulin dependent diabetes in 90 per cent of those who are diabetic and hypertension in 60 per cent of those afflicted with that disease. High success rates are also reported with pickwickian syndrome, sleep apnea, cardiac failure, pseudotumor cerebri, arthritis, and infertility. The rate of rehabilitation to jobs or further schooling is high. Whether the gastroplasty provides equally good control of diabetes is not yet clear.

REFERENCES

Burton BT, Foster WR. Health implications of obesity. National Institutes of Health Consensus Development Conference. Ann Intern Med *103*(Pt 2):981–1073, 1985.

Deitel M (ed): Surgery for the Morbidly Obese Patient. Philadelphia, Lea & Febiger, 1989, p 400.

Foster WR, Burton BT, Hubbard VS. Gastrointestinal surgery for severe obesity. Proceedings of a National Institutes of Health Consensus Development Conference. Am J Clin Nutr *55*(suppl):615S–619S, 1992.

Methods for Voluntary Weight Loss and Control. National Institutes of Health Technology Assessment Conference Statement, March 30 – April 1, 1992.

Pories WJ: Why does the gastric bypass control type 2 diabetes mellitus? Obesity Surg *2*:303–313, 1992.

30

APPENDICITIS

DAVID C. SABISTON, Jr., M.D.

Appendicitis is a common disorder and one about which all physicians should have a thorough knowledge. While most patients with acute appendicitis can be easily diagnosed, there are many in whom the signs and symptoms are so variable that a firm clinical diagnosis may be difficult. It is for this reason that the diagnosis is made rather *liberally* with the full expectation that some patients will be operated upon and found to have a normal appendix. It is far preferable to maintain the indications broad, as this tends to include the group of patients with protean signs and symptoms who actually have the disease but do not fulfill the classical criteria for the diagnosis. If this course is followed, patients who might proceed to perforation, with a host of possible secondary complications, are spared that fate. Therefore, it is generally agreed that 10 to 15 per cent of patients having a diagnosis of acute appendicitis by acceptable standards will actually be found at operation to have a normal appendix.

HISTORIC ASPECTS

Although there were earlier reports of inflammation in and around the appendix termed *perityphlitis*, it is clear that Reginald Fitz deserves the credit for the first accurate description of acute appendicitis. He carefully described the clinical history, physical findings, and pathologic aspects and the fact that appendectomy is the appropriate treatment. He reported these findings in a classic paper published in 1886. Following this description, others rapidly accepted his concepts and urged that appendectomy be done prior to rupture of the appendix. Although appendicitis was formerly associated with a relatively high morbidity and mortality, today the vast majority of patients with acute ap-

pendicitis are diagnosed early in the course of the disease and undergo early appendectomy with excellent results.

ANATOMY

The vermiform appendix rises from the cecum and is generally 6 to 10 cm in length. It has a separate mesoappendix with an appendicular artery and vein that are branches of the ileocolic vessels. The appendix is lined with colonic epithelium characterized by numerous lymph follicles numbering approximately 200, highest in the 10- to 20-year-old age group. After age 30, the number of lymph follicles is reduced to a trace, with total absence of lymphoid tissue occurring after the age of 60. The appendix may lie in a number of locations, essentially any position on a clockwise rotation from the base of the cecum. It is important to emphasize that the *anatomic* position of the appendix determines the symptoms and the site of the muscular spasm and tenderness when the appendix becomes inflamed.

PATHOPHYSIOLOGY

Appendicitis occurs primarily as a result of *obstruction* of the appendiceal lumen. The commonest pathologic cause of this obstruction is marked *hyperplasia* of the lymphoid follicles, which blocks the lumen and occurs in approximately 60 per cent of patients, most of whom are in the younger age groups. The presence of a fecalith may also be a cause of obstruction and occurs in some 35 per cent of patients. In the remainder, foreign bodies, inflammatory strictures, and other

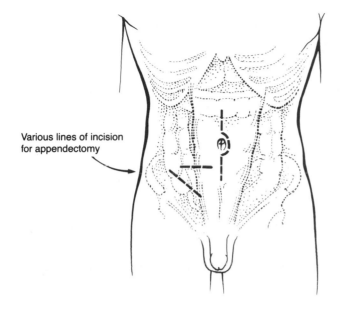

Various lines of incision for appendectomy

Figure 1. The incision for appendectomy can be a midline incision, a right lower quadrant transverse incision overlying the rectus muscle with reflection of the muscle medially, or a gridiron, muscle-splitting incision. (From Sabiston DC Jr [ed]: Atlas of General Surgery. Philadelphia, WB Saunders Company [in press], with permission.)

rare causes are responsible. At times, no specific inciting cause can be found, and in some of these patients it is probable that a fecalith initiated the inflammation and peristalsis propelled it into the lumen of the cecum.

Following obstruction of the appendiceal lumen, mucus continues to be secreted into the lumen. Stasis is created by the obstruction, and bacteria multiply and secrete exotoxins and endotoxins which damage the epithelium and ulcerate the mucosa. Bacteria can then penetrate through the ulcerated base into the muscular layers of the appendix and establish an inflammatory process. The increased pressure within the lumen also elevates the interstitial pressure in the wall of the appendix impeding arterial blood flow and creating a state of ischemia with ultimate infarction and gangrene of the appendix. As the muscular layers become necrotic, perforation of the appendix occurs. Depending upon the time interval involved in the inflammatory process, either a walled-off abscess occurs at the site or, if the pathologic process has advanced rapidly, the perforation may occur free into the peritoneal cavity and cause generalized peritonitis. If the latter occurs, a very serious clinical situation ensues and multiple intraperitoneal abscesses may follow at various sites in the pelvis and subhepatic and subdiaphragmatic spaces.

Figure 2. The appendix is located at the junction of the taeniae of the colonic wall at the tip of the cecum. It is supplied by the appendiceal artery, which must be ligated during removal of the appendix. It may be located in nearly any position, including retrocecal and extending upward toward the hepatic flexure of the colon. (From Sabiston DC Jr [ed]: Atlas of General Surgery. Philadelphia, WB Saunders Company [in press], with permission.)

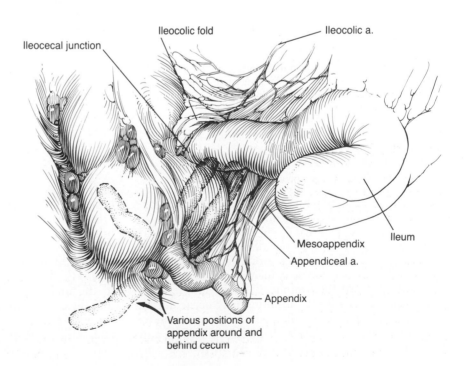

Ileocolic fold

Ileocolic a.

Ileocecal junction

Mesoappendix

Ileum

Appendiceal a.

Appendix

Various positions of appendix around and behind cecum

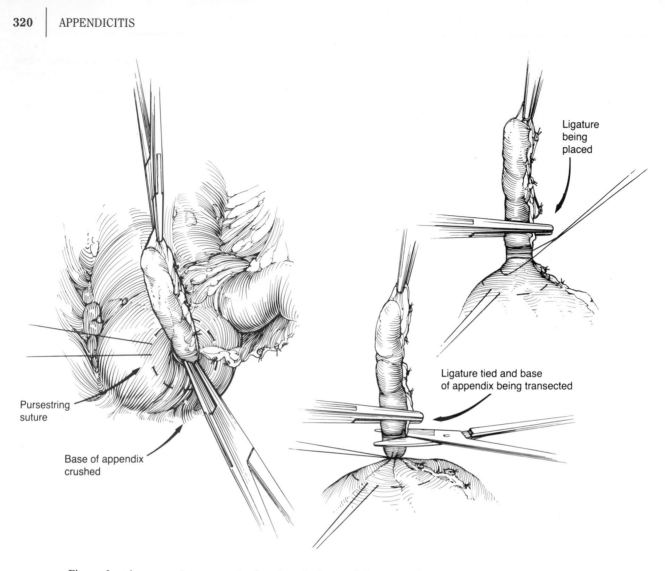

Figure 3.   A pursestring suture is placed at the base of the appendix approximately 1.0 cm from the junction to allow invagination of the stump. Two hemostats are placed at the base of the appendix to crush the tissue. The lower hemostat is removed, and an 0 chromic catgut ligature is placed. (From Sabiston DC Jr [ed]: Atlas of General Surgery. Philadelphia, WB Saunders Company [in press], with permission.)

CLINICAL DIAGNOSIS

The diagnosis of acute appendicitis is made primarily on the basis of the history and the physical findings with additional assistance from laboratory examinations. The *typical* history is one of onset of generalized abdominal pain followed by anorexia and nausea. The pain then becomes most prominent in the epigastrium and moves toward the umbilicus, finally localizing in the right lower quadrant. Vomiting may occur during this time. Examination of the abdomen is apt to show diminished bowel sounds with direct tenderness and spasm in the right lower quadrant. As the process con-

tinues, the amount of spasm increases with the appearance of rebound tenderness. The temperature is usually mildly elevated (approximately 38°C) and rises in the event of perforation. Direct tenderness is usually present in the right lower quadrant and may involve other parts of the abdomen, particularly if perforation has occurred. The appendix is usually situated at or around McBurney's point (a point one third of the way on a line drawn from the anterior superior spine to the umbilicus). However, it must be emphasized that the exact *anatomic location* of the appendix is the site where the pain and tenderness are usually maximal, and varies from patient to patient.

Rovsing's sign, elicited when pressure applied in the

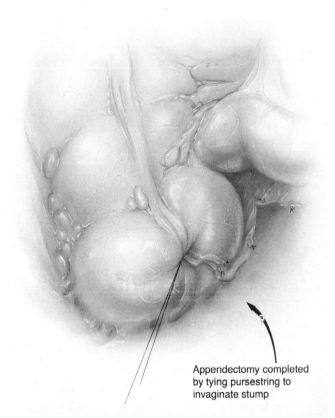

Appendectomy completed
by tying pursestring to
invaginate stump

Figure 4. The appendix is divided and the stump is invaginated by tying the pursestring suture. (From Sabiston DC Jr [ed]: Atlas of General Surgery. Philadelphia, WB Saunders Company [in press], with permission.)

left lower quadrant reflects pain to the right lower quadrant, is often present. Rectal examination generally elicits tenderness at the site of the inflamed appendix in the right lower quadrant. If the appendix ruptures, abdominal pain becomes intense and more diffuse, the muscular spasm increases, and there is a simultaneous increase in the heart rate above 100 with a rise in temperature to 39° or 40°C. At this time, the patient appears toxic and it becomes obvious that the clinical situation has deteriorated.

LABORATORY DATA

The majority of patients with acute appendicitis have an elevated leukocyte count of 10,000 to 20,000. For those in whom the level is normal, there is generally a shift to the left in the differential leukocyte count indicating inflammation. However, it should be emphasized that a number of patients have a *normal* leukocyte count, especially the elderly. Urinary analysis may show a few red cells, indicating some inflam-

matory contact with ureter or urinary bladder, while a significant number of erythrocytes in the urine indicates a primary disorder of the urinary tract.

Radiographic studies are not indicated in classical cases of acute appendicitis, but may be useful when the diagnosis is in doubt. Plain films of the abdomen may show a dilated cecum and fluid level and occasionally a calcified fecalith or foreign body. Barium enema may show an absence of filling of the appendix, which is suggestive of acute appendicitis. If the lumen of the appendix fills with barium, appendicitis is quite unlikely. *Ultrasound* examination is sometimes helpful and may show signs indicating an enlarged appendix or an abscess. Similarly, a computed tomography (CT) scan of the abdomen may be helpful, particularly in establishing the presence of an abscess. However, it should be emphasized that in the *vast* majority of patients, these special studies are unnecessary and delay surgical therapy. It should also be mentioned that laparoscopic examination is frequently used to establish the diagnosis and, in appropriate instances, for appendectomy.

DIFFERENTIAL DIAGNOSIS

Many specific disorders producing signs and symptoms similar to those of acute appendicitis enter the differential diagnosis. These are primarily acute gastroenteritis, cholecystitis, pyelitis, salpingitis, tuboovarian abscess, and ruptured ovarian cysts. While diarrhea may occur with acute appendicitis, it is much more common with gastroenteritis. In young children, intussusception enters the differential diagnosis. Other less common differential disorders include ureteral stones, cystitis, and perforated peptic ulcer. Ectopic pregnancy may also simulate acute appendicitis, as may acute regional enteritis, particularly during the first attack. In males, disorders of testis and epididymis, including epididymitis and testicular torsion, may simulate appendicitis. The important point is that if a patient persists in having pain in the right lower quadrant which cannot be explained by some other definitive diagnosis, the patient should be considered to have acute appendicitis and operated upon or at least very carefully observed, preferably by the same observer.

TREATMENT

Management of the vast majority of patients with a diagnosis of acute appendicitis is appendectomy. For patients with simple acute appendicitis, intravenous fluids should be initiated as well as an antibiotic agent effective against both aerobic and anaerobic organ-

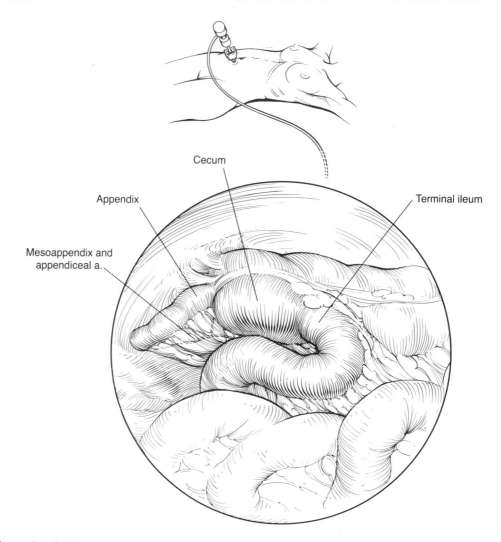

Cecum

Appendix

Terminal ileum

Mesoappendix and
appendiceal a.

Figure 5. A 10-mm trocar is placed in the left lower quadrant in a tangential manner, thereby obviating the need for closure of the fascia at the completion of the procedure. The abdomen is visually explored, and appendicitis is confirmed. An Endoloop is placed through a 5-mm trocar, and the end of the appendix is snared for retraction. The mesoappendix is then easily visualized. (From Sabiston DC Jr [ed]: Atlas of General Surgery. Philadelphia, WB Saunders Company [in press], with permission.)

isms. Therefore, all patients are begun on antibiotics preoperatively and maintained postoperatively as needed. If the appendix is unruptured and not gangrenous, antibiotics may be discontinued after 24 hours. While many agents are effective, cefoxitin is frequently selected as the agent of choice.

SURGICAL MANAGEMENT

After appropriate preoperative preparation, a decision is made as to whether the appendix is to be removed by the *open* or the *laparoscopic* approach. If the open operation is to be done, anesthesia is administered and a transverse incision in the skin lines is made in the right lower quadrant. The appendix is exposed through a gridiron, muscle-splitting incision (Fig. 1). If peritoneal fluid or exudate is present upon opening the peritoneum, the fluid should be cultured and the appendix exposed. Careful observation is made of the pathologic state and especially of the site of perforation or abscess formation. The appendix is then removed as illustrated in Figures 2, 3, and 4. If an abscess is present, it may be drained, but if *generalized* peritonitis is present, this is usually unnecessary.

If a normal appendix is found, additional explora-

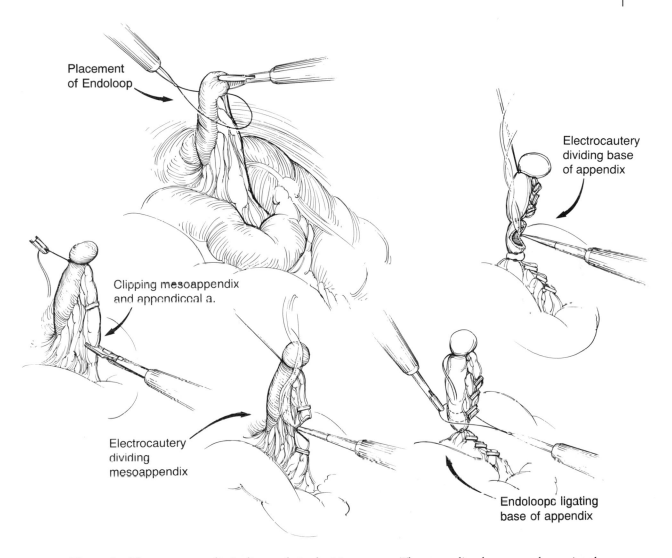

Placement
of Endoloop

Electrocautery
dividing base
of appendix

Clipping mesoappendix
and appendiceal a.

Electrocautery
dividing
mesoappendix

Endoloope ligating
base of appendix

Figure 6. The mesoappendix is dissected via the 10-mm port. The appendiceal artery and associated fat are controlled with the electrocautery and clips. When the base of the appendix is easily seen, three additional Endoloops are placed sequentially on the appendix. Two are placed on the cecal side, and one is placed on the side of the specimen. The specimen is transected. Alternately, an endoscopic linear stapler can be used through a 12-mm port in the left lower quadrant to control both the appendiceal stump and appendiceal artery. The electrocautery is used to cauterize the mucosa on the appendiceal stump. (From Sabiston DC Jr [ed]: Atlas of General Surgery. Philadelphia, WB Saunders Company [in press], with permission.)

tion should follow to eliminate other possible causes, including inspection of the cecum and colon for inflammatory or neoplastic lesions, the terminal ileum for a Meckel's diverticulum, and the gallbladder and duodenum for primary disease. If further evidence of intra-abdominal disease is present, it may be necessary to enlarge the incision or perform a midline incision for more adequate exposure.

The laparoscopic approach may be chosen for selected patients. When the diagnosis is uncertain, this approach is helpful in achieving a more thorough examination of the abdominal contents. This procedure is shown in Figures 5 and 6.

NONSURGICAL MANAGEMENT OF APPENDICEAL ABSCESS

If a patient with appendiceal perforation is seen late in the course of the disease and has a walled-off abscess in the right lower quadrant, the process may be subsiding with minimal systemic findings. In this situation, it may be appropriate to treat the patient with antibiotics and intravenous fluids and careful observation. When the process is resolved, usually requiring 6 weeks to 3 months, an interval appendectomy should be performed because the likelihood of recurrent appendicitis is quite high. Under these circumstances, it is preferable to remove the appendix electively at a later date rather than as an emergency.

The problem of *incidental* appendectomy during the course of other abdominal operations has been raised and opinion is divided. Elective appendectomy is probably performed most often in conjunction with gynecologic procedures. Removal of the appendix in these circumstances eliminates the possibility of postoperative acute appendicitis in these patients who may later develop problems in the right lower quadrant. If the appendix has been removed, it eliminates this possibility. However, most surgeons do not electively remove a normal appendix during the course of general surgical procedures.

SPECIAL FEATURES OF ACUTE APPENDICITIS

There are certain special situations in which the diagnosis of acute appendicitis may differ from the classical clinical manifestations. Appendicitis in infants and young children is very difficult to diagnose preoperatively, since these patients cannot provide a history. Therefore, it is unusual to make a firm diagnosis in a patient under the age of 1 year unless perforation has occurred. Acute appendicitis during pregnancy also presents diagnostic problems because during the third trimester, the uterus is rapidly enlarging and causes displacement of the cecum and appendix into the right upper abdomen. Thus, acute appendicitis in these patients causes symptoms and signs higher and more lateral during the third trimester. Appendicitis in young women also introduces a number of specific differential diagnoses, particularly those involving the tube/ovarian disorders. For these, *culdoscopy* or *laparoscopy* may be helpful in revealing the problem.

Appendicitis in the elderly may also present different clinical manifestations than in younger patients with a general tendency for the *inflammatory* components to be less pronounced. For example, the temperature is usually lower as is the leukocyte count, and there is frequently less pain and tenderness. At times the appendix in this age group may perforate with an abscess without causing the patient a significant earlier problem.

CARCINOMA OF THE APPENDIX

Carcinoma of the appendix is an unusual neoplasm. In one series of 5000 appendices, 41 cases of adenocarcinoma were found. The most common lesion is a carcinoid and accounts for some 90 per cent of all primary tumors of the appendix. Malignant mucoceles are regarded as being well-differentiated adenocarcinomas. The clinical presentation of most patients with appendiceal carcinomas is typical of that for acute appendicitis. In many instances, the appendix is perforated with a localized appendiceal abscess that requires drainage. The management of appendiceal tumors of less than 1.5 cm in diameter without metastases to mesenteric lymph nodes is routine appendectomy. For larger tumors, and those associated with lymphatic spread or invasion of the ileum, a right hemicolectomy is appropriate.

REFERENCES

Andersson A, Bergdahl L, Boquist L: Primary carcinoma of the appendix. Ann Surg *183*:53, 1976.
Arnbjörnsson E: Management of appendiceal abscess. Curr Surg *41*: 4, 1984.
Fitz RH: Perforating inflammation of the vermiform appendix; with special reference to its early diagnosis and treatment. Trans Assoc Am Phys *1*:107, 1886.
Gomez A, Wood M: Acute appendicitis during pregnancy. Am J Surg *137*:180, 1979.
Hayes RJ: Incidental appendectomies. Current teaching. JAMA *238*: 31, 1977.
Hobson T, Rosenman LD: Acute appendicitis — when is it right to be wrong? Am J Surg *108*:306, 1964.
Lewis FR, Holcroft JW, Boey J, Dunphy JE: Appendicitis: A critical review of diagnosis and treatment in 1000 cases. Arch Surg *110*: 677, 1975.

31

THE COLON AND RECTUM

H. KIM LYERLY, M.D.   BRYAN M. CLARY, M.D.

Colon and rectal diseases include disorders that are inflammatory, vascular, infectious, and traumatic in origin as well as benign and malignant neoplasms. The evaluation of patients with diseases of the colon and rectum requires knowledge of the anatomy and pathophysiology of these disorders as well as knowledge concerning the advantages and disadvantages of specific diagnostic studies used to evaluate them. Increasing information about the biology of these problems must be integrated with current knowledge of the multimodality therapy of colon and rectal disease to optimize management of these patients.

ANATOMY

The colon is approximately 1.5 meters in length and extends from the ileocecal valve, located at the junction of the terminal ileum and the cecum, to the anus (Fig. 1). The best way to understand the anatomic relations of the colon in the adult is to review its embryonic development. The midgut gives rise to the proximal colon including the cecum, ascending colon, hepatic flexure, and proximal two thirds of the transverse colon. In contrast, the distal colon, including the remainder of the transverse colon, splenic flexure, descending colon, sigmoid colon, and rectum, is derived from the primitive hindgut. The midgut rotates counterclockwise around the axis of the superior mesenteric artery during gestation, subsequently descending and causing the cecum to lie in the right lower quadrant. Incomplete rotation may occur (termed malrotation), which causes the cecum to lie in an aberrant position in the right or left upper quadrants.

The ascending and descending colon are usually fixed by retroperitoneal attachments, although the ascending colon and cecum exhibit variable degrees of mobility, rendering this segment susceptible to volvulus. The transverse colon with its supporting mesentery traverses the abdominal cavity horizontally; however, it may be found extending down into the lower abdomen, depending on its length. The splenic flexure is fixed by the phrenocolic and splenocolic ligaments, which are important when dissecting the left colon. The sigmoid colon, which is usually 10 to 30 cm in length, courses in the left lower quadrant to the peritoneal reflection. It may frequently become elongated and redundant in older patients, rendering it also susceptible to volvulus. The rectum begins at the peritoneal reflection and is devoid of peritoneal investment distally and thus is extraperitoneal.

Histologic examination of the colonic wall reveals four distinct layers: the serosa, muscularis, submucosa, and mucosa (Fig. 2). The mucosa is composed of columnar epithelium but, in contrast to that of the small intestine, does not have villi. The anal canal, beginning inferior to the puborectalis muscle, is lined proximally by columnar epithelium but, at the dentate (pectinate) line, changes gradually to stratified squamous epithelium. The muscularis mucosa is composed of circular muscle. The outer longitudinal muscular layer incompletely encircles the colon, being separated into three distinct bands termed the *taeniae coli*. These bands help distinguish the large and small intestine. In contrast, the rectum is distinct as these layers fan out and completely encircle it. The serosa layer is absent.

Other external features of the colon include the haustra and appendices epiploicae. Haustra, separated by transient incomplete internal folds (plicae semilunares), are external sacculations that give the colon a segmented appearance. Fatty appendages of the serosa (appendices epiploicae) are present, with increasing numbers distally.

325

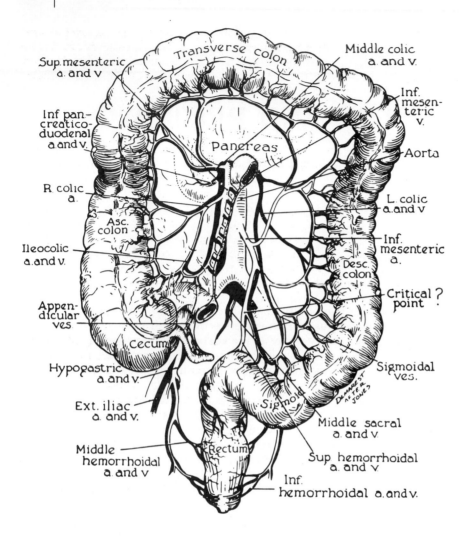

Figure 1. The colon: its anatomical divisions and its blood supply. The veins are shown in broken black. (Modified from Jones T, Shepherd WC: A Manual of Surgical Anatomy. Philadelphia, WB Saunders Company, 1945, with permission.)

Vascular Supply and Lymphatic Drainage

Derived from the embryonic midgut, the cecum, ascending colon, hepatic flexure, and proximal transverse colon receive their blood supply from the ileocolic, right colic, and middle colic branches of the superior mesenteric artery (Fig. 1). The inferior mesenteric artery branches into the left colic, sigmoidal, and superior hemorrhoidal arteries that supply the distal transverse and descending colon, sigmoid colon, and proximal third of the rectum, respectively. Vascular arcades originating at the bifurcation of the main arteries 1 to 2 cm from the mesenteric border form a continuous anastomosing vessel termed the *marginal artery of Drummond*. This supplies collateral flow from the main arterial supplies to the colon. The vascular arcades also provide an anastomosis between the superior and inferior mesenteric arteries, which constitutes the arc of Riolan. The distal bowel is not supplied by the mesenteric arteries, but rather by branches

of the internal iliac arteries. The middle third of the rectum is supplied by the middle hemorrhoidal artery (a branch of the internal iliac artery), and the distal third of the rectum is supplied by the inferior hemorrhoidal artery (from the pudendal artery).

Venous drainage accompanies the arterial blood supply, with the confluence of the superior mesenteric and splenic veins forming the portal vein. The inferior mesenteric vein drains into the splenic vein prior to its junction with the superior mesenteric vein. The rectum is drained by an extensive plexus of venous anastomosis predominantly into the portal system.

The lymphatic channels follow the course of the main vessels and are of important clinical significance in tumor metastases and inflammatory diseases of the colon (Fig. 3). These channels drain to paracolic nodes along the course of the marginal artery of Drummond and to the preaortic nodes. The lymphatic drainage of the superior rectum follows that of the sigmoid to the inferior mesenteric nodes. The middle rectum lym-

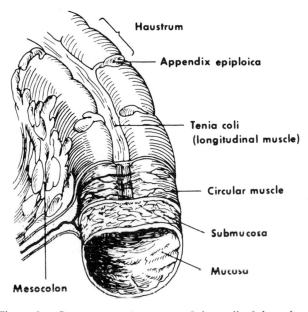

Figure 2. Gross anatomic aspects of the wall of the colon. (From Hardy JD [ed]: Hardy's Textbook of Surgery. Philadelphia, WB Saunders Company, 1983, with permission.)

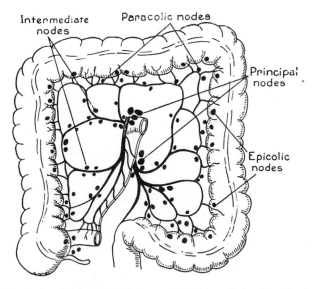

Figure 3. Diagrammatic representation of the lymphatic drainage of the large intestine showing the epicolic, pericolic, intermediate, and principle lymph node groups accompanying the vessels of the colon. (From Grinnell RS: Lymphatic metastases of carcinoid of the colon and rectum. Ann Surg 131:494, 1950, with permission.)

phatic drainage follows the inferior rectal arterial supply to the internal iliac nodes and the nodes of the most distal rectum and anus descend to the skin and superficial fascia of the perineum and to the superficial inguinal nodes.

Innervation

The colon receives neuronal input from both the sympathetic and parasympathetic nervous systems. Sympathetic nerve fibers arise from T10 to T12 and pass in the thoracic splanchnic nerves to the preaortic and superior mesenteric plexuses where they synapse with the postganglionic neurons, which are distributed along the superior mesenteric artery to innervate the right colon. Preganglionic nerve fibers from L1 to L3 synapse in the paravertebral ganglia with postganglionic nerve fibers along the inferior mesenteric artery to innervate the left colon. The rectum receives its sympathetic supply from the presacral nerves, which arise within the preaortic plexuses.

Impairment of the sympathetic innervation of the distal colon from the sacral plexus is thought to be the cause of pseudo-obstruction of the colon (Ogilvie's syndrome). The clinical significance of pseudo-obstruction is the risk of colonic rupture associated with dilatation, which greatly increases when the bowel is distended beyond a diameter of 9 to 10 cm. This condition occurs in association with a variety of conditions including dementia, sepsis, diabetes mellitus, narcotic use, renal failure, electrolyte abnormalities, and following operation. According to this hypothesis, the unopposed parasympathetic innervation to the distal colon causes hypersegmentation of this segment and dilatation of bowel proximally. Treatment involves colonoscopic decompression with placement of a rectal tube to prevent rupture in the acute setting and correction of underlying medical problems.

Parasympathetic innervation for the right and transverse colon arises from right vagal fibers that pass by the celiac plexus and along the superior mesenteric vessels to synapse within the enteric plexuses. Preganglionic parasympathetic fibers that innervate the descending colon, sigmoid colon, and rectum are derived from S2 to S4 and pass through the pelvic plexus and join the sympathetic fibers in the inferior mesenteric ganglion before reaching the enteric plexuses.

Plexuses within the bowel wall are present in the submucosa (Meissner's) and between the muscular layers (Auerbach's or myenteric). Sympathetic innervation inhibits colonic motility and produces internal anal sphincter contraction, whereas parasympathetic stimulation causes the opposite. In the event of spinal cord transection or vagotomy, bowel function remains essentially normal. Absence of ganglion cells in the submucosal and myenteric plexuses causes a neurogenic form of intestinal obstruction known as *Hirschsprung's disease*. Aganglionosis in 80 per cent of patients begins at the anorectal line extending to involve only the rectosigmoid. In 10 per cent, the entire colon and distal ileum may be involved. The loss of parasympathetic innervation causes failure of relaxation of the internal anal sphincter, causing a form of obstruction that in most patients is symptomatic at birth with delayed passage of meconium.

PHYSIOLOGY

The colon and rectum can be considered as having four primary functions: (1) absorption of sodium and water, (2) secretion of potassium and bicarbonate, (3) storage of fecal contents, and (4) elimination of intestinal waste. Absorption of sodium is an active transfer process influenced by pH, osmolarity, mineralocorticoids, glucocorticoids, bile acids, fatty acids, and mucosal cyclic adenosine monophosphate (cAMP) levels. The hormones vasoactive intestinal peptide (VIP) and serotonin reduce absorption of sodium and chloride. An electrical potential is generated across the colonic wall, which in turn leads to absorption of chloride and secretion of potassium. Absorption of water is a passive process secondary to the absorption of solute. Although water can be absorbed throughout the colon, most absorption occurs in the ascending colon. Of the approximately 1500 ml/day of ileal effluent, only 100 to 150 ml/day is excreted after passage through the colon, and the total amount of stool is almost 200 gm.

The colon is also involved in the enterohepatic circulation, although the absorption of bile acids occurs to a greater extent in the ileum. In those with decreased absorption in the ileum, this function is of increasing importance. Conversion of primary bile acids to secondary bile acids also occurs in the colon. Potassium and bicarbonate are thought to be secreted by active processes, potassium secretion being stimulated by mineralocorticoids and with secretion in mucus. Disease states in which there is excessive colonic production of mucus, such as the presence of a large villous adenoma, can lead to large potassium losses.

The primary motor functions of the colon include mixing, storage, and elimination, and are achieved through segmentation, retrograde peristalsis, and mass movements with varying frequencies in the different regions of the colon. The enteric nervous system, consisting of the myenteric and submucosal plexuses, coordinates the various patterns of motility within the colon. A variety of neurohormonal transmitters have been postulated to be involved in this regulatory process, including somatostatin, substance P, neuropeptide Y, VIP, serotonin, and cholecystokinin (CCK), in addition to adrenergic and cholinergic mediation.

Segmentation is caused by annular contractions that propel feces over short distances and occur in both directions. This form of motility predominates in the transverse and descending colon. Retrograde peristalsis occurring within the right colon serves to mix the column of ileal effluent with the column of existing colonic contents. Displacement of contents into the transverse colon occurs with the continued entry of ileal effluent into the cecum. Mass movements are strong propulsive contractions that move contents over longer distances, occurring infrequently and predominantly in the transverse and descending colon. These movements are most commonly associated with the ingestion of meals, with dietary fat as the principal stimulus.

The act of defecation is thought to be initiated by the stimulation of mechanoreceptors within the wall of the anorectum by the passage of feces from the descending and sigmoid colon into the rectum. Defecation requires relaxation of the internal and external sphincters, colonic contraction, and other external processes including increased abdominal pressure and relaxation of the pelvic floor.

CLINICAL EVALUATION

The evaluation of colonic disturbances begins with a thorough history and physical examination. Important clinical information to be gathered is the frequency of bowel movements; changes in the character of the stool (caliber, color, consistency, odor); the presence of hematochezia, tenesmus, abdominal and rectal pain, diarrhea, constipation, obstipation, associated gastrointestinal symptoms (nausea, vomiting); and systemic symptoms including weight loss, fatigue, malaise, fever, night sweats, and anorexia. Some disorders, including intestinal polyps or early stage colon cancers, may be asymptomatic and are incidentally detected by routine examinations or screening tests. A history of familial carcinomas or intestinal polyps is important, as are details of prior operations, medications, and medical problems.

A systematic examination of the abdomen with evaluation of each quadrant is performed. Relaxation of the rectus muscles ensures the adequate palpation of the intra-abdominal contents, including hepatosplenomegaly and signs of peritoneal irritation. Visual inspection of the anus and digital examination of the rectum with testing for occult blood are also performed.

DIAGNOSTIC TESTS

Many diagnostic tests assist in the evaluation of a colonic problem. With longstanding colonic complaints, electrolyte imbalances should be sought as well as a baseline nutritional assessment. Anemia may be present in many, especially colon cancer and ulcerative colitis. Liver function studies are useful in the evaluation of carcinoma of the colon. Examination of the stools with testing for occult blood, fecal fat, white blood cells, and the presence of pathologic organisms (bacterial, viral, parasitic) and/or their products is often done.

RADIOGRAPHIC EVALUATION

Plain films of the abdomen and the large intestine provide substantial information in certain disease processes (Table 1). Although abnormal gas patterns demonstrating dilated bowel with air-fluid levels suggest intestinal obstruction and free intraperitoneal air suggests intestinal perforation, few specific diagnoses can be made with plain abdominal films. Displacement of the normal architecture by tumor masses and abdominal calcifications may be detected, and if so, further diagnostic studies are usually indicated.

The lumen of the colon may be outlined by contrast, most commonly barium or a water-soluble contrast medium such as Gastrografin. Barium studies are usually superior to Gastrografin, but given its insoluble nature, barium should not be used if intestinal perforation is suspected. A barium enema may show colonic obstruction, intraluminal masses, diverticulae, and abnormal mucosal patterns. Air contrast barium enemas are more sensitive in the detection of small mucosal lesions and polyps. Barium studies may not detect superficial mucosal and rectal lesions in the wall of the colon.

Endoscopy

As part of the initial evaluation of suspected colonic disease, anoscopy or proctoscopy permits visualization within 8 to 10 cm of the anal verge. Internal hemorrhoids, proctitis, and rectal masses are detected with this minimally invasive technique. Sigmoidoscopy may be performed with rigid or flexible instruments. Rigid sigmoidoscopy permits visualization of the distal 20 to 25 cm of colon. Flexible sigmoidoscopes may be advanced to visualize the distal 60 cm of colon and permit biopsy, cauterization, and excision of polyps. Sigmoidoscopy is technically less demanding than colonoscopy and usually does not require sedation, but the proximal colon is not visualized. As many as 50 per cent of colonic malignancies can be detected by flexible sigmoidoscopy.

Colonoscopy is the most accurate means of evaluating the proximal colon and its mucosa. The scope can usually be advanced to visualize the colon and cecum, but patient sedation is usually required. Indications for colonoscopy include screening of the general population and high-risk individuals for malignancies and the evaluation of patients with occult blood in the stool. Colonoscopy may also complement barium enema and sigmoidoscopy, allowing a detailed examination of the entire colonic mucosa with the capability of biopsy and polypectomy. Colonoscopy can be indicated in the evaluation of lower gastrointestinal bleeding, as angiodysplastic lesions in the colon can sometimes be detected.

Therapeutic indications for colonic endoscopy include reduction of colonic intussusception, retrieval of foreign bodies, polypectomy, detorsion of volvulus, and the management of lower gastrointestinal bleeding. Although it has been shown to be a relatively safe procedure with minimal mortality or morbidity, contraindications include suspected colonic perforation, peritonitis with a secondary paralytic ileus, acute fulminating inflammatory bowel disease, and the inability to obtain an adequately prepared bowel. Sedation is usually required in the performance of colonoscopy, and comorbid conditions in patients with significant medical problems must be considered. Evacuation of the lumen prior to examination is required for accurate colonoscopic evaluation. This may be accomplished by methods utilized for the mechanical cleansing of the bowel and usually involves oral ingestion of a polyethylene glycol–containing solution.

Nuclear Scanning

Nuclear scanning is useful in the evaluation of the patient with lower gastrointestinal hemorrhage to detect significant intraluminal bleeding. Radioisotope scanning is performed with ^{99m}technetium-labeled sulfur colloid or red blood cells. Sulfur colloid is cleared from the circulation by the liver, spleen, and bone marrow within several minutes. Colloid that extravasates into the intestinal lumen is not reabsorbed and thus remains, allowing the detection of pooling of the labeled colloid. Labeled red blood cells have a much longer half-life, and scanning may be repeated if the initial scan is negative with detection of intermittently bleeding sites.

Nuclear scanning can detect bleeding rates as low as 0.1 ml/min, but they are often inaccurate in the localization of bleeding, as the pooled intraluminal blood acts as a cathartic and may not remain stationary. Superimposition of upper gastrointestinal bleeding sites on the colon may also provide the false impression of a colonic source. Therefore, nuclear scanning is useful as the initial diagnostic study of stable patients with lower gastrointestinal bleeding as a screening test to determine the feasibility of selective

TABLE 1. RADIOGRAPHIC AND ENDOSCOPIC EVALUATION OF THE COLON

Procedure	Advantages	Disadvantages
Plain abdominal film	Identifies gas and calcifications, upright films may demonstrate air-fluid levels and free intra-abdominal air	Few specific features
Tc-RBC scan	Detection of active bleeding in an intermittently bleeding lesion	Poor anatomic definition and localization of intermittent bleeding lesion
Angiography	Demonstration and localization of actively bleeding lesion Options for therapeutic intervention Definition of vascularity of mass lesions	Bleeding lesions are only visualized if blood loss exceeds 0.5 ml/min Large dose of IV contrast needed, and cannot be performed repeatedly due to the contrast load
Barium enema	Shows polyps, tumors, fistulas, diverticula, and structural changes Water-soluble contrast agent can be used	May miss superficial mucosal and rectal lesions, and cannot visualize angioplastic lesion Requires competent anal sphincter
Ultrasonography	Best for fluid-filled lesions, bile ducts, gallstones Real-time examination, Doppler can show flow Can be used intraoperatively and intraluminally	Bowel gas obscures examination, bowel is poorly visualized
CT of the abdomen	Excellent anatomic definition, visualized bowel thickness, mesentery, retroperitoneum, aorta well Density changes may indicate nature of diffuse parenchymal disease Can perform needle aspiration and drainage	Possible reactions to iodinated intravenous contrast Radiation exposure Bowel may not be well visualized without contrast Fat planes are needed for optimal visualization
MRI of the abdomen	Excellent anatomic definition, sensitive detection of hepatic tumors Identifies patency and flow in vessels No radiation	Patient must be cooperative
Flexible sigmoidoscopy	Direct visualization of rectum sigmoid and distal descending colon Permits biopsy and polypectomy	Misses lesions in proximal colon
Colonoscopy	Direct visualization of entire colon Permits biopsy, polypectomy, electrocautery, and laser treatment of bleeding May identify angiodysplastic lesions	Requires bowel prep and sedation Active gastrointestinal bleeding limits examination
Laparoscopy	Direct visualization of the intra-abdominal contents May perform therapeutic procedure	Invasive, requires general anesthesia

Abbreviations: Tc-RBC = ^{99m}technetium-labeled sulfur colloid or red blood cells, IV = intravenous, CT = computed tomography, MRI = magnetic resonance imaging.

angiography. Because colonic bleeding is often intermittent, a negative nuclear scan usually indicates that the amount of bleeding at that moment is insufficient to be visualized by angiography. A positive scan may by followed by angiography, which is used to define the anatomic location of the bleeding.

Angiography

The use of angiography in colonic disease concerns the management of intestinal hemorrhage, which can be identified if a site is bleeding at a rate of at least 0.5 ml/min. Angiography is 40 to 60 per cent accurate in detecting the site of bleeding. However, if it is performed following the documentation of ongoing hemorrhage by a positive nuclear scan or by detecting gross bleeding, its accuracy can be increased to 70 to 100 per cent. Relative contraindications to the performance of selective angiography include renal insufficiency and contrast allergy. Administration of methylprednisolone prior to contrast injection may prevent the latter. Adequate hydration following the administration of intravenous contrast during these studies is fundamental in preventing or minimizing acute tubular necrosis and further impairment of renal function.

Angiography should not be repeated frequently due to the amount of dye required. Therefore, its use is generally limited to episodes of documented hemorrhage, or for detection of a specific lesion such as a suspected arteriovenous malformation. An advantage of angiography, in addition to localization of the bleeding site, is that therapeutic intervention can be considered, including infusion of vasoactive substances or the embolization of specific arteries. Rarely, angiography is contraindicated because the patient is hemodynamically unstable due to persistent bleeding, and urgent surgical exploration should be considered.

Other Diagnostic Studies

Computed tomographic (CT) scans and magnetic resonance imaging (MRI) are used in the evaluation of metastatic and locally advanced colorectal cancer and have been used in the assessment of resectability of rectal tumors. Magnetic resonance imaging does not require the use of contrast agents, and can be used to assess the patency of blood vessels. Computed tomographic scanning is often useful in the evaluation of a patient with a suspected intra-abdominal inflammatory mass, and CT guidance can be used for needle aspiration of fluid collections and drainage of intra-abdominal abscess. The addition of celiac angiography to CT scanning has improved the detection and evaluation of hepatic metastasis.

In patients with large malignant lesions, preoperative identification of the ureters by intravenous pyelography may be considered, with cystoscopy and ureteral stent placement if indicated. Ultrasound has the advantage of real time evaluation and can detect fluid-filled lesions. Bowel gas may obstruct the view of the probe; however, intraoperative probes can be used for evaluation of hepatic lesions. Endorectal ultrasound is now being utilized to stage invasion of the bowel wall in rectal carcinomas, which may have implications for local excision and sphincter-preserving procedures.

INTESTINAL ANTISEPSIS AND MECHANICAL BOWEL PREPARATION

Shortly after birth, the sterile colon of the fetus becomes colonized with bacterial flora. The colon is estimated to contain over 400 bacterial species in a concentration of approximately 10^{12} colony-forming units (CFU) per milliliter. This is in distinct contrast to the small bowel, in which the concentration of bacteria is fewer than 10^5 CFU/ml. The magnitude of the bacterial content of stool is best illustrated by emphasizing that nearly one third of the dry weight of feces consists of bacteria, 99 per cent of which are anaerobic. The most common anaerobic bacterial species include *Bacteroides, Fusobacterium, Bifidobacterium*, and *Clostridia*. Among the aerobic bacterial species are coliforms, *Streptococcus*, and *Lactobacillus*. Of note, *Methanobrevibacter smithii* is the predominant methane-producing organism in human feces. The flora contribute to many normal physiologic processes including deconjugation of bile salts, production of vitamin K, and the prevention of colonization of pathogenic organisms.

Of great significance is the role of the normal intestinal flora in the pathogenesis of surgical infections including postoperative wound complications. The incidence of bacterial contamination parallels the magnitude of bacterial content of the stool, being maximal in the rectum and left colon and minimal in the right colon and cecum. To minimize the incidence of postoperative infectious complications such as wound infection, intra-abdominal abscess, and anastomotic dehiscence, methods of intestinal antisepsis are available to reduce the bacterial content of the colon preoperatively. Mechanical cleansing and enteral or parenteral antibiotic administration are fundamental features of this process.

Without mechanical cleansing, the rate of wound infection following operations on the left colon is approximately 75 per cent. Mechanical cleansing serves to reduce the bulk of feces and bacteria within the colon, commonly by the administration of a clear liquid diet for 3 days combined with laxatives and cleansing enemas. More recently, single-day regimens have been effectively used and currently include colonic lavage by the oral ingestion of a polyethylene glycol–containing electrolyte solution. Typically, 4 L of this solution are administered on the day prior to operation, with effective evacuation.

Enteral antibiotic prophylaxis is combined with the mechanical cleansing and is usually given in the form of nonabsorbable, orally administered, broad-spectrum antimicrobial agents. Although in a randomized prospective study the addition of a parenteral antibiotic to mechanical cleansing and oral antibiotics was shown to be of limited benefit, these agents are commonly administered preoperatively. The choice of prophylactic antimicrobial agent is based on a number of desired characteristics including: (1) broad suppression of aerobic and anaerobic organism, (2) minimal toxicity, (3) ease of administration, and (4) low cost. The most common oral regimens are neomycin and erythromycin-base given as 1 gm each at 1:00 p.m., 2:00 p.m., and 11:00 p.m. on the day prior to operation (18, 17, and 8 hours prior to operation); or metronidazole, 750 mg every 8 hours for 72 hours prior to surgery.

Second-generation cephalosporins effective against gram-negative and anaerobic bacteria are commonly used as prophylactic parenteral agents. Multiple drug regimens including metronidazole or clindamycin in combination with an aminoglycoside have no demonstrable advantage to single-drug regimens utilizing broad-spectrum agents.

OPERATIVE PRINCIPLES

When a colon resection is planned, certain specific factors are considered in addition to achieving an adequate mechanical and antibiotic bowel preparation. In patients with perforated or near obstructing colonic lesions, an adequate preparation may not be possible, and the implications of gross fecal soilage and unprepared intestinal contents must be considered prior to operation.

In addition, it is essential to ensure adequate perfusion to the bowel wall at all colonic anastomoses. The surgeon should be able to palpate pulsating vessels in the colonic mesentery and note active bleeding from the divided edges of the bowel that is to be anastomosed. To minimize tension on an anastomosis, which may compromise capillary flow and impede healing, the colon must be adequately mobilized, which frequently requires division of the peritoneal attachments of the colon including the splenocolic or hepatocolic ligaments.

When resection of the colon is indicated and a primary anastomosis is not advised due to associated inflammation and/or intra-abdominal sepsis, a procedure not involving an intra-abdominal colonic anastomosis is often performed. The three-stage procedure (Fig. 4) involves proximal diversion with a temporary diverting colostomy (or ileostomy), followed by a second operation with resection and primary anastomosis of the diseased segment. Finally, a third operation is required for closure of the colostomy at a later date. Although the three-stage procedure is infrequently used today, it may be utilized to decompress obstructing colon lesions, especially when comorbid conditions are present, precluding more definitive procedures during the initial operation.

The term *colostomy* refers to the creation of a stoma that is usually an opening of the bowel on the surface of the abdomen. Colostomies, whether temporary or permanent, are performed for a number of indications in patients with colonic and gastrointestinal disorders. General purposes for which a colostomy is created include: to function as the site of the elimination of feces when the distal colon or rectum has been removed, to divert the fecal stream to protect a distal anastomosis, or to divert the fecal stream from a pathologic process that will be definitively managed at a later date.

The ideal temporary colostomy should provide adequate fecal diversion, be safe to construct, and easily reconstructed when gastrointestinal continuity is restored. A loop or double-barrel colostomy is typically performed when the requirement for diversion is limited to weeks or months. This is often achieved by exteriorizing a segment of the colon and making an opening in a loop of bowel through the tinea, a relatively straightforward procedure that can be performed as an open procedure or laparoscopically without significant manipulation or dissection.

Because the creation of a colostomy only serves to divert the fecal stream and does nothing to correct the

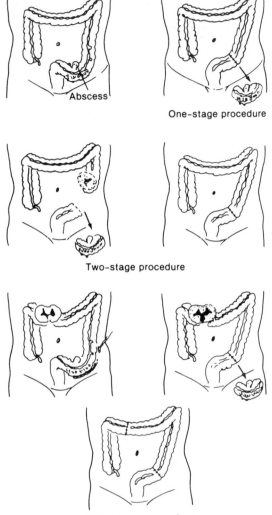

Figure 4. Schematic illustration of the options in the surgical treatment of colonic diseases. A one-stage procedure is noted at the top for management of an intra-abdominal abscess. This demonstrates resection of the diseased segment of colon with primary anastomosis. This is generally not advocated for sigmoid colon lesions. In the second row, a more common two-stage procedure is depicted. This shows a resection of the diseased segment with formation of a temporary end-colostomy as a Hartmann's procedure. The second stage of the procedure includes closure of the colostomy with reconstitution of colonic continuity. The bottom panels demonstrate a three-stage procedure. Initially, simple drainage of the diseased region occurs with formation of a proximal diverting colostomy. Next, a resection of the diseased segment is performed after an interval with a primary reanastomosis. The colostomy is left intact at that point. Finally, the third stage includes closure of the colostomy with reconstitution of intestinal continuity. (Redrawn from Rege RV, Narwhal DL: Diverticular diseases. Curr Probl Surg 26:136, 1989, with permission.)

lesion, three-stage procedures are infrequently used. More commonly, a two-stage procedure is performed if possible, involving resection of the diseased segment of colon with a temporary end-colostomy and subsequent closure of the colostomy and reanastomosis at a later date. Takedown of the colostomy and reanastomosis is often deferred for weeks to months. Common indications for a two-stage procedure include traumatic injury with significant spoilage, resection of the rectum or descending colon in which the bowel has not been adequately prepared, and management of obstructing lesions.

The Hartmann procedure involves sigmoid resection with closure of the distal rectal pouch and creation of an end-colostomy. It is generally temporary, and an elective colostomy takedown with a descending colon-to-rectum anastomosis is performed after a period of weeks to months after resolution of the intra-abdominal inflammation. Resection of the segment with primary anastomosis with creation of a proximal protecting diverting colostomy (or ileostomy) and subsequent closure of the colostomy is another example of a two-stage procedure. This is most commonly performed to protect a distal anastomosis, such as following an ileoanal pull-through procedure.

Colostomy takedown with restoration of gastrointestinal continuity is not an innocuous procedure and has been associated with significant morbidity. Before colostomy closure, the patient should undergo radiographic or endoscopic evaluation and bowel preparation. These procedures should be approached and managed with the same concern and principles that govern primary colon resections and anastomosis. Because of the inherent morbidity associated with colostomy and colostomy takedown, when possible, it is preferable to perform a one-stage colon resection.

Resection with primary reanastomosis is referred to as a one-stage procedure and is usually performed in the colon following an adequate mechanical and antibiotic bowel preparation. It may also be considered for lesions of the ascending colon when there has been minimal soilage. The indications for colon resection are many and usually include elective operations of the left colon and the rectum, but may include neoplastic disease, inflammatory bowel disease, lower intestinal bleeding, diverticulosis, and trauma involving the right colon. As the risk of complications is directly related to the urgency of resection and ability to obtain an adequate bowel preparation, the timing and method of reanastomosis following resection must be selected for each specific situation.

The basic principles of wide local excision to achieve local extirpation of tumors with en bloc extirpation of regional lymph nodes apply to tumors involving the colon. In the context of tumors involving the large intestine, adherence to these principles requires removal of the lymphatics, which follow a course parallel to the blood supply of involved segment of bowel. Therefore, en bloc resection of the colon and the draining lymphatics involves ligation of the appropriate vessels at their origin.

Laparoscopic-assisted colectomy is being used in management of selected disorders of the colon. In principle, the operation performed with laparoscopic assistance is identical to the procedure performed by open laparotomy. Following laparoscopic mobilization, the diseased segment is exteriorized through an incision in the abdominal wall, and the anastomosis is performed under direct external supervision.

Diverticulosis

Diverticulosis of the colon and its associated complications constitute a major problem of western civilization. Some 50 per cent of individuals over the age of 50 have acquired diverticula of the colon. An estimated 15 to 30 per cent experience the complication of infection or hemorrhage at some point.

Diverticula are sac-like protrusions of the colonic wall that are variable in size, ranging from a few millimeters to several centimeters. True diverticula involve all layers of the normal colonic wall and are congenital in origin. In contrast to true diverticula, which are quite uncommon, false diverticula are herniations of the mucosa through the muscular layer of the bowel wall. They are by far the predominant type of diverticula in the colon and are acquired. Most false diverticula form at points of weakness in the bowel wall where perforating vessels (vasa recti) penetrate the circular muscle layer (Fig. 5). This occurs along the mesenteric taeniae and the mesenteric border of the two antimesenteric taeniae. The sigmoid colon is the most common site of diverticula, with involvement in over 95 per cent of individuals with diverticulosis. Confinement to the sigmoid colon occurs in 65 per cent of patients, whereas only 2 to 10 per cent have disease limited to the transverse or ascending colon.

The prevalence of diverticulosis has markedly increased, and while the estimated incidence in 1910 was 5 per cent, it is now 35 to 50 per cent. The incidence of diverticulosis is related to age, with 5 per cent at age 40, 30 per cent by age 60, and 65 per cent of 80-year-olds being afflicted. Diverticular disease is relatively uncommon in less developed regions in comparison to the United States and Western Europe. The reasons for this may relate to different dietary habits, and studies have implicated low-fiber diets in the pathogenesis of diverticulosis.

Alterations in colonic motility as a consequence of this type of diet are thought to predispose to the formation of these diverticula. One hypothesis advanced to explain the relation of low-fiber diets to diverticula

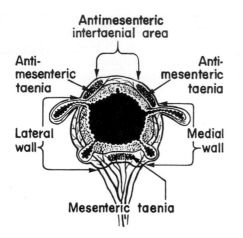

Figure 5. Transverse section of the colon, demonstrating the relationship of diverticula to the colonic tenia, and vasculature. (From Goligher JC: Diverticulosis and diverticulitis of the colon. *In* Duffy H, Nixon H [eds]: Surgery of the Anus, Rectum, and Colon. London, Bailliere, 1984, p 1083, with permission.)

is that individuals with low volumes of stool (low-fiber diets) show an exaggerated pattern of segmentation. Colonic contents are normally transported through the colon by coordinated segmental muscular contractions. The colon contracts, causing a propagation of feces through the relaxed distal colon. An abnormal pattern of contraction with failure of relaxation distally causing occlusion at both ends produces increased pressure within the segment of colon. This predisposes to herniation of mucosa through the bowel wall. Individuals on low-fiber diets have a decreased stool volume and, thus, a more narrowed colon. This colonic narrowing is thought to enhance the distal obstruction during segmentation and produce increased intraluminal pressure, causing diverticulosis. Diverticulosis in most patients remains asymptomatic, but the complications of diverticulitis and diverticular hemorrhage occur in 10 to 25 per cent and 15 per cent, respectively.

LOWER GASTROINTESTINAL HEMORRHAGE

Diverticular hemorrhage causes 30 to 50 per cent of massive lower intestinal bleeding. Upper gastrointestinal hemorrhage from peptic ulcer disease, esophageal varices, and angiodysplasia of both the colon and small intestine are the more common of the remaining causes of lower intestinal bleeding. Although fewer diverticula occur in the right colon, most diverticular bleeds arise in this region.

The proposed mechanism of diverticular hemor-

rhage is thought to be injury or erosion and subsequent rupture of vessels adjacent to the diverticulum. As the diverticulum grows, the vessel becomes separated from the colonic lumen by only a thin layer of mucosa. The predominance of bleeding in the right colon may be due to its thinner wall, thus rendering the vessels more susceptible to damage. Diverticular hemorrhage infrequently occurs in the setting of diverticulitis. Two thirds of patients present with minor or occult bleeding, and the remainder present with massive hemorrhage. Morbidity and mortality associated with diverticular hemorrhage approaches 10 to 20 per cent and is due in part to the presence of comorbid conditions in the elderly population.

Diagnosis

The initial evaluation and management of massive lower intestinal hemorrhage focuses on appropriate resuscitative measures and careful observation (Fig. 6). Patients with active bleeding or hemodynamic compromise are usually evaluated in acute-care settings. The characteristics of the bleeding are determined, as bright red blood is more likely to be from a lower gastrointestinal source than is melena. A history of upper gastrointestinal bleeding, vomiting, peptic ulcer disease, anti-inflammatory drug use, and alcohol abuse should be sought. Patients with prosthetic aortic arterial grafts should immediately be evaluated for the presence of an aortic enteric fistula. Over half of patients with massive diverticular hemorrhage have a history of previous episodes. Physical examination and laboratory studies rarely contribute to the identification of the source of bleeding and the etiology but are important for resuscitation and planning diagnostic and therapeutic studies.

Initial diagnostic measures are directed to defining the site of the bleeding, which is critical to rational management. A nasogastric tube is placed, as withdrawal of blood documents an upper intestinal site of bleeding. A negative aspirate does not, however, exclude the stomach or duodenum as a source of the bleeding, which requires upper gastrointestinal endoscopy. Proctoscopy can exclude the rectum as a source, and further diagnostic studies include radioisotope scanning, selective mesenteric arteriography, esophagogastroduodenoscopy, and colonoscopy.

Radioisotope scanning is performed with either labeled sulfur colloid or red blood cells. Tagged red blood cells have a longer half-life and may be useful in the evaluation of intermittent bleeding, as the patient can be scanned repeatedly if necessary. Radioisotope scanning can detect a bleeding rate of less than 0.1 ml/min, which is identified when the tagged carrier extravasates into the intestinal lumen. Localization with this study remains poor secondary to the mobility

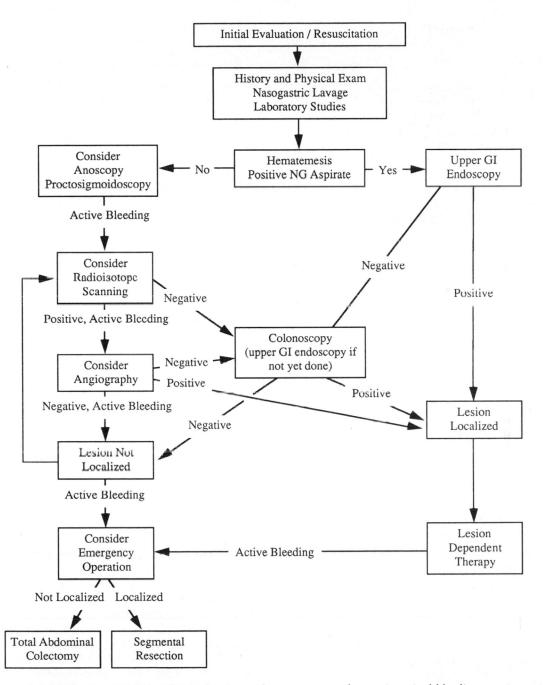

Figure 6. Algorithm for evaluation and management of gastrointestinal bleeding.

of the red blood cells or colloid once inside the lumen. Therefore, radioisotope scanning is frequently utilized as a screening study prior to selective mesenteric arteriography.

Arteriography can detect bleeding rates of over 0.5 ml/min and are thus less sensitive, successfully identifying the bleeding source in 40 to 60 per cent. In patients with continuing hemorrhage documented by ra-

dioisotope scanning, this diagnostic yield increases to 70 to 100 per cent. Identification of the source of bleeding should be followed by consideration for therapeutic intervention while the catheter is appropriately placed. If active bleeding persists despite attempts at localization, an emergency operation should be considered.

Colonoscopy is often difficult to perform in patients

with active, massive hemorrhage because visualization is poor. In situations where colonic lavage is possible, colonoscopy can be effective in localizing the site of bleeding, but attempts at colonoscopy should be abandoned if active bleeding persists. In most patients with spontaneous resolution of hemorrhage, elective colonoscopy following an adequate preparation of the bowel is essential to identify mucosal and angiodysplastic lesions of the colon.

Treatment

Following the initial resuscitative measures and correction of coagulation deficiencies, 70 to 80 per cent of patients with lower gastrointestinal hemorrhage spontaneously cease bleeding. In 15 per cent with massive diverticular hemorrhage, emergent surgical therapy is necessary prior to the performance of further diagnostic studies. In this group in whom the location of the bleeding site is not identified, the mortality approaches 30 to 50 per cent.

Selective intra-arterial infusion of vasopressin controls the hemorrhage in over 90 per cent of patients with an identifiable site of bleeding on arteriography. Contraindications to vasopressin infusion include allergy and evidence of myocardial ischemia. Unfortunately, successful vasopressin infusion is associated with a rebleeding rate of 50 per cent and, in a few patients, may cause serious side effects including catheter-related embolic, thrombotic, and septic events; arrhythmias; hypertension; hypervolemia; and myocardial, mesenteric, and cerebral ischemia.

Embolization therapy with absorbable gelatin or autologous blood clot is a controversial alternative and has been associated with a postembolic colon infarction rate of 13 per cent. Embolization may be attempted in those with a high operative risk due to comorbid conditions such as recent myocardial infarction where vasopressin and general anesthesia are usually avoided. Diverticular hemorrhage is not usually amenable to endoscopic therapy.

Indications for emergent surgical intervention include persistent hemodynamic instability, a large transfusion requirement, and recurrent hemorrhage. It is critical to identify the source and location of bleeding prior to operation, because in instances where the bleeding site has not been identified, a total abdominal colectomy is the preferred surgical treatment and has an operative mortality of 30 to 50 per cent. Segmental resection and hemicolectomy are inappropriate without preoperative localization of the bleeding and are associated with a rebleeding rate of up to 50 per cent if performed. In those who have ceased bleeding and present with a second episode, an elective colon resection should be performed.

DIVERTICULITIS

Although diverticula are confined to the sigmoid in only 65 per cent of patients, diverticulitis is limited to this segment of the colon in 90 per cent. Diverticulitis is unusual in the right colon, presenting in only 5 per cent of patients. This preponderance for the left colon may be explained by the pathophysiologic mechanisms of diverticulitis, which involve perforation of the diverticulum. Perforation is thought to follow erosion of the diverticular wall by increased intraluminal pressure or inspissated particles within the diverticulum, events more likely to occur in the descending or sigmoid colon. The perforation leads to a localized inflammatory process that is usually restricted, as an abscess, by the pericolic fat and surrounding mesentery. Diverticulitis is usually characterized by local inflammation or microabscess formation, but larger abscesses that involve the mesentery or adjacent organs can occur.

Common clinical manifestations of diverticulitis include abdominal pain and tenderness, constipation, diarrhea, abdominal distention, fever, and leukocytosis. Pain in the left lower quadrant is present in over 70 per cent of patients, although pain can occur in other locations. A tender mass is occasionally palpable in the abdomen, rectum, or vagina, and involvement of the bladder by the inflammatory process may cause dysuria, urgency, and frequency. In contrast to noninflamed diverticulosis, bleeding is rarely found in association with diverticulitis.

Diagnosis

The clinical presentation of diverticulitis must be differentiated from colonic spasm associated with diverticulosis as well as perforated colon cancer, acute appendicitis, perforated peptic ulcer, inflammatory bowel disease, ischemic colitis, and adnexal disease. The history and clinical manifestations are usually sufficient to make the diagnosis, as diverticulitis typically is manifested by left lower quadrant pain in older patients, but this should be confirmed with appropriate diagnostic studies. Plain abdominal films are usually unremarkable, as the microperforations associated with diverticulitis infrequently show free intraperitoneal air. However, plain films may demonstrate air in the retroperitoneum suggestive of a paracolic abscess, or intraperitoneal air if gross perforation occurs.

Contrast enemas are usually withheld in the initial period to avoid the risk of rupture of a peridiverticular abscess with extravasation into the peritoneal cavity. Computed tomography is as accurate as barium enema in establishing a diagnosis of diverticulitis and, in addition, can demonstrate other intra-abdominal conditions such as abscesses and phlegmons. Needle aspiration of intra-abdominal fluid collections can also be performed under CT guidance. Following resolution of the acute inflammatory process, patients with diverticulitis usually have an elective evaluation with barium enema and colonoscopy to clearly define the extent of the disease and identify coexistent lesions.

Treatment

Following evaluation and a diagnosis of diverticulitis, a management plan must be developed. Patients with minor symptoms may be treated as outpatients with oral antibiotics and clear liquid diet. Metronidazole and sulfamethoxazole/trimethoprim is a common oral regimen. For patients with more significant clinical symptoms or who have recurrent symptoms during treatment, bowel rest, intravenous fluid resuscitation, analgesics, and intravenous antibiotics are indicated. Appropriate parenteral antibiotic regimens include an aminoglycoside in combination with clindamycin or metronidazole. Most patients respond to intense medical therapy and should be evaluated by barium enema or colonoscopy following resolution of the acute episode. A diet high in fiber to promote a large volume of stool and avoidance of constipation is appropriate following resolution of acute diverticulitis.

Some 20 per cent of patients fail to respond to medical therapy and require emergent surgical intervention. Computed tomography–guided aspiration of known diverticular abscess may be utilized as a stabilizing measure in critically ill patients, but is considered only a temporizing procedure. Patients who fail to respond or deteriorate after 24 to 48 hours of intense medical therapy require urgent exploration. An adequate bowel preparation is not usually possible. The goals of surgical exploration are fecal diversion, drainage of any abscess and fecal soilage, and resection of the diseased colon, which is often accomplished by primary resection of the colon, proximal end-colostomy, and mucous fistula formation or a Hartmann procedure. The patient's condition, the presence and extent of intra-abdominal contamination and inflammation, and the ability to evaluate underlying structures, such as the ureters, must be considered by the surgeon in selecting optimal operation. Three-stage procedures are generally not performed, as simple drainage and proximal colostomy has a significantly higher morbidity and mortality than colon resection and proximal colostomy.

Surgical intervention is also indicated in the management of the complications of diverticulitis, which may develop in up to 25 per cent of patients. The management of intra-abdominal abscesses, including peridiverticular, retroperitoneal, mesenteric, or pelvic, accounts for 40 to 50 per cent of operations for diverticulitis. Abscess extension to adjacent structures including the abdominal wall, thigh, and hip can occur. Resection of the involved segment, drainage of the abscess, and fecal diversion are usually employed to manage an undrained abscess, although successful CT-guided aspiration and drainage of the abscess may be used to stabilize the patient and allow an elective resection and primary anastomosis at a later date.

The appearance of fistulas is a less common complication and usually involves the sigmoid colon. Colovesical fistulas, more common in males, account for two thirds of cases, usually presenting with urinary symptoms including urgency, dysuria, and frequency. Pneumaturia and fecaluria occur in 75 per cent of patients and are pathognomonic findings. However, further evaluation of a patient with a colovesical fistula by cystoscopy and barium enema is indicated to identify the underlying cause of the fistulas. Cystoscopy has a diagnostic accuracy of 80 to 95 per cent and usually reveals localized inflammation and edema of the bladder wall. Although the barium enema may demonstrate evidence of diverticular disease in most cases, the fistula tract is identified in less than 30 per cent. Colocutaneous fistulas are the second most common type of fistula followed by colovaginal and colocutaneous fistulas. Elective segmental colon resection, primary bladder repair, and primary colon anastomosis can be safely performed in most patients with colovesical fistula following adequate preparation of the bowel. Patients with generalized peritonitis due to free perforation of the colon require emergent surgical intervention. Resection of the perforated segment with proximal colostomy is combined with copious irrigation of the peritoneal cavity. The overall mortality is high due to complications of septic shock and multiple organ system failure.

Chronic colonic stricture may complicate diverticulitis and may be difficult to differentiate from carcinoma of the colon. A history of previous episodes of diverticulitis, abdominal pain, and the absence of rectal bleeding are suggestive of stricture secondary to diverticulitis, but biopsy and segmental colon resection should be performed to exclude carcinoma. Intestinal obstruction due to stricture is another indication for operation. Surgical management involves primary resection of the involved segment with colostomy or primary anastomosis, if an adequate bowel preparation was obtained. On occasion, a segment of small bowel may become adherent to the inflammatory process, causing obstruction.

Elective colon resection must be considered in patients with recurrent episodes of acute diverticulitis. After a second episode of diverticulitis, the incidence of complications approaches 50 per cent, and the associated mortality is twice that associated with the initial attack. In contradistinction to urgent operation required for acute complications of diverticulitis, elective surgical management with bowel preparation usually includes resection of the involved segment of colon with primary anastomosis and is associated with a low mortality and morbidity. Therefore, elective colonic resection may be indicated in patients following a second episode of diverticulitis. Although patients under 40 constitute only 2 to 4 per cent of patients with diverticulitis, 70 per cent of these eventually require surgical intervention for recurrence. Therefore, some advocate the use of early elective colon resection in young patients.

ULCERATIVE COLITIS

Chronic ulcerative colitis is a diffuse inflammatory disease primarily involving the mucosal lining of the colon and rectum. In contrast, granulomatous transmural ileocolitis (Crohn's disease) is a characteristically transmural granulomatous enteritis that may involve any part of the intestinal tract, but primarily the small intestine. Ulcerative colitis is characterized by bloody diarrhea that exacerbates and abates without apparent cause and is of unknown etiology. The inflammation involves the mucosa and submucosa of the bowel wall and may involve the entire colon (pancolitis).

In the United States, between 200,000 and 400,000 individuals suffer from inflammatory bowel disease, with 30,000 cases diagnosed annually. Ulcerative colitis affects females more often than males and has a bimodal age distribution, with a first peak incidence between the ages of 15 and 20 and a second smaller peak at 55 to 60.

The cause of ulcerative colitis remains unknown despite intensive work by many investigators. Examination of bacterial and viral agents continues, although there is uncertainty as to the role of infectious agents in the pathogenesis. Genetic factors appear to have a role, as the disease is approximately 50 per cent less frequent in the nonwhite population. Psychological factors may have a role in exacerbation of disease.

There has been considerable speculation that ulcerative colitis is an immunologically mediated disease, and evidence has supported this concept. There is currently much interest in the role of cytokines, immunoregulatory molecules, and control of the immune response in patients with inflammatory bowel disease. Circulating anticolon and antilymphocyte antibodies have been described in ulcerative colitis, but their significance and that of circulating immune complexes is currently unknown. Other studies have suggested that ulcerative colitis is an energy-deficit disease of the colonic epithelium.

Pathology

The pathologic changes that occur with ulcerative colitis are nonspecific but involve the mucosa. Unlike the segmental lesions of Crohn's disease, the mucosa is inflamed continuously (Table 2). Some of the features of ulcerative colitis represent attempts of the colon to regenerate destroyed crypts, which are diminished in number, distorted, and contain goblet cells. The process of ulceration and granulation followed by reepithelialization may lead to polypoid excrescencies forming inflammatory polyps that are not neoplastic and are referred to as pseudopolyps.

Clinical Manifestations

Ulcerative colitis usually presents with bloody diarrhea, abdominal pain, and fever. Occasionally arthritis, iritis, hepatic dysfunction, skin lesions, or other systemic manifestations may predominate. The disease begins as a chronic, relatively low-grade disorder in about half of the patients, characterized by malaise, lower abdominal pain, diarrhea, and rectal bleeding. The mortality is low, and the prognosis favorable. A more abrupt onset of the disease, associated with diarrhea and bloody stools, occurs in about a third of patients. This moderate form of ulcerative colitis is characterized by severe abdominal cramps that may awaken the patient from sleep, low-grade fever, fatigue, and malaise, as well as anorexia and weight loss.

In 15 per cent of patients, ulcerative colitis has an acute and fulminating course, characterized by frequent bloody bowel movements, high fever, and abdominal pain. Abdominal cramps, rectal urgency, and profound weakness are present with nausea and anorexia. Physical findings are directly related to the duration and presentation of the disease. Weight loss and pallor are usually present. These patients appear acutely ill, with tachycardia and hypotension with signs of an acute abdomen accompanied by fever and decreased bowel sounds. Rarely, shock may be present, and in these patients, toxic megacolon with severe abdominal distention may be present. This allows intraluminal pressure to distend the colon beyond the normal diameter, and bacterial overgrowth can produce toxins that contribute to mucosal inflammation and systemic toxicity after absorption.

Clinical signs of toxic megacolon include fever, tachycardia, dehydration abdominal distention and tenderness, and the loss of bowel signs. Plain abdominal films reveal a dilated colon, and leukocytosis, hypokalemia, anemia, and hypoalbuminemia are frequently present. The mortality of patients with toxic megacolon may be a high as 20 to 30 per cent, and aggressive resuscitation with colectomy within 24 hours is mandatory.

TABLE 2.   FEATURES OF INFLAMMATORY BOWEL DISEASE

Feature	Ulcerative Colitis	Crohn's Colitis
Epidemiologic Features		
Incidence	2 to 7 cases per 100,000	2 to 4 cases per 100,000
Sex distribution	Females > males	Males = females
Age of peak incidence	15 to 20 and 55 to 60	10 to 30
Ethnic propensity	Jews > non Jews > blacks	Jews > non-Jews > blacks
Clinical Features		
Malaise, fever	Uncommon	Common
Abdominal tenderness	May be present	Common
Abdominal mass	Not present	Very common, especially with ileocolitis
Abdominal pain	Unusual	Very common
Abdominal wall and internal fistulas	Rare	Very common
Endoscopic Findings		
Diffuse, continuous, symmetric involvement	Very common	Uncommon
Aphthous or linear ulcers	Rare	Common
Friability	Rare	Rare
Radiologic Findings		
Continuous disease	Very common	Rare
Asymmetry	Rare	Very common
Strictures	Rare	Common
Fistulas	Rare	Very common
Pathologic Features		
Discontinuity	Rare	Common
Intense vascularity	Common	Rare
Transmural involvement	Rare	Common
Lymphoid aggregates	Uncommon	Common
Crypt abscesses	Very common	Rare
Granulomas	Rare	Common
Linear clefts	Rare	Common
Ileal Involvement		
Ileal disease on radiologic exam	Rare	Very common
Ileal disease of pathologic exam	Rare	Common
Rectal Involvement		
Rectal bleeding	Common	Intermittent about 50%
Rectal disease on endoscopic exam	Almost 100%	About 20%
Rectal disease of pathologic exam	Common	Rare
Risk of Carcinoma of the Colon	20 to 30% within 20 years	Elevated
Surgical Treatment	Proctocolectomy with ileostomy Abdominal colectomy, rectal mucosectomy, and ileoanal pull through	Subtotal or total colectomy, rectum frequently preserved
Results of Surgical Treatment	Curative	Not curative

Evaluation and Treatment

Sigmoidoscopy is useful in establishing a diagnosis, as the disease involves the distal colon and rectum in over 90 per cent of patients. The mucosa is erythematous and friable and may appear hyperemic. The normal colonic vascular markings may be lost, and the intracolonic haustra are thick and blunted with superficial ulcerations. In advanced disease the areas of ulceration may surround areas of granulation tissue and edematous mucosa and are termed *pseudopolyps*. The use of flexible sigmoidoscopy has improved diagnostic accuracy, and colonoscopy may be useful in determin-

ing the extent and activity of the disease, particularly when the diagnosis is unclear or if cancer is suspected.

Plain abdominal films may show colonic dilatation with toxic megacolon in approximately 5 per cent of patients. Dilatation of the transverse colon is often present, and there may be free air within the peritoneal cavity from perforation of the diseased colon. A barium enema is useful in most patients, although it is potentially dangerous with toxic megacolon. Radiographic signs suggesting ulcerative colitis on barium enema (Fig. 7) include loss of haustral markings and irregularities of the colon wall, which represent small ulcerations. Later in the course of the disease, pseu-

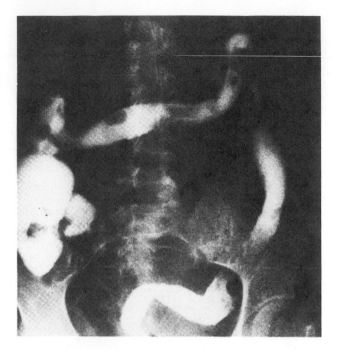

Figure 7. The contracted stovepipe appearance of the colon, as viewed by barium rectogram, is typical of advanced ulcerative colitis in its chronic phase. The large lucid areas in the barium column probably represent fecal matter, whereas the smaller, more subtle shadows along the left colon are most likely pseudopolyps.

dopolyps may be identified. In longstanding chronic ulcerative colitis, the colon assumes the appearance of a rigid contracted tube.

In all patients presenting initially, it is necessary to exclude infectious causes of the enterocolitis. Therefore, stool specimens should be obtained for smears and cultures to exclude colitis due to viruses, bacterial pathogens, and parasites. It may be difficult to differentiate ulcerative colitis from Crohn's disease. Crohn's disease of the colon compared with ulcerative colitis would be suggested by the findings of small-bowel involvement, rectal sparing, absence or infrequency of gross bleeding, perianal disease, focal lesions, segmental distributions or skip lesions, asymmetric involvement, fistulization, granulomas or transmural involvement on biopsy, and a distinct endoscopic appearance.

Medical Management

Most patients with ulcerative colitis are managed medically. The treatment of ulcerative colitis and Crohn's disease is similar because both disorders require long-term treatment using the same or related drugs. In addition, anemia and other nutritional and systemic disorders are treated similarly. However, the surgical management and the prognosis of each of these illnesses is distinct, as ulcerative colitis can be completely cured with colectomy.

Ulcerative colitis is usually treated by sulfasalazine, related derivatives of pyridine-acetylsalicylic acid, antibacterial compounds, corticosteroids, and symptom-controlling medications. In severe cases, immunosuppressants such as azathioprine, 6-mercaptopurine, and cyclosporine are used. Mild to moderate colitis usually responds to supportive measures supplemented by 3 to 4 gm/day of sulfasalazine. Sulfasalazine is hydrolyzed by bacteria in the colon to yield sulfapyridine and 5-aminosalicylate (5-ASA), which is felt to be the active agent in the control of symptoms. Corticosteroids are usually added if sulfasalazine provides inadequate control. Corticosteroids are usually given in doses from 20 to 60 mg/day, then tapered if possible. Left-sided colitis can be managed by the local delivery of corticosteroids including enemas. Once symptoms are controlled, patients are usually continued on maintenance therapy of sulfasalazine or some 5-ASA derivative.

Toxic megacolon occurs in approximately 5 per cent of patients with ulcerative colitis. If toxic colitis with megacolon does not improve within 24 hours, an emergency operation is indicated. The choice of the operation in this setting is abdominal colectomy with a Brooke ileostomy and Hartmann closure of the rectal stump. Emergency operation for acute toxic megacolon has a high morbidity and mortality, which appear to be higher following a total proctocolectomy than following abdominal subtotal colectomy.

The indications for elective operation include the risk of colorectal carcinoma or the failure of medical management. Patients with ulcerative colitis have a 20 to 30 per cent risk of developing carcinoma of the colon within 20 years of the diagnosis. The likelihood of carcinoma in patients with ulcerative colitis appears to relate to both the extent of colonic involvement and the duration of the disease. The time of colectomy for cancer prophylaxis remains controversial. After 10 years of follow-up, prophylactic colectomy should be considered because of the accelerating risk of cancer. The role of colorectal biopsy in directing the timing of colectomy is also controversial. Patients followed for more than 5 to 7 years should undergo annual colonoscopy and biopsies for detection of epithelial dysplasia. Severe dysplasia is associated with a high incidence of cancer of the colon, and prophylactic colectomy is indicated.

The most common indication for operation remains intractable disease, and elective procedures include total proctocolectomy and Brooke ileostomy (Fig. 8), subtotal colectomy with ileostomy or ileorectal anastomosis, and colectomy with mucosal proctectomy and ileal pouch–anal anastomosis (Fig. 9). Because of the availability of a sphincter-saving operation, pa-

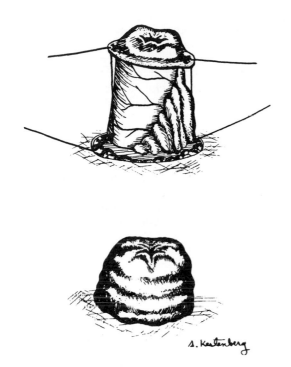

Figure 8. Technique of construction of an end-ileostomy as described by Brooke. The ileum is brought through an abdominal defect ensuring 5 cm of length external to the abdominal wall, and then everted and sutured to the dermis to "mature" the ileostomy. (From Becker JM, Moody FG: Ulcerative colitis. *In* Sabiston DC Jr [ed]: Textbook of Surgery: The Biological Basis of Modern Surgical Practice, ed 14. Philadelphia, WB Saunders Company, 1991, p 935, with permission.)

tients are now electing surgical therapy for intractability earlier.

CROHN'S DISEASE

Medical management of Crohn's disease is similar to the management of ulcerative colitis, with sulfasalazine and corticosteroids being the primary agents. Crohn's disease generally responds to treatment more slowly, with frequent remissions, and surgical treatment is not curative and is avoided because the disease may recur. Surgical intervention is reserved for the management of the complications, including relief of intestinal obstruction, drainage of abscesses, treatment of bleeding, and correction of fistulas.

ISCHEMIC COLITIS

Ischemic injury to the colon may be caused by advanced atherosclerosis or interruption of the colonic blood supply during operation as in resection of an abdominal aortic aneurysm, with ligation of the inferior mesenteric artery. Ischemic injury may also occur following shock, hypercoagulable states, amyloidosis, vasculitis, or the use of oral contraceptive agents. In addition, nonocclusive colonic ischemia may occur in states of low cardiac output, or hypoxia, particularly when aggravated by other metabolic conditions such as dehydration or renal acidosis. The syndrome of ischemic colitis may vary in its extent, severity, and prognosis; however, extensive infarction and perforation appear to be infrequent. More commonly, localized or segmental ischemia is present, particularly affecting those areas of the colon between two adjacent arterial supplies.

These patients are often elderly and present with acute onset of lower abdominal cramping pain, rectal bleeding, vomiting, and fever. Some have a history of

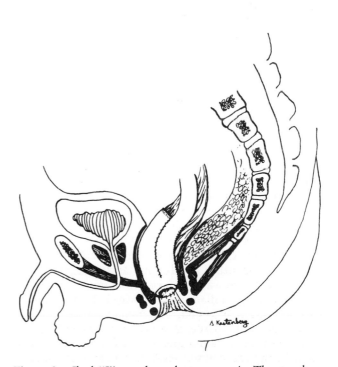

Figure 9. Ileal "J"-pouch anal anastomosis. The two-loop ileal pouch is simple to construct, provides adequate storage capacity, and is evacuated spontaneously. End-to-end ileoanal anastomosis following colectomy, mucosal proctectomy, and endorectal ileoanal pull-through is shown. After abdominal colectomy, the rectal mucosa is circumferentially dissected from the rectal muscle in the anal sphincter. The ileum is then extended down into the pelvis endorectally and anastomosed to the dentate line of the anus. (From Becker JM, Moody FG: Ulcerative colitis. *In* Sabiston DC Jr [ed]: Textbook of Surgery: The Biological Basis of Modern Surgical Practice, ed 14. Philadelphia, WB Saunders Company, 1991, p 937, with permission.)

similar symptoms occurring previously for weeks or months. Left-sided abdominal tenderness and peritoneal signs may be present, and ischemic colitis should be suspected in any elderly patient who suddenly develops rectal bleeding.

Evaluation includes plain abdominal films that show thickening of the bowel wall with edema and fluid. Diffuse abdominal pain may be listed on physical examination if peritoneal irritation is present. Definitive diagnosis requires endoscopic examination. Sigmoidoscopy may be normal, with evidence of mild nonspecific proctitis, or it may reveal multiple discrete ulcers, submucosal blebs, and pseudomembranes. Biopsy documents evidence of ischemic colitis. The differentiation of ischemic colitis from colonic infections, diverticulitis, or idiopathic inflammatory bowel disease may be difficult. Barium enemas may show narrowing of the bowel lumen and a thumb-print configuration in the splenic flexure, the descending colon, or the sigmoid. Thumb-printing is the indentation of the barium column due to submucosal hemorrhage or edema.

The initial treatment consists of general supportive measures including antibiotics with appropriate intravenous fluids. The goals are to restore perfusion to the intestine, reverse ischemia and tissue hypoxia, and prevent infarction. Most patients improve without operation, but for those in whom perforation or infarction of the viscus appears likely, emergency surgical exploration is required.

PSEUDOMEMBRANOUS COLITIS

Pseudomembranous colitis is a disease characterized by exudate or plaques on the intestinal mucosa, commonly involving the colon. It is usually found in association with other conditions, and recognized risk factors include intestinal obstruction, uremia, Hirschsprung's disease, inflammatory bowel disease, shigellosis, intestinal ischemia, and neonatal enterocolitis. During the past decade, the disease has been most often recognized as a complication of antibiotics, with lesions generally confined to the colon. *Clostridium difficile* is the pathogen responsible for most of these cases and is found in the colonic flora of 3 per cent of healthy adults. Although the mechanism of pseudomembranous colitis is not clear, it appears to be a toxin-mediated disease, in which the integrity of the bowel mucosa is impaired due to the release of a toxin from *C. difficile*. The clinical manifestations are diarrhea, fever, abdominal pain, distention, and shock due to fluid loss and bacterial invasion.

The diagnosis can be made by detection of the *C. difficile* toxin in the stool. Colonoscopy reveals punctate, raised, yellowish white plaques with skipped ar-

eas of normal mucosa. Microscopic examination shows epithelial necrosis, goblet cells distended with mucus, and an infiltrative lamina propria, with polymorphonuclear cells and an eosinophilic exudate. The pseudomembrane is attached to the surface of the epithelium and is composed of fibromucin and polymorphonuclear cells.

The most important therapeutic decision is discontinuation of the implicated antibiotic. Specific therapy for diarrhea caused by *C. difficile* is the administration of oral vancomycin or oral or intravenous metronidazole. More seriously ill patients have a mortality of 10 to 30 per cent, but early institution of anti–*C. difficile* antibiotics is usually followed by a prompt symptomatic response.

NEUTROPENIC COLITIS

Colitis may occur in granulocytopenic patients and cause abdominal pain, diarrhea, and fever. Broad-spectrum antibiotic therapy and thorough evaluation are indicated to exclude other causes of intra-abdominal pain such as acalculous cholecystitis. Because many patients have recovery of bone marrow with resolution of the neutropenia and the subsequent colitis, medical management and supportive care are appropriate. Surgical intervention is indicated in patients with perforation or intractable hemorrhage. Rarely, toxic megacolon occurs in this setting and is managed by urgent colectomy with ileostomy.

RADIATION COLITIS

Because of the rapid renewal of the epithelial lining, the colon is particularly susceptible to radiation injury, and mucosal inflammation and atrophy not uncommonly follow acute radiation exposure. The clinical features resemble idiopathic ulcerative colitis with a limited response to local steroids. Radiation enteritis and colitis occurring months or years after radiation therapy may be secondary to obliterative enteritis of submucosal arterioles and appear unrelated to the acute mucosal injury. The colonic wall develops fibrosis and edema, producing strictures, obstruction, and secondary mucosal lesions, leading to ulceration. The tissue dose usually required to produce intestinal colitis is in the range of 4000 rad or more.

Barium contrast studies of the colon show the extent of the disease and localize the site of strictures. Radiation injury usually follows radiation of the cervix, uterus, bladder, or ovaries. Therapy consists of intermittent dilatation, which may relieve symptoms, and progressive obstruction may require a diverting colostomy. Occasionally, resection of the stricture with reanastomosis is indicated.

A rectovaginal fistula may occur secondary to recurrent carcinoma of the cervix with tumor necrosis. A diverting colostomy is the treatment of choice.

VOLVULUS OF THE COLON

Volvulus is the abnormal twisting or rotation of a segment of the bowel about the mesentery. Colonic volvulus generally occurs with a large redundant colonic segment that has a narrow mesenteric base. The redundant segment is freely mobile, whereas the points of fixation are quite close and serve as a focus for the development of twisting the bowel. Compromise of the bowel lumen follows with obstruction, as shown in Figure 10, and vascular compromise may also occur due to obstruction of the blood supply, with subsequent ischemia and gangrene.

The sigmoid colon is most commonly involved, followed by the cecum. Rarely, the right colon, transverse colon, and splenic flexure may undergo volvulus. If untreated, volvulus generally progresses rapidly from colonic obstruction to strangulation and gangrene.

Sigmoid Volvulus

Approximately 75 per cent of large-bowel volvulus involves the sigmoid colon. The age and sex distribution of these patients has two distinct patterns, with patients in Iran, Africa, and Eastern Europe being predominantly middle-aged males and having a pathogenesis ascribed to an acquired redundancy of sigmoid colon. In the United States, Australia, the United Kingdom, and Canada, sigmoid volvulus occurs in elderly individuals of both sexes, with most patients having a long history of altered bowel habits. Many patients are referred from chronic care facilities with Parkinson's and Alzheimer's disease, multiple sclerosis, paralysis, chronic schizophrenia, pseudobulbar palsy, and senility. The patients are often bedridden and take various neuropsychotropic drugs known to alter bowel motility.

Acute sigmoid volvulus generally presents with sudden onset of severe colicky abdominal pain, obstipation, and abdominal distention. Generalized abdominal pain, tenderness, fever, and hypovolemia suggest strangulation.

Plain abdominal radiographs often reveal a dilated colon forming the *bent inner tube* or *omega loop* sign. The convexity of the loop points toward the right up-

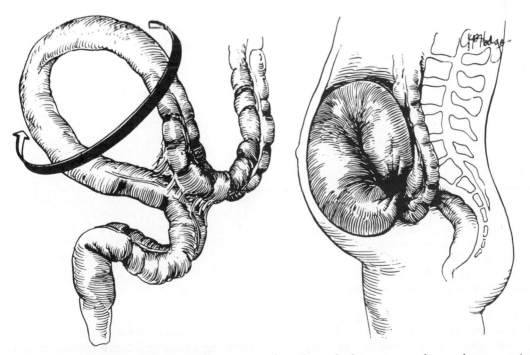

Figure 10. Predisposing factors usually necessary for colon volvulus to occur almost always consist of a segment of redundant mobile colon and a relatively fixed point or points about which the volvulus may occur. (From Kerry RI, Ransom HK: Volvulus of the colon. Arch Surg 99:215, 1969, by permission of the American Medical Association.)

per quadrant or away from the point of obstruction. The narrowed segment of the colon, referred to as the *bird's beak*, generally points toward the site of obstruction. Barium enema is usually not necessary for diagnosis and is contraindicated whenever strangulation is suspected.

The initial treatment of sigmoid volvulus consists of attempted endoscopic reduction by proctoscopy and placement of a rectal tube, which is successful in 70 to 80 per cent of patients. Detorsion permits mechanical and antibiotic preparation of the colon and an elective primary resection of the sigmoid colon with primary anastomosis.

Operative detorsion is performed in patients who fail nonoperative reduction, but as many as 40 per cent of these patients have a recurrence. Other procedures include tube sigmoidostomy, extraperitonealization of the sigmoid colon (Mikulicz procedure), sigmoidopexy, and resection with end-colostomy. If gangrene is present at the time of laparotomy, resection is mandatory with an end-colostomy and a mucous fistula or the Hartmann procedure.

The main determinant of patient mortality from sigmoid volvulus is viability of the colon. Successful nonoperative reduction followed by elective resection has an expected mortality of 6 to 10 per cent, whereas patients operated upon for gangrenous bowel have a mortality of 50 to 70 per cent.

Cecal Volvulus

A mobile cecum is the prerequisite for the development of cecal volvulus and is present in 20 to 40 per cent of cases with volvulus. Approximately 90 per cent of patients with cecal volvulus have a twist of a segment of the proximal colon or the entire right colon. In the remainder, there is a cephalad fold of the cecum across the ascending colon. As many as two thirds of the patients have undergone previous abdominal procedures. Colonic distention following distal obstruction has also been implicated in the development of cecal volvulus and should be excluded.

Cecal volvulus presents with the acute onset of severe colicky pain, nausea, vomiting, and obstipation with a compressible mass extending from the right lower quadrant to the midabdominal region. Abdominal films reveal marked distention of the cecum, and a contrast enema may show narrowing of the bowel lumen.

Nonoperative techniques for the reduction of cecal volvulus are much less successful than for sigmoid volvulus. Approximately 25 per cent of patients are found to have gangrenous changes at the time of laparotomy, and the mortality approaches 40 per cent. Therefore, when a diagnosis of cecal volvulus is made, surgical intervention is appropriate. If the cecum is found to be gangrenous, resection is mandatory, usually with ileotransverse colostomy. If the cecum is viable, the possible procedures of choice include right hemicolectomy and detorsion with cecopexy or cecostomy.

Volvulus of the Transverse Colon or Splenic Flexure

More unusual cases of volvulus include the transverse colon and the splenic flexure. Although patients with transverse colon volvulus present with the typical signs and symptoms of colonic obstruction, the diagnosis of volvulus of the transverse colon is difficult by plain abdominal films and is often not suspected preoperatively. Attempts at a nonoperative reduction have been few and are generally unsuccessful. Urgent surgical intervention is necessary, and if gangrenous bowel is encountered, resection is performed. In patients with viable colon, detorsion alone is associated with a high recurrence and mortality. Transverse colectomy, colopexy, and transverse tube colostomy have been used successfully.

Volvulus of the splenic flexure is rare. Congenital absence or iatrogenic division of the gastrocolic, splenocolic, or phrenocolic ligaments may predispose to volvulus of the splenic flexure. Most of the reported patients have undergone prior abdominal surgical procedures. Urgent surgical intervention is recommended with resection of the involved bowel in most instances.

NEOPLASMS OF THE COLON

Colorectal neoplasms are quite common, with 150,000 new cases occurring in the United States annually, making it the second most frequent cancer. Aggressive approaches to identify patients at high risk and those with premalignant lesions is essential to improve the mortality of this disease. The vast majority of these tumors are adenocarcinomas, some of which arise from adenomatous polyps. The evaluation and management of patients with adenomatous polyps is clearly an important aspect of the prevention of colorectal malignancies.

Colonic Polyps

Polyps originate from the mucosal surface and may occur sporadically or represent manifestations of a dominantly transmitted polyposis syndrome as depicted in Table 3. Hyperplastic polyps are not premalignant. Juvenile or retention polyps occur mainly in children and are considered to be hamartomas and

TABLE 3. POLYPS OF THE COLON

Neoplastic Polyps
   Benign adenomatous polyps (tubular, mixed, or villous)
      Random occurrences
      Familial:
         Familial adenomatous polyposis
         Gardner's syndrome
         Turcot's syndrome
         Family cancer syndrome
   Malignant polyps-carcinomatous changes, in situ and invasive
Nonneoplastic Polyps
   Inflammatory "pseudopolyps"
   Peutz-Jeghers syndrome (hamartomas)
   Juvenile polyps
   Cronkhite-Canada syndrome (hamartomas)
   Mucosal polyps with normal epithelium

consist of large mucus-filled glands. They do not appear to be premalignant; however, patients with the juvenile polyposis syndrome have an increased incidence of adenomatous polyps. In the multiple juvenile polyposis syndrome there is an increased incidence of adenocarcinoma arising from coexistent adenomatous polyps. Neoplastic or adenomatous polyps are relatively common and occur in 10 per cent of adults, with an increase in incidence with advancing age. These polyps may be classified as tubular or villous depending on the glandular pattern. Whereas tubular adenomas occur throughout the colon, villous adenomas occur predominantly in the sigmoid colon and rectum.

Familial syndromes characterized by multiple neoplastic colonic polyps are shown in Table 4. Whereas hundreds of polyps must be present for the diagnosis of these syndromes, the mean number present is about 1000. Familial polyposis coli, Gardner's syndrome, and Turcot's syndrome are examples of familial syndromes characterized by multiple adenomatous colonic polyps. Gardner's and Turcot's syndromes are also associated with a number of extracolonic features including osteomas of the mandible; exostoses of the long bones; soft-tissue tumors such as lipomas, fibromas, or desmoid tumors; and adenomatous lesions elsewhere in the gastrointestinal tract. Malignant degeneration of these colonic polyps is considered to occur in most, and prophylactic resection of the colon is recommended.

Cronkhite-Canada syndrome is a nonfamilial condition characterized by diffuse hamartomatous polyps throughout the gastrointestinal tract. It is characterized by accompanying dystrophy of the nails, alopecia, and cutaneous hyperpigmentation. Weight loss, diarrhea, and malnutrition may occur, and therapy is supportive and directed toward nutritional replacement.

Peutz-Jeghers syndrome is characterized by diffuse hamartomatous polyps throughout the gastrointestinal tract with associated melena and pigmentation about the face, mouth, and lips. Rarely, exostoses,

ovarian tumors, and polyps of the bladder occur. The most frequent complications are bleeding, obstruction, and intussusception. Removal of gastric and small intestinal polyps is performed to manage complications. There is an increased risk for carcinoma of the small bowel due to the presence of associated adenomatous polyps, and colonic polyps occurring in the colon may represent true adenomas and should be endoscopically removed.

Clinical Management

Adenomatous polyps are considered premalignant. Characteristics associated with an increased malignant potential include increasing size, villous histology, severe dysplasia, and ulceration. The frequency of cancer in adenomas less than 1 cm in size is less than 1 per cent, in adenomas larger than 1 cm but less than 2 cm in size it is 10 per cent, and in adenomas greater than 2 cm in size it may be as high as 50 per cent.

Although polyps may cause symptoms related to blood loss from an ulcerated surface, they are most frequently occult and are detected by barium enema or proctosigmoidoscopy or colonoscopy. Very large polyps may cause abdominal pain from partial intestinal obstruction, or may be the lead point in colonic intussusception in an adult. Villous adenomas may occasionally induce watery diarrhea, causing potassium depletion or an excessive secretion of mucus with loss of protein, which rarely causes hypoalbuminemia.

Polyps may be pedunculated (on a stalk) or sessile (broad based), making them accessible to removal by colonoscopy and cautery excision. Following endoscopic polypectomy, the patient should have routine colonoscopic surveillance to detect new or additional lesions. If multiple lesions are present, follow-up is more frequent. With large polyps with a high risk of malignant change, such as a large villous adenoma, a segmental colectomy is often indicated. Villous adenomas have a marked predilection for malignant degeneration and complete excision is required.

Carcinomas occurring in adenomas are usually well differentiated and occur most commonly at the tip of the adenoma. If there is no invasion, these represent in situ carcinomas that rarely metastasize and are adequately treated by polypectomy. In some cases, cancers in adenomas may invade the muscularis mucosa and potentially invade lymphatics and metastasize. Therefore, if the lesion has penetrated the muscularis mucosa and invaded lymphatics, if the cancer is poorly differentiated, or if it extends to the margin of the excision, then segmental resection as used routinely for the treatment of adenocarcinoma of the colon is indicated.

The management of the polyposis syndromes is different than the management of sporadic polyps be-

TABLE 4. POLYPOSIS SYNDROMES

Disorder	Inheritance	Clinical Manifestations	Associated Malignancy	Treatment
Familial adenomatous polyposis coli	Autosomal dominant	Multiple adenomas of the colon	Colorectal carcinomas by age 40	Total or near total colectomy Survey family members
Gardner's syndrome	Autosomal dominant	Multiple adenomas of the colon, some in the stomach and small bowel Osteomas Soft-tissue tumors (lipomas, sebaceous cysts, fibromas, fibrosarcomas) Mesenteric fibromatosis Supernumerary teeth and mandibular cysts Epidermoid cysts of the testes	Colorectal carcinomas by age 40 Other neoplasms of the thyroid, adrenal, and pancreaticoduodenal area	Total or near total colectomy Survey family members
Turcot's syndrome	Autosomal recessive	Adenomas of the colon Tumors of the central nervous system (medulloblastomas, ependymomas, glioblastomas)	Colorectal carcinomas	Total or near total colectomy Survey family members
Peutz-Jeghers syndrome	Autosomal dominant	Multiple intestinal polyposis (hamartomas of the stomach, small bowel, and colon) Mucocutaneous pigmentation Nasal and bronchial polyps Rarely, exostoses, ovarian tumors, and bladder polyps	Carcinoma of the proximal intestine	Removal polyps of upper GI tract for complications Remove adenomatous polyps if they occur in the colon
Juvenile polyposis	Autosomal dominant	Multiple intestinal hamartomas	None	Remove polyps for complications or diagnosis
Cronkhite-Canada syndrome	None	Generalized intestinal polyposis (hamartomas) Dystrophy of the finger nails, alopecia, and cutaneous hyperpigmentation	None	Treatment of symptoms

Abbreviation: GI = gastrointestinal.

cause the familial syndromes may be associated with hundreds or thousands of colonic polyps that are premalignant. Total colectomy with ileostomy eliminates the risk of malignancy, but a consequent creation of a permanent abdominal stoma and loss of continence makes this procedure unacceptable to many patients. Total abdominal colectomy (which leaves the rectal mucosa at risk for polyps and malignant degeneration) mandates continued endoscopic surveillance of the retained rectum. Unfortunately, even though residual rectal polyps may regress transiently, the risk of malignancy is not eliminated. In the management of premalignant polyposis syndromes and ulcerative colitis, resection of the rectal mucosa is required if the procedure is to be considered curative.

Until recently, total proctocolectomy with Brooke ileostomy was the procedure of choice, but there are several alternatives, including abdominal colectomy with ileorectal anastomosis. Because a segment of rectum with its mucosa is retained, the risk for carcinoma of the colon remains and the patient must be followed closely by proctoscopy and digital examination. Another alternative is proctocolectomy with creation of a continent ileostomy. The continent ileostomy or Kock pouch involves creation of an intestinal reservoir composed of ileum with an ileal conduit leading to a cutaneous stoma. Intussusception of the terminal ileum into the pouch for 3 to 4 cm further improves continence. Drainage of these pouches is accomplished by passing a tube through the valve into the pouch via the stoma.

In 1947 Ravitch and Sabiston described abdominal colectomy, mucosal proctectomy, and ileoanal pullthrough and anastomosis, which in modified form has become a frequently used procedure (Fig. 9). After abdominal colectomy, the rectal mucosa is circumferentially dissected from the rectal muscle and anal sphincter. An ileal reservoir is then created by folding the ileum upon itself and, with a stapling device, eliminating the common wall of the folded segments. The terminal ileum is then anastomosed to the dentate line of the anus.

Other Colonic Neoplasms

A variety of submucosal lesions that occur throughout the colon and rectum include lipomas, fibromas, leiomyomas, and carcinoids. Many are asymptomatic, but problems do occur, including blood loss secondary to ulceration or obstruction. Angiodysplasia or arteriovenous malformations may occur anywhere in the gastrointestinal tract. The most frequently encountered subset is an acquired lesion that tends to localize in the right colon. These malformations are thought to develop secondary to altered vascular dynamics in the bowel wall. They occur primarily in older patients, and there may also be an increased incidence in patients with aortic valvular disease and chronic renal failure. Angiodysplasias may cause chronic blood loss with anemia or acute hemorrhage and constitute the second leading cause of lower gastrointestinal hemorrhage in adults. Diagnosis of these lesions may be difficult, with angiography or endoscopy being most useful. When they have been identified, endoscopic coagulation or laser photoablation may be effective. Segmental resection is reserved for failure of endoscopic therapy, particularly in the presence of ongoing hemorrhage when definitive localization has been accomplished.

Gastrointestinal hemangiomas are less frequent than angiodysplasias and are most frequently of the cavernous type. They may be associated with similar lesions in the central nervous system or other organs. Because of their vascularity endoscopic coagulation should not be attempted. Segmental resection is the definitive treatment.

Kaposi's sarcoma is a neoplastic lesion associated with acquired immunodeficiency syndrome. Half of these lesions occur in the gastrointestinal tract, with most in the duodenum. Treatment is resection for relief of symptomatic lesions.

COLORECTAL MALIGNANCIES

Carcinoma of the colon and rectum is generally a disease of older individuals with equal incidence in males and females. In the general population the incidence of colon cancer begins to rise significantly after the age of 40 to 45 and increases each decade thereafter until it peaks at age 75.

Etiology

Several factors are associated with an increase in the incidence of colorectal malignancies as seen in Table

TABLE 5. RISK FACTORS FOR CARCINOMA OF THE COLON

Increasing age
Inflammatory bowel disease
Personal history of colonic carcinoma or adenoma
Family history of colonic carcinoma
Familial polyposis syndromes
History of breast of female genital carcinoma
Peutz-Jeghers syndrome

5 and include familial polyposis, as previously discussed, and ulcerative colitis. The incidence of colon cancer is five to ten times higher in colitis than in the general population, increasing about 10 years after the onset of the disease, and is estimated to be about 20 to 30 per cent at 20 years. High-risk groups include those with the onset of disease before the age of 25 and those with pancolitis and unremitting disease. Patients with longstanding colitis are often advised to undergo prophylactic colectomy. If colectomy is refused, aggressive colonoscopic surveillance with periodic biopsy is indicated. Granulomatous colitis is also generally associated with a higher risk of colon cancer, especially if onset is before the age of 21. Additional risk factors include a history of a previous colon cancer or adenoma. Families with a high incidence of carcinoma in other anatomic sites, such as the endometrium, ovary, and breast, also have a greater-than-average risk of colorectal carcinoma.

A number of environmental risk factors have been suggested to be related to the development of colorectal carcinoma. This is suggested by studies of those who immigrate from an area of low incidence, such as Japan, to an area of higher incidence, such as the United States. These individuals have a likelihood of developing colorectal cancer similar to that of the population of the new country, suggesting environmental and dietary influences. Dietary factors associated with a higher incidence of colorectal carcinoma include those with low dietary fiber and high dietary fat and sugar. Recent data regarding the pathogenesis of colorectal cancer at the molecular level have provided a greater understanding of the biology of these neoplasms. They provide possible explanations of the influence of diet and changes in the bowel microenvironment that lead to genetic changes required for malignant transformation.

Pathogenesis

A fundamental question in the development of colorectal neoplasms is the origin of the malignant cell. Colorectal neoplasias consist of different types of cellular elements, including the neoplastic epithelial cell, as well as a variety of interstitial elements and cell types such as blood vessels, leukocytes, and fibroblasts. Colorectal neoplasms have proven to be an excellent model for the study of the biology of cancer because they develop through clinically and histologically defined stages. Typically, colorectal neoplasias progress from normal epithelium to adenomas to invasive carcinomas. This sequential histologic progression forms the basis of the current clinical management of adenomatous polyps, in which they are removed to prevent progression to carcinoma.

In addition to the sequential histologic progression of tumor development, there are also well-described inherited syndromes associated with a high incidence of colorectal adenomas in addition to carcinomas. Therefore, these neoplasms constitute an ideal system for studying the genetic alterations responsible for tumor initiation and progression. Studies of tumors of various sizes and stages have revealed several basic principles underlying colorectal tumorigenesis, most notably the accumulation of somatically acquired mutations in colorectal adenomas and carcinomas that parallel the histologic progression of tumorigenesis. The paradigm of colorectal tumorigenesis is depicted in Table 6.

The basic principle in the development of colorectal neoplasia is the presence and accumulation of genetic changes, which were first noted by cytogenetic studies that often revealed chromosomal abnormalities, particularly involving chromosome 17 and 18. The importance of the presence of genetic changes was also supported by study of the allotype of neoplastic cells, which provides a molecular survey of a genome for allelic deletion. The detection of restriction fragment length polymorphisms (RFLPs) was used to determine whether one of the two parenteral alleles that were present in the DNA from the nonneoplastic mucosa was lost in DNA from the tumor. The absence of one band on the DNA blot has been called *allelic loss, allelic deletion, loss of heterozygosity* (LOH), or *reduction to homozygosity.*

Allelic loss was noted to be common, as one of the alleles of each chromosomal arm tested was lost in at least some colorectal carcinomas, while some tumors had losses from more than half of their loci. Two chromosomal regions, one, the short arm of chromosome 17 (17p), and the other, the long arm of chromosome 18 (18q), were found to be lost in over 75 per cent of colorectal carcinomas, and at least six additional loci were each lost in more than a quarter of the carcinomas. The deletions were noted to occur in neoplastic cells and were thought to be somatically acquired, rather than being inherited germ-line mutations present in normal tissue as well as neoplastic tissue.

Conceptually, the importance of the accumulation of genetic events is dependent on tumorigenesis being considered as a number of distinct cellular processes. Initiation of events that cause a single epithelial cell to become neoplastic are considered distinct events that can be followed by progression. Progression includes those additional changes that allow or propel the clonal population of neoplastic cells to increase their number and to behave more aggressively. Metastasis can also be considered a distinct event, as certain genetic alterations appear to be associated with the metastatic phenotype.

Each of the events appears to follow accumulated changes in both oncogenes and tumor suppressor genes. This concept is supported by data demonstrat-

TABLE 6. A GENETIC MODEL FOR COLORECTAL TUMORIGENESIS

Histologic Progression	Chromosome	Gene	Tumors with Mutations	Function
Normal epithelium	5	APC	> 70%	Tumor suppressor gene, unknown function
Hyperproliferative epithelium	Various	DNA hypomethylation	> 50%	Epigenetic event, may produce alterations in gene expression and chromatin structure
	18	DCC	> 70%	Tumor suppressor gene, cell adhesion molecule
Early adenoma	17	P53	> 70%	Tumor suppressor gene, regulates gene activity
	12	K-ras	50%	Oncogene, intracellular signaling molecule
Late adenoma	2	FCC	15%	Maintains DNA replication accuracy
	Various	Cyclins	4%	Oncogene, helps regulate cell cycle
Carcinoma	17	neu/erb-B2	2%	Oncogene, growth factor receptor
	8	myc	2%	Oncogene, regulates gene activity
Metastasis	Other chromosome loss			

Abbreviations: APC = adenomatous polyposis coli, DCC = deleted in colorectal carcinoma, FCC = familial colon cancer.

ing that adenomas have few allelic deletions, while many individual carcinomas have lost four to six markers, consistent with the estimates that this number of mutations was required for carcinoma formation. The theoretic basis for understanding allelic deletion lies in the hypothesis that some genes had a role in suppressing the occurrence of neoplasms. Mutations in such genes are recessive in that the neoplastic phenotype is not fully manifest until the occurrence of a second genetic event that inactivated the remaining wild type allele. In the complex regulation of cell growth, this inactivation may consist of an actual deletion or could follow the mutation of the remaining allele or other events in other genes that cause the functional inactivation of the remaining allele. The second event of chromosomal loss can be easily detected by RFLP analysis, since probes from any part of a lost chromosome region can reveal this event even when the relevant tumor suppressor gene is not yet known.

The natural extension of these observations was to determine the nature of the lost loci and the determination of the actual genes that are lost or mutated in colorectal carcinoma. This characterization has formed the basis of much of that currently known about colorectal neoplasia. Unfortunately, a homogeneous and restricted pattern of chromosome loss was not seen in all colorectal cancers studied, although there were some frequent regions lost on chromosome 17p and 18q. This heterogeneity likely underlies the biologic heterogeneity of colorectal carcinoma with respect to a myriad of parameters, such as response to therapy, nodal and distant metastases, tumor growth rate and so forth. A brief discussion of the genetic changes important in the initiation and progression of colorectal neoplasia and genes associated with colorectal neoplasia follows, beginning with the tumor suppressor genes found on chromosome 17p and 18q, which have now been identified as p53 and the *deleted in colorectal carcinoma* (DCC) gene.

The p53 Gene

The p53 gene on chromosome 17 was originally studied as a tumor-associated antigen, and its specific function is currently not well characterized. In adenomas and carcinomas with an allelic loss of 17p, there was variation of both the size and boundaries of the deleted area. However, a region of DNA was identified that formed the consensus deletion, which happened to contain the p53 locus. To definitely exclude or implicate p53 as a critical target, functional deletion of the remaining allele via mutation needed to be documented. This functional deletion is consistent with the hypothesis that both copies of a putative tumor suppressor gene must be deleted to confer the malig-

nant phenotype. To test this hypothesis, the remaining copies of p53 from colorectal tumors were studied and found to contain point mutations at one or more sites. Further tests confirm the absence of these mutations in the normal DNA of the patients, demonstrating that the point mutations in p53 were somatic mutations selected for during tumor progression.

Sequencing of the p53 gene from a variety of human tumor types has subsequently shown p53 point mutations to be common among carcinomas in which one allele has been removed by allelic deletion. The p53 mutations in colorectal, breast, lung, brain, and other tumors are clustered in four hot spots that coincide with the four most evolutionary preserved regions of the gene. Confirming its presumptive classification as a tumor suppressor gene, transfection (introduction of DNA into cells) of the wild type p53 gene has been recently found to suppress the growth of human colorectal carcinoma cells in vitro, as well as in rodent cells transfected with various oncogenes.

The DCC Gene

The DCC gene was discovered following intensive study of the consensus region of deletion in 18q. In one case, a tumor had lost not only one but both the normal allelic markers detected by a DNA probe. Such homozygous deletions are rare but usually occur at sites of ostensible tumor suppressor genes, including the retinoblastoma gene. Eventually the gene was cloned and named DCC.

Once the DCC gene was identified, additional somatic alterations of the gene were found in colorectal carcinomas, further implicating it in the tumorigenic process. Moreover, it was found that the gene was expressed in nearly all normal adult tissues, including the colon and rectum, but that the expression was reduced or absent in most colorectal carcinomas consistent with a normal suppressor role. The DCC gene encodes a protein with sequence similarity to the cell adhesion protein N-CAM, as well as to other related cell surface proteins. It is provocative that alteration in a cell adhesion molecule might have a role in tumorigenesis. Neoplasia is often associated with alterations of such cell interactions, and intracellular adhesion mediated by cellular adhesion molecules can influence cellular differentiation. One form of Lynch syndrome (nonpolyposis hereditary colon cancer) has been genetically linked to the Kidd blood group, which was located near the DCC gene on 18q. This has suggested that germ-line mutations in the DCC gene might be responsible for predisposition to this form of inherited colon cancer.

Other genes felt to be important in the progression to malignancy in the colon include the *adenematous polyposis coli* (APC) gene, the DCC gene, the p53 gene, DNA hypomethylation, and K-*ras* mutations, the FCC gene, cyclins, the *neu*/erb-B2 gene, and *myc* genes, some of which are discussed below.

The APC Gene

The gene responsible for familial APC has been mapped to chromosome 5q. In cases of APC, the colon and rectum generally develop hundreds of adenomas often carpeting the luminal surface of the bowel. If the large intestine is not surgically removed within the first few decades of life, 100 per cent of these patients develop carcinoma. The APC gene was localized following the report of a man having both APC and mental retardation. Retardation in association with inherited syndromes often indicates the loss of a significant amount of chromosomal material, which could be detected by karyotyping, and the patient was found to have a deletion on the long arm of chromosome 5. This stimulated confirmation and refinement of the gene localization through linkage analysis with a number of DNA markers on chromosome 5q. Allelic losses of the region of chromosome 5q containing the APC gene were found in approximately 35 per cent of sporadic carcinomas.

The *ras* Gene

The *ras* gene is the only oncogene noted to be involved in a large fraction of colorectal tumors. The three major members of the *ras* gene family in normal human cells are termed K-*ras*, H-*ras*, and N-*ras* proto-oncogenes. Mutant forms of *ras* genes, termed *ras* oncogenes, were initially found by transfection experiments in which DNA from tumors introduced into murine fibroblast cells caused the transformation to a tumorigenic phenotype. Transfection, however, proved to be an insensitive method for the detection of *ras* oncogenes, especially the larger K-*ras* gene. Consequently, the initial studies of colorectal carcinomas did not detect *ras* mutations. Their detection awaited a discovery of more sensitive techniques, such as polymerase chain reaction (PCR), allele-specific oligonucleotide hybridization, and RNA mismatched cleavage.

Codons 12 and 13 of the human K-*ras* gene were found to be frequent targets for point mutation, and such mutations are found in approximately 50 per cent of the intermediate- and late-stage adenomas, as well as in carcinomas. Their low frequency in small adenomas, however, has indicated that while *ras* mutations are involved in the progression of adenomas, they do not often have a role in their initiation. Nor have *ras* mutations held promise for prognostic applications: their occurrence has not been associated with

pathologic classification or the malignant potential of colorectal carcinomas. This was as expected: genetic alterations that occur relatively early in tumorigenesis might be less likely to affect the metastatic capability of tumors than those mutations occurring late in the process, such as those involving p53 or DCC. A recent case-control study and meta-analysis investigating the associations between rare mutant alleles in the H-*ras*-1 minisatellite locus and various forms of cancer revealed that these alleles represent a major risk factor for colorectal carcinoma.

DNA Hypomethylation

DNA is consistently hypomethylated in colorectal tumors of all stages and, therefore, is a very early event in neoplasia. The methylation state of DNA can be studied through two methods, by a chemical assay or by observation of changes in the ability of some restriction enzymes to cleave DNA that is methylated. The degree of loss in colorectal carcinomas is in the range of 10 to 20 million methyl groups per cell. Methylation changes are referred to as epigenetic events. They do not change the sequence of base pairs, but may produce alterations in gene expression and chromatin structure. There is some evidence that hypomethylation is associated with increased stickiness of chromatin during mitosis-impairing segregation. Thus, hypomethylation in tumors has been proposed to promote aberrant segregation of chromosomal regions, leading to the loss of wild-type tumor suppressor genes.

The Familial Colon Cancer Gene

In 1993, a gene was discovered that was postulated to confer susceptibility to colon cancer and was named the *familial colon cancer* (FCC) gene. It was initially estimated to be carried by one person in every 200 in western populations and was thought to have a novel way of functioning, unlike the traditional oncogenes or tumor suppressor genes. Investigators had noted that cells from some colon cancers display a high degree of genetic instability, marked by numerous mutations throughout the genome. This implies that the FCC gene causes the instability.

Researchers used probes developed to detect microsatellite DNA (short, repetitive DNA sequences) that are interspersed throughout the genome. These sequences may vary in length from one individual to the other, which makes them informative as markers for genetic linkage studies. After testing close to 350 markers, researchers linked a microsatellite marker on chromosome 2 to the FCC gene. This was unexpected because until this point, there had not been a suspicion of a genetic link to colon cancer at that location. In addition, researchers found that the microsatellite DNA at the chromosome 2 marker site varied in length from tumor to tumor, indicating that it had lost or gained nucleotides. Taken together, this suggested that mutation in the regions were widespread in the genome. Although a number of fundamental biologic questions may be answered by an understanding of how this gene functions, knowledge regarding the mere presence of the gene may be useful in the near future. Once the gene itself is isolated, it may be possible to screen populations to determine individuals at high-risk. Surveillance and surgical management of these high-risk populations may identify, and permit the treatment of, precancerous lesions and, indeed, reduce the death rate attributed to colon cancer.

Order of Accumulated Mutations

The genetic alterations noted above occur in a preferential order. Hypoproliferation of the nonneoplastic mucosa may precede the formation of adenomas as shown by in situ DNA labeling of colonic epithelium. In tumorigenesis, hypomethylation and FCC mutations may be very early and *ras* mutations and chromosome 5q allelic losses generally precede 18q allelic losses, which in turn precede 17p allelic deletion. Studies of the coincident presence of *ras* mutations and allelic deletions of chromosomes 5q, 17p, and 18q reveal that only 9 per cent of small adenomas have more than one mutation, while more than 90 per cent of carcinomas have two or more alterations. Middle- and late-stage adenomas had accumulated the number of mutations intermediate between that of small adenomas and carcinomas. However, the order of these mutations with respect to one another is not invariant, as shown by study of different stages of neoplasia present in the same tumor. Thus, detailed analysis at different stages of tumor development strongly suggests that it is the total accumulation of changes, not their order with respect to one another, that is most important.

The studies noted above have provided a theoretic framework for understanding the nature of colorectal neoplasia. Each adenoma appears to arise from a single epithelial cell of a mucosal crypt, and tumor progression represents the selection for a clonal predominance of those cells that have acquired certain additional mutations. The acquisition of multiple changes in an adenoma increases the likelihood of its progression to the carcinoma, whereas in a carcinoma, the more advanced degrees of genetic change are associated with metastatic behavior.

Clinical Features

The clinical features of colorectal carcinomas are related to the tumor size and location. Some 70 to 80 per cent of these lesions are located below the mid-descending colon. Tumors in this location are often infiltrating or annular and may cause obstructive symptoms, changes in bowel habits, or bleeding. Due to the semisolid or solid contents and the small diameter in this location, gas pains, a decrease in caliber of the stool, and the use of laxatives are common symptoms.

In the right colon, large bulky tumors are more common, due perhaps to the wide diameter of the colon and its liquid contents, which allow growth into the lumen without symptoms of obstruction. Patients may complain of abdominal pain that may be confused with gallbladder or peptic ulcer disease, or may have bleeding, weight loss, or anemia.

Screening

The American Gastroenterologic Association supports the following recommendations for screening for colorectal carcinoma: digital rectal examination and testing for fecal occult blood annually beginning at age 40, with flexible sigmoidoscopy beginning at age 50 for individuals at average risk. A negative endoscopy in 2 consecutive years is followed by endoscopy every 3 years thereafter. Patients in high-risk groups include those with ulcerative colitis, Crohn's disease, previous colorectal carcinoma, familial colon cancer, Gardner's syndrome, and familial polyposis, and these require earlier and more frequent endoscopic examination.

Diagnosis

The diagnosis of colorectal carcinomas requires a high index of suspicion and evaluation of all symptoms, especially in high-risk patients. Tests for fecal blood is usually accomplished using Hemoccult guaiac-impregnated paper. Proctosigmoidoscopy is an important diagnostic tool in the symptomatic patient, and flexible instruments have much better patient tolerance and a marked increase in diagnostic accuracy.

Colonoscopy is frequently used to evaluate all patients with symptoms or occult fecal blood, as lesions can be detected and biopsied or excised. Limitations include failure to evaluate the splenic or hepatic flexure or cecum. However, these technical considerations depend on having a well-trained endoscopist perform the procedure. Barium enema with air contrast is complementary to colonoscopy and usually detects all colonic lesions that are at least 5 mm in diameter (Fig. 11). Contraindications include acute, severe inflammatory bowel disease, suspected perforation, and recent injury to the bowel wall.

The entire colon must be evaluated for synchronous lesions when a tumor is found. Complete blood count,

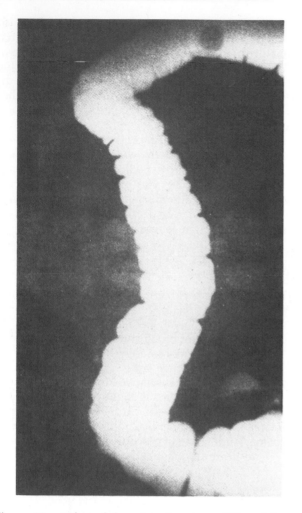

Figure 11. Polyp of the colon showing a filling defect on barium enema. (From Block GE, Lichty RD: Large intestine. *In* Lichty RD, Soper RT [eds]: Synopsis of Surgery. St Louis, CB Mosby Company, 1980, with permission.)

blood chemistries, chest films, liver function studies, urinalysis, and carcinoembryonic antigen (CEA) titer are routinely obtained preoperatively. If symptoms are present or if results of the blood tests suggest further studies, they can be obtained, including abdominal CT scan, MRI, or intravenous pyelogram.

The true extent of disease can be determined only after resection and examination of the specimen with staging. Carcinoma of the colon and rectum extends by six routes: intramucosal extension, direct invasion of adjacent structures, lymphatic spread, hematogenous spread, intraperitoneal spread, and anastomotic implantation. The modes and routes of spread must be considered in deciding on the appropriate surgical extirpation to provide the highest cure rate and to appropriately stage the patient.

Treatment

The objective of therapy is excision of the primary lesion with adequate margins of normal tissue. Almost 90 per cent of patients have tumors that can be resected completely, and the mortality ranges from 2 to 10 per cent. The critical determinant of success is the degree to which the tumor has spread at the time of operation. The principles of surgical resection include excision of the primary lesion with adequate margins, restoration of continuity of the intestine, and maintenance of function whenever possible with minimal morbidity and mortality. The various routes of tumor spread must be considered, including neural, venous, implantation, and direct extension.

The exact surgical procedure is dependent on location of the tumor in the colon. Preoperatively, the patient undergoes bowel preparation. Patients should be psychologically prepared if either a temporary or permanent colostomy is anticipated. They also should be counseled about postoperative sexual dysfunction if extensive pelvic dissection is anticipated. Wide margins surrounding the primary tumor must be removed with an en bloc resection of the draining lymphatics. This necessity to remove the draining lymphatics necessitates interruption of blood supply to a region of the colon, as the lymphatic drainage parallels the blood supply.

Employing the principles described above, the standard treatment of neoplasms of the cecum and ascending colon is right colectomy, which includes a segment of the terminal ileum, the cecum, and the right half of the transverse colon and removal of the corresponding mesocolon and a space around the superior mesenteric artery at the origin of the middle colic vessels (Fig. 12). Carcinomas of the splenic flexure or descending colon are treated by excision of the distal transverse, descending, and sigmoid colon, together with the associated mesocolon excised to the aorta (Fig. 13). For tumors of the sigmoid colon, the proximal resection can be limited, and the transverse colon need not necessarily be removed (Fig. 14). For carcinomas in the upper rectum, an anterior resection and reanastomosis can be performed; however, preservation of the distal rectum to provide continence is extremely important, and a detailed discussion follows regarding the preservation of the rectum for mid and low rectal carcinomas.

In tumors involving the upper rectum, a low anterior colon resection may be performed with a distal margin of 2 inches or 5 cm as seen in Figure 15. Distal intramural spread of cancer is usually restricted, and a 5 cm segment of normal colon or rectum is adequate as a resection margin. Although lymphatic spread may occur downward, it has been shown that upward and lateral displacement through superior, hemorrhoidal, mortality between the two approaches, with a slightly superior survival rate in patients having anterior resections, although it is probably related to the smaller tumor size in those having anterior resections. Local recurrence rates have ranged from 7 to 20 per cent for patients with LAR and APR.

New combined-treatment modalities have allowed some surgeons to perform sphincter-sparing operations for rectal carcinomas that would have previously been managed by APR. These modalities include preoperative radiotherapy combined with chemotherapy. The response of the tumor mass may allow previously unresectable lesions to be removed and may permit LAR to be performed rather than an APR. Long-term follow-up studies demonstrating an improvement in survival have not yet been performed, but short-term results suggest that a decrease in the local recurrence rate may be achieved by neoadjuvant therapy in selected patients.

As an alternative to both LAR or APR, local excision has been advocated by some workers in patients with small, well-differentiated lesions limited to the

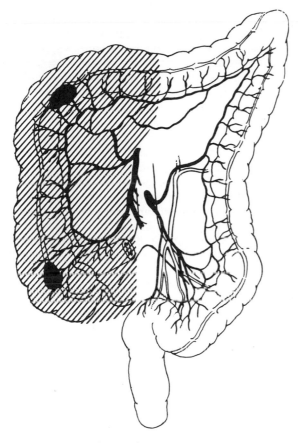

Figure 12. Right hemicolectomy. (From Stearns M, Schottenfeld D: Techniques for the surgical management of colon. Cancer 28:165, 1971, with permission.)

and inferior mesenteric lymphatics is by far the most important type of spread. Therefore, the decision to perform an *abdominoperineal resection* (APR) or a *low anterior resection* (LAR) is determined primarily by the distance of the lower border of the cancer from the anus. The lateral pelvic extension of the two operations, both of which remove the upper lymphatic drainage areas, is essentially the same.

In general, tumors within 7 to 8 cm of the anal verge are treated by APR, whereas those greater than 12 cm from the anal verge are adequately managed by LAR. Lesions lying between 7 and 11 cm from the anal verge may be managed by either procedure, depending on the size of the lesion, the size of the pelvis, and the differentiation of the tumor. In general, a lesion that is easily palpated with the examining finger is often removed by APR. However, if the neoplasm can be delivered to the level of the abdominal incision following mobilization of the rectum, an adequate resection may be performed. The use of circumferential stapling devices greatly facilitates the construction of the LAR.

In many series, there is no difference in operative

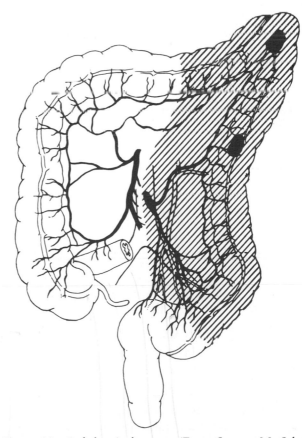

Figure 13. Left hemicolectomy. (From Stearns M, Schottenfeld D: Techniques for the surgical management of colon. Cancer 28:167, 1971, with permission.)

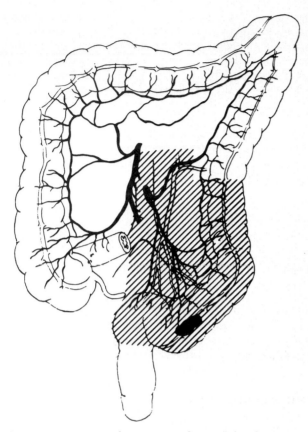

Figure 14. Segmental resection of sigmoid colon. (From Stearns M, Schottenfeld D: Techniques for the surgical management of colon. Cancer 28:177, 1971, with permission.)

mucosa (T1 lesions). In patients with compromised cardiovascular status or other comorbid conditions, selective local therapy may be considered in lesions with favorable characteristics. Whereas a number of techniques have been described for improving the results of surgical excision and preservation of the sphincter in these patients, data are sparse as to their true efficacy. Neoadjuvant therapy including preoperative chemotherapy and preoperative radiotherapy is being evaluated at this time to determine its role for carcinoma of the rectum.

Complicated Colon Cancers

Complete intestinal obstruction occurs in 8 to 23 per cent of patients with colorectal cancer and usually presents with abdominal pain. Patients with obstructing cancers have a generally poor prognosis with overall mortality rate of 15 per cent and a higher postoperative complication rate. The high perioperative mortality is probably due to the inability to perform an adequate bowel preparation, as the patients who survive operation compare with patients' survival fol-

lowing elective colon resection. The most critical determinant of long-term survival after a successful emergency operation is the pathologic stage of the lesion.

In contradistinction to colonic obstruction, colonic perforation tends to increase operative and perioperative morbidity and mortality and decrease long-term survival. Operative mortalities of over 30 per cent with 5-year survivals less than 10 per cent have been reported. This may be related to peritoneal seeding of colon cancer cells following perforation. Surgical management of acute obstruction or perforation due to carcinoma of the colon must rely on the judgment and experience of the surgeon who must consider the dilation and viability of the bowel, the physical status of the patient with associated comorbidities, and the degree of contamination. Usually a resection of the primary carcinoma can be accomplished with a proximal diverting colostomy. Resection is preferable if more than minimal survival is expected, because large fungating colon cancers may bleed, possibly requiring more invasive intervention.

Direct extension of colon and rectal cancer to adjacent organs necessitates en bloc resection of these organs, as the adhesions are usually filled with tumor cells. Although the number of patients in whom extended surgical procedures for colon cancer is relatively small, several features should be considered when extensive lesions are encountered. It has been established that the size of the primary lesion is not a determinant of regional metastases; thus, finding a direct extension of a cancer into an adjacent organ is not statistically a more adverse prognostic sign than regional lymph node metastasis. In fact, advanced colorectal tumors that have invaded other organs but have not metastasized to the lymph nodes may have favorable biologic characteristics. A series of patients with extended resections that usually include colectomy and partial or total excision of an invaded organ has been reported advocating an aggressive approach to locally advanced disease. Response of the tumor to preoperative radiotherapy may allow tumors fixed to adjacent bony structures to be resected.

Bilateral oophorectomy is recommended in all postmenopausal women with carcinoma of the colon to decrease the morbidity of neoplastic change. It should be considered in all premenopausal women with ovarian abnormalities at operation or in the presence of peritoneal implants.

Pathologic Staging and Survival

The original system was developed by Dukes and was further modified by Astler and Collier in 1954. Most recently the TNM system has been recommended by the American Joint Committee on Cancer

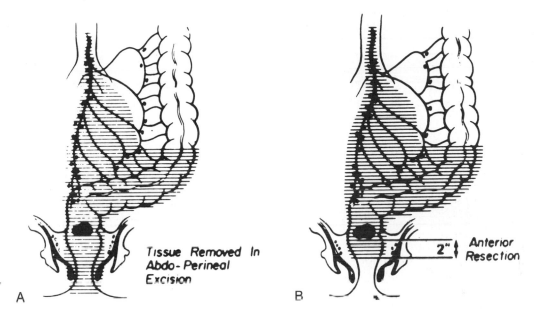

Figure 15. The shaded area shows the extent of removal for carcinoma of the upper rectum by abdominal perineal resection (*A*), and by anterior resection (*B*). Note the necessity for a 2-inch or 5-cm margin to the lesion in an anterior resection. If this cannot be accomplished, an abdominoperineal resection of the rectum should be performed. (From Butcher HR Jr: Carcinoma of the rectum: Choice between anterior resection and abdominoperineal resection of the rectum. Cancer 28:204, 1971, with permission.)

(Table 7). A number of new technologies are being applied to these tumors in the hope of obtaining better prognostic information. A comparison of current staging systems with their associated 5-year survival is depicted in Table 8.

TABLE 7.   TNM CANCER CLASSIFICATION SYSTEM

Primary Tumor (T)

Tx	Primary tumor cannot be assessed
T0	No evidence of primary tumor
Tis	Carcinoma in situ
T1	Tumor invades submucosa
T2	Tumor invades muscularis propria
T3	Tumor invades through the muscularis propria into the subserosa or into nonperitonealized pericolic or perirectal tissue
T4	Tumor perforates the visceral peritoneum or directly invades other organs or structures (including invasion of other segments of the colon across serosa)

Regional Lymph Node (N)

NX	Regional lymph nodes cannot be assessed
N0	No regional lymph node metastasis
N1	Metastasis to 1 to 3 pericolic or perirectal lymph nodes
N2	Metastasis to 4 or more pericolic or perirectal lymph nodes
N3	Metastasis to any lymph node along the course of a named vascular trunk

Distant Metastases (M)

MX	Presence of distant metastasis cannot be assessed
M0	No distant metastasis
M1	Distant metastasis

Postoperative Follow-up

Colonoscopy or barium enema for imaging the entire colon is recommended in the postoperative period usually within 2 to 3 months. Colonoscopy should be repeated annually for at least the first 4 years following the resection. Routine physical examination with complete blood count and liver function tests should be obtained every 3 months for 2 years, then every 6 months for 2 years, then annually. A chest film should be obtained every 6 months for 3 years, then annually. Carcinoembryonic antigen levels should be assessed every 3 months for 2 years, then every 4 months for 2 years, then annually.

Operations for Metastatic Disease

Despite complete preoperative evaluation, the identification of metastatic disease at the time of laparotomy is not uncommon. Excision of the primary lesion is desirable if only for prevention of obstruction in the future, even in the presence of widespread metastatic disease. If resection is not possible, proximal diverting colostomy is indicated. In patients with rectal lesions and accompanying tenesmus or bleeding, abdominoperineal resection can be used as a palliative procedure.

A single small hepatic metastatic lesion can be considered for resection at the time of treatment of the

TABLE 8. COMPARISON OF CURRENT STAGE GROUPING

Stage Grouping				5-Year Survival	Dukes Stage	Description of Astler-Coller Modification of Dukes Classification of Colon Carcinoma	5-Year Survival
Stage 0	Tis	N0	M0				
Stage I	T1	N0	M0	70%	Stage A	Limited to mucosa	93–100%
	T2	N0	M0		Stage B1	Extending to muscularis propria but not through it; negative lymph nodes	67–85%
Stage II	T3	N0	M0	58%	Stage B2	Penetrating muscularis propria and extending into serosa; negative lymph nodes	54–63%
	T4	N0	M0				
Stage III	T1,T2	Any N	M0	25–33%	Stage C1	Extending to muscularis propria but not through it; positive lymph nodes	43–55%
	T3,T4	Any N	M0		Stage C2	Penetrating muscularis propria and extending into serosa; positive lymph nodes	23–28%
Stage IV	Any T	Any N	M1	6%	Stage D	Distant metastasis	0–6%

primary tumor. This can be accomplished with a wedge resection and minimal morbidity. The performance of a hepatic lobectomy concurrently with a colon resection is not indicated. Identification of a single large hepatic metastasis should prompt a curative colon procedure to be followed by complete imaging work-up and possible hepatic resection at a later date. Although it seems likely that operative resection of metastatic disease would have minimal impact on long-term survival, many authors have demonstrated that the judicious application of resection for metastatic colon cancer can prolong life. In general, the metastases must be confined to one organ, and single lesions are associated with a better prognosis than multiple lesions.

It is usually not necessary to perform formal anatomic liver resections to remove metastatic liver disease; however, a margin of uninvolved liver should be excised along with the tumor. Patients with unresectable hepatic metastases have been treated with a number of modalities including hepatic intra-arterial chemotherapy. However, because of toxicity of therapy and the inability to demonstrate a clear survival advantage from intra-arterial 5-fluorouracil (5-FU), this approach remains investigational. Other forms of therapy for hepatic metastases include cryotherapy for nonresectable lesions.

Isolated pulmonary metastases occur in less than 10 per cent of patients with metastases, but 5-year relapse-free survivals have been reported following pulmonary resection confined to the lungs. Patients considered for these procedures must have no evidence of hepatic metastases, and often a laparoscopy is advocated prior to thoracotomy to examine the liver. If enteroabdominal disease is not present, a thoracotomy as planned is continued.

In the presence of multiple unresectable metastases, the management of the primary colon cancer consists of resection of the primary lesion. Although the survival is determined by the metastases, it has been demonstrated that those who undergo primary resection have a more favorable course due to the prevention of anemia, protein loss, obstruction, and pain. Anastomotic recurrences represent a major form of treatment failure and occur in 2 to 15 per cent of all curative resections. Reexploration is necessary to determine resectability. Patients who develop local recurrence after LAR usually may need to undergo APR for achievement of local control.

Adjuvant Therapy

Both radiation therapy and chemotherapy have been used in the adjuvant setting following resection of colon cancer with high risks of recurrence. Radiation therapy has been used to minimize local regional recurrence. While radiation therapy directed at reducing regional recurrence has met with some success, data on whole abdominal radiation for patients is equivocal.

Adjuvant Systemic Therapy

Some 50 to 60 per cent of patients with colorectal cancer have tumors that penetrate the serosa or involve the regional lymph nodes. Most tumors in this category eventually recur and end fatally. Therefore, adjuvant therapy to improve the mortality was sought for this group of patients. *5-Fluorouracil* is the most active drug used against colon cancer, but it achieves only a 10 to 20 per cent response in patients with advanced disease. *Levamisole* is thought to be an immunomodulating agent in advanced colorectal carcinoma. Randomized controlled trials of 5-FU with levamisole, levamisole alone, and surgery in patients with Dukes B2 or C colon cancer were performed and demonstrated that levamisole plus 5-FU and levamisole improve disease-free survival for patients with Dukes B and C lesions. Subsequent analysis demonstrated that Dukes C patients receiving levamisole and 5-FU also had slightly prolonged survival.

A larger, confirmatory intergroup trial was launched that demonstrated that in patients with Dukes C carcinomas of the colon, adjuvant treatment for 1 year with levamisole combined with 5-FU reduced the risk of cancer recurrence by 41 per cent, with overall mortality reduced by 33 per cent, but the results in patients with Dukes B2 disease was equivocal.

Current recommendations for adjuvant therapy are based on the efficacy of adjuvant therapy and the risk of treatment failure. Patients with stage I or Dukes A and B1 disease are at low risk of recurrence and should not receive adjuvant treatment. Optional adjuvant therapy for stage II and stage III colon cancer has been advised due to the higher risk of recurrence. Based on the current clinical trial data, stage III or Dukes C patients unable to enter clinical trials should be offered adjuvant 5-FU and levamisole, as it was administered by the intergroup trial. Specific adjuvant therapy for Dukes 2 or B2 patients has not been recommended by the National Institutes of Health outside of clinical trials. However, ongoing and further trials are apt to modify these recommendations.

Adjuvant Liver Infusion Therapy

Since the liver is the predominant site of distal failure in colon cancer, eradication of micrometastases in the liver in the perioperative period is felt to be a reasonable approach to the treatment of colon cancer. Studies have shown improved survival and decreased liver recurrence following portal vein infusion of 5-FU beginning within 5 days of operation. Other confirmatory trials have revealed a uniform lack of benefit in reducing liver recurrence. Adjuvant portal vein infusion may be a complex way to deliver systemic therapy and is not recommended outside of a clinical trial setting at this time.

Preoperative Radiotherapy of Rectal Cancer

Because neither APR nor LAR resection eliminate local recurrence in the pelvis, especially in patients with stage III or Dukes C disease, investigators have attempted to add other treatments to improve local control of rectal cancer. In theory, administration of preoperative radiotherapy has the advantage that undisturbed oxygenated tissues are more susceptible to ionizing radiation than the vascular planes created by operation and treated with postoperative radiation. Furthermore, more than two thirds of nodal metastases are less than 4 mm in diameter and may be controlled by radiotherapy.

The results of preoperative radiotherapy include significant downstaging of regional disease. However, there has not been any significant improvement in local control or survival in randomized trials of preoperative radiotherapy using relatively low doses to the tumor and pelvis. Therefore, higher doses of radiotherapy have been applied where 40 to 50 Gy have been used, with the performance of sphincter-saving operations for low and midrectal carcinomas with good results. Relatively few patients have undergone local excision after preoperative radiotherapy, possibly because healing in the irradiated field was difficult.

While preoperative radiotherapy may decrease local recurrence, some feel that it may downstage the disease and hinder healing. Further clinical trials may resolve the utility of preoperative radiotherapy, and clinical trials are currently in progress to evaluate the role of radiotherapy combined with chemotherapy in the treatment of rectal carcinomas.

Postoperative Radiotherapy of Rectal Cancer

Although the role of neoadjuvant therapy for rectal carcinoma is being investigated, radiotherapy should be part of the postoperative adjuvant therapy for rectal cancer that has penetrated the rectal wall or metastasized to regional nodes. Postoperative radiotherapy combined with chemotherapy using 5-FU and methyl CCNU (semustine) significantly decreases local recurrence in patients with stage II and III or Dukes B2 and C lesions in the rectum. This has translated into a significant improvement in survival. Thus, the standard of practice for adenocarcinomas of the rectum that penetrate the rectal wall or involve regional lymph nodes is radical resection followed by chemotherapy and radiotherapy.

Limited Resection of Rectal Carcinoma

Although the role of combined therapy has been directed toward prolonging survival and reducing recurrences, preservation of organs and function is also considered a goal of cancer therapy. With this perspective, limited resection to preserve the anus and continence has been advocated. In the narrow confines of the pelvis, a local excision of a primary carcinoma with en bloc removal of mesorectal fat may have a lateral margin that is comparable to that of a standard radical resection. In patients that were carefully selected to minimize the chance of lymph node metastasis, it may be possible to locally excise rectal carcinomas and achieve cure rates similar to those of radical resection. With this policy, T1 and T2 low rectal cancers have been locally excised, with survival rates at 2 years that are comparable to those achieved with radical resection. Excision is usually performed by the transanal approach. However, other sphincter-preserving approaches may be utilized, including transsacral resection. Low resections with coloanal anastomosis are also used to preserve continence. Long-term follow-up to determine the role of these lesions is required. The roles of adjuvant chemotherapy and radiotherapy, along with local excision and sphincter-sparing operations, `are currently being studied.

Squamous Cell Carcinoma of the Anus

Anal carcinoma is relatively uncommon, but squamous cell carcinoma comprises about 70 per cent of all anal cases. The most common treatment for these lesions has been surgical excision by APR, but the results have been disappointing, with 5-year survival rates of 24 to 62 per cent. Combination therapy using radiation therapy and chemotherapy has improved the survival to up to 83 per cent and is now the treatment of choice for this disease. The area of the primary lesion is biopsied, and the patient begins radiotherapy to the pelvis. If inguinal lymph nodes are enlarged, they are also biopsied, usually by fine-needle aspiration, and if positive, they are included in the field of radiation.

Following radiation therapy, the patients receive intravenous 5-FU and mitomycin C. Following treatment, a biopsy of the lesion is obtained. If residual tumor is present, salvage radiotherapy and chemotherapy is given. A biopsy of the tumor site is repeated, and if negative, no further treatment is given. If residual tumor is present, an APR is performed. If enlarged lymph nodes remain after treatment, a node dissection on the side of the abnormality is indicated.

Patients who fail therapy have limited options, including additional chemotherapy or radiotherapy. Salvage therapy may also include APR, lymphadenectomy, or a diverting colostomy, depending on the nature of the recurrence.

DISEASES OF THE RECTUM AND ANUS

Hemorrhoids

Internal hemorrhoids are dilated veins of the superior and middle rectal plexuses that occur above the dentate line and underlying mucosa. External hemorrhoids are dilated inferior rectal veins that lie below the dentate line and are covered by squamous epithelium. The most common causes of hemorrhoids are those that increase pressure in the venous plexuses and include constipation, straining at stool, hereditary varicose tendencies, pregnancy, prolonged upright position, abdominal or pelvic tumors, and portal hypertension. The usual symptoms of hemorrhoids include protrusion, bleeding, dull pain, and pruritus. Thrombosis or acute prolapse with edema and ulceration is extremely painful. Internal hemorrhoids are asymptomatic except when they prolapse and become strangulated. The only significant sign caused by internal hemorrhoids is painless bright red bleeding per rectum during or after defecation.

Hemorrhoidal thrombosis is a common event and can occur in the external anal plexus under the squamous mucosa. External anal thrombosis of hemorrhoids is common and is often seen in patients with no other stigmata of hemorrhoids and may be due to the high venous pressure that develops during excessive straining efforts, leading to distention and stasis. The patient may notice an acute swelling at the anal verge that may be extremely painful. The pain may continue for several days and then gradually subside; however, edema may be present for 3 to 4 weeks. The treatment of thrombosis is usually symptomatic, as the condition usually resolves in a relatively short time. However, the hemorrhoid may be incised with enucleation of the clot under local anesthesia for relief of severe pain and is usually instantly successful. Thrombosis of the internal hemorrhoidal plexus is usually manifest by severe anal pain followed by protrusion of the thrombosed area. This pain may be severe, acute, and prolonged, lasting as long as 1 week. The edema may gradually subside, and the thrombosis is absorbed. Surgical therapy is reserved for severe symptoms.

The treatment of hemorrhoids involves a variety of techniques listed in Table 9. The common rationale behind all of these treatments is to ablate the dilated hemorrhoidal venous plexus, either by reducing traction due to straining at defecation or by causing fibrosis or necrosis of the tissue surrounding the hemorrhoid or the mucosa overlying the hemorrhoid. Operative therapy is generally reserved for those patients who have permanent descent of the anal mucosa coupled with gross hemorrhoidal protrusion in defecation.

Hemorrhoidectomy may be complicated by bleeding, which is usually secondary to a technical error in establishing hemostasis. Urinary retention is not infrequent and may be due to spasm, overhydration, excess sedation, or prostatic obstruction. Fecal impaction may occasionally occur, usually due to the patient's fear of pain on defecation.

Anal Fissures

Anal fissures are ulcers in the anal mucosa that commonly arise from trauma secondary to constipation, hard feces, cryptitis (in which the anal crypts become

TABLE 9. TREATMENT OF HEMORRHOIDS

Treatment	Rationale
Bowel Regulation A firm bulky stool can be accomplished by dietary manipulation increasing fiber or the use of bulk laxative	This will relieve straining on defecation preventing descent of the pelvic floor, weakening of the sphincter and rectal muscles, and gynecologic prolapse
Injection Therapy 5% phenol and vegetable oil or 5% quinine urea hydrochloride is injected around the pedicle of each hemorrhoid; the injection is placed in the submucosa of the upper anal canal above the sensitive squamous epithelium	Injection therapy should cause sclerosis in the surrounding tissue, resulting in fibrosis of these tissues and obliteration of the hemorrhoid
Rubber Band Ligation The upper portion of the mucocutaneous line is grasped and a small rubber band is slipped over the hemorrhoid; the tissue distal to the rubber band undergoes necrosis; if the rubber band is too close to the dentate line, pain results and immediate removal and reapplication of the rubber band slightly higher is necessary	Excess mucosa in the upper canal is removed and the lower anal mucosa is reduced by fibrosis, which also causes adherence of the mucosa to the underlying muscle
Cryotherapy The upper portion of the mucocutaneous line is grasped and the hemorrhoid tissue is frozen using a liquid nitrogen probe; the tissue that is frozen undergoes necrosis	Excess mucosa in the upper canal is removed and the lower anal mucosa is reduced by fibrosis, which also causes adherence of the mucosa to the underlying muscle
Operative Therapy The base of the hemorrhoidal mass is grasped with a clamp and retracted; an elliptical excision is made through the skin and mucosa about the hemorrhoidal plexus, which is dissected and excised en masse; the mucosa and anal skin are closed longitudinally with a running absorbable suture	All of the vascular hemorrhoidal tissue in the submucosa is removed as is all the prolapsed rectal mucosa; excision of the tissue is coupled with the reconstruction of the deformed mucosa; this is usually the only therapy that is effective if hemorrhoidal protrusion is associated with permanent descent of the anal mucosa

inflamed and subsequently develop a mucosal break), and ulceration of mucosa covering a thrombosed hemorrhoid. Spasm of the internal sphincters sustains these fissures. Excruciating pain during and after defecation is the most common symptom and may be associated with varying degrees of bleeding. Gentle examination of the anus usually reveals the fissure, and anoscopy after local anesthesia may confirm the diagnosis.

Anal fissures are usually treated by anal hygiene, hot sitz baths, and stool softeners. If the fissure does not heal within a few weeks, anesthesia followed by sphincter dilatation, fissurectomy, and partial sectioning of the internal sphincter or subcutaneous portion of the external sphincter are operative options. These relax the sphincter mechanism that sustains the fissure. Surgical excision is probably the most common method to manage anal fissures. The anal canal is gradually dilated, and an elliptical incision is made about the fissure to include the sentinel pile, anal fissure, papilla, crypt, or internal hemorrhoid, which is then excised. The mucosa is dissected from the internal sphincter before closing the wound transversely.

Anal Abscesses and Fistulas

Perianal abscesses are usually caused by infected anal glands eroding into underlying tissue secondary to infection with *Escherichia coli*. Laxatives and re-

gional enteritis are common factors leading to anal abscesses. Uncommonly, tuberculosis, actinomycoses, or other fungal diseases, pelvic inflammatory disease, prostatitis, or cancer may be responsible. Symptoms of dull rectal aching and mild stomach complaints progress to severe, throbbing perianal pain with fever, chills, and malaise. Because the perianal skin is often thick, a fluctuant area may not be apparent. Usually, redness, tenderness, and a generalized protrusion are found. Prompt incision and drainage after needle aspiration prevents serious extension of these infections (Figs. 16 and 17). Delay in operative treatment causes further destruction of tissue, and multiple extensions can extend into the thigh, scrotum, or even the abdominal wall if operative therapy is deferred. The surgical treatment usually involves anesthesia with internal and external digital or sigmoidoscopic examination. The area of the abscess is identified, and a large-bore needle is inserted to confirm the presence and the site of purulent material. This is followed by a simple excision with a digital exploration of the abscess cavity and its surrounding tissue, which must be opened and drained.

Perirectal Fistula

Usually, perirectal abscesses drain and heal with no sequelae; however, those that fail to heal may evolve into a perirectal fistula. The external opening may

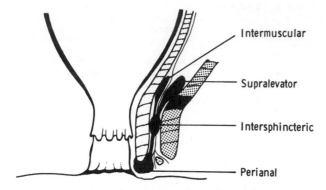

Figure 16. Upward and downward vertical spread of infection from an intersphincteric abscess. (From Parks AG, Thompson JPS: Abscess and fistula. *In* Thompson JPS, Nichols RJ, Williams CR [eds]: Colorectal Disease. Copyright © 1981, William Heinemann Medical Books, London, with permission.)

close temporarily only to reopen when pus accumulates in the tract, and eventually the tract becomes lined with epithelium. Extensions may be directed into the urinary tract, the perianal area, thighs, or bone, and often multiple openings can be seen. Fistulous tracts usually follow a variable course. The primary internal opening is usually found in the anal crypts, mostly on the posterior midline. If the continuous opening is anterior to a transverse line drawn through the anus, the internal opening is on a radial line directly into the anal rectum. If the continuous opening is posterior to this line, the internal opening is probably in the posterior midline. Symptoms are usually

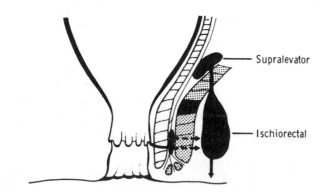

Figure 17. Horizontal spread of infection, medially into the anal canal, and laterally into the ischiorectal fossa. The level at which the primary tract crosses the external sphincter may not be the same as the level of the internal opening. Vertical spread of infection may then occur across the levator ani muscle. (From Parks AG, Thompson JPS: Abscess and fistula. *In* Thompson JPS, Nichols RJ, Williams CR [eds]: Colorectal Disease. Copyright © 1981, William Heinemann Medical Books, London, with permission.)

confined to intermittent swelling drainage and pruritus. A cutaneous opening is characteristically slightly raised, gray-pink, with granulation tissue. A probe can usually be passed through the fistula to the pectinate line.

The operative goal is to incise over the fistulous tract, allowing it to granulate. This is usually accomplished by placing a probe through both openings of the fistula and incising under the probe, with anesthesia. If the fistula follows a course that necessitates division of the sphincter, then the incision must divide the muscle fibers perpendicularly in only one level. Incontinence may follow if the muscle is divided at more than one site. The primary disease must receive appropriate treatment if the lesion is secondary to carcinoma, tuberculosis, Crohn's disease, or colitis.

Prolapse of the Rectum

The three types of rectal prolapse include mucosal prolapse, rectal intussusception, and true prolapse. Mucosal prolapse occurs when an intact sphincter involves an extrusion of rectal mucosa alone through the anus. It becomes symptomatic because of irritation and ulceration of the prolapsed tissue, and soiling following mucosal secretions. This condition is usually present in infants and almost invariably disappears by the age of 5. A radial incision similar to hemorrhoidectomy incisions can be used, which cause scarring that shrinks and holds the redundant mucosa in place.

Rectal intussusception involves protrusion of the entire rectal wall. This usually begins above the pectinate line, and the full thickness of the tissue in the prolapsed portion in concentric folds distinguish it from mucosal prolapse. This is usually considered to be an incomplete prolapse.

True prolapse of the rectum follows herniation of the pelvic peritoneum through the pelvic diaphragm, the anterior rectal wall, and the anus. This is usually associated with poor anal sphincter tone, and may be seen in infants, males in their 20s or 30s, and females at any age. It usually represents a congenital weakness in males because the prostate and seminal vesicles lend inadequate support anteriorly to prevent herniation. With repeated and prolonged protrusion, the anal sphincter becomes relaxed, stretched, and paralyzed.

Many surgical procedures have been described to treat rectal prolapse, but no standard procedure is agreed upon. Operations are used to control this condition by resection of the prolapse and redundant bowel, reduction in the size of the anus, and reinforcement of the perineal floor with transabdominal suspension and fixation of the prolapsed bowel to the pelvis. Obliteration of the cul-de-sac or repair of a perineal sliding hernia is also required.

Pilonidal Sinus

Although not arising from the anorectum, pilonidal sinus often enters the differential diagnosis of anorectal disease. Pilonidal sinuses appear as small openings in the intergluteal fold of the sacrococcygeal area, about 3 to 5 cm superior to the anal orifice. They are usually thought to be due to hairs penetrating first into the dermis and eliciting a foreign body reaction, while others maintain that the condition is congenital. Ingrown hair is almost invariably found within these sinus tracts, and hair scales pointing away from the root are apparently driven inward by rolling action between the buttocks. Hair follicles or other skin appendages are not found within the sinus walls. These lesions occur in the intergluteal region of young hirsute males and, less commonly, in females. It rarely occurs in patients 45 years of age or older. Infection with rupture through the skin, chronicity, and recurrence are the usual findings with this condition. For acutely inflamed sinuses, simple incision and drainage are appropriate. When possible, the ideal treatment is total excision and primary closure or leaving the wound open with healing by packing and formation of granulation tissue with ultimate epithelialization.

REFERENCES

Allen-Merch TG: Pilonidal sinus: Finding the right track for treatment. Br J Surg 77:123–132, 1990.

Broder S: Molecular foundations of oncology. Baltimore, Williams & Wilkins, 1991.

Conden RE, Bartlett JG, Greenlee H, et al: Efficacy of oral and systemic antibiotic prophylaxis in colorectal operations. Arch Surg 118:496–502, 1983.

Dozois RR, Kelly KA, Welling DR, et al: Ileal pouch—anal anastommosis: Comparison of results in familial adenomatous polyposis and chronic ulcerative colitis. Ann Surg 210:268–273, 1989.

Fleites RA, Marshall JB, Eckhauser ML, et al: The efficacy of polyethylene glycol-electrolyte lavage solution versus traditional mechanical bowel preparation for elective colonic surgery: A randomized, prospective, blinded clinical trial. Surgery 98:708–717, 1985.

Friedman JD, Odlin MD, Burbick MP: Experience with the colonic volvulus. Dis Colon Rectum 32:409–416, 1989.

Hughes LL, Rich TA, Delclos L, et al: Radiotherapy for anal carcinoma: Experience from 1979 to 1987. Int J Radiat Oncol Biol Phys 17.1153–1160, 1989.

Kodner IJ, Shemesh EI, Fry RD, et al: Preoperative irradiation for rectal cancer. Ann Surg 209:194–199, 1989.

Mazier WP, Wolkomir AF: Hemorrhoids. Semin Colon Rectal Surg 1(12):197–206. 1990.

Sabiston DC Jr (ed): Textbook of Surgery: The Biological Basis for Modern Surgical Practice, ed 14. Philadelphia, WB Saunders Company, 1991.

Veidenheimer MD, Roberts PL: Colonic diverticular disease. Cambridge, Blackwell Scientific Publications, 1991.

Waldron RP, Donovan IA: Mortality in patients with obstructing colorectal cancer. Ann R Coll Surg Engl 68:219–221, 1986.

32
THE LIVER

TIMOTHY J. BABINEAU, M.D.   ALBERT BOTHE, Jr., M.D.
GLENN STEELE, Jr., M.D., Ph.D

HISTORY

During the past three decades, an enhanced understanding of the anatomy and function of the liver has made the organ more amenable to surgical procedures.

The earliest surgical interventions on the liver were described by Hippocrates in the fifth century BC and involved the draining of hepatic abscesses. Sporadic accounts involved the attempt to repair hepatic trauma, but it was not until the 19th century, however, that elective hepatic resection for removal of a malignancy was performed. In 1886, Luis reported an unsuccessful case of hepatic resection for adenoma, and soon thereafter the first successful elective hepatic resection was done by Langenbuch. He performed a "wedge" resection of the left lobe of the liver to remove a hepatocellular carcinoma.

The last 50 years of hepatic surgery has advanced primarily due to a refined understanding of the segmental anatomy of the liver, better perioperative care, and improved anesthetic and surgical techniques. Until the late 19th century, the liver was believed to be divided into right and left lobes by the falciform ligament. In 1898 Cantlie described the true cleavage plane between right and left lobes of the liver as extending from the gallbladder fossa anteriorly to the inferior vena cava posteriorly. More recently, better technical aspects of liver surgery including vascular isolation, improved blood salvage, and modifications of "finger-fracture" technique, with a better appreciation of the biologic and prognostic implications of liver tumor resection have all made hepatic surgery a realistic option for many patients. In 1963, Starzl performed the first human liver transplant in a patient with biliary atresia, thus beginning the current era of hepatic surgery.

ANATOMY

The complex architecture of the liver and its dual blood supply create surgical problems. Lying in the right upper quadrant beneath the diaphragm, the liver is juxtaposed with the superior and inferior vena cava, right adrenal gland, right kidney, the first and second portions of the duodenum, the head of the pancreas, esophagus, stomach, and colon. Thus, a complete understanding of the surgical anatomy of the liver is as complicated as it is necessary.

The majority of the liver is surrounded by the visceral peritoneum, which is fused to the fibrous capsule of the liver called Glisson's capsule. In the simplest classification, the liver contains four lobes: *right, left, quadrate,* and *caudate.* The division of the right and left lobes is a plane that extends from the gallbladder fossa anteroinferiorly to the inferior vena cava posteriorly. This is in contrast to the historic view, which divided the liver into right and left lobes based on the falciform ligament. Subsequently known, the true right lobe is divided into anterior and posterior segments by a segmental fissure (not readily visible), while the left lobe is divided into medial and lateral segments by the falciform ligament. Within the falciform ligament lies the *ligamentum teres,* which contains the obliterated embryologic remnant of the left umbilical vein, which may be patent in patients with portal hypertension.

There are four peritoneal folds (the falciform, coronary, and two triangular ligaments) that suspend the liver to the anterior abdominal wall and the diaphragm. These folds are divided when the liver is mobilized surgically. The falciform ligament attaches the liver to the anterior abdominal wall. The anterior and posterior right and left coronary ligaments (which are continuous with the falciform ligament) connect the diaphragm to the liver. Laterally, the coronary ligaments give rise to the triangular ligaments, and the area bounded by the falciform, coronary, and triangular ligaments is referred to as the bare area of the liver.

The porta hepatis, which contains the common hepatic duct, portal vein, and hepatic artery, is found within the free edge of the lesser omentum. Also contained within the lesser omentum are the hepatic branches of the anterior and posterior vagus nerves (parasympathetic nerve supply), lymphatics, and occasionally anomalous branches of the left and right hepatic arteries. The liver receives its sympathetic nerve supply from the celiac ganglion surrounding the celiac arterial trunk. Experience with liver transplantation has shown that the entire nerve supply to the liver can be transected without any obvious detrimental effect on liver function.

In 1957, Couinaud divided the liver into eight segments based primarily on the vascular supply as demonstrated by model casts produced from injections of the hepatic artery, portal vein, and bile ducts (Fig. 1). The right lobe contains segments 5 through 8, while the left lobe contains segments 1 through 4. These anatomic subdivisions can be quite variable due to the extensive arborization of the intrahepatic vasculature. Surgical resections involve removal of the liver using either the right and left lobe classification or the segmental classification of Couinaud.

Microscopically, the liver consists of lobules that are separated by the portal triads. These triads contain the terminal branches of the hepatic artery, portal vein, and bile duct. Blood flows from the branches of the portal vein and hepatic artery, through the vascular sinusoids toward the central veins. These central veins form the three major hepatic veins.

BILIARY SYSTEM

Most of the surgically important anatomic variation within the biliary system is extrahepatic, and the intrahepatic biliary drainage is relatively constant. The right anterior and posterior hepatic lobes are drained by major segmental ducts that join to form the right hepatic duct. The medial and lateral lobes are drained by two other major segmental ducts that form the left hepatic duct. Both the right and left hepatic ducts subsequently join, usually extrahepatically, to form the common hepatic duct. Finally, the cystic duct joins the hepatic duct at a variable location to form the com-

mon bile duct. The advent of laparoscopic cholecystectomy has created a compelling need to understand hepatic ductal anatomy, as most injuries to these structures can be avoided if the surgical anatomy is thoroughly understood.

BLOOD SUPPLY

The blood supply to the liver is profuse, and total hepatic blood flow averages approximately 1500 ml/min/m². The liver has dual blood inflow that reaches the liver through the porta hepatis. The oxygenated hepatic arterial blood comprises approximately 25 per cent of total hepatic flow, while the nutrient-rich portal blood contributes approximately 75 per cent. Visualizing the porta hepatis anteriorly (as it is viewed during operation), the portal vein is located posteriorly with the hepatic artery lying anteromedial and the common bile duct anterolateral. The efferent circulatory drainage of the liver is primarily by the three major (right, left, and middle) hepatic veins, which emerge from the liver directly posterior and drain into the inferior vena cava.

The arterial supply of the liver can be quite variable. The common hepatic artery is the largest branch of the celiac artery that, after giving rise to the right gastric and gastroduodenal branches, continues toward the hilum of the liver and divides into the right and left hepatic branches. In 10 to 20 per cent of patients, the right hepatic artery may be "replaced," arising instead from the superior mesenteric artery. Less frequently (in approximately 10 per cent), the left hepatic artery may also be "replaced," arising instead from the left gastric artery. The cystic artery is usually an extrahepatic branch of the right hepatic artery but can also have many anatomic variations.

The portal venous system contains no valves and is formed by the confluence of the superior mesenteric, splenic, and inferior mesenteric veins. Within the hepatoduodenal ligament (porta hepatis) the portal vein divides into its right and left branches.

The major hepatic venous drainage is by the right, middle, and left hepatic veins that enter directly into the inferior vena cava behind the liver. These veins can be difficult to control surgically due to the retrohepatic position. The right hepatic vein usually drains most of the right lobe, the left hepatic vein drains most of the left lobe, and the middle hepatic vein drains the inferior portions of the left medial and right anterior lobes. However, variability occurs in the venous drainage pattern, making surgical control of these vessels, particularly during emergency procedures, even more challenging.

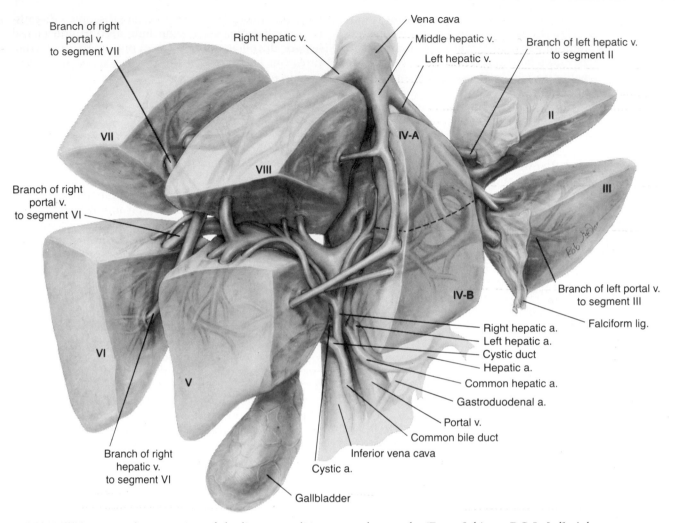

Figure 1. Segmentation of the liver according to vascular supply. (From Sabiston DC Jr [ed]: Atlas of General Surgery. Philadelphia, WB Saunders Company, in press, with permission.)

LIVER FUNCTION AND PHYSIOLOGY

The liver performs many functions, most of which are essential for life. The complexity and importance of these functions is evidenced by the fact that unlike the kidneys, heart, and lung, there is no artificial support device that can replace the liver. Some of the more crucial metabolic functions that the liver performs include glucose production and storage, urea formation, synthesis of proteins and clotting factors, and detoxification of drugs and other substances. The liver influences the substrate formation and utilization of most other organs, and finally, in addition to regulating these metabolic parameters, the liver with its extensive reticuloendothelial system provides a major defense mechanism for the host against infection.

Liver Function Tests

The collection of tests used to characterize liver function has traditionally included the enzymes alkaline phosphatase, serum glutamic-oxaloacetic transaminase (SGOT), serum glutamate pyruvate transaminase (SGPT), and lactic acid dehydrogenase (LDH). Levels of certain plasma proteins such as albumin, fibrinogen, haptoglobin, and ceruloplasmin have been used to assess hepatic synthetic function, and the prothrombin time (PT) is perhaps the most sensitive test for hepatic reserve because it accurately reflects the synthetic ability of the liver.

Alkaline phosphatase is a sensitive measure of biliary obstruction, and its serum level rises with impairment of bile outflow from either benign or malignant causes. It may also be elevated when there is hepatocellular damage or a space-occupying lesion within the liver. Elevated values (from nonhepatic sources) may be noted with increased osteoblastic activity within bones. Distinguishing the source of an elevation in serum alkaline phosphatase is possible by fractionating the isoenzymes based on their heat sensitivity or obtaining a γ-glutamyltransferase level.

Serum levels of SGPT and/or SGOT are also elevated in hepatic disease. In addition to the liver, SGOT is also found in large quantities within heart, muscle, skeletal, and kidney tissue, while SGPT is found in greatest quantities within the liver. Therefore, while the SGOT may be elevated in nonhepatic diseases, an elevated SGPT is highly suggestive of hepatocellular injury. Both enzymes reach their highest serum levels in acute hepatocellular damage. The etiology of the damage can be from any cause, but most commonly originates from infectious etiologies such as hepatitis or "low-flow" phenomena such as shock or ischemic injury. Finally, serum LDH, which is also found in a variety of tissues other than liver, is elevated with hepatic injury.

Approximately 10 gm of albumin are synthesized daily in the normal liver. Albumin has a half-life of approximately 21 days. With hepatic injury (or simply during a severe metabolic stress), the liver undergoes a reprioritization of its functions. The synthesis of acute-phase reactants increases, and the amount of albumin produced decreases. In addition, an increase in albumin degradation and a redistribution of the total body albumin pool serve to further lower the serum value. Although often used as a marker for malnutrition, serum albumin more closely reflects the severity of illness rather than the true nutritional status in most hospitalized patients. Moreover, supplementation with exogenous albumin has little justification in the absence of severe anasarca secondary to a low total protein level and may be harmful.

Defects in the coagulation cascade are multifactorial and commonly occur in both moderate and severe liver dysfunction. A prolongation in clotting time, as measured by the PT, usually is due to either a decrease in vitamin K availability secondary to obstructive jaundice or decreased enterohepatic absorption, or hepatocellular dysfunction and decreased synthesis of prothrombin. In the absence of sepsis or disseminated intravascular coagulopathy (DIC), a prolonged PT that does not respond to the intramuscular injection of 10 mg of vitamin K is a sign of severe liver impairment. Replacement of clotting factors with fresh frozen plasma is often necessary prior to invasive procedures in such patients who have a risk of bleeding.

Physiology

Most of the body's metabolic needs are regulated (either directly or indirectly) by the liver. The numerous metabolic functions that the liver performs are directly related to and dependent on the overall health of the patient. Approximately 20 per cent of the basal metabolic rate (BMR) of a patient is due to the metabolic activities of the liver. Since the BMR is a primary contributor to total energy expenditure (TEE), it is apparent that the liver is involved in both energy production and energy consumption. The principal functions of the liver are performed primarily by two cell types: the *hepatocytes* (or parenchymal cells) and the *macrophages* (or Kupffer cells). Although intimately related through a series of intercellular and intracellular communications, these two cell types perform distinctly different functions. The metabolic functions of the hepatocytes are grouped according to five major activities: (1) provision of energy-fuel substrates, (2) regulation of blood amino acid concentration, (3) synthesis of hepatic secretory and structural proteins, (4) bile acid and bilirubin production, and (5) detoxification of drugs and toxic substances. The hepatic macrophages, conversely, are specialized endothelial cells located within the sinusoids of the liver that constitute (along with splenic macrophages) approximately 90 per cent of the reticuloendothelial system (RES).

While the intake of food is intermittent, the need for a supply of substrates necessary for cellular processes is continuous and must be constantly available for body metabolism. As such, the liver serves as an endogenous reserve of both energy substrates and amino acids. Specifically, the liver contributes to glucose production by conversion of exogenously supplied galactose and fructose, synthesis from lactate and carbon skeletons (gluconeogenesis), and synthesis and storage of glycogen. In the early postabsorptive state, maintenance of blood glucose concentration depends primarily on the liver stores of glycogen. The blood glucose concentration is normally maintained within a relatively narrow range, and the average normal adult requires between 150 and 200 gm of glucose daily. If provided as an exogenous supply such as dextrose-containing intravenous solutions, the rate of infusion that the liver can metabolize with the greatest efficiency is 2 to 4 mg/kg/min. Infusion rates in excess of this (>400 gm of dextrose per day) cause hepatic lipogenesis and possible RES dysfunction. During times of fasting, hepatic gluconeogenesis and glycogenolysis balance the varying rates of glucose absorption, transport, and oxidation of the body's tissues to maintain a steady-state blood glucose level.

The liver also regulates energy production through control of fatty acid and triglyceride metabolism. Degradation of fatty acids into smaller fragments (ketones) through β-oxidation is an energy-producing process, and synthesis of triglycerides from excess glucose concentration is an energy-consuming process.

These two metabolic pathways are the principal means by which the liver coordinates fatty acid metabolism to energy needs. When blood insulin levels fall, as during a fast or hypoglycemia, fatty acids stored as triglycerides in adipose tissue are mobilized, transported to the liver, enter the mitochondria (dependent on the carnitine shuttle), and are oxidized. Conversely, triglycerides are produced in the liver whenever the available carbohydrate supply exceeds the ability of the liver to convert the supply to glycogen or oxidize it. These triglycerides are subsequently transported from the liver primarily as very-low-density lipoprotein (VLDL) to be stored in adipose tissue. Occasionally, as with the excessive caloric intake that occurs with excessive administration of central venous hyperalimentation, these triglycerides may be deposited within the hepatocytes, causing the so-called *fatty liver*. In extreme situations, this preventable process can impair liver function, elevate liver enzymes, and rarely lead to hepatic failure, usually in the pediatric age group.

The protein and amino acid stores of the body are in a constant state of flux described in the process of *protein turnover*. Approximately 300 to 400 gm of protein is produced and broken down (i.e., "turns over") daily in a normal individual. Small amounts of protein in nearly all of the body's tissues are constantly being hydrolyzed only to be immediately replaced by the same structural proteins. This dynamic equilibrium between production and breakdown is closely regulated by the liver. Normally, amino acids that are absorbed following digestion of protein within the intestine are sufficient to satisfy the needs for most of protein synthesis, while excesses are removed through degradation, deamination, and formation of urea. However, during periods of fasting or stress when an exogenous supply of amino acids is not available, the liver, by its regulation of protein turnover, ensures an adequate supply for needy tissues such as bone marrow, visceral organs, and healing wounds. During normal fasting, visceral protein stores are degraded, while skeletal muscle protein is relatively preserved. In a critically ill or stressed patient, the reverse often occurs, with degradation of skeletal muscle providing free amino acids and carbon skeletons necessary for energy production. If allowed to proceed unopposed (i.e., through lack of nutritional support), this catabolic process may potentially provide the initiating factor for multisystem organ failure, as both visceral and skeletal protein stores are depleted.

Ammonia derived from amino acid metabolism is detoxified through its conversion into urea within the liver. This energy-requiring process that produces approximately 10 to 20 gm of urea nitrogen per day is one of the most teleologically primitive functions of the liver. Together with glucose production, it is among the last functions of the liver to fail. An omi-nous sign in a critically ill patient is profound hypoglycemia in conjunction with a diminishing blood urea nitrogen (BUN) and often precedes fulminant hepatic failure.

Most protein synthesis occurs within the functioning liver. The daily net production of new protein by the liver averages approximately 50 gm/day. Among the more important proteins that are secreted by the liver are albumin, fibrinogen, transferrin, haptoglobin, α-globulins, and lipoproteins. Production of albumin, which is closely regulated by colloid osmotic pressure, reaches around 200 mg/kg/day. In health, the supply of amino acids determines the rate at which hepatic protein synthesis occurs. In stress or starvation, the liver undergoes a reprioritization of protein synthesis due to cytokine and hormonal influences such as glucagon, cortisol, and epinephrine. Acute-phase reactants and cytokines (such as tumor necrosis factor [TNF] and interleukin 1 [IL-1]) may increase while synthesis of proteins such as albumin often decrease.

The liver synthesizes 11 proteins that are critical for hemostasis. In addition, vitamin K, a fat-soluble vitamin and therefore dependent on bile acid formation, is necessary for the extrinsic clotting pathway, which is measured by the PT. Therefore, the administration of vitamin K often differentiates patients who have malabsorptive-type coagulopathies seen commonly with obstructive jaundices from those with impaired synthesis of clotting factors, which are commonly seen with parenchymal diseases. Platelet function is also necessary for clotting and is dependent on liver function. Although thrombocytopenia is not commonly associated with liver disease, patients with portal hypertension and hypersplenism may have increased platelet sequestration within the spleen, which heightens the potential for bleeding complications.

Hepatic macrophage function is primarily associated with host defense rather than metabolic homeostasis. It has been well demonstrated that when bacteria are injected into the bloodstream under normal conditions, a functioning reticuloendothelial system (RES) is capable of clearing the bacteria within 4 to 5 minutes. Various disease states including viral infections, cirrhosis, or overwhelming sepsis may hamper the efficiency with which the liver performs this vital task.

Because of their unique location within the portal triads, these macrophages rapidly remove blood-borne bacteria and endotoxin from the portal circulation. This system represents the last line of defense against widespread dissemination of bacteria when the body has failed elsewhere to limit microbial invasion. When liver parenchymal function becomes impaired in sepsis, phagocytic activity may also be impaired, which further worsens the septic state. Finally, it has been demonstrated that the excessive administration of intravenous lipid emulsions may have deleterious effects on the RES and macrophage function.

The liver is the site of bile formation, which is an active, energy-dependent process that occurs along the canalicular membrane of the hepatocyte and the bile ductules. Bile is primarily composed of conjugated bile acids, cholesterol, phospholipids, and bile pigments. Bile acids are synthesized only in the liver. The primary bile acids, cholic and chenodeoxycholic acid, are synthesized from cholesterol. The formation of these bile acids is directly controlled by the amount of bile that returns to the liver by the enterohepatic circulation. Secondary bile acids, deoxycholic and lithocholic acid, are formed by the dehydroxylation of primary bile acids by intestinal bacteria.

Bile acids are conjugated within the liver to the amino acids taurine or glycine, forming bile salts (Fig. 2). These bile salts are excreted into the bile canaliculi and ultimately into the intestine. Within the intestine, bile salts aid in the absorption of lipids through micelle formation. When bile salts reach the terminal ileum and proximal colon, they are rehydrolyzed to bile acids and amino acids. The bile acids are then absorbed by an active process within the terminal ileum, enter the portal venous circulation, return to the liver,

and are once again taken up by the hepatocytes. Subsequent de novo synthesis of bile acids is under negative feedback control. This enterohepatic circulation of bile acids occurs 5 to 15 times daily.

Bilirubin is the end-product of the breakdown of hemoglobin and is excreted almost entirely in the bile. Depending on the amount of hemoglobin broken down, up to 30 mg of bilirubin daily may be produced within the reticuloendothelial cells and secreted into bile. Unconjugated bilirubin is nonpolar, lipid soluble, and is transported (bound to albumin) in the plasma to the liver. Within the liver it is converted to a polar, water soluble compound that allows its excretion into the aqueous bile. This process requires the enzyme bilirubin *uridine diphosphate* (UDP) *glucuronyl transferase*, which is low or absent in neonates and patients with Gilbert's syndrome. The evaluation of the jaundiced patient depends on whether the bilirubin is conjugated (direct) or unconjugated (indirect).

Within the intestine, bilirubin is broken down into urobilinogen, which is excreted primarily in the stool and to a lesser extent in the urine. A fraction of urobilinogen is oxidized to urobilin, a brown pigment that gives stool its characteristic color. With many types of biliary obstruction, bilirubin excretion into the intestine is decreased, leading to a subsequent decrease in urobilinogen and urobilin formation that causes *clay-colored stools*. The amount of urobilinogen in urine often increases, which gives the urine a characteristic dark appearance. The combination of dark urine and clay-colored stools is highly suspicious for extrahepatic biliary obstruction, usually from a stone or a neoplasm.

Bile flow begins within the biliary ductules and proceeds to the major hepatic ducts. During its course through the biliary tree, bile is modified by the secretion and absorption of both water and electrolytes. This process occurs primarily in the epithelial cells that line the biliary tract. The primary function of the gallbladder is to store and concentrate bile of up to 50 times its hepatic concentration during periods of fasting. Under normal conditions, the liver excretes approximately 500 to 1000 ml of isosmotic bile daily, with considerable variation. The electrolyte composition of bile closely approximates that of serum.

DIAGNOSTIC IMAGING OF THE LIVER

Radiologic diagnostic imaging of the liver is performed primarily for the detection of tumors as well as aiding in the differential diagnosis of these tumors. In addition, anatomic landmarks such as major vascular and biliary structures can be seen as they relate to the tumor. During the past two decades, the devel-

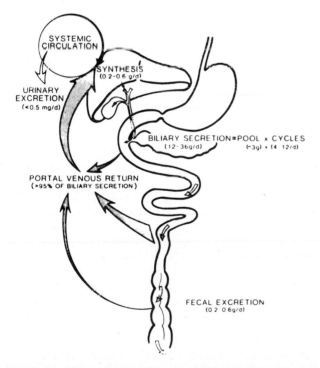

Figure 2. The enterohepatic circulation of bile salts with some general kinetic values for man. (From Carey MC: The enterohepatic circulation. *In* Arias I, et al [eds]: The Liver: Biology and Pathobiology. New York, Raven Press, 1982, pp 429–465, with permission.)

opment of computed tomography (CT) scanning, magnetic resonance imaging (MRI), conventional (external) and intraoperative ultrasonography (US), and, most recently, laparoscopy and translaparoscopic ultrasonography have revolutionized the manner in which the liver is imaged. For primary screening, MRI is considered by many to be superior to CT scanning because of its specificity in discriminating hemangiomas and cysts from malignant neoplasms without the need for iodinated contrast material. Once a malignant tumor is suspected, further staging is often best performed by CT scanning with vascular enhancement. More invasive methods of staging include intraoperative ultrasonography and diagnostic laparoscopy. Finally, the development of endoscopic retrograde cholangiopancreatography (ERCP) has greatly added to the preoperative assessment and treatment of the jaundiced patient.

The CT scan in a patient with suspected liver disease provides information to the surgeon contemplating operative intervention (Fig. 3). In addition to defining normal anatomy, various metabolic and infectious conditions affecting the liver and impacting on operability may be detected. Fatty infiltration characteristic of cirrhosis or increased iron storage from hemochromatosis can be detected on many CT scans. Hepatitis, however, has few if any characteristic CT scan findings. Space-occupying lesions within the liver, such as a pyogenic abscess, echinococcal cyst, malignant neoplasm (both primary and metastatic), or benign tumors (fibroadenomas, hemangiomas, or focal nodular hyperplasia), are all depicted but not differentially diagnosed by the CT scan. When indicated, biopsy of mass lesions may be accomplished under CT scan guidance except for suspected hemangioma.

Despite the results achieved by CT scan, ultrasonography is often the first diagnostic test in the radiologic evaluation of hepatic disease. It is safe, relatively inexpensive and noninvasive, and its greatest efficacy lies in identifying space-occupying lesions within the liver and differentiating mechanical from metabolic causes of jaundice. Dilatation of the intrahepatic and/or extrahepatic bile system is often detected by ultrasound and is highly suggestive of a mechanical cause of jaundice. Conversely, normal-caliber bile ducts by ultrasonography would suggest a metabolic or infectious etiology for jaundice, except in the case of extensive hepatic infiltration of a cancer such as cholangiocarcinoma.

During the past several years, laparoscopy and intraoperative ultrasonography have found a role in the surgical management of hepatic malignancies. These two diagnostic modalities can be joined to determine the resectability of either a primary or metastatic hepatic malignancy. Although neither of these can be used as "screening" tests, both are capable of detecting

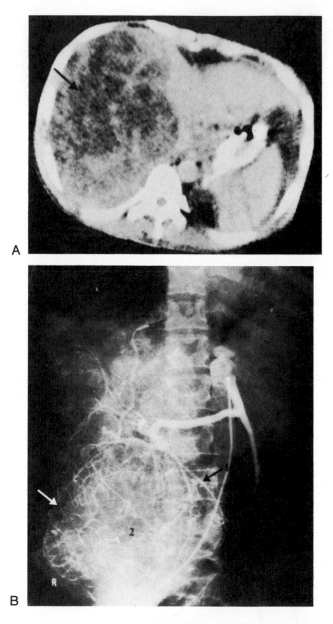

A

B

Figure 3. Computed tomogram (A) and arteriogram (B) of a moderately vascular hepatoma of right lobe of liver. Note displacement of vessels (1) and neovascularity (2) in B. (From Sherlock S, Summerfield JA [eds]: Color Atlas of Liver Disease. Chicago, Year Book Medical Publishers, 1978, with permission.)

lesions not appreciated preoperatively or, with ultrasonography, intraoperatively either visually or through palpation. This is particularly true for satellite lesions smaller than 1 to 1.5 cm or lesions centrally located deep within liver parenchyma. Because the resectability of both primary and metastatic hepatic malignancies is dependent on the ability to remove all of the neoplastic tissues, intraoperative ultrasonography may demonstrate occult lesions that preclude resection. Laparoscopy is useful in demonstrating unsuspected cirrhosis preoperatively, identifying satellite tumor deposits in the liver, and revealing previously unsuspected extrahepatic metastases. These situations obviate any benefit to a major liver resection.

HEPATIC ABSCESSES

Pyogenic Abscess

Although their existence has been long recognized, the diagnosis and treatment of liver abscesses remains a challenge. Improvements in imaging techniques and in antibiotic therapy have helped in the treatment of this difficult disorder. The presentation of liver abscess continues to remain quite subtle and the index of suspicion must be high. There are two main types of liver abscess, *pyogenic* (or bacterial) and *amebic* (from amebiasis). Pyogenic abscesses comprise nearly 90 per cent of liver abscesses that occur in the United States. Although pyogenic and amebic abscess have common features, the diagnosis, treatment, and etiologies are quite different.

The incidence of both types of hepatic abscess has not changed significantly over the past 50 years. Each is quite rare, with only 5 to 15 cases per 100,000 hospital admissions being reported annually. Hepatic abscesses may be single, multiple, amebic, pyogenic, or fungal. Males appear to be affected slightly more frequently than females, and the average age of patients with hepatic abscess is between 60 and 70. The right lobe is more often involved with solitary pyogenic abscesses.

Certain conditions predispose to the development of a pyogenic abscess, and the more important clinical processes are biliary tract disease and infections at sites drained by the portal circulation such as diverticulitis, appendicitis, or perforated intestinal neoplasms. Less frequently, bacteremic seeding, trauma, or contiguous suppurative infections may lead to the development of pyogenic abscess. Before antibiotics were used routinely, appendicitis was the most common predisposing factor for the development of pyogenic liver abscess. With the current use of antibiotics, appendicitis is now rarely complicated by liver abscess, and biliary tract disease, such as cholangitis and acute cholecystitis, represents the most common cause of pyogenic liver abscess. Infections in areas drained by the portal vein are the second leading cause of hepatic abscess. *Cryptogenic* abscesses are those abscesses in which no etiology is found.

For a liver abscess to develop, there is usually pre-existing parenchymal damage. As a normally functioning reticuloendothelial system is capable of clearing most infectious challenges, portal bacteremia alone appears to be an insufficient cause for development of an abscess. Some type of hepatic injury (i.e., ischemic, traumatic, or obstructive), together with a bacterial insult, appears necessary to create an environment for an abscess to develop. Infarcted areas of liver are particularly susceptible to bacterial seeding and abscess formation.

The presenting symptoms and physical findings of hepatic abscess are often varied and nonspecific, and the duration of presentation may range from days to months. The most common presenting complaints are fever (80 to 95 per cent), abdominal pain (50 to 95 per cent), anorexia and vomiting (20 to 60 per cent), fatigue, and weight loss. The physical examination is usually unrewarding with abdominal tenderness, hepatomegaly, or a right upper quadrant mass present in only 20 to 60 per cent. Most patients have leukocytosis, with a significant increase in the percentage of immature leukocytes. Liver chemistries vary, with significant elevation of alkaline phosphatase and mild elevation in transaminase levels.

Until recent advances in hepatic imaging, the radiologic diagnosis of pyogenic hepatic abscess was difficult. Plain abdominal films and chest film findings were subtle and nonspecific and were abnormal approximately 50 per cent of the time. Ultrasonography and CT scanning, however, have increased the diagnostic accuracy to almost 100 per cent. In addition, these two diagnostic modalities can be used to guide percutaneous abscess drainage and monitor therapy. Although MRI scanning may provide additional information, ultrasound and CT scan remain the diagnostic procedures of choice for suspected hepatic abscess.

In 70 to 100 per cent of cases, cultures from a pyogenic abscess are positive for bacteria, and blood cultures are positive in almost 50 per cent of patients. Enteric gram-negative bacilli, most commonly *Escherichia coli* and *Klebsiella* species are the organisms most commonly found in these abscesses. Other organisms include streptococcal species, *Staphylococcus aureus*, *Candida albicans*, *Pseudomonas aeruginosa*, and anaerobic bacteria such as *Bacteroides fragilis* and *Fusobacterium* species. Approximately 20 to 50 per cent of abscesses are polymicrobial, reinforcing the importance of broad-spectrum antibiotic coverage even when a single organism has been cultured.

The underlying principle in the treatment of pyogenic liver abscess remains drainage. While open surgical drainage of the abscess with appropriate perioperative antibiotic coverage has been preferred, recently percutaneous drainage using ultrasound or CT scan guidance has achieved comparable results with few complications. Percutaneous drainage should be attempted initially in patients with abscesses accessible to this procedure and for whom surgical management is not required to correct the predisposing etiology (i.e., perforated colon carcinoma). However, if the patient has a condition that requires operation, if the number and location of the abscesses preclude a percutaneous approach, or if the patient fails to respond to antibiotics and percutaneous drainage, surgical exploration should be performed. Antibiotic therapy alone without aspiration or drainage of the abscess is effective only in the therapy of multiple small abscesses associated with bacterial seeding of the liver from a distant infected source (e.g., with acute *S. aureus* endocarditis).

Formerly, the mortality from pyogenic liver abscess exceeded 50 per cent, but recent series reported an 8 to 22 per cent mortality. The complications of liver abscesses are usually related to rupture of the abscess into an adjacent structure or the dissemination of organisms to other organs causing multisystem organ failure. However, heightened awareness of the diagnosis, aggressive antibiotic treatment, and early drainage should lead to fewer complications and lower mortality.

Amebic Abscess

The protozoa *Entamoeba histolytica* occurs in two forms and causes an intestinal infection through its invasive motile trophozoite. Unlike the cystic form, the motile trophozoite form lives in either the wall or lumen of the colon. Conversely, the cystic form is excreted in the stool and can live outside the body (unlike the trophozoite form). Once ingested, the cyst breaks down to release the active trophozoites. The most common extraintestinal complication of infection with *E. histolytica* is an amebic liver abscess, as trophozoites frequently enter the portal circulation, invade the liver, and produce hepatic necrosis and formation of an abscess.

Patients who present with this disease in the United States usually have emigrated from or traveled through regions with endemic amebic disease. Some 85 per cent present with a solitary lesion, and 70 per cent of these are within the right lobe of the liver. Unlike pyogenic abscesses, amebic liver abscesses do not appear to require predisposing hepatic dysfunction or underlying parenchymal damage other than the necrosis created by trophozoite invasion of the liver. Most patients with amebic abscess are male and in the 20- to 50-year age range.

The presentation of patients with amebic abscess is similar to those with pyogenic abscess, with fever, pain, fatigue, and nausea. Surprisingly, diarrhea is infrequent and many patients report no prior history of amebic dysentery. Parasites are not detectable in the stools of the vast majority. In addition, the physical examination is often unrevealing, with only a few patients demonstrating a right upper quadrant mass or tenderness. Laboratory tests show a leukocytosis without eosinophilia and nonspecific elevation of liver chemistries. Ultrasonography is diagnostic in 90 to 95 per cent of cases, and a CT scan may be unnecessary. Finally, serologic tests of an antibody to *E. histolytica* are available and detect antibody in patients with invasive intestinal amebiasis as well as those with extraintestinal amebic infections.

Although percutaneous diagnostic aspiration was performed routinely in the past, a positive ultrasound coupled with positive serology has decreased the role for aspiration. In patients with bacterial superinfection or in whom the abscess cavity is greater than 10 cm and rupture seems imminent, aspiration and culture may be useful. When the abscess is aspirated, the fluid obtained has various characteristics, but "anchovy paste" is the one most commonly described. Amoebae are seen on wet mount examinations in less than 50 per cent of aspirates.

The treatment of choice for amebic liver abscess is metronidazole, 750 mg every 8 hours for 10 days. This regimen is effective for 85 to 100 per cent of patients. Patients who do not respond to this treatment may require surgical drainage or alternative medical therapy (dehydroemetine and chloroquine). A surgical procedure is used as the primary treatment only to treat or prevent abscess rupture, although an attempt at percutaneous drainage is probably warranted initially. In the absence of superinfection or rupture, survival with amebic liver abscess is nearly 100 per cent.

CYSTS AND BENIGN NEOPLASMS

Cysts

Solitary liver cysts are rare, occurring in as few as 1 in 1000 patients. They are benign, slow growing, usually multilocular, rarely symptomatic, and if small, require no treatment. However, occasionally large cysts cause dull, vague, right upper quadrant pain and, rarely, present with hemorrhage or infection of the cyst. If the cysts are large and symptomatic, surgical management offers the best results, as aspiration is associated with a high rate of recurrence. If approached surgically, the cyst is excised and the wall sent for frozen section examination to exclude the presence of malignancy. If excision cannot be performed safely (due to the proximity of major vascular structures), unroofing and drainage into the abdominal cavity represents an acceptable alternative.

Unlike simple cysts, congenital polycystic disease of the liver is more a systemic disease, often associated with renal malformations, and is genetically transmitted. Approximately 50 per cent of patients with adult polycystic liver disease have renal involvement, while 15 to 75 per cent of patients who present with polycystic kidney disease eventually develop hepatic cystic disease. In hepatic polycystic disease, the cysts are usually located throughout both lobes and range in size from less than 1 cm to greater than 20 cm in diameter. Like solitary cysts, polycystic disease is frequently asymptomatic and undiagnosed. It may be discovered incidentally at laparotomy for other reasons. Symptomatic patients usually present with epigastric fullness, pain, or nausea. Occasionally, progressive kidney failure or a cerebrovascular accident secondary to an associated "berry aneurysm" may be the only presenting symptom. Surgical management is indicated for severe symptoms or complications such as rupture, infection, or hemorrhage. Percutaneous aspiration of multiple cysts is associated with a nearly 100 per cent risk of recurrence. When performed, the goal is to remove or unroof as many cysts as possible. Occasionally, this requires resection of a complete lobe. Without renal involvement, the prognosis is usually excellent.

Caroli's disease is an unusual form of cystic disease in which multiple dilatations of the intrahepatic biliary system cause the formation of biliary lakes or cysts. This syndrome often occurs in conjunction with congenital hepatic fibrosis. Patients usually present with recurrent attacks of cholangitis and are best managed with surgical débridement and drainage. Endoscopic therapy may also have a therapeutic role.

Echinococcal Cysts

Echinococcal cystic disease of the liver is endemic in much of the world where sheep are raised but is relatively uncommon in North America. Infection is caused by *Echinococcus granulosus*, although rarely it may be caused by *Echinococcus multilocularis*. For patients with symptomatic echinococcal ("hydatid") liver disease, surgical therapy is the treatment of choice. Just as with hepatic abscesses, in most echinococcal infections, approximately 70 per cent of cysts are found in the right lobe.

The wall of the cyst (or hydatid) consists of an outer ectocyst and an inner endocyst. Over the years, the cysts expand because the endocyst secretes a clear fluid that contains daughter cysts. As the cyst expands, vague abdominal pain is the most common symptom. Once suspected, the diagnosis is made by indirect hemagglutination and serum immunoelectrophoresis. The Casoni skin test is associated with significant false-positive results.

Surgical therapy should be considered for all patients once the diagnosis is made. Anthelmintics such as mebendazole have met with limited success. The surgical approach varies depending on the number and location of the cysts. At laparotomy and prior to attempted excision, the surgeon must first neutralize the daughter cysts, usually by injecting 3 per cent hypertonic saline directly into the largest cyst. Following this, the cyst may be unroofed, the contents evacuated, and the cyst removed. Spillage of the contents is avoided, as any viable daughter cysts may cause widespread dissemination and/or anaphylaxis.

Benign Tumors

Like cysts, benign tumors of the liver are relatively uncommon. Most of these hepatic neoplasms are hemangiomas, adenomas, focal nodular hyperplasia (FNH), or bile duct hamartomas. As with most space-occupying lesions of the liver, the diagnosis is usually made by CT scan or ultrasonography. Magnetic resonance imaging scanning may provide additional information concerning the relation of the lesion to major vascular structures. When resection is expected, angiography may be necessary to further define the anatomy, although this modality is now being combined with MRI in many centers. Laboratory tests are often unrevealing, as liver function tests are commonly within normal limits. Serologic and tumor serum markers may help differentiate a benign lesion from an infectious process or malignant neoplasm. Preoperative percutaneous biopsy is controversial, fraught with hazard, but occasionally necessary.

Hemangiomas are the most common benign liver tumor. Small capillary hemangiomas are frequently discovered incidentally at laparotomy, have no age or sex predilection, are more common than the larger cavernous hemangioma, and require no treatment. Conversely, cavernous hemangiomas occur most frequently in the third to fifth decades of life among women and may eventually require treatment. The precise etiology of cavernous hemangiomas is not clear. Malignant transformation of a cavernous hemangioma has not been reported, and until they reach large size (>10 cm), most remain asymptomatic. Spontaneous rupture is a rare presenting complaint. Rather, most patients complain of vague abdominal discomfort. Surgical treatment consisting of complete excision is indicated when significant symptoms, pain and discomfort, are present, as most series suggest that the natural history of untreated hemangiomas does not include a significant risk of spontaneous rupture. Occasionally, embolization of the hepatic artery or intraoperative ligation may be done as an emergency measure to control exsanguinating hemorrhage due to spontaneous rupture. Once hemorrhage is controlled, subsequent excision of the lesion is recommended.

Unlike hemangiomas, the incidence of hepatic ade-

10% EtOH cirr → CA
20% viral hep cirr → CA

nomas appears to be increasing, probably related to the increased use of estrogen-containing oral contraceptives among women. One series reports that 90 per cent of women with hepatic adenomas had once used oral contraceptives. Moreover, some hepatic adenomas have regressed following the cessation of oral contraceptives, although others have progressed. The surgical management of patients with suspected adenomas can be challenging, and those who are symptomatic or have complications such as intraperitoneal bleeding should be considered for surgical resection. Asymptomatic patients without history of hormonal use should also be considered for resection, as differentiation from hepatocellular carcinoma on biopsy alone is difficult. Asymptomatic patients with a history of oral contraceptive use may be observed for a period while hormonal therapy is discontinued. The point at which excision is indicated for a lesion that does not regress must be individualized to the patient.

Unlike adenomas, FNH does not appear to be related to oral contraceptives. Patients with FNH are usually asymptomatic, and hemorrhage is rare. Distinguishing FNH from hepatic adenoma based on microscopic appearance is difficult. A characteristic central stellate scar, however, is usually seen with FNH, but not with adenomas. Purportedly, the best test to differentiate the adenoma from FNH is the technetium sulfur colloid liver-spleen scan. If the diagnosis of FNH can be made with certainty, this condition is best managed conservatively unless symptoms, complications, or progression in size occurs.

HEPATIC MALIGNANCY

Primary Lesions

Hepatocellular carcinoma is one of the most common malignancies worldwide, yet it remains relatively uncommon in the United States. As such, only a few centers in North America have developed a significant experience with these tumors. Survival rates for unresectable lesions are generally dismal, with a 4- to 6-month average life expectancy from the time of diagnosis. When diagnosed, the only chance for cure is surgical resection, although there is question as to whether there is any survival plateau even in early lesions completely resected. Cholangiocarcinoma (bile duct carcinoma) also occurs in the liver, although less frequently than primary hepatocellular carcinoma.

The epidemiology and etiology of primary hepatocellular carcinoma is multifactorial and has been related to hepatitis, cirrhosis, and dietary factors including the ingestion of aflatoxins from contaminated grain supplies. It has been estimated that cirrhosis secondary to excessive alcohol intake has an approximate 10 per cent lifetime risk for the development of hepatocellular carcinoma, while cirrhosis secondary to viral hepatitis has an approximate 20 per cent risk. Similarly, cirrhosis secondary to hemochromatosis is also associated with an increased risk of hepatocellular carcinoma.

Hepatocellular carcinoma may develop within the liver as a diffuse process, a multinodular process, or a discrete solitary lesion. Although it usually arises in a background of cirrhosis, *fibrolamellar* hepatocellular carcinoma has recently been described and is not associated with cirrhosis and has improved long-term survival. Hepatocellular carcinoma has a tendency to grow in the vicinity of major vascular structures in the liver, particularly the portal and hepatic veins. Such regional extension is now documentable preoperatively by dynamic CT scan.

Frequently, the diagnosis of hepatocellular carcinoma is obscured by the underlying symptoms of cirrhosis. When cirrhosis is not present, the evaluation of pain, right upper quadrant mass, decrease in liver function, or development of ascites may demonstrate a hepatic malignancy. When hepatocellular carcinoma is suspected, the diagnostic work-up should attempt to differentiate worsening cirrhosis from the onset of cancer through radiologic studies that can define a mass. In addition, although elevation of the serum marker alpha-fetoprotein is highly suggestive of hepatocellular malignancy, it is not excluded by a normal value. Occasionally, angiography may demonstrate the characteristic hypervascular appearance of hepatocellular carcinoma. Preoperative percutaneous biopsy is not recommended due to the highly vascular nature of these cancers and the risk of massive bleeding requiring emergency surgical intervention.

Once the diagnosis of hepatocellular carcinoma is made, the patient should be considered for surgical resection if feasible. Extrahepatic metastatic disease, multifocality within the liver (not manageable with a standard resection), or advanced cirrhosis render patients unresectable. Although surgeons have operated on patients with cirrhosis in the past, the results have been uniformly dismal and most now consider cirrhosis a contraindication to hepatic resection. The reasons for the poor results in cirrhotic patients are multifactorial but relate to the inability of the liver to regenerate following resection and bleeding diatheses. The most suitable candidate for resection is a patient with a solitary lesion arising within a normal liver. Only approximately 30 per cent of patients who are explored are resectable at laparotomy, and of those resected, only 30 per cent are "cured" (i.e., have durable disease-free survival). Diagnostic laparoscopy may decrease the number of laparotomies by identifying unsuspected cirrhosis or extrahepatic metastatic spread.

Cholangiocarcinoma is much less common than primary hepatocellular carcinoma and accounts for only 5 to 30 per cent of all hepatic malignancies. There does not appear to be an association with cirrhosis, and most patients present with obstructive jaundice. The prognosis for these lesions is quite poor, as most present at an advanced, unresectable stage. Extrahepatic bile duct cancers can arise anywhere along the biliary tree, extend proximally or distally for a variable length, and may invade the hepatic parenchyma. Only approximately 20 to 25 per cent of bile duct cancers are found to be resectable at the time of laparotomy. When patients present with earlier lesions of the hepatic bifurcation, so-called *Klatskin tumors*, the resection rates may be only slightly higher. Despite these facts, surgical resection remains the treatment of choice. Fifteen to 30 per cent of patients resected for cure are alive at 5 years, and more cures are achieved with distal than with proximal lesions. Unlike primary hepatocellular carcinoma, unresectable cholangiocarcinomas require either a surgical or endoscopic palliative procedure to relieve the obstructive jaundice.

Metastatic Lesions

Although any solid tumor has the propensity to metastasize to the liver, it is primary carcinoma of the colon and rectum (and some islet cell tumors of the pancreas) that make metastatic lesions amenable to surgical resection (Table 1). When patients with carcinoma of the colon have a pattern of recurrence in the liver alone, which occurs in 3 to 6 per cent of patients with colon resection, hepatic resection offers

a chance for cure. In patients who undergo curative hepatic resection for colorectal metastases, 5-year survivals of 25 to 45 per cent have been reported (Fig. 4). Of all patients with resection of hepatic metastases from colorectal cancer, approximately 50 per cent are found to be resectable at operation. Favorable prognostic signs in these patients are a long disease-free interval (between colonic resection and appearance of hepatic metastasis), hepatic metastases that are few in number, a low preoperative carcinoembryonic antigen (CEA) level, a primary colon cancer of stage II rather than stage III, and, the important prognostic factor, adequate surgical margins (1 to 2 cm).

The presentation of colorectal cancer metastatic to the liver is variable but usually has one of three forms: (1) discovered at initial laparotomy for primary cancer resection, (2) identified as a cause of symptoms, or (3) identified by an elevated CEA level. If liver metastases are discovered at the time of initial laparotomy for colonic cancer (8 to 25 per cent), the primary colon tumor should be resected and the patient should undergo a postoperative evaluation to determine the resectability of the hepatic metastatic disease. An exception is when there is a single liver metastasis, the colonic operation has gone smoothly, and the hepatic resection represents a relatively minor additional procedure (i.e., *wedge resection*). Other primary cancers that rarely have liver metastases amenable to surgical resection include islet cell cancers of the pancreas, carcinoid tumors, and leiomyosarcomas. Rarely, palliative resection of metastatic carcinoid tumors of the liver may be indicated even in the presence of extrahepatic spread.

TABLE 1.   MOST COMMON NONLYMPHOMA MALIGNANT TUMORS METASTATIC TO THE LIVER*

Tumor	Number of Primary Tumors	Number with Hepatic Metastases	Percentage with Hepatic Metastases	Percentage of Patients with Hepatic Metastases Who Were Icteric
Bronchogenic	682	285	41.8	9
Colon	323	181	56.0	34
Pancreas	179	126	70.4	51
Breast	218	116	53.2	30
Stomach	159	70	44.0	60
Unknown primary	102	59	57.0	35
Ovary	97	47	48.0	0
Prostate	333	42	12.6	0
Gallbladder	49	38	77.6	60
Cervix	107	34	31.7	10
Kidney	142	34	23.9	15
Melanoma	50	25	50.0	13
Urinary bladder and ureter	66	25	37.9	11
Esophagus	66	20	30.3	29
Testis	45	20	44.4	14
Endometrial	54	17	31.5	< 20
Thyroid	70	12	17.1	14

*Data obtained at Los Angeles County University of Southern California Medical Center and John Wesley County Hospital. From Edmondson HA, Peters RL: Neoplasms of the liver. *In* Schiff L, Schiff ER (eds): Diseases of the Liver, ed 5. Philadelphia, JB Lippincott Company, 1982, pp 1101–1157, with permission.

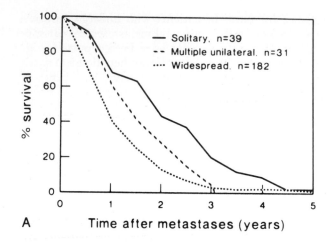

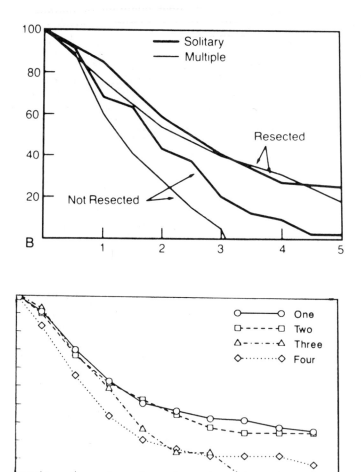

Figure 4. Survival graphs for colorectal cancer patients with *A*, unresected hepatic metastases; *B*, unresected versus resected hepatic metastases; and *C*, 1 to 4 resected hepatic metastases. (*A* from Wagner JS et al: Ann Surg *199*:502, 1984, by permission of the Mayo Foundation.)

HEMOBILIA

Hemobilia is an unusual manifestation of liver disease in which gastrointestinal hemorrhage occurs secondary to biliary tract bleeding. It may originate from almost any site along the biliary system including the liver parenchyma itself or the intrahepatic and extrahepatic bile ducts, including the gallbladder. Although the blood supply to the liver does not communicate directly with the biliary system, certain conditions such as trauma, infection, or tumor may create hemorrhage within the biliary tree. Penetrating or blunt trauma to the liver may cause hemobilia. However, most cases in the United States arise from the iatrogenic trauma of liver biopsy, ERCP, or stent placement. Most recently, transjugular intrahepatic portosystemic shunt (TIPS) procedures have been associated with acute hemobilia. Infection, gallstones, and tumors account for the remaining cases.

Clinically, hemobilia may appear early in the disease or quite late. The extent of bleeding may be massive with hematemesis and shock or minimal with only guaiac-positive stools. Classically, the triad of right upper quadrant pain, jaundice, and gastrointestinal tract bleeding suggests hemobilia.

The diagnosis of hemobilia is best made by arteriography. Occasionally, when a distal bile duct source is suspected, ERCP or percutaneous transhepatic cholangiography (PTC) may be useful. However, both procedures may cause hemobilia and obscure the diagnosis. In addition to its diagnostic use, arteriography with selective hepatic artery embolization is the initial treatment of choice for hemobilia. Because most hemobilia originates from an arterial rather than a venous source, selectively placed radiologic catheters can usually identify and embolize the bleeding source. However, if significant bleeding continues following embolization, operative intervention is mandatory.

HEPATIC RESECTION

Perioperative Care

Hepatic resection remains the treatment of choice for most primary and many metastatic hepatic malignancies. Improvements in surgical technique, perioperative management, and anesthetic monitoring have allowed hepatic resections to be performed with low mortality in many major centers. For hepatic excision to be successful, the surgeon must adequately assess and prepare the patient preoperatively, give meticulous attention to detail intraoperatively, and be capable of managing the potential complications postoperatively.

Patients must be carefully selected to exclude those with unresectable disease in the liver or extrahepatic metastatic spread. Advanced age is not an absolute contraindication. Often the *physiologic* age and performance status of the patient are better measures of operability. Most surgeons agree that cirrhosis is a contraindication to major hepatic resection due to the decreased regenerative capacity of the cirrhotic liver and bleeding complications.

Preoperative testing should include a complete history and physical examination, complete blood count, liver function tests, chest film, electrocardiogram, and coagulation studies. Any coagulation defect should be corrected preoperatively with vitamin K, fresh frozen plasma, or both. Resectability may be determined by a CT scan, ultrasonography, or MRI, with attention to the number and location of lesions, relation of the lesions to major vascular structures, and evidence of extrahepatic spread. Particular attention should be focused on the nutritional status of the patient, because preoperative nutritional support may decrease postoperative complications in severely malnourished patients. Laparoscopic examination is often diagnostic of resectability and should be used in the course to prevent the need for other studies, especially ultrasonography, and biopsy can often be obtained.

Most major hepatic resections require arterial and central venous monitoring. Bleeding is the most common and lethal intraoperative complication and occurs in approximately 5 to 10 per cent of patients. Improved intraoperative blood salvage with the *cell saver* together with preoperative autologous blood banking has decreased the amount of banked blood required during hepatic resection. The postoperative course is often directly correlated with the amount of intraoperative blood loss.

Postoperatively, patients may have massive "third-space" requirements with major extracellular fluid sequestration. Metabolic alkalosis is a common problem when large amounts of blood products are given and, if severe, may rarely need correction with central venous administration of 0.1 N hydrochloric acid. The most common postoperative complication is sepsis involving the wound, lungs, or abdomen. Bleeding, bile leak, and hepatic failure are the other major complications. A transient rise usually occurs in the serum bilirubin and other liver function tests postoperatively, but they should return to baseline within 7 to 10 days. A persistently elevated bilirubin suggests biliary obstruction and warrants further diagnostic evaluation. Persistent elevations in hepatocellular enzymes suggest an infectious complication or vascular injury. Serum albumin levels also transiently fall, but there is no beneficial effect of supplemental albumin administration.

Surgical Resection

Although there are eight segmental divisions of the liver, resection primarily involves four distinct seg-

ments: the anatomic right lobe, the anatomic left lobe, the medial segment of the left lobe in conjunction with the right lobe (a right trisegmentectomy), and the lateral segment of the left lobe (Fig. 5). Attempts to divide the liver along other planes may be hazardous and associated with considerable blood loss. The type of hepatic resection required is determined by the precise anatomic location of the lesions(s). There is increased survival for both primary and metastatic lesions in patients whose resection margins are greater than 1 cm. Heroic attempts to extend resections beyond normal anatomic boundaries as in advanced metastatic disease are rarely warranted due to poor outcome.

Laparoscopy may assist in staging the patient prior to operation. If deemed resectable, most patients are explored through a right upper quadrant or midline incision. Occasionally, with large tumors involving the right hepatic lobe, an extension of the incision into the right chest may be necessary to obtain vascular control. After excluding extrahepatic metastases, the liver is mobilized by dividing its ligamentous attachments. Intraoperative ultrasonography may be used to determine the presence of unsuspected lesions deep within the liver that would preclude curative resection.

After completing the ultrasonographic and visual assessment, the appropriate type of resection necessary to remove the lesion(s) is selected. The porta hepatis is dissected to isolate the hepatic artery, portal vein, and bile duct. After the *inflow* to the liver is isolated, control of the hepatic venous anatomy takes priority. Gaining access to the three hepatic veins constitutes

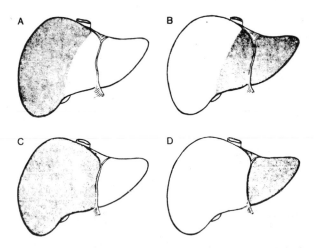

Figure 5. Four classic major hepatic resections: *A*, right hepatic lobectomy; *B*, left hepatic lobectomy; *C*, right trisegmentectomy; and *D*, left lateral segmentectomy. (From Meyers WC: Neoplasms of the liver. *In* Sabiston DC Jr [ed]: Textbook of Surgery: The Biological Basis of Modern Surgical Practice, ed 14. Philadelphia, WB Saunders Company, 1991, p 1008, with permission.)

the most technically demanding part of the operation, and the various techniques for control are well described elsewhere. Following the hepatic venous dissection, transection of the liver may be performed in different ways, but most prefer the *finger fracture* technique. The liver capsule is scored with cautery, and the parenchyma is fractured away by the fingers, exposing the veins, ducts, and arteries, which are subsequently ligated. Following transection of the liver fragment, hemostasis is meticulously obtained and multiple closed suction devices are left in place for 3 to 7 days postoperatively, depending on the drainage.

If severe hemorrhage occurs intraoperatively from a technical misadventure, the liver can be completely isolated by applying a vascular clamp across the porta hepatis (Pringle's maneuver), and the vena cava can be compressed above and below the liver. Warm ischemia is tolerated by the liver for as long as 1 hour. This vascular isolation technique often provides time to define the extent of the technical problem and achieve correction. The cardiac index remains remarkably stable in most patients despite complete vascular exclusion of the liver by vena caval occlusion.

Occasionally, hepatic wedge resection is indicated if the lesion is superficial. The lesion is excised with approximately 1 to 3 cm of surrounding normal liver tissue.

Finally, some lesions may be treated with *cryosurgery*, which destroys tumor in situ using subzero temperatures. This technique involves ultrasonographic localization of the hepatic lesion, placement of an encased liquid nitrogen probe within the lesion, and lowering of the tissue temperature to approximately $-35°C$ for several minutes followed by slow rewarming, repeating this cycle several times. Tumor destruction by cryosurgery has been achieved and is used as primary therapy or in conjunction with surgical resection of another lesion.

REFERENCES

Cady B (ed): Liver Surgery. Surg Clin North Am 69(2):179–445, 1989.

McDermott WV Jr (ed): Surgery of the Liver. Boston, Blackwell Scientific Publications, 1989.

Meyers WC: The liver. *In* Sabiston DC Jr (ed): Textbook of Surgery: The Biological Basis of Modern Surgical Practice, ed 14. Philadelphia, WB Saunders Company, 1991.

Meyers WC, Jones RS: Textbook of Liver and Biliary Surgery. Philadelphia, JB Lippincott Company, 1990.

Steele G, Ravikumar TS: Resection of hepatic metastases from colorectal cancer. Ann Surg 210(2):127–138, 1989.

Warren KW, Jenkins RL, Steele GD (eds): Atlas of Surgery of the Liver, Pancreas, and Biliary Tract. Norwalk, CT, Appleton & Lange, 1991.

33
THE BILIARY SYSTEM

SEAN J. MULVIHILL, M.D.

HISTORY

The first documented evidence of biliary tract disease was the finding of gallstones in an Egyptian mummy dated about 1000 BC. Few records exist documenting an awareness of the syndromes associated with biliary tract disease until the clinical features of jaundice were accurately described by Soranus of Ephesus about 100 AD. The Roman physician and anatomist Galen is credited with the first accurate description of the gallbladder. The pathophysiologic significance of gallstones was not understood until the fifth century AD, when Trallianus of Greece described bile duct calculi. Bobbs is credited with the first biliary tract operation in 1867, when he performed a successful cholecystotomy with extraction of gallstones. Langenbuch performed the first successful cholecystectomy in 1882. The first successful common bile duct operation was probably performed by Courvoisier in 1890, with removal of an obstructing bile duct stone. He subsequently has become well known for his description of enlargement of the gallbladder due to obstruction of the bile ducts by carcinoma of the pancreas (Courvoisier's sign).

A major advancement in the management of patients with suspected biliary tract disease occurred in the early 1920s, when Graham and Cole developed the radiologic technique of cholecystography to image the gallbladder. They discovered that an iodinated phenolphthalein compound was concentrated in gallbladder bile in the fasting state and could be visualized on plain abdominal radiographs. This imaging technique allowed clear identification of gallbladder stones. Direct operative cholangiography was described shortly thereafter by Mirizzi and Losada. Their technique permitted visualization of the intrahepatic

and extrahepatic biliary ductal system and reliable intraoperative detection of choledocholithiasis. Percutaneous transhepatic cholangiography and endoscopic retrograde cholangiography were developed in the 1950s, enabling preoperative evaluation of biliary ductal anatomy and identification of lesions such as tumors or stones with minimal risk. In addition to aiding in preoperative assessment of patients with biliary tract disorders, these imaging techniques also led to the rapid development of therapeutic radiologic and endoscopic procedures. Endoscopic sphincterotomy, for example, was first described in 1974 and, in less than 20 years, has become an important part of the management of a wide spectrum of biliary tract disorders, and many problems previously requiring operation can be managed with these less invasive methods. In modern surgical history, few techniques have been introduced with more rapid and widespread acceptance than *laparoscopic cholecystectomy*. This operation was probably first performed by Mouret in 1987 and represented a radical departure from the traditional abdominal operative techniques. By 1992, most general surgeons in the western world were trained in this technique, and it had become the standard form of management of patients with gallbladder disease.

ANATOMY

The biliary tract is the excretory system of the liver and includes: (1) the *intrahepatic ducts* that collect bile from each hepatic segment and coalesce into the *right and left hepatic ducts*; (2) the *common hepatic duct*, which is formed by the junction of the right and left hepatic ducts in the hilum of the liver; (3) the *gallbladder*, which serves as a reservoir for bile; (4) the *cystic duct*, which joins the gallbladder to the common hepatic duct; and (5) the *common bile duct*, which begins at the junction of the cystic duct and common hepatic duct and ends at the duodenal lumen. The biliary tract is derived from foregut endoderm, initially as a ventral outpouching destined to become the liver. This tissue is first identifiable at about 5 weeks' gestation in the human fetus. The gallbladder is formed as a secondary hollow outgrowth on the posterior edge of the liver diverticulum and can be recognized by about 8 weeks' gestation. The gallbladder is attached to the liver in a shallow fossa that lies at the junction of the right and left hepatic lobes. The extrahepatic biliary ducts are formed by the constriction of the original communication of the liver bud and the future duodenum. The epithelium lining the biliary tract is columnar, which in the gallbladder is expanded with fine rugal folds.

On gross inspection, the gallbladder is a pear-shaped organ with a capacity of approximately 30 to 50 ml (Fig. 1). The bulbous end is termed the *fundus*. The cystic duct arises from the narrow end, or *infundibulum* where, in diseased states, a dilatation known as *Hartmann's pouch* occurs. The cystic duct is usually 2 to 3 cm long and is characterized by crescentic folds in its epithelial lining termed *spiral valves of Heister*. The gallbladder is absent in certain mammals, such as horses and mice and, teleologically, may have evolved in response to a need to store bile in species such as carnivores, in whom food is ingested episodically.

The common bile duct is usually about 6 mm in diameter and passes behind the duodenum about 1 cm to the right of the gastroduodenal artery, traversing the head of the pancreas before it enters the second portion of the duodenum. The common bile duct may be obstructed at this point by pancreatic tumors. At the duodenum, the bile duct generally shares a common channel with the main pancreatic duct, and at their termination, these ducts are enveloped in specialized smooth muscle known as the *sphincter of Oddi* and empty into the duodenum at the *ampulla of Vater*. The sphincter of Oddi is responsible for partitioning the lumens of the intestinal tract, which contains bacteria, from the biliary tract, which is normally sterile. This sphincter relaxes in response to the same stimuli, such as cholecystokinin, that cause contraction of the gallbladder.

The arterial blood supply to the gallbladder is via the *cystic artery*, usually a branch of the right hepatic artery. The biliary ducts receive blood supply from small unnamed branches of the hepatic artery and from small retroperitoneal vessels. The venous drainage of the gallbladder and extrahepatic biliary ducts is into the portal vein. Lymphatics from the gallbladder drain into a cystic duct node found in the space between the cystic duct and the common hepatic duct. Other regional lymph node groups include hepatic or *portal nodes* in the posterior aspect of the hepatoduodenal ligament and those near the pylorus, left gastric artery, and head of the pancreas. The gallbladder and sphincter of Oddi are innervated by neurons of the *enteric nervous system* (ENS). The ENS is best regarded as the third component of the autonomic nervous system, complementing the sympathetic and parasympathetic divisions and is comprised of neurons whose cell bodies lie in gut ganglia. The function of these neurons, most of which use peptides as neurotransmitters, is influenced by input from preganglionic fibers of the sympathetic and parasympathetic nervous systems. Afferent fibers probably contribute to reflex control of gallbladder and sphincter function and are responsible for the pain characteristic of some biliary tract disorders.

The porta hepatis is an important anatomic area bounded by the cystic duct, common hepatic duct, and undersurface of the liver and is known as the *hepatocystic triangle* or *triangle of Calot* (Fig. 2). This small-but-critical region contains the cystic artery, right hepatic artery, cystic node, and an occasional aberrant right segmental bile duct, and must be carefully dissected during cholecystectomy to avoid inadvertent ductal injuries. The structures of the *hepatoduodenal ligament* include the extrahepatic biliary ducts, the hepatic artery, and the portal vein. The bile duct usually lies anterior and toward the right in the hepatoduodenal ligament with the hepatic artery anterior and toward the left. The third structure of the portal triad, the portal vein, lies posterior to the hepatic artery and bile duct. The *foramen of Winslow* is a passage between the abdominal cavity and the lesser sac posterior to the hepatoduodenal ligament that allows the portal structures to be encircled. The *Pringle maneuver* refers to digital compression between the thumb and forefinger of the structures of the hepatoduodenal ligament through the foramen of Winslow, which aids in control of hemorrhage from the liver after traumatic injury and may be performed during elective liver resection to reduce blood loss.

The gastroduodenal artery is usually palpable just distal to the pylorus at the superior aspect of the duodenal bulb. In the setting of severe portal inflammation, the gastroduodenal artery is a useful landmark to aid in determining the location of the supraduodenal bile duct, which lies just to the right. Additionally, division of the gastroduodenal artery opens the retroperitoneal space anterior to the portal vein at the neck of the pancreas. This plane must be identified and dissected to separate the portal vein from the pancreas during pancreaticoduodenectomy.

Anomalies of ductal and arterial anatomy in this

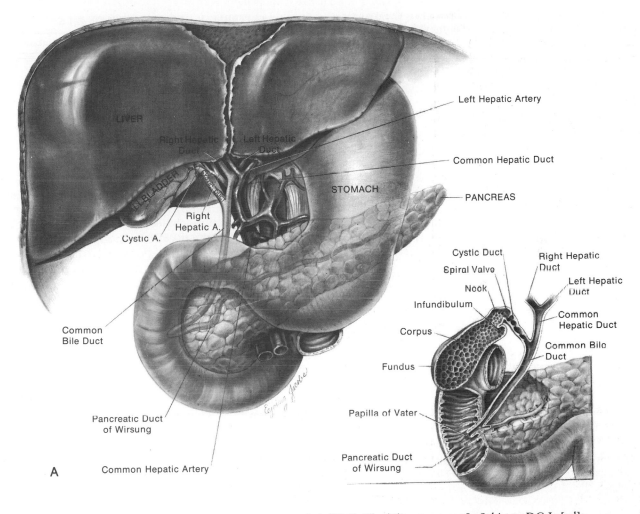

Figure 1. Anatomy of the biliary tract. (From Orloff MJ: The biliary system. *In* Sabiston DC Jr [ed]: Davis-Christopher Textbook of Surgery. Philadelphia, WB Saunders Company, 1981, chapter 36, with permission.)

region are common. The cystic duct normally enters the bile duct at its midportion, but may enter the common bile duct more distally, even in the retroduodenal portion. The cystic duct and bile duct occasionally parallel each other, may share a common wall over a variable distance, and may join in a spiral manner, with the cystic duct entering the bile duct on the left, possibly leading to confusion and misidentification of the common bile duct for the cystic duct. In other patients, the cystic duct may insert into the bile duct high in the porta hepatis, occasionally even into the right hepatic duct. Confusion between the cystic duct and a right posterior segmental hepatic duct may occur when the latter inserts as a separate branch extrahepatically rather than within the liver substance (Fig. 3).

PHYSIOLOGY

Bile Formation

Bile is the combined secretory product of both the hepatocyte and the biliary duct epithelial cell and has three main functions: (1) to solubilize and enhance absorption of enteral fat and fat-soluble vitamins; (2) to provide an excretory pathway for bilirubin, immunoglobulin A (IgA), and some drugs and toxins; and (3) to maintain duodenal alkalinization. The hepatocyte secretes bilirubin, cholesterol, bile acids, lecithin, electrolytes, and water continuously into the bile canaliculus (Table 1). The ductular cells produce mainly water and electrolytes, and their combined output ranges from 500 to 1500 ml/day. While secretion from the

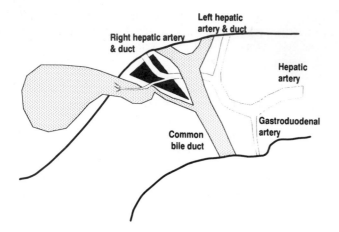

Figure 2. Structures of the porta hepatis. The hepatocystic triangle (*dark shaded area*) contains the cystic and right hepatic arteries. During cholecystectomy, clear identification of the structures in this area is required.

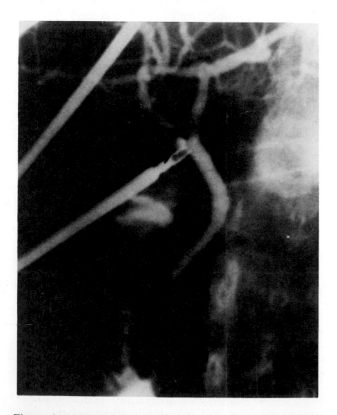

Figure 3. Unusual low and separate insertion of the right posterior segmental duct into the hepatic duct identified during cholangiography. This segmental duct (*arrow*) is adjacent to and may be mistaken for the cystic duct (*double arrows*) during cholecystectomy.

TABLE 1.   COMPOSITION OF BILE

Component	Approximate Concentration
Bilirubin	1–2 mM
Bile acids	3–45 mM
Lecithin	150–800 mg/dl
Cholesterol	100–300 mg/dl
Sodium	145 mM
Potassium	4 mM
Chloride	90 mM
Bicarbonate	25 mM

hepatocyte is mainly constitutive, the ductal cells are subject to regulation by neuroendocrine factors. Vagal stimulation, secretin, cholecystokinin (CCK), and gastrin stimulate ductular cell secretion and increase bile flow. Bile acids provide a positive feedback stimulation to enhance further choleresis via an unclear mechanism.

Bile Acid Metabolism

Bile acids such as cholate and chenodeoxycholate are synthesized within the hepatocyte from the precursor molecule, cholesterol, and are secreted in bile where they aggregate with lecithin and cholesterol to form micelles, which, in the small intestine, facilitate absorption of fat-soluble molecules. About 95 per cent of excreted bile acids are deconjugated in the intestine and reabsorbed in the ileum. Bile acids are then absorbed from the portal circulation at the level of the central lobular veins by hepatocytes. This cycling of bile acids has been termed *enterohepatic circulation*. A marked gradient of bile acid concentration exists between portal venous blood and systemic venous blood. Uptake of some bile acids, such as taurocholate, appears to be dependent upon concurrent sodium uptake by the hepatocyte at the basolateral or sinusoidal membrane, and additional sodium-independent pathways of uptake probably exist. The mechanisms of intracellular transport of bile acids from the basolateral membrane to the canalicular membrane are unclear. Secretion of bile acids by the hepatocyte into the canaliculus appears to be carrier mediated. Bile acid–binding carrier proteins have been isolated from both basolateral and canalicular membranes.

Bilirubin Metabolism

Bilirubin is the metabolic waste product of heme, which is itself the product of red blood cell destruction. The daily production of bilirubin in humans is about 4 mg/kg body weight. When red blood cells are destroyed, the heme is converted initially to biliverdin by the microsomal enzyme heme oxygenase in reticuloendothelial cells, and the biliverdin is rapidly converted to water-insoluble unconjugated bilirubin, which circulates in the bloodstream bound to albumin. Bilirubin is extracted from the bloodstream by the hepatocyte, bound to cytosolic proteins, and conjugated to the water-soluble bilirubin glucuronide. Conjugated bilirubin is then excreted across the canalicular membrane into bile. In the ileum, bilirubin is deconjugated by bacterial enzymes into urobilinogen, of which approximately 20 per cent is absorbed. The absorbed urobilinogen is either reexcreted in bile or excreted in urine. Conjugated bilirubin may be measured *directly* using diazoreagents, and total bilirubin, including the unconjugated fraction, is determined in the same assay with the use of additional substances to accelerate the reaction. The amount of *indirect* or unconjugated bilirubin is thus determined by subtraction of the direct component from the total amount.

Regulation of Gallbladder Function

The gallbladder is not simply a passive storage organ for bile that concentrates bile salts, pigments, and cholesterol up to ten-fold through absorption of water. The gallbladder mucosa secretes mucus that may prevent mucosal damage by bile salts. In response to a meal, the gallbladder contracts, emptying its contents into the duodenum to aid digestion. The regulation of this emptying is mainly hormonal, through the action of CCK. The main stimulant for the release of CCK from duodenal endocrine cells is intraluminal fat and amino acids. Evidence is now accruing that this stimulation of CCK release by fat and amino acids is indirect, and mediated by the release and action of a small, trypsin-sensitive duodenal peptide that has been termed CCK *releasing factor*. Vagal cholinergic fibers have a minor role in regulating gallbladder contraction. After truncal vagotomy, gallbladder emptying is impaired and gallstones are more prevalent. Gallbladder filling during fasting is facilitated by its relaxation and contraction of the sphincter of Oddi. In preparations of gallbladder muscle strips in vitro, vasoactive intestinal peptide (VIP) potently produces relaxation. Somatostatin is an inhibitory peptide that reduces gallbladder contractility. The risk of gallstone formation is increased in patients treated with octreotide, an analog of somatostatin, as well as in states of prolonged fasting, in which lack of CCK stimulation leads to gallbladder stasis.

Regulation of Sphincter of Oddi Function

Basal tone of the sphincter of Oddi is maintained at 5 to 10 mm Hg greater than duodenal pressure and is augmented both by intermittent and by sustained increases in pressure to 15 to 20 mm Hg above baseline.

Additionally, the sphincter exhibits phasic contractions up to 100 to 150 mm Hg approximately four times per minute. Control of sphincter function is due to interaction between both hormonal and neural factors. A major hormonal regulatory factor appears to be CCK, which produces relaxation of the sphincter muscle indirectly, via stimulation of inhibitory neurons. In animal models, evidence points to vasoactive intestinal polypeptide as an important inhibitory, or relaxant, neuropeptide on sphincter smooth muscle. Both adrenergic and cholinergic neurons of the sympathetic and parasympathetic nervous systems influence sphincter function through their interaction with neurons intrinsic to the sphincter itself.

CONGENITAL LESIONS

Gallbladder

Congenital lesions of the gallbladder are rare, with absence of the gallbladder (*gallbladder agenesis*) being reported in about 400 cases. Many patients are asymptomatic, but in about one half, the anomaly is discovered because of symptoms referable to the biliary tract. A genetic predisposition has been suggested, as several clusters within families have been identified. Gallbladder agenesis is associated with sclerosing cholangitis and bile duct carcinoma. Gallbladder duplications have also been reported. They may share a common cystic duct or, more rarely, be drained independently. The gallbladder may occur in ectopic locations, usually within the liver parenchyma and, occasionally, may be found suspended on a mesentery from the liver, rather than intimately bound in the gallbladder fossa. This anatomic arrangement predisposes to torsion of the gallbladder.

Bile Ducts

The main congenital abnormalities of the bile ducts may be divided into hypoplastic and cystic lesions. The main hypoplastic lesion is characterized by the absence of the bile ducts (biliary atresia). *Choledochal* cysts are congenital dilatations of the biliary tract, often reaching enormous size. Several types of choledochal cysts have been described, and a classification scheme has been proposed by Alonzo-Lej and Todani. The most common type is a large, fusiform dilatation of the common bile duct. Other types include diverticula of the bile ducts and localized saccular dilatations of the intraduodenal portion of the common bile duct (*choledochocele*). Rarely, children present with multiple, diffuse cysts in both the intrahepatic and extrahepatic ducts. When the cysts are limited to the intrahepatic ducts, the disorder is known as *Caroli's dis-*

ease. The incidence of Caroli's disease is greater in females than males by a ratio of 4:1. The etiology of choledochal cysts is unclear. A long common channel between the pancreatic and common bile ducts has been observed in most instances, but it is not known if this contributes to the formation of the cysts. Most patients with choledochal cysts present in infancy or childhood with jaundice, cholangitis, or a palpable abdominal mass. Liver function tests invariably reveal an elevated alkaline phosphatase and variable elevations in serum bilirubin. Ultrasonography generally confirms the diagnosis, but cholangiography is useful for an accurate assessment of the biliary anatomy. Choledochal cysts have a high likelihood of future development of carcinoma. Optimal management of the most common type I choledochal cyst is excision with Roux-en-Y hepaticojejunostomy reconstruction, which provides optimal biliary drainage and eliminates future risk of carcinoma in the cyst wall.

CHOLELITHIASIS AND BILIARY COLIC

Gallstones are a common disorder that affects about 20 million people in the United States. Worldwide, the prevalence is greatest in western societies, especially Scandinavia, and lowest in Africa and Asia. Certain defined populations have extraordinarily high risk for the development of gallstones. Adult female Pima Indians in the southwestern United States have a gallstone prevalence of approximately 70 per cent. Besides race, a number of other factors influence gallstone occurrence. Gallstones are uncommon in childhood, and the risk increases with increasing age. Women of reproductive age have a much greater risk than age-matched men. This gender difference is reduced, but still present, in women over age 60. Postmenopausal use of estrogen supplements and high-estrogen oral contraceptive agents also appear to increase the risk. Increasing parity has a modest effect in increasing gallstone risk. Obesity is a significant risk factor for gallstones. Curiously, rapid weight loss in the morbidly obese poses an even greater risk for their development. Gallstones occur frequently in patients with disorders of the terminal ileum, such as Crohn's disease, by a mechanism involving depletion of bile salts. Similarly, some lipid-lowering agents such as clofibrate significantly increase the risk of gallstone development. Gallstones are a common complication of long-term fasting with total parenteral nutrition and, finally, commonly occur in patients with chronic hemolysis.

Pathogenesis of Gallstones

Gallstones are generally classified according to their composition. The most common, composed of a mix-

ture of cholesterol, calcium carbonate, and some bile pigment, have been termed *predominantly cholesterol* or *mixed stones* and are usually yellow to green in color. Rarely, when stones are formed purely of cholesterol they are white and have the appearance of pearls. So-called *pigment* stones occur in two forms. Some are found mainly in the gallbladder and are multiple, black, comprised predominantly of an insoluble polymer of bilirubinate, and are associated with cirrhosis, biliary infections, and hemolysis. Other pigment stones, brown and earthy in appearance, are comprised mainly of calcium bilirubinate, are associated with biliary tract infection in conditions such as bile duct stricture and Oriental cholangiohepatitis, and commonly form within the bile ducts rather than the gallbladder.

Cholesterol and mixed stones form through a combination of three factors: (1) supersaturation of cholesterol within gallbladder bile, (2) a nucleating event, and (3) incomplete gallbladder emptying (Fig. 4). Supersaturation of cholesterol within gallbladder bile occurs through an imbalance in the components of bile, its primary constituents being water, electrolytes, cholesterol, phospholipid, bile salts, and bile pigments. Cholesterol and phospholipid (mainly lecithin) are insoluble in water and are maintained in solution in bile by bile salt micelle formation. Bile is *lithogenic* when the ratios of lecithin and bile salts are insufficient to maintain cholesterol in solution, a condition that can be induced when one or any combination of the following is present: decreased bile salt secretion, decreased biliary phospholipid concentration, and increased biliary cholesterol secretion (Fig. 5). Stone formation additionally requires nucleation with bacteria, cellular debris, mucus, or other substances within the gallbladder. Growth of the stone presum-

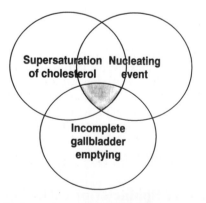

Figure 4. Pathogenesis of cholesterol gallstones. A combination of factors, including supersaturation of bile cholesterol, incomplete gallbladder emptying, and a nucleating event, are probably all required for gallstone formation and growth (*shaded area*).

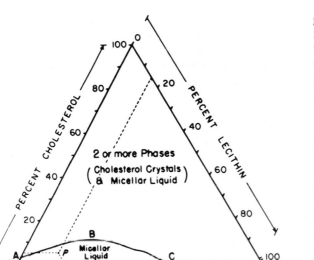

Figure 5. Solubility of biliary cholesterol. The components of bile are listed on separate axes. The area under curved line ABC defines a solution in which cholesterol is soluble and stone formation will not occur. The area above line ABC represents a solution in which cholesterol may exist in several phases, including crystals. Point P contains 80 mol/dl of bile salts, 18 mol/dl of lecithin, and 5 mol/dl of cholesterol, an equilibrium that allows cholesterol solubility in a micellar phase. (From Small DM: N Engl J Med 279:588, 1968, with permission.)

ably requires incomplete gallbladder evacuation in response to a meal.

The pathogenesis of pigment stones is incompletely understood, but involves secretion of an excess of unconjugated bilirubin in the bile. Another factor may be increased activity of the enzyme β-glucuronidase, which hydrolyzes soluble bilirubin glucuronide to insoluble unconjugated bilirubin and glucuronic acid. Bacteria in the biliary tract may contribute to increased β-glucuronidase activity. Unconjugated bilirubin is probably solubilized by bile salts; however, it may precipitate as calcium bilirubinate and form stones in the presence of nucleating factors such as bacteria. Bacteria have been identified by electron microscopy in the interior of the majority of pigment stones, particularly brown, earthy stones.

Biliary Colic: Clinical and Pathologic Findings

Biliary colic is the pain typical of intermittent obstruction of the cystic duct by a gallstone and is the most common presenting symptom of patients with gallstones. Most patients with biliary colic complain of recurrent attacks of right upper quadrant or epi-

gastric abdominal pain following a heavy meal, and nausea is common. The pain is colicky in the sense that it comes and goes and recurs again at intervals ranging from days to months. A single episode of pain generally lasts no longer than 6 hours, and pain that lasts longer is suggestive of acute cholecystitis. Often, the pain radiates around the chest wall to the tip of the right scapula. Other symptoms, such as flatulence, bloating, and excessive gas may be due to gallbladder disease, but are not as reliable as biliary colic. Physical examination of the patient with biliary colic generally reveals mild right upper quadrant tenderness with or without guarding. Jaundice, fever, and peritoneal signs are absent. The gallbladder is not palpable and the liver edge is not tender. Laboratory examination reveals a normal white blood count, liver function tests, and amylase. The gallbladders of most but not all patients with biliary colic show chronic inflammation and fibrosis termed *chronic cholecystitis*. Adhesions of the gallbladder to omentum, duodenum, and transverse colon are commonly found at operation for chronic cholecystitis. Additional pathologic findings of chronic cholecystitis include invaginations of the mucosal lining termed *Rokitansky-Aschoff* sinuses. Occasionally, gallstones are associated with *cholesterolosis*, or punctate deposition of cholesterol in histiocytes of the gallbladder wall.

Radiologic Evaluation

Ultrasound is the most sensitive, specific, and cost effective technique for the radiologic confirmation of cholelithiasis. Ultrasonography has a diagnostic accuracy of 95 per cent or more in experienced hands. It should be recognized, however, that occasional patients with gallstone disease are missed by ultrasound, and ancillary tests may be required. The main criteria for diagnosis of gallstones by ultrasound are mobile echogenic foci within the gallbladder that produce acoustic shadowing (Fig. 6). Other tests include plain abdominal radiographs, which detect only about 15 per cent of gallstones, and oral or intravenous cholecystography. Oral cholecystography was formerly a widely used technique for the diagnosis of cholelithiasis. Its major disadvantages compared to ultrasound include (1) the necessity for oral administration of iopanoic acid, as well as its enteral absorption and hepatic excretion into bile; and (2) the need for ionizing radiation to visualize the opacified gallbladder. It remains, however, a useful test when ultrasonographic examination is equivocal and when determination of cystic duct patency is required.

Treatment

Advances in medical, radiologic, and surgical therapy of gallstones have broadened the treatment op-

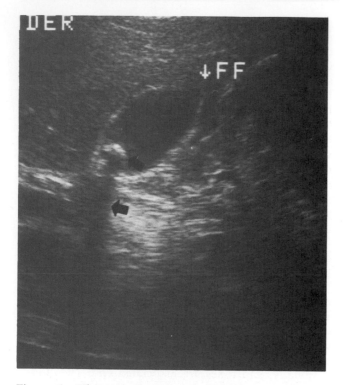

Figure 6. Ultrasonic features of cholelithiasis. The gallbladder is a pear-shaped structure filled with sonolucent bile. Gallstones are identified by their high echogenicity, mobility within the gallbladder, and acoustic shadowing (*arrows*).

on radiographic examination and their buoyancy in bile during oral cholecystography. Efficacy of dissolution therapy markedly decreases in patients with stone diameters larger than 5 to 10 mm and in those with a large total burden of stones. The cystic duct must be patent to allow for filling and emptying of unsaturated bile. This is usually determined by visualization of the gallbladder on oral cholecystography. Finally, oral dissolution therapy is only warranted for patients with uncomplicated, mild attacks of biliary colic. Patients with jaundice, acute cholecystitis, or pancreatitis must be excluded. Within these constraints, 30 to 50 per cent of appropriately selected patients have complete stone dissolution within 2 years with ursodeoxycholic acid treatment, as determined by follow-up ultrasonography. A major drawback of this treatment, however, is the risk of stone recurrence following withdrawal of oral dissolution agents. About 50 per cent of patients in whom stones are successfully dissolved will recur within 5 years.

Contact dissolution of cholesterol gallstones is possible with ether-based compounds administered directly into the gallbladder via a catheter placed percutaneously. Methyl tert-butyl ether (MTBE) is the most widely used agent. It remains under investigation in the United States. In small reported series, 50 to 90 per cent of treated patients are rendered free of stones within 3 to 4 days of treatment. Complications relate both to the placement of the percutaneous catheter and to overdose or extravasation of the MTBE. This therapy is expected to have the same problems with long-term stone recurrence as oral dissolution agents, and it has not yet been approved for use outside clinical trials.

Lithotripsy

As with renal stones, gallstones may be fragmented by focused, extracorporeally generated shock waves. These acoustic waves may be generated by an electrohydraulic spark-gap, piezoelectric crystals, or an electromagnetic membrane. They travel through water and body tissues unimpeded, but release energy on impact with stones, causing fragmentation. Adjuvant bile acid treatment aids in the dissolution of the fragments. Patient selection is similar to that for oral dissolution agents. Patients with arrhythmias and pacemakers are excluded, as the shock wave administration is gated to the electrocardiogram. Up to 90 per cent of selected patients are rendered free of gallstones within 2 years, although multiple lithotripsy sessions may be required. Common bile duct calculi have also successfully been treated with lithotripsy. Complications such as severe hematuria, bile duct obstruction with fragments, or pancreatitis are uncommon. Recurrence of gallstones, however, occurs in about 50 per cent of patients

tions currently available. Therapies with proven efficacy include dissolution agents, lithotripsy, and cholecystectomy. Alterations in diet have little or no effect in preventing symptoms from gallstones or in inducing spontaneous gallstone dissolution. Two main classes of agents are available for dissolution of cholesterol gallstones, oral bile acids and contact dissolution with ether-based compounds. Oral dissolution agents include chenodeoxycholic acid (chenodiol) and ursodeoxycholic acid (ursodiol). These agents both reduce biliary cholesterol secretion, promoting solubilization of crystalline cholesterol from the gallstones. The mechanism of action of chenodiol appears to involve inhibition of hydroxymethylglutaryl-CoA reductase, the rate-limiting enzyme responsible for the hepatic synthesis of cholesterol. Ursodiol, in contrast, inhibits intestinal cholesterol absorption. Side effects of chenodiol, including diarrhea and hepatic toxicity, have limited its use as a single agent. Ursodiol lacks these side effects and is the most widely used agent, either alone or in combination with chenodiol.

Several factors influence outcome in patients treated with oral dissolution agents. Only stones high in cholesterol content are likely to dissolve. This factor is determined indirectly by the lucency of the gallstones within 5 years, and recent U.S. trials suggest that the efficacy and cost of lithotripsy compare poorly with cholecystectomy.

Cholecystectomy

Cholecystectomy remains the most appropriate option for the majority of patients with biliary colic, and *laparoscopic cholecystectomy* has supplanted the open approach in most patients. In this technique, carbon dioxide is infused into the abdominal cavity to create a space (pneumoperitoneum) in which to work. Four trocars are placed through 5- to 10-mm incisions to allow access for the necessary instruments. The surgeon and assistants view the operative field on video monitors that relay images from a telescope and camera. The cystic duct and artery are identified, controlled with small metal clips, and divided. Fluoroscopic cholangiography via the cystic duct may be performed if desired (Fig. 7). The gallbladder is dissected off of the liver fossa, aspirated to evacuate bile and stones, and removed. Postoperative pain, ileus, and disability are all markedly decreased in patients who undergo laparoscopic cholecystectomy when compared to those who undergo open cholecystectomy via a laparotomy incision. Most patients are discharged from the hospital the day following the operation and return to full activity and employment within 1 week. Cholecystectomy substantially relieves or cures symptoms in about 95 per cent of patients. The results are better in patients with definite biliary colic and gallstones than in those with nonspecific dyspepsia or microlithiasis. The risk of death from cholecystectomy is low, especially in the elective setting. The overall risk of death in 42,474 patients undergoing cholecystectomy in California and Maryland in 1989 was 0.17 per cent. The risk of postoperative death is increased in advanced age. Patients under age 65, for example, have a mortality rate for cholecystectomy of 0.03 per cent, whereas the rate in those over age 65 is 0.5 per cent. Most mortality is linked to cardiovascular complications, particularly myocardial infarction.

The overall complication rate of cholecystectomy is 4 to 5 per cent. Most complications are relatively minor, such as wound infections or seromas, urinary retention or infection, and atelectasis. Complications related directly to cholecystectomy include bile leak, bile duct injury, and acute pancreatitis, bile duct injury being most serious. The rate of bile duct injury during cholecystectomy is not precisely known, but is estimated to be 1 per 600 cases, and the risk appears to be modestly higher for laparoscopic cholecystectomy (Table 2).

Postcholecystectomy Syndrome

Postcholecystectomy syndrome refers to a spectrum of conditions causing symptoms referable to the biliary tract following cholecystectomy. Significant symptoms occur in 5 to 10 per cent of patients in long-term follow-up. Causes for pain independent of the biliary tract, including angina, peptic ulcer disease, and irritable bowel syndrome, must be excluded. In patients with recurrent biliary tract pain, the most common findings include common bile duct stones, bile duct stricture, residual stones or neuromas in the cystic duct stump, and sphincter of Oddi dysfunction. Evaluation and management of patients with postcholecystectomy complaints require careful attention to these possibilities.

Special Problems

Asymptomatic Gallstones

Gallstones are occasionally discovered accidentally in patients who do not have symptoms referable to the biliary tract. Decisions regarding management of these stones is predicated on a knowledge of the natural history of the condition. Once gallstones develop, they rarely, if ever, resolve spontaneously. Early studies suggested that the majority of patients with asymptomatic gallstones eventually developed symptoms or complications related to the stones. More recent data, however, suggest that the rate of developing symptoms is only 1 to 2 per cent per year (Fig. 8) and that serious complications or deaths related to asymptomatic gallstones are rare. Decision analysis calculations indicate that the risks of cholecystectomy approximate the potential benefit in preventing complications of asymptomatic gallstones. The average patient should be counseled that gallstones discovered incidentally require no special treatment or follow-up and that therapy can be initiated if and when symptoms such as biliary colic develop. Formerly, it was thought that asymptomatic gallstones in the diabetic population posed special risks and that prophylactic operation was warranted. Critical analysis of the data does not support this position, thus the advice outlined above also applies to the diabetic. In certain situations, prophylactic cholecystectomy does appear warranted. Native American Indians, for example, have a high incidence of gallstone-associated gallbladder carcinoma. Prophylactic cholecystectomy appears warranted in this small group of patients to prevent the development of gallbladder cancer. Similar rationale applies to patients with large gallstones (>2.5 cm diameter) and those with calcification of the gallbladder wall (porcelain gallbladder). In patients undergoing laparotomy for other conditions, incidental cholecystec-

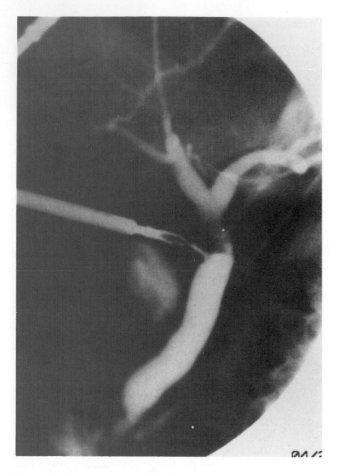

Figure 7. Intraoperative cholangiography. A 4-Fr catheter (*arrow*) is laparoscopically inserted into the cystic duct and secured with a clamp. Dye is injected under fluoroscopic guidance to ensure filling of the entire intrahepatic and extrahepatic ductal system. Free flow of dye is noted into the duodenum (*double arrows*).

tomy for asymptomatic gallstones does not markedly increase operative risk and prevents later symptomatic gallbladder disease as well as the difficult problem of postoperative acute cholecystitis. Cholecystectomy is warranted if the primary operation proceeds smoothly and exposure is adequate.

Biliary Colic in Pregnancy

Gallstones occasionally become evident during pregnancy, and the most common symptoms are upper abdominal pain and nausea compatible with biliary colic. Jaundice and pancreatitis are, fortunately, uncommon. Radiologic evaluation of symptoms suggestive of biliary tract disease can almost always be limited to sonography. If gallstones are identified, the clinician must weigh the severity of the symptoms and stage of gestation to determine if cholecystectomy can be deferred until after parturition. Recent advances in anesthetic management and tocolytic therapy have made cholecystectomy during pregnancy safe regardless of the trimester of gestation. In selected cases, cholecystectomy may be performed laparoscopically. Oral dissolution agents and/or gallstone lithotripsy are contraindicated during pregnancy.

Biliary Colic in the Absence of Gallstones

Occasionally, patients present with symptoms compatible with biliary colic, although gallstones are not identified on screening ultrasonography. Pain in these patients may be due to (1) gallstones missed by ultrasonography, (2) microlithiasis, or (3) disease unrelated to the gallbladder. The approach to such a patient should include repeat ultrasonography or oral cholecystography in an attempt to identify occult stones. Failing this, if the clinical suspicion of gallbladder disease is high, endoscopic retrograde cholangiography with collection of bile for microscopic identification of cholesterol crystals is warranted. If crystals are identified, recent studies suggest that two thirds of patients have relief of their symptoms following cholecystectomy. Upper gastrointestinal tract endoscopy and/or contrast studies and, rarely, computed tomography (CT) of the upper abdomen may be required to exclude peptic ulcer disease, gastroesophageal reflux, or an occult neoplasm as the cause of the pain.

Gallstone Ileus

Gallstone ileus is intestinal obstruction caused by a large gallstone impacted in the intestinal lumen. The

TABLE 2. OUTCOME OF LAPAROSCOPIC CHOLECYSTECTOMY FOR BILIARY COLIC: EARLY SERIES

Group	Year	Number of Patients	Mortality Rate (%)	Bile Duct Injury (%)	Conversion Rate* (%)
Southern Surgeons Club	1991	1516	0.07	0.5	4.7
European	1991	1236	0	0.3	3.6
Louisville	1992	1983	0.1	0.25	4.5
SAGES	1992	1771	0.06	0.2	4.6
Canadian	1992	2201	0	0.14	4.3

* Conversion rate refers to the percentage of patients requiring conversion from a laparoscopic procedure to an open procedure.
Abbreviation: SAGES = Society of American Gastrointestinal Endoscopic Surgeons.

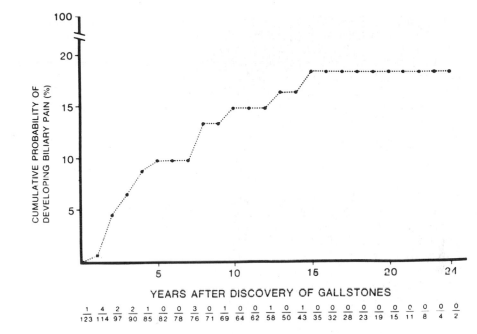

Figure 8. Natural history of asymptomatic gallstones. In a cohort of 123 faculty members of the University of Michigan with asymptomatic gallstones, the probability of developing biliary pain averaged 1 per cent per year of follow-up. (From Gracie WA, Ransohoff DF: N Engl J Med *307*:798, 1982, with permission.)

term is a misnomer in that the symptoms relate to a true mechanical obstruction rather than decreased peristaltic activity. The pathophysiology of gallstone ileus involves erosion of a gallstone through the gallbladder wall and into the intestine, commonly the duodenum, via a cholecystoenteric fistula. Most patients are elderly and complain of intermittent crampy abdominal pain, distention, and vomiting. The symptoms tend to vary as the stone progresses distally. Complete obstruction characteristically occurs in the ileum. Abdominal radiographs reveal an obstructive pattern, but the gallstone is visible in only a small minority of patients. Pneumobilia, if present in the setting of intestinal obstruction, is highly suggestive of gallstone ileus. Ultrasonography is useful to identify cholelithiasis and may suggest the presence of the cholecystoenteric fistula. Initial management is directed at correction of the fluid and electrolyte abnormalities associated with the intestinal obstruction. At laparotomy, the obstruction is relieved by removal of the stone through a small enterotomy, and any additional enteric gallstones should also be removed. Correction of the cholecystoenteric fistula is not required, as it usually closes spontaneously. Cholecystectomy should be performed only if symptoms of chronic cholecystitis persist. The mortality of all patients with gallstone ileus is high, around 20 per cent, and recurrent gallstone ileus occurs in about 5 per cent of patients.

Mirizzi Syndrome

This syndrome refers to common hepatic duct obstruction due to compression by a gallstone impacted in the cystic duct. Commonly, the associated inflammatory changes cause a hepatic duct stricture that may be difficult to differentiate from carcinoma. Most patients present with repeated bouts of pain, fever, and jaundice. Endoscopic retrograde cholangiopancreatography is useful to delineate the ductal stricture. Treatment is individualized, depending on the nature of the lesion, and biliary reconstruction is often required to cure the stricture.

Gallstones in Childhood

Gallstones are uncommon in childhood except in special circumstances, such as chronic hemolysis (as with sickle-cell diseases) and short-bowel syndrome with chronic total parenteral nutrition. Cholecystectomy is indicated for all symptomatic patients and in asymptomatic patients with pigment stones. Laparoscopic cholecystectomy is also feasible in children.

ACUTE CHOLECYSTITIS

Acute Calculous Cholecystitis

Pathophysiology

Acute cholecystitis, an inflammatory condition of the gallbladder, usually follows obstruction of the cystic duct by a gallstone and is the most commonly encountered complication of gallstones. The pathophysiology of acute cholecystitis is not completely understood, but appears to be initiated by impaction of a gallstone in Hartmann's pouch or the cystic duct with obstruction of gallbladder emptying. The obstruction initiates an acute inflammatory response in the gallbladder wall, which is followed by gallbladder wall ischemia from acute distention, pressure necrosis, and venous outflow obstruction. Additionally, mucosal injury occurs due to toxic chemical constituents of the entrapped bile. Bacterial superinfection supervenes in about 75 per cent of cases, but does not appear to play an initiating role in the process. If the obstructing stimulus is relieved (either spontaneously or through external catheter drainage of the gallbladder), the inflammatory response subsides within 6 weeks. In approximately 10 per cent of patients, however, complications of acute cholecystitis supervene, including empyema (intraluminal abscess formation), perforation (with resultant bile peritonitis or pericholecystic abscess), and fistulization to adjacent hollow organs (especially the duodenum, colon, or stomach). Some patients present with hydrops of the gallbladder, a condition in which chronic obstruction of the cystic duct in the absence of infection leads to accumulation of gallbladder mucus within the lumen (white bile).

Diagnosis

The majority of patients with acute calculous cholecystitis present with acute or gradual onset of right upper quadrant pain that initially is indistinguishable from biliary colic. Unlike biliary colic, however, the pain gradually worsens, with nausea, vomiting, and moderate fever being common. Septic shock is uncommon and usually implies the presence of a serious complication, such as perforation. Examination reveals right upper quadrant guarding and tenderness with localized peritonitis. *Murphy's sign*, or inspiratory arrest during gentle palpation of the right upper quadrant over the gallbladder, is usually present, while diffuse signs of peritoneal irritation are usually absent. The gallbladder is seldom palpable, and jaundice is rare. Fever and marked abdominal tenderness may be deceptively absent in three groups of patients: the elderly, the immunocompromised, and those treated with steroids. The clinician must maintain a high degree of suspicion that acute cholecystitis may be the cause of clinical deterioration in these patients, even in the absence of dramatic physical findings. Laboratory examination of patients with acute cholecystitis is significant for leukocytosis, which sometimes helps distinguish this condition from biliary colic. Serum amylase should be measured to differentiate acute cholecystitis (in which the levels are usually normal) from acute pancreatitis (in which the levels of amylase are elevated). Liver function tests are usually normal or minimally elevated in a nonspecific pattern. Some pa-

tients have mildly elevated bilirubin levels (<4 mg/dl), probably due to partial blockage of the common bile duct from edema related to the inflammation in the gallbladder wall. A chest radiograph should be obtained to exclude other diagnoses such as perforated duodenal ulcer or right lower lobe pneumonia. Plain abdominal radiographs reveal opaque gallstones in only about 15 per cent of cases. Rarely, gas is seen in the gallbladder wall, which is diagnostic of an advanced form of necrotizing cholecystitis (*emphysematous cholecystitis*). The mainstay of imaging modalities is ultrasound, which rapidly, accurately, and noninvasively confirms the diagnosis in the majority of patients. Ultrasonographic features of acute calculous cholecystitis include cholelithiasis, gallbladder wall thickening, the presence of pericholecystic (inflammatory) fluid, and gallbladder wall tenderness (the sonographic Murphy's sign). If ultrasonography is equivocal, radionuclide cholescintigraphy with technetium-99m–labeled dimethyliminodiacetic acid (^{99m}Tc-HIDA) may be used to determine cystic duct patency. Absence of gallbladder filling is highly suggestive of acute cholecystitis. False-positive examinations occasionally occur in the fasted patient with a distended gallbladder.

Management

Initial management of the patient with acute calculous cholecystitis includes rehydration and correction of electrolyte deficits. Nasogastric tube decompression of the stomach is valuable if vomiting is prominent, but it is probably unnecessary otherwise. Antibiotics directed against gram-negative enteric organisms are useful in all but the mildest of cases. Anaerobic coverage with agents such as metronidazole should be added for severely ill patients in whom necrotizing or gangrenous cholecystitis is suspected. Following initial resuscitation, cholecystectomy is indicated for most patients. The optimal timing of cholecystectomy in the setting of acute cholecystitis has been studied in at least four randomized, prospective trials. These trials have convincingly shown that early cholecystectomy, within 72 hours of the onset of symptoms, has several advantages over the strategy of delaying surgery for 6 weeks (Table 3). Although delayed surgery allows resolution of the acute inflammation in most patients, about 20 per cent suffer a recurrent attack of acute cholecystitis prior to the planned surgery. The total hospital stay, complication rate, and duration of disability all favor the strategy of early surgery. Recent experience has demonstrated the feasibility of laparoscopic cholecystectomy in most cases of acute cholecystitis. In some patients, the degree of inflammation in the right upper quadrant makes safe dissection of the gallbladder and porta he-

TABLE 3. COMPARISON OF EARLY VERSUS DELAYED CHOLECYSTECTOMY IN ACUTE CHOLECYSTITIS:
COMBINED RESULTS OF RANDOMIZED TRIALS

Timing of Cholecystectomy	Number of Patients	Mortality Rate	Bile Duct Injuries	Total Mean Hospital Stay (days)	Failure of Treatment*
Early	215	0%	0	10.9	—
Late	192	2.6%	0	20.1	19%

*Defined as progressive acute symptoms requiring early surgery.

patis impossible. In these cases, decompression of the gallbladder with evacuation of bile, pus, and stones via a tube cholecystostomy is the preferred approach. In high-risk patients for whom the operative risk is excessive, a tube cholecystostomy may be placed percutaneously, and following resolution of the inflammatory process, cholangiography is performed prior to removal of the tube. Residual stones are removed, if possible, with fluoroscopic guidance. Delayed cholecystectomy is indicated for fit patients.

Acalculous Cholecystitis

In about 5 per cent of cases of acute cholecystitis, gallstones are absent, a condition termed acalculous cholecystitis. This form of cholecystitis generally occurs in patients hospitalized for other reasons, including major vascular and cardiac surgery, trauma, burns, and those receiving total parenteral nutrition or large volumes of blood transfusion. The pathophysiology of acalculous cholecystitis probably involves gallbladder stasis rather than obstruction. The subsequent events leading to the acute inflammatory response are unclear. In many patients, the diagnosis of acalculous cholecystitis is delayed both because of the inability to obtain an accurate history of new abdominal pain and because abdominal findings are obscured by incisional tenderness and analgesic use. Ultrasonography should be performed when the clinical suspicion of acalculous cholecystitis is raised. Findings suggestive of acalculous cholecystitis include marked gallbladder distention, the presence of thick "sludge," gallbladder wall thickening and tenderness, and the presence of pericholecystic fluid. Specificity of ultrasonography in the diagnosis of acalculous cholecystitis varies from 60 to 95 per cent in reported series. If the diagnosis remains uncertain, ^{99m}Tc-HIDA radionuclide scintigraphy may be performed; however, a major drawback of this procedure, as in acute calculous cholecystitis, is the high frequency of false-positive scans. Management options for the patient with acalculous cholecystitis include percutaneous cholecystostomy and cholecystectomy, depending on the fitness of the patient for surgery. Perforation and gangrene commonly complicate the course of patients with acalculous cholecystitis, and mortality rates in recent reported series average 10 to 15 per cent and reflect the serious nature of these patients' underlying illnesses.

CHOLEDOCHOLITHIASIS

Incidence

Choledocholithiasis is the presence of gallstones within the common bile duct or hepatic ducts. Overall, choledocholithiasis is identified in 10 to 15 per cent of patients with cholelithiasis. The risk of common duct stones varies with age, with younger patients being at lowest risk. The incidence of common duct stones in association with gallstones in patients over age 60 is estimated to be 25 per cent.

Pathophysiology

Common bile duct stones are of two types. Most, originating in the gallbladder and passing via the cystic duct into the common bile duct, are cholesterol stones and are invariably associated with cholelithiasis. In a small minority of patients, the stones form de novo in the common bile duct, and have been termed primary *common bile duct stones*. They are usually formed of calcium bilirubinate and are associated with bacteria and stasis. Many patients have associated common bile duct pathology, such as stricture or sclerosing cholangitis. In the Orient, primary hepatic duct stones are commonly found in association with parasitic infections such as *Clonorchis sinensis* and bacterial colonization of the ducts, a condition that has been termed *Oriental cholangiohepatitis*. The natural history of patients with choledocholithiasis is incompletely understood. Some patients appear to harbor common duct stones for long periods of time without symptoms; however, it is also true that some of the most devastating complications of gallstones occur after stone migration into the common bile duct. The rate at which these complications occur in a population of asymptomatic patients with choledocholithiasis is not known with certainty, but appears significant. The most common complication of choledocholithiasis is *obstructive jaundice*, which is usually due to impaction of a stone in the distal common bile duct, near the sphincter of Oddi. This obstruction prevents excretion of bile, and jaundice ensues. In the presence of bacteria in the duct, unrelieved obstruction progresses to a serious infection termed acute cholangitis. Some stones spontaneously pass from the common bile duct through the sphincter of Oddi into the duodenum. During this passage, transient obstruction of the pancreatic duct may lead to gallstone pancreatitis. In a minority of patients, intermittent pain is the only indication of choledocholithiasis. The pain associated with common bile duct stones mimics biliary colic and probably occurs because of intermittent obstruction of the distal duct.

Diagnostic Evaluation

The diagnostic evaluation of a patient with suspected choledocholithiasis begins with an evaluation of liver function tests. Liver function tests are abnormal in the majority of patients with choledocholithiasis. The pattern of the tests aids in distinguishing ductal stones from other conditions such as hepatitis and acute pancreatitis (Table 4). In up to 5 per cent of patients undergoing cholecystectomy, common bile duct stones are present in the absence of abnormalities in liver function tests. As a screening tool, measurement of serum alkaline phosphatase appears to have the highest diagnostic accuracy. The initial radiologic examination in a patient with suspected choledocholithiasis is usually ultrasonography. Although common bile duct calculi are not reliably detected by ultrasonography, indirect signs such as cholelithiasis and dilatation of the intrahepatic and extrahepatic biliary ducts are helpful in differentiating choledocholithiasis from other icteric conditions such as hepatitis. Accurate evaluation of the ductal anatomy is possible via *endoscopic retrograde cholangiopancreatography* (ERCP). In this procedure, the ampulla of Vater is cannulated endoscopically and the ducts are examined with retrograde injection of dilute contrast material. In addition to visualization of the biliary tree, the pancreatic ductal system may be examined, if desired, and the endoscopist can directly examine the periampullary area to exclude obstructing lesions, such as neo-

plasms. An alternative to ERCP is *transhepatic cholangiography* (THC), wherein an interventional radiologist cannulates an intrahepatic biliary duct with a thin needle under fluoroscopic guidance. *Intraoperative cholangiography* may be performed during laparoscopic or open cholecystectomy to visualize the ductal system with direct injection of contrast material via the cystic duct. This procedure adds little risk or cost to cholecystectomy and aids in the identification of unsuspected common bile duct stones and variations in biliary ductal anatomy (Fig. 7).

Treatment

As a general principle, common bile duct stones should be removed when discovered to avoid complications such as pancreatitis, obstructive jaundice, and cholangitis. In patients presenting with obstructive jaundice due to choledocholithiasis, there are two main management strategies: (1) endoscopic sphincterotomy with stone extraction, or (2) cholecystectomy with *common bile duct exploration* (CBDE). In the hands of experienced endoscopists, the former technique is technically successful in clearing the duct in about 85 per cent of patients. Potential complications include bleeding, pancreatitis, and duodenal perforation, which occur in 5 to 7 per cent of patients. The overall mortality in recent published series averages 1.5 per cent. Common bile duct exploration is successful at clearing the duct in about 95 per cent of patients. Recent series of both open and laparoscopic CBDE indicate that the procedure can be performed in selected patients, with a mortality rate of less than 1 per cent. Technically, the duct is explored through a longitudinal incision, termed a *choledochotomy*. Direct visualization of the ductal stones is possible via *choledochoscopy*, and a variety of instruments are available for stone extraction. Once the duct is cleared, the choledochotomy is closed over a *T-tube*, which is removed in about 4 weeks after a follow-up cholangiogram confirms that no residual stones are present. Patients with retained stones identified on follow-up T-tube cholangiography are best treated with stone extraction via the T-tube tract under fluoro-

TABLE 4.   LIVER FUNCTION TESTS IN SELECTED ICTERIC CONDITIONS

| Condition | Bilirubin | | | Alkaline Phosphatase | Transaminases |
	Total	Direct	Indirect		
Hemolysis	↑	N	↑	N	N
Gilbert's syndrome	↑	N	↑	N	N
Acute hepatitis	↑↑	↑	↑↑	↑	↑↑↑
Choledocholithiasis	↑↑	↑↑	↑	↑↑	↑
Bile duct carcinoma	↑↑↑	↑↑↑	↑	↑↑↑	↑

Abbreviation: N = within the normal range.

scopic guidance. If no T-tube is present, patients with retained stones undergo endoscopic sphincterotomy and stone removal.

During cholecystectomy, unsuspected stones are found by routine cholangiography in about 5 per cent of cases. In other patients, stones are suspected preoperatively because of historical features of the patient's illness, laboratory findings, or intraoperative findings. Common bile duct exploration is clearly indicated in patients with the following features: (1) choledocholithiasis identified by cholangiography, (2) palpable ductal stones, (3) the presence of a markedly dilated common bile duct, or (4) overt jaundice. Relative indications for CBDE include a history of antecedent jaundice, pancreatitis, or cholangitis, a single faceted stone or multiple small stones within the gallbladder, and a mildly dilated common bile duct. Today, rather than proceeding directly to CBDE, most surgeons manage patients with these relative indications for exploration by operative cholangiography as a screening method. Laparoscopic CBDE is possible in some centers. Alternatives include conversion to an open CBDE or completion of the laparoscopic cholecystectomy with postoperative endoscopic sphincterotomy. An algorithm of unsuspected choledocholithiasis identified during the course of laparoscopic cholecystectomy is shown in Figure 9. The strategy chosen depends on the skill of the surgeon and endoscopist, the general condition of the patient, and the number and size of calculi present in the bile duct.

Patients with severe gallstone pancreatitis benefit from early endoscopic sphincterotomy and stone ex-

traction. In most patients, this should be followed by elective laparoscopic cholecystectomy. High-risk, elderly patients may be managed with the gallbladder left in situ; however, about 15 per cent develop further biliary tract symptoms requiring cholecystectomy. This risk is greater for those with an obstructed cystic duct at ERCP. Patients with mild gallstone pancreatitis are best treated with laparoscopic cholecystectomy and operative cholangiography during the same hospitalization following resolution of the clinical pancreatitis.

ACUTE CHOLANGITIS

Pathophysiology

Acute cholangitis is an infection of the bile ducts associated with biliary obstruction. *Charcot's triad* describes the most common clinical findings: fever with chills, jaundice, and right upper quadrant pain and, in severe cases, septic shock and altered mental status. Cholangitis always occurs in conjunction with some obstructive lesion of the bile ducts. The obstruction allows bacterial proliferation and, as intraductal pressure rises, *cholangiovenous reflux* occurs at the level of the hepatic sinusoid. This translocation of bacteria from the bile canaliculus into the vascular system accounts for the dramatic septic picture noted in severely affected patients. The bacteria most commonly involved are gut flora, particularly gram-negative aerobic rods such as *Escherichia coli, Klebsiella pneumon-*

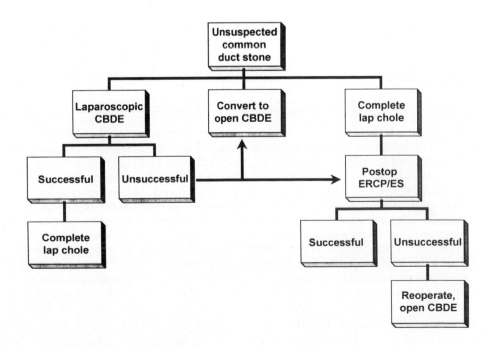

Figure 9. Management of unsuspected choledocholithiasis identified during laparoscopic cholecystectomy.

iae, and *Enterococcus* species. Anaerobic organisms such as *Bacteroides fragilis* are found in about 25 per cent of cases. Biliary tract conditions associated with cholangitis include choledocholithiasis, bile duct or biliary anastamotic stricture, parasitic infestations of the bile ducts, and bile duct tumors. Of these, choledocholithiasis is the most common. Cholangitis is a common complication of instrumentation of the bile ducts. For this reason, antibiotic prophylaxis is warranted before diagnostic or therapeutic procedures are performed on the bile ducts, particularly in the presence of obstruction or foreign bodies, as these predispose to bacteribilia. Parasites such as *Clonorchis sinensis*, *Trichuris trichiura*, and *Ascaris lumbricoides* are associated with inflammatory bile duct strictures, obstruction, and cholangitis, particularly in the Orient and among Oriental immigrants to the United States. Bacterial superinfection of the bile ducts is invariably present.

Diagnostic Evaluation

Cholangitis is a clinical diagnosis based on the symptoms and signs outlined by Charcot. Approximately 70 per cent of patients with cholangitis exhibit these classic features, while the remaining patients nearly always have fever and, even if jaundice is not present, liver function tests are abnormal. The abdominal pain of cholangitis is not severe. Physical findings range from mild right upper quadrant tenderness in a patient who otherwise appears well to florid septic shock with obtundation. Peritonitis is uncommon. Laboratory studies are significant for leukocytosis with a left shift, hyperbilirubinemia, and elevated alkaline phosphatase. Blood cultures grow bacteria in about half of all cases.

Management

The initial management of patients with cholangitis includes intravenous fluids, antibiotics directed against the expected bacterial flora, and close observation. Optimal antibiotic treatment includes ampicillin, an aminoglycoside such as gentamicin, and metronidazole. An ultrasound examination of the right upper quadrant should be performed to assess biliary ductal dilatation, determine the presence of gallstones, and exclude possible confounding conditions such as hepatic abscess. Most patients with cholangitis respond promptly to antibiotic therapy. Endoscopic sphincterotomy with stone extraction or nasobiliary stenting, or transhepatic biliary decompression should be performed in those patients who fail to improve with antibiotics alone. Once the septic picture of cholangitis is controlled, attention is turned toward identification

and correction of the underlying obstructive lesion. Cholangiography is necessary in virtually all patients to define the pathology. If choledocholithiasis is present and the gallbladder is still in place, the main options in management include endoscopic sphincterotomy and clearance of the bile duct followed by laparoscopic cholecystectomy or cholecystectomy and common bile duct exploration. In some centers, the latter can be undertaken successfully laparoscopically. If choledocholithiasis is present and the gallbladder has been previously removed, endoscopic sphincterotomy with stone clearance is probably the best option. If an isolated stricture or malignancy is present, surgical resection and reconstruction is performed. Palliative stenting of a stricture or tumor is an appropriate option for patients at high risk for surgery or those with metastatic tumors.

The mortality of patients with cholangitis varies according to the severity of presentation. Today, the most severely affected patients have a predicted mortality of 20 to 25 per cent. Successful long-term management of the patient with cholangitis depends on complete correction of the underlying obstructive lesion. This is usually possible in patients with choledocholithiasis, isolated strictures, or tumors. More complex patients with sclerosing cholangitis or Oriental cholangiohepatitis typically develop recurrent strictures and further episodes of cholangitis.

BILIARY STRICTURE

Benign Biliary Stricture

Biliary stricture is an uncommon problem, and about 90 per cent of cases are the result of iatrogenic injury during the course of a cholecystectomy. Rarely, common bile duct injury occurs during gastrectomy or as a consequence of common bile duct exploration. Other causes of biliary stricture include chronic pancreatitis, choledocholithiasis, sclerosing cholangitis, and trauma. Strictures due to biliary tract injury during cholecystectomy may present early in the postoperative period or become manifest months or years later. When untreated, the natural history of persistent biliary obstruction is progressive cirrhosis with portal hypertension and liver failure. The typical symptoms of a patient with a bile duct stricture are those of obstructive jaundice with scleral and cutaneous icterus, darkening of the urine, and clay-colored stools. In most patients, this is accompanied by intermittent fever and upper abdominal pain characteristic of cholangitis. Pruritis may be prominent. Laboratory evaluation should include liver function tests, which show a pattern of obstructive jaundice. A leukocytosis is present in most patients with associated cholangitis.

Radiographic evaluation of the patient with a suspected bile duct stricture generally begins with ultrasonography to confirm the presence of dilated ducts. Cholangiography is necessary to define the lesion and its location. In order to plan the subsequent repair, the proximal extent of the stricture must be accurately identified. For this reason, percutaneous transhepatic cholangiography is usually preferred over endoscopic retrograde cholangiography. Percutaneous biliary drainage with external or internal catheters may be performed to acutely treat the obstruction, especially if cholangitis is present. It may be difficult to differentiate benign strictures from those due to malignancy on the basis of cholangiogram. Cholangiocarcinoma, gallbladder carcinoma with extension to the common bile duct, external compression of the bile duct due to metastatic carcinoma in portal lymph nodes, and the Mirrizzi syndrome should all be considered in the differential diagnosis of a bile duct stricture.

Optimal management of patients with benign biliary stricture includes resection of the strictured segment and end-to-side Roux-en-Y hepaticojejunostomy. Direct mucosa-to-mucosa approximation of the jejunum to uninvolved bile duct well proximal to the strictured segment with fine, absorbable sutures gives the best long-term results. Resection of the stricture with direct duct-to-duct anastomosis has been attempted; however, the rate of recurrent stricture formation with this technique is unacceptably high. In selected patients with stricture due to chronic pancreatitis, choledochoduodenostomy gives satisfactory results. Under proper circumstances, 90 per cent of patients are cured of bile duct stricture by surgical repair. The mortality of this complex surgery averages 2 per cent. Most mortality is related to underlying factors such as cirrhosis, renal failure, uncontrolled cholangitis, malnutrition, and old age. For high-risk patients, endoscopic or percutaneous balloon dilatation with stent placement is an alternative. The long-term results of this approach, however, are poorer than with surgical repair.

Sclerosing Cholangitis

Sclerosing cholangitis is an idiopathic inflammatory disease of the bile ducts that causes fibrosis and multiple strictures. Interestingly, the gallbladder is generally spared and there is no association with cholelithiasis. No clear etiology has been described, but it is known that about 70 per cent of afflicted patients have preexisting ulcerative colitis. Males are more frequently affected than females, and most patients are relatively young at the time of onset of symptoms, with an average age of about 40 years. The fibrosis and stricture process is usually most prominent at the hepatic duct bifurcation in the hilum of the liver. With

persistent obstruction, biliary cirrhosis ensues. In late stages, portal hypertension, esophageal variceal hemorrhage, and hepatic parenchymal failure develop. The initial presentation of patients with sclerosing cholangitis is usually painless jaundice and pruritus. The symptoms typical of ulcerative colitis (particularly diarrhea) may be present, and in most patients, this diagnosis has been previously established. No physical findings specific to sclerosing cholangitis exist, but in late stages, the features of portal hypertension, including ascites, caput medusae, and spider angiomata, may be prominent. Laboratory investigation reveals elevations in alkaline phosphatase in nearly all patients. Unlike patients with hepatitis, the transaminases are only minimally elevated. Serologic evidence of autoimmune dysfunction such as the presence of antimitochondrial, antinuclear, and antismooth muscle antibodies is absent.

The diagnosis of sclerosing cholangitis is established by cholangiography, performed endoscopically or percutaneously. Significant radiologic features of sclerosing cholangitis include multiple beaded strictures and a "pruned tree" appearance of the intrahepatic ducts. A rare patient demonstrates only an isolated stricture. Because of the extensive ductal fibrosis, marked dilation of intrahepatic ducts does not occur. Liver biopsy is required to assess the degree of cirrhosis present. Management strategies to halt the underlying fibrotic process, including steroids and immunosuppressants, have been largely unsuccessful, but antibiotics are useful for those patients with recurrent cholangitis. Early studies suggest that ursodeoxycholic acid and methotrexate may be of value. Although in the past surgery played a major role in bypassing strictured segments and providing chronic access to the biliary tract through the placement of U-tubes or other stents, interventional radiologic and endoscopic techniques currently provide similar results. Some patients with extensive extrahepatic strictures and relative sparing of the intrahepatic and proximal extrahepatic ducts benefit from Roux-en-Y hepaticojejunostomy. Recurrent cholangitis is common following any intervention in the biliary tract for sclerosing cholangitis, as not all strictured lesions can be bypassed. Liver transplantation provides definitive management of patients with end-stage sclerosing cholangitis complicated by liver failure.

CARCINOMA OF THE BILIARY TRACT

Gallbladder Carcinoma

Carcinoma of the gallbladder is a rare tumor with poor prognosis. Data from the National Cancer Institute's Surveillance, Epidemiology, and End-Results

(SEER) program suggest that this tumor represents only about 0.5 per cent of all newly diagnosed carcinomas, with the annual incidence estimated to be about 6000 cases per year in the United States. Most occur in elderly patients, and over 70 per cent are associated with cholelithiasis. Women are affected three times more commonly than men. Certain racial groups, including native American Indians, Alaskan natives, and Hispanics, have increased risk for the development of gallbladder carcinoma. Other risk factors include large gallstones (>2.5 cm), calcification in the gallbladder wall (*porcelain gallbladder*), and cholecystenteric fistula. The vast majority of gallbladder malignancies are adenocarcinomas. Their pattern of spread includes direct extension into the liver, regional metastases to lymph nodes, and distant metastases to liver and peritoneal surfaces within the abdomen (*carcinomatosis*). The incidence of gallbladder carcinoma found at autopsy or during cholecystectomy for gallstones is 0.5 to 1.0 per cent. The majority of patients with gallbladder cancer present late in the course of their illness, and when symptoms arise, they generally are initially attributed to gallstones. Pain in patients with gallbladder carcinoma may be continuous, rather than intermittent, as in biliary colic. A history of recent weight loss is common. Physical examination of patients with gallbladder carcinoma is usually unrevealing except in advanced illness, when a palpable gallbladder, ascites, or pelvic metastasis may be detected. Jaundice may develop from direct obstruction of the common hepatic duct, portal lymphadenopathy, or diffuse liver metastases. If the diagnosis of gallbladder carcinoma is suspected, ultrasound or CT examination of the upper abdomen should be performed to identify a gallbladder mass and exclude the presence of liver metastases or ascites. Angiography is helpful to exclude involvement of the hepatic artery or portal vein.

Management of patients with gallbladder carcinoma includes resection of the tumor, if localized. Unfortunately, in most patients these tumors are unresectable for cure by virtue of local invasion, extensive lymphadenopathy, or distant metastases. The majority of patients cured of gallbladder carcinoma have unsuspected, small lesions confined to the mucosa or muscularis resected incidentally at the time of cholecystectomy for symptomatic cholelithiasis. Some patients with larger lesions confined to the gallbladder appear to benefit from radical cholecystectomy, including partial hepatectomy of the gallbladder fossa and regional lymphadenectomy. Palliative options for patients with unresectable disease include systemic chemotherapy with or without regional radiotherapy. Response rates, however, are low. Obstructive jaundice can generally be relieved with percutaneous or endoscopic biliary stent placement. For all patients with gallbladder carcinoma, 5-year survival is about 5 per cent and median survival is 4 to 6 months.

Bile Duct Carcinoma

Carcinoma of the bile ducts is less common than gallbladder carcinoma and tends to present at an earlier stage. Because of the proximity of the bile ducts to liver parenchyma, the hepatic artery, and portal vein, however, even small lesions may be unresectable. Unlike gallbladder carcinoma, no gender differences in incidence are evident. Most are sporadic, but some are associated with other illnesses such as ulcerative colitis, sclerosing cholangitis, and choledochal cysts. In the Orient, bile duct carcinoma is associated with infestation with the parasite *Clonorchis sinensis*. The histology of bile duct carcinoma is almost always adenocarcinoma, but it has been given the special term, *cholangiocarcinoma*. A few patients present with bulky papillary variants that have better prognosis than the average tumor. Most patients with bile duct carcinoma present with painless jaundice. Upon careful questioning, it is also determined that vague right upper quadrant or back pain may be present in up to half of patients. While weight loss and pruritus are common, cholangitis is uncommon and more suggestive of choledocholithiasis. Physical examination is generally remarkable only for jaundice. The liver may be palpable and somewhat tender, but the primary tumor cannot be palpated. If the level of obstruction is in the common bile duct, the gallbladder may be distended and palpable (*Courvoisier's sign*). Liver function tests are compatible with obstructive jaundice with elevated bilirubin (mostly direct) and alkaline phosphatase levels, but relatively normal transaminases. Most patients with malignant obstruction of the biliary tract present with a total serum bilirubin greater than 10 mg/dl, whereas those with obstruction due to a common bile duct stone typically have hyperbilirubinemia less than 10 mg/dl.

Evaluation of a patient with suspected bile duct carcinoma optimally begins with CT or ultrasound examination of the upper abdomen to assess (1) the presence or absence of dilated bile ducts; (2) the level of obstruction (i.e., intrahepatic bile duct dilatation alone or intrahepatic *and* extrahepatic bile duct dilatation); and (3) the presence of liver metastases or ascites. As the primary tumor can seldom be identified because of its small size, further evaluation is directed at imaging the bile duct obstruction. If the level of the obstruction is near the duodenum, endoscopic retrograde cholangiography is performed to identify the tumor. Biopsies of ampullary lesions or brushings of the distal bile duct for cytologic examination may confirm the diagnosis of carcinoma. If the level of the obstruction is near the hepatic hilum, percutaneous transhepatic cholangiography is performed to identify the proximal extent of the lesion. Angiography may be helpful to exclude direct extension of the tumor into the hepatic artery or portal vein. Optimal management of patients with bile duct carcinoma is surgical resection. If the lesion originates at the bifurcation of the hepatic ducts (*Klatskin tumor*), partial hepatectomy may be required. Recent evidence suggests that these bifurcation lesions are commonly asymmetric and that the addition of left or right hepatectomy to bile duct resection improves the margins of resection and increases survival rates. For distal lesions within the pancreas, sometimes difficult to distinguish from primary pancreatic adenocarcinomas, pancreaticoduodenectomy (*Whipple procedure*) is performed. Unresectable lesions may be palliated with percutaneous or endoscopic stent placement to relieve bile duct obstruction. Surgical resection and Roux-en-Y hepaticojejunostomy achieves more durable palliation of biliary obstruction than do percutaneous or endoscopic stents. Radiation therapy with or without chemotherapy sometimes shrinks unresectable lesions; however, the duration of response is short. The prognosis depends on the stage of the lesion and its location, and the best prognosis is for distal bile duct cancers, with 5-year survival rates of 40 per cent in most series. Lesions in the middle third of the bile duct have an intermediate prognosis, with an approximate 5-year survival of 25 per cent, and proximal lesions at the hepatic bifurcation are seldom cured, with 5-year survival rates of about 5 per cent.

REFERENCES

Beal JM: Historical perspective of gallstone disease. Surg Gynecol Obstet *158*:181–189, 1984.

Cotton PB, Lehman G, Vennes J, Geenen JE, Russell RCG, Meyers WC, Ligoury C, Nickl N: Endoscopic sphincterotomy complications and their management: An attempt at consensus. Gastrointest Endosc 37:383–393, 1991.

Johnston DE, Kaplan MM: Pathogenesis and treatment of gallstones. N Engl J Med *328*:412–421, 1993.

Lai ECS, Mok FPT, Tan ESY, Lo CM, Fan ST, You KT, Wong J: Endoscopic biliary drainage for severe acute cholangitis. N Engl J Med *326*:1582–1586, 1992.

O'Connor KW, Snodgrass PJ, Swonda JE, Mahoney S, Burt R, Cockerill EM, Lumeng L: A blinded prospective study comparing four current non-invasive approaches in the differential diagnosis of medical versus surgical jaundice. Gastroenterology *84*:1498, 1983.

Roslyn JJ, Binns GS, Hughes EFX, Saunders-Kirkwood K, Zinner MJ, Cates JA: Open cholecystectomy: A contemporary analysis of 42,474 patients. Ann Surg *218*:129–137, 1993.

Silk YN, Douglass HO Jr, Nava HR, Driscoll DL, Tartarian G: Carcinoma of the gallbladder. The Roswell Park experience. Ann Surg *210*:751–757, 1989.

The Southern Surgeons Club. A prospective analysis of 1518 laparoscopic cholecystectomies. N Engl J Med *324*:1073–1078, 1991.

Vauthey JN, Lerut J, Martini M, Becker C, Gertsch P, Blumgart LH: Indications and limitations of percutaneous cholecystostomy for acute cholecystitis. Surg Gynecol Obstet *176*:49–54, 1993.

34
PORTAL HYPERTENSION

J. MICHAEL HENDERSON, M.B., Ch.B., F.R.C.S.

Portal hypertension consists of an increase in pressure in the portal venous system that may be caused by many different pathologic states. The main clinical presentations are variceal bleeding, ascites and, in patients with advanced liver disease, liver failure. The following actions are taken in patients with portal hypertension: (1) the etiology is defined, (2) the patient is evaluated for risks of bleeding and liver failure, and (3) management is selected based on a full evaluation. Medical management of patients with portal hypertension requires a multidisciplinary approach including specialty consultations from the areas of hepatology, surgery, radiology, and pathology. Overall patient management may require many other support personnel and access to treatment choices including diet, drugs, endoscopy, interventional radiology, and surgery.

Clinically significant portal hypertension is present when the pressure difference between the portal vein and inferior vena cava exceeds 12 mm Hg, and it can be divided into *prehepatic* and *intrahepatic* causes. Prehepatic causes are usually caused by thrombosis of the portal vein and account for less than 10 per cent of cases of portal hypertension. Thrombosis may occur in the neonate secondary to umbilical vein sepsis, may be secondary to a hematologic hypercoagulable state, or may be caused by tumor/trauma compression or invasion. Intrahepatic causes of portal hypertension may be due to presinusoidal, sinusoidal, or postsinusoidal obstruction as shown in Table 1. Cirrhosis, the most common cause of portal hypertension in the United States and Europe, has multiple etiologies and is characterized by lobule collapse, fibrosis, and regenerating nodules. An accurate etiologic diagnosis is important in the prognosis as is a knowledge of the natural history of each type of cirrhosis.

PATHOPHYSIOLOGY

A *block* to portal flow and increased splanchnic inflow both have a role in the development and maintenance of portal hypertension. The *backward* theory of portal hypertension implicates a prehepatic or intrahepatic obstruction to portal flow as the major pathology. While it is now clear that such a block is an important initiating event, it has also been shown that the *forward* component of increased splanchnic blood flow contributes to the maintenance and, perhaps, worsening of portal hypertension.

EVALUATION

Patients with portal hypertension require full evaluation that must define etiology, assess the risk of complications and, in patients with liver disease, define severity. The main points in evaluation are summarized in Table 2. From a management point of view, the aim at this evaluation is to define the likely course of disease for a given patient and to choose therapy. The most useful combination of clinical and laboratory assessments used to determine the status of the patient are albumin, bilirubin, prothrombin time, ascites, and encephalopathy. These are combined into a grading system, shown in Table 3.

TREATMENT

The choices of therapy for portal hypertension and its complications include the following:

Pharmacologic therapy can lower portal hypertension by pitressin combined with nitroglycerin admin-

TABLE 1. INTRAHEPATIC CAUSES OF PORTAL HYPERTENSION

Presinusoidal
    Schistosomiasis
    Congenital hepatic fibrosis
Sinusoidal
    Cirrhosis caused by:
        Hepatitis
        Alcoholism
        Biliary cirrhosis
        Sclerosing cholangitis
        Other
Postsinusoidal
    Budd-Chiari syndrome
    Veno-occlusive disease

TABLE 3. CHILD-PUGH CLASSIFICATION OF THE SEVERITY OF LIVER DISEASE*

	1 Point	2 Points	3 Points
Bilirubin (mg/dl)	<2	2–3	>3
Albumin (gm/dl)	>3.5	2.8–3.5	<2.8
Prothrombin time†	1–3	4–6	>6
Ascites	None	Slight	Moderate
Encephalopathy	None	1–2	3–4

*Grades: A, 5–6 points; B, 7–9 points; C, 10–15 points.
†Expressed in seconds above normal.

istered by continuous intravenous infusion for acute variceal bleeding. Oral administration of propranolol reduces portal hypertension through both reduction in splanchnic inflow by lower cardiac output and by a direct splanchnic effect. It is used to reduce the risk of the initial bleed as well as to lower the risk of rebleeding.

Endoscopic sclerotherapy is a direct attempt to either produce thrombosis of varices or create fibrosis over them. It is performed through a flexible endoscope with either intravariceal or paravariceal injection of a sclerosing solution. This technique is effective in control of acute bleeding episodes and reduces the risk of rebleeding.

Decompressive shunt placement. There are three different types of shunts:

1. Total portal systemic shunts are anastomoses of 10 mm or greater diameter between the portal and systemic venous systems. They correct portal hypertension and are very effective in stopping variceal bleeding and controlling ascites, but divert all portal blood flow away from the liver and accelerate liver failure and are indicated in some circumstances (see below), but their use is limited (Fig. 1).

2. Partial portal systemic shunts are 8 to 10 mm in size between the portal and systemic venous systems. At 8 mm diameter, such a shunt reduces portal

TABLE 2. EVALUATION OF PORTAL HYPERTENSION

Bleeding risk
    Endoscopy
Hemodynamic changes
    Angiography
    Doppler/ultrasound
    Cardiac output
Liver failure risk
    Clinical
    Standard lab tests
    Biopsy
    Quantitative tests

pressure to 12 mm Hg, maintains prograde portal flow in 80 per cent of patients, and controls variceal bleeding. Liver failure is less of a problem than with total shunts.

3. Selective variceal decompression is achieved by a distal splenorenal shunt (Fig. 2). Gastroesophageal varices and the spleen are decompressed by the splenorenal anastomosis, while portal hypertension and portal flow to the liver are maintained in the superior mesenteric and portal veins. Variceal bleeding is controlled and liver failure is *not* accelerated, and this is the most widely used shunt for control of variceal bleeding.

The shunts discussed above all involve surgical operations. There is also interest in placing intrahepatic shunts under radiologic control with a transjugular in-

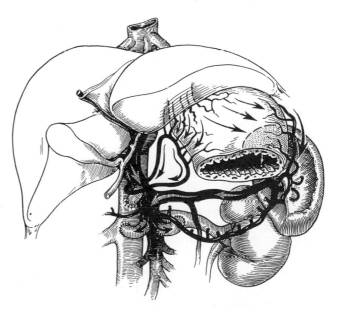

Figure 1. Side-to-side interposition shunts—portacaval, mesocaval, mesorenal—totally relieve portal hypertension and divert all portal flow away from the liver when they are more than 10 mm in diameter. (From Henderson JM, Warren WD: Portal hypertension. Curr Probl Surg 25:174, 1988, with permission.)

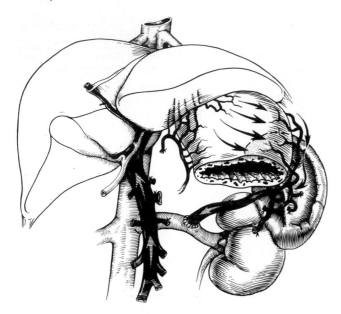

Figure 2. Distal splenorenal shunt selectively decompresses gastroesophageal varices and the spleen. Portal hypertension is maintained in the superior mesenteric and portal veins, keeping prograde portal flow to the liver. (From Henderson JM, Warren WD: Portal hypertension. Curr Probl Surg 25: 177, 1988, with permission.)

trahepatic portal systemic shunt (TIPS) (Fig. 3). Physiologically, this shunt is similar to the total and partial

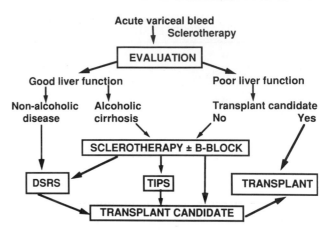

Figure 4. Algorithm for management of variceal bleeding.

portal systemic shunts, depending on the diameter to which the stent is dilated. Data are preliminary, but suggest a role for it in management of acute bleeding not controlled by sclerotherapy. Stenosis and occlusion with small shunts and encephalopathy with larger shunts appear to be significant complications. *Devascularization* procedures aim to reduce the risk of variceal bleeding by reduction of inflow to the varices. Splenectomy, gastric and esophageal devascularization, and esophageal transection are the components of such operations. Such procedures are useful when there are no other viable options.

Figure 3. Transjugular intrahepatic shunt (TIPS) may serve as a total or partial side-to-side portal systemic shunt depending on diameter greater or less than 10 mm.

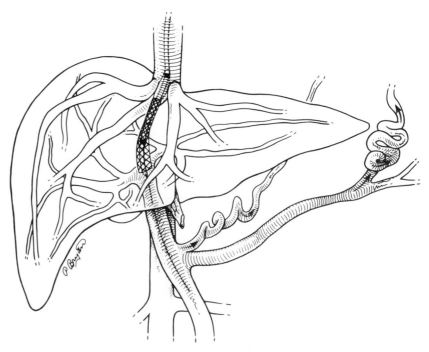

In *liver transplantation*, the cirrhotic liver is removed and replaced with a normal liver, portal hypertension is relieved, and liver function is restored. However, the perioperative risk of the procedure and the risk of lifelong immunosuppression dictate that transplant only be used for patients with end-stage liver disease.

MANAGEMENT STRATEGIES FOR VARICEAL BLEEDING

Portal hypertension develops in approximately 50 per cent of patients with cirrhosis. Once varices have developed, the risk of bleeding from them is 30 per cent, and the mortality of an acute variceal bleed is about 30 per cent. The risk of rebleeding from varices once there has been an initial bleed is 70 per cent. These facts, defined from population studies and randomized controlled trials, set the scene for management strategies at various time points.

Prophylactic therapy to prevent the initial bleed must have low morbidity, as only 30 per cent of patients are at risk of bleeding. Current recommendation is for a nonselective β-blocker, administered in a dose to reduce the pulse to less than or equal to 60 beats per minute. Surgery and sclerotherapy are not indicated for prophylaxis prior to the first bleed.

Acute variceal bleeding should be managed by endoscopic sclerotherapy, which should be done emergently at the time of the initial diagnostic endoscopy. Adjunctive therapy with pitressin and nitroglycerin is indicated by severe bleeding. Decompressive shunt may be required for continued bleeding through sclerotherapy or repeat rebleeding. The goal at this time is to stabilize the patient to allow a full evaluation.

Prevention of recurrent bleeding is a problem of long-term management. As indicated in the algorithm in Figure 4, the major factor in deciding is the status of the liver. Each of the therapies discussed may be required by different patients, or at different times by the same patient. The important step is to develop management strategies based on locally available expertise. Ideally, this combines drug therapy, endoscopic sclerosis, shunt surgery, and liver transplantation.

MANAGEMENT STRATEGIES FOR ASCITES AND LIVER FAILURE

The main question to be answered for these patients is whether or not they are candidates for liver transplantation. If so, a transplant is appropriate therapy. Some patients with ascites and adequate preservation of liver function may be managed by a side-to-side portal systemic shunt such as TIPS, or by a peritoneovenous shunt.

REFERENCES

Groszmann RJ, Grace ND: Complications of portal hypertension: Esophagogastric varices and ascites. Gastroenterol Clin North Am 21:1–276, 1992.
Henderson JM, Gilmore GT, Hooks MA, et al: Selective shunt in the management of variceal bleeding in the era of liver transplantation. Ann Surg 216:248–255, 1992.
Transjugular intrahepatic portal systemic shunts. Abstr Hepatol 16:80A, 85A, 1992.
The W. Dean Warren memorial issue. Am J Surg 160:1–138, 1990.

35
THE PANCREAS

I
The Pancreas

DANA K. ANDERSEN, M.D.

The pancreas is a very important organ, with endocrine and exocrine functions of considerable metabolic significance. It is also the site of a number of developmental, inflammatory, and neoplastic processes.

EMBRYOLOGY

During early fetal development, the pancreas originates from two primordial structures, a *ventral bud* or outpouching arising from the hepatic diverticulum, and a *dorsal* portion arising directly from the developing duodenum. At about the fifth week of life, the ventral pancreatic bud and biliary duct rotate clockwise behind the duodenum, until the ventral structures fuse with the dorsal pancreatic tissue. Each of these pancreatic structures contains ductular elements. As the ventral portion forms the head and uncinate process of the gland, its duct becomes the *duct of Wirsung,* or main pancreatic duct, which fuses with the ductular portion of the dorsal portion and usually becomes the predominant ductular system for the entire gland. The proximal duct of the dorsal portion becomes the *duct of Santorini,* or lesser duct, and usually persists, complete with a lesser or accessory duodenal papilla lying just proximal to the main papilla of Vater. The separate embryologic origins of the pancreatic head and body are reflected in certain anatomic and functional properties of the gland, and abnormalities in the proper rotation or fusion of the developing pancreas may cause specific congenital disorders.

The patency of the lesser papilla, the degree of development of the lesser duct, and the degree of its communication with the main duct are variable. Rarely, the lesser duct is the principal route of drainage of the body and tail, due to incomplete fusion of the ventral pancreatic duct with the dorsal duct during fetal development. This anomaly is termed *pancreas divisum* and occurs in 5 to 10 per cent of patients. When the lesser papilla becomes obstructed or stenotic, persistent symptoms may occur, and *endoscopic retrograde cholangiopancreatography* (ERCP) usually reveals a shortened duct of Wirsung that only drains the uncinate process of the gland. The lesser papilla must be sought to document the cause of symptoms, and a sphincterotomy or sphincteroplasty of the lesser papilla may be necessary to relieve the obstruction.

A ring or collar of pancreatic tissue that completely encircles the second portion of the duodenum is termed *annular pancreas* and is thought to result from abnormal embryologic fusion of dorsal and ventral pancreatic segments. This condition usually causes stenosis of the duodenum and is seen in about 1 in 7000 autopsies. Complete duodenal obstruction is the usual presentation of annular pancreas in the neonate. However, half of the reported instances have been in adults, with some remaining undiagnosed until the eighth decade of life. Peptic ulcer disease occurs in one fifth of adults with this lesion, probably as a consequence of duodenal stasis. Bypass of the stenotic or obstructing segment is the treatment of choice, and duodenojejunostomy or gastrojejunostomy is usually performed.

The presence of pancreatic tissue that lacks anatomic or vascular continuity with the main body of the pancreas is called *ectopic pancreas*, also termed *aberrant pancreas* or *heterotopic pancreas*. It is relatively common, found in 1 to 5 per cent of autopsies. The lesion, which causes either no symptoms or recurrent pain, usually presents as a button of tissue 1 to 4 cm in diameter, on either the mucosal or serosal surface of the stomach or duodenum, or it may present as a pedunculated duodenal polyp. When ectopic pancreatic tissue occurs in the distal small bowel, it is usually present in the fundus of a Meckel's diverticulum of the ileum. Histologically, ectopic pancreatic tissue contains normal elements of acinar, ductular, and islet tissue, but may contain malignancies arising from these tissues in rare instances.

ANATOMY

Size and Location

The pancreas is a soft, yellowish, fleshy (Greek: *pan*—all; *kreas*—flesh), finely lobulated organ that lies behind the posterior peritoneal membrane and extends from the concavity of the duodenum to the hilum of the spleen at the level of the second lumbar vertebra (Fig. 1). It is generally 15 to 20 cm long and weighs from 75 to 100 gm. The regions of the pancreas are described as the *head* (and uncinate process), which is bordered by the duodenal C-loop; the *neck*, which overlies the superior mesenteric vessels; and the remaining distal portion of the gland, which is divided into the *body* and *tail*. The head is the thickest part of the organ (3 to 3.5 cm), and the gland tapers pro-

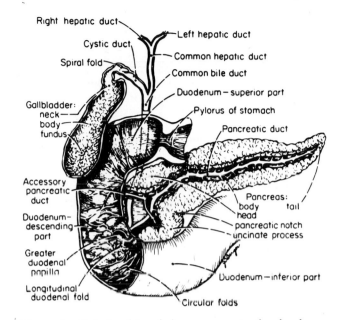

Figure 1. Relationship of the pancreas to the duodenum and extrahepatic biliary system. (From Woodburne RT: Essentials of Human Anatomy. New York, Oxford University Press, 1973, with permission.)

gressively toward the tail. The neck divides the pancreas into sections of approximately equal mass.

Behind the pancreatic head are the inferior vena cava, the renal veins, and the right renal artery. The medial portion of the uncinate process lies just anterior to the aorta, below the origin of the superior mesenteric artery. The body of the pancreas lies just anterior to the left adrenal gland, and the tail ends in the lower splenic hilar area. The splenic vein generally lies within an actual groove along this posterior surface of the gland and receives many delicate pancreatic branches. The common bile duct descends behind the upper duodenum and passes into the posterior surface of the pancreatic head before ending jointly with the main pancreatic duct at the ampulla of Vater in the medial wall of the duodenum.

Pancreatic Ducts

The main pancreatic duct, which begins at the tail of the gland and passes through the center of the gland toward the head, may reside somewhat anteriorly or posteriorly, but is nearly always midway between the superior and inferior borders of the body and tail. After passing the neck of the gland, the main duct turns inferiorly and dorsally and joins the distal common bile duct at the ampulla of Vater. Generally, the pancreatic duct enters the region of the ampulla inferomedially and often appears as a separate orifice on the distal medial wall of the common bile duct. When the common bile duct and pancreatic duct join together prior to entering the ampulla, a short *common channel* results. The lesser pancreatic duct generally drains the head of the pancreas, and enters the duodenum through a smaller accessory papilla located 2 to 2.5 cm proximal and slightly anterior to the ampulla of Vater. The lesser duct usually joins the main duct at the level of the head or neck of the pancreas, but this is not a consistent finding. The main pancreatic duct varies in diameter from 2 to 3.5 mm as it courses through the body of the gland and from 1 to 2 mm in the region of the tail of the pancreas. Approximately 20 secondary branches drain into the duct throughout the body and tail, and the delicate pattern of these secondary ducts and the tertiary ductules that create them forms an important radiologic criterion for the diagnosis of disease. The sphincter of Oddi represents a complex set of muscular fibers surrounding the common bile duct, pancreatic duct, and the common channel of both ducts within the ampulla of Vater. This sphincter, which is regulated by neural and hormonal factors, controls the output of pancreatic and biliary secretions and serves to prevent reflux of duodenal contents into these ductular systems. Normal fasting common duct pressure has been found to range from 7 to 17 mm Hg, while main pancreatic duct pressure ranges from 15 to 30 mm Hg.

Arterial Supply

Both the celiac and mesenteric arterial trunks supply branches to the pancreas, and numerous communications exist within the gland between the arteries arising from these two systems. The head of the pancreas is supplied superiorly by the anterior and posterior superior pancreaticoduodenal arteries, which generally arise from the gastroduodenal artery. Inferiorly, the head is supplied by the anterior and posterior inferior pancreaticoduodenal arteries, which originate from the superior mesenteric artery. The splenic artery gives rise to several arterial branches to the body and tail of the pancreas, including the dorsal pancreatic artery, the inferior pancreatic artery, and the artery pancreatic magna. The network of arteries serving the head of the pancreas also provides the arterial supply to the duodenum. Therefore, it is not possible to resect the entire pancreatic head without causing severe ischemia to the duodenum. Several anomalies of the splanchnic arterial system are known to occur in up to 20 per cent of patients, and may cause variations of pancreatic blood flow. The common hepatic, right hepatic, or gastroduodenal arteries may arise from the superior mesenteric artery and can pass anterior or posterior to the pancreatic head or, very rarely, directly through the pancreatic head.

Venous Drainage

The venous drainage of the head of the pancreas is directed superiorly through the anterior and posterior superior pancreaticoduodenal veins, which enter the suprapancreatic portion of the portal vein directly, lie adjacent to their corresponding arteries, and receive branches from the pancreas and duodenum. Venous drainage of the head is directed inferiorly through the anterior inferior pancreaticoduodenal vein and the right gastroepiploic vein, which generally combine with the right colic vein to form a common venous trunk (called the gastrocolic or Henle's trunk) before entering the superior mesenteric vein at the inferior border of the neck of the pancreas. The posterior inferior pancreaticoduodenal vein drains directly into the superior mesenteric vein, or joins with the first jejunal vein. The splenic vein receives many small pancreatic branches from the posterior surface of the pancreas and from the inferior pancreatic vein, the caudal pancreatic vein, and the great pancreatic vein arising from the body of the gland. The inferior mesenteric vein may also receive small pancreatic venous branches, may join the splenic vein directly, the superior mesenteric vein directly, or may combine with each of these major veins to form a "tripod" origin of the portal vein behind the neck of the pancreas.

Lymphatic Drainage

The pancreatic lymphatic system is abundant and is made diffuse by the absence of a peritoneal barrier on the posterior surface of the gland. Direct lymphatic connections with retroperitoneal tissues exist, and there are intrapancreatic lymph nodes as well. The predominant lymphatic groups that receive drainage from the pancreas are the celiac and superior mesenteric nodes, but other regional lymphatic groups include the splenic, transverse mesocolic, subpyloric, and hepatic lymph nodes. In addition, lymph nodes in the lesser gastric omentum, along the greater curve of the stomach, and in the jejunal and colonic mesentery may also receive lymph drainage from the pancreas. It has been documented that the surgically resectable region around the entire pancreas contains roughly 70 lymph nodes, while resection of the head of the pancreas together with the duodenum (Whipple procedure) removes about one half that number.

Innervation

The pancreas receives both sympathetic innervation via the splanchnic nerves, and cholinergic innervation via the vagal fibers. The splanchnic nerves travel in the para-aortic area and send predominantly sympathetic fibers to the pancreas along the celiac axis and splenic artery. Vagal fibers traverse the lesser gastric omentum and innervate the area of the duodenum and pancreatic head, after which they communicate with all regions of the gland. Intrapancreatic fibers of both sympathetic and cholinergic origin give rise to periacinar plexuses, which send neural fibers to the base of acinar cell groups. Similar plexuses exist around the pancreatic islets, and terminal fibers form a particularly rich network that innervates the islets and communicates directly with the endocrine cells. Afferent sensory fibers travel from the pancreas to the celiac plexus, then accompany the sympathetic para-aortic fibers before reaching the afferent neuronal cell bodies in the dorsal root ganglia of T5 to T12. Thus, intrinsic pancreatic pain may be noted in the epigastrium, may be felt in the right or left hypochondrium, or may present as lower thoracic backache.

STRUCTURE AND HISTOLOGY

Exocrine Structure

The elements of the exocrine portion of the pancreas comprise 80 to 90 per cent of the total volume of the gland and are divided into the acinar and ductular systems. Twenty to 40 acinar cells form the functional unit called the *acinus*, and from each acinus emerges a small *intercalated duct* (Fig. 2). The pyramid-shaped acinar cells are oriented with their apex facing the lumen of the acinus. The luminal membrane contains numerous microvilli, and large, darkly staining zymogen granules are seen in the apical portion of each cell, while the large nucleus is in the central or basilar portion. An elaborate network of endoplasmic reticulum and microtubules supports the vigorous synthetic and secretory functions of these cells. The *centroacinar cells* line the lumen of the acinus, and contain specific enzymes such as carbonic anhydrase that are required for bicarbonate and electrolyte transport, and are specifically responsible for fluid and electrolyte secretion by the pancreas. The *intercalated ducts* from several acini combine to form *interlobular ducts*, which combine to form secondary ducts leading to the main ductular system of the pancreas. While the secondary ducts and main ducts may contribute a small amount of water and electrolyte secretion, most of this function is performed by the centroacinar cells and the interlobular duct cells.

Endocrine Structure

The islets of Langerhans form the endocrine, or ductless, portion of the pancreas, and comprise only 2 to 3 per cent of the total volume of the gland. The islets measure 100 to 600 μm in diameter, and each

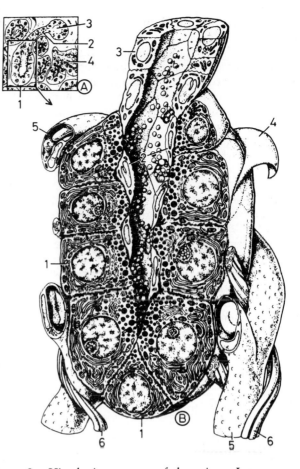

Figure 2. Histologic anatomy of the acinus. Lower magnification view (*A*) shows (1) a single acinus, (2) intercalated duct, (3) intralobular duct, and (4) centroacinar cells. Higher magnification view of single acinus (*B*) shows (1) acinar cells releasing contents of zymogen granules into the acinar lumen, (2) centroacinar cells, (3) intercalated duct cell, (4) acinar basement membrane, (5) capillary, and (6) periacinar neural fibers. (From Krstic RV: Die Gewebe des Menschen und der Saugetiere. Heidelberg, Springer-Verlag, 1978, with permission.)

contains an average of 3000 cells. It has been estimated that the adult pancreas contains about 1 million islets scattered uniformly throughout the pancreas. Islets normally contain four specific cell types, the alpha, beta, delta, and pancreatic polypeptide cells, which contain the hormones glucagon, insulin, somatostatin, and pancreatic polypeptide, respectively. While the islets themselves are uniformly present, the distribution of the individual hormone-containing cells varies within the pancreas. The insulin-containing beta cells are most prevalent throughout the pancreas, and comprise 70 to 75 per cent of all endocrine cells. The glucagon-containing alpha cells comprise roughly 10 to 12 per cent of all endocrine cells throughout the pancreas, but are found almost exclusively in the dorsal portion. Conversely, the pancreatic polypeptide–secreting cells are found almost exclusively in the ventral portion of the pancreas, but still comprise 15 to 20 per cent of the total endocrine cells present in the entire pancreas. The somatostatin-containing cells are distributed uniformly throughout the pancreas and comprise approximately 5 per cent of all endocrine cells (Fig. 3). The arrangement of the hormone-secreting cells within each islet is also specific: beta cells occupy the central portion of each islet, and nonbeta cells are generally present around the periphery. Immunohistochemical studies suggest that small numbers of additional hormone-containing cells are present in the islets. These include D_1 cells, which contain the hormone vasoactive intestinal polypeptide (VIP), and enterochromaffin (EC) cells, which contain numerous amines including 5-hydroxytryptamine (5-HT), or serotonin. The presence of occasional gastrin-containing G cells has been proposed by some studies, but their presence in normal islets remains unconfirmed.

Vascular Pattern

The distribution of blood flow within the pancreas provides arterial supply to the islets preferentially. Although the islets comprise only 2 per cent of the pancreatic mass, they receive 20 to 30 per cent of the pancreatic arteriolar flow. Blood flow can be redistributed after a meal and can be redirected to different areas of the pancreas. The collecting vessels draining all but the largest islets also perfuse the acinar tissue, which allows endocrine regulation of the exocrine pancreas, but this *insuloacinar portal system* may also account for the exocrine pancreas being more susceptible to ischemia than the endocrine portion of the gland. The arteriolar distribution of the islets themselves is also organized in a specific pattern. Rather than a nonspecific "glomerular" network of arterial supply to the entire islet, arterioles appear to enter each islet directly into the beta cell mass, after which collecting venules supply the nonbeta cell mantle or periphery of the islet. This pattern of distribution of blood flow allows insulin secretion to modulate other endocrine cell populations.

PHYSIOLOGY

Exocrine Function

Pancreatic juice contains two major components, alkaline fluid and digestive enzymes. Between 500 and 800 ml/day are secreted into the duodenum, and the high levels of bicarbonate serve to neutralize gastric acid. The enzymatic portion of this juice contains the necessary enzymes for digestion of carbohydrates, proteins, and fats. The products of digestion regulate pancreatic secretion in a negative feedback manner.

Bicarbonate Secretion

Fluid secreted by the centroacinar cells and by ductular epithelium contains 20 mM bicarbonate in the resting state and as much as 150 mM under maximal stimulation. The pH of this fluid ranges from 7.6 to almost 9.0. Sodium and potassium concentrations in pancreatic fluid remain relatively constant and reflect their concentration in the plasma. As bicarbonate secretion increases, the concentration of chloride decreases. The total concentration of anions therefore stays constant, and the osmotic pressure of the pancreatic fluid remains the same as that of plasma. The exchange of bicarbonate and chloride occurs in the intercalated and interlobular ducts, with almost no secretion or exchange occurring in the main ducts. The major stimulus for the secretion of bicarbonate is the activation of intracellular cyclic adenosine monophosphate (cAMP) formation by the hormone secretin. Secretin is secreted by cells located throughout the duodenal mucosa and is present in highest concentrations in the duodenal bulb. The secretin-containing cells release this peptide into the bloodstream in response to acid entering the duodenum in direct proportion to the amount of acid presented. Above a pH of 3.0, secretin release decreases and ceases entirely when the pH reaches 5.0. Cholecystokinin (CCK), also produced by specific duodenal mucosal cells, greatly augments the action of secretin but, by itself, is a weak stimulant of bicarbonate secretion. In contrast to the minimal response of secretin to ingested nutrients, CCK release occurs promptly after the entry of fatty acids or protein into the duodenum and is mediated by the secretion of CCK-releasing factor (CCK-RF) from separate duodenal mucosal cells. Cholecystokinin augments the bicarbonate response to even low levels of secretin, and bicarbonate secretion may be stimulated in the absence of duodenal acidification. Although acetylcholine is a poor stimulant of bicarbonate secretion, bicarbonate secretion is inhibited by atropine and is reduced by up to 90 per cent following truncal vagotomy. These and other pancreatic functions can be assessed by standard tests (Table 1).

The fluid and bicarbonate content of pancreatic juice is probably most important as a vehicle for pancreatic enzyme secretion and as a mechanism for preventing the activation of proteolytic enzymes until they are delivered to the intestinal lumen. The maintenance of a high pH in the pancreatic duct fluid therefore prevents premature proteolysis of the pancreatic tissues. Major digestive disturbances occur not as a result of the loss of pancreatic fluid or bicarbonate

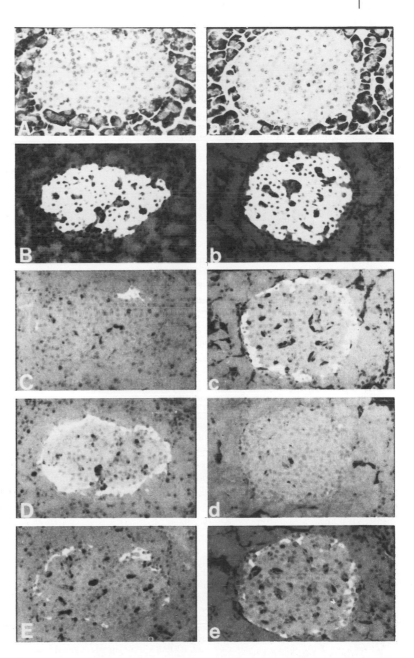

Figure 3. Histologic anatomy of the islet. Serial sections of a representative islet found in the head or ventral portion (*left panels A–E*) and tail or dorsal portion (*right panels a–e*) of the pancreas. *Panels A,a,* Stained with hematoxylin-eosin. *Panels B,b,* Immunohistochemically stained with anti-insulin antisera show beta cells. *Panels C,c,* Stained with antiglucagon antisera show alpha cells. *Panels D,d,* Stained with antipancreatic polypeptide antisera show PP cells. *Panels E,e,* Stained with antisomatostatin antisera show delta cells. (Adapted from Orci L: Macro- and microdomains in the endocrine pancreas. Diabetes *31*:538, 1982, with permission.)

secretion alone, but as a consequence of absent enzyme secretion.

Enzyme Secretion

Pancreatic juice contains three major enzyme groups: amylases, lipases, and proteases, secreted by the acinar cells in multiple forms called *isoenzymes,* together with a small amount of electrolyte-containing fluid. Human pancreatic *amylase* is an α-amylase, which splits the 1,4-α-glycosidic bond of starches to produce glucose, maltose, maltotriose, and a mixture of dextrins. Amylase is secreted in the active state and is stable over a relatively wide range of pH. At least three *lipolytic enzymes* are secreted by the acinar cells. Lipase hydrolyzes insoluble *esters of glycerol* with the help of emulsifiers such as bile salts and colipase, which is also secreted in pancreatic juice. Another lipase hydrolyzes *alcohol esters,* such as those of cholesterol and also requires bile salts as a cofactor. A third lipase hydrolyzes *water-soluble esters.* Phospholipase A is also secreted and is activated by trypsin to cata-

TABLE 1. TESTS OF PANCREATIC FUNCTION

Test	Indications	Technique	Normal Values
Exocrine studies:			
Fecal fat test	Quantify pancreatic insufficiency; guide enzyme replacement therapy	24-hr stool collection	<20 gm fat per 24 hr
Triolein breath test	Quantify pancreatic insufficiency; guide enzyme replacement therapy	Breath samples 4–6 hr after 5 pCi ^{14}C-triolein (corn oil) PO	>3% ^{14}C exhaled per hr
PABA test	Confirm severe pancreatic insufficiency or chronic pancreatitis	6-hr urine collection after 1 gm BT-PABA PO	>60% excretion
Lundh test	Confirm severe pancreatic insufficiency or chronic pancreatitis	Duodenal tube aspirate(s) × 2 hr after test meal	>61 IU/L trypsin output
Secretin test	Evaluate benign versus malignant cause of pancreatic insufficiency	Duodenal tube aspirate(s) × 80 min after 1 U/kg secretin IV	2–4 ml/kg total volume* 90–130 mEq/L bicarbonate 6–8 U/kg amylase
Endocrine studies:			
IV glucose tolerance test (IVGTT)	Evaluate insulin response to hyperglycemia[†]	Every 5–10 min blood samples × 1 hr after 0.5 gm glucose per kg IV	"K" value (% glucose disappearance per min) >1.5
Oral glucose tolerance test (OGTT)	Evaluate insulin response to hyperglycemia[‡]	Every 30 min blood samples × 2–5 hr after 40 gm glucose per m² PO	Basal glucose <115 mg/dl All values <200 mg/dl 2-hr value <140 mg/dl
Tolbutamide response test	Rule out insulinoma, somatostatinoma	Every 10 min blood samples × 1 hr after 1 gm tolbutamide IV	Glucose nadir at 30 min = 50–75% fasting value plasma somatostatin levels <150% basal
Arginine infusion test	Rule out glucagonoma	Every 10 min blood samples during/after 30 min infusion 0.5 gm arginine per kg	<twofold increase in plasma IR-glucagon
Calcium infusion test	Rule out islet cell tumor (insulinoma, gastrinoma, carcinoid)	Every 10 min blood samples during/after 3 hr infusion 4 mg Ca^{++} per kg/hr	<twofold increase in plasma hormone
Pentagastrin stimulation test	Rule out carcinoid tumor	0-, 1-, 3-, 5-, 10-, and 15-min blood samples after 0.6 μg pentagastrin per kg IV	<40% (or <50% ng/ml) increase in IR-serotonin (5-HT) level
Secretin test	Rule out gastrinoma	0-, 1-, 3-, 5-, 10-, 15-, 30-min blood samples after 2 U secretin per kg IV	<200 pg/ml increase in plasma IR-gastrin
Intra-arterial injection (IAI) with hepatic vein sampling (HVS)	Rule out gastrinoma (IAI of 0.3 U secretin per kg) Rule out insulinoma* (IAI of 1.0 mg Ca^{++} per kg)	HVS at 0.5 and 1.0 min after IAI into celiac, gastroduodenal, superior mesenteric, and splenic arteries	<30% increase at 0.5 min, or <100% increase at 1.0 min in plasma hormone compared to basal values

*Local standards or guidelines usually established.
[†]The sum of insulin secretion and tissue responsiveness to insulin.
[‡]The sum of glucose transport and absorption, gut hormone (incretin) secretion, insulin secretion, and tissue responsiveness to insulin.
Abbreviations: PABA = *para*-aminobenzoic acid, BT-PABA = N-benzoyl-L-tryrosyl-*para*-aminobenzoic acid.

lyze the hydrolysis of lecithin to lysolecithin. Lipases function optimally in a pH range of 7.0 to 9.0. Therefore, gastric hypersecretory states that cause duodenal and jejunal acidification may cause inadequate fat digestion and absorption and thereby produce steatorrhea.

Proteolytic enzymes are secreted by the acinar cells in an inactive precursor form. Trypsinogen is activated to form trypsin either through its own dissociation, which occurs as the pH decreases to 7.0 or below, or through the action of *enterokinase*. Enterokinase in an enzyme located on intestinal mucosal cells that resists digestion by the secreted proteases due to its heavy polysaccharide content. Enterokinase specifically converts trypsinogen to trypsin, and the trypsin further activates the chymotrypsins, phospholipase, carboxypeptidases, and elastase, which are also secreted in precursor form. While gastric pepsin contributes to protein digestion, its presence is not essential, as the activated proteases of pancreatic juice are capable of complete protein digestion in the absence of gastric secretion.

In addition to the nucleolytic enzymes ribonuclease and deoxyribonuclease, the acinar cells also synthesize a small amount of trypsin inhibitor. This *antiproteolytic enzyme* binds directly with trypsin and inactivates it. It is thought to protect the pancreatic tissue from trypsin, which may become activated in small amounts within the duct fluid, but the concentration of trypsinogen greatly exceeds that of the trypsin inhibitor protein. When full activation of the trypsinogen occurs, the relatively small quantity of inhibitor becomes ineffective and is digested.

The enzyme precursors are contained within the *zymogen granules* that are in the apical portion of these cells. After release into the lumen of the acinus, the zymogen granules remain intact until the pH of the duct fluid rises above 7.0 as a consequence of bicarbonate secretion. At this pH, the granules dissolve, discharging the enzyme precursors into the duct fluid. With the sustained stimulation of the acinar cells, enzyme synthesis and secretion continues without demonstrable granule formation. However, the secretion of these enzymes does not occur in an absolutely fixed ratio, and alterations in the dietary composition of nutrients may cause corresponding changes in the relative amounts of secretion of amylase, lipases, and proteases. Regulation of enzyme secretion may be mediated through the release of corresponding islet hormones (insulin or glucagon) via the *insuloacinar portal system*. These findings demonstrate that pancreatic enzyme secretion is a rather finely regulated process. Hormonal and neural factors serve as the principal stimuli to enzyme secretion. Cholecystokinin stimulates the acinar cells as well as vagal afferent fibers that mediate acinar function by binding with specific membrane-bound receptors, causing the transport and accumulation of cytosolic calcium within the acinar cell and the intracellular production of cyclic guanosine monophosphate (cGMP). Acetylcholine is also a major stimulant of the acinar cells and is released from postganglionic fibers of the pancreatic plexus. Acetylcholine and CCK act synergistically, and pancreatic enzyme secretion may be reduced as much as 50 per cent after truncal vagotomy. Secretin and VIP are also capable of stimulating acinar cells, but augment the responses to CCK and acetylcholine by increasing intracellular cAMP production.

Endocrine Function

Insulin

Insulin consists of a 21–amino acid A chain connected to a 30–amino acid B chain by two disulfide bridges. The molecule is synthesized as an 81–amino acid precursor peptide termed *proinsulin*, from which a 30–amino acid connecting peptide, or *C-peptide*, is cleaved. This cleavage occurs in the secretory granules of the beta cell, and the C-peptide fragment is secreted together with insulin on an equimolar basis. The structure of insulin varies slightly from species to species, and administration of different insulin preparations can provoke the development of antibodies. Insulin binds to specific receptor proteins on cell membranes and promotes the transport of glucose into most cells. Only beta cells, hepatocytes, and cells of the central nervous system do not require insulin for glucose transport. The interaction of insulin with its receptor sites is a dynamic process: when insulin concentrations change over a period of time, the availability of receptor sites and their binding affinity for the molecule compensate in an opposite manner to allow continued stable rates of glucose transport. When receptor number or affinity decrease, *insulin resistance* results. This compensatory relationship is a ubiquitous characteristic of endocrine systems.

Insulin is metabolized primarily by the liver, and 40 to 50 per cent of the insulin entering the portal system is removed on its passage through the liver. Insulin suppresses glycogenolysis and accelerates nucleic acid formation and protein synthesis. It is also antilipolytic and prevents the breakdown of fatty acids and inhibits the formation of ketones produced by fatty-acid oxidation. Therefore, severe insulin deficiency causes the progressive accumulation of glucose in the blood, as well as the appearance of ketone, which causes *diabetic ketoacidosis*. Insulin excess, or an exaggerated hepatic or peripheral effect of insulin, causes hypoglycemia.

The secretion of insulin is primarily regulated by the concentration of glucose presented to the beta cell and, therefore, by the rate of intracellular glucose metabolism. Glucose transport across cell membranes is facilitated by 59-kd proteins called *glucose transporters*. In the beta cell, the GLUT-2 transporter protein has a low affinity, or high K value, for glucose. This causes progressively higher rates of glucose transport into the beta cell as the glucose concentration rises, which causes increased insulin secretion. Hormonal and neural factors also mediate the beta cell, and intestinal hormones such as gastric inhibitory polypeptide (GIP) and glucagon-like peptide I (GLP-I) enhance the insulin response to glucose. This regulatory effect of the gut on beta cell function is termed the *enteroinsular axis*. Cholinergic stimulation augments insulin release, while sympathetic stimulation inhibits insulin secretion. In the normal pancreas, considerable functional reserve of insulin secretion is present, and destruction or removal of over 80 per cent of the beta cell mass is required before diabetes mellitus becomes apparent.

Glucagon

Glucagon is a 29–amino acid peptide that is similar in amino acid composition to secretin. Multiple forms of glucagon exist in the gastrointestinal tract, and larger glucagon-like peptides in the small intestine are called *enteroglucagon*. Pancreatic glucagon functions in a reciprocal manner to insulin. Its release from the alpha cell is stimulated by hypoglycemia and suppressed by hyperglycemia and hyperinsulinemia. Glucagon activates the breakdown by glycogen through the dephosphorylation of glucose-1-phosphate and accelerates gluconeogenesis, thereby causing endogenous glucose production to increase and plasma glucose levels to rise. In situations of physiologic stress or increased metabolic demand, this process is beneficial and provides additional metabolic fuel for all tissues. Glucagon secretion increases during acute stress, along with cortisol, growth hormone, and catechols. When these "stress hormones" are stimulated by hypoglycemia, they are referred to as *counterregulatory hormones* as they cause a reversal of the decline in plasma glucose. Secretion of glucagon is also stimulated by amino acids, particularly arginine and alanine, and by norepinephrine, while free fatty acids inhibit glucagon release. In normal humans, carbohydrate feeding or a mixed meal produces a modest decline in glucagon levels as insulin release occurs. However, with diabetes mellitus, the glucagon response to these nutrients is paradoxically increased, which contributes to the resulting hyperglycemia. Glucagon is lipolytic and accelerates fatty-acid mobilization, contributing to ketoacidosis in uncontrolled diabetes. In pharmacologic doses, glucagon demonstrates an inotropic effect on the heart, slows gastric and duodenal peristalsis, and relaxes the sphincter of Oddi. Metabolism of glucagon occurs in the kidney and, to a lesser degree, in the liver.

Somatostatin

In 1973, Brazeau and colleagues isolated a hypothalamic peptide that inhibited the release of growth hormone. Because of its antisomatotropin action, this 14–amino acid peptide was named *somatostatin*. Somatostatin is also a potent and reversible inhibitor of the release of insulin, as well as virtually all known pancreatic and intestinal peptide hormones. It also inhibits gastric, pancreatic, and biliary secretion. Immunohistochemical studies demonstrate the presence of somatostatin in the pancreatic delta cell. The release of somatostatin by the isolated pancreas and the demonstration of a nutrient-induced rise in somatostatin levels in pancreatic venous blood in vivo confirm its role as an islet hormone. Somatostatin is also localized to specific cells in the gastric fundus and, to a lesser extent, throughout the gastrointestinal tract. Because of its presence in both the central nervous system (CNS) and the intestinal tract, somatostatin is a prime example of a hormonal link between these diverse organ systems. Termed the *brain-gut axis*, this relationship includes several hormones that interact with, or reside within, the pancreas.

Pancreatic Polypeptide

This 36–amino acid polypeptide is localized to an islet cell distinct from alpha, beta, or delta cells, now referred to histologically as the pancreatic polypeptide (PP) cell. The specific distribution of PP cells has been reviewed previously, and the localization of PP to the pancreas is specific: following total pancreatectomy, plasma levels of PP in humans are undetectable. Pancreatic polypeptide inhibits pancreatic enzyme and bicarbonate secretion, as well as choleresis and gallbladder emptying. Recent studies also suggest a role of PP in nutrient or glucose homeostasis. Carbohydrates, proteins, and fats stimulate PP release when ingested, but not when administered intravenously. Therefore, it is thought that one or more intestinal signals cause the release of PP. Cholecystokinin appears to best fulfill the role of a hormonal stimulant of PP, and vagal innervation is crucial to PP release. Pancreatic polypeptide responses are markedly reduced after vagotomy and after antrectomy. Circulating levels of PP are increased in diabetes, and hyperplasia of islet PP cells has been documented in diabetic subjects. Pancreatic polypeptide also increases with normal aging, which suggests a compensatory response to changes in nutrient metabolism or other hormonal functions.

PATHOLOGY

Acute Pancreatitis

Acute pancreatitis, one of the most common abdominal disorders accounting for hospital admissions, occurs in all socioeconomic and age groups, and is marked by a wide spectrum of clinical severity ranging from a mild, self-limited, transient disorder, to a fulminating, catastrophic process, with an overall mortality of 10 per cent. While multiple etiologies are known or suspected, the disease develops when metabolic or mechanical factors cause a disruption of the physiologic mechanism that normally protect against intrapancreatic activation of proteolytic enzymes (Fig. 4).

Etiology and Pathophysiology

Multiple metabolic, vascular, or mechanical factors can cause acute inflammation of the pancreas.

ALCOHOL. Large studies indicate that 55 to 65 per cent of North American patients with acute pancreatitis have a history of heavy alcohol ingestion or recent significant alcohol abuse. It has been stated that 10 to 15 per cent of alcoholics have evidence of pancreatitis, but the pathophysiology of alcohol-induced pancreatitis remains unclear. Sarles et al. demonstrated the de-

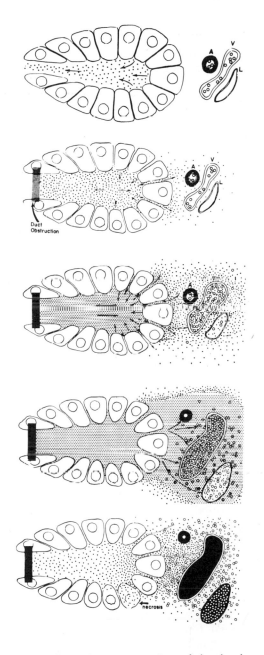

Figure 4. Schematic representation of the development of severe acute pancreatitis due to obstruction of pancreatic duct. *Top figure*, Normal acinar secretion with adjacent artery, vein, and lymphatic duct. *Second figure*, Duct obstruction causes dilated acinar lumen with pericellular leak of secretory products into interstitial tissues. *Third figure*, Increased secretion from acinar cells, with increased interstitial extravasation, edema, and venous engorgement. *Fourth figure*, Massive interstitial edema, arterial spasm, local hemorrhage, and engorged veins. *Bottom figure*, Cellular necrosis, hemorrhage, thrombosis of vessels, and extravasation of blood and secretory products into lymphatic ducts. (From Anderson MC, et al: Circulatory changes in acute pancreatitis. Surg Clin North Am 47:127, 1967, with permission.)

velopment of increased pancreatic protein secretion following chronic ethanol administration and noted the development of protein precipitates in the pancreatic ducts that may cause ductular obstruction. Other possible mechanisms include an increased permeability of ductular epithelium following ethanol ingestion that allows reflux of pancreatic enzymes into the surrounding parenchyma, and the effect of chronically elevated levels of secretory hormones stimulated by alcohol. Once acute pancreatitis has occurred, repeated episodes of alcohol-associated pancreatitis are common if total abstention is not achieved.

GALLSTONES. The second most common cause of acute pancreatitis is *biliary tract disease*. Calculus formation may cause an impacted common duct stone at the level of the ampulla with trauma or obstruction of the main pancreatic duct or regurgitation of bile into the pancreas due to an obstructed common channel. The association of an obstructed common channel was first described in autopsy findings by Opie in 1901 and was initially thought to be the major cause of pancreatitis. Biliary disease occurs in 5 to 50 per cent of patients in North American series of acute pancreatitis, but varies considerably depending on the socioeconomic characteristics of the population studied. In patients with acute pancreatitis associated with cholelithiasis, the risk of subsequent episodes of pancreatitis ranges from 36 to 63 per cent if the cholelithiasis is allowed to persist. Following cholecystectomy, however, the risk of repeated attacks falls to 2 to 8 per cent, which strongly implicates calculus disease as the etiologic factor.

HYPERLIPIDEMIA. There is a strong association of hyperlipidemia with the development of pancreatitis, and patients with the most common form of the disorder, type IV or hypertriglyceridemia, have about a 15 per cent incidence of pancreatitis. The pathophysiologic mechanism is unclear, but it has been suggested that pancreatic lipases may convert increased tissue levels of triglycerides into free fatty acids, which may then cause ductular or parenchymal injury. While the severity of pancreatitis associated with hyperlipidemia is usually mild, severe, chronic, or even fatal episodes have been reported.

TRAUMA. External accidental trauma represents an important mechanical cause of pancreatitis, and operative trauma constitutes a significant cause of acute inflammation, with pancreatitis occurring following gastric or biliary procedures in a small percentage of patients. The insult is usually not noticed at the time of surgery and may be caused by direct blunt or sharp injury or trauma to the region of the ampulla. A related cause of pancreatitis, occurring in 2 to 3 per cent of patients following ERCP, may involve ductal trauma or inoculation of the duct with contaminated material.

DRUGS. A number of drugs have been implicated in the development of acute pancreatitis, but none has been proven to cause the disease. Steroid administration, particularly in children or young adults, has been associated with pancreatitis, but frequently the condition for which the steroids are administered is also a possible factor. Diuretics, azathioprine (Imuran), azulfidine, L-asparaginase, and estrogen preparations have been reported to be possible etiologic factors, although the mechanisms responsible are unknown. The combined use of steroids and azathioprine following renal transplantation may account for the relatively high incidence of pancreatitis in that setting.

INFECTION. Viral infections, particularly mumps and coxsackie virus infection, are associated with acute pancreatitis, and a transient elevation in serum amylase is not unusual during mumps infection. Other viral illnesses such as mononucleosis and cytomegalovirus disease have been suspected but not proven as etiologic factors.

VASCULITIS AND VASCULAR INSUFFICIENCY. Ischemia is an established model of acute pancreatitis experimentally and is thought to contribute to the disorder clinically in patients with atherosclerotic disease of the pancreatic vessels, as well as in patients with systemic vasculitis. Arterial insufficiency due to low cardiac output or as a consequence of cardiopulmonary bypass is also thought to cause acute pancreatitis postoperatively in as many as 1 to 2 per cent of patients who undergo these procedures.

MISCELLANEOUS CAUSES. Hypercalcemia due to hyperparathyroidism has been suggested as a cause of pancreatitis, and the sting of a particular species of scorpion endemic to Trinidad and Venezuela, *Tityus trinitatis*, is frequently followed by acute pancreatitis. The precise etiology related to these factors is unknown. Hereditary factors may also be involved in the development of the disease, as several clusters of children and adults with pancreatitis have been reported within single families. Finally, a significant number of acute, even severe, episodes of pancreatitis occur idiopathically and are unassociated with any of the above.

Clinical Presentation and Diagnosis

The diagnosis of acute pancreatitis is made on the basis of clinical findings and frequently involves the exclusion of other possibilities. No single finding is pathognomonic of the disease, and laboratory data should be regarded as supportive or confirmatory, but not as conclusive proof of the presence or absence of the disorder.

SYMPTOMS. *Pain* is nearly always the presenting complaint and may be epigastric, lower abdominal, or localized to the posterior thoracic or lumbar area. The pain may be noted in the right or left hypochondrium or diffusely present throughout the entire abdomen, and may be mild or severe, but is usually *steady* and not cramping in nature. *Nausea* and *vomiting* frequently occur and *anorexia* is common. Low-grade *fever* may accompany these symptoms, and mild *hypertension* is commonly seen unless dehydration or hypovolemia is present. Frequently, these symptoms have occurred 1 to 3 days after a bout of heavy alcohol ingestion.

PHYSICAL FINDINGS. The patient is frequently uncomfortable in the supine position and prefers to sit up or lie on one side. Midepigastric tenderness is usually present, and a mass may be palpable within the upper abdomen. Bowel sounds are quiet or hypoactive, jaundice is occasionally present, and signs of peritonitis are usually absent, but may occur. The patient may appear dehydrated and hypotensive, and diffuse abdominal fullness or mild distention is frequently present.

LABORATORY FINDINGS. The most commonly observed abnormality is hyperamylasemia, but this is neither a specific nor sensitive finding. Large studies have shown that 20 to 30 per cent of patients with documented acute pancreatitis have normal amylase levels, and 35 per cent of patients with hyperamylasemia have an illness other than pancreatitis. Alternative causes of elevated serum amylase include bowel obstruction, ectopic pregnancy, renal failure, and hepatic disorders, as well as the normal variant of macroamylasemia. Urinary amylase levels are usually elevated for 2 to 5 days after hyperamylasemia subsides. The excretion of amylase depends upon the glomerular filtration rate, however, and the calculation of the amylase/creatinine clearance ratio is the best assessment of increased amylase secretion. In addition to amylase, serum lipase levels also rise during acute pancreatitis, and this is a more specific test for the disorder. Other laboratory findings may include an elevated white blood cell count, a hemoglobin or hematocrit that is either elevated (due to volume contraction) or low (due to retroperitoneal hemorrhage), an increased blood urea nitrogen and creatinine, elevated hepatic enzymes and bilirubin, as well as a metabolic acidosis or mixed metabolic and respiratory acidosis associated with hypoxia. Plasma glucose levels may be elevated due to loss of insulin-secreting ability, but are rarely at the diabetic ketoacidosis level. Plasma calcium may be low due to sequestration of calcium by fat necrosis with saponification, and hypocalcemia may cause signs of tetany. Plain radiography, sonography, and computed tomography (CT) scans of the abdomen may also indicate an enlarged, edematous pancreas, as well as signs of ileus, abscess, or cyst formation.

Clinical Course and Complications

Pathologic changes in acute pancreatitis range from interstitial edema with mild inflammatory cell infiltrates to necrosis of acinar elements, focal hemorrhage and massive edema, to extensive coagulation necrosis of whole areas of the gland with necrosis of peripancreatic tissues and blood vessels causing massive retroperitoneal hemorrhage. The most common cause of morbidity and mortality is *sepsis*, as areas of necrosis become secondarily infected. In addition to abscess and pseudocyst formation and the development of pancreatic fluid extravasation, several other complications occur as the pathologic changes progress. Adjacent structures including the stomach, duodenum, and biliary ducts may become involved in regional edema and necrosis, causing obstruction or local hemorrhage. Splenic or portal vein thrombosis may occur and may cause variceal hemorrhage with preexisting portal hypertension. Pulmonary insufficiency is common and may involve only pleural effusion and atelectasis, pneumonia, or florid adult respiratory distress syndrome. Oliguria, azotemia, or renal vessel thrombosis may cause renal failure, and disseminated intravascular coagulation, pericardial effusion, or refractory circulatory collapse may occur. To assess which patients have severe pancreatitis and are at high risk for the development of one or more of the above complications, Ranson et al. determined five criteria observed at the time of initial diagnosis and six criteria based on the clinical course of the patient in the subsequent 48 hours that correlate particularly well with the ultimate risk of morbidity and mortality (Table 2). It should be noted that the presence or degree of hyperamylasemia is *not* a useful index of the severity of the disease. The correlation between the number of positive criteria and the risk of mortality and morbidity is linear and dramatic: patients with three or more positive signs (defined as severe pancreatitis) have an average mortality of 28 per cent.

Treatment

In 75 to 80 per cent of patients, acute pancreatitis is mild (fewer than three criteria positive), and a successful outcome is usually achieved with nonoperative, supportive therapy. Surgical intervention is indicated only when a definitive diagnosis of pancreatitis cannot be made but signs of an upper abdominal catastrophe persist, when pancreatic abscess is suspected or proven, or when complications or etiologic factors require operative intervention.

SUPPORTIVE THERAPY. The first priority is to *put the gland at rest*. The patient is given *nothing by mouth*, and a *nasogastric tube* is strongly recommended. The removal of gastric acid and the elimi-

TABLE 2. EARLY OBJECTIVE FINDINGS THAT CORRELATE WITH THE RISK OF MAJOR COMPLICATIONS OR DEATH IN ACUTE PANCREATITIS*

At admission or diagnosis
1. Age >55 years
2. White blood cell count >16,000/mm^3
3. Blood glucose level >200 mg/dl
4. Serum lactic dehydrogenase (LDH) concentration >350 IU/L
5. Serum glutamic oxaloacetic transaminase (SGOT) >250 Sigma-Frankel U/dl

During initial 48 hours
6. Hematocrit decrease >10 percentage points
7. Blood urea nitrogen increase >5 mg/dl
8. Serum calcium level <8 mg/dl
9. Arterial Po$_2$ <60 mm Hg
10. Base deficit >4 mEq/L
11. Estimated fluid sequestration (IV fluid replacement required) >6000 ml

Definition of severity

0–2	Signs present:	Mild pancreatitis
3–5	Signs present:	Moderately severe pancreatitis
6+	Signs present:	Severe or "catastrophic" pancreatitis

*From Ranson JHC, et al: Surg Gynecol Obstet 139:69, 1974, with permission.

nation of gastric distention reduce the neural and hormonal stimulation of the exocrine pancreas and help to prevent aspiration due to vomiting. *Analgesics* are prescribed for patient comfort and to reduce stress-induced neural stimulation of gastric and pancreatic secretion. Meperidine (Demerol) is used in place of morphine, as the latter may induce spasm of the sphincter of Oddi. Additional agents intended to reduce pancreatic stimulation such as anticholinergics (atropine or Robinul), trypsin inhibitors (aprotinin), or hormones that have been shown experimentally to inhibit exocrine secretion (glucagon or somatostatin) have not been found to be useful or require further evaluation before their routine use can be recommended. The second priority of supportive therapy is to *prevent potential complications*. Because the major cause of death is sepsis, *antibiotics* are usually prescribed. Their routine application has not been proven to be significantly beneficial; however, clinical studies usually contain only a small number of patients with moderate or severe pancreatitis in whom the risk of sepsis is high. *Antacids* are usually prescribed both to reduce gastric acid output to the duodenum and to reduce the risk of bleeding secondary to gastritis or duodenitis. In all but the mildest forms of pancreatitis, retroperitoneal fluid sequestration and hypovolemia occur and require *intravenous fluid administration*. Hypocalcemia and other ion deficiencies require intravenous replacement, and nutritional support usually requires *parenteral alimentation* with careful monitoring of blood glucose levels. *Ventilatory support* is frequently needed in severe cases, and the common occurrence of hypoxia and pulmonary infiltrates usually requires mechanical ventilatory assistance. *Peritoneal lavage* has proven to be an effective measure that frequently produces dramatic improvement in the symptoms and signs of moderately severe pancreatitis. However, the risk of subsequent sepsis remains high in these patients and the overall time course of the illness is relatively unchanged. Careful attention must still be paid to possible septic complications, and early refeeding of the patient with seeming resolution of symptoms is to be avoided.

SURGICAL INTERVENTION. Extensive drainage of the peripancreatic tissues is hazardous in milder forms of acute pancreatitis and may actually contribute to increased morbidity and mortality. In severe pancreatitis, however, extensive lavage and sump drainage of the region of the pancreas improves survival and should be considered if retroperitoneal necrosis is present. In advanced pancreatic necrosis, resection or débridment of the necrotic gland with extensive open drainage of the region (marsupialization of the pancreas) may offer the only hope of survival. Operative therapy may be required in acute pancreatitis associated with biliary calculus disease. If cholecystitis or common duct obstruction does not respond to conservative management during the first 48 hours, cholecystostomy, cholecystectomy, or common duct decompression may be required to reverse a progressively severe clinical course. Frequently, the coexistence of gangrenous cholecystitis or cholangitis is difficult to exclude in these patients, and early surgical intervention may be required. In general, however, conservative management is advised until the pancreatitis has resolved, whereupon necessary biliary tract procedures may be undertaken with a greater margin of safety.

Pancreatic Abscess

General Description and Pathophysiology

The development of a pancreatic abscess represents a severe, life-threatening complication for the patient with pancreatitis. The mortality for pancreatic abscesses that are *not* treated by operative drainage is virtually 100 per cent, and the most successful series of surgical treatment still show a 30 to 50 per cent mortality. Pancreatic abscess can accompany acute pancreatitis caused by virtually any etiologic factor or can occur as a complication of chronic pancreatitis accompanied by ductular obstruction or pseudocyst disease. The etiology of the infection is thought to be due to either reflux of enteric flora into the pancreas or hematogenous seeding of a pancreatic phlegmon during a septic episode. Bacteria isolated from pancreatic abscesses include a wide range of organisms but are predominantly gram-negative enteric species. The septic state produced by a pancreatic abscess is particularly severe due to the relatively unconfined retroperitoneal location of the abscess, the exuberant vascular and lymphatic supply to the area, and the accompanying tissue damage and necrosis that is caused by the liberation of proteolytic enzymes in the area.

Clinical Presentation

The diagnosis is usually made when the clinical course of the patient with acute pancreatitis fails to reveal significant improvement during supportive therapy and when physical and laboratory parameters are consistent with possible sepsis. Noninvasive radiologic studies such as sonograms and CT scanning may reveal a heterogeneous mass in the region of the pancreas with evidence of entrapped air or liquified debris. Occasionally, such clear-cut radiographic findings are not evident and the decision to proceed with surgical intervention must be made on a purely clinical basis.

Treatment

The treatment of a pancreatic abscess should provide thorough drainage and débridement of necrotic tissue. Multiple sump and irrigation drains are inserted into the abscess and brought out of the abdominal cavity at various sites. Despite this vigorous approach, several reoperations may be required to maintain adequate drainage, and clinical signs of progressive or recurrent sepsis are indications for reexploration. Some surgeons recommend débridement and open packing, or marsupialization, of pancreatic abscesses, leaving the abdominal wound open to allow frequent removal and replacement of the packing material. Despite its seemingly radical nature, the beneficial results obtained with the technique warrant its use in selected patients when pancreatic necrosis is widespread. The clinical course of the patient with a successfully treated pancreatic abscess is still protracted and frequently complicated, and aggressive and meticulous attention to the metabolic and nutritional needs of the patient are essential for a satisfactory outcome.

Chronic Pancreatitis

General Description

Recurrent episodes of acute pancreatitis or persistent inflammation within the pancreas may ultimately cause a chronic disorder characterized by fibrosis, calculus formation, and cystic changes within the gland. Chronic pancreatitis usually presents in males between the ages of 35 and 50, but may occur in patients of either sex from the second to the eighth decade of life. The disease is usually progressive and while symptoms may be controlled by medical therapy or, in selected patients, resolved by surgical treatment, the histologic changes are irreversible.

Etiology and Pathophysiology

The usual etiologic factor associated with the development of chronic pancreatitis is alcohol abuse, but chronic inflammation and fibrosis may be caused by a variety of factors including trauma, biliary tract disease, or hypercalcemia. Alcoholism is the most common cause of *calcific* pancreatitis, in which calcium carbonate calculi form within the ducts and parenchymal calcium deposits are seen. These changes occur in one third of patients with advanced chronic pancreatitis. Progressive fibrosis leads to distortion of the parenchyma with loss of acinar tissue, a reduced number of islets, disruption of normal vascular supply, and distortion or obliteration of various portions of the ductular system. Ductular pathology occurs in several forms and may include proximal (periampullary) obstruction due to stricture or stone formation with resultant distal duct dilatation, intermittent areas of stenosis and dilatation throughout the ductular system ("chain-of-lakes" appearance), or complete stenosis or sclerosis of the ducts, with or without parenchymal cyst formation. Fibrosis may involve adjacent structures such as the distal common bile duct or duodenum, and low-grade obstructive jaundice is frequently seen. The loss of acinar tissue causes clinically apparent exocrine insufficiency (steatorrhea) when enzyme secretion decreases to less than 10 per cent of normal capacity. Similarly, the progressive loss of islet tissue causes a deterioration of glucose tolerance, and clinically demonstrable diabetes mellitus is seen in as many as one third of patients with chronic pancreatitis. Laënnec's cirrhosis occurs in patients with a history of alcoholism, but the coexistence of chronic pancreatitis and severe cirrhosis is less than might otherwise be expected.

Clinical Presentation and Diagnosis

Patients present with persistent abdominal pain that is usually localized to the midepigastrium and may penetrate through to the posterior thoracolumbar region. The pain is usually *steady*, and it may be exacerbated by eating or may occur as separate crises of pain associated with bouts of heavy alcohol ingestion. While nausea and vomiting may occur, there is less hemodynamic instability than is present with acute pancreatitis. Abdominal examination usually reveals moderate *tenderness* in the midepigastrium, and upper abdominal fullness or a *palpable mass* may be present. A history consistent with *steatorrhea* may be present, although demonstrable exocrine deficiency may be present in patients who nonetheless report unremarkable bowel function. Laboratory studies usually reveal normal or only modestly elevated serum amylase levels and white blood cell counts. *Hyperglycemia* is common, as are low-grade elevations of bilirubin and alkaline phosphatase. Liver enzyme elevations are frequently seen, as are laboratory parameters of *malnutrition*. The diagnosis is usually confirmed by characteristic findings on radiologic studies such as plain radiographs of the abdomen (which may reveal diffuse calcification in the region of the pancreas), sonograms and CT scans (which demonstrate ductular dilatation, cyst disease, and calcification), or ERCP (which shows ductular distortion, dilatation, stenosis, or obstruction). Functional tests of exocrine function (secretin test, Lundh meal, *para*-aminobenzoic acid [PABA] test, or triolein breath test) or endocrine function (oral glucose tolerance test) provide additional criteria for the diagnosis of chronic pancreatic disease (Table 1).

Clinical Course and Complications

The natural history of chronic pancreatitis is that of persistent pain associated with progressive signs and symptoms of exocrine and endocrine insufficiency. Acute exacerbations of severe pain are associated with duct obstruction and cyst formation. When intraductular pressure rises 15 to 20 cm H_2O above normal, pain usually occurs or increases. Patients demonstrate progressive malnutrition and general debilitation and frequently exhibit heavy dependence on analgesics. Splanchnic and gastrointestinal complications include biliary tract disease (with calculus formation or common duct stenosis), portal hypertension, splenic vein thrombosis, gastritis, duodenitis, as well as complications of pseudocyst disease. Sepsis may occur, but is relatively infrequent.

Treatment

Supportive therapy during episodes of acute exacerbation of pain is similar to that of acute pancreatitis, with the addition of enteral pancreatic enzyme replacement. The medical therapy of progressive chronic pancreatitis includes the removal of precipitating factors such as alcohol, drugs, or hypercalcemia, with appropriate treatment of pain, steatorrhea, weight loss, and diabetes. The management of the patient with pancreatogenic diabetes is directed toward the control of blood glucose levels, but with particular attention to the avoidance of hypoglycemia. While nonoperative therapy may control the exocrine and endocrine deficiency, the persistence of severe pain or jaundice is an indication for surgical therapy. No single operation is advocated for patients with chronic pancreatitis, and the choice of a suitable surgical procedure depends on the specific anatomic considerations in each patient. Biliary and pancreatic ductular anatomy is carefully evaluated by CT scanning and ERCP to determine the location and extent of the disease process. When ERCP is unsuccessful, cholangiography and operative pancreatograms form the basis for surgical decision making.

Biliary tract procedures may be required to treat cholelithiasis or choledocholithiasis. In a few patients, significant stenosis or obstruction of the ampulla responds to *sphincteroplasty*, in which the ampulla of Vater is enlarged and the sphincter of Oddi sewn open to prevent obstruction. More commonly, the predominant ductular pathology consists of either generalized dilation behind a proximal obstruction in the region of the head or uncinate process, or diffuse sclerosis of the ductular system. A dilated, obstructed pancreatic duct is best treated with internal drainage into a Roux-en-Y loop of jejunum, originally described by Puestow and Gillesby in 1958. This procedure required splenectomy and resection of the pancreatic tail, and has been supplanted by the Partington and Rochelle modification of the Puestow procedure described in 1960, in which a long (10- to 12-cm) longitudinal opening of the anterior aspect of the pancreatic duct is anastomosed to a similar longitudinal enterotomy in the jejunal limb. The operative morbidity and mortality are generally low, and 70 to 80 per cent of patients have good to excellent pain relief following this procedure.

When the main pancreatic duct is not dilated but is sclerotic, a decompression procedure is infeasible. Resection of most or all of the diseased portion of the gland may then provide relief of pain. In general, the procedure that offers the best likelihood of relieving pain with the lowest risk of operative or postoperative morbidity and mortality is preferred. Each resectional procedure carries specific drawbacks, however. While partial distal pancreatectomy is usually the safest procedure to perform, it is associated with only a 50 to 60 per cent incidence of prolonged relief of pain. Conversely, while subtotal distal and total pancreatic resection provide improved relief of pain, they are invariably accompanied by severe exocrine deficiency and a particularly brittle form of diabetes mellitus. Proximal pancreatectomy (and duodenectomy) is indicated only in the unusual situation of severe sclerotic disease limited to the head of the pancreas. Therefore, resectional procedures are chosen with considerable caution and only in carefully selected patients, and demonstrated failure of aggressive nonoperative management of chronic pancreatitis is an absolute prerequisite before these procedures are performed. Recent attempts have been made to reduce or eliminate the obligatory endocrine disease that accompanies subtotal or total pancreatectomy by performing isolated autologous islet transplantation at the time of resection. Technical problems have limited its success due to poor islet yields from the resected portion of pancreas. However, the method offers considerable promise, and clinical experience with these techniques continues to grow at a number of specialized surgical centers.

Pancreatic Neoplasms

General Description

Tumors of the pancreas represent a wide spectrum of diagnostic and therapeutic challenges. The most common malignancy, ductular adenocarcinoma, is a particularly insidious disease and continues to be associated with a poor prognosis of an overall 5-year survival of less than 1 per cent. The rare islet cell tumors can be treated successfully, however, and have contributed greatly to an understanding of endocrine physiology through documentation of the effects of their excessive hormone secretion.

Exocrine Tumors

Benign tumors of exocrine cell origin are rare and include *acinar cell* and *ductular cell adenomas* and connective tissue tumors such as *hemangiomas, lymphangiomas*, and *desmoid* tumors. *Serous cystadenomas* (arising from acinar cells) and *mucinous cystadenomas* (arising from ductular cells), while histologically benign, are thought to have the capacity to degenerate into cystadenocarcinomas. Large, cystic lesions may resemble pseudocysts and are detected because of their increasing size. Smaller lesions are diagnosed on the basis of investigation of complaints of vague or intermittent abdominal discomfort or when the lesions arise near the ampulla or distal common bile duct and cause obstructive jaundice. Once the tumor has been identified by radiologic studies or at the time of operation, it is usually impossible to discriminate between the rare benign exocrine tumors and their more common malignant counterparts, and resection is the treatment of choice when feasible.

Malignant exocrine tumors include a wide spectrum of ductular, acinar cells, and connective tissue tumors, but over 90 per cent of patients have *ductular adenocarcinoma*. Its etiology remains obscure, and the incidence rises progressively from the third decade of life. Multiple intrapancreatic foci of carcinoma are present in 10 to 20 per cent of patients, and the malignancy is characterized by an aggressive pattern of regional and distant metastasis. While the diagnosis of carcinoma is usually made from histologic examination of a biopsy or surgically resected specimen, attempts have been made to identify specific *tumor markers* that may provide an early indication of the disease. A variety of proteins are present in normal embryologic tissues, and occasionally their synthesis is activated by the malignant process. These are referred to as *oncofetal antigens* or oncofetal proteins. *Carcinoembryonic antigen* (CEA) is the most widely studied, but the lack of sensitivity and specificity of this marker for pancreatic cancer precludes its use as a reliable marker. *Pancreatic oncofetal antigen* (POA) is seen in highest levels in patients with pancreatic adenocarcinoma, but the presence of modestly elevated levels of POA can occur in a variety of benign and malignant conditions. *CA 19-9* and *DUPAN-2* are oncofetal antigens detected by monoclonal antibodies and have been found to have greater sensitivity and specificity for pancreatic carcinoma. Elevations in these antigens that occur after surgical resection of a malignancy can be a useful indicator of the presence of recurrent or metastatic disease.

Patients with pancreatic adenocarcinoma usually manifest symptoms of *weight loss* and *vague abdominal discomfort* and may present with *obstructive jaundice* if the tumor arises in the head of the pancreas. *Pain penetrating into the back* is frequently noted, and there is a greater-than-expected association of psychiatric disturbances such as depression and psychosis. When distal common bile duct obstruction occurs, a dilated palpable gallbladder may be present (Courvoisier's sign). The presence of the tumor may be confirmed by contrast or scanning radiography, and evidence of metastatic disease is present in more than half of patients with adenocarcinoma. When the tumor is well localized by ERCP or other studies and when metastatic disease is not detected, arteriography is frequently performed to evaluate potential resectability. The findings of *encasement* or obliteration of major vessels, or of angiographically demonstrable metastases assists in the identification of those patients in whom a surgical approach on the lesion is unwarranted. The angiographic finding of *compression* or mild displacement of the superior mesenteric or portal vein is not a consistent sign of the lack of resectability, as edema and inflammation around the tumor rather than the tumor itself may produce these findings. Final assessment of resectability is made by surgical exploration, and some 20 per cent of patients are found to have a lesion that can be successfully resected in hopes of cure or long-term survival. Surgically resectable adenocarcinomas are usually located in the head of the pancreas, as distal lesions almost always demonstrate metastases by the time the diagnosis is made. The most widely performed procedure is the *pancreaticoduodenectomy* (Whipple procedure) (Fig. 5). Total pancreatectomy is advocated by some authorities, but is generally avoided due to the great degree of postoperative morbidity secondary to the metabolic and nutritional abnormalities that accompany this operation.

In less than 10 per cent of patients with resectable exocrine malignancy, the lesion is found to be a *cystadenocarcinoma* of the *papillary* or *serous* type. This lesion is *less* aggressive in its capacity to metastasize early compared to ductular adenocarcinoma; therefore, surgical resection is associated with a significant 5-year survival in the range of 10 to 20 per cent. The tumor is frequently found to arise in the body or tail of the pancreas, and a *subtotal distal pancreatectomy* may be performed. Absolute exocrine and endocrine deficiency is usually avoided if 10 to 20 per cent of the pancreatic mass is preserved.

Other malignancies of nonendocrine origin include lymphomas, various sarcomas, and tumors whose origin lies in the duodenal or biliary duct epithelium of the ampulla. Well-localized lesions, particularly in the region of the ampulla, are resected as described above, and significant, albeit modest, rates of long-term survival may be achieved.

Endocrine Tumors

Benign lesions of islet cell origin include disorders of *hyperplasia*, and *adenoma* formation. *Islet cell tumors* have been described for each of the four principal islet cell types, as well as for a variety of additional hormone-secreting tumors of pancreatic origin (Table 3). Islet cell tumors (adenomas or adenocarcinomas) may be nonfunctional and associated with no detectable elevation of known hormones, but usually secrete at least one hormone product in sufficient excess to cause significant signs and symptoms. Occasionally, these tumors are *pleuripotential*, and secrete more than one hormone either simultaneously or sequentially over a period of months to years. Rarely, islet cell adenomas (particularly those that secrete gastrin) are associated with hyperplasia or adenomatosis of other endocrine tissue such as the parathyroids, pituitary, and adrenals, and may form part of the multiple endocrine neoplasia type I (MEN-I) syndrome. The histologic differentiation of adenoma from adenocarcinoma is frequently difficult in these lesions, and the designation of malignancy is often dependent upon the presence of grossly apparent metastases.

Islet Cell Hyperplasia and Nesidioblastosis

Islet cell hyperplasia occurs in a variety of conditions, including obesity, following oral hypoglycemic agent therapy, and in some patients with hypergastrinemia (Zollinger-Ellison syndrome) and secretory diarrhea (Verner-Morrison syndrome). Very rarely, the

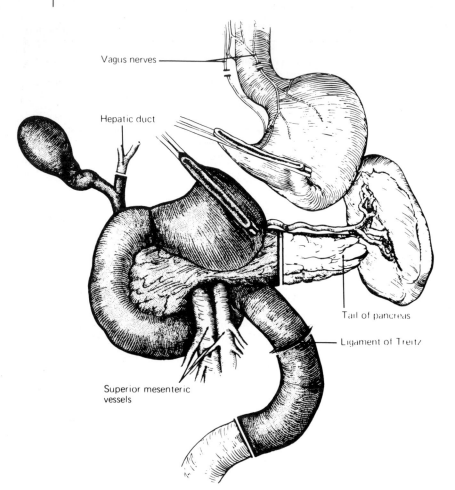

Vagus nerves

Hepatic duct

Tail of pancreas

Ligament of Treitz

Superior mesenteric vessels

Figure 5. Pancreaticoduodenectomy (Whipple procedure). The tissues shaded are resected en bloc. Reconstruction consists of an end-to-end pancreaticojejunostomy, an end-to-side choledochojejunostomy, and a loop gastrojejunostomy. (From Frey CF: *In* Malt RA [ed]: Surgical Techniques Illustrated, Philadelphia, WB Saunders Company, 1985, p 432, with permission.)

hypersecretion of insulin or VIP associated with diffuse islet cell hyperplasia may warrant subtotal or even total pancreatectomy to control the resulting disease. A related disorder is that of *nesidioblastosis*, in which islets become hyperplastic or adenomatous and tufts of islet cells develop around the ductular epithelium. While this appearance is occasionally noted incidentally in pancreatic tissue resected from adults, it can cause a life-threatening illness in infants. *Neonatal hyperinsulinism* due to nesidioblastosis may cause profound hypoglycemia and may require pancreatic resection for control. This etiology of hyperinsulinism is characterized by a marked sensitivity of the beta cells to infusion of *leucine*, and a dramatic rise in insulin following such a challenge suggests this histologic abnormality.

INSULINOMA. The largest number of islet cell tumors reported to date are those of beta cell origin associated with hyperinsulinism and hypoglycemia. The classic triad, described by Whipple in 1935, of *neurologic dysfunction*, documented fasting *hypoglyce-mia*, and *reversal of symptoms* following glucose administration, still stands as a hallmark of the disease. Patients commonly describe a prolonged history of vague or nonspecific symptoms, including altered mental status, prior to the documentation of hypoglycemia. However, because a number of conditions may cause hypoglycemia, specific studies are required for the diagnosis of insulinoma, including (1) the response to a *72-hour* fast (which reveals inappropriately elevated levels of insulin occurring during hypoglycemia), (2) a *tolbutamide response test* or calcium infusion test (which demonstrates exaggerated insulin release and hypoglycemia), (3) elevated circulating levels of proinsulin or C peptide, (4) identification of a tumor mass (by CT scanning or arteriography), or (5) localization of a focus of excess insulin secretion by percutaneous transhepatic venous sampling. Factitious hypoglycemia due to exogenous insulin or sulfonylurea administration should be excluded and can be identified by the presence of low levels of C peptide, detectable levels of anti-insulin antibodies, or the presence of sul-

TABLE 3. ISLET CELL TUMOR SYNDROMES

Syndrome	Excess Hormone	Cell Type	Signs and Symptoms*	Diagnostic Studies†
Insulinoma	Insulin (+ Proinsulin and C peptide)	Beta	*Hypoglycemia, altered mental status,* syncope, dizziness	72-hr fast, tolbutamide test, calcium infusion
Gastrinoma (Zollinger-Ellison)	Gastrin	Gamma	*Gastric acid hypersecretion, peptic ulceration,* diarrhea (steatorrhea), weight loss	Secretin test, calcium infusion, test meal, evidence of MEN-I‡
Glucagonoma	Glucagon	Alpha	*Hyperglycemia, diabetes mellitus, skin rash (MNE),* glossitis, thrombophlebitis, weight loss	Skin biopsy, arginine infusion
Somatostatinoma	Somatostatin	Delta	*Diabetes mellitus, gallstones, hypochlorhydria,* steatorrhea, weight loss	Test meal, tolbutamide test
WDHA (Verner-Morrison)	VIP (or PGE₁)	Delta₁	*Watery diarrhea, hypokalemia, achlorhydria,* dehydration, psychosis	Improvement in symptoms with trial of prostaglandin-synthesis inhibitor (indomethacin) therapy or steroid therapy
Carcinoid	Serotonin (substance P)	EC	*Flushing, diarrhea,* tachycardia, abdominal pain	Calcium infusion, pentagastrin test
PP-OMA	Pancreatic polypeptide	PP	*Weight loss,* abdominal discomfort, diarrhea	Evidence of MEN-I‡

*Signs and symptoms which occur in greater than two thirds of cases are italicized.
†In addition to documented elevated levels of hormone, CT scanning, arteriography, and in selected cases, transhepatic portal venous sampling.
‡Multiple endocrine neoplasia type I—pituitary, parathyroid, and/or adrenal cortical adenomas.
Abbreviations: PGE = prostaglandin E₁, MNE = migratory necrolytic erythema, EC = enterochromaffin cell, PP = pancreatic polypeptide, VIP = vasoactive intestinal polypeptide, WDHA = water diarrhea with hypokalemia and achlorhydria, MEN-I = multiple endocrine neoplasia type I syndrome.

fonylurea compounds in blood or urine. Most beta cell tumors are less than 2 cm in diameter and radiologic studies may fail to reveal them. Therefore, surgical exploration is frequently required for definitive localization. About 80 per cent of insulinomas are single, benign adenomas, which allow surgical cure in most patients by either resection or "shelling out" of the small encapsulated tumor.

GASTRINOMA. The next most widely reported islet cell tumor, but probably one that occurs most frequently, is that originally described in 1955 by Zollinger and Ellison. Histologically distinct gamma or G cells are rarely identifiable in normal islets, but under pathologic conditions, they may comprise a pancreatic or peripancreatic adenoma or adenocarcinoma that is characterized by a high rate of secretion of gastrin. Hypergastrinemia causes dramatic hypersecretion of gastric acid and subsequent peptic ulceration of the upper gastrointestinal tract. Gastrinomas have been detected in patients of all ages, but are most commonly seen in the third to fifth decade. Persistent and

complicated ulcer disease that is refractory to normal therapy occurs in most of these patients, but as many as one third may demonstrate a relatively unremarkable history of peptic disease. Twenty to 25 per cent of incidences have been familial or manifest evidence of the MEN-I syndrome. Gastric hypersecretion may cause diarrhea or steatorrhea (due to mucosal injury and digestion of exocrine enzymes by the increased acid production), and significant weight loss is commonly reported. The diagnosis is made by the documentation of plasma levels of gastrin, which are elevated 2- to 100-fold and which respond paradoxically to feeding (in which the elevated basal levels of gastrin remain unchanged) or to intravenous secretin administration (in which the plasma gastrin rises abruptly by over 200 pg/ml or to levels that are at least twice basal). The tumor may be localized by the radiologic means described for insulinoma, and metastatic disease is often apparent.

While the majority of gastrinomas are malignant, the tumor is typically a slow-growing one, and the principal cause of morbidity and mortality other than the progression of the malignancy itself is related to the complications of the resulting peptic ulcer disease. Treatment is therefore directed toward surgically removing a solitary resectable tumor when present or, in most patients in whom the tumor is unresectable, the absolute prevention of gastric acid secretion. This can be accomplished by performing a total gastrectomy with a Roux-en-Y esophagojejunostomy. This procedure is generally well tolerated by patients with gastrinoma whose disease has been controlled preoperatively through the use of type II histamine (H_2) receptor antagonists (e.g., cimetidine, ranitidine). An alternative approach is to maintain these patients on long-term H_2-receptor antagonist or omeprazole therapy indefinitely. The ultimate safety and success of this nonsurgical approach is being studied.

GLUCAGONOMA. While patients with diabetes mellitus frequently show paradoxic elevations in fasting or postprandial levels of glucagon, the diabetic state is occasionally the direct consequence of excess production of glucagon by an alpha cell adenoma or adenocarcinoma. These patients may appear essentially indistinguishable from those with common forms of diabetes unless they demonstrate the characteristic dermatologic finding of *migratory necrolytic erythema.* This circular, reddish, occasionally psoriatic-appearing rash may be present over the trunk, limbs, and in intertriginous areas. Other manifestations of hyperglucagonemia include glossitis, anemia, hypoaminoacidemia, and repeated episodes of thrombophlebitis. A skin biopsy frequently reveals the characteristic dermatologic pathology, and elevated levels of glucagon that are at least three to five times the norm strongly suggest the presence of this pancreatic lesion. The tumor is usually localized through radiologic scanning studies and arteriography, and surgical excision is attempted when widespread metastatic disease is not apparent. Frequently, these lesions are diagnosed rather late in their course, and the disease is usually at a metastatic level when the diagnosis is made. When a glucagonoma is strongly suspected, the diagnosis may be confirmed through the use of provocative testing such as the *arginine infusion test*, or with localization procedures such as percutaneous transhepatic *portal venous sampling*.

SOMATOSTATIN. With the elucidation of the presence and physiologic properties of somatostatin in the early 1970s, numerous investigators sought to identify a delta cell adenoma or adenocarcinoma secreting excess quantities of the hormone. This was first documented by Larsson and colleagues in 1977, and subsequent reports have verified that this lesion is usually associated with both diabetes (due to inhibition of insulin secretion) and gallstones (due to cholestasis). The finding of a pancreatic tumor in association with these common conditions is an indication for determination of plasma levels of somatostatin. Provocative studies that may demonstrate exaggerated secretion include the tolbutamide response test, as well as a test meal study. Localization procedures as described for other islet cell tumors may be performed to define a resectable lesion, although these tumors are also frequently metastatic at the time of diagnosis.

WATERY DIARRHEA, HYPOKALEMIA, AND ACHLORHYDRIA. Three years after Zollinger and Ellison described the gastrinoma syndrome, Verner and Morrison reported a syndrome associated with islet cell tumors that consisted of *watery diarrhea, Hypokalemia*, and *achlorhydria* (WDHA). The profuse secretory diarrhea of more than 3 L/day suggested the alternative name of *pancreatic cholera*. This diarrhea led to both severe potassium loss and dehydration and frequently caused renal failure. Histologically, the islet-cell adenoma associated with the syndrome was found to be distinct from that which secretes gastrin, and two hormones have been identified as causative agents in the development of the WDHA syndrome. The most frequently documented hormonal product is VIP, which was isolated and characterized by Said and Mutt in 1970 and is found in gastrointestinal and neural tissues throughout the abdomen. VIP-containing cells are extremely scarce in the normal pancreas, but these cells, identified as $delta_1$ cells, may form the adenoma that causes the WDHA syndrome. Occasionally, the WDHA syndrome may occur in patients with normal VIP levels, and in 1977, Jaffe et al. demonstrated that prostaglandin E_1 (PGE_1) may also mediate the syndrome when secreted in excess by an islet cell tumor. These adenomas are frequently less than 1 cm in diameter and may elude standard radiologic imaging techniques. They may be localized by portal venous sampling studies, but are frequently identified at the time of careful surgical exploration of the pancreas. Because these lesions are usually solitary and benign, surgical resection commonly achieves relief of all symptoms.

CARCINOID SYNDROME. Most carcinoid tumors are located in the distal small intestine and colon, but these lesions may arise as a rare islet cell tumor as well. Through the effects of excess secretion of serotonin (5-HT) and other neuropeptides such as *substance P*, these tumors produce their characteristic syndrome of diarrhea, cutaneous flushing, tachycardia, and abdominal discomfort. High plasma levels of serotonin may be measured directly or may be implied by excess urinary excretion of the serotonin metabolite, 5-hydroxyindoleacetic acid (5-HIAA). Provocative studies such as calcium or pentagastrin infusion may exacerbate symptoms and abruptly increase the levels of serotonin. While localization studies are of help in planning treatment, islet cell carcinoid tumors are frequently metastatic when first diagnosed. Surgical resection of the tumor, or "debulking" of the metastatic tissue, provides the best likelihood of cure or control of symptoms.

MISCELLANEOUS SYNDROMES. A variety of other peptide hormone products are associated with islet cell tumors of the pancreas. Pancreatic polypeptide may be secreted in excess by islet cell tumors, and provides a useful marker for an otherwise occult pancreatic tumor. Elevated levels of PP may be the only indication of an islet cell tumor arising as part of the MEN-I syndrome and should be documented in patients with these disorders. A variety of pituitary hormones may be secreted by pancreatic tumors, including adrenocorticotropic hormone (ACTH), melanocyte-stimulating hormone (MSH), antidiuretic hormone (ADH), and related releasing factors. The tremendous potential for peptide secretion by adenomas or adenocarcinomas of the pancreas underscores the complex regulatory role of this organ.

REFERENCES

Grendel JH, Cello JP: Chronic pancreatitis. *In* Sleisenger MH, Fordtran JS (eds): Gastrointestinal Disease, ed 4. Philadelphia. WB Saunders Company, 1989, pp 1842–1872.

Jordan GL Jr: Pancreatic resection for pancreatic cancer. *In* Howard JM, Jordan GL Jr, Reber HA (eds): Surgical Diseases of the Pancreas. Philadelphia, Lea & Febiger, 1987, pp 666–714.

Ranson JHC: Acute pancreatitis: Surgical management. *In* Go VL, Gardner JD, Brooks FP, et al (eds): The Exocrine Pancreas. New York, Raven Press, 1986, pp 503–511.

Seymour NE, Andersen DK: Endocrine tumors of the pancreas. *In* Braasch JW, Tompkins RK (eds): Surgical Disease of the Biliary Tract and Pancreas. Chicago, Mosby Year Book Publishers, 1993 (in press).

Warshaw AL: The relationship between pancreas divisum and pancreatitis: Surgical aspects. *In* Burns GP, Banks S (eds): Disorders of the Pancreas. New York, McGraw-Hill, 1992, pp 159–171.

II
Pancreatic Pseudocysts

PAUL M. AHEARNE, M.D.

Pancreatic pseudocysts are collections of pancreatic fluid bounded by the peritoneum and by the pancreas. Since the fluid collection is not totally surrounded by an epithelial lining, it is therefore not a *true* cyst. Pancreatic pseudocysts occur in association with pancreatitis, cholelithiasis, and biliary tract disease, and as a result of blunt abdominal trauma. The mechanism of formation of these pseudocysts is probably associated with pancreatic duct obstruction with subsequent increased intraductal pressure, ductal rupture, and extravasation of pancreatic juice into the surrounding soft tissues with autodigestion. The diagnosis is usually made by ultrasonography or a computed tomography (CT) scan (Fig. 1).

The clinical manifestations of pancreatic pseudocysts include upper abdominal pain, tenderness, jaundice, and in some cases an epigastric mass. Nausea and vomiting may occur. Rarely, pancreatic ascites or a pancreatic pleural effusion is present. The diagnosis of these complications is supported by demonstrating an albumin content greater than 3.0 gm/dl and an amylase content more than 1000 IU/ml. Octreotide, a somatostatin analogue, may be useful in reducing pancreatic secretion, thereby reducing the effusion.

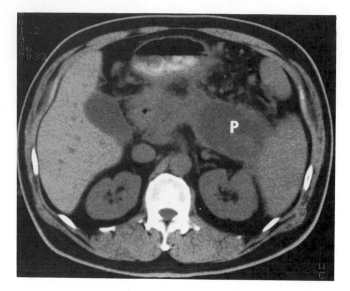

Figure 1. Computed tomography (CT) scan of a patient with a pseudocyst (P) in the body and tail of the pancreas that developed after an episode of acute pancreatitis. (From Sabiston DC Jr [ed]: Textbook of Surgery: The Biological Basis of Modern Surgical Practice, ed 14. Philadelphia, WB Saunders Company, 1991, p 1091, with permission.)

The management of pancreatic pseudocysts has previously been a choice between close observation and surgical drainage. More recently, other forms of less invasive therapy have been introduced. The current management is dependent upon several factors, including the symptoms, size of the pseudocyst, and the relative risks involved. Infection or hemorrhage can be life threatening, and such complications require urgent intervention. However, if the patient is asymptomatic, observation for a period of 6 to 8 weeks is appropriate to follow the size of the pseudocyst. It has been shown that many of these lesions spontaneously resolve in the first 6 weeks following discovery.

If the symptoms and the abdominal mass persist longer than 6 to 8 weeks, interventional therapy must be considered, especially if the mass is greater than 5 cm in diameter. The specific therapies include surgical or percutaneous procedures. Surgical options include external drainage, internal drainage, or resection. If external drainage is performed, a fistula between the pseudocyst and the abdominal wall follows and usually closes spontaneously. This approach is most frequently used when the cyst in infected or when the lining is not sufficiently developed for suturing for internal drainage. The preferred method of surgical management is internal drainage, suturing the wall of the pseudocyst to the stomach, duodenum, or jejunum. The most frequent procedure is cystogastrostomy, as the cyst is usually quite adherent to the posterior wall of the stomach and a cystogastrostomy

can be quite easily performed. If the location of the cyst is not appropriate for a cystogastrostomy, a cystoduodenostomy or a cystojejunostomy can be performed. These procedures are usually followed by collapse and ultimate disappearance of the pseudocyst (Fig. 2). For pseudocysts located in the tail of the pancreas, resection of the lesion is an option.

Advances in radiology have led to CT- or ultrasound-guided percutaneous drainage and is a much simpler procedure when feasible. While a single aspiration may effect a cure, failure rates are high with this approach (Table 1). However, if a catheter is placed into the cyst for *continuous* drainage, the failure rates range between 8 and 30 per cent, with an average complication rate of about 16 per cent. *Endoscopic* drainage has occasionally been performed creating a communication between the pseudocyst and the stomach or duodenum. However, experience

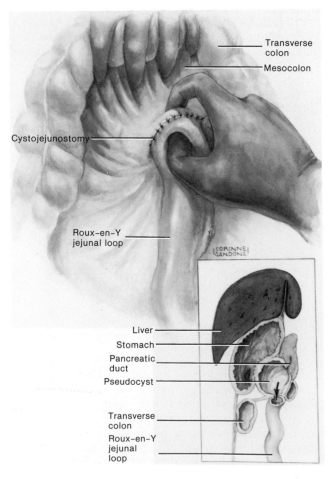

Figure 2. Illustration of internal drainage of a pancreatic pseudocyst by Roux-en-Y cystojejunostomy through the base of the transverse mesocolon. (From Cameron JL: Atlas of Surgery, vol 1. Toronto, BC Decker, 1990, p 379, with permission.)

TABLE 1.   COMPARISON OF SURGICAL MANAGEMENT WITH PERCUTANEOUS DRAINAGE OF PANCREATIC PSEUDOCYSTS*

| | Surgical Management | | Percutaneous | |
	Total	Internal Drainage	Single Drainage	Continuous Catheter
Recurrence or treatment failure[†]	9%	8%	63%	19%
Complications	35%	25%	0%	16%
Mortality	9%	6%	0%	2.6%

*Based on data reviewed by Gumaste and Ahearne.
[†]Treatment failure was defined as a pseudocyst not amenable to percutaneous drainage with or without the need for surgical therapy.

with this technique is limited. In some patients the administration of octreotide, an analog of secretin, may sufficiently decrease the pancreatic secretion to achieve symptomatic relief. Moreover, if a pancreatic pseudocyst has been drained percutaneously, the amount of drainage may be reduced by the administration of octreotide. In urgent situations such as hemorrhage, arterial embolization by radiologic catheterization can be effective. If this is not successful, open surgical control of the hemorrhage may be necessary.

Endoscopic retrograde cholangiopancreatography (ERCP) may be useful in delineating the anatomic as-

pects of the pancreatic duct. In a study of 102 patients, can algorithm that was applied retrospectively allocated treatment according to the ERCP-defined anatomy of the pancreatic duct. Patients with a normal pancreatic duct were more likely to have pseudocysts amenable to percutaneous drainage than those with a stricture of the duct or a communication between the duct and the pseudocyst. The study showed that such an algorithm may be the best predictor in the management of pancreatic pseudocysts.

An algorithm utilizing the basic principles is depicted in Figure 3. In nonelective or emergent cases, bleeding or infection is immediately treated, with sub-

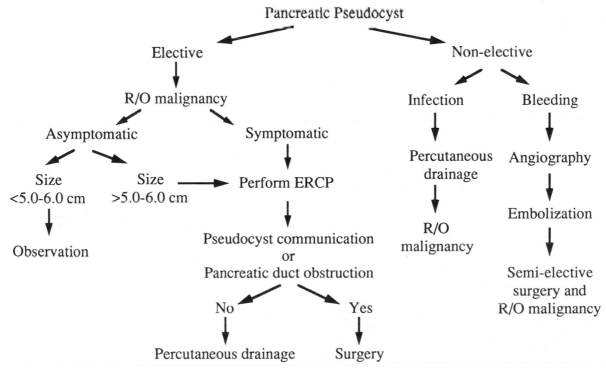

Figure 3.   Comprehensive pseudocyst treatment algorithm.

sequent therapy being determined by the underlying etiology. In patients who present electively, the first consideration is to determine whether the pseudocyst is due to a malignant process, and the next move is dependent upon the presence or absence of symptoms and the size of the pancreatic pseudocyst.

In summary, pancreatic pseudocysts represent a significant clinical problem and are usually the result of gallbladder disease, alcoholic pancreatitis, or blunt abdominal trauma. The diagnosis can usually be established without difficulty, and the current management depends upon the severity of symptoms and the size of the pseudocysts. Specific therapy includes percutaneous drainage, open drainage, or drainage of the cyst into the stomach, duodenum, or small intestine. The results are usually quite favorable.

REFERENCES

Ahearne PM, Baillie JM, Cotton PB, Baker ME, Meyers WC, Pappas TN: An endoscopic retrograde cholangiopancreatography (ERCP)-based algorithm for the management of pancreatic pseudocysts. Am J Surg *163*:111–116, 1992.

Bradley EL, Clements JL Jr, Gonzalez AC: The natural history of pancreatic pseudocysts: A unified concept of management. Am J Surg *137*:135–141, 1979.

D'egidio A, Schein M: Pancreatic pseudocysts: A proposed classification and its management implications. Br J Surg 78:981–984, 1991.

Gumaste VV, Dave PB: Editorial: Pancreatic pseudocyst drainage—the needle or the scalp? J Clin Gastroenterol *13*(5):500–505, 1991.

Yeo CJ, Bastidas JA, Lynch-Nyhan A, Fishman EK, Zinner MJ, Cameron JL: The natural history of pancreatic pseudocysts documented by computed tomography. Surg Gynecol Obstet *170*: 411–417, 1990.

36
THE SPLEEN

JAMES G. NORMAN, M.D.   LARRY C. CAREY, M.D.

ANATOMY

The spleen is situated in the left upper quadrant of the abdomen, where its position is maintained by suspensory ligaments attached to neighboring structures. With the fundus of the stomach medially, the splenic flexure of the colon inferiorly, the left kidney and adrenal gland posteriorly, and the diaphragm superiorly, the attachments provide protection and support for this organ. With the exception of the gastrosplenic ligament, which contains the short gastric vessels, the splenic ligaments are normally thin and avascular. In pathologic conditions such as portal hypertension, collateral vessels may develop in these attachments. Division of these thin ligaments allows the spleen to be mobilized medially and anteriorly quite easily. The arterial supply is via the splenic artery, a branch of the celiac trunk that follows a tortuous course along the superior edge of the pancreas to enter the splenic hilum on its most medial aspect (Fig. 1). The venous drainage is through the splenic vein, which leaves the hilum to course posterior to the pancreas, eventually joining the superior mesenteric vein to form the portal vein. The parenchyma of the spleen is divided into three distinct regions: *red pulp, white pulp,* and an interfacing *marginal zone.* The red pulp is made of large, branching, thin-walled vessels, the *splenic sinuses* or *sinusoids.* The white pulp consists of many small white zones scattered throughout the red pulp and contains lymphocytes, plasma cells, and macrophages, and resembles numerous small lymph nodes in structure and function. The marginal zone is the ill-defined vascular space that serves to connect the white pulp with the surrounding red pulp.

FUNCTION

The spleen has several major functions, including hematopoiesis in the fetus, the filtering of blood, and immune processing of blood-borne foreign antigens. The microcirculation of the spleen is ideally structured for its role in the management of the cellular components of circulating blood. The numerous types of leukocytes found in the white pulp provide an excellent setting for antigen processing. When the spleen is removed, some of these functions are lost. Despite its relatively small size, the spleen receives a large amount of blood flow, with a typical red blood cell passing through its sinusoids as many as 1000 times a day. These red blood cells may undergo repair by having surface abnormalities such as spurs and pits removed. Reticulocytes pass through the splenic sinusoids more slowly than mature red cells, probably because they are less pliable and do not conform to the walls of the sinusoids as well. This slow passage enables the spleen to remove the nuclear remnants and excess cell membrane found in these immature cells, an important step in the maturation of normal erythrocytes. Abnormal blood cells are also filtered and removed by the normally functioning spleen. Erythrocytes with abnormal architectures such as those found in spherocytosis and sickle-cell disease are trapped within the red pulp where they can be removed by free macrophages and other cells of the reticuloendothelial system. Aged red blood cells that have been circulating for approximately 120 days are removed from the circulation by this same process.

Although the spleen is a reservoir of red blood cells in many animals, it does not have this function in humans and contains only about 1 per cent of the total red cell mass. In contrast, the human spleen can har-

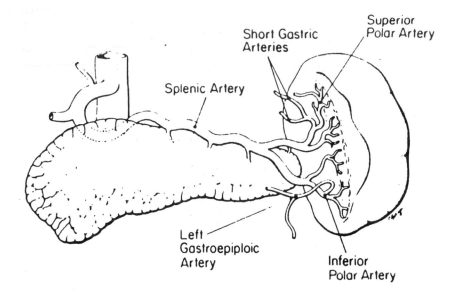

Short Gastric
Arteries

Superior
Polar Artery

Splenic Artery

Left
Gastroepiploic
Artery

Inferior
Polar Artery

Figure 1. Major branches of the splenic artery. These branches lie behind the tail of the pancreas. (From Perry JF: Anatomy of the spleen splenectomy, and excision of accessory spleens. *In* Nyhus LM, Baker RJ [eds]: Mastery of Surgery. Boston, Little, Brown & Co, 1984, p 824 with permission.)

bor as much as 30 per cent of the total circulating platelets, but is clinically significant in only a few pathologic conditions. Another important role of the spleen is its active participation in the specific and nonspecific immune responses. Macrophages and histiocytes within the spleen remove foreign cells and are especially effective in removing bacteria coated with antibody. The splenic white pulp provides an excellent environment for these captured foreign antigens to be processed, ultimately leading to the production of specific antibody, especially immunoglobulin M(IgM).

INDICATIONS FOR SPLENECTOMY

Despite the important and varied roles of the spleen, it is not essential for life, and the vast majority of those who have had their spleens removed function quite well. The indications for splenectomy have slowly changed with the improved understanding of immune anemia and the role of the spleen in many hematologic diseases. The most frequent indications for splenectomy now are *traumatic injury, immune thrombocytopenic purpura, hypersplenism, and hereditary sperocystosis.*

Trauma

The spleen is the most common organ injured secondary to blunt abdominal trauma, and is frequently injured in penetrating abdominal injuries. Splenic injury should be suspected in any patient with abdominal pain following blunt trauma, especially if the pain is in the left upper quadrant. Additionally, the spleen

must be considered the most likely source of hemorrhage in patients with hypotension after a blunt injury to the abdomen or left hemithorax. If a splenic injury is suspected, the patient must be admitted to the hospital for observation, and a careful history and physical examination is performed to determine if the mechanism and the symptoms are consistent with splenic damage. The usual injury is to the left upper abdomen or lower thorax associated with fractured ribs. If the patient is in shock and shows evidence of abdominal trauma and intra-abdominal bleeding, the diagnosis of splenic injury is best made at the time of abdominal exploration. In hemodynamically stable patients, the symptoms of splenic trauma are those of generalized and nonspecific abdominal pain, often more intense in the left upper quadrant. Occasionally, the pain may be referred to the top of the left shoulder (Kehr's sign) because of irritation of the left diaphragm, and this is a useful diagnostic symptom. It is rare to be able to palpate the injured spleen, but tenderness in the left upper quadrant is almost always present. The hemoglobin and hematocrit generally are decreased following splenic injury, and other factors contribute to the acute anemia such as concurrent injuries and the volume of intravenous fluids used for resuscitation. Isolated splenic trauma may be difficult to prove with physical examination and routine laboratory testing alone, and other studies are useful if the diagnosis is in question. If intra-abdominal bleeding is suspected, diagnostic peritoneal lavage is easily performed and is highly reliable. If blood is found within the peritoneal cavity, laparotomy is performed to diagnose and treat all bleeding organs, including the spleen. The computed tomography (CT) scan is a method of diagnosis of splenic trauma and is the diagnostic test of choice in children. An additional benefit of CT scanning is that it provides information about other abdominal organs. Treatment of splenic injuries has changed in recent years as the immunologic functions of the spleen have been clarified and the danger of serious bacterial infections in asplenic patients has been established. The emphasis has shifted from simple splenectomy to operations designed to retain all or as much of the spleen as possible. Whenever feasible, every effort is made to avoid removing the spleen, often requiring the use of several different techniques designed to preserve this soft and fragile organ. The avoidance of splenectomy for minor splenic injuries is most important in children, and nonoperative therapy has evolved as a relatively safe alternative, but requires hospitalization for as long as a week to observe continued or delayed bleeding. The surgeon must be aware of the possibility of concomitant intra-abdominal injuries that may go undetected in patients managed nonoperatively. Finally, the risks associated with blood transfusion are of major concern and must be judged against the relatively low risks associated with operation and the rare incidence of postsplenectomy infections.

Immune Thrombocytopenic Purpura

Immune thrombocytopenic purpura (ITP) is a hemorrhagic syndrome characterized by a persistently low platelet count and a shortened platelet lifespan and is currently the most frequent hematologic indication for splenectomy. The thrombocytopenia is caused by platelet destruction within the spleen. The thrombocytes become coated with a circulating antiplatelet factor, usually an immunoglobulin of the IgG subtype directed toward a platelet surface antigen making them susceptible to destruction. The decrease in platelets causes a prolonged bleeding time and poor clot retraction, but coagulation times remain normal. Because the problem lies with platelet destruction and not production, abundant megakaryocytes are seen in the bone marrow. The signs of ITP are bleeding and easy bruising. Bleeding is unlikely with platelet counts above 50,000. When platelet counts fall below 50,000/mm^3, bruising and excessive bleeding following minor trauma is common. With counts of 20,000/mm^3 or less, spontaneous bleeding with purpura, petechiae, epistaxis, menorrhagia, and gingival bleeding is common. At these very low platelet levels, life-threatening events such as intracranial hemorrhage become a concern. The diagnosis of ITP requires the exclusion of drug-induced antibodies formed against the cellular elements of blood as the cause of platelet destruction. Collagen vascular diseases such as systemic lupus erythematosus can mimic the symptoms of ITP, and the presence of these diseases must be in-

vestigated. The exclusion of all other diseases and conditions associated with thrombocytopenia is essential prior to a definitive diagnosis of ITP. The onset of symptoms may be acute or chronic, the acute form being more common in children. Overall, the chronic form is much more common and can be seen at any age; however, the vast majority occur in young women in their mid to late 30s. Typically, patients experience symptoms for several months prior to seeking medical advice. Immune thrombocytopenic purpura has recently been associated with the acquired immunodeficiency syndrome (AIDS) and in persons infected with the human immunodeficiency virus (HIV). This association has caused an increase in the incidence of ITP over the past several years and provides a challenge in management for these immunocompromised patients.

The treatment for ITP depends on the severity of symptoms, age of the patient, presence of underlying diseases, and general health. The goal of therapy is to achieve a sustained remission and eliminate the risks of significant hemorrhage. Patients with minimal symptoms often require no specific therapy and are advised to adjust their lifestyle to decrease exposure to minor trauma. Corticosteroid therapy is indicated in symptomatic patients, with most responding within 1 week. Despite this favorable response, only a minority of adults achieve complete remission with steroid therapy, and splenectomy produces the highest cure rate. It is indicated in patients who have failed to achieve a sustained remission on steroid therapy, require large or prolonged doses of steroids, or have a contraindication to the use of steroids. Sustained remission rates of 80 per cent can be expected after splenectomy and are more likely to occur in patients who have shown a response to steroids. Most achieve platelet counts over 100,000/mm^3 within the first several days following removal of the spleen, with 90 per cent sustaining normal platelet counts after 1 week. Occasionally, the platelet count rises to 1,000,000/mm^3 or higher, and an antiplatelet drug such as aspirin is indicated until the thrombocytosis resolves.

The childhood form of the disease often appears following a viral upper respiratory illness. Spontaneous remission without specific therapy is common and the need for splenectomy is rare. Because of the active lifestyle of children, they must be watched closely to prevent a small bump from becoming a life-threatening hemorrhage, especially during the first month of the illness when platelet counts are at their lowest.

Thrombotic Thrombocytopenic Purpura

Thrombotic thrombocytopenic purpura (TTP) is a syndrome of unknown etiology characterized by widespread deposition of platelet aggregates that lodge in the capillary beds of various organs. The pentad of clinical features includes fever, microangiopathic hemolytic anemia, fluctuating neurologic abnormalities, renal failure, and thrombocytopenia. The symptoms are caused by the ischemic damage produced as capillary beds are blocked by small platelet clots. Thrombotic thrombocytopenic purpura is quite rare and occurs much less frequently than ITP. Similar to ITP, however, TTP can be initiated by various stimuli such as drugs or serious infections and is associated with some of the collagen vascular diseases and, more recently, with AIDS and the HIV virus. The prognosis for patients with TTP is poor, with mortality as high as 90 per cent for untreated patients. Death usually follows renal failure or cerebral bleeding. Recently, combination treatment with plasmapheresis, fresh frozen plasma, steroids, and antiplatelet drugs such as aspirin allow a remission to be achieved in most patients. The role of splenectomy is poorly established, but seems warranted in patients who do not respond favorably to combined therapies or in whom relapse occurs. Removal of the spleen in a patient in this group is occasionally followed by a sudden and dramatic improvement.

Hypersplenism

A patient who has symptoms attributable to exaggerated activity of normal splenic function is said to have *hypersplenism*, usually manifested by a decrease in one or more of the cellular elements of blood as the hyperfunctioning spleen becomes the site of destruction of normal blood cells. Other essential components of the disease include a compensatory hyperplastic bone marrow and splenomegaly, but the diagnosis still is not proven until the patient shows improvement following removal of the enlarged spleen.

Hypersplenism is classified as *primary* when no underlying disease or pathologic process can be identified that could account for the splenic enlargement and hyperfunction. Most patients with primary hypersplenism are women. The symptoms at presentation depend on which cell line is depressed and include the fatigue and malaise associated with anemia, recurrent infections associated with leukopenia, and easy bruising and prolonged bleeding associated with thrombocytopenia. It is important to note that primary hypersplenism is a very rare condition and diagnosis can only be made after an extensive search for other causes. *Secondary* hypersplenism is a term given to overactivity of the spleen secondary to splenomegaly from a known cause. Portal venous hypertension associated with intrahepatic or extrahepatic obstruction to portal blood flow or obstruction of the splenic vein is the most common cause of venous engorgement of the spleen. About 60 per cent of patients with cirrhosis develop splenomegaly, but only a small number develop hypersplenism and even fewer ever require splenectomy. If a portacaval shunt is required for bleeding esophageal or gastric varices, the reduction in portal pressure is usually followed by a decrease in the passive splenomegaly and an improvement in the degree of hypersplenism. Common findings in venous hypertension associated with splenic vein thrombosis ("left-sided portal hypertension") are splenomegaly and hypersplenism in addition to esophageal and gastric varices. Patients with these symptoms can expect excellent relief following splenectomy, and this is the treatment of choice. Various other diseases or conditions are associated with splenomegaly and secondary hypersplenism (Table 1). Most are uncommon, and some are extremely rare.

The treatment of hypersplenism varies greatly with the nature of the underlying disease. When no etiology can be identified, the treatment for symptomatic patients with primary hypersplenism is splenectomy. Treatment of the inciting disease state may provide relief for some patients with secondary hypersplenism, such as in cases of malaria. In those with self-limited diseases such as infectious mononucleosis, resolution of the disease over a period of time causes normalization of the splenic dysfunction. Splenectomy is indicated in symptomatic patients resistant to medical therapies or in those for whom direct therapy is not available, such as the hemolytic anemias.

Hodgkin's Disease

Hodgkin's disease is a malignant lymphoma characterized by the presence of multinucleated giant cells known as *Reed-Sternberg cells*. The presence of these cells is important in the diagnosis. The disease has a bimodal incidence with a peak in the patient's mid 20s, decreasing until the mid 40s, and increasing slowly with age thereafter. Asymptomatic lymphadenopathy is the usual presenting symptom, with cervical adenopathy being most common, followed by axillary adenopathy, and then inguinal adenopathy. Constitutional symptoms such as fevers, night sweats, and weight loss are common and usually indicate widespread disease and a worse prognosis.

TABLE 1. ETIOLOGY OF SECONDARY HYPERSPLENISM

Congestive	Cirrhosis, portal hypertension, splenic vein thrombosis
Neoplastic	Lymphoma, leukemia, metastatic carcinoma
Infiltrative	Sarcoidosis, amyloidosis, Gaucher's disease
Inflammatory	Lupus erythematosus, Felty's syndrome
Infectious	Mononucleosis, tuberculosis, malaria
Chronic hemolytic diseases	Thalassemia, spherocytosis, G6PD deficiency
Myeloproliferative disorders	Myelofibrosis with myeloid metaplasia

Hodgkin's disease often involves more than one group of lymph nodes, allowing for a staging system based upon the sampling of lymph nodes to determine the extent of disease and providing the basis for some types of therapies. The concept of staging intra-abdominal organs and lymph node groups by laparotomy was introduced to determine the extent of the disease. This knowledge is important because localized disease is best treated with local irradiation, while diffuse disease is usually treated with systemic chemotherapy. In addition to staging the disease according to anatomic location and extent (Table 2), patients are classified as *A* (without) or *B* (with) constitutional symptoms, an important prognostic indicator. Staging laparotomy is used much less today than it was several years ago because of improved accuracy of CT scans in evaluating intrathoracic and intra-abdominal adenopathy. The procedure of staging laparotomy is an organized approach to sampling of representative tissues and consists of splenectomy, liver biopsy, and the removal of multiple abdominal and pelvic lymph nodes. Currently, this procedure is necessary in only a few patients for whom a significant chance exists that the stage of disease might be changed causing a change of therapy.

Non-Hodgkin's Lymphoma

Lymphomas of non-Hodgkin's variety are a group of malignancies originating in lymphoreticular tissue. Non-Hodgkin's lymphomas are more variable in their clinical course than Hodgkin's disease, and their behavior is much less predictable. Additionally, one fourth to one third of these patients have disease outside the lymphoreticular system, a characteristic that rarely accompanies Hodgkin's disease. Because the location of the primary site and the extent of disease are unpredictable and variable, the symptoms of non-Hodgkin's lymphoma differ widely, with constitutional symptoms of fever, anorexia, and weight loss most common. The incidence is greatest in the patient's mid 50s, with no preference to gender. As with Hodgkin's disease, the treatment of non-Hodgkin's lymphoma is radiation and chemotherapy. Staging

laparotomy is rarely indicated, as most patients have diffuse disease and constitutional symptoms at the time of diagnosis. Non-Hodgkin's lymphoma is often associated with splenomegaly, occasionally leading to secondary hypersplenism and pancytopenia, much less common in Hodgkin's disease. Splenectomy is indicated in those few patients who suffer from symptomatic hypersplenism, with the vast majority gaining a significant and rapid improvement in their pancytopenia.

Leukemias

The leukemias are a diverse group of malignancies originating within blood leukocytes, often involving the lymphatic system, the type being determined by the predominant cell type and degree of maturation. *Chronic lymphocytic leukemia* (CLL) occurs primarily in the elderly and is characterized by the accumulation of abnormal lymphocytes within the blood and lymphatic tissues, causing lymphadenopathy and splenomegaly. Therapy for CLL includes chemotherapy and occasionally radiation therapy, with splenectomy being reserved for patients with significant symptoms of secondary hypersplenism. *Chronic myeloid leukemia* (CML) is characterized by an abundance of myeloid cells in all stages of maturation present in the blood. The incidence of CML increases with age and is more common in men. Approximately 90 per cent of patients with CML have a characteristic chromosomal abnormality, the Philadelphia chromosome, which is associated with a more favorable prognosis. Splenomegaly is the most common physical finding, but generalized lymphadenopathy and hepatomegaly are also common. Splenectomy may be of benefit in some CML patients with secondary hypersplenism to relieve thrombocytopenia and anemia, but it does not influence the overall prognosis of the disease. *Hairy cell leukemia* (HCL) is an uncommon form of leukemia with characteristic mononuclear cells in the blood associated with pancytopenia and splenomegaly but rarely involving the lymph nodes. The malignant mononuclear cells of HCL have irregular, filamentous projections of their cell surface that gives them a hairy appearance on light microscopy and are thought to be a cause of the splenomegaly, as these irregular cells get caught within the splenic sinusoids. Often, the initial complaint is abdominal fullness associated with the large spleen in addition to nonspecific complaints related to the associated anemias. Splenectomy is indicated in HCL as in the other leukemias when the symptoms of secondary hypersplenism become uncontrollable. Additionally, splenic infarctions occur in these patients due to the blockage of the sinusoids by the hairy cells and may be an indication for splenectomy for relief of pain. New chemotherapeutic agents

TABLE 2. ANN ARBOR STAGING FOR
HODGKIN'S DISEASE

Stage	Definition
0	No detectable disease following excisional biopsy
I	Single node or nodal group
II	Two nodal groups on the same side of the diaphragm
III	Two nodal groups on different sides of the diaphragm
IV	Disease spread to organs other than lymph nodes or spleen (liver, skin, gastrointestinal tract, lungs, central nervous system)

have made the need for splenectomy nearly obsolete in HCL.

SPLENECTOMY FOR ANEMIA

Anemia resulting from increased destruction of red blood cells is termed *hemolytic anemia*. The numerous causes for this abnormal destruction are either genetic, which are due to a structural abnormality within the erythrocyte itself, or acquired, in which normal red cells are destroyed. The acquired disease is more common in a mild form that is often undetected and requires no therapy. The severe forms of hemolytic anemias are usually hereditary in nature, with the initial complaints associated with the degree of anemia causing variable levels of fatigue and pallor and the enlarged spleen often causing abdominal discomfort. Metabolism of hemoglobin, the major product of red cell destruction, may cause jaundice as serum levels rise. In addition, the frequency of gallstones increases due to the excess hemoglobin breakdown. It is important to obtain a detailed family history from these patients to determine the possibility of an inherited disorder and to identify other family members who are at risk. A careful search for inciting medications or a history of a recent illness is also important to separate those hemolytic anemias that are acquired in nature. The laboratory findings are similar in most hemolytic anemias, with reticulocytosis (> 10 per cent), elevation of indirect (free) bilirubin, and hyperplasia of the bone marrow.

Hereditary Spherocytosis

Hereditary spherocytosis is the most common form of congenital hemolytic anemia. The red cell defect is located within the cell membrane where spectrin, the most important structural protein, is deficient, causing the cells to be smaller, more dense, and round. These characteristics make the cells less pliable and more fragile, leading to their destruction, as they have difficulty traversing the splenic sinusoids. The red cell's lack of deformability leads to slowing of transit through the spleen, and this delay leads to a decrease in glucose available to the red cell, making its abnormal membranes more vulnerable to destruction by the reticuloendothelial system. Although the disease is transmitted in an autosomal dominant manner, at least 20 per cent of cases occur sporadically. The severity of symptoms are variable depending on the degree of red cell destruction. Jaundice due to hemolysis is common, and gallstones are to be expected with longstanding disease. Nearly all patients with hereditary spherocytosis should undergo splenectomy, but it

is preferable to wait until at least 6 years of age. The destruction of red cells is alleviated following splenectomy, with red cell survival returning to normal. Because the intrinsic defect within the cell membrane is not corrected, however, the cells remain as spherocytes on peripheral smears for the remainder of the patient's life.

Hereditary Elliptocytosis

Hereditary elliptocytosis is a disorder of the red cell membrane causing the cells to maintain an elliptical shape instead of the usual biconcave disk. The cells tend to be somewhat more deformable and less fragile than those associated with hereditary spherocytosis and thus traverse the splenic sinusoids with less difficulty. The hemolytic anemia is usually mild, and most patients are asymptomatic. Splenectomy is indicated in those with symptomatic anemia, after which the normal red cell survival returns to normal.

Hereditary Nonspherocytic Hemolytic Anemia

The red blood cell is vulnerable to increased destruction by the reticuloendothelial system from hereditary deficiencies associated with enzyme abnormalities within the cytoplasm as well as structural abnormalities within the cell membrane. Pyruvate kinase (PK) deficiency, the most common of these enzyme deficiencies, causes decreased adenosine triphosphate (ATP) generation, with subsequent cell membrane injury. The damaged cell is destroyed as it passes through the spleen, leading to a typical hemolytic anemia. Splenectomy produces symptomatic improvement, but the damaged cells still have a shortened lifespan and the anemia persists, although it is less severe. Splenectomy is not indicated for all of the hereditary enzymatic deficiencies present in red blood cells. A good example is glucose-6-phosphate dehydrogenase (G6PD) deficiency in which red cell destruction takes place outside of the spleen. Hemolysis is initiated by acute illnesses and infections as well as ingestion of fava beans, causing lysis of the energy-deficient cells, and is not affected by splenectomy.

Thalassemia

The *thalassemias* are a group of hereditary anemias caused by a defect in hemoglobin synthesis in which an insufficient amount of one of the two hemoglobin polypeptides is produced. The α, β, δ, or γ chain may be lacking, depending on which gene is defective. β-Thalassemia has an insufficient quantity of the β hemoglobin peptide chain and is the most common of the thalassemias. Thalassemias are further divided into major and minor categories according to the presence of homozygous or heterozygous genetic defects, respectively. When one of the hemoglobin peptide chains is produced in insufficient amounts, the normal chain is overproduced, leading to precipitation within the red cell cytoplasm and premature cell death.

Thalassemia major causes a severe anemia usually obvious within the first year of life. Patients require frequent blood transfusions because of the inability of the bone marrow to keep pace with red cell destruction. Hepatosplenomegaly and gallstones are common. Thalassemia minor, however, is associated with a mild anemia, and most patients are asymptomatic. Splenectomy is indicated for the relief of the discomfort associated with massive splenomegaly in some patients with thalassemia major. Iron chelation is the mainstay of treatment to delay or prevent the systemic effects of iron overload caused by the extensive turnover of hemoglobin peptides.

Autoimmune Hemolytic Anemia

Autoimmune hemolytic anemia (AIHA) is an acquired hemolytic anemia in which antibodies are formed against antigens present on the red cell surface. The symptoms are typical of the hemolytic anemias discussed earlier and include fatigue and a mild to moderate degree of splenomegaly. The presence of antibodies coating the surface of otherwise normal erythrocytes produces a positive direct Coombs' test and helps distinguish this type of hemolytic anemia from all others. Many times, the inciting event can be linked to the presence of drugs such as penicillin, streptomycin, methyldopa (Aldomet), and quinidine. Autoimmune hemolytic anemia can also occur following, or in association with, other acute or chronic diseases such as leukemia, lymphoma, lupus erythematosus, mycoplasma pneumonia, infectious mononucleosis, and AIDS. Similar to the autoimmune destruction of platelets seen with ITP, the destruction of red cells in AIHA can be slowed or stopped with steroid therapy. Splenectomy is reserved for those patients who fail to respond to steroids or require prolonged high doses of steroids. The response rates expected following removal of the spleen are good, with up to 80 per cent of properly selected patients achieving normal red cell survival.

Cysts and Tumors of the Spleen

Tumors of the spleen are rare, but must be considered in patients with an enlarged spleen or an unidentified left upper quadrant mass. Most primary cancers are of blood vessel origin, such as the angiosarcoma, which is rare. Lymphoma may also originate in the

spleen as discussed in previous sections. Despite its role as a filter, the spleen is rarely the site of metastatic cancer. Interestingly, the splenic capsule is frequently the site of metastases in patients with diffuse intraperitoneal gastrointestinal cancer, yet the splenic pulp very rarely is involved.

Splenic cysts may be parasitic or nonparasitic, and the parasitic variety are most often echinococcal. The hydatid disease associated with echinococcal cysts is endemic to South America and parts of Australia and Europe, but is quite uncommon in the United States. Nonparasitic cysts are much more common in North America. As the cysts found elsewhere, those of the spleen that are nonparasitic are classified as true cysts when they contain a true epithelial lining, or pseudocysts when they do not. Pseudocysts are found much more frequently than true cysts and are usually the result of splenic infarctions and hematomas. The symptoms of all types of splenic cysts are similar, with vague left upper quadrant pain predominating due to associated splenomegaly and compression of adjacent abdominal viscera. Once the etiology of these cysts has been determined by various radiologic studies, the treatment is usually internal surgical drainage. Total splenectomy is indicated for most large cysts and those of undetermined etiology.

OPERATIONS ON THE SPLEEN

Preoperative Preparation

Once the decision to remove the spleen has been made, certain steps are taken preoperatively to reduce the possibility of both early and late complications. Central to this preparation is ensuring the availability of sufficient and appropriate blood products for replacement. Frequently, the spleen is extremely large, making the vascular pedicle difficult to control and increasing the possibility of significant blood loss. Additionally, the splenomegaly itself is usually associated with some type of blood component deficiency such as anemia or thrombocytopenia. These deficiencies should be strongly considered and sufficient intravenous access ensured to permit quick transfusions. Polyvalent pneumococcal vaccine should be administered prior to splenectomy.

Removal of the Spleen

The spleen can be removed by one of two techniques, depending on the indication and the size. For the normal sized spleen, the dissection is begun by detaching it from its surrounding and supporting organs by incising the splenic ligaments, allowing the spleen to be mobilized medially and anteriorly on its pedicle into the wound where it is easy to see and manipulate. This technique is especially helpful in the injured spleen, where repair may be attempted rather than removal (Fig. 2) and allows clear visualization of the tail of the pancreas. In splenectomy, the vascular structures within the splenic pedicle are isolated and ligated individually, allowing the organ to be removed. With a massively enlarged spleen, it is often easier and safer to isolate the splenic artery and vein prior to its mobilization, accomplished by entering the lesser peritoneal sac and ligating the splenic vessels as they course along the superior edge of the pancreas. By obtaining control of most of the blood supply to the enlarged spleen prior to its mobilization, the risk of uncontrolled hemorrhage is greatly reduced, thus permitting a more careful and deliberate isolation of the individual vessels within the splenic hilum, which can be technically difficult if the spleen is massively enlarged.

Postsplenectomy Sepsis and Other Complications

Complications following splenectomy include atelectasis, especially involving the left lower lobe. Pancreatitis and subphrenic abscess also occur after the removal of the spleen, but occur much less often. Postsplenectomy thrombocytosis is a frequent event and should be expected in all patients following splenectomy. Specific therapy including antiplatelet drugs such as aspirin is usually not warranted if platelet counts are below $1,000,000/mm^3$. A syndrome of rapidly progressive sepsis has been recognized for many years. This complication continues to be a concern for all asplenic patients, usually occurring within 3 years following removal of the spleen but, at times, occurring as many as 10 or 12 years later. Children are more susceptible to this problem than adults, with the incidence declining sharply beyond the early teenage years. The overall incidence is quite rare, with only about 1 per cent of asplenic children developing severe infection, most being young when the spleen is removed and undergoing splenectomy because of a reticuloendothelial disease. Postsplenectomy sepsis often begins insidiously with fever and signs of an upper respiratory infection. There is a rapidly progressive septic course with death in 24 to 48 hours in 50 per cent of patients. *Streptococcus pneumoniae* occurs in approximately half of patients, with *Haemophilus* and *Meningococcus* species, also common pathogens. The awareness of this rare but lethal complication has led to aggressive attempts at splenic repair following trauma.

All physicians should consider the possibility of sepsis in any patients who become ill with a history of splenectomy. Prophylaxis against pneumococcal sepsis can be accomplished by pneumococcal vaccine, although it does not impart immunity to all strains of this organism. Therefore, even vaccinated patients may develop overwhelming sepsis due to the pneumococcus, albeit at a significantly decreased rate. Immunization against *Haemophilus* organisms has recently become available and is recommended in all children. Vaccinated patients may develop a fatal infection with a number of *other* organisms for which vaccines are not available.

The risk of overwhelming postsplenectomy sepsis is less following splenectomy for *trauma* than for *hematologic disorders*. The reason for this is unknown but is probably related to an underlying defect in immune processing in patients who require splenectomy for hematologic diseases. Since splenic processing of blood-borne antigens seems to play an important role for these particular organisms, it has been recommended that the pneumococcal vaccine be given prior to splenectomy whenever possible. When splenectomy is performed for trauma, vaccination immediately postoperatively is recommended.

A 2- or 3-year course of prophylactic antibiotics is usually given to young children following splenectomy to guard against *H. influenzae* as well as pneumococcus during this very vulnerable period. To decrease the incidence of this fulminant infection, splenectomy in children should be delayed until at least age 4 unless the hematologic disease is unusually severe and requires urgent treatment.

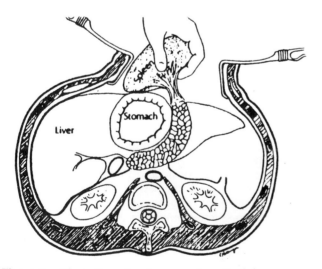

Figure 2. Blunt dissection between the tail of the pancreas and the left kidney allows the spleen to be elevated anteriorly and the posterior aspect of the splenic hilus to be exposed. (From Perry JF: Anatomy of the spleen, splenectomy, and excision of accessory spleens. *In* Nyhus LM, Baker RJ [eds]: Mastery of Surgery. Boston, Little, Brown & Co, 1984, p 826 with permission.)

REFERENCES

Akwari OE, Itani KMF, Coleman RE, Rosse WF: Splenectomy for primary and recurrent immune thrombocytopenia purpura (ITP). Ann Surg *206*:529–541, 1987.

Lucas CE: Splenic trauma. Ann Surg *213*:98–112, 1991.

Moormeir JA, Williams SF, Golomb HM: The staging of Hodgkin's Disease. Hematol Oncol Clin North Am 3:237–251, 1989.

Vevon PA, Ellison EC, Carey LC: Splenectomy for hematologic disease. Adv Surg *22*:105–140, 1989.

Wilhelm MC, Jones RE, McGhee R, Mitchner JS, Sandusky WR, Hess CE: Splenectomy in hematologic disorders. Ann Surg *207*(5): 581–589, 1988.

37

HERNIAS

DAVID C. SABISTON, Jr., M.D.

HISTORIC ASPECTS

Hernias were described in the earliest medical writings, but only in the last century have the anatomic variations been understood and appreciated. Surgeons then devised operative procedures to correct these anatomic defects and to prevent their recurrence. A century ago, recurrence rates within a year of surgical operation for hernias was 30 to 40 per cent. In 1889, Bassini was the first to describe an anatomically appropriate surgical correction for inguinal hernias. Soon thereafter, Halsted independently described a quite similar procedure. These two surgical pioneers are due much credit for their careful anatomic dissections and descriptions of the basic pathologic features of the musculofascial defects in the inguinal region.

Most *hernias* are caused by defects in the *fascial* tissues of the abdominal wall. These defects allow the peritoneum by intra-abdominal pressure to penetrate to the subcutaneous tissue of the abdominal wall. A hernial *sac* of peritoneum is the result with the subcutaneous fatty tissue beneath the skin. In many instances, the hernial sac contains viscera, particularly the small intestine. The *neck* of the hernial sac is frequently smaller in diameter than the hernial sac, and this may present a problem in reduction of the hernia into the peritoneal cavity. The appropriate treatment for the vast majority of hernias is *surgical* correction to prevent serious, even fatal, complications.

By far the commonest of the hernias of the abdominal wall are those which occur in the inguinal region, accounting for some 75 per cent of the total. *Ventral* hernias are those that involve the abdominal wall except for those in the inguinal region and include *epigastric* and *incisional* hernias that occur through pre-

vious abdominal incisions and have not healed completely.

Most hernias are reducible, meaning that their contents can be replaced by appropriate manipulation into the peritoneal cavity. When a hernia is not reducible, it is termed *incarcerated*. While this state is not necessarily a clinical problem, since it is not associated with intestinal ischemia or gangrene of the hernial contents, nevertheless, it is a reason for more urgent surgical correction. If intestinal ischemia or gangrene develop, the incarcerated hernia is considered *strangulated*, and an emergency operation to reduce the hernia and correct the defect is mandatory. Because a strangulated hernia is usually one in which bowel and adjoining mesentery become edematous from the increase in the venous pressure, interstitial edema follows with further increase in interstitial pressure that ultimately impedes arterial inflow with ensuing ischemia and gangrene. As the hernial sac and its contents are at that time considerably enlarged, an *incarcerated* hernia can seldom be reduced through the neck of the sac because the latter is generally smaller in diameter than the hernia itself. Under very rare circumstances, a strangulated hernia can be reduced, but this is quite uncommon. For this reason, if a hernia is found to be incarcerated, all appropriate attempts are usually made to reduce the hernia to prevent an emergency operation.

ANATOMIC ASPECTS

Because the surgical correction of hernias depends on a full understanding of the anatomic aspects of hernial defects, this aspect is of great importance in the pathogenesis of hernias. The general principles of surgical correction consist primarily of careful dissection of the hernial sac with closure at its neck and excision of the excess sac. This is followed by careful assessment of the tissues surrounding the hernial defect and mobilization of the *fascial* structures, primarily the fascia of the rectus abdominis and external oblique muscles (conjoined tendon), and suturing these strong tissues to either the inguinal ligament or to Cooper's ligament. Particular care is taken to avoid approximation of muscle to these ligaments, since muscle does not hold sutures well and a recurrence of the hernia is apt to occur.

INGUINAL HERNIAS

Three quarters of all hernias occur in the inguinal region. Most are indirect hernias of congenital origin and occur as a failure of obliteration of the processus vaginalis as it descends through the abdominal wall into the scrotum in embryologic life. If the sac passes into the inguinal canal and extends into the scrotum, it is termed a *complete* hernia. The differentiation of a *direct* versus *indirect* hernia is an *anatomic* one and depends on the relationship of the hernia defect to the deep epigastric artery. With indirect hernias, the defect is lateral to the deep epigastric artery, and in direct hernias, this vessel lies medially. While it is very difficult to be certain preoperatively by clinical examination whether a hernia is indirect or direct, the physical findings usually make it possible to draw an appropriate conclusion. The final classification is made at operation.

The *clinical* diagnosis of an inguinal hernia is made by the presence of a bulge in the inguinal region or an actual mass that descends into the inguinal region or into the scrotum. By inversion of the scrotal skin into the inguinal canal, the defect can usually be palpated in the abdominal wall. As the hernial sac protrudes against the examining finger, it is accentuated when the patient coughs. Inguinal hernias are much more common in males than in females and more often occur on the right rather than the left side. Etiologic factors include congenital failure of closure of the internal ring embryologically as well as a variety of factors that cause increased intra-abdominal pressure, predisposing to the development of a hernia. These include chronic cough, pregnancy, ascites, and intra-abdominal masses. One of the most common presenting features is a history of an episode of heavy straining as during lifting of heavy objects that is followed by the feeling of weakness or a mass in the groin. As the hernia enlarges, patients are apt to complain of a heaviness in the groin and of a dull pain that is relieved in the reclining position or following manual reduction of the hernia. If the hernia descends into the scrotum, it is more likely to be an indirect hernia. Inguinal hernias can at times be confused with enlarged inguinal lymph nodes, a femoral hernia, varicocele, a benign tumor, or a hematoma.

The therapy of inguinal hernias is straightforward in most patients because spontaneous cures do not occur. Therefore, surgical correction is nearly always indicated unless some severe underlying coexisting serious medical disorder precludes therapy. Formerly, many patients were advised to wear a truss, but such advice is rarely given today. Inguinal herniorraphy is a straightforward procedure attended by few complications and excellent results. The correction of inguinal hernia is usually done by approximation of the fascial structures of the rectus abdominis and internal oblique muscles (conjoined tendon) to the inguinal ligament. For femoral and some large indirect hernias, this fascia is sutured to Cooper's ligament. The results are excellent, and the recurrence rate is generally less than 5 per cent.

The majority of patients are able to successfully reduce their own hernias. However, should a hernia become incarcerated and the patient unable to reduce it, the physician is often able to accomplish it with special maneuvers. Reduction is indicated because if the hernia can be reduced, the surgical procedure can then be done electively *rather than emergently.* To reduce an incarcerated hernia, gentle pressure is applied overlying the hernia directing it toward the neck of the sac to reduce it into the peritoneal cavity. Lowering the head (Trendelenburg position) is helpful while pressure is constantly applied to the incarcerated hernia. The administration of analgesic agents to relieve discomfort is also advisable. With persistent pressure over a period of 5 to 10 minutes or longer, hernias can usually be successfully reduced. It is important to avoid excessively forceful pressure, as it is possible on very rare occasions to reduce a strangulated hernia. If this is thought to be a possibility, the patient should be closely monitored. If peritoneal signs develop, an emergency operation is indicated. Otherwise, the patient can be electively scheduled for correction of the hernia. The reason that a strangulated hernia can rarely be reduced is the marked edema of the contents and the difficulty in reducing such a swollen mass through the small neck of the sac. A correction of an inguinal hernia is depicted in Figure 1. *Bilateral* inguinal hernias, both direct and indirect, are often present simultaneously. If quite large, they may be separately corrected. However, the majority can be corrected simultaneously with a good clinical result.

An alternate technique for correction of inguinal hernias is by the laparoscopic method, for which only small incisions in the abdominal wall are necessary. A piece of prosthetic material is placed over the defect and sutured to the abdominal wall. This approach causes less postoperative discomfort, but long-term

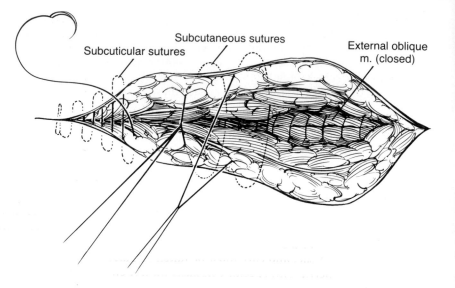

Figure 1. A correction of an inguinal hernia. (From Sabiston DC Jr [ed]: Atlas of General Surgery. Philadelphia, WB Saunders Company [in press], with permission.)

postoperation data for the laparoscopic approach are not yet available.

POSTOPERATIVE COMPLICATIONS

Significant postoperative complications following inguinal herniorraphy are uncommon. Wound infections may occur (< 2 per cent) as well as hematomas (< 1 per cent). Scrotal swelling, testicular atrophy, and postoperative hydroceles occur rarely. Scrotal bleeding may occur and require reoperation for control. Urinary retention may be a problem requiring catheterization and is occasionally followed by a urinary tract infection requiring antibiotics.

FEMORAL HERNIAS

Femoral hernias occur in the groin and are bounded by the femoral vein laterally and the lacunar ligament medially. These hernias are more apt to present with incarceration (~ 25 per cent) and are more common in males than in females.

A diagnosis of a femoral hernia is made by the presence of a mass, often tender, in the femoral triangle. A cystogram may demonstrate part of the urinary bladder filling the hernial sac. Appropriate *therapy* is surgical by the McVay technique. It is important to understand that suturing these structures to the *inguinal* ligament fails to correct hernial defect, and Cooper's ligament must be utilized.

UMBILICAL HERNIAS

Umbilical hernias are usually *congenital* in origin and are present at birth. Nearly all of these hernias close spontaneously for reasons that are poorly understood but well recognized. Therefore, it is only rarely necessary to surgically correct congenital umbilical defects except in the very rare incidences when they become incarcerated in childhood. Therefore, most advise that umbilical hernias be observed in this age group until the child is 4 years of age. Acquired umbilical hernias may occur in women following pregnancy. These should be surgically corrected, as they do not close spontaneously. Another factor that causes development of umbilical hernias is an increase in abdominal pressure due to ascites, abdominal masses, or obesity. In adults, surgical correction by direct approximation of the edges of the hernial defect is usually curative, and recurrence is quite unusual.

INCISIONAL HERNIA (VENTRAL HERNIA)

Incisional or ventral hernias generally are the result of previous incisions that have healed poorly or those that have undergone considerable strain. While most of these hernias are small, nevertheless, they can be quite extensive, particularly if caused by a postoperative wound infection in the incision. Most patients complain of a dull ache, and these hernias frequently become incarcerated. Surgical management is generally recommended, and closure is usually straightforward. However, in very large defects, it may be necessary to intensively mobilize the adjoining fascia or use prosthetic material in order to adequately close them.

SLIDING INGUINAL HERNIAS

Sliding inguinal hernias are a special anatomic group in which the neck of the hernial sac is formed both by peritoneum and by a segment of bowel or the urinary bladder. In order for this somewhat complex anatomic variation to be fully appreciated, it is best understood by careful observation at the time of operation. For sliding hernias on the *right* side, the cecum usually forms a part of the sac, while on the *left* side the sigmoid colon forms a portion of the hernial sac. The presence of a sliding hernia is clearly defined on opening of the sac, and care must be taken to place the sutures properly, with special emphasis on not entering the bowel or the urinary bladder.

Epigastric Hernias

Epigastric hernias occur in the linea alba between the xiphoid process and the umbilicus. Generally, these are quite small defects, usually less than 1 cm in diameter. They usually contain preperitoneal fat, which may become quite tender and cause the patient discomfort and anxiety. If the defect is 1 cm or more in diameter or if it is smaller and quite symptomatic, surgical correction is recommended. The defect is closed by dissection of the ring and direct closure.

RICHTER'S HERNIA

Richter's hernia is a special type of hernia in which only a portion of the circumference of the bowel is involved, usually the antimesenteric border. These hernias can be quite serious because, if not promptly treated, ischemia of the herniated portion of the bowel is apt to occur, with the development of gangrene and perforation. Some 15 per cent of incarcerated hernias are of the Richter's type, most occurring in femoral hernias, and operation is indicated.

LITTRE'S HERNIA

Occasionally, a Meckel's diverticulum occurs in a hernial sac, and this is defined as a *Littre's* hernia. Most of these are in the inguinal and femoral regions and are apt to become incarcerated. Because the signs and symptoms are not significantly different from other hernias in these locations, the diagnosis is established at the time of operation.

SPIGELIAN HERNIA

Within the abdominal cavity, the *semilunar* line is the anatomic site at which the transversus abdominis muscle becomes an aponeurosis. This line curves outward and extends from the midportion of the costal margin to the pubic tubercle. The line is located lateral to the lateral edge of the rectus abdominis muscle, and the area between the semilunar line and the lateral edge of the rectus abdominis is termed the spigelian fascia. A hernia through this fascia is a *spigelian* hernia. With this defect, patients, many of whom are obese, often complain of pain in the region as well as a mass. A definitive diagnosis can be established by a computed tomography (CT) scan that delineates the defect in the abdominal wall. The sac of these hernias often includes omentum and intestine. They should be closed by direct suture.

OBTURATOR HERNIA

When a hernial sac appears in the pelvis in the obturator canal, it exits the abdominal cavity at the site of the obturator vessels and nerve and penetrates the obturator membrane through the obturator foramen. When symptoms appear, they usually consist of nausea, vomiting, and abdominal pain of the type characteristic of intestinal obstruction. A helpful sign is pain along the course of the obturator nerve that provides the sensory innervation to the upper and medial portion of the thigh. Pain referred along this nerve is called the Howship-Romberg sign. These hernias may also be diagnosed by CT scan. Many are incarcerated or strangulated at the time of operation, and the patients require careful preparation prior to emergency surgery.

LUMBAR (DORSAL) HERNIA

Hernias occasionally occur in the flank and are termed *lumbar* or *dorsal* hernias. They are seen in the superior (Grynfeltt's) and inferior (Petit's) triangles. A mass located in either of these sites may be associated with discomfort and tenderness. Generally, these hernias are reducible, but may become incarcerated. The differential diagnosis includes lipomas, fibromas, hematomas, and herniated muscle. A definite defect can often be established by CT scan.

PERINEAL HERNIA

The muscles in the perineal floor occasionally are the site of a hernia. Uncommonly, it may be primary, but secondary perineal hernias follow surgical procedures such as prostatectomy, abdominoperineal resection, and other pelvic operations. Correction is achieved by combined abdominoperineal approach with closure of the fascia.

SCIATIC HERNIA

A hernia through the *greater sciatic foramen* occurs rarely and is seldom symptomatic until incarcerated. An abdominal approach is used for correction with or without the necessity to remove ischemic bowel. The defect is closed by direct suture.

PERISTOMAL HERNIA

When a colostomy or ileostomy is created, a *peristomal hernia* may later develop at the site where the bowel passes through the abdominal wall. Prevention is the most important feature of these hernias, but when they occur, they may require surgical correction. Primary indications for herniorraphy include the presence of a large protruding mass, especially if the fascial defect is a small one or if incarceration or strangulation are present and require operation. Occasionally a patient requests correction for cosmetic reasons.

REFERENCES

Andrews NJ: Presentation and outcome of strangulated external hernia in a district general hospital. Br J Surg 68:329, 1981.

Condon RE, Nyhus LM: Complications of groin hernia and hernial repair. Surg Clin North Am 51:1325, 1971.

McVay CB: Surgical Anatomy, ed 6. Philadelphia, WB Saunders Company, 1984.

Nyhus LM, Condon RE (eds): Hernia, ed 3. Philadelphia, JB Lippincott Company, 1989.

Wantz GE: Complications of inguinal hernia repair. Surg Clin North Am 64(2):287, 1984.

38
PEDIATRIC SURGERY

SAMUEL M. MAHAFFEY, M.D.

Many common general surgical problems are seen in the pediatric age group, but pediatric surgery is much more than just general surgery for children. Abnormal embryogenesis, unique physiologic response patterns of the preterm and term infant, size considerations, and possible sequelae of therapeutic interventions on long-term growth and development all present major intellectual challenges to the satisfactory surgical management of this patient population. From the pioneering efforts of Ladd and Gross earlier this century, the realm of pediatric surgery has grown to include the correction of complex congenital anomalies, innovative management of trauma, treatment of malignant neoplasms, solid-organ transplantation, extracorporeal life support techniques, and fetal surgery. Much of the success achieved in dealing with these problems is the result of improved techniques of supportive care. Specialized intensive care units, downsizing of medical devices, development of pressure-controlled assisted ventilation, improved anesthesia care and monitoring techniques, improved prenatal diagnosis and obstetric care, and development of parenteral hyperalimentation for nutritional support are just a few of the factors contributing to substantially improved outcome for disease entities that formerly carried high morbidity and mortality. This chapter is devoted to developmental abnormalities, physiology, and disease processes unique to infants and children.

THE SURGICAL NEWBORN

Physiology

Cardiovascular

During intrauterine life, minimal blood flow is required to the unaerated lungs. Pulmonary vascular resistance is high, causing higher pressures in the right side of the heart and pulmonary artery compared to the left side of the heart. Therefore, oxygenated blood returning from the placenta through the ductus venosus enters the right atrium, is shunted through the foramen ovale to the left atrium, and is then circulated systemically. Oxygenated blood ejected from the right ventricle flows from the pulmonary artery into the aorta through the ductus arteriosus, also the result of suprasystemic pressure in the pulmonary artery. Two major cardiovascular events are associated with birth: (1) the low-resistance placenta is removed from the systemic circuit, causing increased systemic arterial pressure; and (2) with the baby's first breath, lung expansion produces decreased pulmonary vascular resistance. Pressures in the right heart and pulmonary artery fall below systemic pressures, and the foramen ovale functionally closes. With exposure to increased oxygen tension, the ductus arteriosus constricts and is usually obliterated within 24 hours. These changes produce an adult circulatory pattern: unoxygenated blood returns from the body to be circulated through the right heart to the lungs for gas exchange, then returns to the left heart for circulation throughout the body.

A number of pathologic processes, including pulmonary hypoplasia, aspiration of meconium, and sepsis can cause persistence of the fetal circulatory pattern, known as *persistent fetal circulation* (PFC) or *persistent pulmonary hypertension of the newborn* (PPHN). Increased pulmonary vascular resistance and suprasystemic pressure causes unoxygenated blood returning to the right heart to be shunted across the foramen ovale or through the patent ductus arteriosus, causing systemic arterial desaturation, decreased oxygen delivery to the tissues, progressive metabolic acidosis, and ultimately cellular failure and death. The mediators of the pulmonary vasomotor response are not well understood. However, animal studies have demonstrated increased pulmonary vascular resistance due to acidosis, hypercarbia, and hypoxia. Therefore, alkalinization, hyperventilation, and maintenance of satisfactory arterial oxygen saturation are the mainstays of treatment. Pharmacologic interventions, including vasodilators such as tolazoline and Thorazine are limited by the nonselectivity of the vasodilator response, which often causes systemic hypotension. Neonatal cardiovascular responses differ from the adult in other aspects. In particular, the neonate has limited ability to increase stroke volume. Therefore, when increased oxygen demand requires an increase in cardiac output, this is usually accomplished by an increase in heart rate.

Respiratory

Pulmonary maturation is incomplete at the time of birth. New pulmonary units (terminal bronchioles and alveoli) are added until 8 years of age. The more immature the infant, the fewer the number of pulmonary units present. In particular, the premature infant has fewer type II pneumocytes, causing insufficient synthesis of pulmonary surfactant, which predisposes the premature infant to alveolar collapse, hyaline membrane formation, and insufficient pulmonary gas exchange. High ventilatory pressures and oxygen concentration required for satisfactory gas exchange may cause injury to the pulmonary parenchyma, pneumothoraces, and ultimately pulmonary fibrosis. The recent development of artificial surfactants has resulted in marked improvement in respiratory function in many premature infants.

Renal

The immature kidney has limitations compared to adult renal function. Glomerular filtration rate in a term newborn is only 20 ml/min per 1.73 m^2. The immature kidney has a poorly established cortical-medullary concentration gradient and can only concentrate urine to a maximum of approximately 600 mOsm. The term infant also has increased total body water content compared to the adult, approximately 75 per cent of body weight. In the first week of life, there is a dramatic 5 to 10 per cent decrease in total body water, which then slowly decreases over the next 12 to 18 months of life to near-adult levels. This diuresis occurs despite limited glomerular and tubular function. These factors make fluid and electrolyte management of the neonate extremely challenging, particularly when they occur commensurate with fluid shifts associated with operative procedures.

Hepatic

Hepatocyte function is also immature at birth. Maturation of hepatocyte function involves structural changes in membranes, incorporation of carrier proteins, formation of intracellular binding proteins, and maintenance of energy supply. Inadequate function of bilirubin conjugating enzymes may cause accumulation of unconjugated bilirubin, which is toxic to the central nervous system. Premature infants are particularly susceptible to central nervous system damage due to bilirubin. Immaturity of hepatic elimination and detoxifying enzyme systems, particularly those of the cytochrome P-450 family, has considerable pharmacodynamic implications, including possible toxic accumulation of drugs.

Endocrine

Endocrine function, including the stress response to injury or operation, is largely intact at birth. Endocrine effects accomplish two goals: maintenance of satisfactory intravascular volume and maintenance of energy substrate. Intravascular volume may be depleted by ongoing unreplaced fluid losses, hemorrhage, or redistribution of fluid from the intravascular space ("third space"). Adequate circulation and oxygen delivery are enhanced by endogenous catecholamine secretion, which increases contractility, heart rate, and vasomotor tone. Intravascular volume is further preserved by decreased excretion of sodium and water, mediated by secretion of mineralocorticoids and antidiuretic hormone (ADH), respectively.

The neonate has limited energy stores. Significant deposition of glycogen in liver and skeletal muscle occurs late in gestation. Even then, glycogen stores are quite limited and are quickly consumed. In the absence of exogenous glucose intake, the neonate rapidly becomes hypoglycemic. In addition, the infant has limited stores of available fat and nonessential protein for gluconeogenesis.

Management Considerations

Temperature Regulation

The newborn infant has difficulty maintaining temperature stability due to its relatively large surface area/body mass ratio. Heat loss occurs through evaporation, conduction, convection, or radiation. Infants produce heat by increasing metabolic activity, primarily through nonshivering thermogenesis utilizing brown fat. Nutritional depletion, or inaccessibility of brown fat due to blockage by certain drugs, may rapidly overwhelm the capability of the infant to maintain temperature stability. The infant is optimally maintained in a thermoneutral environment, the range of ambient temperatures in which the newborn can maintain normal body temperature with a minimal metabolic rate. The appropriate ambient temperature is determined by the patient's weight and postnatal age. Double-walled incubators offer the best thermoneutral environment, although accessibility is compromised. Radiant warmers improve accessibility for patient care, but cause increased convective heat loss and higher insensible water loss due to evaporation.

Fluid and Electrolyte Therapy

Intravenous fluid therapy can be conveniently subdivided into three major categories: maintenance therapy, replacement of ongoing losses, and replacement of existing deficits. Maintenance therapy consists of the fluid and electrolyte supplementation required to replace obligatory losses. These losses include sensible (measurable) water losses such as urine, and insensible losses including evaporation from the skin and respiratory system. An infant in a thermoneutral environment requires approximately 1500 to 1800 ml/m^2/day to replace combined sensible and insensible losses. Due to the obligatory diuresis within the first days of life discussed previously, most clinicians decrease maintenance fluid by one third on the first day of life, and by one fourth on the second day of life. Maintenance therapy also includes sodium (3 to 5 mEq/kg/day) and potassium (2 to 3 mEq/kg/day). Due to the marginal hepatic and skeletal muscle glycogen stores, the infant who does not receive enteral feedings also requires continuous infusion of glucose to maintain normoglycemia. The newborn may also require calcium supplementation due to decreased calcium stores, immature renal function, and relative hypoparathyroidism secondary to suppression by high fetal calcium level. Infants at risk for hypocalcemia are also at risk for hypomagnesemia. Symptoms of hypocalcemia and hypomagnesemia are nonspecific and include jitteriness or seizures. Acute hypocalcemia is corrected with 10 per cent calcium gluconate solution, 1 to 2 ml/kg. Asymptomatic hypocalcemia is corrected by the addition of 50 mg/kg/day elemental calcium (5.5 ml of 10 per cent calcium gluconate) to the maintenance solution. Hypomagnesemia is corrected by intravenous infusion of diluted 50 per cent magnesium sulfate solution, 0.2 mg/kg. Replacement therapy includes replacement of ongoing measurable losses. This may include nasogastric aspirate or drainage from a tube thoracostomy or abdominal drain. The fluid should be replaced milliliter per milliliter with a solution of comparable composition (Table 1). Pleural or peritoneal fluid losses may cause substantial loss of protein, causing hypoproteinemia if these losses are not appropriately replaced.

TABLE 1. COMPOSITION OF BODY FLUIDS AND REPLACEMENT SOLUTIONS

	Na$^+$ (mEq/L)	K$^+$ (mEq/L)	Cl$^-$ (mEq/L)	HCO$_3^-$ (mEq/L)	Protein (gm/dl)
Body Fluids					
Gastric aspirate	60	10	130	—	—
Duodenum/bile	140	5	80–100	35	—
Pancreatic	145	5	75	115	—
Ileal	140	5	100	30	—
Pleural/peritoneal	140	5	100	25	6
Replacement Solutions					
Lactated Ringer's*	130	4	109	28	—
0.9% NaCl	154	—	154	—	—
3.0% NaCl	513	—	513	—	—
Plasmanate	130–160	<2.0			4.7–6.3

*Lactated Ringer's also contains 2.7 mEq/L Ca^{++}.

Replacement of existing deficits is the most difficult aspect of fluid therapy. A complete history provides clues to the nature and magnitude of fluid and electrolyte deficits (e.g., duration of illness, vomiting, diarrhea). Physical examination is critically important. Dry mucous membranes (oropharyngeal mucosa, tears), tenting of the skin, and tachycardia are signs of mild to moderate intravascular volume depletion. Hypotension is a manifestation of profound intravascular volume depletion (30 to 40 per cent), and is associated with deteriorating end-organ function including obtundation and anuria. Critical intravascular volume depletion requires immediate resuscitation. It is usually appropriate to infuse a 10- to 20-ml/kg bolus of isotonic fluid (lactated Ringer's or normal saline), which should be repeated if ineffective. If the intravascular volume loss is due to hemorrhage, resuscitation with blood products may be appropriate to maintain adequate hematocrit and satisfactory oxygen-carrying capacity. Infusion of 10 ml/kg of packed red blood cells increases hematocrit by approximately 3 per cent. Less severe volume depletion is corrected over several hours. Deficit therapy is provided in addition to maintenance therapy and replacement of ongoing losses. It is critical that volume and electrolyte resuscitation be complete prior to any operative procedure because induction of anesthesia and rapid fluid shifts associated with a major operation may cause cardiovascular collapse if the resuscitation is inadequate.

Assisted Ventilation

Infants with respiratory distress who are unable to maintain satisfactory gas exchange require intubation and assisted ventilation. Due to the small sizes involved, endotracheal intubation should always be performed by someone with expertise. Infant endotracheal tubes, due to their small size, are uncuffed and do not provide infallible protection against aspiration. Unlike the volume-controlled ventilators usually used in adults, infant ventilators are pressure controlled. The tidal volume delivered is a function of the total lung compliance. This mode of ventilation prevents generation of high ventilatory pressures, which may occur during volume ventilation when compliance changes rapidly. Generation of high pressures may lead to barotrauma, pneumothorax, pneumopericardium, or interstitial air, known as pulmonary interstitial emphysema (PIE).

Nutritional Support

Infants with satisfactory gastrointestinal function should be fed enterally. The ideal formula for this purpose is, of course, breast milk. If breast milk is not available, commercial formulas may be substituted. Most commercial formulas are formulated to provide 20 kcal/oz, although caloric density may be increased to supply energy demands if the additional fluid load cannot be tolerated. Commercial formulas can be broadly classified into three categories:

1. Standard formulas (Enfamil, Similac, SMA) are similar in composition to breast milk, providing carbohydrate as lactose, and protein from casein and whey. These are satisfactory under most circumstances.

2. Soy formulas (Prosobee, Isomil) are advantageous in that they are lactose free (corn syrup solids and sucrose). Disaccharidase activity in the intestinal mucosa is decreased after periods of disuse. Lactose intolerance may lead to malabsorption, bacterial overgrowth, and diarrhea. Under these circumstances, it may be advantageous to use a lactose-free formula. In addition, many surgeons feel that soy-based formulas form smaller curds and provide an advantage following anastomosis or other manipulation of the gastrointestinal tract, where large curds may lead to mechanical obstruction.

3. Elemental formulas (Pregestimil, Nutramigen) are also lactose free (corn syrup solids and tapioca starch). Protein is usually provided from casein hydrolysate for easy absorption. Lipid is provided as corn oil and medium-chain triglycerides, which are also readily absorbed. Elemental formulas are useful when the absorptive surface of the small intestine has been severely compromised, or when a large portion of the absorptive area has been resected.

Total parenteral nutrition (TPN) refers to the delivery of hyperosmolar solutions of dextrose, amino acids, lipid emulsion, vitamins, and minerals directly into the circulation, obviating the need for a functional gastrointestinal tract (Table 2). Total parenteral nutrition allows survival, with normal growth and de-

velopment, of infants with gastrointestinal catastrophes or prolonged gastrointestinal dysfunction. Hyperosmolarity of the solutions requires that they be delivered into the central circulation, usually by placement of a central venous catheter for long-term access. Placement requires a small operative procedure, utilizing venous cutdown on the external jugular, common facial, cephalic, or saphenous veins as entry points into the central circulation. In larger infants and older children, the subclavian vein may be accessed percutaneously by the Seldinger technique. Although these catheters provide satisfactory long-term access, they are intravascular foreign bodies that put the patient at risk for infectious complications, thrombosis, and catheter dysfunction.

Extracorporeal Life Support

Extracorporeal life support (ECLS) is a technique of prolonged cardiopulmonary bypass that has proven useful in the management of infants and children with severe respiratory failure. Infants with reversible respiratory insufficiency, such as that following meconium aspiration, sepsis, and idiopathic pulmonary hypertension of the newborn, respond dramatically to extracorporeal support, with survival rates greater than 90 per cent. Patients with parenchymal lung disease or pulmonary hypoplasia may benefit from ECLS, but the survival rates are not as dramatically improved. This technique is discussed in detail in Chapter 48L.

Intrauterine Surgery

With improved diagnostic ultrasound and obstetric care, potentially catastrophic congenital anomalies are being discovered early in gestation. It seems reasonable that intrauterine correction of anatomic abnormalities would then allow normal development of the affected organ. However, the technical feasibility of intrauterine repair must be tempered by the risks of repair to the fetus and to the mother. Selected centers have attempted intrauterine repair of anomalies that are associated with high morbidity and mortality, such as congenital diaphragmatic hernia and congenital cystic adenomatoid malformation. These lesions cause pulmonary hypoplasia, and it has been demonstrated in animal models that intrauterine correction allows more normal development of the affected lung. Early attempts at intrauterine repair were hindered by technical complications, which have been largely worked out. However, initiation of premature labor following the operative repair remains a major problem. Pending the development of adequate tocolytic therapy, intrauterine repair continues to play a limited role in the management of these anomalies. An interesting aspect

TABLE 2. PARENTERAL HYPERALIMENTATION IN INFANTS AND CHILDREN

Step 1	Estimate energy requirements (guideline only; Provide adequate energy for weight gain of 15–30 gm/day)	Neonate (birth–6 mo) Infant (6–24 mo) Child Adolescent	100–120 kcal/kg/day 90–100 kcal/kg/day 60–90 kcal/kg/day 30–60 kcal/kg/day
Step 2	Estimate protein requirements	Neonate Infant Child Adolescent	2.2–2.5 gm/kg/day 2.2–2.5 gm/kg/day 2.0–2.5 gm/kg/day 1.5–2.0 gm/kg/day
Step 3	Determine distribution of energy	Lipid emulsion should usually provide 25–30% of the total energy (American diet is 40–60% lipid), and should not exceed 60% of total energy or 4.0 gm/kg/day The increased caloric density of lipid emulsion may be advantageous when fluid restriction is necessary Hyperphosphatemia, hyperbilirubinemia and thrombocytopenia are relative contraindications to the use of lipid emulsion	
Step 4	Determine water requirements	Insensible loss only: 600 ml/m²/day Total: 1500–1800 ml/m²/day	
Step 5	Determine dextrose concentration	$\dfrac{Total\ Energy \times \%\ CHO}{3.4\ kcal/gm\ dextrose} \times \dfrac{1}{L\ H_2O/day} = Dextrose\ Concentration$	
Step 6	Determine amino acid concentration	$\dfrac{Protein\ (gm/day)}{L\ H_2O/day} = gm/L\ TPN$	
Step 7	Add electrolytes	NaCl MgSO₄ Ca⁺⁺ P (as K-phos) K⁺	3.0–5.0 mEq/100 kcal energy/day 0.5–1.0 mEq/100 kcal energy/day 1.0–2.0 mEq/100 kcal energy/day (1 mEq Ca⁺⁺ = 200 mg Ca gluconate) 1.0–1.5 mM/100 kcal energy/day (1 mM K-phos = 1.47 mEq K⁺) Add remaining K⁺ as chloride or acetate to total 2.5–3.0 mEq/100 kcal energy/day
Step 8	Add vitamins	Check formulation for recommended amount	
Step 9	Add trace elements	Check formulation for recommended amount	
Step 10	Order lipid emulsion (10% = 1.1 kcal/ml, 20% = 2.0 kcal/ml)	$\dfrac{Total\ Energy \times \%\ Lipid}{1.1\ kcal/ml\ or\ 2.0\ kcal/ml} = ml\ Lipid\ Emulsion/day*$	

of this work was the discovery that wounds created in the fetus healed without scarring. This has created an entirely new area of investigation into the biology of fetal wound healing that may dramatically affect cosmetic and functional outcomes of adult wounds.

DEVELOPMENTAL ANOMALIES OF THE HEAD AND NECK

Branchial Cleft Cysts and Sinus Tracts

Branchial cleft anomalies are remnants of the paired embryonic arches, clefts, and pouches. The lesions may present as cysts, sinus tracts, or cartilaginous rests. The first branchial cleft sinus presents with a small opening just anterior to the ear which connects with the eustachian tube. Second branchial cleft remnants are the most common and may present any-

where along the anterior border of the sternocleidomastoid muscle from the angle of the jaw to the lower third of the neck. The associated sinus tract passes under the digastric muscle, through the bifurcation of the carotid artery, and under the hypoglossal nerve to end in the tonsillar fossa. The third and fourth branchial clefts develop into the lower and upper parathyroid glands, respectively. Maldevelopment may present as a pharyngeal pouch deficiency syndrome, characterized by absent parathyroids, absent or depleted thymus leading to immunosuppression, and parathyroid insufficiency causing hypocalcemia.

Cystic Hygroma

Cystic hygromas are developmental lymphangiomas. They occur most commonly in the neck, with 10 per cent extending into the axilla or mediastinum. Complete excision is the therapy of choice, although this may not be feasible, since these lesions tend to extensively intertwine around associated blood vessels and nerves.

Thyroglossal Duct Anomalies

Anomalies of the thyroglossal duct are midline lesions that originate at the base of the tongue and pass through the central portion of the hyoid bone. Due to the connection with the base of the tongue, the midline mass moves with deglutition and protrusion of the tongue. Infection of the cyst is the most common complication. When asymptomatic, the lesion should be resected, including the central portion of the hyoid bone and the complete sinus tract up to the base of the tongue (Sistrunk procedure). If the cyst is infected, incision and drainage should be performed, deferring the Sistrunk procedure until the inflammation has subsided.

Torticollis

Torticollis refers to a hard, spindle-shaped fibrous tumor within the sternocleidomastoid muscle. The mass is usually detected within the first month of life, and may be the result of birth injury. Clinical presentation includes a hard mass within the sternocleidomastoid muscle, often causing shortening of the muscle and inability to straighten or rotate the head. In the majority of patients, the mass responds to conservative therapy, including massage and range-of-motion exercises. The remaining patients require division of the affected muscle below the level of the spinal accessory nerve.

DEVELOPMENTAL ABNORMALITIES OF THE GASTROINTESTINAL TRACT

Signs and Symptoms of Gastrointestinal Obstruction

A number of developmental anomalies and perinatal events cause mechanical intestinal obstruction. Prenatal intestinal obstruction may alter amniotic fluid dynamics, causing accumulation of excessive amounts of amniotic fluid known as polyhydramnios. Polyhydramnios may occur if the obstruction is located proximal to the omphalomesenteric duct. Bilious vomiting is always pathologic and demands immediate investigation. The bilious nature of the vomitus implies obstruction distal to the ampulla of Vater. The most common cause of bilious vomiting in the newborn is adynamic ileus associated with sepsis. Other entities, such as midgut volvulus, must be immediately ex-

cluded to avoid catastrophic sequelae that may be preventable by early operative intervention. Abdominal distention may occur with distal gastrointestinal obstruction. When the obstruction is very proximal, the distal gastrointestinal tract is usually decompressed and abdominal distention may not be present. Failure to pass normal meconium may also be a sign of intestinal obstruction. The gastrointestinal tract distal to an obstruction continues to secrete mucus and cellular debris. Therefore, meconium may be passed even when there is complete obstruction. Failure to pass meconium within the first 24 hours of life is considered abnormal and demands further evaluation.

Duplications and Cysts

Enteric duplications may occur anywhere along the alimentary tract, although they occur most commonly in the small intestine. Enteric duplications share a common mesenteric blood supply and bowel wall with normal intestine. The lesions may be cystic or tubular, and in approximately 20 per cent the duplication communicates with the lumen of the normal intestine. The duplication cyst may contain ectopic gastric mucosa or pancreatic tissue. Duplications may cause cramping abdominal pain or vomiting due to partial obstruction of the intestinal lumen. Gastrointestinal hemorrhage may result from peptic ulceration due to ectopic gastric mucosa. On examination, a duplication of the small intestine presents as a shifting abdominal mass due to its mesenteric attachment. The diagnosis can usually be confirmed by ultrasound examination and ^{99m}technetium scanning, which demonstrates ectopic gastric mucosa. The therapy of choice is resection of the cyst. If a long segment of the intestine is involved, the mucosal lining may be stripped to remove potential sites of ectopic mucosa, and the duplication joined, side wall to side wall, with normal bowel to avoid extensive bowel resection.

Esophageal Atresia and Tracheoesophageal Fistula

During normal development, lateral ingrowths divide the common foregut into the trachea anteriorly and the esophagus posteriorly. Abnormalities of this septation process may cause esophageal atresia and various combinations of connections between the esophageal remnants and the tracheobronchial tree. Most often, this causes esophageal atresia with a blind proximal esophageal pouch, the distal esophagus connected to the tracheobronchial tree just above the carina or on the right mainstem bronchus (Fig. 1). The incidence of this anomaly is 1 in 1500 to 3000 live births, with both sexes equally affected. Sixty to 70

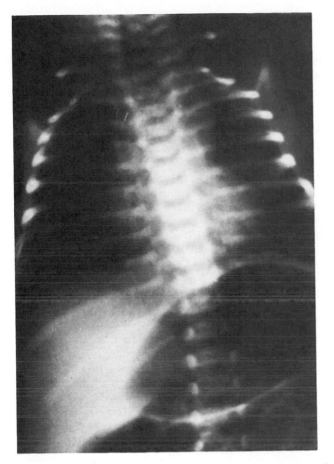

Figure 1. Esophageal atresia with distal tracheoesophageal fistula. Note the orogastric tube curled in the blind upper esophageal pouch and the gastric distention caused by air forced through the fistula.

per cent have associated anomalies involving the gastrointestinal, cardiac, genitourinary, musculoskeletal, and central nervous systems. A common association of congenital anomalies is the VACTERL association including *v*ertebral anomalies, *a*norectal anomalies, *c*ardiac anomalies, *t*racheoesophageal fistula, *e*sophageal atresia, *r*enal anomalies, and *l*imb anomalies, most commonly radial dysplasia.

Infants with esophageal atresia present with respiratory distress and excessive salivation. Choking, coughing, and cyanosis are noted on the first attempt at feeding. The diagnosis is confirmed by attempting to pass a nasogastric tube into the stomach. When a distal tracheoesophageal fistula is present, air is forced through the fistula into the gastrointestinal tract. This may cause acute gastric distention and can precipitate aspiration of gastric contents and a chemical pneumonitis.

Emergency management of the infant includes insertion of a suction catheter in the proximal pouch to control oral secretions and placement of an intravenous catheter. The patient should be quickly assessed for other anomalies. In particular, echocardiography should be obtained to evaluate structural heart defects and to ascertain the position of the aortic arch. Stable patients may be candidates for primary repair. This is usually accomplished through the right chest, using an extrapleural dissection. The proximal blind esophageal pouch has a longitudinal blood supply and can be extensively mobilized to narrow the gap. The distal esophagus has a segmental blood supply. Extensive mobilization of the distal esophagus may cause ischemia, and traction on the distal esophagus may promote gastroesophageal reflux. If satisfactory length to narrow the gap cannot be obtained by mobilization of the proximal pouch, circular myotomies can be performed through the esophageal wall, leaving a mucosal sleeve between the divided muscle fibers. With this technique, sufficient length can usually be gained for end-to-end anastomosis after the fistula to the trachobronchial tree is divided and oversewn.

Patients with significant congenital heart defects, respiratory distress, or pulmonary insufficiency due to aspiration pneumonia are not satisfactory candidates for primary repair. These infants benefit from a staged procedure that is accomplished by placement of a temporary gastrostomy to decompress the stomach and prevent aspiration. Infants with esophageal atresia with no connection to the tracheobronchial tree also benefit from staged repair. These lesions are associated with a long gap between the atretic segments. With growth of the patient, there may be concomitant growth of the proximal esophageal segment, narrowing the gap. Mechanical dilatation of the upper esophageal pouch is of unproven benefit.

Pyloric Atresia

Pyloric atresia is an uncommon cause of alimentary tract obstruction in the newborn. Affected infants present with vomiting of gastric juice or feedings. Maternal polyhydramnios is common. Plain radiographs usually reveal a single upper abdominal gas bubble or a gastric air-fluid level. Persistent vomiting may cause a hypochloremic metabolic alkalosis. Preoperative management includes placement of an orogastric tube to decompress the stomach and intravenous fluids to correct existing fluid deficit or electrolyte abnormality. The lesion is commonly a mucosal web that can be excised with pyloroplasty. Occasionally, there is complete separation of the distal stomach and duodenum, requiring a gastroduodenostomy.

Duodenal Obstruction

Duodenal obstruction occurs during intrauterine life as a result of failure of recannulization of the duodenal lumen. Duodenal obstruction usually takes the form of in-continuity mucosal atresia, although occasionally membranes and webs may cause duodenal obstruction. In most cases, the obstruction occurs just distal to the ampulla of Vater and the infant presents with bilious vomiting. Polyhydramnios is noted in up to one half of the patients. There is a high incidence of associated anomalies, including trisomy 21, cardiac, renal, and other gastrointestinal anomalies. The diagnosis is confirmed by a characteristic radiographic picture known as a double bubble, with one air bubble in the stomach and the second in the proximal duodenum (Fig. 2). Preoperative stabilization includes gastric decompression, correction of fluid and electrolyte deficits, and evaluation for associated anomalies. When stable, the infant undergoes laparotomy through a transverse right upper quadrant incision. Excision of the mucosal atresia is dangerous due to the possibility of injury to the ampulla. Side-to-side anastomosis between the proximal and distal duodenal segments is the preferred operative approach. Due to the distention and atony of the stomach and proximal duodenum, the return of adequate gastric emptying may be significantly delayed.

Intestinal Atresia

Unlike duodenal atresia, small-intestinal atresia occurs due to late mesenteric vascular accidents that cause ischemic injury. Atresias occur more commonly in the jejunum than in the ileum. Most are single, although 10 to 15 per cent of patients have multiple atresias. Ten to 12 per cent of atresias occur in infants with cystic fibrosis; therefore, sweat chloride determination should be obtained in each case. Atresias may occur as mucosal webs or diaphragms; with an atretic cord between two blind ends of the bowel with an intact mesentery; with blind ends of the bowel separated by a V-shaped mesenteric defect; or in the so-called apple peel or Christmas tree deformity, in which the distal bowel receives its blood supply in a retrograde manner from the ileocolic or right colic artery. In this circumstance, the bowel spirals around the supplying blood vessel, which forms its central axis. Multiple atresias are characterized by a "string-of-sausages" appearance.

Infants with distal intestinal atresias present with abdominal distention, bilious vomiting, and failure to pass meconium. Plain radiographs may reveal dilated intestinal loops with air-fluid levels. A barium enema examination should be obtained to exclude distal obstruction. Typically, the enema demonstrates a small unused "microcolon."

Preoperative stabilization includes gastric decompression and correction of fluid and electrolyte abnormalities. The infant should undergo abdominal exploration promptly, usually through a transverse supraumbilical incision. The objective of the operative procedure is to restore intestinal continuity while preserving adequate absorptive area. The proximal intestine may be very dilated and the infant may benefit from a tapering enteroplasty, which is performed along the antimesenteric border. This helps correct size disparities between the dilated proximal intestine and the smaller, atrophic distal intestine, and may shorten the period of time required for return of gastrointestinal function.

Meconium Syndromes

Meconium ileus is a unique form of congenital intestinal obstruction that occurs almost exclusively in infants with cystic fibrosis. Deficiency of pancreatic enzyme secretion and abnormal composition of the meconium produce thick, tenacious meconium that becomes impacted in the distal ileum, causing obstruction. Viscid meconium mixed with air appears on plain radiographs as ground glass or soap bubbles.

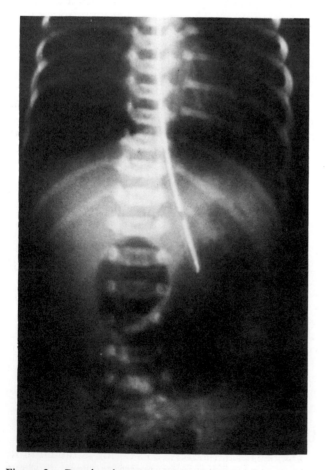

Figure 2. Duodenal atresia. Air in the stomach and proximal duodenal segment create the "double bubble."

Contrast enema examinations usually demonstrate a microcolon. Meconium ileus may be broadly classified as simple or complicated. In cases of simple meconium ileus, up to three fourths of the infants may be managed nonoperatively. Hyperosmolar contrast enemas are used to draw water into the thick meconium. This separates the thick meconium pellets from the bowel wall, allowing them to be passed and relieving the obstruction. Careful attention to fluid balance is essential to this technique. Complicated meconium ileus includes associated atresia, volvulus of the dilated loops, perforation, or formation of a giant meconium cyst. These infants, as well as infants who do not respond to nonoperative management, require laparotomy. An enterotomy may be performed to irrigate the intestinal lumen and flush the meconium into the colon. Resection with primary anastomosis, or resection with exteriorization, may be required in complicated cases. Family counseling, appropriate diet and enzyme supplementation, and management of pulmonary complications of cystic fibrosis are essential to a satisfactory outcome. In older children and young adults with cystic fibrosis, inadequate enzyme replacement may lead to inspissation of fecal material and development of intraluminal obstruction, known as meconium ileus equivalent. In most cases, these patients respond to hyperosmolar contrast enemas and operation can be avoided.

Meconium plug syndrome is unrelated to meconium ileus and is usually not a sequela of cystic fibrosis. These infants typically present with abdominal distention and failure to pass meconium in the first 24 hours of life. Plain radiographs again demonstrate many loops of distended bowel with air-fluid levels. Contrast enema examinations demonstrate a distal microcolon, up to a point in the descending or transverse colon where the bowel becomes dilated and thick meconium plugs are encountered. The contrast enema is often diagnostic and therapeutic. The meconium plugs are usually passed, and the obstruction is relieved. Hirschsprung's disease may be associated with the meconium plug syndrome, and mucosal suction rectal biopsies should be performed to exclude Hirschsprung's disease.

Malrotation and Midgut Volvulus

From the 5th through 12th week of fetal development, the developing gastrointestinal tract is herniated out into the umbilical cord. Upon its return to the abdomen, the intestine rotates 270 degrees in a counterclockwise direction around the central axis of the superior mesenteric artery. With the return of the intestine, the duodenum and right and left colon become fixed to the posterior abdominal wall in a retroperitoneal position, and the mesentery develops a broad base between the ligament of Treitz in the left upper quadrant and the cecum in the right lower quadrant. When the bowel fails to rotate and fix properly, the intestine is left hanging from a narrow pedicle based on the superior mesenteric artery and vein. Abnormal fibrous bands, known as Ladd's bands, develop between the cecum and the right lateral abdominal wall. These bands, coursing over the second portion of the duodenum, may cause partial or complete duodenal obstruction. Of more concern, however, is the potential for twisting of the intestine on the narrow mesenteric pedicle. When such twisting occurs, the blood supply to the entire midgut can be compromised, causing massive intestinal infarction. This is known as midgut volvulus.

Approximately one third of cases of volvulus occur in the first week of life, and the vast majority occur by 1 year of age. Infants present with the abrupt onset of bilious vomiting and rapidly become quite ill. If not recognized and treated, midgut infarction ensues and causes death or massive enterectomy. Therefore, bilious vomiting in any infant requires immediate evaluation. The abdomen may be distended, but in many infants, the physical examination is deceptively benign. Plain radiographs are also not particularly helpful. Contrast examinations are required to make the diagnosis. Both a barium enema and upper gastrointestinal series may be useful in establishing the diagnosis. On upper gastrointestinal contrast study, obstruction is demonstrated at the second to third portion of the duodenum, with a characteristic tapering of the lumen (bird's beak or corkscrew effect). The infant should be rapidly fluid resuscitated during the evaluation and immediately taken to the operating room.

At laparotomy, the volvulus is identified and reduced. Although the bowel may appear dusky, it usually recovers rapidly. Any obviously infarcted intestine is resected. Intestine of questionable viability should be left in place with plans for a second-look procedure in approximately 24 hours. To complete the procedure, any abnormal bands across the duodenum are divided, the small intestine is placed on the right side of the abdomen, straightening the duodenum, and the colon is placed on the left side of the abdomen. Taking these steps broadens the base of the mesentery and prevents recurrent volvulus. The appendix is removed because the cecum will be left in an atypical location. Because a midgut volvulus can occur at any time, this procedure should be performed whenever malrotation is identified either as the primary diagnosis or at the time of laparotomy for another condition.

Omphalomesenteric Remnants

The omphalomesenteric duct connects the distal ileum to the umbilicus. Persistence of portions of the duct produces various omphalomesenteric remnants, the most common form being a diverticulum from the antimesenteric border of the distal ileum, known as Meckel's diverticulum. Other omphalomesenteric duct abnormalities include persistence of the duct, which presents as a fistula draining to the umbilicus; fibrous band connecting the ileum to the undersurface of the umbilicus, causing twisting and obstruction; or an omphalomesenteric cyst located just beneath the umbilicus.

Meckel's diverticulum is a true diverticulum containing all layers of the intestinal wall. Ectopic tissue is commonly noted in these lesions, particularly gastric and pancreatic. The most common complication of Meckel's diverticulum occurs due to the ectopic gastric mucosa. The acid produced causes peptic ulceration of the adjacent ileal mucosa, causing gastrointestinal hemorrhage and painless bleeding per rectum. Other complications include inflammation (Meckel's diverticulitis), and intussusception with a Meckel's diverticulum acting as a lead point.

Diagnostic evaluation begins with a ^{99m}technetium pertechnetate scan. This isotope is concentrated in gastric mucosa. The treatment of choice is resection of the Meckel's diverticulum, and this is usually accomplished by wedge excision along the antimesenteric border.

Colonic Atresia

Isolated atresia of the colon is uncommon, accounting for only 5 per cent of intestinal atresias. Clinical manifestations include failure to pass meconium, abdominal distention, and bilious vomiting due to distal intestinal obstruction. The diagnosis is confirmed by contrast enema that demonstrates a blind ending distal microcolon and dilated loops of proximal intestine. Colonic atresia may be managed by resection and primary anastomosis or by preliminary diverting colostomy in the newborn, with subsequent closure at age 3 to 6 months of age.

Aganglionic Megacolon (Hirschsprung's Disease)

Aganglionic megacolon is a form of intestinal obstruction caused by absence of ganglion cells in the myenteric and submucosal plexuses. The absence of parasympathetic innervation causes failure of relaxation of the involved intestine, and neurogenic intestinal obstruction follows. Aganglionosis begins at the anorectal line and extends to the rectosigmoid in 80 per cent of patients, to the splenic flexure in 10 per cent, and through the entire colon and into the ileum in approximately 10 per cent. Most infants with Hirschsprung's disease present with delayed passage of meconium. Abdominal distention and bilious vomiting result from distal obstruction. In approximately 10 per cent of cases, the infants develop severe diarrhea alternating with constipation. This protein-losing enteropathy is known as enterocolitis of Hirschsprung's disease and is associated with increased morbidity and mortality.

The diagnosis of aganglionic megacolon may be made by barium enema examination. The site of the "transition zone" between innervated and noninnervated intestine is marked by proximal dilation of the bowel. In infants, this transition zone may not be definitively demonstrated. Another characteristic radiographic finding is failure to pass the barium within 24 to 48 hours. It is essential that late follow-up films are obtained. The diagnosis is confirmed by rectal biopsy. Submucosal suction rectal biopsy is adequate in the majority of patients. Characteristic pathologic findings are absence of ganglion cells and hypertrophy of the nerve fibers within the intestinal wall.

The operative procedure of choice in the neonatal period is temporary decompressing colostomy proximal to the transition zone. The site should be evaluated to confirm the presence of ganglion cells by seromuscular biopsy. At 9 months to 1 year of age, the definitive operation can be performed and involves pull-through of the innervated intestine to the anus. Three procedures are performed regularly: (1) Soave endorectal pull-through, in which the innervated intestine is brought through the residual muscular sleeve after removal of the rectal mucosa; (2) Duhamel procedure, in which the innervated intestine is brought down through the avascular presacral plane and a long side-to-side anastomosis is performed with the native rectum; and (3) Swenson operation, a rectosigmoidectomy, with anastomosis of the innervated intestine to the anus.

In cases of total colonic aganglionosis, anastomosis of the innervated small intestine to the anus may prove unsatisfactory due to malabsorption, particularly due to loss of the water-absorptive capabilities of the colon. Several modified operations have been developed, including a modified Duhamel operation with a long side-to-side anastomosis between the ileum and the colon from the anus to the splenic flexure, and the use of vascularized patches of right colon placed on the antimesenteric border of the ileum.

Survival is quite good in infants with Hirschsprung's disease. Rare deaths are usually the result of enterocolitis and sepsis. Enterocolitis may occur after pull-through procedures and can cause severe sepsis and shock. Overall, survival is achieved in more than 90 per cent of the patients. Most patients are continent, although constipation and fecal soiling may cause long-term problems.

Anorectal Anomalies

Abnormalities of anorectal development cover a broad spectrum, from simple membranes covering the anal orifice to rectal agenesis. An international symposium held in 1984 resulted in a unified classification of anomalies known as the Wingspread classification. Anal atresia refers to inappropriate ascent of the proctodeum, which produces a thin membrane covering the normal anal canal. This can usually be managed simply by puncturing the skin membrane, with subsequent anal dilatations. Anorectal anomalies are categorized as low, intermediate, or high, according to whether the rectal pouch has descended below the puborectalis sling, is at the level of the puborectalis, or remains above that level. Some 85 to 90 per cent of infants with rectal atresia have an associated fistula tract from the rectal segment. In males, the tract usually extends to the perineum in low lesions, or to the prostatic urethra in intermediate or high lesions. In females, low lesions may cause fistulas to the perineum or vestibule; intermediate lesions may form fistulas to the posterior fourchette of the vagina; high lesions may form fistulas to the upper portion of the vagina.

High lesions in both sexes are usually managed in the neonatal period by creation of a diverting ostomy. The definitive operation is performed at approximately 1 year of age. Most commonly, the procedure performed is the posterior sagittal anorectoplasty, which involves a careful midline perineal dissection. Keeping the dissection in the midline preserves the innervation of the muscles of continence. The rectal pouch is identified, fistula tracts are divided, and the mobilized rectal pouch is brought down to the perineum, with careful closure of the wound in layers.

Low and intermediate lesions can usually be managed in infancy. Lesions with fistulas to the perineum are managed by perineal anoplasty, whereas fistulas to the posterior fourchette or lower vagina are best managed by transplantation of the fistula to a site within the circular fibers of the external sphincter. Long-term outcomes are reasonably good. Newborns undergoing perineal anoplasties have excellent continence. The higher the level of atresia, the poorer the long-term outcome. Perfect continence may never be achieved in these cases due to the absence of adequate neuromuscular function. Many children with anorectal anomalies have associated spinal dysraphism which should be evaluated by ultrasound examination or magnetic resonance imaging. Anorectal anomalies are also seen in the VACTERL association, thus patients should be evaluated for vertebral, cardiac, tracheoesophageal, renal, and limb abnormalities.

POSTNATAL GASTROINTESTINAL ABNORMALITIES

Infantile Hypertrophic Pyloric Stenosis

Pyloric stenosis is a condition of unknown etiology. Pyloric obstruction results from hypertrophy of the smooth muscle of the pylorus and is more common in male infants. Pyloric obstruction causes progressive, often projectile, nonbilious vomiting following feedings. The onset is usually between the second and third weeks of life, with increasing frequency and force of vomiting. On physical examination, gastric peristalsis may be visible across the upper abdomen. The diagnosis can be definitively established by palpation of the pyloric mass (olive shaped) in the midline midway between the xiphoid and umbilicus. If the mass cannot be palpated, ultrasound examination may demonstrate the elongated pyloric channel and thickened muscle wall. Persistent vomiting may cause severe dehydration and shock, and a characteristic hypokalemic/hypochloremic metabolic alkalosis. The infant must be adequately volume resuscitated, and the electrolyte abnormalities must be corrected prior to the operative procedure. Operative correction is by incision of the hypertrophic pyloric musculature, known as a pyloromyotomy or Ramstedt-Fredet procedure. This can be accomplished through a small, transverse right upper abdominal incision. Postoperatively, feedings can usually be resumed within 8 hours. Early postoperative vomiting is not uncommon but is usually self-limited.

Necrotizing Enterocolitis

Necrotizing enterocolitis is a life-threatening intra-abdominal catastrophe. A number of inciting events precipitate a common pathophysiologic insult involving vasoconstriction of the splanchnic vascular bed, decreased oxygen delivery to the gut, mucosal injury, and invasion by luminal bacteria. Inciting events include shock, hypoxia, sepsis, hyperviscosity syndromes, exchange transfusions, hyperosmolar feedings, and cyanotic congenital heart disease causing hypoperfusion. Unfortunately, the most commonly affected infants are the extremely premature and low-birth-weight infants.

Early signs and symptoms include apnea and bradycardia and increased gastric residuals. With progression of the disease, abdominal distention develops, associated with vomiting, lethargy, and mucosal hemorrhage causing rectal bleeding. In the late stages of the disease, the patient may develop an abdominal mass, erythema of the abdominal wall, and shock.

Any suggestion of necrotizing enterocolitis in an infant at risk should prompt cessation of feedings, and immediate evaluation including careful physical examination, plain radiographs of the abdomen, and laboratory evaluation. Plain radiographs may reveal air in the intestinal wall, known as pneumatosis intestinalis, which is pathognomonic of necrotizing enterocolitis. Other radiographic findings include fixed dilated intestinal loops, air within the portal vein, and free intraperitoneal air, which is diagnostic of full-thickness injury and perforation of the bowel wall. Laboratory findings may include leukocytosis or leukopenia, thrombocytopenia, electrolyte disturbances, and a persistent metabolic acidosis. Evidence of diffuse intravascular coagulation may also be present.

Initial management of the infant with necrotizing enterocolitis includes nasogastric decompression, intravascular volume resuscitation with crystalloid and blood products as necessary, ventilatory support as required, and administration of broad-spectrum systemic antibiotics. Approximately three fourths of the affected infants respond to nonoperative therapy and recover from the intestinal injury within 7 to 14 days. Free intraperitoneal air on abdominal radiographs (intestinal perforation), abdominal wall erythema (perforation and abscess), or failure to respond to appropriate medical management requires operative intervention. The surgical management must be individualized according to the findings noted in each case. Obviously necrotic intestine is resected with exteriorization of the ends. When the intestinal involvement is extensive, a second-look laparotomy in 24 to 48 hours may be helpful to allow further delineation of the injury and preservation of viable bowel. Postoperative complications are common, usually resulting from ongoing sepsis. Infants who survive the perioperative period require reoperation to establish intestinal continuity in 6 to 12 weeks. Stenotic lesions may develop in the distal intestine after the first resection, and a contrast examination should be performed prior to reanastomosis. These stenotic lesions more commonly occur in the colon. Many infants suffer severe malabsorption due to the resection of large lengths of the intestine and may require prolonged parenteral hyperalimentation.

Gastroesophageal Reflux

Gastroesophageal reflux is a common entity in the pediatric age group, particularly among the neurologically impaired population, infants and children with chronic pulmonary conditions, infants with esophageal atresia, following repair of abdominal wall defects, or in disorders associated with diaphragmatic distortion. Common presenting findings include failure to thrive due to persistent vomiting and repeated episodes of aspiration that may cause recurrent lung infections, apnea and bradycardia, choking, reactive airway disease, and coughing or choking at night. Gastroesophageal reflux has also been implicated as an etiologic factor in the sudden infant death syndrome (SIDS). In the neurologically impaired population, where placement of a gastrostomy for nutritional support is frequently required, gastroesophageal reflux will develop with high frequency after placement of the gastrostomy. Therefore, it has become common practice to perform an antireflux procedure along with the gastrostomy in this patient population.

Many patients with gastroesophageal reflux can be managed nonoperatively by elevation of the head of the bed, small frequent feedings, and thickening of the feedings. In some cases, feeding through a transpyloric tube may be utilized to correct severe nutritional deficits, although it is difficult to keep these tubes in place long term. Indications for operative intervention include failure to thrive, peptic esophagitis and stricture, or evidence of aspiration such as recurrent respiratory infection or apnea and bradycardia in association with decreased esophageal pH, best demonstrated by 24-hour esophageal pH probe. A number of antireflux operations are used to control gastroesophageal reflux. The most popular is the Nissen fundoplication, in which a 360-degree wrap of fundus is placed around the distal esophagus. If there is evidence of delayed gastric emptying preoperatively, a pyloroplasty should also be performed. In neurologically impaired children, a gastrostomy is desirable for nutritional support. In neurologically normal infants, the gastrostomy is usually not necessary. Significant postoperative complications are observed in over 30 per cent of patients. The most frequent complication involves the wrap itself, with wrap breakdown or herniation causing recurrent symptoms. Gagging and retching, difficulty vomiting or belching, and bloating are noted in a significant number of patients, and may be related to altered motility in the esophagus and stomach.

Intussusception

Intussusception occurs when the intestine becomes invaginated into itself. The proximal lead point is carried downstream by peristalsis, dragging more and more intestine and its mesentery into the intussusception, causing luminal compromise and obstructive symptoms and eventual compromise of venous and arterial flow to the intussuscepted bowel, finally causing infarction. The majority of cases are observed between the ages of 3 months and 2 years. Most cases in small children occur in the ileocolic region, and no definite lead point for the intussusception is identified. However, a Meckel's diverticulum, lymphoma, polyp, or hemangioma of the small intestine may serve as a lead point for the development of intussusception.

The clinical presentation is characterized by the sudden onset of colicky abdominal pain, manifested in small children by their drawing up their legs and crying out. Complete obstruction causes abdominal distention and vomiting. When the mucosa becomes compromised, gastrointestinal hemorrhage produces a typical "current jelly" stool consisting of blood mixed with mucus. A sausage-shaped mass may be palpated in the right mid to upper abdomen, and the right lower quadrant may feel empty (Dances' sign).

Initial management includes nasogastric decompression and correction of intravascular fluid deficits. When satisfactorily resuscitated, the patient is taken to the radiology department for barium enema examination. The barium enema may be both diagnostic and therapeutic. A 90-cm column provides adequate hydrostatic pressure to reduce the intussusception in the majority of cases, without risk of perforation of the normal colon. Recently, air reduction of intussusception has been performed in a number of centers. The air pressure must be monitored, using a maximum of 110 mm Hg. If perforation occurs during attempted reduction, or if nonoperative reduction is unsuccessful, the patient should undergo laparotomy through a right lower quadrant transverse incision. Manual reduction is attempted using a milking technique to squeeze the mass retrograde. In rare cases where there is necrosis of the intussuscepted bowel, resection and anastomosis will be required. Postoperative complications include prolonged ileus, wound infection, and high fevers. Recurrent intussusception should be considered when obstructive symptoms persist. The reported incidence of recurrence after hydrostatic reduction is 8 to 12 per cent. Recurrences are also reported after surgical reduction, although the incidence is lower.

Mesenteric and Omental Cysts

Mesenteric and omental cysts probably result from abnormalities of the lymphatics. Cysts have a fibrous wall lined by a single layer of endothelial cells. Omental cysts frequently present as large asymptomatic abdominal masses. Cysts within the mesentery may cause luminal compromise or obstruction, causing abdominal pain, vomiting, distention, or volvulus. The diagnosis is usually made easily by ultrasound examination that demonstrates a sonolucent mass with a smooth wall. The treatment of choice is resection which, in the case of mesenteric cysts, may require resection of a segment of adjacent intestine.

Chemical Injury of the Esophagus

Small children are naturally curious, and potentially injurious material left within their reach may be in-

gested. Alkaline materials are much more likely to cause corrosive injury than acid chemicals. Commonly available products such as commercial drain cleaners, lye solutions, and strong dishwasher detergents contain agents that often produce necrosis of the esophagus. Dry materials are likely to stick to the oropharyngeal mucosa and may not be swallowed. However, liquid materials are slippery and easily progress into the esophagus where extensive injury may occur. The depth of the burn injury is directly related to the development of circumferential scarring, causing stricture of the involved areas.

The injury to the esophagus occurs almost instantaneously; therefore, there is no practical first aid. Rigid esophagoscopy should be performed to document the extent of esophageal injury. Antibiotics and steroid administration to minimize scarring are not beneficial. Esophageal stenosis can be managed by progressive dilation. The injured esophagus is at risk for the development of squamous carcinoma. In cases of severe stenosis with significant malignant potential, esophageal replacement offers a better alternative.

Appendicitis

Acute appendicitis is one of the most common causes of an acute abdomen in children. It is often caused by obstruction of the appendiceal lumen by a fecalith, causing distention, eventual vascular congestion and thrombosis, mucosal injury, and bacterial invasion. Untreated, the inflammatory process progresses rapidly and may cause perforation and intra-abdominal soilage as early as 12 hours after the onset of pain. Perforation may cause a localized periappendiceal abscess. In young children who are unable to wall-off the process due to the short, flimsy omentum, free perforation and peritonitis is usual. The classic presentation includes epigastric or periumbilical abdominal pain, followed by anorexia, nausea, and vomiting. The pain then migrates to the right lower quadrant, becoming more localized and intense. Careful evaluation of other systems is important, including the possibility of urinary tract infection, lower lobe pneumonia, and pelvic inflammatory disease in the adolescent female. Inflammation of the appendix in the retrocecal position may cause irritation of the psoas muscle, presenting as hip pain, or pain upon extension of the hip.

Laboratory evaluation is not particularly helpful in confirming the diagnosis. A moderate leukocytosis is often noted; however, the white count may be normal and should not delay surgical intervention. Urinalysis and chest radiograph may be helpful. Plain abdominal films may demonstrate a calcified appendicolith, which is consistent with the diagnosis. Barium enema examination is not useful. Some centers have gained experience with ultrasound imaging, but this has not been universally of value. Preoperative evaluation includes correction of intravascular volume deficits and antibiotic prophylaxis. Exploration is performed through a muscle-splitting right lower quadrant incision. In cases of simple inflammation, the appendix is removed and the cauterized appendiceal stump is inverted into the cecum. When a localized periappendiceal abscess is encountered, the abscess should be drained. Removal of the appendix may be performed. However, when there is extensive inflammation, it may be prudent to simply drain the abscess, treat the patient with antibiotics, and perform an appendectomy in 4 to 6 weeks.

In as many as half of the young children, the appendix will be perforated with peritonitis at the time of presentation. In this circumstance, the appendix should be removed and the abdominal cavity irrigated to reduce the contamination. Drainage of the peritoneal cavity is not of value. The patient will require volume resuscitation and a prolonged course of broad-spectrum antibiotics (10 to 14 days). There may be an associated ileus that requires nasogastric decompression. The layers of the abdominal wall should be closed, but the skin should be packed open, with possible delayed primary closure in several days. This management protocol has reduced the incidence of intra-abdominal and wound infectious complications.

Inflammatory Bowel Disease

Crohn's disease may occur in childhood or adolescence. Crohn's disease causes transmural inflammation of the intestine, most often affecting the distal ileum and right colon. In rare cases, the colon alone or the duodenum may be involved. These patients present with growth failure, cramping abdominal pain, diarrhea, perianal inflammatory disease, or strictures that cause intestinal obstruction. Diagnosis is usually made by barium contrast studies. Nonoperative therapy includes the use of Azulfidine and steroids. Surgical intervention is required for growth failure, intestinal obstruction, or transmural perforation with the development of internal fistulas. Limited resection of obviously involved segments with anastomosis is the operative procedure of choice. Recurrence following surgical intervention occurs in up to one half of the patients.

Chronic ulcerative colitis is also seen in the pediatric age group. As in adults, these patients present with abdominal pain and bloody diarrhea. The diagnosis is made by contrast studies and endoscopy, demonstrating characteristic mucosal ulcerations and crypt abscesses. Pediatric patients also develop toxic megacolon, which may require urgent operative intervention and colon resection. Long term, the potential for ma-

lignant transformation within the abnormal mucosa justifies removal of all the involved mucosa, accomplished by proctocolectomy with construction of a permanent ileostomy. The social consequences of permanent ileostomy are unacceptable to most young people. Therefore, a reconstructive operation was designed to allow more normal functional reconstruction. This includes total abdominal colectomy, mucosal proctectomy (which removes the involved mucosa and leaves the muscular sleeve of the rectum intact), and pull-through of the uninvolved ileum through the muscular sleeve of the rectum for anorectal anastomosis. This may be accomplished with or without construction of a reservoir from the ileum. Although stooling frequency may be increased, this reconstruction removes the risk of colon carcinoma and generally effects satisfactory continence and maintenance of lifestyle.

LIVER AND BILIARY TRACT

Cholestasis

Neonatal jaundice is common and is considered physiologic, the result of immaturity of the enzyme glucuronyl transferase, which is responsible for the conjugation of bilirubin. Jaundice persisting more than 2 weeks is pathologic and demands further evaluation.

The differential diagnosis of persistent jaundice is extensive. When unconjugated bilirubin predominates, hemolytic disorders such as Rh and ABO incompatibility and hereditary spherocytosis must be considered. When more than 20 per cent of the total bilirubin is conjugated, cholestasis due to biliary obstruction must be considered. The causes of obstruction include metabolic conditions; hepatic infections such as cytomegalovirus, herpes virus, hepatitis B and other viruses; sepsis; cholestatic jaundice associated with total parenteral nutrition; intrahepatic disorders such as arteriohepatic dysplasia (Alagille syndrome); and extrahepatic biliary obstruction (biliary atresia, biliary hypoplasia, bile duct stenosis, inspissated bile syndrome). Evaluation of the jaundiced infant should include sweat chloride determination, viral screen (TORCH), metabolic screen for aminoacidurias, and determination of α_1-antitrypsin level.

Extrahepatic Biliary Atresia

Atresia of the extrahepatic bile ducts is probably related to an intrauterine inflammatory process leading to fibrosis of both the intrahepatic and extrahepatic biliary tree. Some reports suggest a viral etiology, although this has not been confirmed. A sense of urgency is important in the evaluation of the jaundiced infant who may have biliary atresia. Recent reports suggest a much higher success rate when operative correction is performed in the first 2 months of life and further suggest that operation is probably of no value after 3 months of age due to progressive ductular fibrosis. The patient should initially undergo metabolic screening as described above. An ultrasound examination of the extrahepatic biliary tree may demonstrate the presence of a gallbladder or malformation of the extrahepatic biliary system. [99m]Technetium disida scan should be obtained. If the radioisotope appears in the intestine, extrahepatic biliary obstruction is excluded. Failure of hepatic clearance indicates obstruction. Percutaneous needle biopsy of the liver may be helpful in the differentiation of biliary atresia (bile duct proliferation) from idiopathic neonatal hepatitis (giant cells in focal areas of necrosis).

The operative procedure of choice for correction of extrahepatic biliary atresia is the Kasai hepatoportoenterostomy. At the time of exploration, fibrous obliteration of the gallbladder and extrahepatic bile ducts will usually be noted. The fibrous cord representing the bile duct is dissected up to the portal vein. If microscopic bile ductules are demonstrated, a Roux-en-Y hepatoportoenterostomy is performed. The Roux limb may be brought out as a temporary ostomy to evaluate bile flow and perhaps reduce the incidence and severity of postoperative cholangitis. Some surgeons prefer to establish an antireflux intussuscepted valve in the limb, while others have used a vascularized pedicle of appendix as a conduit between the porta hepatis and duodenum.

Successful outcome is related to the age of the patient (<2 months), the severity of the liver disease, and the presence of microscopic bile ducts at the porta hepatis. When there is adequate bile flow and complete resolution of the jaundice, good long-term survival can be anticipated. Satisfactory outcome is anticipated in 30 per cent of patients. The 30 per cent long-term success rate justifies performance of hepatoportoenterostomy, as this precludes the need for transplantation, long-term immunosuppression, and its sequelae. If the bile flow is moderate but the infant remains jaundiced and liver disease is stabilized, extended survival is expected, but the child will likely eventually develop progressive hepatic insufficiency and will require liver transplantation. Delaying the transplant improves the success rate and accessibility to donor organs. When no bile flow is achieved and the infant's liver disease is rapidly progressive, the patient becomes a candidate for early liver transplantation.

Choledochal Anomalies

Cystic enlargement of the common bile duct is known as a choledochal cyst. A number of variants

have been identified, including fusiform dilation of the common hepatic and common bile duct, lateral saccular dilations, cystic change of the intraduodenal portion of the common bile duct, or combinations of intrahepatic and extrahepatic cysts (Fig. 3). The lesions are more common in females. Most patients present with jaundice, a right upper quadrant mass, and abdominal pain.

Preoperative percutaneous transhepatic cholangiography and endoscopic retrograde cholangiopancreatography may demonstrate the anatomy of the biliary system but are probably unnecessary in most cases. At operation, a cholangiogram should be performed through the gallbladder or cyst wall to delineate the anatomy. Internal drainage procedures such as cystoduodenostomy and cystojejunostomy are not satisfactory because the cyst is devoid of epithelium and the fibrous wall fails to contract, leading to poor emptying and bile stasis. The operation of choice is complete resection of the cyst and Roux-en-Y hepaticojejunostomy. If significant inflammation is present, the cyst can be resected, leaving the outer layer of the cyst wall

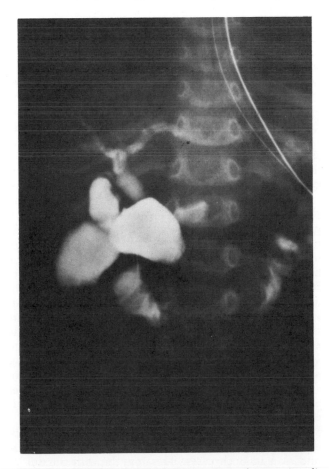

Figure 3. Type IV choledochal cyst. Note the massive dilation of the common bile duct and the main hepatic ducts.

in place on the portal vein. Postoperative complications are rare, although cholangitis, anastomotic stricture, progressive hepatic insufficiency, and carcinoma have been reported. Therefore, long-term follow-up is important.

ABNORMALITIES OF THE ABDOMINAL WALL

Omphalocele and Gastroschisis

Omphalocele is a midline defect resulting from failure of closure of the umbilical ring. The defect is covered by a sac of amnion and peritoneum. More than 50 per cent of patients have associated anomalies, most commonly structural congenital heart disease. There are a number of associated syndromes, including the Beckwith-Wiedemann syndrome, chromosomal abnormalities, extrophia of the bladder or cloaca, and the pentalogy of Cantrell (omphalocele, anterior diaphragmatic hernia, sternal cleft, ectopia cordis, and cardiac defects). The sac may include only bowel; however, the liver and the entire gastrointestinal tract may be contained within the sac. The location of the viscera within the sac leads to a small abdominal cavity that makes reduction and primary repair difficult.

Gastroschisis is a defect of the anterior abdominal wall that occurs lateral to the umbilicus, usually to the right. There is no peritoneal sac; thus the eviscerated bowel is exposed to amniotic fluid that causes a chemical serositis and produces a thick, exudative membrane. The bowel is congested and shortened. Associated anomalies are rare, although atresias of the bowel may be associated with intrauterine volvulus or interruption of the blood supply by a tight defect in the abdominal wall. The diagnosis of omphalocele or gastroschisis may be made prenatally by ultrasound examination. Ideally, the infant should be delivered in a center prepared to manage the defect. Delivery by cesarean section has not been shown to have a particular advantage over vaginal delivery. Emergency management of infants with omphalocele and gastroschisis includes insertion of an orogastric tube to prevent further distention of the bowel due to swallowed air. The omphalocele sac or exposed bowel should be covered with a sterile dressing that is kept moist, and the infant should be placed in a plastic bag to minimize evaporative losses of water and heat. Ongoing fluid losses are considerable, and adequate intravenous fluid is essential.

Ideally, the viscera should be returned to the abdominal cavity with the primary closure of the fascia and skin in both cases. This may be difficult due to the thickening and edema of the bowel wall and the small size of the abdominal cavity. Stretching of the abdominal wall and evacuation of the gastrointestinal tract may allow complete reduction and primary closure. However, the increased intra-abdominal pressure may cause compromised venous return from the lower extremities, compromised motion of the diaphragm leading to hypoventilation, or compromised intestinal blood flow. Under those circumstances, staged closure using a Dacron-reinforced Silastic silo is the preferred management. The bowel is contained within the silo, which is sutured to the edge of the defect. The contents of the silo are gradually reduced over a period of days, and the baby is returned to the operating room for removal of the silo and closure of the abdominal wall. Postoperatively, the patients may have a prolonged adynamic ileus requiring total parenteral nutrition for weeks. Overall, survival of infants with omphalocele and gastroschisis is quite good. Most mortality is the result of associated anomalies, particularly congenital heart defects.

Umbilical Hernia

Umbilical hernia is a defect of the umbilical ring with a peritoneal sac covered by umbilical skin. It is more common in females and black children, and the incidence of complications is low. The natural history of umbilical hernia is spontaneous resolution in more than three fourths of the patients. Therefore, it is reasonable to observe the hernia until the patient is 4 to 5 years of age. If the hernia persists beyond that time, repair of the fascial defect with suture inversion of the umbilical skin is the preferred operative management.

Inguinal Hernia and Hydrocele

Inguinal herniorrhaphy is the most common operative procedure performed in the pediatric age group. In the process of testicular descent, a peritoneal evagination known as the processus vaginalis accompanies the testis as it migrates through the anterior abdominal wall into the scrotum. Persistence of all or part of the processus vaginalis may cause an inguinal hernia, hydrocele of the spermatic cord, or hydrocele of the tunica vaginalis (Fig. 4). The incidence of inguinal hernias is increased in preterm infants, and in infants with increased intra-abdominal pressure due to concomitant lung disease, closure of an abdominal wall defect such as omphalocele or gastroschisis, congenital diaphragmatic hernia, and in patients in whom the peritoneal cavity is used for fluid absorption such as drainage of hydrocephalus by ventriculoperitoneal shunt or peritoneal dialysis.

The major risk factor in inguinal hernia is the possibility of incarceration and strangulation of the bowel. The risk of incarceration is higher in prema-

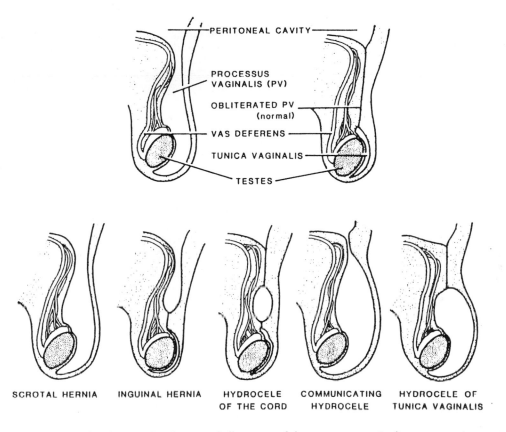

PERITONEAL CAVITY

PROCESSUS VAGINALIS (PV)

OBLITERATED PV (normal)

VAS DEFERENS

TUNICA VAGINALIS

TESTES

SCROTAL HERNIA INGUINAL HERNIA HYDROCELE OF THE CORD COMMUNICATING HYDROCELE HYDROCELE OF TUNICA VAGINALIS

Figure 4. Testicular descent. Persistence of all or part of the processus vaginalis causes various anomalies of the inguinal canal. (From Grosfeld JL: Current concept in inguinal hernia in infants and children. World J Surg 13:506, 1989, with permission.)

ture infants and in infants in the first year of life. The risk of incarceration and a 10- to 20-fold increase in postoperative complication rate suggest that repair of an inguinal hernia in infancy should be performed expediently after making the diagnosis. Most patients are successfully managed by careful dissection of the hernia sac from the adjacent vascular structures and vas deferens. A high ligation of the hernia sac at the level of the internal ring is usually all that is required. Routine exploration of the contralateral side remains controversial. In premature infants and patients with increased intra-abdominal pressure, the incidence of bilaterality is quite high and routine contralateral exploration seems justified. Otherwise healthy infants and children can usually undergo the procedure on an outpatient basis. Infants up to 52 weeks' postconceptual age are at risk for postanesthetic apnea and bradycardia and should be admitted overnight for monitoring. In addition, patients with other complicating medical problems may require admission and observation. A hydrocele of the tunica vaginalis may resolve spontaneously. If the hydrocele persists be-

yond 12 months of age, hydrocelectomy is warranted.

Undescended Testes

Undescended testes or cryptorchidism is noted in 1 to 2 per cent of term males. The incidence is much higher in preterm infants. Histologic and morphologic changes are noted in the affected testis, with progressive depletion of germ cells and atrophy of Leydig cells. Orchiopexy is recommended at approximately 1 year of age, to enhance testicular development and bring the testicle into an intrascrotal position where it may be carefully examined. This is necessary because the cryptorchid testis is at an approximately 40-fold higher risk for the development of testicular carcinoma than a normal testis. Orchiopexy is usually accomplished by mobilization of the testicular vessels, which are transposed to the medial side of the inferior epigastric vessels. This straightens the course of the testicular vessels, increasing the useful length and allowing the testicle to be brought down into the scrotum where it is fixed within a pouch of dartos fascia.

SURGICAL ABNORMALITIES OF THE RESPIRATORY SYSTEM

Abnormalities of the Upper Airway

Congenital abnormalities of the upper airway that produce airway obstruction and respiratory distress include micrognathia, choanal atresia or stenosis, tracheomalacia, subglottic stenosis (usually the result of prolonged intubation), laryngeal or tracheal webs, laryngotracheal cleft, and congenital tracheal stenosis. The diagnosis is usually made by careful physical examination, laryngoscopy, and rigid bronchoscopy.

Congenital Cystic Lung Disease

The lung is derived from an outpouching of the primitive foregut. Sequential branching of the outpouching causes the development of respiratory units. Abnormalities of this branching process cause a number of malformations.

Congenital Lobar Emphysema

Congenital lobar emphysema presents in the first few months of life. The usual presentation is respiratory distress that results from compression of adjacent lung tissue by an overdistended, hyperaerated lobe, usually the upper or middle (Fig. 5). Management is by lobectomy of the involved lobe.

Pulmonary Sequestrations

Pulmonary sequestrations are lung masses that have a systemic arterial supply and lack bronchial connection. The lesions may be contained within the normal lung tissue (intralobar), or adjacent to the lung tissue (extralobar). Venous drainage of intralobar sequestrations is usually through the pulmonary veins, whereas extralobar lesions drain into the azygos system. Connection of the sequestration with the esophagus has also been reported. The major complication of pulmonary sequestration is infection. The treatment is thoracotomy and resection.

Congenital Cystic Adenomatoid Malformations

These malformations are the result of overgrowth of elements of lung parenchyma, in particular cartilaginous elements. Air is trapped in large spaces within

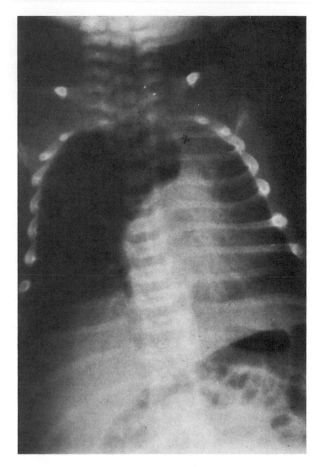

Figure 5. Congenital lobar emphysema. Note the overdistention of the right upper lobe causing a shift of the mediastinum and compression of the normal lung parenchyma.

the lesion, causing overdistention and compression of adjacent normal tissues. Up to one third of the patients are stillborn. In other infants, severe respiratory distress develops shortly after birth marked by persistent pulmonary hypertension with right-to-left shunting and coexistent pulmonary hypoplasia. Some patients are improved by urgent lobectomy. Extracorporeal life support techniques may be beneficial during the period of lung recovery. Prenatal lobectomy has been attempted successfully in infants felt to be at particularly high risk, although the experience is still quite limited.

Congenital Diaphragmatic Hernia

Congenital posterolateral diaphragmatic hernia (foramen of Bochdalek) is a defect in the normal separation of the pleural and peritoneal cavities by invagination of the pleuroperitoneal folds. The abdominal viscera herniate through the defect to occupy the involved hemithorax. This prevents normal lung development, causing varying degrees of pulmonary hypoplasia. The defect is on the left side in the vast majority of cases, although right-sided defects have been noted postnatally, particularly in association with bacterial pneumonias. Histologic changes in the hypoplastic lung include decreased numbers of alveoli and smooth muscle hypertrophy in the branches of the pulmonary artery. These histologic changes are also noted in the contralateral lung. Depending on the severity of pulmonary hypoplasia, the infant may develop respiratory distress immediately after delivery or shortly thereafter. Wide swings in oxygenation are sometimes observed, suggesting that vasospasm in the pulmonary vascular bed causing increased pulmonary artery pressures and right-to-left shunting of unsaturated blood may be partially responsible for the hypoxia that ensues.

The traditional approach to operative management was immediate operation with reduction of the abdominal viscera and closure of the diaphragmatic defect. However, this approach does not address the problem of pulmonary hypoplasia, and mortality rates throughout this century have remained approximately 60 per cent. Recently, a period of preoperative stabilization has been advocated. Treatment should include adequate volume resuscitation; nasogastric decompression to avoid distention of the intrathoracic viscera and further compression of the lung parenchyma; and hyperventilation and alkalinization, which have been demonstrated to lower pulmonary vascular resistance. The timing of operation and the use of extracorporeal life support are still controversial. The author's current preference is to attempt preoperative stabilization. Failing that, the baby is placed on ECLS support, and the repair is performed approximately 24 hours later while the baby is on bypass. This can be accomplished safely, although meticulous technique is required, since the baby is anticoagulated for ECLS support. The baby is then weaned from ECLS support as tolerated. Alternatively, if the baby can be stabilized for 48 to 72 hours, the repair may be performed in the usual manner using a transabdominal approach. If the baby deteriorates postoperatively, ECLS can be used for rescue.

Unfortunately, although ECLS support has benefited many infants with congenital diaphragmatic hernia, some infants have such severe pulmonary hypoplasia that stabilization with ECLS only postpones their demise but does not prevent it. Currently, no good, objective criteria are known that reliably identify infants who do not benefit from ECLS support. Severely affected babies may require very long periods of ECLS support, which is ultimately withdrawn due to technical complications, or they are weaned from extracorporeal support but cannot be weaned from assisted ventilation and develop chronic lung injury to

which they ultimately succumb. The role of intrauterine repair is similarly unclear. At selected centers infants felt to be at high risk have been offered intrauterine repair. The first attempts were fraught with technical complications, particularly kinking of the umbilical vein that resulted in fetal demise. The technical aspects of intrauterine correction have been largely worked out, although the procedure remains problematic due to the risk of premature labor. Pending the development of adequate tocolytic therapy, intrauterine repair will continue to play a limited role in the management of this disease.

TRAUMA

Accidents are by far the leading cause of death in children. The impact of injuries on somatic and psychosocial growth and development, family dynamics, and lost productivity of caregivers makes the overall morbidity and cost very difficult to estimate. Size is an important consideration in dealing with the injured child. Not only does their small size contribute to the patterns of injury observed, but appropriate management both in the field and in the emergency department requires downsizing of medical equipment and special technical skills by medical personnel in attendance. In many respects, management of the injured child is very similar to that of the injured adult. A rapid initial survey should be performed with attention given to the "ABCs" of trauma management: maintenance of an adequate airway, establishment of adequate respiratory function (breathing), and maintenance of adequate circulation. The large size of the head relative to the body makes infants and small children particularly susceptible to cervical spine injuries. Thus, adequate immobilization of the neck is essential during transport and procedures. If endotracheal intubation is required to satisfactorily maintain the airway, it should be performed with an appropriately sized laryngoscope and endotracheal tube by someone skilled in the procedure. Adequate venous access is almost always a problem in small children. Placement of central venous catheters can be difficult, and is not recommended in the acute situation. If peripheral intravenous access cannot be established, one alternative is the use of the intraosseous infusion device. This special catheter can be placed into a long bone, usually the upper tibia. The fluids are infused into the marrow, where they are absorbed into the rich capillary beds to access the circulation. Although these devices are very useful, there is risk of inappropriate placement, development of osteomyelitis, and fat embolism syndromes. Therefore, these devices should be reserved for situations where adequate peripheral venous access cannot be established in a timely manner.

The secondary survey should then be performed. During the secondary survey, the patient should be completely examined (including the back). Long-bone fractures may be splinted or placed in traction. Assessment of neurovascular function distal to a long-bone fracture is essential.

Management of Nonpenetrating Abdominal Trauma

In injured adults, exploratory laparotomy is generally indicated for intra-abdominal injury associated with nonpenetrating trauma. As early as the 1940s it was recognized that many children recovered uneventfully following fracture of the spleen. This nonoperative approach to management of the injured spleen assumed particular importance when it was recognized that children are at particularly high risk for overwhelming postsplenectomy sepsis. The septic event is usually related to infection with encapsulated organisms, such as *Streptococcus pneumoniae* and *Haemophilus influenzae*. These infections may be so severe that death occurs within 24 hours of the onset of symptoms. Conservation of functional splenic tissue is therefore a worthwhile goal.

As more experience was gained with nonoperative management of splenic injuries, it became apparent that this management technique could also be applied to injuries of the liver and kidneys. Currently, most children with injuries of solid viscera who are hemodynamically stable can be managed nonoperatively. Hemodynamic stability requires emphasis—hemodynamic instability, suggesting ongoing hemorrhage, demands immediate operative intervention.

Since a hemoperitoneum is not necessarily an indication for exploration, diagnostic peritoneal lavage is not particularly useful in hemodynamically stable patients. Computed tomography (CT) has become the diagnostic procedure of choice (Fig. 6). Management of a child with documented injury of a solid viscus includes careful observation in an intensive care unit setting and serial hematocrit determinations. Transfusion is rarely required. The surgical team must be immediately available if there is any evidence of ongoing or recurrent hemorrhage. Patients who remain stable are usually kept at bed rest for 7 to 10 days, followed by 3 months of restricted activity. Indications for operative intervention include ongoing hemorrhage from solid visceral injury, hollow visceral injury causing perforation, or evidence of pancreatic duct injury.

A blow to the epigastrium is a common mechanism of injury that may cause crush injury of fixed retroperitoneal structures including the duodenum and pancreas between the vertebral column and the im-

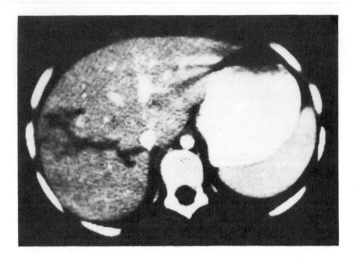

Figure 6. Liver fracture secondary to nonpenetrating abdominal trauma. This injury was managed without operation.

pacting force. Development of a hematoma within the wall of the duodenum may cause transient luminal obstruction that can be managed nonoperatively (Fig. 7). Duodenal transection and pancreatic injury involving the pancreatic duct require operative intervention.

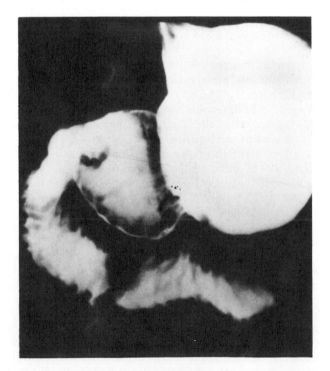

Figure 7. Duodenal hematoma resulting from a blow to the epigastrium. The symptoms of duodenal obstruction resolved after 2 weeks of nasogastric decompression and parenteral nutritional support.

Child Abuse

Physical abuse and neglect are trauma mechanisms that are, unfortunately, too commonly seen in the pediatric age group. Multiple bruises, multiple long-bone fractures (particularly those of varying ages), burns, evidence of sexual abuse, and injury patterns inconsistent with the history of injury should all suggest the possibility of abuse. It is the responsibility of medical personnel to report any suspected abuse, and to protect the child from further injury. Most pediatric institutions now have child protection teams that are responsible for investigating suspected cases of abuse and reporting such cases to appropriate authorities.

Burns

Thermal and electrical injury are also common in the pediatric age group. Burns from hot liquids are particularly common. These may be seen when the child is bathed in hot water or in the kitchen setting where cups and pans of hot liquids abound. As in adults, the depth of injury is related to contact time; thus the child whose clothing becomes soaked with a hot liquid is more likely to develop full-thickness injury than the child who is simply splashed.

The general principles of burn management are very similar to those in adults. When estimating the percentage of total body surface area injured, the head and trunk represent a greater percentage of surface area in the infant and small child than in the adult. Burn charts are available specifically for infants and children. Appropriate volume resuscitation should be administered. The injured areas should be carefully débrided and dressed with an appropriate antimicrobial. Silver sulfadiazine cream is appropriate for most injuries, although sulfamylon may be preferable for the ears, since it is concentrated in cartilage, and Neosporin may be more appropriate for the face. Injuries that occur within a closed space suggest the possibility of inhalation injury. Careful physical examination of the oropharynx as well as determination of carboxyhemoglobin levels should be performed. Fiberoptic bronchoscopy should be performed if inhalation injury is considered a possibility.

Early excision and split-thickness skin grafting is appropriate for areas of full-thickness injury. Maintenance of satisfactory nutrition is essential for a good outcome. The author has found placement of a transpyloric feeding tube useful for nutritional support. In patients with extensive burn injury, a multidisciplinary team consisting of physicians, nurses, occupational therapists, physical therapists, and dieticians is essential to a satisfactory functional and cosmetic outcome.

NEOPLASMS

Nephroblastoma (Wilms' Tumor)

Nephroblastoma is an embryonal tumor of renal origin. The majority of patients present between 1 and 4 years of age, and the most common presenting symptom is an abdominal mass, although hematuria or hypertension may be associated. Nephroblastoma may be associated with aniridia, hemihypertrophy, or the Beckwith-Wiedemann syndrome. On physical examination, the tumor presents as a round, smooth mass arising from the flank. Ultrasonography or CT demonstrates an intrinsic renal mass, causing distortion of the collecting system. The tumor may extend into the collecting system and down the ureter or, more commonly, into the renal vein with extension up the inferior vena cava, occasionally into the right atrium (Fig. 8). The lung is the most common site of metastasis, and adequate chest radiograph and/or CT of the chest is essential.

Nephroblastoma is managed according to protocols of the National Wilms' Tumor Study Group, including a combination of surgical resection and chemotherapy. Operative management must include radical excision of the involved kidney, with adequate sampling of regional lymph nodes. An important part of the procedure is careful examination of all surfaces of the contralateral kidney, as bilateral nephroblastoma is not uncommon. In cases of bilateral disease where extensive resection would not leave adequate functioning renal parenchyma, biopsy of both lesions may be appropriate. Following chemotherapy and reduction in

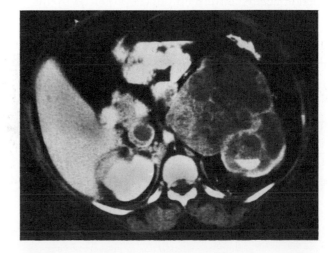

Figure 8. Nephroblastoma (Wilms' tumor). Note the renal mass, distortion of the calyceal system, and tumor thrombus in the inferior vena cava surrounded by an enhanced crescent of intravascular contrast.

tumor size, definitive resection may be attempted in a second procedure.

The two major factors determining outcome are the stage of disease (Table 3), and the histologic subtype. Histologic type is divided into favorable (89 per cent), characterized by blastemal, epithelial, mixed and glomerular elements; and unfavorable (11 per cent), which is further subgrouped into anaplastic, clear cell, and rhabdoid variants (Table 4). The overall survival for patients with favorable histology tumors is 90 per cent for all stages. Patients with anaplastic tumor that is completely resected with no regional or distant spread (stage I) have excellent survival, in excess of 90 per cent. However, in patients with unfavorable histology, advanced stage of disease negatively impacts survival, which decreases to 80 per cent with stage III disease and 60 per cent in patients with distant metastases.

Neuroblastoma

Neuroblastoma is an embryonal tumor of neural crest origin that may arise anywhere in the sympathetic nervous system. Over half the tumors arise in the adrenal medulla. Another 25 per cent arise within the abdomen in the paraspinal ganglia, and the remainder arise in the posterior mediastinum, neck, and pelvis. The vast majority present in young children, over 50 per cent presenting in the first 2 years of life. The tumors may secrete metabolically active products, including catecholamines, vasoactive intestinal peptide, and ferritin.

Signs and symptoms of neuroblastoma may be due to the primary tumor, to metastatic disease, or to the metabolically active by-products produced by the tumor. Abdominal tumors present as an abdominal mass that is firm, nodular, and tender. Extension of paraspinous tumors into the neural foramina may cause spinal cord compression, resulting in muscle weakness

TABLE 3. NEPHROBLASTOMA STAGING: NATIONAL WILMS' TUMOR STUDY GROUP

Stage I	Tumor limited to the kidney and completely excised; no residual tumor apparent beyond the margins of resection
State II	Regional extension of tumor beyond the kidney, but complete resection; includes infiltration of blood vessels or tumor thrombus, previous biopsy, or local spillage
Stage III	Residual nonhematogenous tumor, confined to the abdomen; includes lymph node involvement, gross peritoneal spillage due to tumor rupture, or incomplete resection due to invasion of vital structures
Stage IV	Hematogenous metastases (lung, liver, bone, brain, etc)
Stage V	Bilateral renal involvement

TABLE 4. EFFECT OF TUMOR HISTOLOGY ON OUTCOME: NATIONAL WILMS' TUMOR STUDY-3 (ALL STAGES)

Histologic Subtype	2-Year Relapse-Free Survival (%)	3-Year Survival (%)
Favorable	88	93
Unfavorable		
Anaplasia, diffuse	51	51
Anaplasia, focal	68	79
Clear cell	75	80
Rhabdoid	19	19

or bowel and bladder dysfunction. Thoracic primary tumors may cause a Horner's syndrome, respiratory distress, or dysphagia due to the mass effect of the tumor. Metastatic disease to the orbits may cause proptosis or bilateral orbital ecchymoses. Metastasis to bone cortex may cause pain and difficulty in ambulation. Involvement of bone marrow may cause pancytopenia. Secretion of metabolically active products causes hypertension, profuse watery diarrhea (vasoactive intestinal peptide), and opsoclonus and nystagmus (dancing eye syndrome).

Computed tomography will demonstrate the mass, often with stippled calcification within the mass. Computed tomography scan will almost always allow discrimination from primary renal tumors and will iden-

TABLE 5. CURRENT STATUS STAGING IN NEUROBLASTOMA: PROPOSED INTERNATIONAL STAGING SYSTEM FOR NEUROBLASTOMA (INSS)*

Stage	Description
I	Localized tumor confined to the area of origin; complete gross excision, with or without microscopic residual disease; identifiable ipsilateral and contralateral lymph nodes negative microscopically
IIA	Unilateral tumor with incomplete gross excision; identifiable ipsilateral and contralateral lymph nodes negative microscopically
IIB	Unilateral tumor with complete or incomplete gross excision; with positive ipsilateral regional lymph nodes; identifiable contralateral lymph nodes negative microscopically
III	Tumor infiltrating across the midline with or without regional lymph node involvement; or unilateral tumor with contralateral regional lymph node involvement; or midline tumor with bilateral regional lymph node involvement
IV	Dissemination of tumor to distant lymph nodes, bone, bone marrow, liver, and/or other organs (except as defined in stage 4S)
IVS	Localized primary tumor as defined for stage 1 or 2A with dissemination limited to liver, skin, or bone marrow

*From Smith EI, et al: A surgical perspective on the current staging in neuroblastoma—the international neuroblastoma staging system proposal. J Pediatr Surg 24:386–390, 1989, with permission.

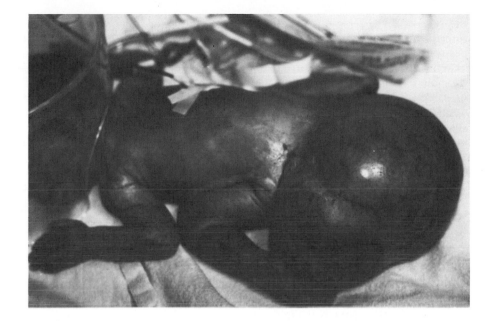

Figure 9. Massive sacrococcygeal teratoma, consisting of fluid-filled cysts and mature neuro-epithelium.

tify the site of origin of the lesion. Bone survey and ^{99m}technetium scintiscan are useful for detecting bone metastasis. A bone marrow aspirate should be obtained to exclude disease disseminated to bone marrow, and 24-hour urine collection for catecholamine levels and serum ferritin determination are important diagnostic adjuncts.

The two key determinants of survival in neuroblastoma are the patient's age and the stage of disease at the time of diagnosis (Table 5). Overall survival for children less than 1 year of age is 76 per cent, versus 32 per cent for those over 1 year of age (independent of clinical stage). Early-stage neuroblastoma (stage I and II) is also associated with good prognosis, as is the IVS group. Advanced-stage disease is associated with poor outcome (20 to 40 per cent), which has not been dramatically influenced by the addition of chemotherapy to treatment regimens. Very aggressive chemotherapy with bone marrow transplantation has shown promise in advanced disease. Other prognostic factors, including DNA ploidy and oncogene amplification (N-*myc* copy number), are under investigation.

Hepatic Tumors

Benign liver tumors in children include hemangiomas, hemangioendotheliomas, mesenchymal hemartoma, and focal nodular hyperplasia. Hemangiomas are the most common benign liver lesions and may be single or multiple. Some infants present with a syndrome of hepatomegaly, cutaneous hemangiomas, cardiac failure due to arteriovenous shunting, and a consumptive coagulopathy due to sequestration

of platelets and coagulation factors (Kasabach-Meritt syndrome). The natural history of liver hemangiomas is spontaneous involution. However, symptomatic patients may require resection or hepatic artery embolization or ligation. Two types of malignant tumors develop within the liver. Hepatoblastoma is a disease of infancy, the majority of cases occurring within the first 3 years of life. Hepatocellular carcinoma is a disease of older children and adolescents, commonly arising in an abnormal liver (metabolic disorder, glycogen storage disease, neonatal hepatitis, biliary atresia, and cryptogenic cirrhosis). Patients usually present with hepatomegaly or a right upper quadrant mass. Computed tomography scan is valuable to delineate the extent of the tumor and often predicts resectability. Serum alpha-fetoprotein and ferritin levels may be elevated and can be used as tumor markers.

The treatment of choice of hepatic malignancies is complete resection. Chemotherapy plays an adjuvant role in the management of these patients. Patients with very large tumors or those initially considered unresectable may respond to preoperative chemotherapy, leading to reduction of tumor size that allows hepatic resection and long-term survival. The overall survival for patients with hepatoblastoma is approximately 50 per cent, but is only 15 per cent for patients with hepatocellular carcinoma.

Teratoma

Teratomas are tumors composed of tissues from all three germ layers (endoderm, ectoderm, and mesoderm). The most common sites of occurrence are in the sacrococcygeal region (Fig. 9) and ovary, but the tumors may also be seen in the mediastinum, retroperitoneum, and within the pericardium. The majority of teratomas seen in infants are benign. Elective resection can usually be performed in the first week of life. In some cases, arteriovenous shunting through the tumor causes high-output cardiac failure and a consumptive coagulopathy that demands emergency resection. Delays in recognition and excision are associated with a higher rate of malignancy. Malignant teratomas are either endodermal sinus tumors or embryonal carcinomas. Serum alpha-fetoprotein and human chorionic gonadotropin levels may be elevated and can be used as tumor markers. In cases of malignancy, the treatment of choice is complete excision with adjuvant chemotherapy.

Rhabdomyosarcoma

Rhabdomyosarcoma is a highly malignant soft-tissue sarcoma of infancy and childhood. In infancy, lesions of the lower genitourinary tract, head and neck, perianal region, and bile duct predominate. In adolescence, tumors of the trunk, extremities, and uterus are more common. Computed tomography and magnetic resonance imaging are important adjuncts to diagnosis. There are no known tumor markers. The most important component of therapy is complete resection of the primary tumor. Adjuvant chemotherapy with vincristine, actinomycin-D, and cyclophosphamide (VAC) has been useful. Survival rate is related to the site of the primary tumor, the stage of disease, the histologic type, and tumor size. Overall survival from a review of 3000 patients treated in the Intragroup Rhabdomyosarcoma Study III was 70 per cent. Although the results in some types of tumors have been encouraging, other sites remain a problem, and overall the results for stage IV disease (distant metastasis) remain dismal.

REFERENCES

Ashcraft KW, Holder TM: Pediatric Surgery, ed 2. Philadelphia, WB Saunders Company, 1993.

Harrison MR, Adzick NS, Longaker MT, Goldberg JD, Rosen MA, Filly RA, Evans MI, Golbus MS: Successful repair *in utero* of a fetal diaphragmatic hernia after removal of herniated viscera from the left thorax. N Engl J Med 322:1582–1584, 1991.

Hays DM: Pediatric Surgical Oncology. Orlando, FL, Grune & Stratton, 1986.

Polin RA, Fox WW: Fetal and Neonatal Physiology. Philadelphia, WB Saunders Company, 1992.

Welch KJ, Randolph JG, Ravitch MM, O'Neill JA, Rowe MI (eds): Pediatric Surgery, ed 4. Chicago, Year Book Medical Publishers, 1986.

39

OTOLARYNGOLOGY: Head and Neck Surgery

RICHARD L. SCHER, M.D.
WILLIAM J. RICHTSMEIER, M.D., Ph.D.

ANATOMY

Otolaryngology is an important specialty in the field of surgery with a number of congenital, inflammatory, traumatic, metabolic, and neoplastic disorders. It is important to understand the anatomy of the cervical fascial compartments and their relationship to the spread of otolaryngologic and head and neck infections. A cross-section of the neck at approximately C6 reveals a central area containing the airway and alimentary tract. Adjacent to this central area are the great vessels, anterior to which is the compartment containing the thyroid gland. The central visceral compartment includes the pharynx, esophagus, and trachea. The visceral compartment extends laterally to a visceral-vascular compartment (including both the viscera and the great vessels). The significance of infection of these spaces is apparent when it is realized that infection can follow these planes longitudinally and dissect to the mediastinum. Once the vascular compartment is involved, infection can extend intravascularly causing thrombosis. Septic microthrombi may well be the initial mechanism by which infections reach the central vascular compartment. Septic thrombi are probably an important mechanism for the spread of infections within the head and neck, particularly from the tonsil or pharynx to the internal jugular vein and from the ethmoid sinus to the orbit. The retropharyngeal space is posterior to the visceral compartment, that is relatively well-defined within the head and neck, and extends from the base of the skull to approximately the thoracic inlet. Deep to the retropharyngeal compartment lies the prevertebral space, and if infection extends through the prevertebral fascia, it permits extension inferiorly along the vertebral column.

In addition to the spaces in the neck, it should be emphasized that the hyoid and the muscles attached to it separate the neck from the head. Infections above the hyoid sling tend to be contained in the oral cavity and submandibular space. Of note is infection of the floor of the mouth above the attachment of the mylohyoid muscle to the mandible, usually caused by a periapical dental abscess. The anaerobic infection that usually occurs is called *Ludwig's angina*. The suprahyoid infection has the potential to cause rapid swelling within the oral cavity, obstructing the airway leading to asphyxiation and death.

Infections that extend from the teeth laterally into the masseteric space can extend to the base of the skull, and inflammation in this area causes spasm of the muscles of mastication with trismus. The dense fascia that surrounds the parotid and submandibular glands tends to contain infections within them and are usually caused by stasis of saliva with obstruction of the glands by either inspissated mucus or stone formation. The microbiology is varied in that the parotid infection tends to be caused by staphylococcus, whereas the submandibular glands tend to be infected with flora of the oral cavity. The cervical deep space infections should be aggressively managed. The risk of airway obstruction is significant and requires close and continuous monitoring, often with the need for endotracheal or tracheostomy tube placement. Once airway obstruction begins, routine airway support may not be possible.

CONGENITAL MALFORMATIONS

The failure of normal embryologic development of the head and neck, particularly of the nasomaxillary complex, can lead to midline facial clefts, which can be of varying degrees of severity from a complete cleft of the lip and palate to components of either. The surgical approach depends on the severity of the cleft and the amount of remaining tissue for repair. Since clefts occur in 1 of every 680 births, management of the problem involves a team of reconstructive head and neck surgeons, otologists, dentists, speech pathologists, audiologists, pediatric geneticists, psychologists, social workers, nurses, and nutritionists. Because of the attachment to the palate of the palatine muscles, which open the eustachian tube, clefts of the soft palate often cause otitis media with effusion.

The branchial arches, clefts, and pouches form the soft tissues, supporting structures, and neurovascular components of the head and neck. Abnormal development of the first and second branchial derivatives, responsible for development of the external and middle ear, can cause alterations in hearing and facial appearance. Similarly, altered fusion of the hillocks that form the ear can cause sinus tracts and cysts of the first branchial cleft. Any sinus tract or cyst in and around the ear may involve the facial nerve, and the surgical approach to these should be planned accordingly. The cysts of the second and third branchial arches present as cystic masses in the anterior cervical triangle and typically connect to the tonsil or the cervical skin by passing over the hypoglossal nerve between the internal and external carotid artery. The third branchial cyst may connect to the piriform sinus or the cervical skin by passing posterior to both branches of the carotid artery and over the hypoglossal nerve. Cystic masses within the neck not in the midline are typically of a second or third branchial origin, and the patient should be counseled as to the risk to the above structures during excision. The thyroid develops from the foramen cecum of the tongue. During embryologic growth it descends to its normal position in the neck just below the cricoid cartilage. Occasionally, it leaves a midline sinus tract termed a thyroglossal duct cyst (Fig. 1). All the cysts mentioned above are potential sites of infection, and treatment involves resection with preservation of normal structures. Once infected, they are much more difficult to dissect from normal structures than they are in the uninflammed state. Care should be taken not to enter the cysts during excision, as this may prevent complete removal. Reoperation for recurrences is often difficult and frustrating. Because a second branchial cleft cyst may connect to the tonsil, it serves as a potential site of entry for actinomycotic organisms to the neck. Persistent drainage from an excised second branchial cleft

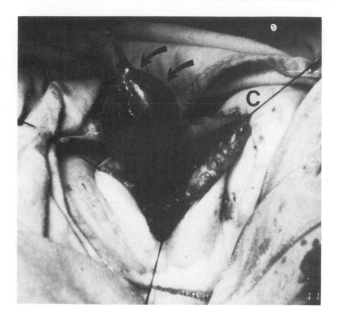

Figure 1. Excision of thyroglossal duct cyst (*arrows*). These cysts develop from remnants of the thyroid primordia and may be located anywhere in the anterior midline neck from the tongue base to the level of the thyroid gland (C denotes the chin).

cyst should alert to the possibility of actinomycotic infection. A direct sinus tract from the pyriform sinus to the thyroid gland may exist as a remnant of the epithelial cells that become the chief cells of the thyroid, and may be a potential site for recurring thyroiditis in certain individuals. Removal of this sinus tract essentially involves a hemithyroidectomy, as the pyriform sinus lies under the thyroid cartilage ala and the approximation of the thyroid gland to this must be dissected preserving the recurrent and superior laryngeal nerves.

Other cystic masses occur in the neck, the most common being hemangiomas and lymphangiomas. Hemangiomas are the most common tumors in children and are often located in this region. Hemangiomas are classified into three main categories. Capillary hemangiomas are composed of endothelial and capillary vessel proliferation with sheets of epithelial cells and small vascular spaces. Cavernous hemangiomas are larger less discrete lesions with large sinusoidal, thin-walled, blood-filled cavities. A third category, the mixed hemangioma, has areas that contain the other two types of hemangiomas. These lesions can involve any portion of the head and neck, including the oral cavity, nasal cavity, larynx, soft tissues of the neck and parotid gland. In most children, these lesions appear during the first few months of life, usually with rapid growth and then eventual involution by the fifth to seventh year. Depending on the location, continued enlargement of a hemangioma can cause significant symptoms. Respiratory stridor, dyspnea, inability to take adequate nutrition, and facial deformity are all sequelae of head and neck hemangiomas. The use of systemic steroids has been reasonably effective in causing stabilization and often decrease in tumor size. Use of laser excision or photodynamic therapy with the laser has been utilized to care for the most aggressive of these lesions, often necessary when involvement of structures such as the larynx causes airway compromise. In most patients, complete involution of the hemangioma does occur, necessitating a conservative approach to therapy. Hemangiomas are also associated with a number of syndromes such as Von Hippel-Lindau disease, Rendu-Osler-Weber syndrome, Beckwith-Wiedemann syndrome, and Klippel-Trenaunay syndrome.

Lymphangiomas are tumors composed of a proliferation of thin-walled lymphatic vessels. Over half of these lesions are present at birth, with 90 per cent manifest by 2 years of age. These lesions most commonly infiltrate the soft tissues of the head and neck, with the floor of mouth and posterior triangle of the neck common sites of occurrence. When located in the neck, these lesions are called cystic hygromas, and with enlargement and extension to surrounding tissues, they may cause respiratory compromise, feeding difficulty, and disfigurement. Because the natural course of these lesions is continued growth without involution, therapy is usually directed toward surgical excision with preservation of vital structures. Recent use of systemic interferon-α has led to dramatic resolution of these lesions as well as other vascular malformations such as hemangioma.

An atresia of the posterior nasal choanae can occur as a unilateral or bilateral phenomenon. It usually presents in the newborn period of a patient who appears to have normal oxygenation with oral respiration and crying but becomes cyanotic with reversion to normal obligate nasal breathing. The child appears to be in respiratory distress. Initial management of this problem involves placement of an oral airway. Surgical management can be approached either transnasally, if there is a minimal amount of bony atresia, or by a variety of approaches including a transpalatal approach for more extensive bony atresias. Because of the potential for reformation, nasal stents are usually placed and secured temporarily to prevent scarring and stenosis.

Hearing loss, either unilateral or bilateral, secondary to a congenital process is important to recognize due to the profound effect it may have on the development of speech. Children with significant congenital sensorineural hearing loss may have no other associated abnormalities. When a child has an abnormally low response to noise or a delayed speech develop-

ment, hearing evaluation should be performed. The placement of an intracochlear electrical stimulator is extremely beneficial for those affected with a profound congenital sensorineural hearing loss.

Airway obstruction in the newborn period can be associated with abnormalities of the laryngotracheal complex. In certain individuals, there is hypoplasia of the subglottic space leading to a subglottic stenotic segment. In others, this may be induced through the placement of endotracheal tubes for airway support in the premature or otherwise ill infant. Regardless of the etiology, the treatment involves opening of the airway and placement of a costochondral graft. Using perichondrium to face toward the airway, the graft serves to increase its diameter at the level of the cricoid cartilage. Depending on the degree of stenosis, one or more grafts may be placed anteriorly and/or posteriorly. Appropriately performed, this procedure has had a high degree of success.

Some infants may have soft laryngeal cartilage at birth allowing the airway to collapse on deep inspiration. When a child cries or fusses, airway obstruction may develop. This condition, termed *laryngomalacia*, usually requires no intervention. With increasing age, the cartilage stiffens and maintains laryngeal patency. This diagnosis is usually made by direct laryngoscopy of the awake infant and should be differentiated from laryngeal clefts and webs that may cause mechanical obstruction and/or potential for aspiration and require operative intervention.

INFECTION AND INFLAMMATION

Infections

Infections arising in the head and neck have as their usual portal of entry the oral cavity or oropharynx. Infected teeth are the most common focus in the modern antibiotic era; however, pharyngitis and tonsillitis, sinusitis, and otitis media continue to cause a significant number of serious infections. Cellulitis and abscess are common results of acute infection. In contrast to the organisms that routinely cause sinusitis and otitis media, infections of dental origin tend to be low virulence, anaerobic, or microaerophilic organisms and often present with a subacute type of presentation. It is important to recognize that among these organisms, *Actinomyces*, which reside in normal healthy tonsils, do not form the typical abscess or cellulitis patterns seen with more aggressive acute infections. For all infections of the head and neck, culture and sensitivity for aerobic and anaerobic organisms is essential. Information can be obtained from Gram stain that permits rapid appropriate antibiotic therapy. Abscesses and/or head and neck masses should also be biopsied, to diagnose infections that are difficult to culture (i.e., actinomycosis) and because regionally metastatic squamous cell carcinoma has the potential to undergo a central necrosis that can be mistaken for purulent infection.

The Pharynx

Infections of the pharynx have been known for centuries, and antibiotics have nearly eradicated the significant renal and cardiac complications of streptococcal pharyngeal infections associated with the antibody response to these organisms. Nevertheless, pharyngeal infections continue to be a significant source of serious illness and morbidity. Infections of the tonsils and adenoids should be considered separate diseases, although they commonly occur simultaneously. The lymphoid tissues of Waldeyer's ring, including the tonsils, adenoids, lateral bands, and lingual tonsils, can participate in the same infectious process whether viral or bacterial.

The adenoids are lymphoid tissue covered by respiratory epithelium and are responsible for secretion of a significant amount of IgA. In contrast to the adenoids, the tonsils are covered by stratified epithelium, which has special cells that participate in antigen processing. The crypts of the tonsils, particularly in older individuals, may provide a reservoir for pathogens that can cause acute pharyngitis and spread to others. Adenoiditis in children tends to cause obstruction of the nasopharynx leading to nasal airway obstruction. Additionally, a significant pathogenic burden (greater than 10^5 organisms/gm of tissue) is associated with an increased incidence of acute otitis media because the orifice of the eustachian tube empties directly into the nasopharynx. Passive obstruction of the eustachian tubes with serous otitis media is an additional complication of enlarged adenoids. Removal of the adenoids is seldom complete and regrowth is common. The procedure appears to be of significant benefit and persists as a key to the management of nasal airway obstruction and otologic infections in children.

Tonsillectomy similarly decreases the pathogenic burden to the patient, and infection may penetrate the capsule surrounding the tonsils to form an abscess in the peritonsillar area. This generally occurs in older children or young adults and should be treated as any abscess, usually by incision and drainage. However, repeat aspiration with appropriate antibiotic coverage can also be effective. Acute tonsillectomy is usually reserved for patients with abscesses that do not respond to typical conservative therapy or those that form in an area difficult to reach in the clinic setting. Patients with a peritonsillar abscess as the only recent pharyngeal infection may well have no recurrent disease. The decision regarding tonsillectomy should be

based on the severity of the illness, presence or absence of other recurrent tonsillar disease, and the general medical health of the patient. While the course of recurrent acute tonsillitis cannot be predicted, it appears that even a significant number of infections observed over 1 or more years spontaneously reverse in many patients. The decision regarding removal of the tonsils for recurrent disease is dependent on the severity of the illness, the patient's access to medical care, the spread of disease to other family members, interference with quality of life, the failure of standard medical therapy, and the medical condition of the patient relating to anesthetic risk.

The Larynx

The airway itself may become infected with cellulitis. Because of the difference in the anatomic drainage, the supraglottis is separated from the glottic and infraglottic laryngeal space. Consequently, infections of the supraglottis tend to remain contained in that area only, occasionally appearing to involve only the anterior, posterior, or hemilarynx. When the anterior portion only is involved, it is typically termed epiglottitis, but all infections of the supraglottis should be treated similarly. The primary flora in young children and adults is *Haemophilus influenzae*, which usually responds rapidly to intravenous antibiotics. A viral etiology cannot be distinguished from the bacterial infection clinically and, therefore, management of the airway is similar regardless of the infectious agent. With a small airway, a significant amount of edema rapidly causes a decreased caliber of the airway, and changes laminar flow to turbulent flow, with airway obstruction. Patients typically present with odynophagia as the initial symptom. In the child who cannot complain specifically of pain on swallowing, the usual presentation includes inability to swallow saliva, tachypnea, and splinting of the airway by maintaining an upright posture. The acute respiratory obstruction, that may be the final result of this disease process can occur quite rapidly. Therefore, once this disease is suspected, the patient should remain under direct observation by both a skilled endoscopist and surgeon until an airway can be established. The diagnosis of acute supraglottitis is usually made in the operating room by direct laryngoscopy under adequate inhalation anesthetic where an airway can be established immediately. By this mechanism, it can be distinguished from "croup" (laryngotracheitis), that can be similar but is primarily a viral inflammation of the subglottis. Croup responds to anti-inflammatory airway management, and the patient may be managed without an artificial airway under the proper circumstances. Unless the managing physician or surgeon has extensive experience, it is better to establish and maintain an artificial airway for 48 hours or until the inflammatory process has resolved . The cooperation of the anesthesiologist, the head and neck surgeon, and the pediatrician is essential to avoid acute airway obstruction in an uncontrolled setting.

The Nasal Cavity and Paranasal Sinuses

Infections of the nasal cavity, sinuses, and ears commonly follow infection with *Streptococcus pneumoniae, Haemophilus influenzae, Branhamella catarrhalis,* and a variety of other bacteria and viruses. While the pathway of infection for the ears is thought to be retrograde through the eustachian tube, infections of the nose and sinuses passed through the nasopharynx can also contribute to otologic disease. Structurally, the sinuses are a complex labyrinth involving mucociliary transport as the essential method of removal of pathogens from these areas. Obstruction of the sinus ostia can occur by a variety of mechanisms. Smoking and other inflammatory conditions can cause loss of cilia motility and thereby allow mucus stasis to obstruct the ostia. Cellulitis, allergy, and anatomical deformities can narrow the ostia causing stasis and obstruction to drainage. Once obstruction occurs, an overgrowth of the pathogens that normally reside within the sinuses is likely. In the acute setting, antibiotics are the primary therapy, and lavage of the nose to allow drainage may be of benefit. Many patients are symptomatically helped by lavage of maxillary sinus. In the chronic setting, topical steroids are often added, but despite these efforts, it is common for the problem to persist. In this setting, surgical opening of the sinuses to allow reestablishment of mucociliary transport may be of value.

The proximity of the contents of the orbit and the base of the skull to the sinuses demands focused study of the techniques to remove diseased tissue from the sinus. The external ethmoidectomy is the standard with regard to surgical safety of the orbit. However, recent use of telescopic endoscopes with improved visualization has led to a general improvement in the intranasal approach to drainage of the sinus, with regard to safety and effectiveness. The endoscopes themselves are of significant use to the head and neck surgeon, because they make possible the diagnosis of discrete sites of infection and inflammation as well as other disorders such as malignancies that can occur in the nose or paranasal sinuses. The techniques for ethmoidectomy, which is the fundamental sinus operation employed due to the central role of ethmoids in drainage of the maxillary and frontal sinuses, are well described. In the acute setting, a procedure that provides safe, adequate drainage should be employed, whether intranasally or externally. In the chronic setting the surgeon has more flexibility in the choice of ap-

proaches. It should be noted that simple aeration of the sinuses is usually not adequate therapy for sinusitis, as mucociliary transport has a specific pattern in the sinuses. Establishment of dependent drainage is important in patients who have no mucociliary transport (i.e., cystic fibrosis or Kartagener's syndrome) and may be of benefit in overcoming the chronic pseudomonal or fungal sinus infection often seen in patients with chronic squamous metaplasia and mucus stasis.

Invasive infection of the sinuses by fungus is rare and requires biopsy of the mucosa for diagnosis, and if positive, amphotericin B should be administered intravenously. Allergy to fungus can lead to an allergic sinusitis, and usually responds to conservative reestablishment of normal sinus function by sinusotomy. Special note should be made of infections of the sinuses caused by the family of organisms that includes *Rhizopus*. These infections, occurring in patients who are either immunosuppressed or suffering from diabetic ketoacidosis, cause an invasive anaerobic infectious vasculitis, which causes infarction of tissues in the sinuses, giving the mucosa a black color. The septic intravascular thrombi that develop can extend rapidly to the orbit and the base of the skull. Wide débridement, intravenous amphotericin B, and hyperbaric oxygen are the therapeutic options. The high mortality associated with this disease requires prompt reversal of ketoacidosis, if present, and aggressive surgical management.

The Ear

Acute otitis media is an infectious process involving the middle ear, often associated with upper respiratory infection, and is usually treated successfully with antibiotic therapy. It occasionally may require incision and drainage of the tympanic membrane in situations where serious complications such as meningitis or facial nerve paralysis are encountered. Myringotomy may also be useful in obtaining a specimen for culture and sensitivity. If the mastoid air cells are unable to drain through the middle ear and eustachian tube, mastoiditis may occur and an incision and drainage of the mastoid through use of a simple mastoidectomy may be indicated. An infection that penetrates the surface of the mastoid sinus and accumulates beneath the skin of the retroauricular space is termed a Bezold's abscess and indicates the presence of significant infection. Obstruction of the eustachian tube causing persistent serous effusion within the middle ear space can be reversed by placement of a ventilation tube through the tympanic membrane. Potential complications include allowing infection to reach the middle ear cleft from the outside, migration of epithelium into the middle ear, or persistent perforation of the tympanic membrane once the tube extrudes. Despite these risks, the ability to reequalize the pressure within the middle ear space provides the advantages of improved hearing as well as prevention of additional chronic or recurrent otitic problems.

Chronic otitis media is the presence of a tympanic membrane perforation caused by secondary infection or trauma and requires tympanoplasty. The presence of keratinizing epithelium in the middle ear cleft, either left as a congenital remnant or acquired as a result of negative pressure within the middle ear space or by growth through a tympanic membrane perforation, is termed cholesteatoma. Cholesteatomas typically occur in the pars flaccida portion of the ear drum in its posterior superior extent where the drum is the weakest and the resistance to medialization is least. Secondary to cytokine (IL-1) secretion, the cholesteoma can erode into the ossicles of the middle ear and otic capsule of the inner ear and lead to impairment of hearing. If the cholesteatoma communicates to the outside, skin contaminants can grow into the cholesteatoma and infection in this site can cause additional inflammatory problem. An ear with a draining tympanic membrane perforation should always be examined thoroughly with a microscope to exclude the presence of cholesteatoma. If cholesteatoma is present, it should be removed. Because of the adjacent facial nerve and involvement of the ossicles, removal usually requires a transmastoid approach. Reestablishment of normal function of the eustachian tube and aeration of the middle ear is essential to preventing a recurrence of chronic ear disease.

Inflammation

There are a variety of primary inflammatory disorders of the head and neck, including inflammation of the joints by connective tissue disorders (Table 1). Probably the most common is temporomandibular joint dysfunction, which can arise from a variety of mechanical causes in addition to autoimmune phenomena. It should be remembered that the articulation of the arytenoid with the cricoid is also a joint, and inflammation of this space, as in rheumatoid arthritis, can lead to vocal cord immobility and airway obstruction.

Autoimmune diseases can also involve the salivary glands, with Sjögren's syndrome being the most common, and may present initially as a mass in a single salivary gland. Should the diagnosis of Sjögren's syndrome be considered, biopsy of a minor salivary gland of the inner lip usually provides pathologic confirmation of the suspected underlying lymphocytic infiltrate, as all salivary glands are affected by this disorder. Autoimmune inner ear disease is also suspected in certain types of sensorineural hearing loss; however, the site

TABLE 1. INFLAMMATORY AND AUTOIMMUNE DISEASES AFFECTING THE HEAD AND NECK*

Disease	Sites of Involvement
Rheumatoid arthritis	Larynx, cervical spine, oral mucosa
Sjögren's syndrome	Salivary glands, lacrimal glands
Wegener's granulomatosis	Larynx, nasal cavity, paranasal sinuses
Giant cell arteritis	Temporal artery, external carotid artery
Sarcoidosis	Salivary glands, facial nerve, paranasal sinuses
Hashimoto's/Graves' thyroiditis	Thyroid, eye
Scleroderma	Esophagus, salivary glands
Pemphigus	Oral mucosa
Relapsing polychondritis	Ear, nose, larynx, trachea

*Adapted from Richtsmeier WJ: Basic allergy and immunology. *In* Cummings CW, et al (eds): Otolaryngology-Head and Neck Surgery, vol 1, ed 2. St. Louis, Mosby, 1993, pp 243–276, with permission.

of the inflammation is not known. Vasculitis such as Wegener's granulomatosis can occur in the head and neck and commonly presents as chondritis with loss of the mucoperichondrial support of the structures of the nose or the laryngotracheal complex. A specific biopsy of these tissues can provide the diagnosis, in conjunction with a work-up for additional systemic involvement. Giant cell arteritis is another disorder marked by vascular inflammation of the branches of the external carotid artery. This disease complex, also termed temporal arteritis, presents with headaches, loss of vision, and claudication of the jaw and usually responds to steroids. There are inflammatory conditions in the head and neck thought to be infectious, but without specific causative agents. One of the most striking is that of presumed viral inflammation of the facial nerve causing Bell's palsy. It typically presents as a facial paralysis, often preceded by an upper respiratory illness, and nearly always resolves with return of facial function. Recovery may take weeks to months and is hastened by steroids. If recovery does not occur, it is not likely to be Bell's palsy, and a more sinister cause of facial nerve involvement, such as from a tumor, should be entertained.

A nonspecific inflammation of the bone of the cochlea and stapes can lead to fixation of the stapes in the oval window causing a conductive hearing loss. The proliferation of bone is known as otosclerosis and appears to have a familial tendency. This disease, which occurs in 10 per cent of adult Caucasians, is usually treated by stapedectomy and prosthetic replacement of the stapes to correct the conductive hearing loss. An inflammatory disease seen frequently in the American population is allergic rhinitis. The deposition of aerosolized mucopolysaccharide antigens in the nasal cavity can combine with IgE adjacent to the nasal mucosa leading to degranulation of mast cells. The acute response associated with histamine release is followed by a delayed response of other inflammatory mediators, causing the symptoms of nasal congestion, sneezing, and rhinorrhea. The primary approach to this problem is avoidance of the allergen. When this is not possible, antihistamines and topical nasal steroids provide significant symptomatic improvement. There is no specific surgical treatment for rhinitis. However, the associated inflammatory response is often seen in conjunction with chronic sinusitis, and treatment of the underlying allergic phenomena is important for control of the chronic sinusitis. In addition, certain patients with nasal polyps have an associated asthmatic-type of chronic obstructive pulmonary disease that appears to worsen when their sinus disease worsens. Surgical control of the chronic sinusitis combined with medical management is indicated.

TRAUMA

Airway Injury

The exposed position of the head, face, and neck makes these regions vulnerable to injury by a number of external forces. Regardless of the mechanism of injury, trauma to the head and neck places the airway at significant risk. Maintenance of adequate respiration and protection of the lungs are foremost concerns in patients with head and neck trauma. Loss of ventilation and airway protection may occur acutely or be delayed, and concern for the airway must be maintained at all times (Table 2).

TABLE 2. CAUSES OF AIRWAY COMPROMISE FROM HEAD AND NECK TRAUMA

Neurologic	Cerebral contusion with obtundation
	Brainstem injury
	Subdural/epidural hematoma
	Toxin effects – alcohol
Soft Tissue Injury	Neck hematoma
	Tongue/oral cavity lacerations
	Stab and gunshot wounds to face and neck
Skeletal Injury	Mandible fractures
	Midface/Le Fort fractures
	Cervical vertebral fractures
Laryngeal Injury	Vocal cord paralysis
	Thyroid/cricoid cartilage fractures
	Laryngotracheal separation
	Laryngeal mucosal laceration and edema
Other	Laryngotracheal and esophageal foreign bodies
	Dislodgment of previously placed endotracheal or tracheotomy tube
	Pneumothorax

Blunt and Penetrating Neck Trauma

Blunt trauma to the neck, as occurs in motor vehicle accidents, causes a number of significant injuries that may compromise the airway. Fractures of the laryngeal cartilages can occur with associated injury to the laryngeal musculature and mucosal lining. Fracture of the cricoid cartilage can cause complete collapse of the airway, as this structure is responsible for maintenance of the laryngotracheal lumen. High-impact injuries confined to a relatively narrow region of the neck, such as with steering wheel impact or "clothes-line"-type injuries, can cause laryngotracheal separation with complete transection of the trachea from the cricoid cartilage. Injury to the soft tissues of the neck can cause soft tissue edema or hematomas that may cause compression of the pharyngeal or laryngotracheal lumen resulting in airway compromise.

Penetrating injuries to the neck such as those occurring with gunshot wounds and stab injuries can also significantly injure the pharyngeal and laryngotracheal complex. Injury to the pharyngeal lumen, vocal cords, recurrent laryngeal and vagus nerves, and great vessels of the neck can occur with resultant impairment of airway mechanics. Gunshot wounds may also cause significant tissue loss and extensive defects requiring not only airway maintenance but eventual reconstruction. Patients with significant injury to the neck may have immediate loss of ventilation requiring emergent establishment of an artificial airway either through tracheostomy or endotracheal intubation. The symptoms of odynophagia, hoarseness, hemoptysis, dyspnea, and tachypnea are often present in those patients who are unable to maintain an airway. Disruption of the mucosal lining with communication to the neck causes subcutaneous emphysema palpable in the soft tissues. Injury to the cervical vasculature can cause rapidly expanding hematomas that are easily seen and palpated. Palpation over the larynx in patients suffering laryngeal trauma reveals significant tenderness and swelling as well as an inability to discern the normal contours of the cartilages. Radiographic imaging with computed tomography (CT) scanning is helpful for delineating both soft tissue and skeletal injury and assessing the presence of airway narrowing or collapse.

Initial management of patients with significant injuries of the head and neck and documented or potential airway compromise involves securing the airway, most often accomplished by the use of tracheostomy or endotracheal intubation. These patients are at risk for cervical spine injury, and appropriate stabilization of the neck must be maintained during manipulation of the airway. Once the airway is secured, direct examination of the pharynx and laryngotracheal complex is performed by direct laryngoscopy, tracheoscopy, and esophagoscopy. Direct repair of mucosal injuries may be necessary and is usually accomplished through an external approach. Any cartilaginous injuries to the laryngotracheal complex can then be addressed, with direct wire fixation used to reestablish skeletal support for larynx and tracheal fractures. Significant risk or concern of vascular or neural injury also necessitates exploration of the carotid sheath, with direct repair accomplished at the time of exploration. Angiography can often be useful to identify potential vascular injury in the cervical vasculature.

Significant sequelae such as glottic and subglottic stenosis, laryngeal webs, and vocal cord paralysis may be caused by either the initial injury or by the therapeutic maneuvers directed at management of the trauma. Laryngeal and tracheal stenoses are significant problems following any injury that disrupts the mucosal lining and cartilaginous support of these structures. In addition, use of endotracheal or tracheostomy tubes is associated with these sequelae in both the setting of trauma and in normal clinical use. Management of these problems usually involves attempts at endoscopic dilatation, laser excision of stenotic areas, excision of stenotic areas with internal splinting, or excision with end-to-end anastomosis of the trachea.

Vocal cord paralysis may be caused by either direct injury to the vocalis muscle of the true vocal cord or from injury to the recurrent laryngeal nerve or vagus nerve. Direct injury to the nerve, either from external forces or from intubation injury, has been recognized and is often associated with poor outcome. Attempts at reinnervation of the larynx have not been successful. Unilateral vocal cord paralysis is associated with hoarseness and aspiration of salivary secretion. Bilateral vocal cord paralysis causes airway obstruction and often necessitates placement of a tracheostomy for maintenance of the airway, with future attempts at correction of the glottic airway directed toward repositioning or removal of an arytenoid cartilage. Augmentation of the paralyzed vocal cord with Teflon injected lateral to the vocalis muscle or placement of an autograft or alloplast wedge lateral to the vocalis muscle to produce medialization has been quite successful. Alternative treatment with either nerve-muscle transplants or nerve repairs for reinnervation of the vocal cord is being investigated. In addition to trauma, vocal cord paralysis can be caused by infectious and neoplastic involvement of the vagus and recurrent laryngeal nerves as well as from degenerative neurologic disorders.

Foreign Bodies

Airway compromise may also occur following the retention of foreign bodies in the larynx, tracheobronchial tree, or esophagus. Foreign body obstruction of the larynx occurs most commonly at the glottic level and often follows aspiration of a bolus of food. Clearance of a foreign body that causes complete airway obstruction may be accomplished by use of the Heimlich maneuver, performing abdominal thrusts that increase the intrathoracic pressure. When this is unsuccessful, emergent tracheostomy may be necessary, with endoscopic removal of the foreign body after the airway is secured. Foreign bodies that pass through the larynx and into the tracheobronchial tree often erode the mucosa of the trachea or bronchus. The right mainstem bronchus is most often involved because of the more acute angulation of the left mainstem bronchus. Children are quite susceptible to aspiration of foreign bodies placed in the mouth, especially objects such as nuts, coins, beans, and plastic toys. Aspiration of foreign bodies is usually manifest initially by spasmodic coughing which subsides quickly. Following this, with failure to diagnose the lesion promptly, obstructive emphysema, pulmonary atelectasis, purulent tracheobronchitis, pneumonitis, lung abscess, and empyema may develop. Physical findings with a tracheobronchial foreign body include expiratory wheezing on chest auscultation, obstructive emphysema visualized radiographically with expiratory views on fluoroscopy, and visualization of a foreign body by radiography if it is nonradiopaque. Immediate extraction of the foreign body must be performed with rigid bronchoscopy under general anesthesia, and complete examination of the tracheobronchial tree distal to the lesion is necessary to be certain that no additional foreign body, obstructing lesions, or purulent material are identified.

Foreign bodies of the esophagus may cause airway obstruction secondary to compression of the posterior tracheal wall. Esophageal foreign bodies most commonly lodge just distal to the cricopharyngeus muscle. Other common sites of impaction of foreign bodies in the esophagus are at the gastroesophageal junction and the narrowing in the region of the aortic arch and left mainstem bronchus. Foreign bodies in the esophagus may cause dysphagia, odynophagia, and subcutaneous emphysema if perforation occurs. Neck and chest radiographs should be obtained, as they may identify and localize radiopaque foreign bodies prior to removal (Fig. 2). Contrast esophagography may be used to demonstrate the point of obstruction from a radiolucent foreign body. Prompt removal of the foreign body is performed using rigid esophagoscopy. The foreign body must be disimpacted from the esophageal wall and retracted into the esophagoscope prior to removal to prevent any further injury to the mucosal lining or muscular wall of the esophagus and pharynx. Perforation of the esophagus is a serious consequence of foreign bodies of the esophagus and may cause mediastinitis, pneumothorax, empyema,

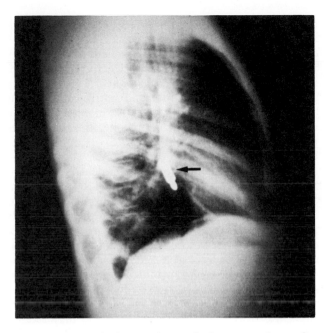

Figure 2. Lateral chest radiograph demonstrating radiopaque foreign body (*arrow*) lodged in the midthoracic esophagus of a child. Rigid esophagoscopy is necessary for safe removal.

sepsis, and vascular injury. Prompt recognition of perforation and treatment with drainage and broad-spectrum antibiotics is necessary to prevent mortality.

Soft Tissue Injury

Lacerations and avulsions of the head and neck may involve both the skin and mucosal surfaces as well as the underlying musculature and neurovascular structures. Because of the rich vascularity of the head and neck, these injuries often present acutely with profuse bleeding and may appear more extensive than they are. Management for these injuries includes control of hemorrhage, usually best accomplished with digital pressure, adequate cleaning of the wound with topical irrigation, judicious and minimal débridement of tissue, ligation of bleeding vessels, and careful approximation and realignment of injured tissues with meticulous suture repair. Every attempt should be made to preserve injured tissue, as even questionably viable skin and mucosa, if managed properly, usually survive. Loss of tissue from avulsion may require repair with the use of local soft tissue augmentation. Local flaps can often be developed from surrounding facial skin or mucosal lining, providing excellent cosmetic and functional results.

Several areas of the head and neck pose unique treatment problems. Lacerations of the lip should be managed by reapproximation of the mucosal, mus-

cular, and cutaneous layers. An adequate cosmetic result necessitates alignment of the vermilion border of the mucosa. Precise approximation of the orbicularis oris muscle produces acceptable functional outcome. In patients with extensive lacerations, adequate oral hygiene with rinsing of the mouth and soft or liquid diet should be maintained for several days after repair to permit healing. Nasal lacerations and avulsions require precise alignment of the mucosa and underlying cartilaginous framework. Loss of cartilage or bone often causes functional deformity, with nasal collapse and airway obstruction requiring secondary reconstruction. Lacerations and avulsions of the ear can be managed by direct closure if tissue appears viable. Complete avulsions of portions of the pinna or the entire pinna may survive with direct reattachment. Microsurgical revascularization procedures have also been utilized to provide survival of major avulsed segments of the ear. Lacerations of the face place the facial nerve in jeopardy of transection. Transections of the nerve posterior to the lateral canthus of the eye and lateral commissure of the mouth should be repaired by direct exploration of the facial nerve branches involved and anastomosis with microsurgical neurorrhaphy. Lacerations of the fine distal branches usually do not require repair, as regeneration produces satisfactory return of function. Treatment for significant avulsions of facial nerve segments includes nerve grafting or facial reanimation with temporalis muscle transposition or microvascular free tissue transfer of reinnervated muscle.

Thermal, chemical, and electrical burns of the head and neck can cause devastating injury. Thermal injuries to the skin of the face should be treated with wound care similar to burns on other portions of the body. Topical antibiotics with judicious débridement of devitalized tissue and eventual reconstruction is indicated. Thermal burn injury in the region of the mouth or nares should alert the physician to the possibility of thermal injury to the pharynx, larynx, and tracheobronchial tree. Continuous inspection of these regions is necessary to avert possible airway compromise. A short course of anti-inflammatory steroids, cool mist, inhalant, and possible intubation with either endotracheal tube or tracheostomy may be necessary. Chemical burns to the mucosa of the oral cavity, pharynx, and esophagus frequently occur after ingestion of caustic materials such as lye. These strong alkalis penetrate the soft tissues, creating significant damage and necrosis, and injuries should be treated aggressively, with copious irrigation to wash away the offending chemicals and decrease any subsequent inflammatory reaction. The use of neutralizing agents, either topical or systemic, should be avoided, as this may worsen the situation. Management of possible sequelae such as infection or perforation should be managed aggressively with antibiotics, systemic cardiovascular support, and surgical drainage. Electrical burns of the lip often occur in children secondary to their chewing on electrical cords, and deep coagulation necrosis can follow the extremely high temperatures produced by the electrical arc. Treatment should be undertaken in a manner similar to that of other burns, with topical antibiotics, prophylactic systemic antibiotics, and limited débridement of nonviable tissue. Significant contracture of the oral commissure can occur secondary to scar formation and may require extensive rehabilitation and reconstructive procedures.

Skeletal Injuries

Temporal Bone Fractures

Fractures of the temporal bone (basal skull fractures) are caused by significant blunt trauma to the skull, especially in the occipital region. These fractures are suspected when there is bleeding from the ear. Blood may be identified behind an intact tympanic membrane, through a rupture of the tympanic membrane, or through a fracture line in the external auditory canal. Fractures of the temporal bone are divided into two types, longitudinal and transverse, based on their orientation to the long axis of the petrous pyramid. Approximately 80 per cent of fractures are longitudinal and are associated with disruption of the external auditory canal, tympanic membrane, and ossicles with resultant conductive hearing loss. Transverse fractures extend across the cochlea and vestibule of the inner ear as well as the facial nerve canal causing profound sensorineural hearing loss, vertigo, and facial nerve paralysis. The same sequelae are also possible with longitudinal fractures. Treatment for these lesions involves prevention of intracranial contamination, correction of conductive hearing loss through tympanic membrane repair and ossicular repair, hearing aid amplification for sensorineural hearing loss, and exploration and repair of the facial nerve for possible restoration of facial function.

Midface Fractures

Fracture of the nasal bones is the most common fracture of the facial skeleton and is usually associated with epistaxis, external nasal deformity, septal deformity, and often mucosal or skin lacerations. Patients present with ecchymoses of the periorbital soft tissues, tenderness to palpation of the nasal dorsum, and palpable deformity and mobility of the nasal bones. Reduction of the nasal fracture is often performed with closed manipulation. Septal reconstruction may be necessary as well to provide an adequate nasal airway.

Soft tissue injuries should be repaired if present. Failure to repair nasal fracture deformity acutely may cause permanent cosmetic and functional deformity that ultimately requires reconstructive septorhinoplasty. Fractures of the nasal bones are often associated with injury to other midfacial and paranasal sinus structures, such as fractures of the maxilla, zygoma, ethmoid complex, and frontal bone. Because of the proximity to the orbit and cranial cavity, injury to the ocular adnexa, globe and optic nerve, brain, and meninges can occur. Cerebrospinal fluid leak is a common finding with significant midfacial trauma and comminution of the naso-ethmoid complex. This usually presents as persistent clear rhinorrhea and may require operative repair by reduction of the naso-ethmoid fracture, endoscopic transnasal patching, or craniotomy. Epistaxis seen with these injuries can be severe and may require prolonged anterior and posterior nasal packing for control. Failure of packing to adequately control bleeding suggests significant disruption of the nasal vascular supply and may require ligation of the ethmoidal and internal maxillary arteries or endovascular embolization to prevent continued hemorrhage.

Fractures of the upper jaw can cause significant cosmetic and functional deformity. Maxillary fractures cause malocclusion and difficulty with mastication and speech. The injuries are often associated with zygomatic bone fractures, which can cause diplopia, visual loss, enophthalmus, and facial deformity with flattening of the malar eminence. Management of these fractures involves alignment of the fracture with fixation by either wires or miniplates. Normal occlusal relationships must be established at the time of fixation to prevent secondary occlusal deformity. Loss of bone because of severe comminution can be addressed by immediate or secondary bone grafting to replace regions important for structural support. Fractures of the midface involving the maxilla and zygoma have been classified as Le Fort I, II, and III fractures. A Le Fort I fracture is a transverse maxillary fracture with the fractured segment containing the maxillary teeth, palate, and lower portions of the pterygoid process and maxillary sinus walls. A Le Fort II fracture is a pyramidal fracture in which the fracture line extends to include the nasal bones and frontal processes of the maxilla bilaterally. A Le Fort III fracture is known as a craniofacial dysjunction in which the entire maxillary, nasal, and zygomatic complex is separated from its attachment to the skull base. These are significant injuries and can present alone or in combination with other facial bony and soft tissue injuries. Open reduction and fixation is required to provide adequate repair. Determination of the type and extent of the fracture is based on physical examination with palpation of all injured regions as well as radiographic study.

CT scans are effective in delineating the extent and location of bony and soft tissue injuries.

Mandibular Fractures

Fractures of the mandible can occur in isolation or in conjunction with other midfacial injuries. The most common sites of fracture of the mandible include the parasymphyseal and angle regions. Often there is more than one fracture site in the mandible, depending on the direction and magnitude of the injuring force. Fracture of the mandible is associated with malocclusion, as the muscles of mastication exert forces that create displacement of the fractured segment of bone. Assessment of mandibular fracture is done by physical examination, with point tenderness, hematoma, and mobility noted at the fracture site. Radiographic imaging with panoramic mandibular x-rays and CT scanning is quite helpful in assessing the extent of injury. Treatment of mandibular fractures can be accomplished by several methods. Determination of the appropriate method depends to a large extent on the patient's age, overall medical condition, association of other facial injuries, and condition of the patient's dentition. In single, isolated, or easily reduced fractures in a patient with good dentition, interdental fixation with wiring of the mandibular to maxillary teeth may be all that is necessary. With multiple fractures, comminuted fractures, or fractures in association with other midfacial injuries, open reduction and internal fixation becomes necessary, usually with the use of plates and interdental fixation. The primary concerns of treatment are reestablishment of the occlusal relationships and adequate fixation and stabilization of the bone to allow normal healing.

Frontal Sinus Fractures

Fractures of the frontal sinus can occur in association with other midfacial injuries or in isolation. Fractures involving only the anterior table of the sinus can be repaired by open reduction and fixation of the fractured segments (Fig. 3). Those involving the posterior table or the region of the nasofrontal ducts requires open exploration with obliteration of the sinus cavity after removal of the mucosa. This is necessary in order to prevent the formation of mucoceles that may develop several years after the injury. Mucoceles can cause chronic infection as well as expansion into and destruction of the surrounding orbital and cranial bone. Obliteration of the sinus with implantation of abdominal fat after removal of the mucous membrane prevents mucocele formation.

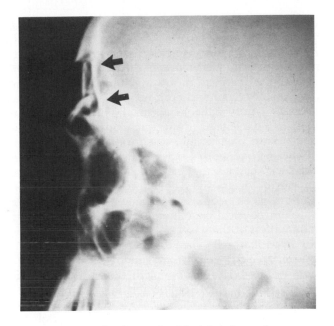

Figure 3. Lateral radiograph of facial skeleton demonstrating comminuted frontal sinus fracture involving only the anterior table (*arrows*). Repair can be accomplished by open reduction and fixation of the fragments.

NEOPLASMS

Structures of the head and neck are composed of the entire spectrum of tissue types derived from the three embryologic germ layers, the ectoderm, mesoderm, and endoderm, and from these a wide array of both benign and malignant tumors develop. The histology of these tumors is representative of the tissues of origin and may demonstrate, singularly or in combination, evidence of epithelial, osseous, neural, vascular, or endocrine features. The development of neoplasia in the head and neck is often associated with alterations in cosmesis and function. Because of the unique relationship of the head and neck to the external environment, tumors which develop in this region affect such important functions as sight, smell, taste, hearing, speech, mastication, and deglutition. Furthermore, extensive tumors may impact on adjacent structures such as the vasculature of the thorax and intracranial compartment, as well as involvement of the brain and the brainstem itself. For these reasons, management of head and neck neoplasms involves a multidisciplinary team approach with involvement by several specialists providing optimal care for the patient.

Benign lesions such as adenomas, hemangiomas, papillomas, chondromas, osteomas, neuromas, and fibromas have all been documented within the various regions of the head and neck. Similarly, malignant neoplasms develop that represent the counterparts to these benign tumors, including adenocarcinomas, chondro- and osteosarcomas, fibrosarcomas, and epidermoid carcinomas. Most of these neoplasms are relatively uncommon; however, their swift recognition and proper treatment means much to the patient. The symptoms of head and neck neoplasia depend on the precise location of the neoplasm and include otorrhea, otalgia, hoarseness, dysphagia, odynophagia, epistaxis, nasal obstruction, or sore throat. In addition, the specific finding of a mass in any region of the head and neck dictates that neoplasia be included in the differential diagnosis. The appropriate diagnosis of head and neck neoplasms is made after performing a thorough physical examination, including endoscopic examination of the nasal cavity, nasopharynx, larynx, and hypopharynx. This assessment, combined with appropriate radiographic imaging by such methods as computed tomography or magnetic resonance imaging, provides a basis for formulating an appropriate differential diagnosis. The definitive diagnosis depends on obtaining histologic or cytologic material for pathologic review. For many lesions of the head and neck, especially those located subcutaneously, a fine needle aspiration (FNA) often provides the diagnosis. A FNA biopsy should be the first step for diagnosis of any neck mass, as incisional biopsy may lead to contamination of surrounding soft tissues by tumor cells or may alter the approach to definitive therapy. For those lesions within the lining of the aerodigestive tract, a tissue biopsy of the lesion is usually sufficient to provide appropriate diagnosis.

Benign Neoplasms

Acoustic Neuroma

Acoustic neuromas are the most common neoplasms involving the base of the skull and account for approximately 7 per cent of all intracranial neoplasms. They are derived from Schwann cells and most commonly arise from the vestibular division of the eighth cranial nerve. These tumors produce symptoms of vertigo, tinnitus, and sensory neural hearing loss, with associated impairment of speech discrimination and loss of acoustic reflexes on audiometric and tympanometric testing. Diagnosis of these tumors is accomplished with brainstem auditory-evoked response testing, which shows increased latency of the neural response to sound transmitted through the eighth cranial nerve. Additionally, magnetic resonance imaging with gadolinium enhancement has been shown to be highly sensitive for detection of extremely small tumors. During their initial development acoustic neuromas are usually confined to the internal auditory meatus. As the tumor increases in size, it begins to protrude into the cerebellopontine angle and may progress to compression of the brainstem and additional cranial nerves. Treatment of these lesions requires microsurgical resection accomplished by one of three temporal bone approaches: translabyrinthine, retrosigmoid, or middle fossa. Selection of technique depends on the presence of useful hearing. For those patients who are too elderly or debilitated to undergo this type of procedure or for those patients with bilateral tumors or in an only-hearing ear with an acoustic neuroma, radiotherapy provided by a gamma knife approach may be utilized.

Glomus Tumors

Glomus tumors are neoplasms that arise from the paraganglionic chemoreceptor cells located throughout the body and are the second most common tumors of the skull base following acoustic neuroma. In the regions of the head and neck these highly specialized cells are located along the vasculature of the great vessels as well as in the mucosa of the upper aerodigestive tract and along many of the cranial nerves. The most common tumors in the head and neck arise in the region of the middle ear, jugular bulb, vagus nerve, and carotid body, and are known respectively as glomus tympanicum, glomus jugulare, glomus vagale, and carotid body tumors. Histologically they are composed of highly vascularized tissue surrounded by epithelioid cells and, depending on the location, may present with pulsatile tinnitus, otorrhea, vertigo, hearing loss, facial nerve paresis, or neck masses. True loss of neural function in those tumors involving cranial nerves is uncommon early in the disease, but may develop with continued growth of the lesion. The diagnosis depends on radiographic imaging that may demonstrate erosion of bone and surrounding structures with extension of the tumors intracranially through the skull base foramina. Arteriography is often useful for confirmation of the diagnosis. Although these neoplasms grow slowly, surgical resection is indicated to prevent prolonged growth with involvement of surrounding structures. When involvement of the base of the skull is present, resection usually includes mastoidectomy and cranial nerve dissection. For those lesions involving the carotid body, careful dissection off of the carotid artery is usually possible with preservation of the extracranial and intracranial blood flow. For patients unable to undergo surgical resection, radiation therapy may be used in an attempt to control the growth of these tumors.

Juvenile Nasopharyngeal Angiofibroma

Juvenile nasopharyngeal angiofibromas are vascular lesions that occur only in pubescent males, arise from the region of the basisphenoid, and may become quite extensive with involvement of the nasal cavity and surrounding paranasal sinuses. Continued growth often leads to involvement of the infratemporal fossa, orbit, and intracranial spaces by direct extension through the skull base foramina. Composed of a fibrous stroma with multiple vascular spaces, these tumors have sensitivity to androgens and rely on these hormones for continued growth. *Epistaxis*, the usual presentation for patients with juvenile nasopharyngeal angiofibroma, can be quite extensive and usually leads to the diagnosis of a mass in the nasopharynx. Confirmation of the diagnosis is usually made with a combination of computed tomography to evaluate the extent of the tumor, and angiography, which usually demonstrates a characteristic vascular blush. In most patients, the vascular supply of these tumors arises from the branches of the internal maxillary artery. Treatment involves complete surgical resection. Even with complete resection of all gross disease, recurrence rates may approach 20 per cent because of microscopic extension to surrounding soft tissues. The resection of these lesions is usually performed with either a transpalatal or transmaxillary approach with removal of soft tissue and involved bone. Preoperative treatment with antitestosterone therapy has been utilized to try to decrease the vascularity of the tumor with a resultant decrease in intraoperative blood loss. Arteriography with embolization is also helpful, and radiation therapy is effective in controlling further growth of recurring tumors or those that are quite extensive with a large intracranial component.

Papillomas

Squamous papillomas are common lesions involving the mucosal surfaces of the head and neck. Thought to be caused by papovavirus infection, they are most common in the nasal cavity and larynx where they appear as warty, exophytic growths. In the nasal cavity, they usually follow a benign course, and local excision is sufficient for cure. Papillomas of the larynx, although benign histologically and biologically, may produce significant sequelae. They often occur in infants and children who present with hoarseness and airway compromise and whose mothers may have had a papilloma of the cervix. Repeated therapy with direct laryngoscopy and laser excision often provides control until such time as the lesion can be ablated or spontaneous resolution occurs. Temporary control is obtained with interferon therapy, but this treatment does not cause long-term remission. Variations of these papillomatous lesions are seen, and in the nasal cavity an inverting papilloma may develop. It is benign histologically but can be quite aggressive, with local invasion and destruction of soft tissue and bone. The lesion most commonly arises from the lateral nasal

wall in the region of the maxillary and ethmoid sinuses, and treatment requires a complete resection with a transnasal or external approach to the sinus cavities. Because these lesions are associated in 5 to 10 per cent of patients with progression to invasive squamous cell carcinoma, careful histologic evaluation of the specimen should be performed. Similarly, occasional cases of invasive laryngeal papillomatosis have been reported, and most are associated with a component of invasive squamous cell carcinoma. Treatment involves wide resection with possible use of additional radiation therapy.

Malignant Neoplasms

Squamous cell carcinoma comprises greater than 90 per cent of all malignant tumors of the head and neck. It occurs in all sites of the head and neck, and although the exact mechanism for the development of the malignant phenotype is not completely understood, alcohol and tobacco abuse are definite etiologic factors. The clinical behavior of squamous cell carcinoma is, to a large extent, dependent on the site of origin of the primary tumor. Squamous carcinoma is capable of local invasion with extension to surrounding soft tissue, cartilage, and bone. Histologically, the tumors may demonstrate nests and sheets of invasive epithelial cells into surrounding stroma, with variations in degree of differentiation from that of a well differentiated malignancy that closely resembles normal epithelium to that of a poorly differentiated lesion. The use of immunohistochemistry to identify epithelial cell antigens can be quite helpful in differentiating poorly differentiated squamous cell carcinoma from other poorly differentiated malignancies such as lymphoma, melanoma, and sarcoma.

Metastatic spread of squamous cell carcinoma is most often to regional lymphatic nodes. It is common to find a cervical mass that is a lymph node metastasis in patients with squamous cell carcinoma of the upper aerodigestive tract. For those sites with a rich lymphatic supply such as the floor of the mouth, tongue, pharyngeal wall, nasopharynx, and supraglottic larynx, the rates of cervical metastasis can range from 40 to 70 per cent. The presence of cervical metastases does not correlate well with the size of the primary tumor, as even small lesions may present with regional metastases. Distant metastases are found more frequently, as improvements in treatment options prolong life, with between 8 and 20 per cent reported in patients with head and neck squamous cell carcinoma. Squamous cell carcinoma of the hypopharynx and esophagus have the highest rates of distant metastatic disease, with metastases to the lung, liver, and skeleton being most common.

Synchronous and metachronous second primary tumors are a significant risk in patients presenting with primary malignancies of the head and neck, especially squamous cell carcinoma. The presence of multiple areas in the aerodigestive tract affected by tobacco and alcohol increases the probability of additional tumors in other areas of the head and neck as well as in the tracheobronchial tree, lung parenchyma, and esophagus. Therefore, adequate work-up of most head and neck malignancies involves careful assessment of these other regions with radiographic studies and endoscopy under general anesthesia.

The process of staging head and neck cancer is designed to provide a means of predicting the behavior of a particular tumor and the probability for patient survival as well as a method of standardizing tumor documentation and treatment approaches. The TNM system following the criteria of the American Joint Committee on Cancer is used (Table 3). Estimates of tumor volume are accomplished either by actual measurement of tumor diameter, as for lesions of the oral cavity and oropharynx, or by delineating tumor extent to adjacent structures as for lesions of the larynx and nasopharynx. The presence of nodal metastases greatly effects patient outcome, and staging of nodal disease is based on the number, size, and location of the nodal metastases to either the ipsilateral, contralateral or both necks. By combining staging of the primary tumor and nodal metastases, an overall stage is determined. Increasing size of the primary tumor to T3 or T4 or the presence of nodal disease places the patient in an advanced stage category (stage III and IV). Recent investigation has sought to determine improved methods of cancer staging by taking into account such factors as genetic alteration and defects in immune function. At this point, however, other methods have not proven to be as useful in the clinical setting as the TNM system.

Therapy for squamous cell carcinoma of the head and neck involves a multimodality approach, especially for advanced stage lesions. Many T1 and T2

lesions are treated with equal success by primary radiotherapy or surgical resection alone. The decision for treatment takes into account morbidity of therapy and functional outcome, as well as patient preference. For advanced stage lesions, therapy is usually surgical resection followed by postoperative radiotherapy. Newer forms of management have been devised to attempt to preserve function of such structures as tongue, pharyngeal wall, and larynx by employing hyperfractionated radiation therapy alone or in combination with chemotherapy. Recent studies have suggested that this protocol may provide preservation of an organ such as the larynx with comparable survival outcome to that seen with total laryngectomy. Presently, the use of chemotherapy for squamous cell carcinoma of the head and neck is experimental, with most protocols involving the use of cisplatinum and 5-fluorouracil in some combination. Presently, there is no standard chemotherapeutic regimen used alone or in an adjuvant setting with radiotherapy and resection for squamous cell carcinoma of the head and neck.

The management of cervical lymph node metastases for squamous cell carcinoma of the head and neck is controversial, and the standard therapy for cervical lymph node disease has been the radical neck dissection. Originally, this procedure involved removal of all of the affected lymphatic tissues in the involved neck with the submandibular gland, sternocleidomastoid muscle, internal jugular vein, and spinal accessory nerve. Recent advances in surgical technique have led to modifications, and the radical neck dissection is now reserved for advanced nodal disease with large lymph nodes having extracapsular spread of tumor. In patients with no nodal involvement or lower staged nodal disease, modified neck dissections are performed, which provides equal survival outcome while improving the functional result of the operative procedure. In these procedures, attempts are made to preserve the sternocleidomastoid muscle, internal jugular vein, and spinal accessory nerve by themselves or in combination. Radiotherapy as the primary treatment for cervical metastases is effective in those patients staged N0 and N1. For nodes greater than 1 to 2 cm in diameter, the recommended therapeutic approach combines neck dissection with radiotherapy. In patients with multiple nodes, extracapsular spread, or gross invasion of surrounding soft tissue, postoperative radiotherapy is usually given following a neck dissection.

TABLE 3.   TNM SYSTEM FOR STAGING OF HEAD AND NECK CANCER*

Stage I	T1 N0 M0
Stage II	T2 N0 M0
Stage III	T3 N0 M0
	T1, T2, or T3 N1 M0
Stage IV	T4 N0 or N1 M0
	Any T N2 or N3 M0
	Any T Any N M1

*Adapted from Beahrs OH, et al [eds]: Manual for Staging of Cancer, ed 4. Philadelphia, American Joint Committee on Cancer, 1992, with permission.
Abbreviations:
   T = Primary tumor extent or size,
   N = Regional lymph node number, size, and location,
   M = Presence or absence of distant metastases.

Squamous Cell Carcinoma of the Skin

Squamous cell carcinoma occurring in the skin of the face is quite common and is usually associated with actinic damage following prolonged exposure to the sun. The most common sites for these lesions to develop are the external nose and the pinna, but all areas of the face and scalp may be involved. Usual treatment involves surgical excision, with pathologic assessment of the surgical margin to be certain that all tumor is resected. For extensive lesions of the pinna involving the external auditory canal, a lateral temporal bone resection is indicated followed by postoperative radiotherapy. Similar involvement of the skeletal structure of the nose, with involvement of the nasal cartilages or bones, requires wide resection often combined with radiotherapy. Adequate resection provides excellent control for most of these lesions.

Squamous Cell Carcinoma of the Oral Cavity

Squamous cell carcinoma comprises 95 per cent of all malignant lesions occurring in the oral cavity. These tumors may involve any of the subsites in the oral cavity including the lip, floor of the mouth, buccal mucosa, tongue, alveolar ridge, and palate. Because there is a rich lymphatic supply to this region, lymph node metastases are frequent. Lesions located in the midline of the palate, tongue, and floor of mouth are also at high risk for bilateral nodal metastases. The etiologic factors associated with oral cavity malignancy include tobacco and alcohol abuse, poor oral hygiene, use of chewing tobacco and snuff, and, with buccal carcinoma, beetle nut chewing. Treatment concerns in this area include maintenance of mastication, phonation, salivation, and respiration. Early stage lesions are often managed with excision or radiotherapy alone. Combined treatment with both modalities is often indicated for advanced stage tumors. These tumors often require extensive resection for complete extirpation, necessitating reconstruction with either skin grafts, local musculocutaneous flaps, distant pedicled musculocutaneous flaps, or microvascular free tissue transfer. Rehabilitation following extensive resection can be quite difficult, and adequate nutritional supplementation may require alternate modes of enteral feeding such as with a gastrostomy tube. Additionally, many patients require temporary diversion of the airway via tracheostomy.

Squamous Cell Carcinoma of the Pharynx

The pharynx is divided into three regions, the nasopharynx, oropharynx, and hypopharynx. The etiologic factors associated with oropharyngeal and hypopharyngeal carcinoma are similar to those for squamous cell carcinoma of the oral cavity. Patients with squamous cell carcinoma of the oropharynx and hypopharynx usually present with symptoms of sore throat, dysphagia, odynophagia, voice change, or otalgia on the side of the tumor. The tonsil and tonsillar fossa are the most common sites for squamous cell carcinoma of the pharynx. Tumors of the oropharynx can often become quite extensive, with involvement of the soft palate, base of tongue, and mandible. Treatment for these tumors requires either extensive resection with postoperative radiotherapy or experimental treatment schema with chemotherapy and radiotherapy in an attempt to preserve function. Hypopharyngeal carcinoma arises from the pyriform sinuses, posterior pharyngeal wall proximal to the esophagus, or the posterior cricoid mucosa and often involves the larynx. They may remain asymptomatic while small, often not detected until they are in the advanced stage. Treatment is resection with total laryngectomy and pharyngectomy and reconstruction with either pedicled gastric transposition or free jejunal microvascular transfer.

Nasopharyngeal carcinoma occurs in younger age groups, with an unusually high incidence among patients of Chinese ancestry. Squamous cell carcinoma of the nasopharynx has immunologic similarities to Burkitt's lymphoma and infectious mononucleosis. Epstein-Barr virus (EBV) titers are noted to be elevated in almost all patients with advanced lesions. EBV titer levels can be utilized to assess the response to therapy as well as to monitor for recurrent disease. These tumors are associated with a high incidence of cervical lymphatic metastases secondary to the rich lymphatic supply of the nasopharynx. Many patients present initially with a neck mass localized to the posterior cervical triangle, and because the nasopharyngeal mass causes eustachian tube obstruction, most present with a serous otitis media. For this reason, adults identified with unilateral otitis media unresponsive to routine antibiotic management should undergo nasopharyngeal examination to exclude the presence of nasopharyngeal carcinoma. Treatment for nasopharyngeal carcinoma involves primary radiotherapy to the nasopharynx and all cervical metastases. These lesions are extremely radiosensitive and usually respond completely to the radiotherapy. Persistent nodal disease can be managed with neck dissection.

Squamous Cell Carcinoma of the Larynx

Squamous cell carcinoma is the most common malignancy involving the laryngeal mucosa and can arise from any part of the laryngeal mucous membrane and is often preceded by the presence of leukoplakia. Most patients present with the symptom of persistent hoarseness, often associated with otalgia and dysphagia. Initial evaluation for laryngeal carcinoma involves the use of flexible fiberoptic laryngoscopy. Findings of laryngeal ulceration or mass, especially in the presence of impaired vocal cord mobility, necessitates biopsy of the lesion for pathologic confirmation of the diagnosis. The biologic behavior of laryngeal cancer is dependent on the site of origin within the larynx. Tumors confined to the true vocal cords rarely metastasize to the cervical lymph nodes, whereas tumors of the supraglottic and infraglottic portions of the larynx have a 35 to 40 per cent incidence of mid- to low-jugular nodal metastases. Early stage lesions, T1 or T2, which are localized to the glottis, can be treated with an 85 to 90 per cent cure rate by either primary radiotherapy or surgical resection. Surgical management for these lesions involves endoscopic laser excision or partial laryngectomy. For more extensive tumors, such as T3 or T4 lesions, a combined therapeutic approach is indicated. Standard therapy includes surgical resection with postoperative radiotherapy, although newer treatment regimens incorporate chemotherapy with cisplatinum and 5-fluorouracil in conjunction with radiotherapy to try to preserve the larynx. Patients who either fail or recur following this therapy or those with extensive tumors with cartilaginous invasion usually require total laryngectomy. Vocal rehabilitation can be undertaken by the use of an electrolarynx, tracheoesophageal prosthesis, or esophageal speech.

Adenocarcinoma

Tumors of glandular epithelial origin are relatively uncommon in the head and neck. They may arise from major and minor salivary gland tissue as well as the submucosal mucus secreting glands located throughout the upper aerodigestive tract. Adenocarcinomas can develop in the middle ear space, nasal cavity, nasopharynx, palate, and larynx. Etiologic factors associated with the development of adenocarcinoma in the nasal cavity and paranasal sinus include exposure to wood dust and nickel compounds, and some salivary tumors have recently been postulated to develop from excessive use of diagnostic x-rays in the region of the oral cavity. These tumors usually behave quite aggressively and have a propensity for lymphatic and hematogenous spread. The finding of adenocarcinoma in a cervical lymph node, especially in the lower jugular chain or supraclavicular region, should prompt a search for a primary site below the clavicles. Adenocarcinomas of the lung, esophagus, stomach, intestines, and genitourinary organs can metastasize to the cervical region. Primary head and neck adenocarcinomas are usually treated with surgical resection followed by radiation therapy. Even with aggressive therapy, local recurrence and distant metastases unfortunately frequently occur.

Esthesioneuroblastoma

Malignant neoplasms arising from the olfactory epithelium in the superior vault of the nasal cavity are also known as esthesioneuroblastomas or olfactory neuroblastomas and behave aggressively with extension into the surrounding paranasal sinuses and erosion superiorly through the cribriform plate into the anterior cranial fossa. No definite etiologic factors have been associated with these tumors. They have been identified in patients of all ages, and usually present with nasal congestion, anosmia, and epistaxis. The diagnosis requires adequate radiographic imaging to determine the full extent of the tumor, along with diagnostic biopsy. Pathologic determination must exclude such neoplasms as melanoma, lymphoma, and undifferentiated carcinoma. Therapy for these lesions involves a combined approach with surgical resection and radiation therapy, with possible chemotherapy for extensive lesions extending beyond the confines of the nasal cavity and paranasal sinuses. The use of a craniofacial resection, with a combined craniotomy and transfacial resection, is advocated for en bloc tumor resection.

Melanoma

Melanoma of the head and neck may occur in both cutaneous and mucosal sites. These lesions, like those in the extremity and trunk, often behave in a capricious manner with a high incidence of lymphatic and distant metastases. The treatment usually involves wide local resection with reconstruction. Postoperative radiotherapeutic protocols have been investigated in an attempt to improve local recurrence rates, and immunotherapeutic methods aimed at augmenting the body's immune response against melanoma are presently being investigated.

Sarcomas

Sarcomatous tumors of the soft tissues and bones are relatively uncommon but can occur. They usually behave quite aggressively, with a high incidence of distant metastases. Rhabdomyosarcoma, the most common in children, is often identified in the nasal cavity and middle ear. Treatment presently involves a multimodality approach with surgical resection in combination with chemotherapy. Survival rates have improved with some of the newer chemotherapeutic regimens as well as with the ability to provide greater clearance of tumor by resection and reconstruction.

Salivary Tumors

Tumors arising in the major and minor salivary glands of the head and neck comprise a wide variety of histologic types. Whereas most parotid neoplasms are benign, tumors located in the sublingual gland and minor salivary glands of the oral cavity and pharynx are usually malignant. Benign tumors include pleomorphic adenoma, which is the most common lesion in children and adults, papillary cystadenoma lymphomatosum (Warthin's tumor), oncocytoma, monomorphic adenomas, hemangioma, and benign lymphoepithelial lesions. Malignant tumors are usually divided into low-grade and high-grade malignancies. Low-grade tumors, which include acinic cell carcinoma and low-grade mucoepidermoid carcinoma, usually present as solitary mass lesions in the parotid, submandibular, or minor salivary glands, and are readily controlled by surgical resection. High-grade salivary malignancies, which include malignant mixed tumor, high-grade mucoepidermoid carcinoma, carcinoma *ex* pleomorphic adenoma, adenoid cystic carcinoma, adenocarcinoma, squamous cell carcinoma, and undifferentiated carcinomas, are much more aggressive. These tumors have a significant incidence of cervical lymphatic metastases and facial nerve invasion with paralysis. A neck mass localized to the periauricular or submandibular region that is associated with pain and neural dysfunction, such as hypesthesia of the tongue or facial nerve paralysis, should be considered to be a malignant salivary neoplasm until proven otherwise. Diagnosis has been aided by the use of fine needle aspiration cytology. For benign tumors or low-grade malignancies of the parotid gland, superficial parotidectomy is the treatment of choice. With evidence of surrounding tissue invasion or for high-grade parotid malignancies, a total parotidectomy with preservation of the facial nerve, if possible, is indicated. Direct invasion of the facial nerve requires resection of the involved portion with immediate reconstruction by nerve graft and neurorrhaphy. Postoperative radiation therapy increases the locoregional control rates in high-grade salivary malignancies. Chemotherapy has not been shown to be of benefit in the management of these lesions, except for palliative therapy.

REFERENCES

Alberti PW, Ruben RJ: Otologic Medicine and Surgery. New York, Churchill Livingstone, 1988.

American Academy of Otolaryngology-Head and Neck Surgery Foundation: Common Problems of the Head and Neck Region. Philadelphia, WB Saunders Company, 1992.

Batsakis JG: Tumors of the Head and Neck. Clinical and Pathological Considerations, ed 2. Baltimore, Williams & Wilkins, 1979.

Cummings CW, Fredrickson JM, Harker LA, Krause CJ, Schuller DE: Otolaryngology-Head and Neck Surgery, vol 1–4, ed 2. St. Louis, Mosby, 1993.

Eisele DW: Complications in Head and Neck Surgery. St. Louis, Mosby, 1993.

Snow JB Jr: Surgical Disorders of the ears, nose, paranasal sinuses, pharynx, and larynx. *In* Sabiston DC Jr (ed): Textbook of Surgery: The Biological Basis of Modern Surgical Practice, ed 14. Philadelphia, WB Saunders Company, 1991, pp 1187–1208.

Thawley SE, Panje WR: Comprehensive Management of Head and Neck Tumors, vol 1 and 2. Philadelphia, WB Saunders Company, 1987.

40
NEUROSURGERY

DENNIS A. TURNER, M.D.

GENERAL PRINCIPLES

The brain and nervous system remained an enigmatic region during the 19th century and proved a challenge to surgical treatment. Refinement in cerebral localization, hemostasis (particularly the Bovie cautery), asepsis, anesthesia, and development of the craniotomy at the close of the 19th century led to the evolution of neurosurgical approaches and the elucidation of basic principles that remain in use today. These basic principles include clinical, radiographic, and physiologic localization of lesions, and determination of the subsequent operative field, including the concept of intracranial masses and their decompression for symptomatic relief.

One critical feature is the *neurologic examination* to localize lesions. As nervous system localization has evolved with increased knowledge of neuroanatomy, common neurosurgical syndromes have been defined that point to specific regions of involvement. These syndromes include level of consciousness with brainstem lesions, lateralization between cerebral hemispheres, and spinal localization. Such definitions are commonly used for both localization and prognosis, possibly indicating either reversible or irreversible damage to focal areas of the central nervous system (CNS). The neurologic examination is usually divided into subsections to reflect its use as a localizing probe (Table 1).

The categories of the examination follow the functional aspects of regions of the nervous system, including the cerebral hemispheres, deep nuclei (such as the basal ganglia), diencephalon (thalamus and hypothalamus), brainstem, cerebellum, and spinal cord. In compromised situations such as the comatose patient, certain limited aspects of the neurologic examination become critical, including the response to verbal and painful stimuli, best motor response, the pupils, and respiration. These critical aspects are grouped into the Glasgow Coma Scale, which is commonly used to rank patients for prognosis and outcome following traumatic injury (Table 2). The neurologic examination remains the most helpful and sensitive technique to follow changes in function of the nervous system, whereas adjuncts such as *intracranial pressure* (ICP) recordings are considerably less sensitive. Unfortunately, the neurologic examination can be clouded by medication and anesthesia, leaving only alternative techniques, such as ICP recording, electrical monitoring, and radiologic scans to infer the status of functional levels. However, these alternative techniques are most useful in concert with the neurologic examination to point to changes in levels of functioning and ultimate prognosis.

Another major neurosurgical principle is the concept of the *intracranial mass* and shifts in the position of the brain, which create secondary pressure on initially uninvolved regions. This form of secondary pressure may cause irreversible changes, but may be differentiated from intrinsic primary damage of the brain, implying functional recovery if the mass and

TABLE 1. NEUROLOGIC EXAMINATION

Cerebral function, including mental status, level of consciousness, and cerebral localization
Cranial nerve examination, including special sensory reflexes
Motor examination, compared to gravity resistance (0–5 scale)
Sensory modalities, including aspects of light touch, vibration, proprioception, and nociception
Reflexes, including brainstem, myotatic, superficial or cutaneous, and pathologic
Cerebellar function, including tone and coordination across joints
Gait, including tandem walking

TABLE 2. GLASGOW COMA SCALE (GCS)

Eye Opening (E)
Spontaneous	4
To speech	3
To pain only	2
No eye opening	1

Best Motor Response (M)
Obeys commands appropriately	6
Localizes to stimulation	5
Withdraws to stimulation	4
Abnormal flexion response	3
Abnormal extension response	2
No motor response	1

Best Verbal Response (V)
Oriented and appropriate	5
Confused conversation	4
Inappropriate words	3
Incomprehensible sounds	2
No verbal response	1

*Total score = sum of eye opening + best motor response + best verbal response (minimum score = 3).

secondary pressure can be surgically relieved in a timely manner. This principle applies particularly to tumors and traumatic hematomas. If such masses are unrelieved, irreversible pressure may ensue due to critical herniation of the brain through fixed dural and cranial apertures, particularly the tentorial notch and the foramen magnum. However, increased intracranial pressure alone is not dangerous in the same sense, as long as there is no significant shift and the cerebral perfusion pressure (mean arterial pressure minus mean intracranial pressure) remains at an acceptable level (> 55 to 60 mm Hg). In benign intracranial hypertension (where a tumor has been excluded and ventricular enlargement has not occurred), intracranial pressures as high as 50 to 55 mm Hg may be well tolerated, except for papilledema and secondary retinal changes, as long as the systemic blood pressure remains elevated to maintain cerebral perfusion pressure. Thus, there is no "absolute" dangerous level of ICP, but shifts cause secondary problems, such as herniation and *cerebrospinal fluid* (CSF) loculation at the ventricular and cisternal level, beginning a vicious cycle that leads to irreversible herniation. This cycle may sometimes be detected by ICP recordings, particularly if the trend of the ICP and the ease of ICP control are used as the critical factors rather than the mean ICP alone.

Operations on the nervous system are rarely exploratory, as the quality of contemporary neuroradiology together with neurologic localization almost always leads to precise localization of a suspected lesion. Thus, operative procedures are usually carefully designed around imaging studies, including computed tomography (CT) and magnetic resonance imaging (MRI) scans for both cranial and spinal diagnosis with myelogram procedures for further spinal diagnosis.

These studies are low in risk, can be rapidly obtained, with such a high yield and resolution (within a few millimeters) that only rarely do patients not have proper diagnosis and localization. However, it may be difficult at times to relate a lesion on one of these studies to an exact localization because of variable scanner angle and positioning; therefore, standard radiologic studies may also be required for confirmation of the level and position. Such detailed studies frequently lead to consultation for the presence of asymptomatic abnormalities, which would not otherwise have been detected. Such asymptomatic lesions may lead to a difficult dilemma, because the risk of surgical treatment may outweigh the risk of spontaneous pathologic changes, as, for example, with berry aneurysms and arteriovenous malformations.

Intraoperative considerations are also determined by the neurosurgical anatomy and procedure. Many nervous system procedures can be performed under local anesthesia, particularly if the compromised function of the region necessitates intraoperative testing to avoid further deterioration. Careful neuroanesthesia is important for those who may suffer deterioration from herniation of an intracranial mass at the time of induction of anesthesia. Operative positioning may often be complex, due to the entry point to the nervous system, such as the posterior fossa. Careful hemostasis is critical in all brain and spinal cord operations to avoid the occurrence of hematomas. Wounds are closed in layers for both hemostasis and closure of the dead space, and the dura is always closed if possible, even with a patch of fascia or other internal material, to avoid later infection and leakage of CSF.

Most operations on the nervous system can be placed in a few general categories. A *craniotomy* is usually performed for supratentorial procedures, such as for tumor resection. This procedure involves a scalp flap designed around the lesion to ensure access and blood supply, an opening of the skull and the dura if needed, and subsequent access to the intracranial contents. Such a craniotomy involves either a *free flap* or an *osteoplastic flap*, the difference being whether or not the muscle is left attached to the skull for vascular supply. The posterior fossa is a much smaller region and is defined by the large transverse venous sinuses superiorly and the foramen magnum inferiorly. Due to this small size and increased risk of tearing the dura, a *craniectomy* or bone removal without replacement is usually performed. Other approaches to the base of the skull are often used, an example being a *transsphenoidal pituitary approach* through the sphenoid sinus. Spinal operations usually involve either a posterior *laminectomy* or an anterior approach when feasible (such as in the cervical spine). Additionally, posterolateral and anterolateral approaches have been developed for the lumbar and thoracic spine, and for the treatment of fractures, tumors, and infections that involve the anterior aspect of the spinal cord. These spinal operations may often be combined with some form of stabilization and fusion to assure mechanical stability postoperatively.

Adjunct techniques that aid in the monitoring, diagnosis, and treatment of nervous system disease include recording of ICP, performed using an intracerebroventricular cannula placed through the frontal bone, or lumbar CSF drains performed through a lumbar puncture. For example, CSF leaks from basilar skull fractures may often be treated with a temporary lumbar CSF drain to decrease the CSF pressure and allow a better inherent seal to form around the fracture with healing. The *electroencephalogram* (EEG) is used to document seizures and regional damage, and the electromyogram and nerve conduction velocities (EMG/NCV) can be monitored for nerve and muscle changes. Peripheral nerve procedures require electrical testing for adequacy of nerve function and localization of abnormalities and can be obtained by electromyographic and nerve conduction studies. Many of these studies may also be extended into the operating room for intraoperative guidance, including ultrasound for localization of lesions, intraoperative electrical monitoring of nervous system function, electrocorticogram for surface EEG recordings of the brain, and other aspects of physiologic monitoring.

CONGENITAL MALFORMATIONS AND DISORDERS OF CSF CIRCULATION

Congenital malformations represent a diverse group of abnormalities of the brain and spinal cord. The severity of these abnormalities may range from anencephaly, in which only a remnant of brain exists and which leads to early postnatal death, to milder anomalies such as occult spinal dysraphism. Many developmental anomalies do not become apparent until postnatal growth. An example is suture growth leading to craniosynostosis. Thus, congenital abnormalities of the nervous system represent a wide range of defects that can be detected at a number of different intrauterine, postnatal, childhood, and adulthood time points. The range of problems encountered include: (1) various types of cranial and spinal developmental abnormalities (such as Chiari malformations, syringomyelia, and myelomeningocele); (2) hydrocephalus, such as that due to aqueductal stenosis; and (3) other bony abnormalities, such as wedge vertebra and arachnoid cysts at various levels of the neuraxis.

Spinal dysraphism occurs very early in the development of the fetus, prior to the time at which pregnancy can be diagnosed (first 3 to 4 weeks), and prophylaxis must be made on a routine basis in women of childbearing age. Current concepts include a number of toxic states that may increase the risk of dysraphism, such as hypervitaminosis A. Exogenous B vitamins are currently recommended in mothers at high risk of conceiving offspring with dysraphism. The severity and level of the dysraphism varies from cranial regions (anencephaly and encephalocele formation) to low spinal areas (syringomyelia and diastematomyelia) (Fig. 1). Generally these defects are related to defects in neural tube closure and/or detachment of the neural tube from overlying epithelial structures. Severe defects appear early in life, but more subtle defects, particularly the occult spinal forms, may not appear until adulthood. The latter is particularly true of such entities as tethered cord, which may express itself as decreased spinal cord function in early adulthood. The more severe defects, particularly those with cutaneous abnormalities, may require surgical closure or other treatment in the first few postnatal days due to the high likelihood of meningitis and other critical infections. Likewise, the associated hydrocephalus may require CSF diversion at an early time if the head is rapidly expanding. Defects associated with later worsening of either brain or spinal cord function may often be best diagnosed with an MRI scan, because all elements can be visualized and the very convenient sagittal plane may be imaged.

Surgical treatment of cranial and spinal dysraphism involves the principles of: (1) stabilizing the neural elements and preventing further compression or stretch such as untethering the spinal cord, (2) closing the dura to prevent CSF leaks and/or secondary infections, and (3) adequately closing the fascia and subcutaneous tissues for future strength. For example, the closure of a meningomyelocele involves gently dissecting the neural placode, the remnant of the spinal cord that had not closed correctly, from the subcutaneous tissues, finding the dural plane and closing it with a patch if necessary, and identifying the remaining bony elements and fascia for a sturdy closure over the dura. Treatment of an encephalocele involves truncating the often damaged brain within the encephalocele sac and closing both the dural defect and the bony defect to prevent reherniation of contents. Inadequate CSF absorption or defects in CSF circulation, such as aqueductal stenosis, requires either an internal CSF shunt, draining ventricular CSF into the cisterna magna at the foramen magnum or, preferably, an external CSF shunt with drainage into the right atrium or the peritoneal cavity.

Hydrocephalus implies an abnormality of CSF circulation, either through an obstruction to flow at some level or through decreased absorption. Many of the situations causing hydrocephalus and increased ventricular size are congenital, such as aqueductal stenosis, in which the aqueduct is either narrowed or

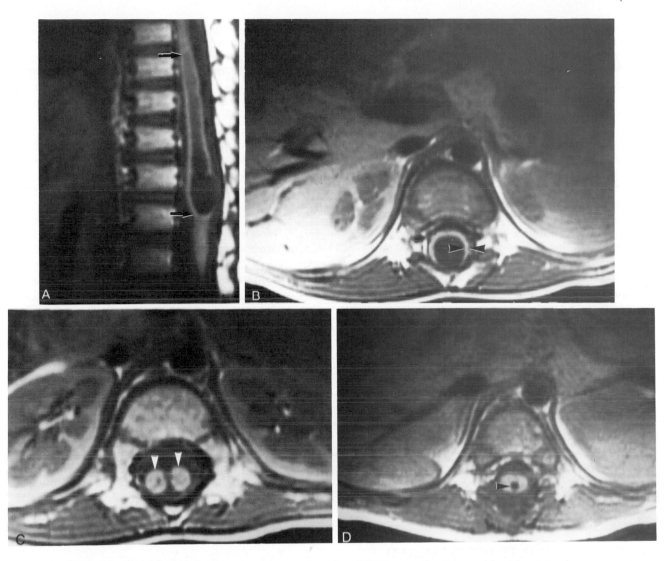

Figure 1. A midsagittal magnetic resonance imaging (MRI) scan of a 3-year-old with minimal neu-rologic difficulties. *A,* The large syrinx within the spinal cord is apparent (*arrows*). *B,* Axial image through the lower portion of the syrinx. The massive enlargement of the syrinx is surrounded by the rim of spinal cord (*arrowheads*). *C,* A somewhat caudal axial section below the syrinx demonstrating diastematomyelia with the two cut sections of the spinal cord seen on end (*arrow*). *D,* Postoperative axial MRI with total collapse of the syrinx cavity around a hollow tube (*arrowhead*) connecting the syrinx with the subarachnoid space. (From Oakes WJ: Congenital Abnormalities. *In* Sabiston DC Jr [ed]: Textbook of Surgery: The Biological Basis of Modern Surgical Practice, ed 14. Philadelphia, WB Saunders Company, 1991, p 1273, with permission.)

forked and imperforate. Mild cases may lead to some CSF flow and may not become symptomatic until early adulthood, at which time greatly enlarged ven-tricles are noted on CT scanning (often with an en-larged cranium, indicating childhood origin). Other types of hydrocephalus are acquired, including that caused by tumors or scarring, which prevent the flow of CSF from lateral to third to fourth ventricle, or at

the exit from the fourth ventricle into the subarach-noid space. These types of symptomatic hydrocephalus are routinely treated by shunting of CSF from the cra-nial ventricles or the lumbar intrathecal space, using a valve system that permits overflow of CSF.

Commonly, however, the CSF absorption pathways are disturbed, such as by infection or subarachnoid hemorrhage, without any more obvious form of obstruction. The pore size of CSF absorption channels at the arachnoid villi are of necessity smaller than blood cells, to prevent the backup of venous blood into CSF and to allow a one-way channel from CSF at higher pressure into veins at slightly lower pressure. Thus, red blood cells effectively block these pores and lead to outflow obstruction, requiring months to resolve. This type of hydrocephalus may demonstrate clearly enlarged ventricles with symptoms, but at the time of diagnosis the mean pressure of the CSF may actually be in the normal range. This is termed *normal pressure hydrocephalus* (NPH). Both increased tension on the ventricular walls associated with dilation (but decreased luminal pressure) and the slow improvement in absorption capability have acted to alter pressure. However, a CSF shunt may often help in terms of symptomatic improvement in NPH patients, with the primary symptoms being ataxia, incontinence, and dementia. Rarely does a CSF shunt lead to improvement in dementia.

Another unusual manifestation of decreased absorption of CSF is benign intracranial hypertension, previously called *pseudotumor cerebri*. This syndrome usually occurs in young females and causes a resting intracranial pressure greater than 25 to 30 mm Hg. The cerebral perfusion pressure is often maintained by a secondary systemic hypertension. Because the brain is also "stiff," the ventricles do not dilate and may often be observed as very small. There are usually no cerebral symptoms, but papilledema commonly follows and the major morbidity lies in blindness or scotoma from papilledema. Treatment consists of a CSF shunt if the pressure is not easily treated by osmotic agents, or intermittent therapeutic lumbar punctures.

SPONTANEOUS INTRACRANIAL AND INTRASPINAL HEMORRHAGE

Spontaneous hemorrhage within a particular anatomic space in the head or spine often provides clues concerning the origin or nature of the hemorrhage. Likewise, the nature of the space determines consequences of the bleeding and the actions required to contain or remove the blood. From superficial to deep, the anatomic spaces involved are shown in Table 3. Spontaneous hemorrhage in the subgaleal space often occurs in the neonate at birth and is termed a *cephalohematoma*. Rarely does this require evacuation, as the blood is absorbed with time. *Epidural* and *subdural* hemorrhage are most commonly associated with trauma, and hemorrhage into these spaces usually forms a mass requiring evacuation. However, *subarachnoid* hemorrhage is usually from rupture of a large intracranial vessel (or from pial oozing in trauma) and rarely forms a mass, since the blood can spread freely to the spinal compartment. *Parenchymal* hemorrhages may often occur spontaneously and form a mass leading to brain shifts. However, *intraventricular* hemorrhage can spread within the CSF space and is often due to rupture of a parenchymal hemorrhage into a ventricle. Spontaneous hemorrhage most often occurs in the subarachnoid and parenchymal spaces.

Subarachnoid hemorrhage often occurs with the spontaneous rupture of *berry aneurysms*, which develop in weak areas at the bifurcation of major intracranial vessels at the base of the brain (Fig. 2). All major vessels must penetrate the subarachnoid space (which normally contains CSF) to reach the brain parenchyma, and thus, the rupture of an aneurysm effectively permits the full arterial pressure to reach the CSF space through free release of blood. Such a rupture can often only be contained if the intracranial pressure approaches the arterial pressure, thus decreasing the cerebral perfusion pressure (CPP) (the mean arterial pressure minus the mean ICP) to near zero. This period of stagnant arterial flow leads to the extremely high mortality (~50 per cent) of a major subarachnoid hemorrhage due to brain anoxia. If a patient survives such a hemorrhage, a cerebral angiogram is performed to identify the location of the berry aneurysm. If the patient is sufficiently stable for an operation, clip ligation of the aneurysm should be considered. This operation effectively prevents further bleeding from the aneurysm but does not in itself improve the patient's neurologic condition, as this requires subsequent recovery of the brain. One consequence of significant blood in the subarachnoid space is that a secondary form of vasospasm occurs, usually with a delay of 5 to 7 days following the hemorrhage. There are numerous hypotheses regarding the etiology of this vasospasm, but one intriguing idea is that access of the CSF to the large arterial vessel wall becomes blocked by the hemorrhage, which lines the outer surface of the vessel. Since intracranial arteries are without vasa vasorum, this blockage leads in effect to vessel ischemia, particularly of the media layer, which may comprise much of the destructive changes in the media with this form of vasospasm.

The treatment of subarachnoid hemorrhage is initially aimed at the prevention of further hemorrhage, which is very likely during the first 48 to 72 hours. During the early period, the vessel wall may be susceptible to treatment with calcium channel antagonists to prevent vasospasm, and nimodipine is currently in clinical use. Pharmacologic approaches to the prevention of *delayed* vasospasm have also focused on the use of such calcium channel antagonists. The blood pressure should be well controlled, and activities such as excitement and straining at the stool should be avoided if the aneurysm is not clipped. During the later period when the possibility of vasospasm is

TABLE 3.   HEMORRHAGE INTO CRANIAL AND SPINAL SPACES

Name of Space (Superficial to Deep):	Type of Hemorrhage
Scalp and subgalea (between the pericranium and galea)	Cephalohematoma
Bone and diploe of the skull	Intradiploic hematoma
Epidural space (between the skull and the dura)	Epidural hematoma
Subdural or intradural space	Subdural hematoma
Subarachnoid space (between the arachnoid and the pia)	Subarachnoid hemorrhage
Parenchyma of the brain (deep to the pia)	Parenchymal hematoma
Intraventricular space (within the cerebral ventricles)	Intraventricular hemorrhage

higher, the cerebral perfusion pressure may be maintained through hypervolemic hypertensive therapy, with monitoring by a Schwann-Ganz catheter. If this fails and neurologic symptoms progress due to vascular narrowing and decreased focal cerebral perfusion, limited success has been achieved with direct transluminal angioplasty of the cerebral arteries involved, including the middle cerebral or anterior cerebral vessels.

A major limitation of therapy for berry aneurysms is the severe consequences of the initial subarachnoid hemorrhage. Occasionally, a patient may experience a *sentinel* hemorrhage, with a severe headache but without neurologic deficits, and at this point, a major deficit may be avoided by early, aggressive evaluation and treatment. Many of these early warning hemorrhages are accompanied by the same severe headache, often described by the patient as "the worst headache of my life." Treatment requires effective triage, often in a busy emergency room setting where further evaluation may not be pursued as it should be. Thus, earlier detection of *symptomatic* berry aneurysms may prevent much of the morbidity associated with the hemorrhage. However, most aneurysms detected in asymptomatic patients cause fewer problems than those that have previously been associated with a hemorrhage. The range is 1.5 to 2.0 per cent annually for likelihood of hemorrhage. Thus, occasionally the prophylactic clipping of an asymptomatic aneurysm may be recommended, especially if the aneurysm is large, lobulated, or otherwise appears likely to rupture.

Parenchymal hemorrhage is often spontaneous and may occur due to a congenital lesion, such as an *arteriovenous malformation* (AVM), amyloid deposits,

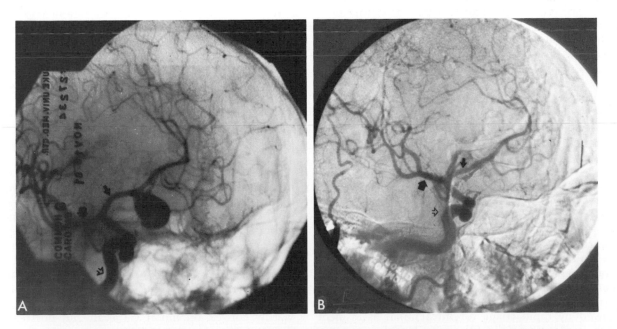

Figure 2.   *A*, Oblique view of a right carotid angiogram demonstrating an aneurysm originating at the anterior communicating artery. *B*, The same angiographic view following surgical ligation of the aneurysm. (From Friedman AH, Wilkins RH: Spontaneous intracranial and intraspinal hemmorhage. *In* Sabiston DC Jr [ed]: Textbook of Surgery: The Biological Basis of Modern Surgical Practice, ed 14. Philadelphia, WB Saunders Company, 1991, p 1248, with permission.)

vessel changes, or various acquired disorders. Hypertension may predispose to both deep (in the basal ganglia or thalamus) and superficial hemorrhages (in the superficial cerebral cortex or cerebellum). These hemorrhages require evacuation only if they lead to severe brain shifts and have a significant mass effect, as intrinsic brain destruction from the hemorrhage is rarely improved by surgical evacuation. Arteriovenous malformations often lead to further hemorrhages, and the removal of these lesions is usually recommended if feasible, in accordance with the location, size, and possible deficits that follow removal. Unless neoplasm is suspected to have led to the hemorrhage or if an AVM is present, the blood resorbs over time, and the main role of surgical evacuation is to relieve a mass effect to avert significant brain herniation during the early phase after the hemorrhage. Additional abnormalities leading to spontaneous hemorrhage include mycotic aneurysms, which occur with direct infection of the arterial wall, and development of a pseudoaneurysm, which may rupture secondarily. Other unusual etiologies for hemorrhage include cavernous and venous angiomas and occult lesions that do not appear on imaging studies.

The treatment of AVMs includes a number of alternatives in addition to direct surgical excision, with the goal being complete obliteration of the direct connection between one or more arteries and draining veins. Alternative treatments include stereotactic radiosurgery for AVMs less than 40 mm in size and particularly those that are in deep areas and cannot be easily excised. Additional treatment includes embolization by the intravascular route, usually combined with surgical resection to effect a cure. Such embolization may greatly decrease the vascularity, leading to an easier resection of the lesion. The operative excision of AVMs is one of the most challenging and formidable neurosurgical procedures, because of the abnormal vessels and the need to preserve functioning brain immediately around the periphery of the lesion.

CRANIOCEREBRAL AND SPINAL INJURIES

Injuries to the brain and spinal cord often involve bony trauma to the skull or the spine. The damage to the nervous system cannot be assessed adequately until systemic stabilization is achieved, including control of the airway and the circulation. Such stabilization is followed by rapid triage for intracranial assessment and treatment, especially if the neurologic function appears to be declining. Current practice involves rapid neurologic screening and, often, emergency CT scan, to determine whether an intracranial mass is developing. Often these masses require time to accumulate

and become apparent on CT scanning, with an evolution of abnormalities over the first few hours after injury. The rapid evaluation of the possibility of nervous system injury is required in the emergency room, and the changes occurring in the neurologic examination are critical. Observation over the first 24 to 48 hours may reveal latent injuries not evident initially.

A number of tissue planes can be involved with serious head injury, as shown in Table 3. Scalp lacerations, cephalohematomas, and linear skull fractures are common following head injuries and usually require only local care and débridement. However, penetrating and/or compound skull injuries, which involve contamination of the intracranial contents with breach of the dura, require exploration for débridement of the brain and closure of the dura and scalp. The purpose of such débridement is to prevent both superficial and deep infection, secondary brain abscess, and meningitis. Unlike the dural lining along the cranial vault, which is very tough and elastic, the dura along the base of the skull is thin and adherent to the bone. Whereas *linear skull fractures* of the vault may lead to a stripping of the dura away from the skull and the development of an epidural hematoma, *basilar skull fractures* often cause tearing of the dura, with a subsequent leak of CSF into a sinus, such as the frontal or the mastoid sinus. This type of CSF leak usually seals over time with conservative management. However, these fractures are a common cause of persistent CSF leaks and recurrent meningitis, and surgical repair is indicated in these instances, usually by craniotomy to seal the leak from the inside.

Common intracranial masses include epidural hematomas, subdural hematomas, and primary parenchymal injuries, which can involve cerebral contusions, shear injury of the white matter, and direct injury to the brainstem. The formation of an epidural hematoma requires the dura to be stripped away from the skull with development of a space permitting epidural bleeding and the progressive formation of a mass (Fig. 3). This is a classic situation in which a *lucid interval* may occur after the injury, during which time the patient appears clear but then rapidly deteriorates, requiring urgent evacuation of the hematoma to prevent herniation and irreversible damage. Acute subdural hematomas occur over a wide area of the hemisphere, often from avulsion of a bridging vein from the cortex to the dura, and may be associated with either cerebral contusions or nearly normal cortex. Such acute subdural hematomas appear outwardly convex on initial CT scan and possess high density (white appearance) with a significant shift (Fig. 4). However, these may increase in size over 10 to 14 days to become lens-shaped chronic subdural hematomas, which are either similar density to the brain or lower density (dark appearance).

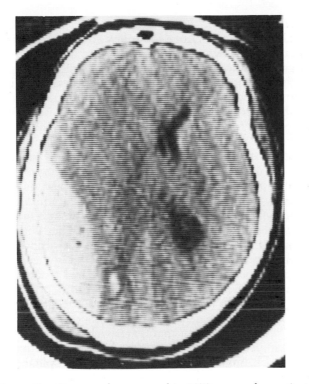

Figure 3. Computed tomographic (CT) scan of a patient who suffered a traumatic epidural hematoma. Note the shift of the ventricles off of the midline. (From Friedman AH: Craniocerebral injuries. *In* Sabiston DC Jr [ed]: Textbook of Surgery: The Biological Basis of Modern Surgical Practice, ed 14. Philadelphia, WB Saunders Company, 1991, p 1256, with permission.)

Parenchymal contusions may often coalesce from "salt and pepper" areas of hemorrhage into large intracerebral hematomas, and evacuation is required if a sufficient mass develops. Due to the rough surfaces of the frontal fossa and the sharp angles at the temporal tip and sphenoid wing, most cerebral contusions occur in the frontal and temporal lobes. The primary treatment of cerebral contusions is to prevent secondary shift and deterioration using ICP recording, along with treatment of the associated metabolic problems (such as profound hyponatremia and seizures). Another common mechanism of injury in addition to intracranial hematomas and cerebral contusions is *shear injury*, which involves small areas of damage in the white matter, often associated with small hemorrhages on the CT scan. This type of injury shows little mass effect (and often minimal ICP elevation), but may lead to considerable neurologic deficit due to the change in the white matter. Such shear injury can involve diffusely the cerebral white matter but may also occur in the brainstem, leading to long-lasting coma following the injury. Furthermore, shear injury and irreversible herniation syndromes may cause a permanent vege-

tative state, in which a patient may appear awake with spontaneous eye opening but show neither consciousness nor meaningful response to the environment.

Management plans for head trauma include defining the primary neurologic damage using indices of neurologic responsiveness, particularly the Glasgow Coma Scale, and identifying the mechanism of injury from the initial CT scan. Immediate evacuation of the hematoma may be required to prevent secondary injury, with follow-up observation for intracranial swelling. Depending on the neurologic condition, the patient may be monitored preferentially by neurologic examination but secondarily by ICP monitoring if the clinical examination is not reliable. However, the ICP may not be elevated if there is no mass, such as with a shear injury, despite severe deficit. The mean ICP may not be sensitive to the presence of a significant mass. However, with elevated intracranial pressure, both ICP recordings and CSF drainage may be helpful in avoiding secondary damage to the brain from shifts

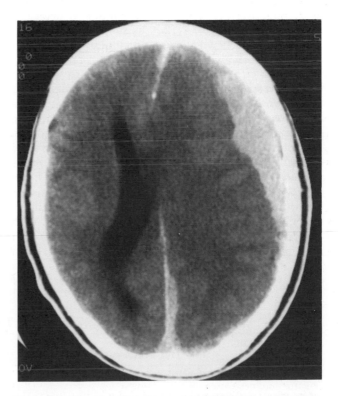

Figure 4. Computed tomographic (CT) scan of a patient who sustained a subdural hematoma from head trauma. The left subdural space in this photograph appears isodense as compared with the adjacent skull. (From Friedman AH: Craniocerebral injuries. *In* Sabiston DC Jr [ed]: Textbook of Surgery: The Biological Basis of Modern Surgical Practice, ed 14. Philadelphia, WB Saunders Company, 1991, p 1257, with permission.)

and herniation (Table 4). The purpose of the ICP recordings is not to maintain the pressure at a "safe" low level, but rather to prevent a rapid loss of intracranial compliance and markedly increased pressure. The latter may compromise the cerebral perfusion pressure and/or lead to intracranial shifts. Thus, ICP drainage is usually set at a completely arbitrary level, such as 20 mm Hg, even though the actual dangerous level may be a sustained ICP of greater than 40 to 45 mm Hg, depending on the systemic arterial blood pressure. If shifts continue unabated despite treatment, herniation syndromes may occur, and lead to irreversible damage (Table 4).

Additional methods to decompress a compromised intracranial space include treatment with mannitol to decrease extracellular fluid in more normal parts of the brain. Hyperventilation for a short duration can decrease arteriolar content by a decreased PCO_2, and furosemide decreases the extracellular fluid compartment. Additional treatment may include anticonvulsants for seizures as required, although prophylaxis does not appear to prevent future development of an epilepsy focus. Nutritional support is needed 5 to 7 days after injury, as well as pulmonary management, particularly when coma precludes adequate control of the airway. However, in some instances, these supportive efforts may not be sufficient to maintain the intracranial and the cerebral perfusion pressure adequate with severe brain injury. Progressive ischemia may arise such that there is no blood flow into the intracranial compartment. This leads to the condition known as *brain death*, in which there is no discernible brain function and the prognosis for recovery is extremely remote. The criteria for diagnosing brain death include: (1) no apparent cortical or brainstem function, including respiration (although spinal reflexes are allowed); (2) no respiratory response with an apnea test and an ending PCO_2 value of at least 60 mm Hg; (3) clear structural diagnosis, such as brain injury on CT; and (4) no interfering factors, such as drug overdose or hypothermia. After declaration of brain death, often by confirmation with a secondary study (such as EEG or blood flow study), the patient legally becomes a cadaver and may be acceptable for organ donation.

Spinal injury often combines a bony canal and/or vertebral body injury with neurologic injury, such as with a fracture-dislocation. However, spinal injury can also occur following soft tissue injuries, such as severe stretch in children or in association with cervical spondylosis or osteoarthritis in adults. The bony injuries are considered for treatment separately from the neurologic injury, although surgical treatment is frequently combined at a single sitting for both. Spinal cord syndromes include complete quadriplegia (above the level of the arms, at C4) or paraplegia, with no function below a thoracic level. Partial syndromes include a central or anterior cord injury in the cervical area with weakness in the arms compared to the legs, a Brown-Sequard syndrome, associated with decreased motor function on the side of injury and contralateral sensory loss, and sensory sparing associated with either quadriparesis or paraparesis. Following spinal cord injury, a number of events occur, particularly spinal shock. *Spinal shock* includes the loss of spinal cord reflex function below the level of the injury acutely, which only slowly recovers with time. However, upon return of local (segmental) function, there is slow onset of involuntary spasticity of the extremities. This type of spinal spasticity can be treated with baclofen for partial relief.

The initial treatment of spinal cord injury requires careful examination concerning the level of injury, the assessment of bony injury at the appropriate level, and often an examination to confirm the neurologic injury, unless it is clear that the bony injury and neurologic injury are concordant. Following a firm diagnosis concerning the etiology of the deficit, high-dose steroids are recommended, as a partial help in functional recovery. If a fracture is present, in many instances it should be reduced, particularly in the cervical spine. If reduction is not complete and/or there appears to be

TABLE 4. SIGNS OF TENTORIAL HERNIATION*

	Consciousness	Pupillary Size, Response to Light	Oculovestibular Reflex	Response to Pain
Uncal (Unilateral) Herniation				
Early third nerve pressure	Drowsy	Dilating, no response	Full, conjugate	Appropriate
Late third nerve pressure	Obtunded	Dilated, no response	Third nerve palsy	Semipurposeful
Midbrain compression	Comatose	Bilateral fixed	Dysconjugate gaze	Posturing
Central (bilateral) herniation				
Early diencephalon pressure	Obtunded	Small, reactive	Conjugate	Appropriate
Late diencephalon pressure	Obtunded to comatose	Small, reactive	Conjugate	Semipurposeful
Midbrain compression	Comatose	Midposition, fixed	Dysconjugate	Posturing

Appropriate implies following commands and fully responsive; *obtunded* indicates very slow to follow commands and requiring effort to arouse; *semipurposeful* motor function indicates moving in some directions that are appropriate but not all; *posturing* implies either flexion or extension posturing reflex, which may vary considerably.

continuing spinal cord injury after attempts at closed reduction are made, an open operative approach is required, which may include elements of both neural decompression and fusion. However, neural decompression is usually performed only if there is indeed function to be gained, although late pain may be reduced by the débridement at an early time. Thus, neural decompression may offer the possibility of late improved rate of recovery, which is difficult to measure, as most incomplete patients continue to improve for up to a year after the injury. Such decompression to help prevent late pain states and other morbidity is considered worthwhile in most instances, particularly if the spinal canal remains severely compromised after the injury.

RUPTURED INTERVERTEBRAL DISK AND DEGENERATIVE JOINT DISEASE OF THE SPINE

The spine demonstrates a complex set of muscular, fascial, and bony planes. Pathologic alterations in the spine include the two interrelated features of neurologic function and mechanical stability. The anatomic location of the spinal cord and segmental nerves directly adjacent to and surrounded by the elements required for bony stability leads to an intertwined but separate status. As an example, spinal cord injury usually includes elements of both bony instability due to fracture and neurologic damage due to either spinal cord or nerve root injury (or both), for which treatment must be considered separately though often at the same time. Thus, neurologic and mechanic considerations must be considered individually.

Separate from infection and traumatic fractures of the spine, the two leading spine disorders are herniated disks and degenerative joint disease of the spine. These can occur at any level, but most commonly are present at segments with increased motion (and stress), particularly the cervical and lumbar levels. There are two primary types of neurologic involvement: (1) central spinal canal impingement, primarily with involvement of the spinal cord or cauda equina, and (2) lateral canal compromise with individual nerve root syndromes. Both central and lateral syndromes occur with either herniated disk or degenerative (spondylitic) changes, although the herniated disks tend to occur in younger individuals and the spondylitic changes occur in older patients. A typical example of a herniated disk of the lumbar spine is shown in Figure 5. The common segmental neurologic signs that can be used to localize the level of a root abnormality are shown in Table 5.

Changes in the central canal cause *myelopathy* in the cervical and thoracic regions, with classic lower

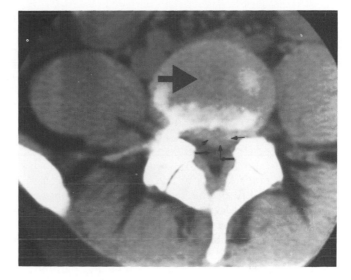

Figure 5. Noncontrast computed tomographic (CT) scan of the lumbar spine at the disk space nicely demonstrates the difference in CT density between the spinal sac filled with cerebrospinal fluid (*medium arrows*) and disk material (*large arrow*). The asymmetric contours of the disk material represent a herniated disk fragment. (From Meisler WJ: Neuroradiology. *In* Sabiston DC Jr [ed]: Textbook of Surgery: The Biological Basis of Modern Surgical Practice, ed 14. Philadelphia, WB Saunders Company, 1991, p 1238, with permission.)

motor neuron changes in the affected levels, such as arm weakness, and upper motor neuron alterations in the lower extremities, with spasticity, increased reflexes, and decreased function. Such "inverse paraplegia" occurs typically with a large central herniated disk in the midcervical region or with *cervical spondylitic myelopathy*. The treatment of either type of myelopathy is through an anterior or posterior surgical approach with decompression, depending upon the number of levels involved and the location of the offending lesion. Thus, a herniated disk at one level leading to a myelopathy is usually best treated with an anterior cervical diskectomy with or without a fusion, whereas the more diffuse spondylitic changes may require an extensive posterior cervical laminectomy (C3 to C7) or one or two focal levels of treatment anteriorly. Occasionally, the anterior involvement is severe and a laminectomy is contraindicated due to the presence of kyphosis, pointing to the need for an anterior cervical multilevel vertebrectomy, often accompanied by a strut graft. This type of procedure usually requires halo immobilization because of the instability created by the decompression.

Most herniated disks leading to spinal cord compressive syndromes occur in the cervical region, as degeneration of the disk is more common with the in-

TABLE 5.   SEGMENTAL ASSESSMENT IN ROOT SYNDROME

Level	Root	Motor Segment	Sensory Level	Reflexes
C4-5	C5	Deltoids, biceps	Shoulder, arm	None
C5-6	C6	Biceps, brachioradialis	Arm, thumb	Biceps
C6-7	C7	Triceps, wrist flexion	Index, middle fingers	Triceps
C7–T1	C8, T1	Intrinsic hand muscles	Ring, small finger	None
L2-3	L3	Psoas, hip flexion	Anterior thigh	None
L3-4	L4	Psoas, quadriceps	Anterior thigh, knee	Knee
L4-5	L5	Ankle dorsiflexion	Dorsum of ankle	None
L5–S1	S1	Ankle plantar flexion	Lateral aspect of ankle	Ankle

creased mobility of the region. However, a thoracic disk herniation occasionally occurs. Due to the small size of the thoracic spinal canal, this may lead to a severe myelopathy. Such thoracic disks may be difficult to expose, particularly by the posterior approach, which requires mobilization of a taut and pathologically stretched spinal cord. For this reason, thoracic disks with myelopathy are usually approached from either a posterolateral or anterolateral direction, where mobilization of the spinal cord is not required. Thus, the major part of the offending lesion is attacked directly if possible by whichever route appears the most appropriate.

In the lumbar region, central canal involvement is accompanied by diffuse cauda equina pressure, which often is manifest as *neurogenic claudication*. This syndrome involves bilateral leg pain, usually when walking, but not with other forms of exercise that do not involve extension of the back, such as bicycle riding. In addition to pain, the patient often experiences "rubbery legs," or diffuse weakness in both lower extremities with no focal deficit that is improved by sitting. The diagnosis is usually apparent on myelography or MRI scanning, which demonstrates a near-complete spinal block due to degenerative bone, ligament, and disk changes at one or more levels, commonly L3-4 and L4-5. Typical of this syndrome are bone spurs from the posterior aspect of the body, enlarged lateral facet joints protruding into the canal, and redundant ligamentum flavum, all contributing to a very small central canal. Decompression in this instance is most commonly performed by posterior laminectomy and full decompression of the dural sac, the levels dictated by the preoperative studies. Often, relief of neurogenic claudication is rapid and this is a highly beneficial procedure.

In addition to central canal stenosis and involvement of either the spinal cord or cauda equina as a whole, a more common problem is lateral herniation, causing impingement on one or more nerve roots. Part of the ligaments that normally contain the soft nucleus pulposus include the posterior longitudinal ligament, which courses along the posterior aspect of the body. This ligament is much more stout in the midline than laterally so that most disk herniations occur in the lateral position. This lateral occurrence naturally leads to individual nerve root compression, at any level of the canal. The level of involvement can be accurately predicted by *localizing signs*, including a segmental assay of the spinal cord and roots at a particular level (Table 5).

Cervical roots proceed laterally to join the intervertebral foramina, crossing the major portion of the disk. For example, this leads to the C5-6 disk impinging on the C6 nerve root, which exits through the C5-6 foramen. Localizing signs for such a radiculopathy include decreased strength in the biceps and brachioradialis muscles, decreased biceps reflex, and decreased sensation over the thumb. The pain follows the distribution expected for the sensory changes, shooting in a lightning-like manner from the neck into the thumb. In contrast, a thoracic radiculopathy from a thoracic herniated disk usually occurs as a radiating, ring-like pain around the thorax, following the distribution of a rib. Common levels of involvement include T4, which is even with the nipple line anteriorly, and T10, which localizes at the umbilicus. In the lumbar region, the spinal roots follow a longer course within the spinal canal, such that the L5 root has a shoulder of exit from the main dural sac above the L4-5 disk, traverses over the disk, and exits around the pedicle of L5. Thus, lumbar disk herniations commonly lead to involvement of the root exiting below the level. An exception is a lateral disc herniation, which may only be apparent on lateral CT scans or an MRI scan. This type of herniation courses either laterally or cephalad and compresses the root above. As an example, an L4-5 herniated disk that protrudes laterally may involve primarily the L4 root. It is critical to recognize such an "anomalous" presentation, because a different surgical approach may be required (Table 5). Herniated disks may also occur in dormant disk spaces such as at S1-S2, or between C1 and C2.

Herniated intervertebral disks cause radicular symptoms in response to chemical irritation, pressure on the root, or stretch of the posterior longitudinal ligament, which also has pain fibers leading to a referred pain syndrome. Most patients treated conservatively (bed rest and analgesics) improve over 6 to 8 weeks, presumably due to decreased root irritation over time. Residual radiculopathy may be best treated with diskectomy and nerve root decompression, although newer and more experimental treatments are being evaluated, such as percutaneous diskectomy techniques. However, patients with myelopathy usually require early and appropriate surgical decompression, to both stabilize the myelopathy and to prevent permanent nerve and muscular injury.

PERIPHERAL NERVE INJURIES

Injuries to peripheral nerves can occur following a variety of causes, including trauma (stretch and frank section), compartment syndromes and anoxia, injections and other forms of local irritants, missile wounds and penetrating injuries, pressure neuropathy, and metabolic insults. Civilian injuries may form a much different spectrum than wartime injuries, although the latter have led to considerable therapeutic improvement in the treatment of such injuries. Depending on the severity of the initial injury, a direct suture and/or partial excision of the traumatized nerve may be required. However, it is often better to allow the injured nerve to demarcate into active and injured zones over a period of 2 to 3 weeks and to resuture the nerve with clean and appropriate margins. This delayed repair also allows any partial nerve injuries to recover, although there may be a considerable lag time until end-organs (muscles and sensory endings) become reinnervated. Many other types of repair may be indicated, particularly cable grafts (with sural nerve), with and without transposition to increase the length of the nerve available. The exact timing of repair remains controversial, although an optimal time appears to be 2 to 3 weeks.

The assessment of peripheral nerve injuries involves a detailed and sequential examination of the extremity involved, a preoperative detailed EMG/NCV for evaluation of the level and extent of the injury, and postoperative studies to assess reinnervation of denervated muscle groups. Often a neurolysis may be initially performed, which involves exploring the nerve and gently releasing it from surrounding perineurium and scar tissue, often accompanied by direct intraoperative nerve recordings to assess the conduction through the segment. Attempts at suture and/or grafting of the nerve may be delayed until it is clear that further recovery is unlikely, although there is a limit to when end-organs, particularly muscle, may be receptive to reinnervation. Thus, in the lower extremity, a high sciatic nerve injury may require over 2 years to reach the distal muscles of the lower extremity, using the guide of approximately 1 inch per month reinnerva-

tion, at which time it is very unlikely that the muscle will be responsive to reinnervation due to atrophy. Thus, early repair (within 6 months) is often recommended if possible. The intraoperative studies may be helpful in demonstrating nerve regrowth across the site of injury, prior to the time at which reinnervation can occur.

INTRACRANIAL AND SPINAL INFECTIONS

Spontaneous, postoperative, and traumatic infections follow the cranial and spinal tissue planes (Table 6). Infections include entities such as cellulitis of the scalp, osteomyelitis of the skull, subdural empyema, meningitis, cerebritis, brain abscess, and encephalitis. Postoperative infections may occur in more than one plane, such as with a combined meningitis and scalp infection. For this reason, the dura is closed tightly to prevent the subsequent spread of infection from one plane to another. Traumatic infections follow the planes contaminated by the trauma. A penetrating infection into the brain may include an element of brain abscess as well as a more superficial infection. The major principles of treatment of infections apply; that is, debridement of contaminated planes, drainage of the infected plane, and in certain cases, closure of the critical planes to facilitate healing. Appropriate antibiotics should also be administered.

Scalp infections are initially treated by open packing until clean edges develop, at which time secondary closure may be attempted, usually with radical debridement of the edges to viable tissue and a one-layer closure with a monofilament suture, with drains infiltrating the antibiotics. Chronic osteomyelitis, such as occurs in bone flaps, requires removal of the infected bone and subsequent closure of the scalp. Infection also particularly occurs in cranioplasty flaps, which are likely to fester until the cranioplasty flap (either metal or plastic) is removed. Subsequent cranioplasty procedures may require endogenous bone replacement, such as rib or half-thickness skull, which is more resistant to further infection than artificial materials.

Infections of the subdural space usually occur following sinusitis, spreading by veins that subsequently thrombose. This infection is termed *subdural empyema* and may lead to further deep venous thrombosis and severe cerebral inflammation. The CT appearance of subdural empyema is typically a small amount of subdural material, which is contrast enhancing, with a diffuse hemispheric mass out of proportion to the subdural material. The subdural infection often is not culture-positive in CSF samples (unlike meningitis) and usually requires a large craniotomy for decompression and drainage in addition to antibiotics. The

TABLE 6.   INFECTION IN CRANIAL AND SPINAL SPACES

Name of Space	Type of Infection
Scalp and subgalea (between the pericranium and galea)	Cellulitis of the scalp
Bone and diploe of the skull	Osteomyelitis of the skull
Epidural space (between the skull and the dura)	Extremely rare
Subdural or intradural space	Subdural empyema
Subarachnoid space (between the arachnoid and the pia)	Leptomeningitis
Parenchyma of the brain (deep to the pia)	Cerebritis and cerebral abscess
	Encephalitis (viral in origin)
Intraventricular space (within the cerebral ventricles)	Ventriculitis

decompression is urgent in nature because of the large area of irritation and because brain dysfunction may rapidly spread to involve the entire hemisphere, through either direct or indirect irritation.

Meningitis is most commonly spontaneous, often with a highly infectious strain of bacteria. The classic symptoms of obtundation and stiff neck should lead to a high degree of suspicion and performance of a lumbar puncture for examination of the CSF. Unusual organisms may be encountered in the postoperative setting, often requiring multiple antibiotics and occasionally intrathecal instillation of gentamicin or systemic chloramphenicol, particularly for a refractory gram-negative infection. Because of the open nature of the subarachnoid space, meningitis rapidly spreads over the entire surface of the brain and spinal cord and can focally affect any part of the central nervous system.

Cerebral or parenchymal bacterial infections lead to an area of inflammation termed *cerebritis*. The site is often diffuse and poorly localized on CT scan. Over a 2- to 3-week period, the brain forms a border around the infected region. If there is a normal reaction, which is often not present in acquired immunodeficiency syndrome (AIDS), this walled-off area becomes a *brain abscess*. Treatment necessitates drainage, often by a stereotactic route with appropriate administration of systemic antibiotics. Only rarely does one or more drainage attempts fail to resolve the abscess. Should the abscess persist, it may necessitate excision. Viral infection of the brain is termed *encephalitis*, and certain areas of the brain show predilection for this involvement. Thus, herpes leads to bitemporal involvement, which, on CT scan shows as large, patchy areas of low density in both temporal lobes that may be contrast enhancing. Early treatment with acyclovir may be helpful in ameliorating the infection, although morbidity from antecedent brain damage may occur.

Spinal infections show similar categories, but because the planes of dissection differ, additional regions of involvement with infection occur. In the spinal region, the epidural space, which usually contains fat and a venous plexus, is more easily dissected. Spontaneous infections, presumably hematogenous, occur in the epidural space, often in patients with a risk factor, such as diabetes mellitus. These infections classically lead to diffuse back pain throughout the region of involvement, severe stiffness and spasm of the paraspinal muscles of the back, and rapidly progressive neurologic involvement. This entity is another requiring urgent neurosurgical evacuation of the abscess to prevent progression of the neurologic deficit. Other spinal infections include hematogenous osteomyelitis, which may lead to adjacent diskitis and with involvement of neural elements through either bony collapse or epidural extension into the spinal canal. The approach to such a bone infection involves a needle biopsy for culture, and if antibiotics prove to be inadequate treatment, open débridement with resection of the sequestrum and possible fusion may be required. Adequate treatment of such a bone infection may require months of antibiotic treatment, and full fusion may require several years.

BENIGN AND MALIGNANT NEOPLASMS OF THE CENTRAL AND PERIPHERAL NERVOUS SYSTEM

Neoplasms occur in both congenital tissue remnants and existing tissue types in the nervous system and its coverings. The two primary groups include: (1) intrinsic tumors of the nervous system and its coverings, and (2) metastatic tumors. Intrinsic tumors consist of neoplasms originating from fetal cellular remnants, neurons, and glial and mesenchymal elements included in the nervous system, such as meningeal cells, endothelial cells, and Schwann cells. Extrinsic tumors include those that have spread hematogenously and/or by direct local invasion, such as from the head and neck region. The systemic principles of diagnosis and debulking apply to the nervous system, but with special precautions. Rarely can a proper removal of a malignant tumor be performed with adequate margins at any level of the nervous system, due to the involvement of multiple layers, including the CSF spaces, and the critical function of elements of the nervous system.

Thus, a wide excision of tumor would remove critical neural tissue and would often cause a significant loss of function without necessarily providing adequate additional margins. As a consequence of the limited margins that may be achieved, tumors are usually treated by debulking or gross removal, with additional reliance being placed on adjunct treatments, such as radiation.

The most common tumors in children are *ependymoma*, which arise from ependymal cells around the ventricles, and *medulloblastoma*, which arise from external granular neurons in the cerebellum. Pediatric tumors also include a number of unusual fetal remnant tissues, such as *germinomas* (Fig. 6), *endodermal sinus tumors*, *neural crest tumors*, including neuroblastoma, and unusual neural tumors, such as *ganglioglioma* and *hemangioblastoma*. These latter tumors may persist into adulthood and show dividing neuronal elements, which normally do not divide in the adult. These tumors are resected aggressively and at times can be cured with removal and chemotherapy. Ordinarily, radiation treatment is withheld in children due to its adverse influence on growing neural tissue. Additional tumors occurring in the pediatric age group include low-grade hypothalamic or optic nerve gliomas, which also may occur in the cerebellum. These tumors may be very slow growing and at times have been followed

for 20 to 30 years with no progression of disease, which is very unusual for gliomas in general. Thus, except for a mural nodule associated with cerebellar cystic gliomas, the tumor is often biopsied but cannot be fully resected due to diffusion of abnormal glial cells beyond a surgical margin.

Tumors in adults consist primarily of gliomas, arising from several different types of glial cells and include astrocytic gliomas, which are usually graded as low-grade, anaplastic, and glioblastoma multiforme, as well as oligodendrogliomas. The current treatment of these tumors is craniotomy and internal decompression and resection to the point where more normal appearing brain tissue is reached at the margins. Often, however, complete debulking cannot be performed due to the threat of severe functional loss, and only partial removal is possible. Tumors of neural origin are uncommon, and increasing age is associated with greater malignancy. Rarely do glial tumors metastasize outside of the CNS, but usually the growth within the CNS is relentless and overall survival is poor. Current treatments include radiation and occasionally chemotherapy protocols, but these remain experimental due to a relatively low efficacy rate. The recurrence of the tumor is often to distal areas within the brain rather than a local recurrence in the operative bed. This diffuse infiltration is characteristic of

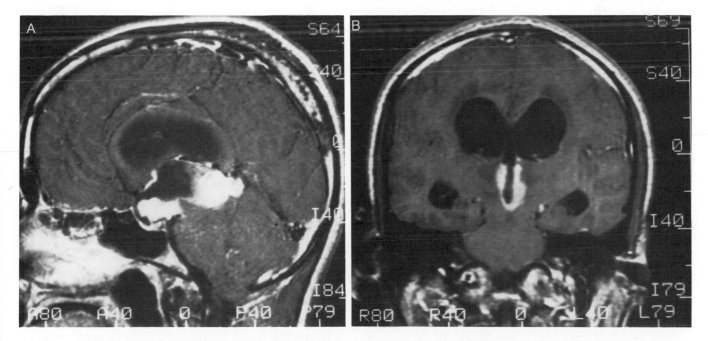

Figure 6. Sagittal (*A*) and coronal (*B*) magnetic resonance images (MRI), showing an enhancing germinoma in the pineal and suprasellar areas with spread along the walls of the third ventricle. Obstructive hydrocephalus is also demonstrated. (From Wilkins RH: Intracranial tumors. *In* Sabiston DC Jr [ed]: Textbook of Surgery: The Biological Basis of Modern Surgical Practice, ed 14. Philadelphia, WB Saunders Company, 1991, p 1243, with permission.)

gliomas in general, as such widespread growth has proven very difficult to control.

Benign tumors in the adult include meningiomas and variant schwannomas, which may occur in several cranial nerves. Meningiomas arise from arachnoid cells, which are predominantly located in the dura. However, these cells may be present in the ventricle and with arachnoid granulations. Therefore, meningiomas need not necessarily be attached to the dura. The usual treatment is aggressive and complete resection if possible. Radiation treatment has an inhibitory or static effect that may prevent these tumors from progressing and can be used for unresectable tumors in special areas such as the cavernous sinus or other deep structures. Schwannomas most commonly occur on the acoustic (VIII) and trigeminal nerves (V) and should be aggressively resected (Fig. 7). However, the growth of these tumors is often very slow, and a partial resection for functional improvement may be acceptable in certain situations, particularly with advanced age and when the morbidity of full resection may be unacceptably high. Usual complications of the removal of these tumors are cranial nerve deficits and occasionally changes in the brainstem.

NEUROSURGICAL RELIEF OF PAIN

The subjective appreciation of *discomfort* may arise in a number of different conditions that can be grouped into general categories (Table 7). Such discomfort may be more or less tightly linked to actual ongoing and incoming pain (nociceptive) signals and may show a dissociation with respect to actual tissue damage. A critical medical assessment for these conditions is current (or past) evidence of either tissue or nervous system damage, and to ensure that the tissue damage is stabilized for optimal healing. Each of these conditions and appropriate treatment schemes will be briefly discussed.

Acute pain states include surgical incisional healing, burns, fractures, and other conditions in which tissue damage has occurred and recovery is expected. Clearly, the tissue damage leads to generation of nociceptive signals that are interpreted as painful, and as the damage heals, these signals should wane. Initial approaches include identification and stabilization of any associated tissue damage to ensure prompt healing, as well as initiation of appropriate medical treatment. For example, adequate treatment of pain associated with vertebral osteomyelitis includes biopsy or débridement, stabilization, and antibiotics. However, healing occurs slowly over many months, and the discomfort decreases slowly. The approach to pain management is suppression at the spinal and central levels with narcotics, which stimulate opioid receptors and

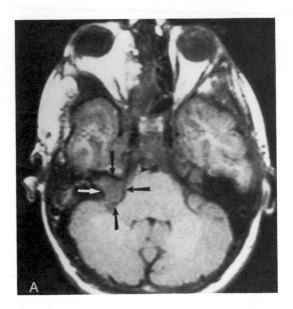

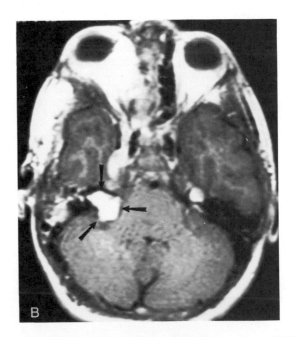

Figure 7. *A*, Noncontrast magnetic resonance image (MRI) of the brain at the level of the cerebellopontine angle cisterns reveals an isointense mass on the right in the region of the internal auditory canal (*arrows*). Note the typical lack of signal exhibited by flowing blood in the basilar artery. *B*, Contrast-enhanced examination at the same level as in *A* indicates that the mass is enhanced uniformly, which proved to be an acoustic neuroma. (From Meisler WJ: Neuroradiology. *In* Sabiston DC Jr [ed]: Textbook of Surgery: The Biological Basis of Modern Surgical Practice, ed 14. Philadelphia, WB Saunders Company, 1991, p 1240, with permission.)

TABLE 7. OUTLINE OF PAIN STATES

Acute pain—active nociception and tissue damage is present
Chronic benign pain—a past episode of tissue damage may be
  prolonged after healing without any current ongoing
  nociception (previous acute pain)
Malignant pain—may include an active component of tissue
  damage and also suffering
Neurogenic pain—associated with lesions of the central or
  peripheral nervous system

partially block the central transmission of nociceptive signals. Rarely is neurosurgical treatment required for acute pain states.

Benign chronic pain is associated with a healed but uncomfortable minor tissue damage. Common examples include diffuse neck pain following a cervical myofascial strain and mechanical low back pain following a strain. Although these injuries clearly heal, the conditions surrounding the injury may in some instances lead to propagation of the discomfort, and the complex soft tissue injuries may only partially heal. Thus, a long-term discomfort may follow, often without any objective basis in terms of demonstrable tissue damage. Without a reason to consider a surgical procedure, such as a clear herniated disk syndrome with associated symptoms and signs, such procedures are contraindicated. Most procedures to control pain often do more harm than good, and the general principle is that operative procedures may either prolong the discomfort or cause a more intense focus of discomfort from the surgical trauma. The best approach to these syndromes is evaluation in a comprehensive pain clinic, including reassurance through adequate studies that the tissue damage is healed and that malignancy is not present. A psychiatric evaluation may also be useful. Treatment may include biofeedback to decrease secondary muscle spasm and associated pain, focal injections, and adjuncts such as stimulators, but surgical procedures are rarely indicated. Often, these types of pain syndromes stabilize over several years, particularly if the patient has received compensation for an associated injury.

Malignant pain states include both ongoing tissue damage from tumor invasion and a significant reaction to the realization of tumor spread, limiting the patient's lifespan. The ongoing tissue damage can often be treated with long-term narcotics, particularly MS-contin, a long-acting form of morphine, and methadone, a synthetic morphine substitute. The tissue damage should be treated and stabilized as much as possible, as in the use of radiation treatments for bone pain due to metastases, and resection of tumor associated with pathologic fractures. Often, tissue invasion cannot be halted by primary medical or surgical approaches, particularly in advanced malignancy,

and there are neurosurgical alternatives to systemic narcotics for treatment of pain. These vary from intrathecal infusions of morphine to various types of nervous system lesions. Intrathecal narcotics are particularly useful for bilateral painful conditions below the cervical region, such as abdominal metastases or pelvic malignancy. An intrathecal test dose of 1.0 mg of morphine is given, and either an external or internal infusion pump can be used for constant infusion. The primary drawback is the eventual tachyphylaxis to narcotics, which may be partially decreased by periods of intermittent withdrawal.

Direct procedures include peripheral nerve section proximal to a malignant lesion or a form of anterolateral cordotomy (spinal cord section). The classical cordotomy is performed percutaneously at C1-2, and produces a contralateral hemihypalgesia, or decreased pain sensation. Unfortunately, due to the high crossing of most cervical pain fibers, the highest level obtainable at C1-2 is usually low cervical, and the main risk of the procedure is decreased respiratory drive during sleep, termed Ondine's curse. Thus, patients with bilateral or midline disease seldom improve, and patients with lung malignancy and decreased contralateral respiratory capacity (on the side of the pain) may have a critically diminished respiratory drive. A higher section of pain fibers is possible at the mesencephalic level and has the advantage of involving the entire hemibody, including the face. This type of cordotomy is performed using stereotaxic techniques, but has the complication of producing secondary oculomotor symptoms because the lesion is close to the oculomotor nucleus and coordinating centers. As suffering may often predominate due to the subjective appreciation of discomfort and the presence of an advanced malignancy, a modified psychosurgical procedure may also be considered, such as making a lesion in the bilateral cingulum. This type of lesion selectively reduces the suffering associated with a malignancy.

Neurogenic pain conditions comprise the most difficult category of pain states and are associated with damage at some level of the nervous system. Because the nervous system acts in many ways as an information or relay system from the body to the brain, lesions along these pathways can give rise to spontaneous sensations of tissue damage without any damage actually existing. An excellent example is a radiculopathy due to root pressure, as commonly occurs in the herniated disk syndrome. The patient experiences extremity discomfort that is highly localized to the area of distribution of the nerve root, yet there is no tissue damage in this distribution. The underlying basis for the discomfort is presumably the spontaneous generation of impulses at the site of the nerve root pressure or irritation, which is signaling to the brain that tissue damage must be present. In a sense, these signals are falsely interpreted as nociceptive in nature. This example emphasizes the general problem in which the brain attempts to interpret such abnormal signals in the context of a relay system. The signals are referred back to the dermatomal distribution associated with the nervous system element. Pain suppression rarely helps these forms of discomfort.

Peripheral nerve damage can lead to such common syndromes as neuroma pain, causalgia, and phantom limb pain, with signals arising from the damaged end of the nerve and/or aberrant regrowth of inappropriate fibers, such as sympathetic afferents. In rare instances, further proximal neurectomy may be helpful, but more likely to be of benefit is proximal stimulation with electrical current, either around the nerve or at the spinal cord level; that is, the *dorsal column stimulator*. Treatment may initially be directed at improving recovery of the nerve, such as by resuture or cable grafting if possible. Root-level irritation or damage may lead to a radiculopathy syndrome. The appropriate initial treatment is to determine if a remediable cause is present, such as nerve root compression by bone or a disk. However, even after adequate decompression, this pain may persist, indicating permanent damage to the nerve, causing spontaneous uncomfortable signals. Treatment of this difficult condition may be with further injections or antidepressant medications such a amitriptyline. Nerve root section or neurolysis is rarely helpful and may worsen any preserved motor or sensory function.

Additional examples of peripheral nerve changes leading to discomfort are pain associated with herpes zoster due to damage in the sensory ganglion, and *tic douloureux*. Tic douloureux is intriguing, as it appears to involve large-fiber abnormalities rather than nociceptive inputs and may be due to "cross-talk" between nerve fibers at the root level, in the posterior fossa. Various types of treatment ameliorate the discomfort of tic douloureux, including traditional anticonvulsants such as carbamazepine and phenytoin. Trigeminal rhizolysis and relief of the compression neuropathy by a direct posterior fossa approach, termed *microvascular decompression*, may also be helpful. Thus, tic douloureux may represent a highly treatable form of neurogenic spontaneous pain syndrome.

Damage to the spinal cord or higher in the CNS may also cause the perception of spontaneous discomfort. An example is phantom pain in the paralyzed lower extremities following traumatic thoracic paraplegia, in which no sensation is preserved. Such phantom discomfort may relate to the nature of the original injury, particularly if associated with complex tissue injury such as crushing. Additional examples include spontaneous pain associated with demyelination, as in multiple sclerosis, and thalamic stroke with a contralateral hemibody perception of discomfort (Dejerine-

Roussy syndrome). These conditions are rarely responsive to medications, but occasionally stimulation of the nervous system may lead to improvement. Interestingly, the lack of sensation itself may also lead to a spontaneous sensation of discomfort, termed *anesthesia dolorosa*. This is a relatively common problem following complete nerve section for tic douloureux, in which the patient experiences "crawling worms" or other uncomfortable sensations in the area of the denervation. In general, the discomfort associated with CNS damage may be very difficult to ameliorate with either medical or surgical treatments and represents a challenge for further research.

NEUROSURGICAL RELIEF OF EPILEPSY

A single convulsion may be differentiated from a chronic, recurring pattern of stereotyped seizures, termed *epilepsy*. A single convulsion may be provoked by a variety of conditions, including common medications such as penicillin or lidocaine, lack of sleep, electric shock therapy, the immediate response to head injury, and so forth. A recurring pattern of seizures is more likely due to a region or multiple regions of abnormalities within the brain, which may be due to structural lesions such as tumors, mesial temporal sclerosis, AVMs, or lesions that may be more diffuse and not recognizable on scans. Several types of epilepsy may show strong genetic tendencies, such as *petit mal*, which may represent a diffuse cortical tendency for decreased inhibition (Table 8). Other types of epilepsy may be due to diffuse structural damage, such as that following intrauterine anoxia. Thus, the critical difference between seizures and epilepsy is the tendency of one or more regions of the cortex to spontaneously express stereotyped seizures rather than respond in a nonspecific manner to generalized insults.

Seizures can be classified into several types, based both on the behavioral features and the electrical manifestations, identified on the EEG. These types include primary generalized seizures, which do not appear to have a focal origin, and various types of focal or partial seizures, such as partial elementary with a motor manifestation or partial complex with multiple behavioral outputs. These various seizure disorders respond in a mixed manner to anticonvulsants, which are more or less specific for each type of seizure. However, many types do not respond well to these drugs, which were developed using animal models with generalized convulsions. One particular seizure that does not respond well to traditional anticonvulsants is *partial complex*. After trying multiple drugs for a period of at least 2 years, the patient may be considered for a focal resection of the area of cortex that appears to be

TABLE 8. CLASSIFICATION OF EPILEPSY TYPES

Partial Seizures
  Partial elementary (no impairment of consciousness)
    Motor symptoms
    With special sensory or somatosensory symptoms
    With autonomic symptoms
    Compound forms of the above
  Partial complex (generally with impairment of consciousness)
    With impairment of consciousness only
    With cognitive symptomatology
    With affective symptomatology
    With psychosensory symptomatology (automatisms)
    With psychomotor symptomatology
  Partial seizures with secondary generalization
Primary Generalized
  Absence (petit mal)
  Bilateral massive epileptic myoclonus
  Infantile spasms
  Clonic seizures
  Tonic seizures
  Tonic-clonic seizures (grand mal)
  Atonic or akinetic seizures
Unilateral seizures (or predominantly unilateral)
Unclassified epileptic seizures (incomplete data)

responsible for the origin of the seizure. Various techniques, both electrical and behavioral, have been used to identify the stereotypical origin of seizures for individual patients, particularly scalp EEG recordings of both interictal (between seizure) activity and ictal onset. If these are not clear, additional invasive techniques may be applied, such as depth electrodes, subdural electrodes, and grids that can be placed directly on the brain or implanted for a period of time. These invasive electrodes overcome many of the problems inherent with scalp electrodes, including measurement of electrical activity in deeper areas of the brain and surface areas not accessible to the scalp, particularly temporal lobe. The rationale for surgical treatment is more thoroughly explained in a National Institutes of Health (NIH) consensus conference on epilepsy surgery.

In many instances the apparent cortical origin of the seizures lies in an area of the brain such as the hippocampus, which can be excised. Other areas of the temporal lobe and frontal and parietal lobes may be similarly managed following these localizing and lateralizing studies. Additional studies that may be helpful in this decision include *positron emission tomography* (PET), which localizes decreased glucose metabolism in focal areas on an interictal basis, particularly in the temporal lobes, and increased metabolism during a seizure, newer nuclear techniques to localize the seizure onset with other radioisotopes, and careful neuropsychologic testing, which may show areas of the cortex that are either damaged or inhibited by ongoing seizure activity. Thus, the confluence of these tests remains critical for the successful surgical

excision of the epileptic region. Such an excision primarily involves temporal lobectomy, usually with removal of the medial temporal structures (the hippocampus and amygdala), although other focal areas may also be excised, including the frontal regions or parietal regions. The ability to excise a focal region of cortex appears to be a choice between the chance of decreasing the critical mass of cortex leading to seizure onset and creating new deficits following excision. Generally, mild deficits such as a quadrantopsia visual field loss are well tolerated and expected following a "standard" right temporal lobectomy. However, more severe deficits such as a hemiparesis, severe memory loss, or a speech defect are not well tolerated and usually provide a contraindication for proceeding with this approach. The success rate with such a focal cortical resection is higher if a focal structural lesion is removed, such as a tumor or area of mesial temporal sclerosis, and lies in the range of one third cured of seizures, one third with a significant decrease in frequency, and one third with no change. The risks of the surgery include approximately 3 to 5 per cent risk of serious morbidity or mortality and the specific risks of producing a cortical deficit according to the area involved.

STEREOTACTIC NEUROSURGERY

Stereotactic procedures involve the use of a fixed frame attached to the skull and guidance of a probe or instrument into a specific part of the brain. Frontal lobotomy for psychosurgery and deep lesions for the alleviation of Parkinson's disease using this approach are examples of *functional neurosurgery*. This includes lesions, stimulation, or transplants in often normal brain circuits to affect the function of other abnormal circuits. Other stereotactic procedures are performed for *structural* lesions, including tumor biopsy. The general principle of localization that evolved was to measure the location of the desired target lesion with respect to a local landmark. Thus, for targets in deep areas, such as with thalamic lesions for movement disorders, the third ventricle is the natural landmark. However, CT and MRI scans have recently become more widely used for localizing targets.

Targets for stereotactic lesions have included lateral thalamotomy for movement disorders, primarily in ventrolateral thalamus, sensory thalamotomy for pain control, mesencephalic lesions for a high cordotomy, frontal lobe lesions for modified psychosurgery, and occasionally lesions for control of epilepsy. The lesions produced for these various disorders have evolved from leukotomy (using a small wire loop, which is rotated), cryolesions using liquid nitrogen, chemical lesions using ethanol injections, and the current most widely used type of lesion, a thermal-controlled radiofrequency lesion. The radiofrequency lesion is basically a well-controlled coagulation, but is very predictable in terms of the size of the lesion and demonstrates decreased risks in terms of vessel encroachment and secondary hemorrhage. Thus, a common protocol for these procedures is imaging with CT and MRI or a contrast ventriculogram, calculation of the location of the lesion, and introduction of a small probe into the target area. Control of the location is usually performed by stimulation through the probe, revealing the functional area of brain in which to properly make the radiofrequency lesion. Additionally, the awake patient can provide feedback as to the proper initial placement of the probe and lesion, before any irreversible effects are produced. Several neurosurgeons have gradually developed maps of the particular function of such deep areas of the brain, particular sensory areas, thus contributing greatly to the overall functional knowledge of the human brain.

As computer-assisted imaging techniques have improved with the advent of CT and MRI scans, it is now possible to directly image both normal structures, such as the cerebral ventricles, as well as lesions including small tumors or other abnormal areas. New frame systems have been developed to localize the lesion in stereotactic space with the use of the imaging techniques, termed *image-guided stereotaxis*, particularly the Brown-Robert-Wells frame. This frame allows prior localization with the frame in place, using either an MRI or a CT scan, and calculation of the coordinates of a lesion with respect to the frame using a small, portable computer. This type of system has been frequently used for the biopsy of small lesions throughout the brain, particularly inaccessible tumors and infectious lesions. The rate of positive diagnosis with the small tissue biopsies is greatly improved by performing frozen sections until abnormal tissue is encountered. This frozen section guidance ensures that sufficient material has been obtained to provide a diagnosis and that the biopsy was performed in the correct location. Such biopsies for specific lesions have eclipsed the former use of this technique, although occasionally a functional lesion may still be managed by stereotaxis.

Newer methods are currently being developed that may eclipse these conventional forms of stereotactic procedures and are termed *frameless stereotaxis*. Although still dependent on digital imaging techniques, these methods use powerful computers to link the skull contours in the operating room to the previous scans, using a form of intraoperative digitization. The digitization techniques under development include line-of-sight digitizers, based on sound-emission or light paths, and mechanical digitizers, particularly a robot arm with position encoders. Thus, the patient in a fixed head holder is aligned with the previous scans using the image-processing computer, and the position of the probe can be visualized directly on the scans and provide feedback concerning the location of the probe. Clearly, this real-time feedback will be quite helpful in confirming the location of the probe, as well as localizing critical structures that cannot be visualized directly.

REFERENCES

Allen GS, Ahn HS, Preziosi TJ, et al: Cerebral arterial vasospasm—a controlled trial of nimodipine in patients with subarachnoid hemorrhage. N Engl J Med 308:619, 1983.

Plum F, Posner JB: The Diagnosis of Stupor and Coma. Philadelphia, FA Davis Company, 1988.

Pomeranz S: Craniospinal Magnetic Resonance Imaging. Philadelphia, WB Saunders Company, 1989.

Schmidek HH, Sweet WH (eds): Operative Neurosurgical Techniques: Indications, Methods and Results. Orlando, FL, Grune & Stratton, 1988.

Surgery for Epilepsy: NIH Consensus Conference. JAMA 264:729–733, 1990.

Wilkins RH, Rengachary SS (eds): Neurosurgery. New York, McGraw-Hill Book Company, 1985.

41
FRACTURES AND DISLOCATIONS

L. SCOTT LEVIN, M.D.

GENERAL PRINCIPLES

The treatment of fractures and dislocations requires knowledge of the anatomy, physiology, and biomechanics of the musculoskeletal system. Although a fracture represents a disruption in the continuity of a bone, there is also a major soft tissue injury in the surrounding area. The surgeon must be aware of the soft tissue structures adjacent to the fracture site and be particularly alert for neurologic and vascular components of the injury.

Fractures

A single fracture line is termed a *simple fracture*. When there are multiple fracture lines and bone fragments, the fracture is termed *comminuted*, and penetrating injury produces a fracture or fracture fragments that protrude through the skin, constituting an *open fracture*. Open fractures are usually contaminated with pyogenic bacteria, and the treatment and prognosis are quite different from those of closed fractures. The direction, or rate of application of a force, predicts the pattern of fracture and associated soft tissue injury. A force applied to the distal end of a bone at a set length from the point of fracture is termed a *bending moment* and usually produces a simple transverse or oblique fracture. When a direct crushing force is applied to bone, comminuted open fractures occur and are accompanied by severe soft tissue injury. Torque force applied to bone often produces a spiral or oblique fracture, while compression forces cause an impacted fracture, usually at the junction between the metaphysis and diaphysis. Violent muscle contractions

that occur with seizure disorders may produce avulsions of portions of bones.

Fractures in children are unique because the thick periosteum is strong and makes their bones more resilient and less brittle than those of adults. Bending forces applied to the bone of a child may cause a *greenstick* fracture, in which there is distraction of the cortex on the convex side and compression of bone on the concave side. Fractures may occur through the physeal plates and cause future growth disturbances.

In the elderly patient with osteoporosis and/or a metabolic bone-wasting disease, the activities of daily living may be sufficient to produce pathologic fractures in diseased bone. The most common causes of pathologic fracture are osteoporosis and metastatic carcinoma. Healthy bone may also fracture with the repetitive application of minor trauma. These fractures are known as *fatigue* or *stress fractures* and commonly occur in the metatarsal bones.

Patient Evaluation

The initial evaluation of a fracture requires careful neurologic and vascular examination, as the proximity of major nerves to bones makes them vulnerable to injury. Direct arterial injury may also occur following laceration of vessels by sharp bone fragments. Bleeding within a closed compartment may cause muscle ischemia, progressing to eventual muscle necrosis, and is termed a *compartment syndrome*. The surgeon must be aware of the compartment syndrome and be prepared to perform a *decompressive fasciotomy*, often as an emergency.

Adjacent organ injury such as lung contusion with

fractures of the ribs may occur. Fractures of the pelvis with disruption of the symphysis pubis may cause rupture of the bladder. With fractures of the femur or pelvis, hemorrhage at the fracture site may be sufficient to produce *hypovolemic shock*. Fat embolism from the bone marrow is a respiratory complication and most frequently occurs in patients who have been in hypovolemic shock with long-bone fractures. Tachypnea and dyspnea occur following decreased pulmonary function, and petechia of the chest and abdomen, as well as in the conjunctiva are transient findings. Serum lipase levels may be elevated and the symptoms may be sudden in onset with rapid fatal deterioration. Ventilatory support with a respirator may be necessary.

Fracture Reduction

Fractures are displaced from trauma and are further displaced by the pull of muscles that cross the fracture site. The first step in fracture reduction is to relieve pain by gentle manipulation of the fracture and administration of analgesics if indicated. The goal of fracture reduction is correction of angular deformity, rotational deformity, and displacement, and reduction may be accomplished by *manipulative reduction* or *continuous traction*. Manipulative reduction usually is appropriate for distal portions of the extremities such as in the distal radius. Fractures that are more proximal, such as in the humerus or femur, may require continuous traction, which is performed by inserting a pin distal to the fracture site and placing the patient in a bed with continuous pull on the pin. As muscle spasm decreases, the fracture becomes realigned.

Certain fractures that are comminuted or widely displaced may require surgical therapy such as open reduction and internal fixation. Some fractures such as comminuted fractures of the patella or radial head require excision of a portion of the bone. Prosthetic replacement may be required in some fractures such as those in the neck and femur due to avascular necrosis that follows these injuries. Furthermore, rehabilitation of the elderly patient may be shortened by prosthetic replacement. Most fractures can be treated by appropriate immobilization using plaster. Increased pressure after cast application is heralded by increasing pain in the extremity and progressive numbness and diminished circulation of the digits, and the cast should be split at the earliest sign of these symptoms.

Open Fractures

An open fracture should be treated as a surgical emergency, for which surgical débridement of the wound is required. Débridement is performed in the operating room as a formal surgical procedure. All devitalized tissue is removed. Appropriate tetanus prophylaxis should be given, and the wound is copiously irrigated. When débridement is completed, fracture stabilization must be addressed. If there is any question regarding viability of muscle tissue to a degree of contamination, the wound is dressed open. The morbidity of delayed closure in 3 to 5 days following initial débridement is minimal compared to the consequences of infection that may follow primary closure. When extensive skin loss has occurred over the fracture site, split-thickness skin grafting, pedicle, or free flap grafting may be required.

Fracture Healing

The proliferation of osteogenic cells and the early primitive bone they produce constitutes the callus of the fracture. When motion is persistent at the fracture site, the differentiation of cartilage progresses. If a cleft develops between layers of cartilage covering each fragment of the fracture, the cells at the periphery of this cleft differentiate into synovial cells, producing a *pseudarthrosis*. If there is excess of distraction at the ends of the fracture, a dense fibrous scar develops between bone, producing a *fibrous nonunion*. Compression of a fracture enhances fracture healing, which is also affected by the blood supply.

Late Complications

The soft tissue injury accompanying a fracture causes scarring of the adjacent muscles, ligaments, and tendons and produces limitation of motion of the adjacent joints. Fractures may require bone grafting to stimulate healing, and the bone can either be autogenous or from a cadaveric donor. Bone is deposited along the osteoinductive and osteoconductive grafts, a process termed *creeping substitution*. *Malunion* results when a fracture heals with unacceptable angulation or rotation. If shortening exceeds half an inch in the lower extremities, a shoe lift may be required.

Certain fractures lose their blood supply and cause avascular necrosis, occurring commonly in the femoral neck in elderly patients, in fracture dislocations of the talus, and fractures through the waist of the carpal navicular bone. Fractures involving the articular surface may ultimately cause traumatic arthritis. Even with anatomic reduction, the articular surface of cartilaginous irregularities may produce arthrosis. This often depends on the degree of joint incongruity.

Summary

The important principles regarding fractures and dislocations include:

1. An appreciation of fracture mechanics is important, and the surgeon must evaluate and treat adjacent soft tissue injury.

2. Recognition of associated injury (such as to other organ systems), hypovolemia, and fat embolism are important.

3. Wound complications can be avoided by débridement, fasciotomy, and appropriate antibiotics.

4. Open fractures are treated emergently and require operative débridement.

5. Fractures heal expeditiously with compression.

6. Complications such as nonunion, malunion, and traumatic arthritis may require further reconstructive surgery.

FRACTURE OF THE SPINE

Fracture of the spine, when associated with concomitant injury of the spinal cord, represents one of the most physically disabling and economically devastating conditions in modern medicine. Approximately 10,000 spinal cord injuries occur annually within the United States, with less than 10 per cent associated with neurologic deficits. Patients presenting with complaints of pain or tenderness in the neck or back following injury must be suspected of having a fracture of the spine until proven otherwise. Trauma may subject the vertebral column to violent force, including flexion extension, axial compression, rotation, and shearing. If these forces are greater than the physiologic range of the spine, a fracture or dislocation occurs. The spinal cord terminates between L1 and L2. In the cervical and thoracic spinal canal the cord occupies approximately 50 per cent of the available space, while in the lumbar area, the cauda equina is the only neural element in the canal and therefore more free space surrounds the neural tube.

The Cervical Spine

When a patient complains of pain in the neck after an injury, a fracture dislocation of the cervical spine must be suspected. Subsequently, a neurologic examination is performed, and cervical spine films are obtained. Plain films should include anteroposterior, lateral, open mouth, odontoid, and trauma oblique views. The patient's head should not be moved for conventional oblique examinations. If these studies are negative, supervised gentle lateral flexion extension views of the cervical spine may be obtained to exclude an unstable cervical spine secondary to soft tissue injury only.

A *Jefferson fracture* occurs in the *atlas* from an axial load on the top of the head. The resultant force is exerted laterally on the ring of C1, and the arch is fractured at the thinnest, weakest points (Fig. 1). Usually, the spinal cord is not damaged because the canal of the atlas is normally large, and with fracture fragments spread away from the center, the dimensions of the neural canal are increased. Computed tomography (CT) is the most appropriate radiograph to evaluate this injury. If the neurologic examination is normal, Jefferson fractures can be managed in a four-poster brace.

Fracture of the Odontoid

Rotation of the atlas around the odontoid process of the axis represents approximately half of the rotatory movement of the head. The dens is held adjacent to the anterior arch of C1 by the transverse and alar ligaments. On the lateral radiograph centered at C2, the predental space is 3 mm or less in the adult. A

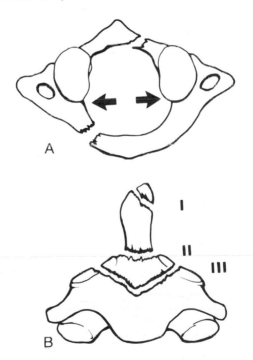

Figure 1. *A,* Jefferson fracture. Fractures of the arch of C1 are secondary to axial loads. The resultant of this force leads to expansion of the ring of C1 as indicated by the arrows, leading to a fracture of the narrow areas of the arch. *B,* Fractures of the odontoid may be type I, oblique fracture of the tip of the odontoid process (dens); type II, which occurs at the waist of the odontoid process; or type III, which extends through the cancellous bone of the C2 vertebral body. (From Hardaker WT Jr, Richardson WJ: Fractures of the spine. *In* Sabiston DC Jr [ed]: Textbook of Surgery: The Biological Basis of Modern Surgical Practice, ed 14. Philadelphia, WB Saunders Company, 1991, p 1295, with permission.)

predental space of greater than 5 mm indicates rupture of the transverse ligaments, and a predental space of 12 mm suggests that all ligaments of the dens have ruptured. Transverse or alar ligament ruptures are uncommon unless there are predisposing factors such as rheumatoid arthritis, posterior pharyngitis, or ankylosing spondylitis. If ruptures occur and the odontoid is intact, cervical myelopathy may be the presenting symptom. Fractures of the odontoid (dens) represent about 10 per cent of cervical spine fractures. Lateral views centered on C2 vertebrae and open mouth views of the odontoid usually allow adequate visualization of the dens. Tomograms may be necessary. *Type 1* dens fractures are oblique, occur at the extreme upper level of the odontoid process, and do not lead to gross instability. *Type 2* fractures, which occur through the junction of the odontoid process in the C2 vertebral body, are the most common odontoid fracture and should be considered unstable. *Type 3* fractures extend through the cancellous bone and the C2 vertebral body. They are rarely unstable and, following 3 months of immobilization in a four-poster brace, usually heal.

Fractures of the Pedicles of the Axis (Hangman's Fracture)

A fracture through the pedicles of C2 usually occurs following a severe extension injury. Compression of the spinal cord is rare because the neural canal is enlarged with forward displacement of the body of C2. The four-poster brace is usually satisfactory as treatment.

Fractures or Dislocations of C3 to C7 Vertebrae

Films of this region should include views from the occiput down to the C7 to T1 junction and may require swimmer's views or CT. Fractures of the lower cervical spine may be stable or unstable and may involve injury of the spinal cord and nerve roots.

Compression Fractures of the Cervical Vertebral Bodies

Compression fractures can follow flexion, axial loading, or coupling of these two forces. If there is minimal comminution and no dislocation at the facet, the fracture is usually stable and can be treated with a hard cervical collar. In contrast, bursting or teardrop fractures represent catastrophic injuries with a high incidence of spinal cord injury. The fragments of the vertebral body are displaced posteriorly into the spinal canal with the resulting injury to the spinal cord. In patients with incomplete neurologic injury and evidence of compression, operative anterior decompression with anterior interior fusion may be indicated.

Dislocations of the cervical spine occur most commonly between C3 and C7 interspaces. The C5 to C6 level is the most frequently involved level and follows a flexion distraction force. These injuries are associated with a variable degree of neurologic loss ranging from none to complete quadriplegia. A 25 per cent anterior listhesis of the vertebral body on the body below observed on a neutral radiograph indicates a probable fracture or dislocation of one of the posterior facet joints. Bilateral dislocation of the facets presents with full subluxation of at least 50 per cent on the lateral radiograph (Fig. 2).

Fractures and dislocations of the cervical spine are managed by prompt realignment. Initially these injuries may require halo traction until reduction is obtained, and the patient is subsequently placed in a halo vest or is treated with open reduction and internal fix-

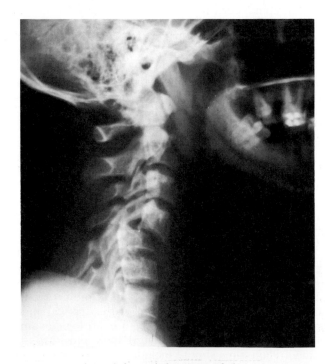

Figure 2. Bilateral facet dislocation of the cervical spine. This is a flexion-distraction injury and is often associated with complete quadriplegia at the level of the injury. Reduction is achieved by skull traction with tongs or halo. Surgical therapy may be necessary to achieve reduction and stabilization. (From Hardaker WT Jr, Richardson WJ: Fractures of the spine. *In* Sabiston DC Jr [ed]: Textbook of Surgery: The Biological Basis of Modern Surgical Practice, ed 14. Philadelphia, WB Saunders Company, 1991, p 1297, with permission.)

ation using wire and fusion techniques with an autogenous bone graft.

Avulsion fractures of the spinous processes are caused by sudden severe muscle contractions (clay shoveler's fracture), and these are not associated with neurologic loss.

The Thoracolumbar Spine

The spinal cord usually terminates at the lower margin of the L1 vertebrae. Caudal to L1, the spinal cord contains only spinal roots (cauda equina), and it occupies 50 per cent of the space in the thoracic area. The neural canal has considerable free space below L1. Moreover, the cauda equina consists of nerve roots that have a greater capacity for recovery following an injury than does the spinal cord. A bursting fracture of the cervical or thoracic lesion may cause devastating neurologic loss, whereas a similar fracture in the lumbar area may produce no permanent neurologic deficit.

Spinal injuries cephalad to T10 involve only the cord, injuries from T10 to L1 involve both the cord and nerve roots, and those caudal to L1 involve only nerve roots. In the osteoporotic patient, a rather minimal incident such as bending or lifting may cause a compression fracture of the spine. Most thoracolumbar fractures are a result of violent forces.

A patient being evaluated for thoracolumbar spine injury requires a neurologic examination, and one designed to determine the motor as well as sensory level of the injury. Inspection for the abrasions, ecchymoses, and distortions of the spinal canal often manifest themselves as step-offs or gibbus deformities. Anal sphincter tone and bulbar cavernous reflexes must be included in the evaluation of the neurologic status. In the sensory testing, particular attention should be given the perianal region because many spinal cord levels are represented in this small cutaneous area. Complete loss of motor and sensory function including perianal sensation during the first 24 hours after injury indicates complete cord injury. The bulbar cavernous reflex easily recovers within the first 24 hours, and recovery together with the presence of complete anesthesia and paralysis is compelling evidence that the patient will not recover functional motor power of the lower extremity muscle groups innervated below the level of the fracture.

A CT scan provides an extremely accurate assessment of the degree of spinal canal compromise. In addition, it provides valuable data for suspected fracture of the posterior elements. Myelography is not necessary in most patients with a significant fracture dislocation in which the results of neurologic examination are consistent with the level of the fracture. When there is no apparent fracture dislocation and neurologic loss is present, the metrizamide myelography is indicated.

Classification and Management

Denis developed a classification system for thoracolumbar spine injuries based on a three-column system, which divides the spine into three longitudinal regions. *Region 1* includes the *anterior* column consisting of the anterior longitudinal ligament and the anterior half of the vertebral body including the annulus fibrosis. *Region 2* includes the *middle* column consisting of the posterior half of the vertebral body, disk elements, and the posterior longitudinal ligament. *Region 3* includes the *posterior* column consisting of the supraspinous and infraspinous ligaments, spinous processes, laminal arch, pedicles, facet joints, and capsule. In general, instability of the spine follows significant disruption in two of the three columns.

Pure flexion injuries are the most common of all thoracolumbar skeletal fractures, and most of these injuries involve only the anterior column and, therefore, are stable. Neurologic loss is uncommon. When there is greater than 50 per cent anterior wedging with multiple contiguous anterior wedge compression fractures, progressive angulation may occur. Paralytic ileus secondary to hemorrhage adjacent to the sympathetic ganglia is common in these injuries. There is an increased incidence of thromboembolic disease, and anticoagulation therapy may be indicated. If the compression is mild, a three-point brace is satisfactory for treatment. In patients with anterior comminution, an iliac crest bone graft may be indicated with stabilization by use of either the Harrington or Cotrel-Dubousset instrumentation.

Lateral compression injuries are relatively uncommon and are usually stable. Axial compression injuries such as burst fractures occur at the thoracolumbar junction, and their character is typically associated with retropulsion of bone into the spinal canal with associated neurologic deficit.

The goal of surgical therapy is to provide an environment for spinal cord recovery. The functional goals are: (1) decompression of the spinal canal to remove impinging bone and disk fragments, (2) restoration of the normal alignment of the spine, and (3) stabilization that enables the height of the vertebral body to be restored. Long-term stabilization of the fracture site with bone grafting is often required. Operative procedures are performed through anterior or posterior approaches, but laminectomy is usually contraindicated because it contributes to further instability of the spine.

Fracture dislocation always involves *translation* of one spinal motion segment or a portion of a segment in relation to the remaining spine, and translation always causes failure in all three columns. Radiographic appearance of these injuries represents the recoiled position of the spine, and greater displacement may have occurred than is apparent on radiography. *Flexion distraction* injuries, which commonly occur over a seat belt when the torso is flexed forward with a restraining belt, may be associated with marked displacement and are very unstable. Open reduction is usually required. The *Chance* fracture is a unique flexion distraction injury in which there is horizontal splitting of the neural arch, the pedicles, and the vertebral body.

FRACTURES AND DISLOCATIONS OF THE SHOULDER, ARM, AND FOREARM

Anterior Dislocation of the Shoulder

The cumulative range of motion of the shoulder is greater than any other joint. The humeral head articulates with the glenoid, a shallow disk with a surface that is one third that of the humeral head. These anatomic peculiarities render this joint susceptible to traumatic dislocation. The humeral head lies retroverted 35 degrees, and the glenoid is anteverted 20 degrees, a configuration that is in part responsible for the more frequent occurrence of anterior dislocations than posterior dislocations. Acute traumatic dislocations occur as a result of forward abduction extension in external rotation of the shoulder. The humeral head is levered over the rim of the glenoid and causes a tear or defect in the glenoid labrum known as a *Bankart lesion*. With repetitive traumatic dislocation a groove forms in the posterior portion of the humeral head (Hill-Sachs lesion). Traumatic dislocations most commonly occur in active adults, while children and adolescents are more likely to have an epiphyseal separation. Some patients habitually dislocate and are voluntary dislocators. This may be associated with collagen diseases such as *Ehlers-Danlos syndrome* or through a psychiatric disturbance.

Following traumatic dislocation of the shoulder the arm is at the side, the acromial process is prominent, and normal fullness of the shoulder is replaced by a concave contour just below the acromium. Injury to the brachial plexus must be sought, particularly to the axillary nerve. Films should include anterior, posterior, tangential scapular, and axillary views. Reduction of the dislocation should be prompt and gentle and accomplished with some sedation. Occasionally, a general anesthetic is needed. Reduction is accomplished by longitudinal traction on the arm with countertraction applied in the axilla. The arm is immobilized in a sling and held in internal rotation for approximately 3 weeks. Range-of-motion exercises are then subsequently initiated, but abduction and external rotation

should be avoided for 3 months. Recurrence is common in younger patients and less so in patients over 40 years of age. Recurrent anterior dislocations may require soft tissue orthopedic procedures on the shoulder to prevent redislocation.

The *dead arm syndrome* is observed in patients suffering recurrent transient subluxation of the shoulder. Posterior shoulder dislocations comprise only 2 per cent of all glenohumeral joint dislocations and may occur as a result of violent seizure. Transaxillary or transcapular lateral radiographs are important for clarifying the diagnosis. The arm should be mobilized in posterior dislocations with moderate abduction and external rotation.

Fractures of the Proximal Humerus

Fractures of the proximal humerus occur more frequently with advancing age. These fractures have been classified by Neer into four types: (1) articular segment or fracture occurring through the anatomic neck, (2) fractures involving the greater tuberosity, (3) fracture involving the lesser tuberosity, and (4) fractures through the metaphyseal region or surgical neck. The classification identifies the fractures as one, two, three, or four-part fractures depending on the number of segments displaced. One centimeter of separation or 45 degrees of angulation of any segment is considered a displaced fragment.

Most humeral fractures are secondary to a fall on an outstretched arm. Treatment consists of external immobilization with a sling and swathe for minimally displaced fractures, which comprise 80 per cent of these injuries. Within 2 to 3 weeks, range-of-motion exercises are begun. Two-part fractures involving the greater tuberosity that cannot be reduced and those displaced more than 1 cm require open reduction internal fixation. Three-part fractures are treated by open reduction and internal fixation. Four-part fractures, because of the disruption of blood supply and the risk for avascular necrosis of the humeral head, may require prosthetic replacement. If a proximal physeal fracture occurs in the adolescent, it should be reduced and pinned.

Fractures and Dislocations of the Clavicle

The clavicle is an S-shaped bone that provides connection between the shoulder girdle and axial skeleton. Proximally, it articulates with the sternum, and stability is maintained by a complex of capsule and sternoclavicular ligaments. Its lateral articulation occurs with the acromial process of the scapula. Stability is provided by strong acromioclavicular and coracoclavicular ligaments. The clavicle is one of the most frequently fractured bones, and 60 per cent of all clavicular fractures occur in children younger than 10 years of age. Fractures are divided by anatomic regions in the proximal, middle, and distal third and can be treated with a figure-of-8 bandage and an arm sling if necessary. It is particularly important to recognize birth fractures, which present as pseudoparalysis of the limb. Association with brachial palsy is to be excluded. Open reduction and internal fixation of clavicle fractures is not usually indicated. Dislocations of the acromioclavicular joint can be treated with a protective sling. Subluxation and complete dislocations of the acromioclavicular joint are easily managed by the application of a Kenny-Howard splint, which reduces the dislocation. Posterior sternoclavicular dislocations should be reduced by use of a towel clip to avoid pressure on major vascular structures. The most frequent complication of clavicle fractures is nonunion, which occasionally can cause irritation of the brachial plexus.

Fractures of the Scapula

The scapula is a broad, flat bone that assists in stabilization of the shoulder girdle by providing contact with the ribs. Scapula fractures are relatively uncommon, rarely require internal fixation, and are usually treated symptomatically with a sling and swathe. A CT scan can be helpful to delineate intra-articular fractures that involve the glenoid.

Fractures of the Shaft of the Humerus

The humeral shaft is cylindric proximally and broad distally. The major neurovascular structures are all medial except the radial nerve. While nondisplaced fractures are usually treated by wrapping the arm to the chest, displaced fractures can be treated by the hanging cast method, which may occasionally cause overdistraction of the fracture and nonunion. Coaptation splint is perhaps the most effective means of mobilizing humeral shaft fractures, although alignment of the fracture is more difficult. Patients with associated vascular injuries may benefit from rapid internal fixation prior to vessel repair. The humerus is the most common site of pathologic fractures, and these can be repaired with intramedullary devices and methyl methacrylate. Complications of humeral fractures include neuropraxia injury to the radial nerve, particularly at the junction of the middle and distal third of the humerus.

Fractures of the Distal Humerus and Elbow

Supracondylar fractures of the humerus represent 50 to 60 per cent of all fractures in the region of the elbow. Fractures around the elbow in children may lead to growth disturbance if not treated appropriately. Anatomically, the humerus is divided into the *lateral condyle*, which consists of the lateral epicondyle, the origin of the extensor muscle, and the capitellum. The *medial condyle* is formed by the medial epicondyle (the origin of the flexor muscle mass) and trochlea. When the elbow is flexed to 90 degrees, an isosceles triangle is formed posteriorly by the landmarks of the lateral epicondyle, the medial epicondyle, and the tip of the olecranon. Displaced fractures involving the elbow joint distort the relationship.

Supracondylar fractures are classified by mechanism of injury (*flexion* or *extension*), with extension-type fractures the most common. Transcondylar and intracondylar fractures may be observed in adults, particularly in the elderly. It is imperative that neurovascular status be observed in distal humerus and supracondylar fractures because of arterial and neurologic injury that often occurs with these injuries. In children, comparison films of the uninvolved distal humerus and the elbow are helpful in making the diagnosis of fracture or dislocation. Measurement of Baumann's angle may be helpful in assuring a normal carrying angle. Any displaced supracondylar fracture in a child should be treated in the operating room under anesthesia and may need to be opened for pinning of fracture fragments that cannot be treated by closed means such as manipulation and percutaneous pinning.

The most serious complication of the supracondylar fracture is Volkmann's ischemic contracture. Varus, valgus, and rotatory malunion do not remodel and may persist. The most common malunion observed is that of cubitus varus (gun stock deformity). If significant, this may require corrective osteotomy. Fractures of the lateral condyle are significant injuries in children and deserve special consideration. The fracture may be misdiagnosed as a minor injury, and a natural fracture is usually Salter type 4 injury. Unlike most children's fractures, these have a tendency to progress to nonunion and should be treated with appropriate reduction and internal fixation. Medial epicondyle fractures displaced more than 5 mm warrant open reduction and internal fixation.

Dislocations of the Elbow

Dislocation is caused by falling on an outstretched arm, and neurovascular structures can be affected. Complications involve dislocation after manipulative reduction, including myositis ossificans. This leads to ossification of surrounding muscle, which may impair motion. Fractures of the olecranon may cause contusion and neuropraxia of the ulnar nerve. Fractures of the olecranon with displacement are treated with open reduction and internal fixation. Comminuted small fragments can be excised. Fractures and dislocations of the radial head are common in children. Radial head dislocations that occur with fracture of the proximal ulna are known as *Monteggia fractures*. In young children, subluxation of the radial head through the annular ligaments is common and referred to as pulled elbow or nursemaid's elbow. Often this injury can be reduced nonoperatively.

Fractures of the Shaft of the Radius and Ulna

Proximal and distal articulations of the radius and ulna allow the radius to rotate around the ulna, providing pronation and supination of the forearm. Proximally, this rotation is through the complex articulation at the radial-ulnar and radial-humeral joints. Distally, the radial-ulnar relationship is maintained by the triangular fibrocartilage complex. The shaft of the radius and ulna are connected by the fibrous interosseous membrane that serves as a hinge allowing the radius to rotate around the ulna. Distortion of the anatomy by fractures or dislocations alter the biomechanics of the forearm and particularly the change in the normal interosseous membrane space. This causes an abnormality of pronation and supination. A distal radius fracture with dislocation of the distal ulna is referred as a Galeazzi or Piedmont fracture.

At times, forearm fractures can present with impaired neurovascular function based on the increased pressure within muscle compartments of the forearm. Swelling with tight muscle compartments of the forearm can cause occlusion of venous and arterial circulation and may cause Volkmann's ischemic contracture. Significant swelling of the forearm compartments associated with pain on passive extension of the fingers should call attention to this possibility.

Treatment of displaced fractures of the shaft of the radius and ulna or those with radial head dislocation are best managed by operative methods. Forearm fractures are best managed by compression plating of the radius and ulna to restore the normal interosseous space. Most forearm fractures in children can be managed by closed methods. However, rotational malalignment does not remodel and must be avoided during treatment of these injuries. The most serious complication of forearm fractures is neurovascular compromise subsequent to Volkmann's ischemic contracture and this must be avoided.

Fractures of the distal forearm include distal ulnar fractures and distal radial fractures. Distal ulnar fractures can be treated usually with a splint. A distal radial fracture, known as a *Colles' fracture*, is a fracture of the distal radial metaphysis with *dorsal* displacement and *volar* angulation. A *Smith fracture* is a fracture with *volar* displacement and *dorsal* angulation. Barton described an intra-articular fracture of the dorsal or volar lip of the distal radius. In all distal radius fractures, median nerve function should be tested because this nerve is the most susceptible to compression or contusion. Intra-articular fractures of the distal radius should be treated by open reduction. Median nerve compression may be a chronic problem related to distal wrist fractures.

FRACTURES OF THE WRIST

The *scaphoid* is the most frequently fractured carpal bone. It is the linkage between the proximal and distal carpal rows through which dorsiflexion and volar flexion occur through both the radiocarpal and intercarpal joints. The axis of normal carpal movement is at the neck of the capitate. The scaphoid bridges the proximal and distal carpal rows. In evaluating the wrist, anteroposterior, posteroanterior, radial and ulnar deviation, flexion, extension, and clenched fist views are often necessary to delineate pathology. The scaphoid is usually injured following a fall on the outstretched hand.

Fracture of the carpal scaphoid produces tenderness to pressure in the anatomic snuff box that is located between extensor pollicis longus and extensor pollicis brevis-abductor pollicis longus compartments (Fig. 3).

Special radiographs can be obtained for scaphoid fractures that include ulnar deviation views. Care must be taken not to be forceful with this maneuver, as severe ulnar deviation can displace nondisplaced scaphoid fractures. Furthermore, if a scaphoid fracture is suspected but not present initially, repeat films should be obtained 10 to 14 days after injury, when the lesion is sometimes demonstrable due to the resorption at the fracture site. Computed tomography scans and bone scans may be helpful in the diagnosis of scaphoid fractures. The major difficulty with treatment of scaphoid fractures relates to lack of early diagnosis and delayed initiation of appropriate treatment. Acute scaphoid fractures that are not displaced should be immobilized in a long arm cast with the thumb included in the cast.

The major blood supply of the scaphoid is from the radial artery. The scaphoid is prone to avascular necrosis of the proximal fragment, due to injury of the dorsal distal–to–proximal arterial arcade that supplies the scaphoid bone. Seventy per cent of scaphoid fractures involve the middle part of the bone, and the healing time is generally 8 to 12 weeks. If the scaphoid fracture fragments are displaced, some degree of carpal instability exists. In these instances, open reduction internal fixation should be employed. In incidences of scaphoid nonunion, iliac crest bone grafting is performed as advocated by Russe.

joints are held in 60 to 80 degrees of flexion, the PIP joint in 10 to 20 degrees of flexion, and the *distal interphalangeal* (DIP) joint in 5 to 10 degrees of flexion. With the metacarpal phalangeal joint and inner phalangeal joints in extension, the collateral ligaments at the respective joints are elongated, thereby decreasing the likelihood of the ligament contracture and subsequent joint stiffness. Each finger has a flexor profundus tendon that inserts into the proximal segment of the distal phalanx and a flexor superficialis tendon that inserts into the middle phalanx. These extrinsic muscles originate in the forearm.

The interosseus muscles abduct and adduct the fingers. The lumbricales that assist in flexing the metacarpal phalangeal joints and extending the IP joints originate within the hand and are termed *intrinsic muscles*. The thumb intrinsics include the opponens pollicis, abductor pollicis brevis, flexor pollicis brevis, and adductor pollicis.

Clinical Examination

A pattern of assessment should be followed consistently, including the patient's age, sex, occupation, hand dominance, and accurate data concerning the injury (when, where, how, and why). Questions to be asked include: What was the interval between the injury and examination? Who treated the injury initially and what was the treatment? Was the injury in a dirty or clean environment? Was it a bite? Did it occur at work? What was the mechanism of the injury (such as crushing, twisting, or direct blow)?

Circulation is tested by compressing the distal pulp adjacent to the nail for capillary refill and observing the color of the digit, as well as comparing the surface temperature with that of the rest of the adjacent digits. Often the digital artery compressing test (Allen's) cannot be performed because of pain or swelling, and capillary refill is particularly helpful. A pale finger usually indicates diminished arterial flow, and a blue finger indicates venous congestion. Elevating the extremity may provide information about venous and arterial flow. After hand injury or fracture, all rings and jewelry should be removed immediately. Sensitivity is tested by determining light touch, deep pressure, two-point discrimination, and sharp point. The sensory deficit may be profound if the digital nerve was lacerated completely or may be minimal if the nerve was only contused. In an open fracture with sensory loss, the assumption is that the digital nerve has been lacerated or severely damaged. The involved digit is examined to determine the site of disruption of bone and soft tissue. The precise areas of tenderness are palpated such as the central slip on the dorsum aspect of the PIP joint, the collateral ligaments on the radial and ulnar side, and the palmar plate, as well as the flexor

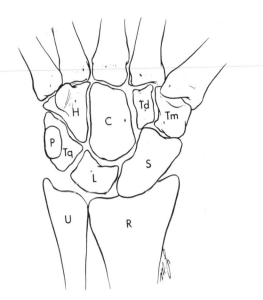

Figure 3. The carpal bones: schaphoid (S); lunate (L); triquetrum (Tq); pisiform (P), which is sesamoid bone within the flexor carpil ulnaris; trapezium (Tm); trapezoid (Td); capitate (C); and hamate (H). Radius (R) and ulna (U) are noted. (From Goldner RD, Ugino MR, Goldner JL: Injuries to carpal bones. *In* Edlich RF, Spyker DA [eds]: Current Emergency Medical Therapy. Norwalk, CT, Appleton-Century-Crofts, 1984, with permission.)

FRACTURES AND DISLOCATIONS OF THE HAND

Fractures of the metacarpals and phalanges represent 10 per cent of all fractures, and of these, fractures of the distal phalanx are most common, followed in order by fractures of the metacarpals, proximal phalanges, and middle phalanges. The individual joints in each digit have a direct effect on the total function of the involved and adjacent digits, with the *proximal interphalangeal* (PIP) joint being the most sensitive to injury, fibrosis, and stiffness.

Each tubular bone is divided anatomically into its base, shaft, neck, and head (articular component). The thumb has one metacarpal, two phalanges, and independent intrinsic muscles, as well as extensors and flexors (extensor and flexor pollicis longus). If the fingers are flexed, their line of action converges with the center of each nail pointed toward the scaphoid. As none of the fingers is flexed in a straight line, the fingers should not be immobilized parallel to the long axis of the hand.

To avoid malrotation, the proper position of digit immobilization is determined by observing the position of flexion of the normal uninjured digits. Splints, plaster, and dressing should pull the digits in intrinsic-plus position; that is, the *metacarpophalangeal* (MCP)

and extensor tendon insertions. Abnormalities regarding alignment are noted, as well as angle and rotation of deformities.

Open wounds are examined cautiously. Both sides of the hand are inspected. Swelling on the dorsum may follow penetration on the volar surface. The examiner should do minimal probing until adequate peripheral anesthesia has been obtained and the patient is in a location where definitive treatment can be completed, such as an operating room.

Terminology provides description of the alignment of fractures. *Dislocation* means that the articular surfaces are not opposed and that the restraining ligaments and probably the joint capsule have been partially or completely torn. *Subluxation* is a partial displacement of one side of the joint onto the other but with less severe distortion than the dislocation. Soft tissue interposition may prevent complete reduction in either instance. Reduction is the action required to obtain anatomic alignment.

Fractures are described as *stable, unstable, displaced, nondisplaced, impacted, comminuted, intra-articular, extra-articular, transverse, oblique,* or *spinal. Angulation* may occur in any direction: *dorsal, volar, radial, ulnar,* or in combinations. *Malrotation* may also occur. If there is no wound, the fracture is *closed*; if the skin is broken, the fracture is termed as *open.* Fractures of the phalanx or intra-articular injury in the digit may be managed by local infiltration or by digital nerve block using lidocaine without epinephrine in the metacarpal area. A digital block is performed by injecting the anesthetic agent into the web space on either side of the metacarpal neck with the needle inserted palmarward toward the digital nerve. In some instances, blocking the median and ulnar nerves, as well as blocking the superficial radial nerve, can be helpful for analgesia.

Antibiotics should be administered for contaminated wounds. A first-generation cephalosporin is given for most open hand fractures. Antibiotics for human bite wounds include penicillin. With extreme contamination such as foreign body injuries, aminoglycosides should be given, as well as cephalosporin and penicillin. The wounds of all open fractures are considered tetanus-prone wounds, and the patient's tetanus immunization should be updated. With crush injuries, a high index of suspicion should be maintained for the development of compartment syndrome.

Distal Phalangeal Fractures

The distal phalanx is frequently fractured by crush from a hammer or heavy object. The fracture can be splinted for 10 to 14 days to decrease discomfort and allow healing. The fingernail may be elevated by hematoma from the fracture, which is extremely painful. This hematoma can be released by a hole made in the center of the nail, using an open paper clip that has been heated with a flame, or by disposable cautery. If the nail bed has been lacerated, the nail plate should be removed and laceration repaired with fine absorbable sutures.

Dorsal avulsion fractures occur when the extensor digitorum communis tendon is avulsed. The superior part of the articular surface may constitute part of the fracture fragment, and loss of extension occurs usually at the distal phalanx, causing a *mallet finger* or *drop finger.* The patient should be splinted after the fracture is reduced for a total of 8 to 12 weeks.

Avulsion fracture from a flexor surface may occur as a result of hyperextension of the distal phalangeal joint following a forcible blow or fall. Pain, swelling, and inability to flex the distal joint are associated with this injury, and operative treatment is required to reattach the flexor tendon to the point of avulsion.

Fractures through the distal portion (neck of the middle phalanx) are likely to have apex palmar angulation because the proximal fragment is flexed by the superficialis tendon. A fracture through the proximal portion (base of the middle phalanx) is likely to have apex dorsal angulation caused by flexion of the distal fragment by the superficialis and extension of the proximal fragment by the central slip of the extensor tendon. Stable fractures can be immobilized initially in a splint followed by adjacent digit taping (buddy taping). Spinal and oblique fractures are well suited for open reduction and internal fixation with screws. Condylar fractures are, by definition, intra-articular and require accurate reduction of the articular surface to avoid joint incongruity and subsequent traumatic arthrosis.

Dorsal dislocations of the PIP joint are classified by location of the middle phalanx in relation to the proximal phalanx, either palmar, dorsal, or lateral. Dorsal dislocation of the middle phalanx with avulsion of the volar plate from the middle phalanx is a common injury. The PIP joint is swollen and may be mistaken for a "sprained" finger. Often, a small volar fragment of the proximal end of the middle phalanx is seen on lateral radiographic film. Treatment consists of splinting the PIP joint in about 20 to 30 degrees of flexion for 2 to 3 weeks. Fractures that involve greater than 40 per cent of the articular surface are usually unstable and require open reduction internal fixation. Occasionally, if the base of the middle phalanx is comminuted, a volar plate arthroplasty is performed. Palmar dislocation of the PIP joint may cause avulsion at the central extensor tendon slip, flexion deformity of the PIP joint, and hyperextension of the DIP joint (boutonnière deformity).

Proximal phalangeal fractures require appropriate splinting relaxation of the extrinsic and intrinsic muscles. Oblique fractures tend to shorten and may require percutaneous pinning or open reduction. Metacarpal phalangeal joint dislocation may follow hyperextension force. The index finger is dislocated most frequently, and the mechanism of injury involves avulsion at the volar plate. This may become trapped between the metacarpal head and the proximal phalanx, and reduction may not be possible by closed methods, requiring open reduction and release of the volar plate that is entrapped.

Metacarpal fractures are divided by region. Fractures of the metacarpal head may be intra-articular and require fixation. Brewerton views are obtained with the metacarpal phalangeal joint flexed 65 degrees. The dorsum of the hand is next to the plate and the radiographic apparatus is angled 15 degrees ulnar to radial, which aids in visualization of fractures of the metacarpal head. Fracture of the neck of the fifth metacarpal is a common injury caused by a direct blow. Termed *boxer's fracture*, it occurs when a dorsal force is applied directly to the metacarpal head. The head is displaced palmarward and the shaft bows dorsally. As much as 40 to 45 degrees of dorsal angulation is acceptable in the fifth metacarpal, and approximately 30 degrees is acceptable in the fourth metacarpal. However, in the index and long metacarpals, anatomic reduction is desirable because of the relative lack of mobility of the shaft of these metacarpals. Angulation of greater than 15 degrees is unacceptable secondary to the lack of compensatory carpal metacarpal motion. Rotational alignment must be restored in all fingers. Transverse and short oblique metacarpal shaft fractures are treated by casting of minimally displaced fragments and may require open reduction internal fixation if any persistent rotational deformity persists.

Metacarpal fractures at the base of the thumb are caused by a fall on the outstretched hand. A common intra-articular fracture to the proximal end of the metacarpal is known as *Bennett's fracture*, and a comminuted intra-articular fracture of the proximal end of the metacarpal is termed *Rolando's fracture*, both of which are usually treated with percutaneous pin fixation of the first metacarpal into the base of the second metacarpal. Occasionally, the metacarpal phalangeal joint of the thumb can be injured when the ulnar collateral ligament is avulsed from the proximal phalanx. Stress radiographs are used to evaluate this injury. If the collateral ligament is torn completely, it can become trapped outside the adductor aponeurosis and may not heal (Stener's lesion). This may require open reduction internal fixation.

Summary

Treatment of hand fractures is directed toward regaining flexible, properly aligned, strong digits with adequate vascular supply and sensibility. One common complication is decreased motion secondary to tendon adhesions or ligament encapsular contracture. This condition is often improved by active exercises and by dynamic splinting. Occasionally, however, these conditions require tenolysis with surgical release of joint capsules or ligaments. Narrowing, malrotation, or angulation can be corrected by osteotomies, and nonunion can be corrected by bone grafting and rigid internal fixation if needed. Infections may occur with open fractures or those fractures treated by open reduction and internal fixation.

FRACTURES OF THE PELVIS, FEMUR, AND KNEE

Pelvic fractures are associated with massive trauma and frequently follow automobile collision with pedestrians. In older patients with osteoporosis, fractures of the pelvis more commonly occur from minor injuries such as from a fall. Major pelvic fractures are life threatening and death occurs in as many as 20 per cent of patients. Injury to many organ systems may occur with the massive trauma that causes pelvic fractures and includes retroperitoneal hemorrhage, neurologic changes from damage to the lumbosacral plexus, and nerve root or genitourinary damage, as well as injury to major arterial trunks.

The pelvis is a rigid ring composed of the pubic rami, ischium acetabulum, ileum, and sacrum, joined by heavy ligaments at the symphysis and the sacroiliac joints. Disruption at one point does not necessarily produce instability. Disruption at two points on the same side of the pelvis may allow displacement as the paravertebral muscles shorten. Either prolonged skeletal traction or open reduction with internal fixation is needed for maintenance of the fracture in position.

Tile has classified pelvic injuries by the mechanism of injury. Anterior posterior compression occurs when the patient is struck from the front with disruption of the symphysis anteriorly and disruption of the anterior ligaments of the sacroiliac joint. The pelvis thus opens as a book opens, leaving the posterior ligaments of the sacroiliac joint intact.

Vertical shear fractures follow axial loading as in a fall from a height. Anteriorly, there may be a fracture of one or both pubic rami with disruption of the symphysis pubis. A vertical shear fracture is usually unstable and is difficult to treat with traction. Open reduction is generally indicated. Minor fractures include the fractures of the ileum, lateral fractures of the pubic rami, and avulsion fractures at points of muscle attachments. Fractures of the anterior superior iliac spine occur in athletes by force of the contracture of the sartorius muscle. Sprinters may avulse at the ischial tuberosity by forceful contraction of the hamstrings.

The most common complication of pelvic fractures

is massive hemorrhage in the retroperitoneal space, which occurs in the plexus of veins and arteries lying in the inner pelvic wall. Most doctors agree that open reduction of unstable pelvic fractures is mandatory to achieve bony union and satisfactory functional position. Persistent pelvic deformity can cause leg length inequality, causing difficulty in walking and other activities. Careful neurologic evaluation should include evaluation of the obturator nerve, which supplies the adductor muscle, the sciatic nerve, and the lumbosacral plexus. Retroperitoneal bleeding may mimic a gastrointestinal trauma, and peritoneal lavage may be necessary to exclude ruptured intra-abdominal organs. Careful examination of the rectum and the vagina may reveal blood in either orifice and is presumptive evidence for open pelvic fractures.

In the event of an anterior posterior compression fracture, the volume in the pelvis is increased approximately four times. The use of an external fixator on the pelvis to close the symphysis or reduce the volume in the pelvis may be needed to reduce retroperitoneal bleeding. If after application of an external fixator the blood pressure is not stabilized, the patient may require arteriography and subsequent embolization of the hypogastric artery. Emergency radiographic evaluation should include an anterior posterior view and 40-degree caudad and cephalad projection of the pelvis. When the acetabulum is fractured, a 45-degree oblique view should be obtained.

Complications of pelvic fracture include hemorrhage and injury to the lower urinary tract. As the bladder extends, it may fill most of the true pelvis and rise above the symphysis where it becomes vulnerable to trauma. Injuries to the lower urinary tract, bladder, and urethra occur in 14 per cent of all pelvic fractures and may be detected by urethrogram, cystogram, and intravenous urogram.

If the urethrogram demonstrates the urethra intact retrograde, cystography should be performed with a 14- or 16-Fr catheter with injection of dye. The passage of a blind catheter without urethrography is not appropriate because it may enter and drain blood from the perivesicular space, simulating extraperitoneal rupture of the bladder. Rupture of bladder and urethra are surgical emergencies requiring immediate urinary diversion and repair. The sciatic nerve is most frequently damaged by fractures of the pelvis that extend into the ileum and to the sciatic notch and may be recognized by failure to contract the hamstrings and to dorsiflex the foot. Paralysis of the obturator nerve may occur and is recognized by the inability to connect the adductor muscles.

All unstable pelvic fractures are best treated by open reduction and internal fixation with plates or screws. Open reduction to reconstruct the weight-bearing surface of the hip joint is usually indicated when the acetabulum is also involved.

Fractures of the Hip and Upper Femur

Fractures of the proximal femur occur most commonly in elderly women but may occur at any age. Before the 20th century, fracture of the femur was almost universally fatal because of pulmonary, renal, and cardiac complications. Advances with the use of side plates, pins, and prosthetic replacement have decreased mortality. In any fracture, healing depends not only on fixation but, more significantly, on blood supply. Blood supply is more subject to damage in that portion of the femur that is intracapsular, which makes the prognosis for these fractures much worse than for those occurring below the intertrochanteric line outside the capsule. Intracapsular fractures include fractures of the head of the femur, impacted subcapital fractures, and displaced subcapital and neck fractures. Because there is no periosteum on the femoral neck, healing is by endosteal callus. Fixation must be rigid and, yet, must allow impaction as the fracture lines resorb. The femoral head receives only a small amount of blood supply from the pelvic side of the joint through the ligamentum teres. The major blood supply is from the vascular ring at the base of the neck, which arises from retinacular arteries that pierce the capsule and supply the femoral head. The arteries may become torn or damaged following head fractures. Fractures of the femoral head occur most often in posterior fracture dislocations of the hip, and manipulation allows for relocation. However, if a portion of the femoral head is trapped in the joint, it needs to be removed operatively. Patients presenting with minor groin pain may have stress fractures of the femoral neck (Fig. 4). Impacted subcapital fractures often slip into an unstable position, and the safest course is to treat them with percutaneous pin fixation. Aseptic necrosis is a complication of femoral head fractures and may develop as late as 5 or 6 years after injury. Displaced subcapital fractures of the neck of the femur are prone more to avascular necrosis. Fractures of the femoral neck can be treated either with percutaneous pins, or in elderly patients with osteoporosis, a screw and side plate. In elderly patients, if a perfect reduction cannot be obtained, replacement with an endoprosthesis or bipolar prosthesis is desirable for quick immobilization of the patient. However, this is to be avoided in young patients.

Intertrochanteric fractures occur below the inferior attachment of the head capsule outside the vascular ring supplying the femoral neck and head. Blood supply is excellent. Stability of intertrochanteric fractures requires both support along the medial calcar and lateral buttress to prevent the femoral shaft from shifting

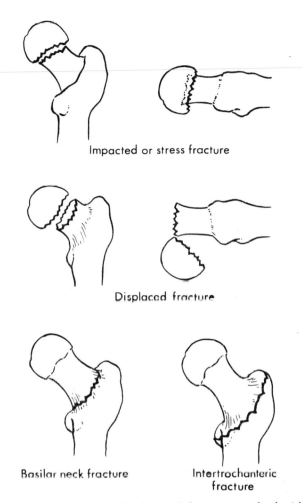

Impacted or stress fracture

Displaced fracture

Basilar neck fracture

Intertrochanteric fracture

Figure 4. The impacted subcapital fracture may heal without intervention, but there is a risk of the head slipping off of the neck during the healing period. In the younger patient, the displaced fracture should be reduced and fixed with multiple pins. In the older patient the displaced fracture is treated with prosthetic replacement. The basilar neck fracture and the intertrochanteric fracture must be fixed with a lag screw, which passes through the trochanter, into the neck and the head, and is attached to the femur by means of a side plate. (From McCollum DE: Fractures of the pelvis, femur, and knee. *In* Sabiston DC Jr [ed]: Textbook of Surgery: The Biological Basis of Modern Surgical Practice, ed 14. Philadelphia, WB Saunders Company, 1991, p 1331, with permission.)

medially as it is drawn by the pull of the adductor muscles. Hip fractures in children are uncommon, but complications are common and include growth disturbance, vascular changes, nonunion, and partial ankylosis. For epiphyseal growth to continue, reduction must be anatomic and fixation secure. These goals can best be met with open reduction internal fixation with screw fixation.

Transepiphyseal fractures may occur with severe

trauma, or minor trauma may cause complete destruction of an epiphyseal line already weakened by chronic slipping capital femoral epiphysis. Fractures of the neck of the femur and shoulder produce a high incidence of avascular necrosis of the femoral head. Pin fixation should be accomplished and anatomic reduction obtained. Subtrochanteric fractures may be managed in the child by traction for an initial period followed by plaster immobilization.

Fractures of the femur can be divided into four areas: subtrochanteric, midshaft or diaphyseal, supracondylar, and condylar. The patient with a fractured femur must be evaluated carefully. Loss of 2 to 3 units of blood within the thigh may not be apparent, and shock may ensue without warning. The hip and knee joints must be radiographically evaluated for association of hip dislocations or supracondylar fractures. Femoral fractures can be treated by cast braces, which rely on hydrodynamic effects of compressed thigh muscles within the cast and cause considerable shortening and perhaps angulation of the fracture. The cast brace has been replaced by the use of the interlocking femoral nail for treatment of fractures of the femoral shaft. Supracondylar fractures of the femur are difficult to treat by closed methods and traction, and are best treated by open reduction internal fixation, which allows early fixation of the knee. Fractures of the patella are often stellate, comminuted, and compound due to the direct nature of the injury. If the extensor retinaculum is torn and inactive and knee extension is not possible, an open reduction is required to restore the extensor mechanism. Comminuted patella fractures often cause *chondromalacia*. Occasionally, the fractures are so comminuted that they may be treated by excision rather than repair. Fractures of the patella must be differentiated from the bipartite patella. When this condition is suspected, radiographs of the opposite knee may reveal the same condition.

In dislocations of the knee, the cruciate ligaments are often torn, as is the joint capsule. Displacement of the tibia may be anterior, posterior, lateral, or medial, but anterior dislocation is most common. The position of the knee may be normal at the time of presentation, and the dislocation may have spontaneously reduced. Absence of deformity can be misleading because severe vascular nerve damage may be present. The greatest cause of morbidity from this injury is nerve and vascular damage. Goldner and Ford found perineal palsy in half the patients, and Shields found vascular damage in 40 per cent of 26 patients. The popliteal artery and vein are subject to injury during hyperextension of the knee or anterior displacement of the tibia. The pulses are diminished, and if there is any question about the continuity of vessels, immediate exploration of the popliteal space should be done. Arteriography is time consuming and probably unnecessary because vascular damage is always within a few inches of the joint line. Replacement by prosthetic artery or vein graft may be necessary.

FRACTURES OF THE TIBIA, FIBULA, ANKLE, AND FOOT

The tibia and fibula are two of the most frequently fractured long bones. High-energy and motor vehicular trauma cause many injuries, often producing open or compound fractures with soft tissue defects. The tibia can be palpated along the medial subcutaneous border of the leg, and the lower end of the tibia is slightly expanded and projects downward as the medial malleolus. The fibula can be divided into three regions: the head, shaft, and lateral malleolus. Tibial fractures can be caused by high- or low-energy injury. The prognosis is determined by the amount of energy absorbed and not necessarily by the location of the fracture. Automobile-pedestrian accidents can impart up to 100,000 foot-pounds of energy to the victim. The fibula can be fractured by direct blow, or the head may fracture with an isolated medial malleolar fracture of the so-called *Maisonneuve's fracture.* Fractures of the proximal tibia, or *tibial plateau fractures,* have been divided into six types depending on the degree of joint incongruity and whether or not the metaphysis is separated from the diaphysis.

Fractures of the tibial shaft are usually classified into thirds, with delays in healing observed commonly in the middle third and the region between the proximal and middle third. Open tibial fractures commonly involve the shaft. Gustilo and Anderson have classified open fractures into three categories that have significance regarding the incidence of fracture union and risk for infection and/or amputation. Grade I fractures are those that have perforation of the skin from the inside; wounds are less than or equal to 1 cm. Grade II open fractures are produced by outside-to-inside forces, with soft tissue injury being greater than 1 cm. Grade III injuries involve significant soft tissue damage. These are further classified into grade IIIA, soft tissue injury without periosteal stripping or vessel damage; grade IIIB, soft tissue damage with periosteal stripping; and grade IIIC, major vascular injury and soft tissue damage. Difficult fractures involving the lower tibia are tibial plafond fractures occurring at the lower tibia and frequently extending into the ankle joint.

Patients with tibial fractures should be suspected of having *compartment syndrome,* defined as an increase in tissue pressure in the closed fascial compartments of the leg, which can occur in open or closed tibial fractures. If intracompartmental pressures exceed capillary pressure, diminished tissue perfusion may cause anoxia and necrosis of tissue within the compartment. Signs include pain on passive stretching of muscles in the compartment, swollen compartments, diminished sensibility, and motor weakness. A variety of methods may be used in measuring compartment pressure. Fasciotomy should be performed if clinical suspicion is high and pressures are elevated with respect to arterial pressure.

The principles of the care of tibial fracture are classic and are: reduction of the fracture, stabilization of the limb to allow healing, and proper care of the soft tissue envelope. Nondisplaced fractures of the tibia may be treated with casting. The long leg casts are initially used to control forces about the knee joint, and when the fracture becomes consolidated, a walking cast can be applied. Disadvantages of cast treatment include the possibility of creating fracture disease, which refers to disuse osteoporosis muscle wasting, joint stiffness, and posttraumatic dystrophy. External fixation is easily applied to open tibial fractures where gross contamination and severe soft tissue injury precludes the use of internal fixation. Plating is occasionally indicated for the treatment of tibial fractures.

Intramedullary devices may be used for stabilization of tibia shaft fractures. These are usually reserved for fractures that are difficult to control with closed methods such as casting. Tibial fractures often involve bone loss that may require bone grafting using either conventional bone grafting, which is autogenous iliac crest, cortical cancellous graft, or vascularized grafting such as free vascularized fibular grafts.

Open fractures of the tibia and fibula usually involve soft tissue injury. Staged soft tissue reconstruction is performed after fracture stabilization. In proximal third injuries, the gastrocnemius is commonly used for coverage. In those of the middle third, the soleus may be rotated. In distal third lesions, there may be a need for soft tissue closure by free tissue transplantation using microsurgical techniques. Infection is the most severe complication of tibial fractures and usually follows open injuries. Aggressive management of soft tissue includes aggressive débridement of nonviable soft tissue. With early coverage of exposed implants and bone, the incidence of infection-related morbidity and chronic osteomyelitis is reduced. Fractures of the fibula that accompany fractures of the tibia are usually not associated with the morbidity of tibia fractures and heal rapidly.

Ankle injuries are among the most frequent conditions treated in orthopedic surgery. Fractures may occur based on several mechanism of injury usually involving external rotation of the foot in the ankle joint. The fibular fracture is in the oblique or spiral plane and is often displaced posteriorly. The medial malleolus also may be fractured. The optimal treatment of ankle fractures should attain several goals. The *talus* must be located in its normal position in the ankle mortis. Even a slight amount of tilt or displacement of the talus can lead to disabling arthritis. *Joint congruity* should be restored in intra-articular fractures. If the requisites for adequate treatment cannot be obtained by closed manipulation of the ankle fracture, open reduction and internal fixation should be used.

Fractures of the foot include displaced fractures of the talar neck, which should be treated with open reduction and internal fixation. There is significant risk for avascular necrosis of the body of the talus. Fractures of the calcaneus can cause many problems, particularly in the subtalar joint due to the intra-articular nature of the injury. The usual plan of treatment restores the calcaneus to its original height and width and restores the articular surface. Fractures in the midfoot include fracture of the navicular cuneiformis and cuboid bones. Dislocation of the tarsal metatarsal joints are usually the result of a direct injury or twisting. This is known as Lisfranc's joint. The spectrum of dislocation at Lisfranc's joint ranges from complete dislocation of all five tarsal metatarsal joints to the dislocation of one or two metatarsals. Fractures of the metatarsals do not require anatomic reduction unless the metatarsal heads are displaced into the plantar surface of the foot. Avulsion of the styloid process at the base of the fifth metatarsal is the result of an inversion force with avulsion following traction by the peroneus brevis tendon. Fractures of the diaphysis of the fifth metatarsal are difficult to treat because of their slow propensity to heal. Immobilization and non–weight-bearing or open reduction internal fixation are required.

Stress and fatigue fractures of the metatarsals are common and should be suspected in any patient who presents with pain and puffiness in the foot following unaccustomed excess activity such as walking or jogging. Fractures of the toe phalanges do not require treatment other than strapping the injured digit to an adjacent toe for comfort.

AMPUTATIONS AND LIMB SUBSTITUTIONS

Amputation is one of the oldest surgical procedures and existed before recorded history. Trauma, diabetes, and vascular conditions are now so common that there are 2 million amputees in the United States. Amputation is usually followed by replacement with a prosthetic device that can restore reasonable function. When timed properly and with consideration of physical rehabilitation, amputation is not a destructive procedure. It is a form of reconstruction that may be

elected whenever the prognosis is such that a well-fitted prostheses provides a better result than can be obtained in a reasonable length of time with further attempts at salvage.

With total-contact plastic sockets the only critical factor in determining the length of an amputation stump is the viability of skin. Almost any length of residual limb can be fitted with a prosthesis. In lower extremity amputees, it is extremely important to save the knee. The presence of an active knee joint markedly decreases the physical exertion of the patient, and may in fact determine whether an elderly patient can ambulate.

If amputation is performed for wet gangrene, osteomyelitis, or severe trauma, the amputation site should be left open. A posterior flap can be fashioned with delayed secondary closure. Amputation in dysvascular or diabetic limbs may be better performed using a fish-mouth incision to avoid long posterior flaps that may be prone to necrosis. Postoperatively, patients should be fitted with terminal devices early, particularly in upper extremity patients. This lessens the psychologic impact of the loss of limb and initiates the rehabilitation phase immediately.

The most commonly prescribed prostheses for the below-knee amputee is the *patella tendon bearing* (PTB) prosthesis. This socket contacts all surfaces of the stump, with weight bearing borne mainly by the medial surface of the tibia, the shaft of the fibula, and the patella tendon. A solid ankle cushioned heel (SACH) is prescribed, whereby ankle motion is simulated by compression of a sponge rubber wedge in the heel. The most common suspension for prostheses is a strap around the supracondylar area of the thigh with or without an additional elastic strap attached to the waist.

The psychologic impact of upper extremity amputations is greater than lower extremity. Patients may be fitted with a conventional body-powered prosthesis or with a myoelectric prosthesis that is activated by contracting residual muscles in the forearm. Ongoing problems of the amputee include loss of socket fit, and they may need evaluation by an orthotist. Other difficulties include neuromas, phantom limb pain, and negative psychiatric response. Occasional problems with skin, such as choke syndrome, may cause painful verrucous hyperplasia of the skin, which may be treated by refitting the prosthesis.

INFECTIONS AND NEOPLASMS OF BONE

The dictum that *every suspected tumor should be cultured and every suspected infection should be biopsied* is definitely applied to bone infections and neoplasms. *Osteomyelitis* is the general term used to denote infection of bone. The most common organism producing this infection is *Staphylococcus aureus*. Tuberculous and nonpyogenic organisms produce a less aggressive granulomatous type of infection in bone.

Suppurative infection of bone occurs in one of two ways. Blood-borne bacteria from an active focus of soft tissue infection, such as a furuncle, or urinary tract infection may become lodged in the bone and form an abscess. This mechanism is referred to as *hematogenous osteomyelitis*, commonly observed in children. If the bacteria reach bone from an external environment, such as in penetrating wounds in open fractures, exogenous osteomyelitis may result. Hematogenous osteomyelitis is primarily a disease of childhood, occurring most frequently between the ages of 5 and 15 years. Males are effected three times more frequently than females. The mechanism for hematogenous osteomyelitis in the child is related to slow blood flow in metaphyseal veins that provide an ideal location for lodgement of bacteria and subsequent infection. Isolated necrotic bone segments within abscess cavities cause sequestrum. Around the periphery of the granulation tissue and sequestrum new host defenses make an effort to isolate the infection. The new bone laid down around this is know as *involucrum*.

Adherence of the periosteum to the metaphysis and the permeability of the physeal plate usually protect the adjacent joint from infection. In infants younger than the age of 12 months, vessels traverse the physeal plate, and osteomyelitis may develop and produce adjacent *pyarthrosis*.

The hip joint in any age group is vulnerable to infection because the capital femoral epiphysis lies within the joint capsule. Ewing's sarcoma and other conditions such as acute rheumatic fever, scurvy, acute septic arthritis, and acute juvenile or rheumatoid arthritis may mimic the clinical pattern of acute osteomyelitis. Acute pyarthrosis produces swelling localized to the joint level, and the patient cannot tolerate any joint motion. The organism most frequently encountered in hematogenous osteomyelitis is *S. aureus*. In neonates and infants *Streptococcus* species may be the etiologic agent. Salmonella osteomyelitis occurs commonly in sickle cell patients.

The principles of surgical treatment of osteomyelitis are the same as treatment for any soft tissue abscess, and consists of incision and drainage, termed *saucerization* when bone is removed. When extent of bony involvement is diffuse and complete sequestrectomy is not possible, multiple sinus tracts may develop and indicate the initiation of chronic osteomyelitis. Infection can be quiescent for many months or even years and may periodically recur with drainage, fever, and swelling. Chronic osteomyelitis occurs over many years and may become lined with squamous epithelium that may undergo metaplasia and develop squamous cell carcinoma, called *Marjolin's ulcer*.

Skeletal tuberculosis may result from hematogenous seeding of tuberculi, tubercle bacilli from preexisting pulmonary or gastrointestinal focus. This organism most frequently involves the joints and adjacent bone rather than the metaphyseal area of long bones. The intervertebral disks at the lower thoracic and upper lumbar spine and adjacent vertebrae are the most frequent sites of skeletal tuberculosis, and the hip and knee joints are the next most frequently affected. The chief radiographic change in tubercular spondylitis is narrowing of the disk space at the affected level, causing the outline of the end plates to become distorted.

When treating acute pyarthrosis, one must remember that the hip joint is most frequently involved. Aspiration of the involved joint under careful sterile conditions may reveal a cloudy turbid synovial flow with cell counts ranging from 50 to 200,000/cm^3. These cells are at least 90 per cent polymorphonuclear neutrophils. Gram stain reveals organisms in about half. Joint fluid should be retained for aerobic and anaerobic cultures, and blood cultures are frequently positive. In the performance of joint aspiration, a large-bore needle should be used. Treatment of pyogenic arthritis constitutes an orthopedic emergency. Surgical incision and drainage should be performed in almost all cases.

Neoplasms of Bone

Primitive mesenchymal tissue produces cartilage, bone, fibrous tissue, and marrow elements, the four basic tissue components of the mature skeleton. Benign and malignant conditions from each of these tissue types may also arise. Although only primary neoplasms of bone are discussed, metastatic disease from sarcomas and carcinomas of the breast, lung, thyroid, kidney, and prostate are the most common neoplasms to present in bone. The common benign and malignant primary skeleton neoplasms are summarized in Table 1. To plan accurate treatment, staging of skeletal lesions is necessary. Accurate determination of the anatomic site and aggressiveness based on histologic grade and radiographic appearance is mandatory. Enneking has described the useful system for staging benign lesions: grade I, inactive lesions, tend to remain static or regress; grade II, active lesions, have potential for continued local growth; and grade III, aggressive lesions, have a potential for rapid growth and further bone destruction. Intracompartmental lesions are designated by the letter A, extracompartmental lesions are designated by the letter B, and histologically low-grade lesions by grade I and high-grade by II. Placement of the biopsy incision includes consideration of the possibility of future resection of the lesion and

TABLE 1.   COMMON SKELETAL NEOPLASMS*

	Cartilage	Bone	Fibrous	Marrow
Benign	Osteochondroma Enchondroma Chondroblastoma	Osteoid osteoma Osteoblastoma	Nonossifying fibroma Giant cell tumor Desmoplastic fibroma	Eosinophilic granuloma
Malignant	Primary chondrosarcoma Secondary chondrosarcoma	Osteosarcoma Periosteal osteosarcoma	Fibrosarcoma Fibrous histiocytoma	Ewing's tumor Lymphoma Myeloma

*From Harrelson JM, Callaghan JJ: Infections and neoplasms of bone. *In* Sabiston DC Jr [ed]: Textbook of Surgery: The Biological Basis of Modern Surgical Practice, ed 14. Philadelphia, WB Saunders Company, 1991, p 1355, with permission.

should allow complete removal of the biopsy site with the specimen. If the lesion is potentially malignant, it is inadvisable to exsanguinate the extremity with an Esmarch bandage before inflating the pneumatic tourniquet. Careful hemostasis and wound closure is mandatory. The pathologist should be consulted prior to the biopsy and should be present in the operating room at the time of the operation (Table 2).

Intralesion removal involves curettage of the lesion from within. Local resection removes the lesion intact through the capsule of the active tissue surrounding it. Wide local excision removes the lesion with a cuff of normal surrounding tissue. Radical excision removes the entire anatomic compartment in which the lesion arises and frequently requires amputation.

Neoplasms

Tumors of cartilaginous origin include *osteochondromas*, which are the most common benign neoplasms of bone, composed of normal osseus and cartilaginous tissue. They are usually discovered during teen years secondary to local mechanical symptoms. The metaphyseal ends of long bones are the most common sites, with 50 per cent occurring in the distal femur. The radiographic appearance is that of a bony stalk arising from the metaphysis and usually pointed away from the adjacent epiphysis. Osteochondromas are probably the result of ectopic epiphyseal cartilage.

Enchondroma is a benign growth of hyaline cartilage within the medullary cavity of a bone that often occurs in the phalanges, metacarpals, and metatarsals, and the pathologic fracture to an existing lesion may be the presenting symptom. The margins of the lesions are well defined, with a sclerotic reactive bone cavity.

Enchondromas may be single and multiple such as in *Ollier's disease* and may be associated with multiple cavernous hemangiomas (*Maffucci's syndrome*). The likelihood of malignant generation and multiple enchondromatosis is higher than in solitary lesions.

Chondroblastomas occur in epiphysis long bones. They have only a slight sclerotic margin and may have central areas of stippling that represent calcification within the substance of the tumor. Although generally considered a benign tumor, chondroblastoma may behave aggressively. *Chondrosarcomas* are the third most common primary malignant neoplasm of bone. It is frequently encountered in central axis bones such as the pelvis, the scapula, and the sacrum. These lesions grow slowly, and the radiographic appearance of the tumor is lobulated with calcifications. Most chondrosarcomas present as stage IA lesions and wide local excision is the treatment of choice.

Osteoid osteoma is a solitary exquisitely painful lesion. Bones of the lower extremity are the most frequently affected. The common presenting symptom is pain that occurs at night and is relieved by the use of aspirin. Treatment is by resection of the osteoid osteoma en bloc.

Osteosarcoma is the most common malignant primary neoplasm of bone with the exception of multiple myeloma. Occurrence is in the metaphyseal ends of long bones, and the distal femur is the most frequent site. The tumor classically produces a sunburst appearance that consists of trabeculae of bone, or it right angles to the cortical surface beneath the periosteum. Adjuvant chemotherapy in conjunction with operative therapy is the treatment.

Nonossifying fibromas are benign tumors but are focal and considered focal developmental defects. This lesion is also known as a benign metaphyseal cortical defect or fibrous cortical defect. It occurs as an incidental finding on radiographs and may be quite large and undergo pathologic fracture, which gradually heals as the patient matures. Curettage and bone grafting are curative.

Giant cell tumors are found in the epiphyseal long bones with subsequent involvement of the adjacent metaphysis. Giant cell tumors can behave in a malignant manner. When possible, wide local resection of

TABLE 2.   STAGING MALIGNANT TUMORS (ENNEKING)*

	Intracompartmental	Extracompartmental
Low-grade	Stage I, A	Stage I, B
High-grade	Stage II, A	Stage II, B

Stage III: any site, any grade, with metastases.

*From Harrelson JM, Callaghan JJ: Infections and neoplasms in bone. *In* Sabiston DC Jr [ed]: Textbook of Surgery: The Biological Basis of Modern Surgical Practice, ed 14. Philadelphia, WB Saunders Company, 1991, p 1356, with permission.

the tumor should be done because of high incidence of recurrence when they are curettaged and bone grafted.

Tumors of marrow-cell origin include *Ewing's sarcoma* that occurs commonly in the first and second decade of life. Patients present with fever, leukocytosis, and increased sedimentation rate. It is often mistaken for osteomyelitis. The radiographic appearance of Ewing's sarcoma in the diaphysis of the long bones is one of periosteal elevation or onion skin appearance as a result of replacement of the cortex by tumor. The lesion radiographically may resemble osteomyelitis. Histochemical staining for glycogen may aid in the differential diagnosis. Some Ewing's sarcomas contain glycogen on *periodic-acid-Schiff* (PAS) staining.

Myeloma is a malignant neoplasm of marrow cell origin and is the most common primary malignant neoplasm of bone. It is seen in the middle decades of life, more frequently in males than in females. Anemia, fever, hypercalcemia and renal failure related to extensive skeletal involvement, and abnormal production of immunoglobulins may be presenting factors. Radiographically, the appearance of a punched-out lesion with no accompanying sclerosis is seen. Diagnosis is by marrow cell aspiration demonstrating abnormal plasma cells. Bence Jones proteins may be found in urine in approximately half, and serum protein electrophoresis demonstrates an abnormal amount of globulins. Chemotherapy is the treatment of choice for this lesion.

Tendon and Joint Repair (The Hand)

Tendon continuity is necessary for transmission of force from muscle tendon units to the hand or digits. Each muscle tendon unit has a vascular supply, a nerve supply, and pulley mechanism, all of which insure good nutrition and smooth activity. Disruption of a tendon causes loss of motion of the digit and diminished grip or pinch. The severity of tendon injury varies according to the location and loss of continuity, the mechanism of injury, the conditions that exist at the time of injury, the particular tendon involved, and the anatomic location of the laceration in relationship to the muscle tendon unit. A tendon laceration directly over a joint is more serious than is an injury at the muscular tendinous junction. Maximal tendon function requires full-thickness skin coverage, epitenon and paratenon to protect the tendon from surrounding adhesions, and muscle bellies of adequate strength.

Tendon Healing

The healing tendon forms a strong bond as fibroblasts realign. Collagen fibers unite, blood vessels invade the area of healing, and fibroblasts migrate from the periphery to the centrum to establish a bond between tendon ends. The modified Verdan system divides the entire length of flexor tendons in the five anatomic areas (Fig. 5). Zone II, which Bunnell termed *no man's land*, is a common area for tendon lacerations and begins proximal to the metacarpal phalangeal joint and extends to the midportion of the middle phalanx. It is in this range that most tendon repairs occur. The flexor retinaculum system consists of a firm fibrous sheath lined by synovium that holds the flexor tendons close to the bone. This strong constraint provides a straight mechanical advantage so that a large excision occurs for a relatively small applied force.

Anatomic Dissection

Anatomic dissections have shown that preservation of the A2 and A4 are necessary for complete tendon excursion. Primary tendon repair of a lacerated tendon is performed within 24 hours after injury. *Delayed repair* refers to a period of up to 1 week after the initial injury, during which time the initial wound heals and repair of the tendon is performed or delayed closure

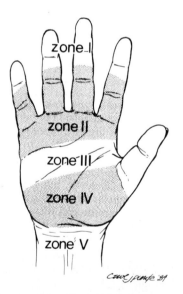

Figure 5. The hand zones are important in differentiating one tendon laceration from another and in determining how to treat single or double tendon lacerations that occur in the different zones. The annular ligaments vary according to the zones. They are most important in effecting postoperative function in zone II. Zone I includes only the insertions of the flexor digitorum profundus, and zone V contains median and ulnar nerves, median and ulnar arteries, the wrist flexor tendons, and all of the flexor digitorum profundus and flexor digitorum superficialis tendons. (From Nunley JA, Goldner JL: The hand. *In* Sabiston DC Jr [ed]: Textbook of Surgery: The Biological Basis of Modern Surgical Practice, ed 14. Philadelphia, WB Saunders Company, 1991, p 1362, with permission.)

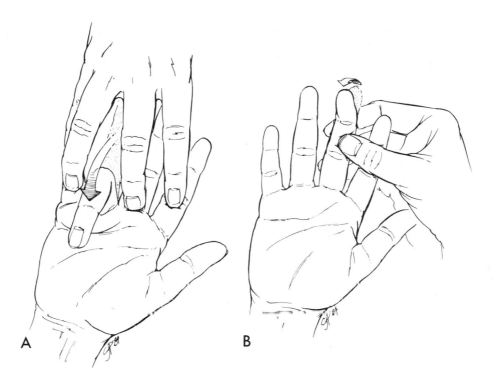

A   B

Figure 6. *A,* This technique is used to determine the strength of each individual flexor digitorum superficialis muscle. The adjacent digits are held in full extension to eliminate the action of the flexor digitorum profundus. The patient then voluntarily attempts to flex the proximal interphalangeal joint. Resistance is applied after flexion has occurred in order to determine the strength of the muscle. The distal phalanx of the same digit is tapped from the extensor side and the flexibility of the joint is determined. If there is no tension on the flexor digitorum profundus and if all of the action is through the flexor digitorum superficialis, then the differentiation of the two tendons in the digits is evident. *B,* A method of testing the strength of the flexor digitorum profundus of the long finger. The proximal interphalangeal joint is maintained in extension, as is the metacarpophalangeal joint. The patient is then asked to voluntarily flex the distal phalanx at the distal joint. Accurate testing of the ulnar three digits requires that the distal joints of the long, ring, and little fingers be flexed simultaneously, after which each digit is tested individually. The thumb and index finger may be tested individually in 85 per cent of the population and simultaneously in the remaining 15 per cent. (From Nunley JA, Goldner JL: The hand. *In* Sabiston DC Jr [ed]: Textbook of Surgery: The Biological Basis of Modern Surgical Practice, ed 14. Philadelphia, WB Saunders Company, 1991, p 1364, with permission.)

of the wound occurs and delayed repair of the tendon is performed at the same time as wound closure. *Secondary repair* refers to any time longer than 1 week after the original injury when all wounds are healed and edema has subsided. *Primary repair* of lacerated flexor tendons has several advantages compared with secondary repair: (1) accurate anatomic alignment, (2) no adhesions at the time the repair is performed, and (3) no delay in initiation of repair recovery. Primary repair is appropriate if the surgeon is experienced in tendon repair, if the wound is exceptionally clean, and if there has been little or no crushing of the tendon or the surrounding tissues. The decision to perform delayed repair is made if the wound is contaminated, if trauma is severe, if the patient's general condition does

not justify a prolonged operative procedure, and if the surgeon is not experienced in performing complicated tendon repair. The delay does not compromise the end result.

Delayed or secondary repair involves initial wound exploration with excision of wound margins and either primary closure or delayed wound closure 3 to 5 days later. The tendon may be repaired at this time. Delayed repair has several advantages as compared to immediate repair, including: (1) the risk of infection is diminished; (2) an experienced physician is available to perform the repair; and (3) vascular or nerve injury should be treated prior to the definitive tendon repair when encountered with multiple tendon injuries that occur with fractures.

Infection

Examination of lacerated tendons is demonstrated in Figure 6. After tendon repair, passive flexion and active extension exercises are done postoperatively. The tendon begins gliding immediately in the flexor sheath, with active extension and active flexion performed by a rubber band to take tension off of the repair. Occasionally it is necessary to perform a tendon graft when the actual tendon itself is damaged beyond repair. The graft is obtained from the palmaris longus tendon or the toe extensor.

Compression Neuropathy of the Hand and Forearm

A trapped nerve is suspected when the patient complains of intermittent tingling, numbness, or function impairment, and if the symptoms are recurrent and affect a particular anatomic area of the hand and forearm. Nerve conduction studies, particularly sensory latency, are helpful in localizing nerve compression agents. Sensory conduction studies are more sensitive than are motor conduction velocities. If electrical studies do not confirm the clinical diagnosis of nerve compression, a lesion may be present that affects the nerve minimally or intermittently. Nonoperative treatment is usually indicated in this instance.

The median nerve is commonly compressed with a carpal canal formed by the transverse carpal ligament on the palmar surface and the carpal bones of the dorsal surface. Females are affected more frequently than males with carpal tunnel syndrome, with a wide age range but usually between 40 and 60 years. The usual complaints are weakness or clumsiness of the hand. Percussion of the median nerve at the wrist proximal to the flexor retinaculum over the carpal ligament or in the palm may cause paresthesias. Tingling may be produced or aggravated by wrist flexion (*Phalen's test*) for 20 to 30 seconds.

Factors that contribute to median nerve compression at the wrist and in the hand include repetitive minor trauma such as grasping, squeezing, twisting, or hitting an object with the heel of the hand. If these motions are performed several hundred times a day and if the frequency increases in an effort to increase production (e.g., on the assembly line), median nerve compression may occur from tenosynovitis or trauma to the nerve from wrist flexion motion.

Other causes include congenital muscular abnormalities and following displacement of a Colles fracture. It can cause immediate damage to the median nerve or delayed nerve compression after the fracture has healed. Treatment of median nerve compression at the wrist includes splinting the wrist in neutral position at night, weight reduction, and decreased repetitive activities of the hand and wrist. Anti-inflammatory medicines may be useful in treating the tenosynovitis, and a diuretic may assist in partially dehydrating synovial sheaths. Soluble corticosteroid mixed with 1 per cent lidocaine may be injected into the tendon sheaths of the flexor digitorum profundus to locally decrease inflammation. If these conservative measures fail, median nerve decompression may be performed by incising the transverse carpal ligament at the wrist.

The median nerve can also be compressed by the pronator teres muscle in the proximal forearm. Compression of the anterior interosseous branch of the median nerve can occur, with reduction of pinch between the thumb and index finger as the presenting symptom. There usually is no sensory deficit.

The ulnar nerve can also be compressed, usually at the cubital tunnel. Compression of the ulnar nerve is caused by repetitive contusion at the elbow, such as resting on chairs. The ulnar nerve can be treated by splinting in extension or, if necessary, transposition anteriorly either under skin or under muscle.

Neuropathy of the radial nerve can occur when there is complete disruption. Clinically, the patient is unable to extend the wrist, thumb, or finger metacarpophalangeal joints. Anesthesia, hypesthesias, or paresthesias of the skin or the dorsal radial surface of the hand may occur. Radial nerve may be compressed by a displaced fracture at the distal third of the humerus or by prolonged external pressure associated with a "Saturday night palsy." The anatomic area of compression may be opposite the humeral midshaft in the radial groove in the distal third of the humerus where the nerve courses from posterior to anterior. The radial nerve injury associated with the proximal or midshaft fracture of the humerus usually follows trauma at the time of injury. In 90 per cent of the patients, these lesions recover spontaneously within a few months after injury. The distal oblique fracture occasionally may entrap the nerve between the fracture fragments and may require operative decompression.

REFERENCES

Chapman MW: Operative Orthopaedics, vol 1–4. Philadelphia, JB Lippincott Company, 1988.

Evarts CM: Surgery of the Musculoskeletal System, ed 2, vol 1–4. New York, Churchill Livingstone, 1989.

Green DP (ed): Operative Hand Surgery. New York, Churchill Livingstone, 1988.

Rockwood CA, Wilkins K, King RE: Fractures in Children, vol 3. Philadelphia, JB Lippincott Company, 1984.

Various authors: Fractures and dislocations. *In* Sabiston DC Jr (ed): Textbook of Surgery: The Biological Basis of Modern Surgical Practice, ed 14. Philadelphia, WB Saunders Company, 1991, pp 1291–1376.

42
THE SKIN

L. SCOTT LEVIN, M.D.

The skin serves as the barrier between the relatively closed system of the human body and the external environment. It is strong, elastic, waterproof, protective, and self-repairing and serves as a sensory organ and an excretory organ. It regulates heat loss by sweat glands and, in some places, by hair. It serves to identify individuals by fingerprints and responds to environmental stress directly by sun tanning and healing.

SKIN FUNCTIONS

One of the main functions of the skin is that it serves as a barrier between the organism and the environment. Bacteria, toxic chemicals, and gases have difficulty penetrating this barrier due to the cells in the stratum corneum layer. The thickness of the stratum corneum is inversely proportional to water loss. Mammals, including humans, possess hairy as well as glabrous skin. Glabrous skin is in constant contact with the environment, and is found on the fingertips, palms, and soles of the feet. There is no hair on glabrous skin, and it is heavily keratinized. Topographically, glabrous skin is organized with highly specialized ridges and grooves in addition to sweat ducts that empty through pores in the papillary ridges.

Glabrous skin contains many sensory end-organs that transmit sensibility to the brain, including free nerve endings, Merkel cell neurite complexes, and Meissner and Pacini corpuscles. Each neural receptor encodes and transmits as a first order afferent, sensory impulses to the brain (Fig. 1). In contrast, hairy skin is less innervated and buffers the organism from the environment because hair dampens tactile stimuli.

The skin is a tough, relatively impenetrable, resilient structure and can tolerate significant mechanical injury due to the collagen within the dermis, ground sub-stance (mucopolysaccharide), and elastin and reticulin (noncellular components of the dermis). The skin is a viscoelastic structure that responds to force by lengthening, and resumes its original shape when force is removed. Force applied beyond maximal tensile strength causes rupture. Skin tension is very important in wound healing and varies at different anatomic sites. Crease lines associated with aging are tension lines, and incisions in surgical procedures should be placed in crease lines, termed the *lines of Langer*.

Skin stretches in response to biologic changes such as weight gain, pregnancy, ascites, or aging. Skin expansion is now being used for a variety of reconstructive procedures as in the use of a silicone bag first inserted into a subcutaneous pocket. This is gradually filled with saline over a period of several weeks, expanding the silicone bag, and stretching the overlying skin. The increased surface area of skin is then advanced into defects after the expander is removed.

The skin serves as an organ that regulates body temperature by dissipation of heat by radiation (60 per cent) and conduction (25 per cent) as influenced by the amount of cutaneous blood flow, ambient temperature, and humidity. Evaporative loss from sweating (15 per cent) is the body's most efficient mechanism for dissipation of heat. Temperature regulation is also controlled by the hypothalamus, which regulates vasomotor tone in cutaneous vessels and subsequently alters heat loss.

The skin also has important immunologic functions with three major cell types present in epidermis. These are keratinocytes (from ectoderm), melanocytes (neuroectoderm) that produce pigment, and Langerhans cells (derived from mesenchyme). Langerhans cells (about 2 to 4 per cent of epithelial cells) express IgA antigens and have receptor sites for the Fc portion of

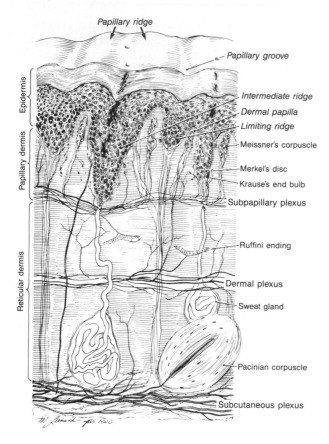

Papillary ridge

Papillary groove

Epidermis

Papillary dermis

Reticular dermis

Intermediate ridge

Dermal papilla

Limiting ridge

Meissner's corpuscle

Merkel's disc

Krause's end bulb

Subpapillary plexus

Ruffini ending

Dermal plexus

Sweat gland

Pacinian corpuscle

Subcutaneous plexus

Figure 1. Cross-section of glabrous skin. Note the intermediate ridge, which acts as a magnifying lever for the transmission of pressure stimuli on the surface of the skin. (From Serafin D: The skin. *In* Sabiston DC Jr [ed]: Textbook of Surgery: The Biological Basis of Modern Surgical Practice, ed 14. Philadelphia, WB Saunders Company, 1991, p 1383, with permission.)

the IgG antibody and complement components (C3). These cells assist in the cutaneous immune response. Ultraviolet (UV) light adversely affects the function of the Langerhans cells, impairing their ability to process antigens. The skin is instrumental in the synthesis of vitamin D, and about 90 per cent of this conversion occurs in the stratum Malpighii after exposure to ultraviolet light. Skin color in humans is due largely to the content of melanin within keratinocytes. The number of melanocytes is the same in the same species for a specific region of skin. Melanin inhibits transmission of radiation through the skin, demonstrated by the up to tenfold decrease in UV light that passes through the negroid epidermis. Moreover, exposure to ultraviolet light is thought to be a principal etiologic factor in the development of human malignant melanoma.

WOUND CLOSURE

Following trauma or disease, open wounds should be closed to prevent entrance of bacteria and infection with restoration of the protective barrier of the skin. Transudative fluid loss can cause loss of proteins, dehydration, and death, such as in burns. Disruption of the skin over bones, tendons, and joints causes tissue desiccation, infection, and functional loss. The goal of wound closure is reestablishment of viable epithelial cells that seal the wound and protect the internal milieu of the organism.

The natural tendency is to close open wounds by the process of epithelialization and wound contraction. Within 24 hours after injury, epithelial cells at the periphery of the wound begin to multiply and migrate toward areas devoid of epithelium. When migrating cells contact each other at the center of the wound, migration ceases due to cellular contact inhibition, and wound closure is achieved. Myofibroblasts also contribute to closure by producing centripetal contractile forces. A reconstructive algorithm should be followed for closure of wounds, and the technique of closure is dependent on the size and depth of the wound. The plan of reconstruction includes:

1. *Excision and primary closure*: The defect is small, wound edges are approximated without excess tension, and the incision should parallel normal skin tension lines.

2. *Local skin flaps*: These contain skin similar to the adjacent defect and are placed into the defect either by rotation or advancement.

3. *Skin grafts*: Partial-thickness or full thickness grafts are used for wounds devoid of dermal elements or too large to allow contraction and epithelialization within a reasonable time. The thickness of graft is determined by the amount of dermis included, and the thicker the graft, the more durable, but healing is slower (Fig. 2).

4. *Skin flaps*: Skin flaps are used on large defects where exposed structures cannot be covered by skin grafts and require increased blood supply. Examples include muscle flaps, fasciocutaneous flaps, and autologous free tissue transplantation.

TUMORS OF THE SKIN

Benign

Epithelial nevi (Table 1) appear at birth or early childhood, should be distinguished from other papillomas such as seborrheic keratosis or verruca vulgaris, and may be treated with topical liquid nitrogen. *Seborrheic keratosis* occur everywhere except on the soles and palms, appear in middle age, may become in-

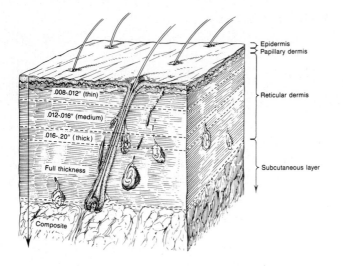

Figure 2. Cross-section of skin indicating the varying thicknesses of skin grafts. Note that a full-thickness graft removes all of the epidermal appendages. Epithelialization is possible only from the periphery of the wound. Usually the donor site of full-thickness grafts are closed primarily. (From Serafin D: The skin. *In* Sabiston DC Jr [ed]: Textbook of Surgery: The Biological Basis of Modern Surgical Practice, ed 14. Philadelphia, WB Saunders Company, 1991, p 1387, with permission.)

fected, and are treated with cryotherapy. *Epidermal* and *dermoid cysts* are slow-growing, intradermal or subcutaneous lesions lined with epidermal cells and contain keratinaceous material. Surgical excision is the treatment of the cysts and wall. *Keratoacanthoma* is a lesion characterized by a horn-filled crater that grows rapidly and may spontaneously involute within a few

TABLE 1. TUMORS OF THE SURFACE EPIDERMIS*

Benign tumors
  Localized linear epidermal nevus
  Inflammatory linear epidermal nevus
  Systematized linear epidermal nevus
  Oral epithelial nevus
  Seborrheic keratosis
  Clear cell acanthoma
  Epidermal, pilar, and dermoid cysts
  Steatocystoma multiplex
  Warty dyskeratoma
  Keratoacanthoma
Precancerous tumors (located largely in situ)
  Solar keratosis
  Leukoplakia
  Oral florid papillomatosis
  Bowen's disease
  Erythroplasia of Queyrat
Carcinomas
  Squamous cell carcinoma
  Paget's disease

*From Lever WF, Schaumburg-Lever G: Histopathology of the Skin, ed 7. Philadelphia, JB Lippincott Company, 1990, p 523–524, with permission.

months, but it must be differentiated from squamous cell carcinoma. They may occur on the lips, necessitating a shave biopsy for diagnosis. *Premalignant tumors* include solar keratosis, leukoplakia, and Bowen's disease. Squamous cell carcinoma may arise from solar keratosis and is treated with 5-fluorouracil (5-FU). *Leukoplakia* occurs on the oral or rectal mucosa, and its histologic appearance is remarkable for anaplasia of basal layers, which distinguishes it from leukokeratosis, which is clinically identical in appearance. Leukoplakia may give rise to carcinoma, and treatment requires removal of the irritant and biopsy if carcinoma is suspected. Bowen's disease is a form of squamous cell carcinoma associated with an increased incidence of visceral cancer and is treated by excision.

Malignant

Squamous Cell Carcinoma

Squamous carcinoma of the skin is a common disorder, and predisposing factors include exposure to the sun, irradiation, and chronic irritation. Approximately 2 per cent of these lesions metastasize, with metastases being greater in those malignancies arising from sinus tracts following osteomyelitis or from irradiated areas. Aggressive surgical resection should be performed for these lesions and those that are poorly differentiated in histologic structure. Tumors of epidermal appendages include benign lesions such as hamartomas, adenomas, and benign epitheliomas. Malignant lesions include carcinoma of sebaceous glands, carcinoma of apocrine glands, and carcinoma of eccrine glands.

Basal Cell Carcinoma

The least differentiated appendage tumors, which almost always occur on hair-bearing skin and rarely metastasize, are the basal cell carcinomas. They are quite common and are associated with exposure to the sun. Treatment usually consists of wide excision and closure.

REFERENCES

Goldsmith LA (ed): Biochemistry and Physiology of the Skin. New York, Oxford, Oxford University Press, 1983.
Lever LS, Schaumburg-Lever WF: Histopathology of the Skin, ed 7. Philadelphia, JB Lippincott Company, 1983.
Mathes SJ, Nahai F: Clinical Applications for Muscles and Musculocutaneous Flaps. St. Louis, CV Mosby, 1982.
McCarthy JG: Plastic Surgery. Philadelphia, WB Saunders Company, 1977.
Peacock EE Jr: Wound Repair, ed 3. Philadelphia, WB Saunders Company, 1984.
Serafin D: The skin: Functional, metabolic, and surgical considerations. *In* Sabiston DC Jr (ed): Textbook of Surgery: The Biological Basis of Modern Surgical Practice, ed 14. Philadelphia, WB Saunders Company, 1991.

43
THE UROGENITAL SYSTEM

W. MARSTON LINEHAN, M.D.

The urinary system comprises the kidneys, ureters, bladder, and urethra, and performs the functions of production, transportation, storage, and elimination of urine. The male genital system includes the testes, epididymides, vas deferens, seminal vesicles, prostate, and penis, with the primary function of reproduction.

ANATOMY AND PHYSIOLOGY

Kidney

The kidneys are paired retroperitoneal organs that lie along the border of the psoas muscle below the diaphragm and are in proximity to the spinal column (Fig. 1). The average kidney is 11.5 cm in length, 150 gm in weight, and is lined by a fibrous capsule. A variable amount of perirenal fat lies around the renal capsule. Surrounding the kidney and perirenal fat is Gerota's fascia, which extends from the diaphragm to the ureter. The kidneys lie between the twelfth thoracic and second lumbar vertebra and are bounded medially by the psoas, posteriorly by the quadratus lumborum, laterally by the abdominal muscles, and superiorly by the diaphragm.

Ureters

The ureters are retroperitoneal conduits connecting the kidney with the bladder. The ureters pass through Gerota's fascia and cross the psoas muscle and common iliac vessels. They course along the posterior aspect of the pelvis, under the vas deferens, and enter the base of the bladder at the trigone. The blood supply of the ureter is from the renal, gonadal, aortic, common iliac, and internal iliac vessels. The lymphatics accompany the arteries and drain into the hypogastric, iliac, and para-aortic nodes. The autonomic

innervation of the wall of the ureter causes peristaltic activity in which rhythmic contractions emanating from a proximal pacemaker control the efficient transport of urine from the renal pelvis to the bladder. The mucosa of the ureter is composed of transitional epithelium, resting on a fibrous lamina propria. Under the lamina propria are the well-developed circular and longitudinal muscle layers and the adventitia.

Bladder

The bladder is a muscular organ that functions as the main reservoir of the urine and has a capacity of 350 to 450 ml. The ureters enter the posteroinferior portion of the bladder at the trigone, and the trigone forms the base of the bladder from the ureteral orifices to the bladder neck. Anterior to the bladder is the space of Retzius, which contains fatty tissue and a plexus of veins, as well as the pubic bone of the pelvis. Posterior to the bladder in the male are the seminal vesicles, vas deferens, ureters, and the rectum. In the female, the vagina and uterus are located between the bladder and the rectum.

Urethra

The urethra (Fig. 2) is the conduit for both urine and the products of the male genital system. The male urethra extends approximately 23 cm from the bladder neck to the meatus and is divided into anterior and posterior portions. The anterior urethra is divided into the bulbar, the penile, and the glandular divisions. The fossa navicularis is a small distal dilation in the glandular urethra. The anterior urethra is surrounded by an erectile body, the corpus spongiosum. The bulbourethral glands, also known as *Cowper's glands*, are located in the urogenital diaphragm and empty into

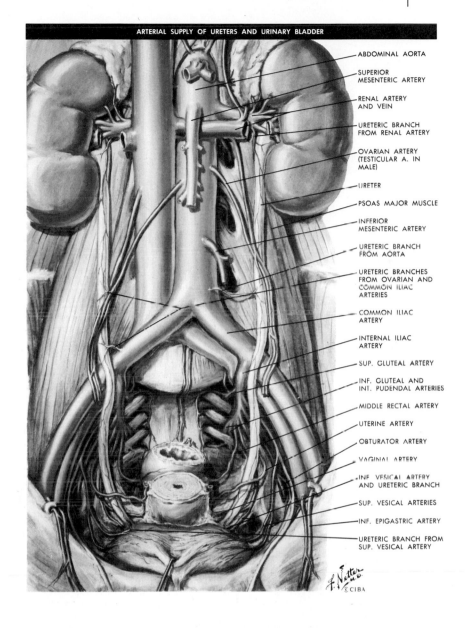

ARTERIAL SUPPLY OF URETERS AND URINARY BLADDER

ABDOMINAL AORTA
SUPERIOR MESENTERIC ARTERY
RENAL ARTERY AND VEIN
URETERIC BRANCH FROM RENAL ARTERY
OVARIAN ARTERY (TESTICULAR A. IN MALE)
URETER
PSOAS MAJOR MUSCLE
INFERIOR MESENTERIC ARTERY
URETERIC BRANCH FROM AORTA
URETERIC BRANCHES FROM OVARIAN AND COMMON ILIAC ARTERIES
COMMON ILIAC ARTERY
INTERNAL ILIAC ARTERY
SUP. GLUTEAL ARTERY
INF. GLUTEAL AND INT. PUDENDAL ARTERIES
MIDDLE RECTAL ARTERY
UTERINE ARTERY
OBTURATOR ARTERY
VAGINAL ARTERY
INF. VESICAL ARTERY AND URETERIC BRANCH
SUP. VESICAL ARTERIES
INF. EPIGASTRIC ARTERY
URETERIC BRANCH FROM SUP. VESICAL ARTERY

Figure 1. The arterial supply and relationship of organs of the urinary tract. (From Netter FH: *In* Ciba Collection of Medical Illustrations, vol 6, Summit, NJ, 1953, with permission.)

the bulbar urethra. The penile urethra is lined by numerous small glands, the glands of Littre. The posterior urethra is composed of the membranous and prostatic urethra.

Prostate

The prostate gland is a fibromuscular organ that surrounds the vesical neck and proximal portion of the urethra in the male. It is approximately 20 gm in weight in the adult male and is composed of an anterior and a posterior portion. Embryologically, the prostate is derived from five epithelial evaginations of the posterior urethra. The blood supply of the prostate is provided by the inferior vesical artery and enters at the posterolateral aspect of the vesical neck. The venous drainage of the prostate is diffuse and empties into the *plexus of Santorini*. The nerve supply of the prostate is predominantly of sympathetic origin from the hypogastric plexus and from fibers arriving from the third and fourth sacral nerves through the sacral plexus. The lymphatic drainage of the prostate is to the obturator, internal iliac, external iliac, and presacral nodes, and is of considerable importance in evaluating the extent of spread of disease from the prostate.

Seminal Vesicle

The seminal vesicles are paired structures located beneath the trigone at the base of the bladder and are

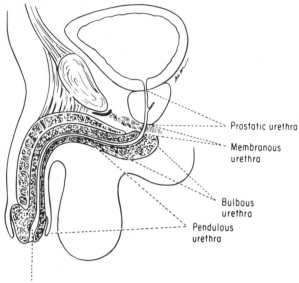

Prostatic urethra

Membranous
urethra

Bulbous
urethra

Pendulous
urethra

Fossa navicularis

Figure 2. The divisions of the male urethra. (From Webster GD: *In* Paulson DF [ed]: Genitourinary Surgery. New York, Churchill Livingstone, 1984, with permission.)

invested posteriorly by Denonvilliers' fascia, separating them from the rectum. The seminal vesicles secrete a viscous fluid that is the source of fructose in the ejaculate. The seminal fluid is formed predominantly by the secretions of sexual accessory tissues, including the epididymides, vasa deferentia, ampullae, seminal vesicles, prostate, Cowper's glands, and the glands of Littre. The main body of the penis is composed of three erectile bodies. The corpus spongiosum is a ventromedial structure that surrounds the urethra. Dorsal and lateral to the midline *corpus spongiosum*, there are two other erectile structures, each known as the corpus cavernosum. Each of these erectile bodies is separately invested with fibrous tissue known as the *tunica albuginea*, and these structures are collectively surrounded by fibrous tissue, termed *Buck's fascia*. Underneath the skin of the penis and scrotum is *Colles' fascia*, a fibrous tissue that extends from the base of the glans to the urogenital diaphragm and is contiguous with Scarpa's fascia of the abdominal wall. The lymphatic drainage of the skin of the penis is to the superficial and deep inguinal lymph nodes, while the lymphatic drainage from the glans penis and urethra is to the deep inguinal and external and internal iliac nodes.

Scrotum

The scrotum is dual chambered and contains the testes, epididymides, and terminal portion of the sper-

matic cord. Beneath the scrotal skin is *Darto's fascia*, which contains elastic fibers, connective tissue, and smooth muscle. The cutaneous innervation to the scrotum is from branches of the ilioinguinal and external spermatic nerves, and lymphatic draining is to the superficial and deep inguinal nodes. The scrotum is formed by the fusion of the genital swellings that form the labia majora in the female.

Spermatic Cord

The spermatic cord, which suspends the testicle, is a fascial-covered structure that contains spermatic arteries and veins, the pampiniform plexus, lymph channels, the autonomic nerve supply to the testicle, and the cremasteric muscle. The contractions of the cremasteric muscle change the position of the testis for regulation of temperature.

Testis

The testes are paired glands located in the scrotum and covered by the tunica albuginea. At the upper pole of the testis is a small pedunculated body termed the *appendix testis*. The tunica vaginalis is a sheath that invests the testes and epididymis. The arterial supply to the testis is provided by the internal spermatic, deferential, and external spermatic arteries, and the veins from the testis and epididymis form the pampiniform plexus. The lymph node drainage from the testes is to the retroperitoneum and to mediastinal and supraclavicular lymph nodes.

Epididymis

The epididymis is a coiled duct that lies posterolateral to the testis and consists of an upper portion, the globus major, and a lower portion, the globus minor. Sperm passes into the epididymis through the efferent ducts from the rete testis and then through the vas deferens into the ampulla.

EVALUATION

In the genitourinary evaluation, it is important to ascertain whether the patient has had previous genitourinary surgical procedures or has a history of congenital abnormalities. Because many genitourinary abnormalities manifest themselves as abnormalities in voiding, careful questioning about patterns, frequency, and character and control of voiding is essential.

Pain

Pain from the kidney is usually felt as a dull ache in the flank or lumbar area and is usually a late finding in a neoplasm involving the kidney. If a renal tumor or infection is extensive and involves the diaphragm, pain can be referred to the shoulder. Pain from the ureter is most commonly secondary to acute obstruction such as from a stone or blood clot, and chronic obstruction and hydronephrosis may be totally asymptomatic. An acutely obstructing stone in the upper ureter is likely to cause pain in the flank or abdomen, and as the stone moves down the ureter, the pain moves progressively toward the groin. Pain in the scrotum may represent referred pain from the ureter, or it may be due to an abnormality of the epididymis or testis. Primary scrotal pain may be due to epididymitis, orchitis, or testicular torsion. Chronic prostatitis can cause a dull ache in the perineum or lower back; acute prostatitis generally presents as pain in the perineum associated with fever. Prostatic carcinoma rarely presents with pain until it is quite advanced.

Abnormalities in Voiding

Hesitancy refers to difficulty starting the urinary stream. Most commonly, this is due to outlet obstruction from an abnormality such as prostatic enlargement or urethral stricture. However, it can also be secondary to neurogenic bladder dysfunction. Decreased caliber and force of urinary stream are symptoms commonly associated with bladder outlet obstruction. This may be secondary to a benign or malignant enlargement of the prostate gland, a urethral stricture, or a neoplastic process involving the urethra. *Frequency* means that the patient voids more often than usual. This may be due to bladder irritation secondary to an infection or other inflammatory process, or it may be due to an unstable or chronically distended, poorly emptying bladder. Urgency signifies an abnormal urge to void and is generally associated with a bladder that is contracting inappropriately. *Urgency* may be secondary to inflammation or to another pathologic condition that causes bladder instability. *Nocturia* indicates that the patient voids an unusual number of times during the night and may be a sign of an unstable bladder in which the normal nocturnal inhibition of the voiding sensation is no longer present. Frequency, urgency, and nocturia are symptoms of bladder instability. *Dysuria* refers to painful voiding and is commonly secondary to a urinary tract infection. A nonbacterial inflammation, a stone, or a tumor can also cause dysuria. *Enuresis* is the involuntary passage of urine at night or while asleep. Enuresis is normal up to a certain age, although, if persistent, it can be secondary to a congenital anatomic abnormality or neurologic dysfunction. *Polyuria* is the voiding of an excessively large volume of urine, and this is most commonly secondary to a primary renal disorder such as an abnormality in the urinary concentrating mechanism. *Incontinence* is the inability to prevent involuntary passage of urine. *Stress incontinence* refers to exertional leaking of urine as a result of coughing, sneezing, or other straining. *Urge incontinence* refers to leaking of urine associated with an uncontrollable urge to void and is usually a sign of an unstable bladder. *Pyuria* indicates the presence of white blood cells in urine and often is associated with a urinary tract infection. *Pneumaturia* means the passage of gas in the urine, and this can be secondary to an infection by a gas-forming organism in the genitourinary system, although it most commonly indicates the presence of a urinary-enteric fistula. *Hematuria* is a term used to define the presence of blood in the urine. With gross hematuria, the blood is plainly visible, but in microscopic hematuria, the presence of blood cells is detected with a microscope. In unexplained cases of either microscopic or gross hematuria, a thorough examination is required. A patient who is receiving chemotherapeutic agents or anticoagulants can also have a bladder tumor, kidney tumor, or other abnormality as a cause of the hematuria, and these possibilities should be excluded. A thorough physical examination is an integral part of the evaluation of a patient with a genitourinary abnormality. Palpation in the right or left upper quadrants and flank may elicit tenderness in the renal fossa. Palpation of the scrotum is performed to detect abnormalities of the spermatic cord, epididymis, or testis. In the penile examination, the foreskin should be retracted and the meatus inspected for position and for the presence of discharge or inflammation. The prostatic examination includes palpation of the prostate as well as examination of the periprostatic tissue and rectal sphincter. Any abnormal prostate nodule found on examination should be evaluated further. The seminal vesicles are normally not palpable. However, seminal vesicles that are invaded by prostatic carcinoma may be hard, whereas seminal vesicles that are inflamed are usually nodular.

RADIOGRAPHIC EVALUATION

Plain Film

The plain film demonstrates bony abnormalities, calcifications, and abnormal fat or gas densities. A calcification on the plain film may indicate the presence of a urinary tract stone, or it may represent a calcification in the substance of the adrenal gland, kidney, collecting system, bladder, or an adjacent lymph node.

Intravenous Pyelogram

The intravenous pyelogram is a radiologic study in which sequential films are taken as the kidneys concentrate and excrete an intravenously injected contrast dye. This study provides anatomic information about the renal parenchyma, pelvis, ureter, and bladder, and can provide information about renal function.

Cystogram

A cystogram is performed by placing a catheter in the bladder and filling the bladder with contrast medium. The cystogram provides information about bladder anatomy and the absence or presence of vesical masses, diverticula, or ureterovesical reflux.

Retrograde Pyelogram

Dye is injected into a catheter placed endoscopically in the ureter. This procedure is very useful in delineating the anatomy of the upper tract when the intravenous pyelogram does not provide sufficient anatomic information, when there is a nonfunctioning kidney, or when it is not possible to perform intravenous pyelogram because of renal insufficiency, obstruction, or dye allergy.

Retrograde Urethrogram

Retrograde ureterography is performed by injecting contrast media into the urethra and obtaining a lateral radiograph of the urethra. This test provides information about the extent and location of strictures, diverticula, stones, or neoplastic disease.

Ultrasound

Ultrasound, a noninvasive procedure that depends on differences in tissue echogenicity, has gained widespread use in the evaluation of genitourinary abnormalities. Renal ultrasound is particularly helpful in differentiating cystic from neoplastic lesions, and it may also be useful in the detection of hydronephrosis. Scrotal ultrasound is quite accurate in differentiating lesions of the epididymis from those in the testis, and in detecting masses within the testes. Recently, *transrectal* ultrasound has been used for detection of prostatic tumors.

Computed Tomography and Magnetic Resonance Imaging

Computed tomography (CT) and magnetic resonance imaging (MRI) scans have become an integral part of the urologic evaluation of many genitourinary abnormalities. The CT scan is very accurate in the differentiation of cystic from solid renal masses, and in some instances, it has replaced the arteriogram. The CT scan is commonly used for preoperative evaluation and staging of patients with testicular and renal carcinoma and for surveillance after treatment.

THE KIDNEY

Anomalies

Renal agenesis, the total absence of a kidney, can be unilateral or bilateral. Unilateral agenesis is usually accompanied by compensatory hypertrophy of the contralateral kidney. In *renal aplasia*, nephrogenic tissue is present but fails to develop. This is generally due to either inadequate stimulation of the metanephros, a ureteral bud of poor quality, or inadequate vascularity of the metanephrogenic blastema. In *renal hypoplasia*, the kidney is normal but small, and there is usually a poorly developed ureter and trigone. A hypoplastic kidney is generally not able to undergo hypertrophy if the opposite kidney is damaged or removed.

A kidney that is not in its normal position is termed an *ectopic kidney*. The ectopic kidney is usually malrotated and may even be on the side with the other kidney, in which case it is termed *crossed renal ectopia*. An ectopic kidney is secondary to persistence of early embryonic vasculature, which presents normal ascent of the kidney during development. Some 85 per cent of the time when there is crossed renal ectopia, there is also fusion with the other kidney. The most common type of fusion is the *horseshoe* kidney, in which the lower poles of the kidneys are fused.

Renal cysts are lesions that predominantly occur in adults, and they may vary in size and may be multiple or bilateral. Use of a renal ultrasound study or abdominal CT scan can often differentiate a benign renal cyst from a neoplastic lesion, although an arteriogram may be required.

Polycystic Kidney Disease

Adult polycystic kidney disease is an autosomal dominant disease in which there are multiple cysts of varying sizes in both the renal medulla and cortex. It generally manifests itself in the third or fourth decade, but there is usually normal renal function until late in life, at which time dialysis or renal transplantation may be required.

Angiomyolipoma is a benign renal tumor that is often mistaken for a malignant lesion. Histologically, this tumor contains vascular and muscle elements and fat cells. Medullary cystic disease can be an isolated occurrence or part of an autosomal dominant disorder. Medullary cystic disease does not often necessitate surgical management and, although small renal stones may form, this disorder is consistent with a normal lifespan. Multicystic kidney is a nonhereditary, developmental anomaly in which there are 20 variable-sized renal cysts that do not communicate with the collecting system. A small renal pelvis is usually present. Idiopathic ureteropelvic junction obstruction is the most common cause of congenital hydronephrosis. Intravenous pyelography typically shows delayed function and a dilated collecting system. Retrograde pyelography often shows an abnormally high insertion of the ureter on the renal pelvis. A perinephric abscess may follow pyelonephritis or the rupture of a renal abscess, or it can occur secondary to hematogenous spread of infection from another part of the body. Perinephric abscess often occurs in patients with chronic urinary tract infection or diabetes mellitus.

Malignant Lesions

Renal cell carcinoma, which is thought to originate in the proximal renal tubule, occurs in over 25,000 patients in the United States each year, with 10,000 deaths annually. Renal carcinoma is predominantly a disease of adults, although it has been reported in patients as young as 6 months of age. This disease often presents in an advanced stage because the kidneys are located in the retroperitoneum and the malignancy can progress undetected. The standard treatment for localized renal carcinoma is radical nephrectomy, which is the removal of the kidney and Gerota's fascia. A transabdominal, flank, or thoracoabdominal incision can be used for the removal of a renal tumor, depending on the size and location of the tumor. Systemic chemotherapy of metastatic renal carcinoma has met with only limited success. The response rate to different chemotherapeutic regimens is 15 to 35 per cent, and long-term survival is uncommon. A new approach to the therapy of cancer has been developed based on the use of a lymphokine, interleukin-2. This therapy has been associated with objective regression in patients with renal carcinoma, and it is approved for use in these patients. Wilms' tumor, or nephroblastoma, is the most common solid mass occurring in children. The peak incidence is during the second year of life and 75 per cent present before the age of 5. The combined use of surgical excision, radiation therapy, and chemotherapy has greatly increased the survival in children with Wilms' tumor.

Renovascular Disorders

Five to 15 per cent of the hypertensive population in the United States has renovascular disease. With an increased understanding of the renin-angiotensin system and improved medical, surgical, and radiographic techniques, there have been great advances in the diagnosis and treatment of this disease. *Atherosclerosis* and *fibrous dysplasia* comprise approximately 90 per cent of renal arterial lesions. Atherosclerotic lesions tend to occur in the proximal third of renal artery, are bilateral in approximately a third of patients, and affect males more often than females. Fibrous dysplasia produces lesions of greater length that are often multiple and bilateral. It affects females more often than males by a ratio of 4:1.

Urinary Tract Calculi

A stone in the genitourinary tract can be due to many causes. Stone formation may be secondary to a primary metabolic disorder or to an obstruction causing urinary stasis and infection, or it can idiopathic. Urinary tract calculi are most commonly composed of calcium oxalate, calcium oxalate plus hydroxyapatite, or magnesium ammonium phosphate (struvite). Uric acid or cystine stones are encountered less frequently. Urinary tract stones can occur in the pelvis of the kidney, in the ureter, in the bladder, or in the urethra. With the introduction of percutaneous ultrasonic lithotripsy, urethroscopy, urethroscopic ultrasonic lithotripsy, and extracorporeal shock wave lithotripsy, the indications for open surgical removal of calculi have dramatically changed. Stones that originate in the kidney and course down the ureter are most likely to lodge at the ureteropelvic junction, at the point where the ureter crosses the iliac vessels, or at the ureterovesical junction. Primary vesical stones are rare in the United States, but are not uncommon in the Middle East and Africa. In the United States, vesical stones are usually secondary to bladder outlet obstruction with infection of residual urine.

Tumors of the Renal Pelvis and Ureter

Tumors can occur in the renal collecting system, pelvis, or ureter either in association with tumors of the bladder or as isolated events. The standard treatment for a high-grade tumor in the renal pelvis or ureter is total nephroureterectomy with the removal of a small cuff of bladder.

THE BLADDER

Anomalies of the Bladder and Ureter

A ureter that enters the bladder in an area other than the trigone is termed *ectopic*. The ureter may enter anywhere in the bladder, vesical neck, prostatic urethra, seminal vesicle, or vas deferens. In the female, the ureter may enter the vagina, cervix, uterus, or rectum. Some 80 per cent of ectopic ureters are associated with a duplicated collecting system. In this case, the ureter from the upper collecting system is most often associated with an ectopic insertion of the ureter. A *ureterocele* is a cystic dilation of the distal portion of the ureter and may be diagnosed by intravenous pyelogram or cystogram. Ureteroceles are commonly associated with duplicated collecting systems and often become obstructed.

Vesicoureteral reflux is a congenital condition caused by a malformation of the ureterovesical junction in which there is lack of a sufficient intramural tunnel to provide the normal antireflux mechanism. Reflux may be mild or severe and is commonly associated with ureteral ectopia. The diagnosis of reflux is made on cystogram.

Bladder abnormalities such as agenesis, hypoplasia, duplication, and *exstrophy* are rare. Exstrophy is a severe congenital malformation that occurs in 1 of 40,000 births and is caused by a failure of the mesoderm structures of the abdominal wall to develop. Exstrophy can present as epispadias, the failure of closure of the dorsal aspect of the urethra, to complete exstrophy with pubic separation and a persistent cloaca.

Bladder Neoplasms

There are over 46,000 new cases of bladder carcinoma, with 10,400 deaths annually in the United States. Both the grade and stage of the bladder tumor are important for planning appropriate treatment (Fig. 3). Bladder tumors are graded from 1 to 3, with grade 1 tumors being the most well differentiated and grade 3 tumors the least differentiated. Stage O represents a mucosal papillary tumor, a stage A tumor has invaded the lamina propria, and stage B signifies that the tumor has invaded either the superficial (B1) or deep (B2) muscle. A stage C tumor has extended beyond the muscle into the perivesical fat, and a stage D tumor has metastasized. Approximately 90 per cent of bladder tumors are transitional cell carcinomas, 7 per cent are squamous cell, 2 per cent are adenocarcinoma, and 1 per cent are undifferentiated. Squamous cell carcinoma of the bladder is often related to longstanding infection or inflammation. Adenocarcinoma may be urachal or nonurachal in origin and is seen in a high percentage of patients with exstrophy. Chronic infection may lead to the development of cystitis glandularis followed by overt adenocarcinoma. Adenocarcinoma is an aggressive lesion in which early invasion and metastases are common.

The clinical staging of a patient with a known or suspected carcinoma of the bladder often includes an intravenous pyelogram, cystourethroscopy, and an abdominal CT scan. A biopsy of the tumor and its base is performed to assess the extent of muscle invasion. Biopsies are also performed in other areas of the bladder to identify unsuspected tumor or carcinoma in situ. Low-grade and superficial tumors are treated by endoscopic resection followed by instillation of intravesical therapy such as bacille Calmette-Guérin (BCG) (Fig. 4). *Radical cystectomy* is the standard treatment of invasive bladder carcinoma. This procedure includes removal of the pelvic lymph nodes and, in the male, the prostate and seminal vesicles. In the female, the ovaries and uterus are generally removed along with a small anterior cuff of vagina. Many surgeons routinely remove the urethra in the male, while others perform a urethrectomy only if carcinoma in situ is present or if the bladder neck or prostatic urethra are involved in the tumor. Partial or segmental cystectomy may be appropriate for invasive transitional cell

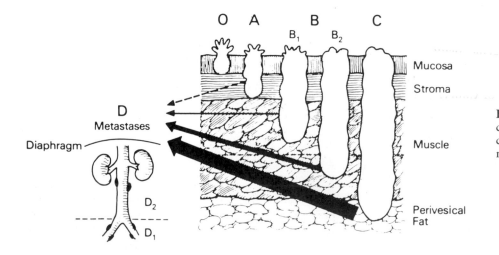

Figure 3. The staging of bladder cancer. (From Skinner DG: Cancer Res 37:2838, 1977, with permission).

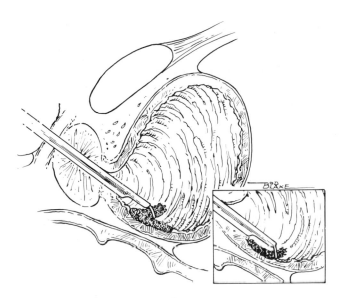

Figure 4. In the transurethral removal of a bladder tumor, the initial superficial resection is followed by a deeper cut to make certain that a portion of the bladder wall is removed so that the depth of invasion by tumor can be properly assessed. (From Benson M, Olsson CA: *In* Paulson DF [ed]: Genitourinary Surgery. New York, Churchill Livingstone, 1984, with permission.)

carcinoma or adenocarcinoma in very specific circumstances.

Carcinoma in situ is a bladder lesion in which there is cellular anaplasia with no papillary component or lamina propria invasion. Histologically, carcinoma in situ is characterized by severe cellular anaplasia with marked variety in size, shape, and staining intensity of nuclei.

Neurogenic Bladder Incontinence

Normal control of micturition is maintained by a complex mechanism involving interaction of the cerebral cortex, spinal cord, bladder, and the vesical sphincter mechanism. Neurogenic bladder disorders are not uncommon in patients with multiple sclerosis, myelodysplasia, spinal cord injury, or diabetes mellitus, or after pelvic operation or injury. The goals of management with neurogenic bladder dysfunction are (1) preservation of renal function, (2) achievement of continence, (3) prevention of upper and lower urinary tract deterioration, and (4) prevention of urinary infection.

Urinary Stress Incontinence

Urinary stress incontinence is an abnormality that involves the involuntary loss of urine associated with an increase in intra-abdominal pressure caused by coughing, sneezing, or straining. On physical examination of a patient with stress incontinence, an assessment of the pelvic floor support and urethral hypermobility is made. With the bladder filled with fluid, the patient is observed for leakage while coughing or straining. When this procedure is repeated, with the examiner providing urethral and bladder support, there should be no leakage.

Cystitis

Cystitis is more frequent in females than in males and is often accompanied by dysuria, urgency, or a low-grade fever. In females, cystitis may be caused by organisms that have colonized the urethra or vagina and may often follow sexual intercourse. Recurrent bacterial cystitis is often encountered in women with diabetes, pregnancy, or congenital anomalies that cause secondary infection. In the male, cystitis is usually secondary to a prostate or kidney infection or to retention of residual urine.

THE PROSTATE

Congenital Anomalies

A small or absent prostate gland is a rare congenital abnormality that may be associated with malformations of the cloaca, urethra, and testes. Asymmetric development of the prostate is often associated with ductus deferens and seminal vesicle abnormalities and the presence of a malformed or absent kidney. Congenital fistulas may develop between the prostatic urethra and the rectum.

Prostatitis

Patients with acute prostatitis present with fever, chills, dysuria, and perineal pain, and may have bladder irritability, hematuria, bladder outlet obstruction, or prostatic abscess formation. Patients with acute prostatitis usually respond dramatically to intravenous antibiotics and hydration. Following the initial treatment, antibiotic treatment for 6 weeks to 6 months is often required to prevent the development of chronic prostatitis. Chronic prostatitis is usually secondary to invasion of bacteria from the urethra, but it may arise from a hematogenous source or may be secondary to inadequate treatment of acute prostatitis. Chronic prostatitis can be caused by a gram-negative organism such as *Escherichia coli* or an agent such as *Chlamydia trachomatis* or *Trichomonas* species.

Benign Prostatic Hypertrophy

Benign prostatic hypertrophy is a disease of older males and is rarely encountered before the age of 40. The normal prostate in man undergoes a slow increase in size from birth to puberty, at which time there is a rapid increase in size, which continues until the late 30s. Midway through the fifth decade, the prostate may undergo hypertrophic changes. Benign prostatic hypertrophy occurs in the periurethral glandular tissue, which is involved with neither essential functions of the prostate nor the origin of malignancy. The periurethral glandular tissue expands, and the portion of the prostate that is compressed is termed the "surgical capsule." Patients with bladder outlet obstruction secondary to benign prostatic hypertrophy may present with difficulty in initiating voiding, incomplete emptying, dribbling, frequency, or total urinary retention with complete inability to void. The enlarging prostate produces urinary obstruction and persistently increased intravesical pressure, which causes detrusor hypertrophy, bladder trabeculation, and formation of diverticula. This process can progress to hydronephrosis and upper tract deterioration.

Neither prostatic size nor degree of outlet obstruction can be accurately determined on physical examination. Urinary retention may occur with a gland that feels normal on rectal examination. Conversely, a gland that seems significantly enlarged may produce no bladder outlet obstructive symptoms. A postvoid catheter residual urine volume aids in determination of inadequate bladder emptying. The normal postvoid residual urine volume in an adult male is approximately 35 ml. Measurement of urinary flow rate is an accurate screening tool for evaluation of bladder outlet obstruction. The average urinary flow rate in a male is 16 ml/sec, and patients with prostatic hypertrophy usually have flow rates less than 10 ml/sec. Cystourethroscopy, a procedure in which a cystoscope with fiberoptic illumination is introduced through the urethra to the bladder, is an important part of the evaluation of patients with suspected benign prostatic hypertrophy. This procedure permits estimation of the size and anatomic configuration of the prostate, as well as the length of the prostatic urethra. At present, there are surgical and nonsurgical forms of therapy for patients with bladder obstruction secondary to benign prostatic hypertrophy. The goal of surgical therapy is to relieve symptoms while preserving anatomic integrity and function. There are four standard surgical approaches to the removal of prostate for benign prostatic hypertrophy: (1) transurethral, (2) transvesical, (3) retropubic, or (4) perineal. Regardless of the surgical approach, the operation is performed to remove the adenomatous portion of the prostate that is located within the surgical capsule.

Transurethral Resection

Transurethral resection of the prostate enables relief of the obstruction with a minimum of morbidity and a relatively short postoperative course. By use of a resectoscope with current from an electrosurgical unit, the surgeon resects prostatic tissue with a wire loop.

Suprapubic Prostatectomy

The suprapubic, transvesical approach is used when there is a large gland with a significant intravesical component. The suprapubic prostatectomy is performed through a low midline abdominal incision, through which the bladder is opened, and the prostatic adenoma is digitally enucleated along the plane of the surgical capsule. The retropubic prostatectomy is performed through a low abdominal approach, and a transverse incision is made through the prostatic capsule. This procedure can be performed very rapidly, with few postoperative complications, and it is best suited to patients who do not have a small, fibrotic gland or who are not significantly obese.

Recently, new forms of nonsurgical management of patients with outlet obstruction secondary to benign prostatic hypertrophy (BPH) have been developed utilizing the 5α-reductase inhibitor *finasteride* and the α-blocker *terazosin*. Finasteride blocks the conversion of testosterone to dihydrotestosterone, which is the active androgen in the prostate that stimulates the development of BPH. Terazosin blocks the α-adrenergic receptors in the bladder neck and prostatic urethra that increase flow rate.

Prostatic Carcinoma

Prostatic carcinoma is the most common malignancy in males and is the second most common cause of cancer death in males over 55 as well as the most common cause of death by cancer in males over 75. There are 130,000 new cases of prostatic carcinoma each year, with over 30,000 deaths annually. Prostatic carcinoma is predominantly a disease of elderly males, with a peak incidence in the late 60s and early 70s. Fewer than 1 per cent are younger than 50 years old.

The etiology of prostatic carcinoma is unknown, but a number of observations suggest a hormonal role. The disease is not found in eunuchs, and there is often marked tumor regression seen after orchiectomy. The fact that vegetarians and Japanese show low rates of prostatic carcinoma has led some investigators to suggest a dietary etiology. Prostatic carcinoma may be divided into four stages:

1. *Stage A* carcinoma is diagnosed by endoscopic resection of the prostate. In *stage A1*, disease, a mi-

croscopic focus of well-differentiated adenocarcinoma is present in fewer than three microscopic foci. In *stage A2*, there is diffuse involvement of the gland.

2. *Stage B1* carcinoma is confined to the prostate in a discrete nodule detected by rectal examination; *stage B2* indicates large or multiple nodules.

3. In *stage C* the carcinoma has grown outside the prostatic capsule to the periprostatic area.

4. *Stage D* is metastatic prostatic carcinoma, *stage D1* indicates metastases to pelvic lymph nodes, and *stage D2* is defined as metastatic disease in bone, distant lymph nodes, or soft tissue.

Histologically, prostatic carcinoma may be well, moderately, or poorly differentiated. Gleason developed a pathologic classification in which histologic characteristics of the tumor are combined to produce a prognostic score of 2 to 10, which may be of use in predicting the course of the disease.

The evaluation and staging of patients with prostatic carcinoma often includes determination of prostate-specific antigen (PSA), bone scan, and abdominal CT scan. Bone is the most frequent site of hematogenous metastases of prostate carcinoma, and the bone scan is a very sensitive test for detecting metastases. The most common bony sites involved are the pelvis, lumbar spine, and femur. A number of therapeutic options are available for treatment of patients with prostatic carcinoma, depending on the stage of the disease, including radical prostatectomy, external beam radiotherapy, and hormone manipulation.

Stage A1 prostatic carcinoma is often managed conservatively, and a repeat resection of the prostate may be performed. Although this type of carcinoma has very little propensity to progress or metastasize and an excellent prognosis some physicians recommend early intervention with surgery or radiation therapy. Stages A2, B1, and B2 carcinoma may be treated by radical prostatectomy, which involves the total removal of the prostate gland, the prostatic capsule, the ampullae, and the seminal vesicles. The two operative approaches used are the radical perineal prostatectomy and the radical retropubic prostatectomy. Stage C carcinoma was previously treated by radical prostatectomy, cystoprostatectomy, radical prostatectomy plus hormone therapy, and external beam radiotherapy. However, it has not been clearly demonstrated that these treatments increase survival, and many clinicians treat an asymptomatic patient with stage C carcinoma conservatively. Huggins and Hodges opened a new era in the treatment of advanced prostatic carcinoma when they reported the use of orchiectomy and diethylstilbestrol (DES) for the treatment of metastatic disease. Since that time, the use of hormonal manipulation for patients with metastatic prostate carcinoma has become widespread. Currently, patients with advanced prostate carcinoma are often treated with either orchiectomy or a luteinizing hormone-releasing hormone (LHRH) analog with the addition of an androgen-blocking agent.

THE SEMINAL VESICLES

Seminal vesicle cysts, which are rare, are usually congenital in origin, although ejaculatory duct obstruction can also cause them. The cysts can be removed transvesically or perineally. Inflammatory disease may affect the seminal vesicles and can cause hematospermia and painful ejaculation. Rectal examination often reveals tenderness and induration in one or both seminal vesicles.

THE PENIS

Phimosis is a condition in which it is not possible to retract the foreskin on the penis. This may be a complication in which too much foreskin is left, or it may be secondary to an infection that occurs under redundant foreskin. This condition commonly follows poor hygiene, and treatment involves local measures to eradicate the infection. A dorsal slit of the prepuce may be necessary. When the acute infection and inflammation resolve, the definitive treatment is circumcision. *Paraphimosis* is a condition in which the foreskin, once retracted behind the glans, cannot be returned to its original position. The foreskin becomes entrapped behind the coronal sulcus by secondary swelling of the glans. This can usually be resolved by gentle pressure. If the glans is left unreduced, continued swelling may render reduction impossible. To treat the acute condition, an incision may be made to incise the constricting lesion. *Balanitis* is an inflammation of the glans penis, and *balanoposthitis* is an inflammation of both the glans and the foreskin. Balanitis is most commonly due to redundant foreskin and poor hygiene. However, a more ominous disease such as squamous cell carcinoma can cause balanoposthitis, and if the inflammation does not clear with good hygiene, further evaluation is necessary. *Erosive balanitis* may be due to an infection of *Borrelia refringens* and *Vibrio* species.

Circumcision

Circumcision is performed in many countries and prevents phimosis, paraphimosis, and balanitis. There are a number of techniques available for circumcision. In the neonate and young infant, circumcision is often performed with the use of a Gomco clamp.

Priapism

Priapism is a rare disorder in which a male experiences a prolonged erection that is unassociated with sexual stimulation and may be painful. In this condition, which may persist for days if left untreated, the corpus cavernosum fills with viscous blood. In 60 per cent of patients, priapism is idiopathic. It also may be associated with leukemia, metastatic carcinoma, local trauma, and sickle cell anemia.

Peyronie's Disease

Peyronie's disease is a fibrotic process of the sheath of the corpus cavernosum that usually begins with pain followed by development of plaque in the sheath. This area then becomes fibrotic and causes curvature during erection. In most, symptoms resolve spontaneously with conservative management. However, in a small percentage, painful erections persist, and the penile curvature may be of such severity that sexual intercourse is not possible. Medical treatment has been unsatisfactory in the treatment of this disorder, and a number of surgical procedures have been developed.

Lymphogranuloma Venereum

Lymphogranuloma venereum is an infectious venereal disease caused by *Chlamydia trachomatis*. A penile lesion typically develops 30 to 60 days after exposure, heals spontaneously, and may be overlooked by the patient. This genital lesion is followed by lymphadenitis and, in the female, by rectal stricture. The involved inguinal nodes suppurate and form multiple sinuses. The diagnosis is made by a positive complement fixation test.

Granuloma Inguinale

Granuloma inguinale is a chronic venereal infection of the skin and subcutaneous tissues involving the genital area, perineum, and inguinal regions. The infectious agent is a bacterium related to *Klebsiella pneumoniae*. The initial genital lesion forms a nodule that fragments and ulcerates. This ulcer is painful, may bleed, and can spread extensively. The diagnosis is made by the identification of Donovan bodies, which are organisms located inside monocytes.

Condyloma Acuminatum

Condylomata acuminata, or *venereal warts*, are caused by a virus that has a propensity for residing in the moist areas in the genital region. Histologically, they are keratin-covered papillary projections from the surface of the penis. The growth down into the stroma is characterized by normal maturation without anaplasia, although there may be some abnormal mitotic activity. When the lesions are on the penis, they are treated with podophyllin. Giant condylomata acuminata of the Buschke-Lowenstein type are characterized by deep tissue penetration. Treatment consists of surgical removal because this entity may represent a type of verrucous carcinoma.

Herpes Progenitalis

Genital herpes, usually caused by herpes virus type II, is characterized by vesiculopustular lesions and may include adenopathy. These lesions, which can be painful and recurrent, often appear on the foreskin or glans penis and coalesce to form a superficial, spontaneously healing ulcer.

Syphilis

Syphilis, caused by the spirochete *Treponema pallidum*, typically produces a painless ulcer 2 to 4 weeks after sexual exposure. The lesions may appear on the glans, corona, foreskin, or shaft of the penis. Histologically, the lesion contains small round cells plus plasma cells and contains neutrophils if there is a secondary infection. The diagnosis is made by finding spirochetes on darkfield examination of serous exudate from the lesion.

Neoplasms

Premalignant Lesions

Erythroplasia in Queyrat's and Bowen's disease are histologically similar lesions that may represent carcinoma in situ. Bowen's disease is associated with a high incidence of internal malignancy that can occur anywhere on the body. When Bowen's disease occurs on the penis, it occurs on the penile shaft, while Queyrat's erythroplasia occurs on the glans or coronal sulcus.

Malignant Lesions

Most tumors of the penis are epithelial and are related to chronic infection and inflammation of the foreskin or glans. Carcinoma of the penis is unusual in countries where neonatal circumcision is practiced, but it is prevalent in areas where circumcision is not routinely performed. Carcinoma of the penis usually arises on the glans or inner surface of the foreskin and may appear as an erythematous plaque or an ulcer. *Stage A* penile carcinoma is restricted to the glans or foreskin. *Stage B* involves the shaft of the penis and/or the corpus cavernosum. *Stage C* involves the inguinal lymph nodes, and *stage D* involves metastasis beyond the inguinal pelvic nodes.

Sexual Dysfunction

The exact mechanism of penile erection is incompletely understood. The stimulus for erection is complex and of both somatic and psychogenic origin. Male sexual dysfunction is a complex phenomenon that can be associated with a number of disorders. *Impotence* is defined as erectile dysfunction that is characterized by the persistent inability to obtain or sustain an erection that is adequate for intercourse. There is a wide range of causes of male sexual dysfunction including vascular, metabolic, and medication-related problems. Vasculogenic causes for impotence can be arterial or venous in origin. A long list of pharmacologic agents have an adverse effect on sexual function in the male. Diabetes is one of the more common causes of impotence in men and is seen in up to 59 per cent of impotent patients. Neurogenic causes can include spinal cord injury, multiple sclerosis, myelodysplasia, and peripheral neuropathy. Endocrine disorders, such as abnormalities of the pituitary testis axis and thyroid dysfunction, account for 10 per cent.

Few forms of medical treatment for impotence have been successful. If an endocrinologic abnormality exists that causes impotence, its correction should allow normal sexual function to return. A patient in whom diabetes is under poor control often regains potency when the diabetes is brought under better control. Neurogenic impotence secondary to a vitamin deficiency or pernicious anemia may also be reversible. A number of surgical procedures are available for the treatment of impotence, especially the insertion of inflatable prostheses, which are often successful.

A pharmacologic strategy has been developed for the management of impotence, which involves the injection of papaverine hydrochloride with phentolamine mesylate directly into the corpus cavernosum of the penis. Both these agents cause vasodilation. Following self-injection of these or other medications, the patient has an erection for approximately 2 hours, during which time intercourse may be performed, often with ejaculation. Intracavernous injection expands the therapeutic options, and in selected patients, provides an alternative to prosthesis implantation, which has a major role in the management of patients with impotence.

Surgical interference with the sympathetic nerves may cause ejaculatory dysfunction. A certain percentage of patients who undergo retroperitoneal node dissection for metastatic testicular carcinoma, sympathectomy for peripheral vascular disease, abdominoperineal resection of the rectum, and aortoiliac surgical procedures experience ejaculatory dysfunction.

THE URETHRA

Urethral Valves

Urethral valves are folds of the mucosa that arise from the floor of the prostatic urethra. Patients with urethral valves may present with mild or moderate obstruction with mild vomiting problems, or they may present with severe obstruction and upper tract deterioration. Obstruction from urethral valves can cause dilation of the prostatic urethra and hypertrophy of the detrusor muscle with concomitant trabeculation and formation of vesical diverticula.

Hypospadias

In hypospadias, which occurs in 8 of 1000 male infants, the urethral meatus is situated in a more proximal position than normal on the ventral aspect of the penis. The meatus can be located as far back as the perineum, but the more distal hypospadias is more common. Hypospadias tends to be familial and is often associated with *chordee*, a ventral curvature of the penis. It may also be associated with undescended or other genitourinary abnormalities. Severe hypospadias is more likely to be associated with other genitourinary anomalies.

Epispadias

In epispadias, an uncommon disorder that occurs in 1 of 120,000 males, the urethral meatus opens on the dorsal aspect of the penis. Epispadias is often associated with exstrophy, and the combination of epispadias and exstrophy occurs in 1 of 30,000 births. Epispadias can be glandular, penile, or penopubic. Surgical repair is most often a multistage procedure, the objective of which is to achieve continence, normal sexual function, and a satisfactory cosmetic result.

Urethral Stricture Disease

Urethral stricture disease is usually secondary to trauma or inflammation. Gonococcal disease is a leading cause of inflammation, and frequent traumatic causes may include pelvic fracture, instrumentation, or long-term urinary catheter drainage. When the mucosa is traumatized, urine tends to extravasate and the scarring that follows causes a stricture. The patient with a stricture may present with a urinary tract infection or a decrease in size and force of urinary stream. In many cases, urethral strictures can be managed by dilation or direct vision internal urethrotomy. In selected patients with short strictures, internal urethrotomy, performed endoscopically with a small cutting instrument, has produced excellent results. When frequent dilation is required, when there are multiple or long strictures, when the dilation is too difficult, or when the stricture presents in a child, open surgical intervention is indicated.

Inflammatory Disease

Neisseria gonorrhoea is a gram-negative organism that is transmitted by sexual contact. The patient typically presents with a discharge, dysuria, and pyuria 2 to 10 days after sexual exposure. The diagnosis is made by culture of the urethral discharge and by identification of gram-negative intracellular diplococci on Gram stain or culture. The gonococcus invades the periurethral glands, and during the healing process, inflammation and fibrosis cause scarring and stricture formation.

THE SCROTUM

Neoplasms

Scrotal tumors are uncommon and appear to be secondary to an occupational exposure to carcinogens such as soot, tar, creosote, or various petroleum products. In the management of a tumor localized to the scrotum, a partial scrotectomy is often sufficient, and when inguinal nodes are involved, a bilateral inguinal lymph node dissection is indicated.

Gangrene

Scrotal gangrene is encountered in a number of different clinical situations. Gangrene of the scrotum can be a sequela of urinary tract extravasation, epididymitis, or prostoseminovesiculitis. Fournier's gangrene is a particularly ominous variant of rapidly advancing inflammatory disease of the scrotum usually seen in middle-aged or older men. This disease undergoes an explosive, fulminant course that presents in the scrotum, may involve the abdominal wall to the axilla within a short period of time and usually requires urgent and extensive drainage with antibiotic therapy.

Hydrocele

A hydrocele is a serous collection of fluid that develops between the visceral and parietal layers of the tunica vaginalis. Primary hydroceles occur in children and are caused by failure of closure of the processus vaginalis, an embryonic peritoneal diverticulum that

traverses the inguinal canal and forms the tunica vaginalis. In a hydrocele that presents in a neonate, operation is often delayed up to 2 years because the patent processus vaginalis usually closes. In adults, secondary hydroceles tend to develop slowly over a period of time and are thought to be secondary to lymphatic outflow obstruction. The diagnosis of hydrocele can be made by transillumination of the scrotum. A hydrocele transilluminates, whereas a hernia, tumor, or enlarged testis from orchitis does not.

THE SPERMATIC CORD

Varicocele

A varicocele is a dilation of the pampiniform plexus of veins. It is a common finding in young males and is most often seen on the left. The pampiniform plexus empties into the internal spermatic vein, which drains into the renal vein on the left and the vena cava on the right. The frequent occurrence of this abnormality on the left side is thought to be related to the fact that the left spermatic vein empties into the renal vein and the combination of upright position and incompetent valves may increase pressure and cause varicocele formation. A varicocele may also be associated with a renal tumor or other retroperitoneal neoplasm.

Neoplasms

Most spermatic cord tumors are benign. Lipoma, fibroma, leiomyoma, and myxofibroma may occur in the spermatic cord and are treated by simple excision. Malignant tumors are usually sarcomas, such as leiomyosarcoma, liposarcoma, or rhabdomyosarcoma, that present in middle age and may initially be mistaken for an inguinal hernia.

THE EPIDIDYMIS

Epididymitis

Epididymitis may be caused by a number of organisms and usually occurs in older males, although it sometimes occurs in younger men. In the male over the age of 35, *E. coli* is the most common cause, and in men under 35, *C. trachomatis* is the most common organism. Epididymitis may occur spontaneously or may follow a surgical procedure such as prostatectomy. In the acute stage, there may be pain, swelling, and low-grade fever. On physical examination, the scrotum is enlarged, spermatic cord tenderness may be present, and palpation reveals a thickened, painful epididymis.

Neoplasms

Three fourths of epididymal tumors are benign. *Adenomatoid tumor*, the most common benign epididymal tumor, appears between the third and sixth decade and is thought to take origin from müllerian mesenchymal elements. Malignant fibrosarcoma and rhabdomyosarcoma occur in the epididymis of younger patients and are treated by radical removal of the cord, epididymis, and testis.

THE TESTIS

Anorchia

Gonadal abnormalities may be divided into anomalies of development and anomalies of position. Testicular absence, termed *anorchia*, is an uncommon finding that occurs in approximately 1 of 5000 births. The fetal testis is essential to the development of the wolffian duct system and for the degeneration of the female müllerian duct system. For a male phenotype to develop, the testis must be present until at least the 16th week of gestation. Therefore, in a normal phenotypic male with an XY karyotype and anorchia, some type of injury must have occurred to the developing gonad after the 16th week, such as torsion of the vessels, infection, or trauma. It must be established whether or not a testis is actually absent or only incompletely descended, because a testis that remains intra-abdominal has a 40-fold greater chance of developing a testicular tumor than a normal testis.

Undescended Testes

There are two types of undescended testes: an *ectopic testis*, which lies outside the normal path of descent, and a *cryptorchid testis*, in which descent has been arrested along the correct pathway before reaching the scrotum. Ectopic testes are thought to be due to an abnormality of the gubernaculum, which normally guides the descent of the testes. Ectopic testes may be found in the superficial inguinal region, over the pubis, in the perineum, or, rarely, under the skin at the base of the penis. Cryptorchidism occurs in 3.4 per cent of full-term infants. Approximately 50 per cent of the time, these testes descend during the first month of life. Cryptorchidism is thought to be due to an intrinsic testicular defect, deficient hormonal stimulation, or an abnormality of the gubernaculum. A cryptorchid testis may be found in the abdomen, upper or lower inguinal canal, or high scrotum. Most of these testes lie in the inguinal canal, although 15 per cent are abdominal.

Torsion

In testicular torsion, a disease of prepubertal and pubertal males, there is incomplete reflection of the tunica vaginalis on the testis and epididymis. This deformity permits the testis to rotate within the tunica vaginalis and causes strangulation of the blood supply. The testis undergoes permanent damage unless the abnormality is promptly corrected. Young males with testicular torsion are typically awakened from sleep with scrotal pain and may present with nausea, vomiting, and scrotal edema. On physical examination, the testis on the affected side is often higher than the opposite side and it may have a transverse position.

Orchitis

Acute infection may reach the testis by a hematogenous route, by lymph channels, or down through the vas deferens. Any agent causing bacteremia can infect the testis, and *E. coli*, *Streptococcus* species, and *Staphylococcus* species are not uncommonly encountered. The most common causes of bacterial orchitis are epididymitis, prostatitis, or urinary tract infection.

Testicular Neoplasms

Carcinoma of the testis has an incidence of 2.8 in 100,000 and is the most common solid neoplasm occurring in males between the ages of 15 and 45. The germ cell tumors that cause 95 per cent of testicular neoplasms include classic seminoma, spermatocytic seminoma, embryonal carcinoma, yolk sac tumor, teratoma, and choriocarcinoma. Testicular tumors tend to spread early to the retroperitoneal lymph nodes. The initial embryologic development of the gonads originates in the area adjacent to the developing nephrogenic tissue, and even though the testis descends to the scrotum, the primary lymphatic drainage remains retroperitoneal. Testicular carcinoma is divided into three stages. *Stage I* is confined to the testis, *stage II* has spread to the retroperitoneum, and *stage III* has metastasized outside the retroperitoneum.

A patient with a suspected testicular tumor should always undergo an inguinal exploration, because a transcrotal approach may spread tumor and complicate future management. In a case of a testicular mass suspected to be malignant, the serum tumor markers alpha-fetoprotein (aFP) and human chorionic gonadotropin (HCG) are determined. These tumor markers are important in the initial evaluation of a suspected testicular tumor and in surveillance after removal of the tumor. Elevated tumor markers may be the earliest indication that the tumor has recurred and are helpful in following response to chemotherapy. An abdominal

CT scan provides information about the presence of retroperitoneal metastases.

Seminomas tend to occur in the fifth and sixth decades of life and represent about 40 per cent of testicular tumors occurring in adults. The prognosis for early-stage seminoma is very good. The treatment for stage I, II, and III seminoma has historically involved radiation therapy. *Spermatocytic seminoma* occurs in men over 65 and is considered a benign tumor. Histologically, these tumors form solid sheets of cells of varying sizes without a lymphocytic infiltrate. Patients with this tumor are often treated conservatively with orchiectomy. A highly malignant tumor, *embryonal carcinoma* represents 20 per cent of testicular tumors in adults. This tumor forms glandular and papillary structures with irregular nuclei, hemorrhage, and necrosis. This tumor characteristically metastasizes rapidly to the retroperitoneum or lungs. The *yolk sac tumor* accounts for 60 per cent of testicular tumors in children. This is a particularly malignant tumor that rarely presents in adults in its pure form but commonly accompanies embryonal carcinoma or teratocarcinoma. Histologically, this tumor consists of anastomosing tubular and acinar structures. *Teratomas* account for 7 per cent of testicular tumors in adults and 40 per cent in children and combine elements of fetal and adult structures originating from three germ cell layers: endoderm, ectoderm, and mesoderm. It is considered benign in children, but a significant number of teratomas metastasize in adults. In its pure form, *choriocarcinoma* is a rare, aggressive tumor. Choriocarcinoma often occurs mixed with other germ cell elements and consists of two cell types, syncytiotrophoblasts and cytotrophoblasts. Serum HCG levels are typically very high with choriocarcinoma. Although *non–germ cell tumors* of stromal origin tend to be benign, 10 per cent are malignant. Leydig cell tumors and Sertoli cell tumors are the most common stromal tumors.

Infertility

Infertility has become an increasingly common problem that affects an increasing number of married couples. The evaluation of an infertile couple includes an examination of both partners, and in approximately 50 per cent the cause of infertility is found in the male. A wide range of abnormalities can have an adverse effect on male fertility, including germ-cell aplasia, a congenital defect in development of the seminal cells, and spermatogenic arrest, a developmental abnormality of maturation. Cryptorchidism is associated with an increased infertility rate. The cryptorchid testis is subjected to a higher temperature than the normal testis and is also likely to have other associated developmental abnormalities in addition to failure of descent. Mumps orchitis or radiation orchitis can

cause damage to the spermatogenic cells. The ductal system can become obstructed by inflammation caused by epididymitis or vasitis, or there can be a congenital absence of the vas deferens. Pituitary abnormalities can also lead to abnormalities in testicular function. In hypogonadism from primary testicular failure, an example of which is Klinefelter's syndrome, poorly formed seminiferous tubules show only marginal function. A varicocele may be associated with a decreased sperm count, an increase in immature forms, and a decrease in motility.

Intersex

A newborn infant who presents with ambiguous genitalia is an urgent problem needing immediate evaluation. An early decision should be made about the gender status, and the choice of gender often depends upon the infant's anatomic characteristics. If there is inadequate phallus, the child may be reared as a female regardless of genetic sex. There are four major intersex abnormalities in newborns: (1) female pseudohermaphroditism, (2) male pseudohermaphroditism, (3) mixed gonadal dysgenesis, and (4) true hermaphroditism.

Female Pseudohermaphroditism

Female pseudohermaphrodites are generally genetic females who have been exposed to endogenous or exogenous androgens during development. In congenital adrenal hyperplasia, the most common type of female pseudohermaphroditism, there is an overproduction of adrenal androgen that virilizes the female fetus. These patients have normal female internal structures with partially masculinized external genitalia.

Male Pseudohermaphroditism

Male pseudohermaphrodites are genetic males with gonads but incompletely masculinized genital ducts and external genitalia. This syndrome can be secondary to (1) failure of testicular differentiation, (2) failure of secretion of müllerian inhibitory factor, (3) failure to target tissue to response to testosterone, or (4) failure of conversion of testosterone to dihydrotestosterone, owing to deficiency of 5α-reductase.

Mixed Gonadal Dysgenesis

Mixed gonadal dysgenesis is the second most common cause of ambiguous genitalia in the newborn. These children often have karyotypic mosaicism, the etiology of which is unknown. They present with asymmetry of ambiguous external genitalia, a dysgenetic testis on one side and a streak gonad on the other side. A uterus, vagina, and at least one fallopian tube are commonly present, and these children are most often reared as females.

True Hermaphroditism

True hermaphroditism is a rare disorder in which both ovarian and testicular tissue is present. There is a variable differentiation of both the internal and external genitalia, and the external genitalia are ambiguous.

REFERENCES

Bennington JL, Beckwith JB: Tumors of the Kidney, Renal Pelvis, and Ureter. Washington, DC, Armed Forces Institute of Pathology, 1975.

Bergman H (ed): The Ureter. New York, Springer-Verlag, 1981.

Bradley WE: Urologic Clinics of North America. Philadelphia, WB Saunders Company, 1978, p 279.

Donahoe PK, Crawford JD: Management of neonates and children with male pseudohermaphroditism. J Pediatr Surg 12:1045, 1977.

Finlayson B, Roth RA: Clinical management of urolithiasis. *In* JA Lippertino (ed): International Prospectives in Urology. Baltimore, Williams & Wilkins, 1983.

Glenn JF (ed): Urologic Surgery. Philadelphia, JB Lippincott Company, 1991.

Javadpour N: Principles and Management of Urologic Cancer. Baltimore, Williams & Wilkins, 1983.

Kaufman JJ: Current Urologic Therapy. Philadelphia, WB Saunders Company, 1986.

Kelalis PP, King LR, Belman AB: Clinical Pediatric Urology. Philadelphia, WB Saunders Company, 1985.

Mostofi FK: Testis, scrotum, and penis. *In* Anderson WAD, Kissane JM (eds): Pathology. St. Louis, CV Mosby Company, 1977.

Paulson DF: Genitourinary Surgery. New York, Churchill Livingstone, 1984.

Smith DR: General Urology. Los Altos, Lange Medical Publications, 1981.

Walsh PC, Retik AB, Stamey TA, Vaughan ED: Campbell's Urology. Philadelphia, WB Saunders Company, 1992.

Williams DI, Johnson TH: Paediatric Urology. London, Butterworth Scientific, 1982.

Witten DM, Myer GH, Utz DC: Emmett's Clinical Urography. Philadelphia, WB Saunders Company, 1977.

Zorgniotti AW, Lefleur RS: Auto-injections of the corpus cavernosum with a vasoactive drug combination for vasculogenic impotence. J Urol 133:39, 1985.

44

DISORDERS OF THE LYMPHATIC SYSTEM

RICHARD L. McCANN, M.D.

HISTORICAL ASPECTS

Lymphatic vessels were first identified by Aselli in 1622. From the study of the mesentery of dogs, he first recognized that the lacteals were vessels rather than cords and that they contained a fluid distinct from blood. Pecquet described the cisterna chyli and the thoracic duct in 1651, and Bartholin first applied the term "lymphatics" to these vessels and recognized their wide distribution in the body. A century later, Mascagni injected mercury into the lymphatics of a human cadaver to enhance their visualization. Hunter, in the mid-18th century, taught that the lymphatic system had the function of fluid absorption throughout the body and transportation of this fluid into the vascular compartment. In the late 19th century, Starling proposed a concept of capillary fluid filtration and reabsorption that remains nearly intact today. The effect of colloid osmotic pressure was added by Pappenheimer and Soto-Riviera in 1948. These views gave the first satisfactory explanation of lymph formation and led the way for investigation of diseases of the lymphatic system. Visualization of lymphatic vessels in a living subject was achieved in 1930 when Hudack and McMaster injected patent blue-violet dye and observed its absorption by dermal and subcutaneous lymphatics. The next important step was the direct cannulation of lymphatic vessels and injection of radiopaque contrast material for the radiographic visualization of lymphatic anatomy by Glenn in 1948 in animals that rapidly led to the development of the technique of lymphangiography in humans.

ANATOMY

An understanding of the embryology and anatomy of the lymphatics is important because most diseases of the lymphatic circulation derive from abnormalities in development. Lymphatic vessels are thought to derive embryologically from venous structures. By the sixth week of human gestation, the lymphatic system consists of paired jugular lymph sacs in the neck and paired iliac sacs in the lumbar region. The iliac vessels coalesce to form a retroperitoneal dorsal collecting sac termed the *cisterna chyli*. The jugular lymph sacs become linked with the subclavian veins producing paired thoracic ducts. Usually the left one becomes dominant and receives lymphatic drainage directly from the cisterna chyli. This is the mechanism whereby lymph fluid returns to the vascular system. Lymphatic capillaries are located throughout the dermis and subcutaneous tissues. The structure of lymphatic capillaries is similar to that of blood capillaries except the basement membrane is less well defined. There are large gaps between adjacent lymphatic endothelial cells, and particles as large as red blood cells and lymphocytes have been observed passing through these gaps. Certain tissues are notable for their lack of lymphatic capillaries. The entire epidermis, the central nervous system, the coats of the eye and skeletal muscle, cartilage, and tendon do not have lymphatic drainage. The dermal lymphatics are valveless channels that drain into one of several superficial lymphatic vessels. These are valved channels that, in the extremities, pass primarily on the medial aspect of the limb toward the groin or axilla where they end in one or more lymph nodes. These vessels maintain a uniform caliber as they ascend and frequently communicate with each other through transverse branches, have a well-defined adventitia, a media containing smooth muscle cells, and an intima. The vessels are innervated, and spasm as well as natural rhythmic contractions have been observed. In the extremities, there is a separate deep lymphatic system. This network closely follows the main vascular pathways deep to the fascia of the skeletal muscles. In normal circumstances there is little, if any, communication between the deep and superficial systems in the periphery.

Lymph nodes are periodically interposed throughout the course of the collecting lymphatic channels. Each node has several efferent channels entering through the capsule. Lymph enters the lymph sinuses, bathes the cortical and medullary areas, and exits by a single efferent channel. Normal lymph node architecture consists of cortical and medullary regions (Fig. 1). The cortical areas contain predominantly lymphocytes that are arranged in follicles separated by trabecular extensions of the capsule. Within the follicles are discrete germinal centers. The medulla may contain macrophages and plasma cells as well as lymphocytes, and these cells are thought to be in dynamic equilibrium within the node. Lymph nodes also have a separate vascular and nervous supply, and it is here that vascular and lymphatic interactions occur. Lymphatic channels draining the lower extremities and abdominal viscera join to form the cisterna chyli adjacent to the aorta in the upper abdomen. The latter structure passes through the diaphragm to become the thoracic duct. Within the thorax, the duct receives the intercostal and thoracic visceral lymph vessels and finally enters the venous system by joining the left subclavian vein in the neck. A separate right lymphatic duct drains the right upper extremity and neck and enters the right subclavian vein.

PHYSIOLOGY

The functions of the lymphatic system are to maintain a continuous exchange of interstitial fluid, to return macromolecules from the interstitial space to the vascular system, and to contribute immunologic protection by transporting bacteria, foreign bodies, and malignant cells to the regional nodes where concentrations of macrophages, plasma cells, and lymphocytes can interact with them, initiating the immune response. Interstitial fluid is formed as a filtrate of plasma across the capillary membrane. Its rate of formation depends on the pressure gradient across this membrane. Starling, in the last century, recognized that a hydrostatic pressure gradient existed between the interstitial space and the vascular compartment. Pappenheimer and Soto-Riviera contributed the concept of semipermeability of the capillary membranes to large, principally protein, molecules. These large molecules trapped within the capillary space exert an osmotic effect, tending to keep fluid volume within the vascular space. Thus, the exchange of fluid between the capillaries and interstitial space depends on a dynamic interaction involving the hydrostatic pressure within the capillary and interstitial space and the osmotic pressure within these two compartments. The oncotic pressure of normal plasma approximates 20 mm Hg, whereas the oncotic pressure of interstitial fluid is usually less than 1 mm Hg. The hydrostatic

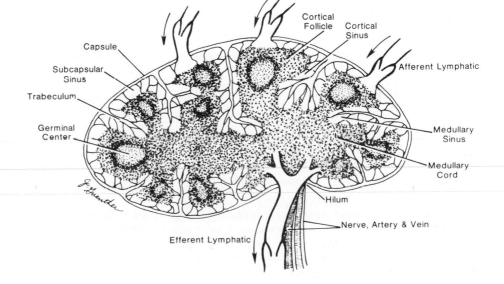

Figure 1. Diagram of typical lymph node architecture. There are multiple afferent lymphatic channels and a single efferent lymphatic duct. The lymph node also has a separate vascular and nervous supply. (From DePalma RG: Disorders of the lymphatic system. *In* Sabiston DC Jr [ed] Textbook of Surgery, ed 14. Philadelphia, WB Saunders Company, 1991, p 1482, with permission.)

pressure at the arteriolar end of a capillary is estimated to be 37 mm Hg and, at the venous end, 17 mm Hg (Fig. 2). The hydrostatic pressure of the interstitial fluid varies in different tissues, being minus 2 mm Hg in subcutaneous tissues and 6 mm Hg in the kidney. There is a net flux of fluid out of the capillary into the interstitial space at the high-pressure arteriolar end of a capillary and a net flux inward at the venular end. The net efflux normally exceeds net influx, and this extra fluid returns to the circulation by way of the lymphatics. Normal lymph flow is 2 to 4 L/day. The rate of flow, however, is greatly influenced by a number of local and systemic factors including protein concentration in the plasma and interstitial fluid, local arterial and venous pressure relationships, and capillary pore size and integrity. *Lymph propulsion* is also a complex process. At rest, the intrinsic rhythmic contraction of the walls of the collecting ducts is thought to propel lymph toward the thoracic duct in a peristaltic fashion. Active skeletal muscle contraction compresses the lymphatic channels and, because of the presence of the competent valves in the lymphatic channels, lymph is propelled cephalad. Increased intra-abdominal pressure, as from coughing or straining, also compresses the lymphatic vessels, accelerating the flow of lymph. The phasic changes in intrathoracic pressure associated with respiration establishes another pumping mechanism to propel lymph through the mediastinum. The rapid flow of blood in the sub-

clavian vein may exert a siphon effect on the thoracic duct.

LYMPHEDEMA

The delicate homeostatic mechanism controlling interstitial fluid volume can fail if an abnormality develops in any of its components. A local or generalized accumulation of excessive interstitial fluid is termed edema and may follow breakdown of any of the factors that influence formation of the interstitial fluid. For example, elevation of the venous pressure causes less interstitial fluid reabsorption and accumulation of interstitial fluid. This may occur from obstruction of the venous system due to acute venous thrombosis or may be due to a more systemic disorder such as heart failure. Lymphedema refers to the accumulation of interstitial fluid caused by an imbalance of interstitial fluid formation and lymph drainage. Conditions causing lymphedema are separated into two categories. *Primary lymphedema* refers to a congenital absence or deficiency of lymphatic channels, a condition that is most common in females and usually affects the lower extremities. For unclear reasons, the left side is more commonly affected than the right. Primary lymphedema is usually due to a deficiency of subcutaneous lymphatic channels. When the deficiency is severe, swelling occurs in the neonatal period and the condition is termed *lymphedema congenita*. When less severe, the swelling occurs at or shortly after the time of puberty, termed *lymphedema praecox*. Lymphedema that appears after the second or third decade is termed *lymphedema tarda*. There is a general correlation between the severity of the syndrome and the time of its onset. The stimulus for provoking the emergence of lymphedema later in life is not clear. In approximately half of the patients, an injury or other defined event precipitates the onset of swelling, which then fails to resolve. *Milroy's disease* refers to an uncommon sex-linked form of lower extremity lymphedema. Congenital lymphedema may also be associated with other conditions such as Turner's syndrome, distichiasis, and lymphangioma.

Secondary lymphedema is due to acquired lymphatic obstruction that may be produced by tumor infiltration of regional nodes such as in Hodgkin's disease or other lymphomas. Obstruction may also be caused by surgical extirpation of regional lymph nodes during operations for malignant disease. Fibrosis and occlusion of lymphatic pathways may also be caused by radiation therapy for malignant disease. Secondary lymphedema was commonly related to radical mastectomy in the past when that procedure was performed more often. Throughout the world, the most common cause of secondary lymphatic obstruction is *filarial in-*

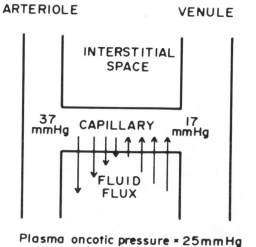

Figure 2. Diagrammatic representation of fluid flux across a capillary membrane. Fluid transfer is dependent upon the net hydrostatic and oncotic pressure gradients. This is usually positive near the arteriolar end leading to net outflow of fluid and negative near the venular end where most of the fluid returns to the vascular space.

festation with *Wuchereria bancrofti* or *malayi*. In this condition, the adult nematode lodges in the lymph nodes and lymph vessels and causes a severe form of lymphedema that may progress to elephantiasis.

LYMPHANGIOGRAPHY

Lymphatic diseases have been classified on the basis of lymphangiographic appearance. Lymphangiography is performed by first identifying the lymphatics on the dorsum of the foot by injecting a blue dye subcutaneously, which outlines the subdermal lymphatic channels. Under local anesthesia, a cutdown is performed on a selected vessel. These vessels are often extremely small, and optical magnification is frequently required. Ethiodized oil contrast medium is slowly injected, and the transit of dye is observed by serial roentgenograms over 24 hours or more. Because the dye eventually enters the venous circulation, it is trapped in pulmonary capillaries. Previous pulmonary radiation may allow the oil to pass through the lungs and enter the systemic circulation. This could cause cerebral oil embolism, and a history of previous pulmonary irradiation is a contraindication to this procedure. Other complications of lymphangiography include allergic reactions and symptomatic pulmonary oil embolism if excessive volumes are injected. If no lymphatics are found in the foot, an inguinal lymph node can be injected directly to visualize the pelvic lymphatic vessels.

Normal lymphangiographic anatomy demonstrates several parallel channels coursing on the medial aspect of the limb. These often branch and intercommunicate, but the diameter remains relatively constant as the vessels ascend. Small ampullae are demonstrated every several centimeters, representing the site of the valves. The deep lymphatics are only rarely seen with a dorsal pedal injection. Normal lymph nodes have a uniform, ground glass appearance and may remain opacified for weeks. Several lymphangiographic patterns can be observed in patients with lymphedema, the most common being hypoplasia seen in over 90 per cent of patients with primary lymphedema (Fig. 3). In these patients, the lymph vessels are small and few in number, with usually less than five trunks entering the inguinal region. The vessels present may be discontinuous, and in severe cases, no major lymphatic trunks may be identified. *Hypoplasia* may be limited to the distal portions of the limb, in which case the edema is usually mild and nonprogressive. Hypoplasia of the proximal lymphatic system in the pelvis usually causes a more severe clinical picture with swelling of the entire limb, which is often progressive. In this condition, dermal backflow frequently occurs in which there is abnormal movement of dye out of the lymphatic chan-

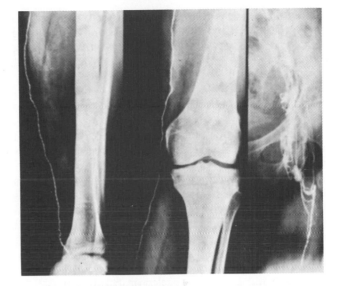

Figure 3. Lymphangiogram in a 43-year-old woman with lymphedema of the feet and ankles. A single lymphatic channel is demonstrated below the groin, but pelvic lymphatics are normal. This is an example of distal hypoplasia. (From Kinmonth JB, Eustace PW: Ann Coll Surg Engl 58:278, 1976, with permission.)

nels into the dermal plexus. The second major lymphangiographic pattern occurring in lymphedema is *hyperplasia*. It is thought that this pattern is caused by lymphatic obstruction at the level of the cisterna chyli or thoracic duct, and thus the disease is always bilateral. Numerous mildly dilated vessels are usually demonstrated in both legs (Fig. 4). This condition is distinct from a rarer unilateral form of hyperplasia termed *megalymphatics*, in which varicose valveless lymphatic vessels are observed, usually in only one

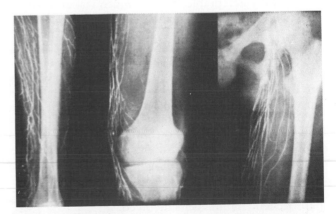

Figure 4. Lymphangiogram demonstrating hyperplasia with multiple channels of normal caliber and with competent valves. (From Gouh MH: Br J Surg 53:917, 1966, with permission.)

limb, and which is frequently associated with cutaneous angiomas. Chylus reflux may be prominent and may present as chylometrorrhea, chylus skin vesicles, or chyluria.

TREATMENT OF LYMPHEDEMA

The majority of patients with lymphedema can be managed nonoperatively. A conservative program of meticulous skin hygiene, external elastic support garments, and intermittent extremity elevation maintains a functional extremity in all but the most severely affected patients. Daily use of mild antiseptic soap and careful nail trimming help in the avoidance of skin and nail infections. Care should be taken to keep the web spaces dry, and use of an antifungal powder may be helpful. An emollient cream may be used to keep the skin soft and to avoid cracks or fissures. If eczema appears, short courses of a steroid-containing cream may be used, but these should not be employed for long periods. Skin ulceration, as frequently observed in severe deep venous insufficiency, is rarely seen in lymphedema. Approximately 25 per cent of patients experience intermittent episodes of cellulitis. The most frequent organisms are *Streptococcus* and *Staphylococcus* species, which are usually sensitive to antibiotics. Therapy with systemic antibiotics, bed rest, and leg elevation should be started promptly, and is usually effective. External compression using an elastic garment is helpful in controlling excessive fluid volume in the moderately lymphedematous limb. Several grades of these stockings are available commercially; however, the most effective are those that are custom manufactured and designed with a built-in pressure gradient from the toe to the groin. Lighter, less well-fitting, mass-produced garments may be more cosmetically acceptable, but are much less effective in controlling edema. It should be remembered that the elastic in these garments stretches with use, and the garment should be conscientiously replaced at 3- to 4-month intervals if they are to maintain their effectiveness. Several types of pneumatic compression devices are available. The simplest of these is a single sleeve (in which the extremity is placed), which is inflated by a compressor at chosen intervals. A more effective device is a sleeve divided into compartments that are serially inflated by the controlling device. These may be applied several times daily and may be used during sleep. Diuretics are of little use in controlling lymphedema fluid because they do not act on the specific pathogenetic mechanisms involved.

Surgical treatment is indicated if the size of the extremity compromises function. Attempts to improve lymphatic drainage by pedicle transfer of lymphatic-bearing omentum, skin, or defunctionalized bowel

have universally met with an unacceptably high incidence of complications, with no convincing evidence of substantial benefit. Excisional therapy was first described by Charles at the turn of the century. In this procedure, the entire skin and subcutaneous tissue, as well as the superficial muscle fascia, are removed circumferentially, except for the plantar surface of the foot (Fig. 5). Originally, split thickness skin grafts were used for coverage, but more recently, full thickness grafts, harvested from the excised tissue when possible, have been found to be more durable and to reduce the risk of subsequent breakdown. In less severe cases where the skin remains adequate, simple staged excision of the thickened fibrotic subcutaneous tissue and superficial muscle fascia beneath 1- to 2-

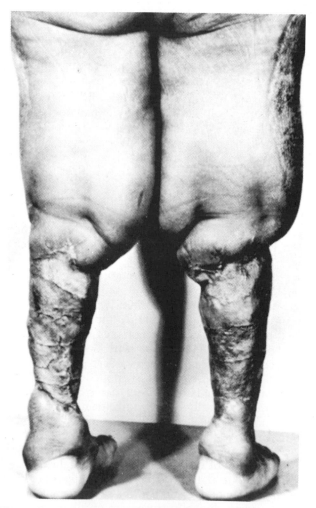

Figure 5. Long-term result after excision of subcutaneous tissue and skin with skin grafting. Note the "plus 4" appearance. (From Bunchmann HH II, Lewis SR: Plast Reconstr Surg 54:64, 1974, with permission.)

cm-thick skin flaps may be the best procedure. This is usually accomplished in a staged manner, with the medial side being done first followed in 3 to 4 months by the lateral side. It is interesting to note that studies have shown that lymph drainage as measured by clearance of subcutaneously injected radioactive albumin increases twofold after this procedure. Microsurgical anastomosis of lymphatic vessels or lymph nodes to local venous structures has been reported. The procedure is most applicable in patients who have proximal lymphatic obstruction, such as that occurring following treatment for breast cancer. Because most patients with primary lymphedema have lymphatic hypoplasia rather than obstruction, this procedure is rarely feasible in that group.

LYMPHATIC TUMORS AND MALFORMATIONS

Lymphangiomas are congenital malformations of the lymphatic vessels that usually are apparent in infancy. These lesions often increase in size and cause symptoms by compressing adjacent normal structures. Although rare, malignant transformation has been reported as well. The lesions may consist of masses of small capillary–size lymphatic channels (lymphangioma simplex), dilated lymphatic vessels (cavernous lymphangioma), or endothelial-lined cysts (hygroma), and may be located anywhere in the body, but the larger cystic lesions are usually found in the neck or the axilla (Fig. 6). Treatment is surgical excision, with preservation of surrounding normal vital structures. If possible, it is beneficial to defer operation until 2 to 3 years of age to minimize the risk of injury to adjacent tissues in the neck. Large lymphangiomas may require staged excision.

CHYLUS SYNDROMES

Chyle is formed in the lacteals of the small intestines by absorption of the products of fat digestion. Chyle is normally transported to the cisterna chyli and then to the thoracic duct and may be found outside of the normal channels if there is an acquired or congenital block of the thoracic duct or incompetence of the lymphatic valves. Fistulization may occur into the peritoneal, pleural, or pericardial cavities. Chylous ascites and chylothorax may respond to treatment with a medium-chain-triglyceride diet. These fats are transported directly to the liver via the portal venous system, thus decreasing chylomicron formation and intestinal lymph volume. Occasionally, direct suture closure of a chylus fistula is indicated if conservative

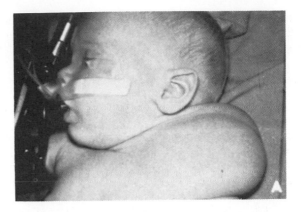

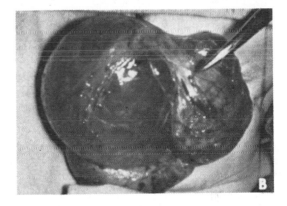

Figure 6. Cystic hygroma. *A*, Gross appearance in a 5-month-old boy. *B*, Appearance at surgery. Clamp points out spinal accessory nerve. (From Fonkalsrud EW: Am J Surg *128*:152, 1974, with permission.)

measures fail. Chylous ascites developing spontaneously in an older patient is nearly always due to an underlying malignancy, and this should be sought prior to initiating therapy.

LYMPHANGIOSARCOMA

Lymphangiosarcoma is a rare lesion that may develop in a lymphedematous extremity regardless of cause. It appears first as purple-red nodules in the skin. Although a very unusual event, it is a rapid-acting fatal lesion.

REFERENCES

DePalma RG: Disorders of the lymphatic system. *In* Sabiston DC Jr (ed): Textbook of Surgery, ed 14. Philadelphia, WB Saunders Company, 1991, pp 1479–1489.

Ersek RA, Danese CA, Howard JM: Hereditary congenital lymphedema (Milroy's disease). Surgery *60*:1098–1103, 1966.

Fonkalsrud EW: Surgical management of congenital malformations of the lymphatic system. Am J Surg *128*:152–159, 1974.

Kobayashi MR, Miller TA: Lymphedema. Clin Plast Surg *14*:303–313, 1987.

Miller TA: How I do it. Surgical management of lymphedema of the extremity. Ann Plast Surg *1*:184–187, 1978.

Savage RC: Collective review. The surgical management of lymphedema. Surg Gynecol Obstet *160*:283–290, 1985.

45
VENOUS DISORDERS

WORTHINGTON G. SCHENK, III, M.D.

PATHOPHYSIOLOGY

The principal function of veins is to serve as a conduit for the return of postcapillary blood to the right heart. Minor secondary functions include blood volume capacitance and thermoregulation. Most of venous blood flow occurs passively, driven by the slight pressure gradient between postcapillary venules and the right heart in this low-resistance circuit. Active propulsion of venous blood is necessary particularly in the lower extremities where the deep veins are within the relatively rigid muscle compartments. Because of the presence of valves, rhythmic contraction/relaxation of the muscles (such as during walking) augments blood flow in an antegrade direction.

The most significant pathophysiology of venous disorders is the tendency toward formation of intraluminal clot. Fibrin deposition within the lumen of veins is a commonplace occurrence, but is opposed by naturally occurring fibrinolytic activity. The development of occlusive clot may be promoted by Virchow's triad of stasis, hypercoagulability, and intimal injury. This can lead to *obstruction* causing increased resistance to venous outflow and sequelae such as edema, pain on exercise, and *postphlebetic syndrome*. Chronic venous insufficiency caused by established outflow obstruction is, fortunately, relatively rare. Postphlebitic venous insufficiency can also be caused by *valvular incompetence*. Deep venous thrombosis typically occurs within venous valves, and after luminal recanalization from thrombolytic activity, the valve leaflets can be scarred, foreshortened, or completely destroyed, leading to retrograde flow with extrinsic compression, effectively destroying the function of the "muscular pump." This sequence of events, while producing anatomically patent venous channels, still causes physi-

ologic outflow obstruction because of the lack of active flow augmentation, causing the same pathophysiologic changes as anatomic obstruction. Release of clot into the lumen of the vein can cause *pulmonary embolism*, a pathophysiology discussed in Chapter 46. The additional pathophysiologic changes of *inflammation*, *infection*, and *dilatation* are less significant and generally non–life threatening. Venous conduits, except when surgically altered and used as arterial substitutes, are not prone to obstructive changes of atherosclerosis. Malformations such as arteriovenous malformations and venous hemangiomas do occur. True neoplasms of veins, and particularly malignancies, are extraordinarily rare.

Pathophysiologic changes in the veins of the lower extremities and most of the venous problems evaluated by surgical consultation are discussed in this chapter. Thrombosis, compression, and obstruction can occur in the upper extremities, great central veins, and portal system. Central venous obstruction or thrombosis (of the subclavian or innominate veins or superior vena cava) related to instrumentation for the insertion and maintenance of central venous catheters is a special case and is not discussed in this chapter. A classification of venous disorders of the lower extremity is shown in Table 1. Paradoxically, a recommendation for surgical intervention is relatively unusual in the entire spectrum of lower extremity venous disorders. Surgical ablation of prominent superficial dilated veins (varicose veins) is effective, but less invasive and less costly measures are often available. Surgical palliation for the sequelae of chronic postphlebitic syndrome can be beneficial, but few patients with chronic postphlebitic changes are identified for whom the risk/benefit analysis for surgical intervention is considered favorable.

543

TABLE 1. VENOUS DISORDERS OF THE LOWER EXTREMITIES

DISORDER	SURGICAL Rx
Varicose veins	Frequently unnecessary
Acute thrombophlebitis	Very rarely indicated
Deep venous thrombus	Very rarely indicated
Acute iliofemoral thrombosis	Last resort; sometimes helpful
Chronic postphlebitic syndrome	Useful palliation in carefully selected cases

DIAGNOSTIC TECHNIQUES FOR EVALUATION OF VENOUS DISORDERS

A classification of the available diagnostic modalities for venous testing is shown in Table 2. The table includes the specific question to be addressed by each study. It is generally advisable and cost-effective to begin with the least-invasive studies, progressing to the more complex noninvasive studies to answer specific clinical questions and to reserve the invasive testing for failure of the noninvasive assessment, or to define specifics of venous anatomy *after* a patient has been considered to be an operative candidate. In particular,

TABLE 2. DIAGNOSTIC MODALITIES FOR EVALUATION OF VENOUS DISORDERS

Test	Utility
Physical examination	
Inspection	Varicosities, ulcers, edema, skin changes
Homans' sign	Thrombophlebitis (low sensitivity and specificity)
Trendelenburg test	Venous filling time; superficial valvular incompetence
Ochsner-Mahorer test	Incompetent perforators
Perthes' test	Venous claudication
Noninvasive testing	
Doppler ultrasound	Deep vein flow, reflux, valvular incompetence
B-mode ultrasound imaging	Thrombosis in deep veins
Impedance plethysmography	Whole-extremity venous outflow rate
Invasive testing	
Ambulatory venous pressure monitoring	Quantitation of "muscle pump" effectiveness
Radionuclide studies	Research applications only in present-day practice
Contrast venography	"Gold standard" for obstruction (clot) in deep veins, but largely replaced by duplex or B-mode ultrasound
Descending venography	Special technique used only for preoperative localization of incompetent valves

contrast venography is not considered routine for screening or initial evaluation of any lower extremity venous disorder.

VARICOSE VEINS

Etiology, Signs, and Symptoms

Varicose veins of the lower extremities is an extremely common affliction, affecting 15 to 20 per cent of the adult population. A familial history may be obtained in about 15 per cent of patients. The affliction is more prevalent among females (the female/male ratio is 5:1), with many women dating the onset of visible and symptomatic varices to the time of pregnancy. Varicose veins are classified as primary and secondary. *Primary varicose veins* is an isolated disorder of the superficial veins of the lower extremities and are not a sequela of deep venous thrombosis. *Secondary varicosities* may be a manifestation of deep venous insufficiency and associated with multiple stigmata of chronic venous insufficiency, including edema, skin change, stasis dermatitis, and ulceration. This condition has a distinctly different pathophysiology from primary varicose veins and should be carefully distinguished because its prognosis and treatment should be approached differently.

Continuous and prolonged overdistention of the relatively thin-walled veins of the lower extremity produces enlargement in both the transverse and longitudinal dimensions. The longitudinal enlargement produces the characteristic tortuosity of the subcutaneous veins, and the transverse distention causes the visible and palpable engorgement responsible for the symptomatic and cosmetic features. This overdistention also produces loss of valvular competence; operative therapy, when indicated, is ablative and consists of destruction or removal of the veins, rather than correction of the valvular incompetence. Factors contributing to the development of varicose veins include congenital weakness or absence of valve leaflets, incompetent perforating veins with reversal of venous blood flow from deep to superficial, volume expansion and hormonal influences of pregnancy, the effects of gravity on hydrostatic pressure (most notably in individuals whose occupations require standing or sitting for prolonged periods without intermittent calf muscle contraction), and occasionally direct trauma to the valves of perforating veins. It is postulated that primary varicose veins propagate from proximal to distal. The combined effects of gravity and volume expansion may first render the valve at the saphenofemoral junction incompetent, causing a longer column of blood acting on the next lower valves, which would become similarly overdistended to the point of incompetence, and so forth. Most patients complain primarily of the cosmetic aspect of multiple visibly distended veins of the lower extremities. Other complaints include a fatigued and heavy sensation, particularly upon standing for a long period, characteristically relieved by elevation of the leg. A more disabling pain may occasionally be noted, and hemorrhage, either spontaneous or from minor trauma, has been reported but is unusual.

The history should include a careful search for previous injury or previous deep venous thrombophlebitis. Previous treatment of varicose veins should also be noted in view of their recurrent nature. The physical examination should include a search for stasis dermatitis, pigmentation, edema, and ulceration, as these may all be evidence of more significant deep venous insufficiency. Whenever any form of therapy is planned, it is important to confirm the patency and competency of the deep venous system. If the patient improves with the application of a well-fitted elastic stocking, patency of the deep venous system is suggested, as compression of the superficial veins in the presence of inadequacy of the deep veins would be expected to make the patient worse. An easy bedside confirmation of this phenomenon is called the *Perthes' test*, wherein the effected extremity is wrapped with a compressive elastic bandage and the patient is asked to walk several hundred yards. Relief of the distention of primary varicose veins from external compression should produce limited symptomatic improvement (negative Perthes' test), whereas compression of the patent superficial channels in the presence of deep venous obstruction causes dramatic worsening of the patient's "venous claudication" (positive Perthes' test). Confirmation of deep venous function should be performed with the Trendelenburg test and venous plethysmography confirming normal deep venous outflow. Contrast venography is not necessary prior to the institution of treatment for primary varicose veins if the noninvasive tests are normal.

Indications for Treatment

Minor involvement should be treated conservatively, symptomatically, and nonoperatively. The first therapeutic approach is avoidance of prolonged standing, encouragement of weight loss and muscular activity such as walking, and reassurance that minor cosmetic concerns are not a health hazard. The use of light comfortable support hose may be quite helpful. Knee-length stockings with a tight elastic top should be avoided because of their tourniquet effect on superficial veins. For more symptomatic patients with significant discomfort and those whose occupation requires them to endure the deleterious effects of gravity, a graded-pressure, custom-fitted, full-length elastic garment should be prescribed. The treatment options for more severe symptomatic and refractory involvement include *excision* and *injection sclerotherapy*. The patient's expectations and anticipated outcome should be carefully considered when the indications for treatment are solely for cosmetic reasons. Many patients with uncomplicated varicose veins can be treated equally well with ligation and stripping or injection sclerotherapy. If a sufficiently symptomatic patient has demonstrable incompetence at the saphenofemoral junction, surgical vein stripping may provide more durable results than injection sclerosis. The numerous collateral branches of the saphenous bulb can be ligated surgically, but treatment by injection sclerosis causes a relatively high recurrence rate.

Sclerotherapy

Nonoperative obliteration of dilated subcutaneous veins has fluctuated in popularity since the time of Hippocrates. The method of sclerosis/compression therapy as described by Fegan and others appears to be successful in properly chosen patients. The method has been used by Sigg and Zelikovski with more than 58,000 patients in Switzerland. With the patient in the upright position, the veins are marked and individually injected through fine-bore needles with 3 per cent sodium dodecylsulfate in benzyl alcohol (Sotradecol). Particular attention is paid to the identification of the location of "blowouts" (i.e., points of incompetent deep venous perforators), so that injections can be made at or close to these sites. The injection of no more than 0.5 ml of sclerosant is made at each site with the leg elevated, although the actual needle insertion may be aided by temporarily allowing the extremity to hang over the side of the examining table. The most distal veins are injected first, and a compressive dressing is applied from below upwards as the injections are made. As many as ten sites can be injected at a single visit, and residual sites can be injected at the follow-up visit 7 days later. It is important that the compressive dressing consisting of elastic bandage reinforced with elastic tape remain in place for 7 days. This immediate compression encourages apposition of the walls of the superficial veins to obliterate them by direct fibrosis rather than thrombosis, and recanalization does not occur. It is also important for the patient to walk for 1 hour each day throughout the treatment period. Compressive hose are prescribed for at least 2 months following the treatment, except for "touch-up" injections of isolated veins. Symptomatic relief and patient satisfaction with the cosmetic result are expected in 90 per cent.

Serious allergic reactions and unsightly skin discoloration or necrosis are much less likely with Sotradecol than with the previously used sclerosing agent sodium morrhuate. Mild allergic reaction is seen in 0.05 per cent, and 10 to 20 per cent of patients have recurrence via persistent or collateral veins. However, the technique is well suited to isolated recurrences, whether following medical or surgical therapy. Efforts at prospective randomized trials comparing operative therapy and sclerotherapy have shown similar results with both techniques.

Vein Stripping

Ligation plus excision, or "vein stripping," constitutes the operative method of removing varicose subcutaneous veins. Preoperatively, the visible and palpable engorged subcutaneous veins should be marked with indelible ink, with the patient standing in an upright position. General or spinal anesthesia is appropriate, and a time-consuming procedure should be anticipated. A unilateral procedure can be done on an ambulatory outpatient basis. The goal of the operation is ligation and removal of the involved subcutaneous veins with ligation of the deep communicating perforators. Isolated varices are excised prior to the stripping of the long and short saphenous veins. These individual veins are meticulously excised through separate small transverse incisions directly over the marked skin. Incisions are closed in layers, and a subcuticular technique is frequently employed.

The entire long saphenous system can be removed by use of the internal vein stripper. This is done last so that a compressive dressing can be applied immediately, thus reducing the risk of subcutaneous bleeding and hematoma formation. The saphenous vein is isolated at the ankle, and available branches are ligated and divided so that the intraluminal stripper can be passed upward from below. Through a groin incision, the entrance of the long saphenous vein into the common femoral vein at the fossa ovalis is identified and all tributary veins to the saphenofemoral junction are carefully identified, doubly ligated, and divided. Finally, the entire length of the greater saphenous vein is removed through its subcutaneous position utilizing an internal vein stripper. The long flexible stripper is passed through the entire vein from the ankle to the groin. On occasion, an additional incision may be necessary to pass the stripper successfully, particularly around the knee. The instrument is somewhat forcibly extracted through the groin incision, while simultaneously a compressive dressing is applied from the ankle upward to reduce subcutaneous bleeding and hematoma formation. The compressive dressing remains in place for several days, and the patient, while permitted to walk several minutes per hour, gradually increasing daily, should be advised to avoid sitting with the extremities in a dependent position, or standing still without walking.

ACUTE THROMBOPHLEBITIS

Acute thrombophlebitis may be *superficial* or *deep*. Superficial thrombophlebitis is generally a benign condition, but deep thrombophlebitis can be a morbid condition. The most severe form is *acute iliofemoral thrombosis*, and there are a number of chronic sequelae that are of considerable consequence.

Superficial Thrombophlebitis

Superficial thrombophlebitis is an intensely painful condition involving intravascular thrombosis and an intense inflammatory reaction in the superficial veins. It is frequently associated with intravenous cannulation sites. The diagnosis is confirmed by the presence of linear erythema visible in the overlying skin, exquisite tenderness to palpation, and, occasionally, a palpable cord. The condition frequently occurs in the upper extremities of hospitalized patients as a complication of intravenous fluid therapy. Careful nursing care of intravenous cannula sites and routine 72-hour rotation of the sites are important prophylactic measures. This condition is not associated with long-term disabling sequelae, nor is it a significant risk factor for pulmonary embolism. The treatment is symptomatic, the indwelling catheter is removed, and the patient should be treated with adequate analgesia, elevation of the affected extremity, application of moist heat, and salicylates. Heparin anticoagulation is unnecessary in most patients. Because this condition involves a serious risk if it extends into the deep venous system, screening with noninvasive studies to exclude deep vein involvement may be employed when the lower extremities are involved. *Suppurative thrombophlebitis*, a rare purulent infection in superficial veins seen almost exclusively in burn patients, may require surgical excision.

Deep Venous Thrombophlebitis

Involvement of the deep venous system produces much less pain and tenderness, and objective signs and symptoms may be subtle. If duplex ultrasound imaging or other noninvasive studies are unequivocally positive, treatment can be initiated on that basis. With a subtle presentation or when the noninvasive studies are equivocal, the diagnosis is usually confirmed by venography. A positive venogram is shown in Figure 1. Treatment consists of therapeutic anticoagulation with intravenous heparin as described in the treatment for acute iliofemoral thrombosis. The goal of treatment is the prevention of pulmonary embolism, protection of the deep veins from further propagation of clot, and prevention of the long-term sequelae of

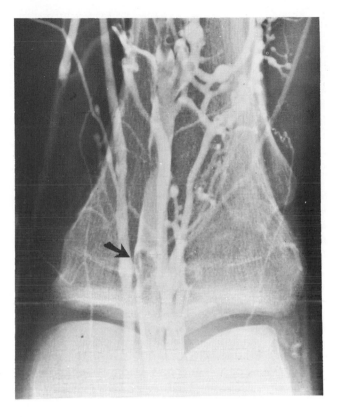

Figure 1. Conventional contrast venogram. A partially occluding thrombus in the popliteal vein appears as a lucent filling defect and is indicated by the arrow.

chronic postphlebitic syndrome. Deep vein thrombosis can also occur in the upper extremity, causing chronic edema, pain, disability, and infrequently, pulmonary embolization. It can occur secondary to trauma, subclavian vein cannulation for central venous access, or occasionally from "effort thrombosis" related to very strenuous physical activity such as wrestling or weight lifting.

Acute Iliofemoral Thrombosis

The recognition of florid acute iliofemoral venous thrombosis is usually straightforward. Edema involves the entire extremity up to the groin, pain may be intense in ambulatory patients, there may be tenderness to palpation because of edema in deep muscle compartments, and the color is likely to be deeper than normal. Subcutaneous collateral veins may appear visibly distended, and mild inflammation and low-grade fever are not unusual. Signs and symptoms are bilateral if both iliofemoral systems or the inferior vena cava is involved. The diagnosis is easily suspected clinically in these florid presentations. However, in as

many as half, iliofemoral thrombosis is asymptomatic and unsuspected, accompanied only by edema of gradual onset frequently in bedridden patients and suspected only on the basis of pulmonary embolization or lower extremity edema. A secure diagnosis must be established before undertaking medical or surgical therapy. Noninvasive studies, including Doppler flow analysis and venous plethysmography, are useful. An unequivocally abnormal Doppler study or duplex ultrasound is sufficient for initiating therapy. If plethysmographic studies are unequivocally normal, no further evaluation is necessary. In other patients, contrast venography remains the standard for diagnosis.

In its most severe form, iliofemoral venous thrombosis can lead to impending or actual gangrene and tissue loss. The venous thrombosis may be accompanied by arterial spasm causing swelling, pain, and pallor of the leg, termed *phlegmasia alba dolens.* This condition, sometimes called "milk leg," was attributed to deposition of milk in the extremity in postpartum women in the 1700s. Iliofemoral thrombosis with accompanying arterial spasm is now known to be the etiology. Prompt recognition and treatment are vital to avoid progression to *phlegmasia cerulea dolens,* which is a more virulent form with a mortality as high as 50 per cent. In this rare but severe form, the leg is not only swollen to the inguinal ligament, but it is also cold and frankly cyanotic and progresses to bullae formation and tissue necrosis. The venous thrombosis is probably more extensive, occluding all venous collaterals, and is associated with arterial spasm.

The standard treatment of iliofemoral thrombosis consists of anticoagulation and, more recently, thrombolytic therapy. Enthusiasm for operative intervention has varied in the past. Thrombectomy is generally reserved for patients with actual or impending tissue loss caused by an associated arterial insufficiency as with phlegmasia cerulea dolens. The usual treatment of acute iliofemoral thrombosis is full therapeutic anticoagulation with heparin, bed rest, and elevation of the affected extremity. Anticoagulation with heparin is initiated promptly with a loading dose of 75 to 100 U/kg followed by continuous infusion of 800 to 1200 U/hr, depending on the patient's weight, and monitored by blood coagulation studies. Maintaining the activated partial thromboplastin time (aPTT) at twice normal is an accepted therapeutic goal. A decrease in pain and edema should be noted within 24 hours, and full therapeutic heparinization is usually continued for 5 to 7 days before conversion to an oral warfarin anticoagulant. Warfarin (Coumadin) anticoagulation to a prothrombin time (PT) of 1 1/2 to 2 times control is sought. Coumadin anticoagulation is continued along with the use of custom-made, graded-pressure stockings for 4 to 6 months. Following this, there is no agreement on long-term therapy, although some surgeons recommend aspirin in a dose of one-half to one tablet once or twice daily. The use of thrombolytic therapy with streptokinase has theoretical advantages over heparin anticoagulation in that it may produce more rapid resolution of intravascular thrombosis. There is some evidence that long-term preservation of venous valvular function may be improved with streptokinase over heparin therapy alone. Streptokinase is most commonly administered as a continuous peripheral infusion. This consists of an infusion of 250,000 U over the first hour and 100,000 U/hr for approximately 72 hours, followed by conversion to heparin anticoagulation and subsequently to warfarin in the manner described earlier. The duration of fibrinolytic therapy may be determined by the use of noninvasive venous studies to confirm reestablishment of deep venous patency. The course of fibrinolytic therapy is rarely less than 48 hours, is usually continued for 72 to 96 hours, but is seldom beneficial if continued beyond 6 days.

Full pharmacologic anticoagulation with either heparin or warfarin is associated with a significant risk of complication, which increases with the duration of treatment. Complications such as gastrointestinal bleeding, hematuria, external hemorrhage from minor trauma, and cerebrovascular stroke underscore the need for careful monitoring. The PT is assessed at least daily while warfarin dosage is being adjusted, weekly when a stable dose is established, and at least biweekly for the duration of treatment. The list of medications that interfere with the actions of warfarin is extensive, and careful patient education is necessary for chronic anticoagulation to be maintained safely. Surgical treatment of acute iliofemoral venous thrombosis remains controversial. Acute results of thrombectomy are often dramatic, but long-term function is frequently disappointing. For these reasons, direct thrombectomy is rarely considered except when there is impending loss of tissue.

CHRONIC VENOUS INSUFFICIENCY AND POSTPHLEBITIC SYNDROME

Pathophysiology

Chronic venous insufficiency follows a mechanical or physiologic interference with venous outflow from the lower extremities. This syndrome requires obstruction or incompetence of the deep venous system. Obliteration of the superficial venous system alone does not produce gross venous insufficiency. Congenitally absent or insufficient deep veins of the lower extremity is extremely uncommon. Iatrogenic or traumatic interruption of main venous channels from the infrarenal inferior vena cava to the common femoral

vein can cause disability, although the establishment of adequate venous return through collaterals is the rule. The syndrome arises most commonly as a consequence of deep venous thrombosis. An episode of symptomatic deep thrombophlebitis can frequently be elicited (as described under "Acute Iliofemoral Thrombosis"). Alternatively, a past episode of silent thrombophlebitis is frequently implied, and a history of trauma, fracture, or transient lower extremity edema may be elicited despite the absence of a recognized diagnosis of thrombophlebitis. Although a properly treated episode of deep vein thrombosis may resolve with normal vein function, the episode may resolve with permanent obliteration of major venous channels, or these channels may recanalize with destroyed or defective valves, subjecting the deep venous system to the gravitational effects of hydrostatic pressure, especially in the upright position. Valvular incompetence must be distinguished from insufficient venous outflow when operative therapy is being considered. Either situation can cause a series of changes ultimately leading to the disability associated with the *postphlebitic syndrome*, in which the deep veins of the lower extremity become overdistended and reversal of flow in the perforating veins occurs and may lead to secondary varicose veins. Dependent edema follows elevation of capillary and postcapillary pressure. Inflammation, fat necrosis, and, eventually, calcification occur in the subdermal soft tissues, a result of pressure necrosis arising from increased pressure from within. Microextravasation of red cells in the dermal and subdermal tissues causes pigment accumulation in the typical reddish brown hyperpigmented appearance of the postphlebitic limb, especially in the supramalleolar area. Full-thickness dermal necrosis produces skin ulceration, which can heal only by epithelialization over the granulation tissue bed. Because of the poor mechanical characteristics of this unsupported epidermis and because the underlying disorder persists, poor wound healing, repeated breakdown and reulceration, chronic recurrent soft tissue infection, and an alarming degree of disability result.

Diagnosis

The history may reveal a clear episode of acute thrombophlebitis. The absence of such a history does not preclude the diagnosis, however, because an episode of silent thrombophlebitis is much more likely than the primary occurrence of symptoms. Physical examination of the lower extremities may reveal edema, ulceration, hyperpigmentation, and the typical inflexible, scarred, woody characteristic of the subcutaneous tissue. The typical appearance of a chronic postphlebitic lower extremity is shown in Figure 2. Accompanying infection, drainage, or cellulitis should be

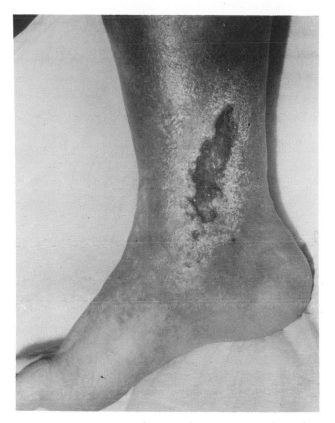

Figure 2. Appearance of a typical venous stasis ulcer. There is brawny edema, thickening of the skin, and pigment deposition. The ulcer is located at and slightly above the medial malleolus, with hypertrophic edges.

noted. The presence of inframalleolar ulceration, pulse deficit, shiny atrophic skin without pigment deposition, or a history of claudication should alert the physician to the possibility of ulceration caused by arterial rather than venous insufficiency. The possibility of concomitant arterial and venous disease should not be overlooked; the noninvasive laboratory tests can be most helpful in this regard with Doppler analysis, sequential pressure measurements, pulse volume recording, and exercise tolerance testing to aid in excluding concomitant arterial insufficiency.

If the patient does not respond to the usual conservative measures as described below, and further surgical intervention is contemplated, additional diagnostic study is necessary. Impedance plethysmography may be helpful in identifying the subset of chronic postphlebitic patients with persistent physiologic outflow obstruction. It is only this group for whom venous bypass is a useful consideration. If Doppler analysis and duplex imaging confirm a diagnosis of deep vein obstruction in the *iliac* or *common femoral vein*, contrast venography is useful preoperatively in plan-

ning the specific anatomy of a venous bypass. Venous Doppler ultrasound analysis is useful in identifying the appropriate patients with deep vein valvular incompetence above the level of the popliteal vein. These patients may be candidates for restoration of valvular competence, and the anatomic diagnosis is further clarified with descending venography as illustrated in Figure 3. Unfortunately, the majority of patients with chronic postphlebitic syndrome have neither of the above-mentioned correctable pathophysiologies and their condition can only be palliated.

Treatment of the Postphlebitic Syndrome

Treatment for the postphlebitic extremity may be begun without contrast venography confirmation of the anatomic extent of pathology, which is reserved to answer specific questions when surgical therapy is considered. Treatment of the postphlebitic lower extremity should be initially conservative and nonoperative. The patient with classic stigmata of chronic venous insufficiency of the lower extremity, including edema, pigment deposition, and ulceration, should be advised of the chronic relapsing and usually incurable nature of this condition. Meticulous skin care, avoidance of local trauma, and the use of compressive stockings should be emphasized. For the atrophic skin of the postphlebitic extremity that progresses to frank ulceration, the use of the Unna's paste boot is frequently employed for outpatient management. This compressive/supportive dressing consists of an absorbent dressing applied directly over the ulcer, followed by wrapping of the leg from the metatarsal heads to the upper calf with gauze impregnated with a gelatin/calamine compound. This semirigid compressive dressing typically remains in place for 5 to 7 days and is reapplied as necessary until the ulcer heals. In refractory cases, hospitalization with continuous elevation of the leg, aggressive wound care, daily whirlpool treatment, and antibiotic therapy when needed nearly always heal the acute ulcers.

Patients in whom healing fails or those who experience multiple recurrences and incapacitation may become candidates for more aggressive surgical therapy. If incompetence of the superficial venous system can be documented in conjunction with a patent deep venous system, ligation and stripping of the greater and lesser saphenous systems may be beneficial. Simple split-thickness skin grafting alone for venous stasis ulcers has a relatively high rate of recurrence because covering the granulating ulcer with epidermis alone has the same recurrence tendency as a spontaneously epithelialized ulcer: the thin epidermis is unsupported by normal underlying dermis and the basic venous insufficiency disorder remains. Rotation flaps, myocutaneous flaps, and composite microvascular free flaps

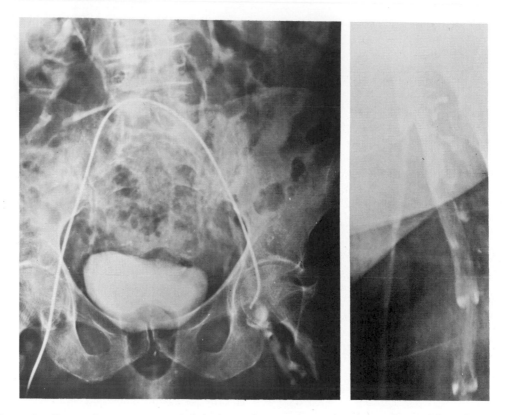

Figure 3. Descending venogram. A left descending venogram has been obtained by advancing a catheter percutaneously through the right common femoral vein, across the confluence at the inferior vena cava, and the tip is positioned in the left common femoral vein. The x-ray table has been tilted into a semiupright position as a bolus of iodinated contrast has been injected. The contrast can be seen to reflux down the femoral vein instead of flowing cephalad to the common iliac vein. The inset demonstrates reflux in both the deep and superficial (great saphenous) veins, and several incompetent valves are identified.

have not been widely used because the creation of a large wound in an extremity in which the primary venous problem remains uncorrected may lead to an even larger nonhealing wound.

In patients for whom direct correction of the venous pathophysiology is not possible, the next step in the surgical management of the postphlebitic syndrome is isolation of the dermis from the deep venous system by ligation of all perforating veins (Linton procedure). In this procedure, longitudinal incisions are made on the medial and lateral aspects of the leg with complete separation of the superficial tissues at the fascial level and identification and ligation of all venous perforators emerging from the muscle fascial level. The procedure frequently must be accompanied by a skin graft over large ulcerated areas. This aggressive procedure is reserved for patients with a disabling and recurrent postphlebitic syndrome despite previous efforts at good nonoperative care.

Since 1975, direct correction of the venous pathophysiology has been approached operatively. These corrective operations involve venous bypass, venous valvular repair, or the interposition of autologous venous valves. Direct repair of the abnormal venous system is intellectually appealing, but because the immediate results are quite variable and the long-term recurrence rate remains high, the use of these corrective operations remains somewhat controversial. These operations are best employed at centers with a specific interest in corrective venous procedures. To consider such an operation, precise anatomic definition of the venous pathology is critical. Chronic venous outflow obstruction must be distinguished from venous valvular incompetence. If chronic venous outflow obstruction is documented by impedance plethysmography and contrast venography corroborates obstruction at the level of the iliac or femoral vein, the patient may be a candidate for a venous bypass procedure. Depending on the anatomy, either autologous vein or a prosthetic conduit can be used to bypass the obstructed area. At the present time, there is no successful means of bypassing obstruction below the level of the popliteal vein. Deep venous valvular incompetence without venous outflow obstruction can be confirmed by appropriate noninvasive studies. Bypass or shunting procedures would obviously be ineffective in this circumstance, but two approaches that have been attempted for direct correction of this condition are *venous valvular repair* and *autologous valve interposition*. For venous valvular repair to be considered, descending venography is first employed to identify the sites of deep vein valves that are present but incompetent. This operation consists of meticulous resuspension of the individual incompetent valve leaflets using microvascular techniques. The details are illustrated by Kistner, who reported 90 per cent symptomatic relief up to 7 years in selected patients. Alternatively, a segment of normal vein containing a competent valve, typically a segment of brachial vein

taken from the arm, can be interposed into the femoral vein to restore venous valvular competence. Taheri and coworkers reported corrected venous flow physiology in 13 of 30 patients undergoing this procedure; 14 retained venous reflex and three developed thrombosis of the femoral vein.

REFERENCES

Gruss JD: Venous bypass for chronic venous insufficiency. *In* Bergan JJ, Yao JST: Venous Disorders. Philadelphia, WB Saunders Company, 1991, pp 316–330.

Kistner RL: Surgical repair of the incompetent femoral vein valve. Arch Surg *110*:1336, 1975.

Sigg K, Zelikovski A: "Quick treatment"—a modified method of sclerotherapy of varicose veins. Vasa *4*:73, 1975.

Thomson H: The surgical anatomy of the superficial and perforating veins of the lower limb. Ann R Coll Surg Engl *61*:198, 1979.

46
PULMONARY EMBOLISM

LEWIS B. SCHWARTZ, M.D.   DAVID C. SABISTON, Jr., M.D.

Acute pulmonary embolism (PE) is a common malady afflicting up to 500,000 Americans annually, causing some 200,000 deaths. It remains the most common preventable cause of hospital mortality and the most common cause of maternal demise associated with live births. For many years it was thought that thrombosis of the pulmonary arteries was a spontaneous event. In 1849, Rudolf Virchow first postulated that blood may clot the deep venous system (deep venous thrombosis [DVT]) and these thrombi could become detached from the vein wall and be swept into the vena cava, right heart, and pulmonary arterial system. In performing postmortem examinations, Virchow stated, "As often as I have found plugs in the pulmonary artery, I have always been able to demonstrate plugs also in the venous system leading thereto." It is now established that essentially 95 per cent of all such emboli originate in the veins of the legs, thighs, and pelvis.

DEEP VENOUS THROMBOSIS

Pathogenesis

Thrombosis within blood vessels occurs following three conditions— (1) stasis of flow, (2) intimal injury, and (3) a hypercoagulable state—and collectively are termed Virchow's classic triad. One or all of these components are present in a variety of medical and surgical conditions and represent the risk factors for the development of DVT and PE (Table 1). For surgical patients, the most important risk factor is the operation itself. Deep venous thrombosis develops following 20 per cent of general surgical procedures and up to 70 per cent of major orthopedic procedures involving the lower extremity. Deep venous thrombosis

may occur in any deep venous system, although the most common vessels involved are the iliac, common femoral, deep femoral, popliteal, and deep veins of the calf.

Diagnosis

The diagnosis of DVT can be difficult, as many patients are entirely asymptomatic. When symptoms occur, the most common is a dull unilateral leg pain aggravated by movement. The most reliable clinical sign is unilateral swelling of the leg, and comparative measurements of calf and thigh circumference with the normal leg can often be diagnostic. Calf pain on dorsiflexion of the ankle (Homans' sign), the presence of a palpable "cord" (a thrombosed superficial vein), and/or calf or thigh tenderness can sometimes be elicited but are nonspecific. Even when the clinical history, complaints, and physical findings are suggestive of DVT, the diagnosis is eventually confirmed in only 50 per cent of patients. Therefore, the most important factor in establishing the presence of DVT is a high index of suspicion.

The least invasive method for confirming the diagnosis of DVT is duplex ultrasonography. These techniques employ B-mode ultrasound to provide a three-dimensional image of the venous system and its flow velocity. Although the test is dependent on the skill of the operator, current data suggest that duplex ultrasonography can detect thrombi between the knee and iliac crest with nearly 90 per cent sensitivity and specificity. Unfortunately, the duplex exam is unreliable for examination of pelvic or calf veins. Other noninvasive methods currently in use include duplex color flow with mapping, venous plethysmography, and ^{125}I-labeled fibrinogen scanning. The ultimate standard for

TABLE 1. RISK FACTORS FOR THE DEVELOPMENT OF DEEP VENOUS THROMBOSIS

Stasis of blood flow
 Obesity
 Surgery
 Trauma
 Lower extremity paralysis
 Cerebrovascular accident
 General or spinal anesthesia
 Long-bone fractures
 Myocardial infarction
Intimal injury
 Surgery
 Trauma
 Indwelling catheters
 Varicose veins
 Advanced age (phlebosclerosis)
 Pacemaker wires
 History of DVT
 Operative manipulation or dilation
Hypercoagulable state
 Malignancy
 Pregnancy
 The puerperium (first 42 days after delivery)
 Oral contraception
 Polycythemia vera
 Thrombocytosis
 Connective tissue disease
 Antithrombin III deficiency
 Protein C deficiency
 Protein S deficiency
 Disseminated intravascular coagulation (DIC)
 Heparin-associated thrombocytopenia and thrombosis (HATT)
 Inflammatory bowel disease
 Nephrotic syndrome
 Myeloproliferative disorders
 Homocystinemia
 Anticardiolipin antibodies
 Paroxysmal nocturnal hemoglobinuria

the diagnosis of DVT remains contrast venography. A small vein in the distal extremity (most often the dorsal vein of the foot) is cannulated, and contrast is injected. Thrombi appear as filling defects in the anteroposterior or lateral planes (Fig. 1). Unfortunately, even venography may fail to demonstrate venous thrombi, especially if clots are nonocclusive or above the iliac crest. For this reason, magnetic resonance imaging (MRI) modalities have recently been used for the diagnosis of DVT, and the early results are quite encouraging (Fig. 2).

Treatment

Deep venous thrombosis is treated by anticoagulation, which is effective in preventing clot propagation, recurrence, and the postphlebitic syndrome. The decision to treat DVT depends on the anatomic location of the venous system involved. About 50 per cent of untreated clots originating in the deep venous system of the thigh and pelvis embolize to the pulmonary

arterial system, and therapy should therefore be initiated. Thrombosis of the deep calf veins is more benign, however. Although propagation and embolization occurs in as many as 20 per cent of patients, the emboli are generally small and usually not associated with significant morbidity or mortality. Anticoagulation for *calf* vein thrombosis, therefore, should be reserved for high-risk patients. Treatment for thrombosis of the subclavian and axillary veins is somewhat controversial, but most authors advocate anticoagulation, since significant PE occurs in 10 to 25 per cent of untreated cases.

Anticoagulation should be initiated with intravenous heparin, which potentiates the effect of antithrombin III, a naturally occurring plasma protein that inactivates factors IX, X, XI, and XII. Although heparin does not dissolve the thrombus, it does prevent clot propagation. The recommended dose of heparin is a bolus of 70 to 100 U/kg followed by a continuous infusion of 15 to 25 U/kg/hr. Monitoring of heparin anticoagulation is accomplished using the partial thromboplastin time (PTT), which should be kept in the range of 1.5 to 2.0 times control. Heparin's half-life is about 90 minutes. Therefore, it is recommended

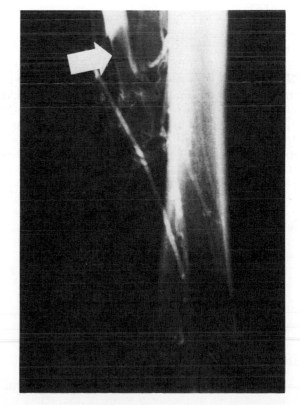

Figure 1. Venographic demonstration of deep venous thrombosis (DVT) involving the left superficial femoral vein. Filling defect (*arrow*) indicates the presence of thrombus.

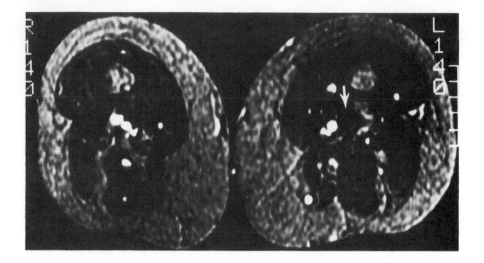

Figure 2. Magnetic resonance imaging (MRI) demonstration of deep venous thrombosis (DVT) from the same patient as in Figure 1. Axial GRE images demonstrate the absence of flow within the left superficial femoral vein (*arrow*). Note also the increased signal in the soft tissues indicating edema. The right venous system is normal.

that the PTT be checked after the first 6 hours, three times during the first 24 hours, and once daily thereafter. In addition, the platelet count must be monitored judiciously, as heparin therapy causes thrombocytopenia in as many as 5 per cent of patients. In rare cases, heparin may also cause paradoxic arterial thrombosis (heparin-associated thrombocytopenia and thrombosis [HATT]), which is life and limb threatening and for which there is no effective treatment except immediate discontinuation of heparin.

Most agree that anticoagulation for DVT should be continued for 3 to 6 months following the diagnosis, but extended therapy and the risk of hemorrhage should be individualized. Following initial treatment with heparin, therapy may be continued with warfarin (Coumadin), an oral inhibitor of the vitamin K–dependent clotting factors II, VII, IX, and X. Warfarin therapy may be begun as soon as the patient is fully anticoagulated with heparin, but the overlap of heparin and warfarin should be at least 4 days, as one of the initial effects of warfarin is to decrease protein C levels (a powerful natural anticoagulant), which could theoretically induce a hypercoagulable state. The dose of warfarin is usually 7.5 mg/day for 2 to 3 days, titrated thereafter to achieve a prothrombin time of 1.2 to 1.5 times control.

PULMONARY EMBOLISM

Pathogenesis

As previously stated, 95 per cent of venous thrombi causing PE arise in the deep veins of the pelvis and thigh. These blood clots may break away from the venous endothelium and embolize to the pulmonary artery. The effects of embolization on pulmonary function are dependent on the size of the embolus, but usually include an increased pulmonary vascular resistance, ventilation-perfusion mismatch with increased dead space and hypoxemia, and decreased pulmonary compliance. These effects are mediated through (1) the mechanical effect of pulmonary artery occlusion, and (2) the immunologic and endothelial response of the pulmonary vasculature. Regarding the mechanical effects, experimental and clinical evidence indicates that acute occlusion of 50 per cent or more of the pulmonary arterial tree is necessary to produce significant pulmonary hypertension. The degree of hypertension is usually linearly related to the amount of angiographically demonstrable obstruction. It is well known, however, that surgical occlusion of up to 50 per cent of the pulmonary arterial tree is well tolerated in most individuals and rarely produces symptoms. During PE, however, symptoms may occur even with minimal embolization, probably caused by the release of humoral factors affecting pulmonary vascular resistance, especially serotonin and thromboxane A_2. The release of these autocrine substances causes vasoconstriction and increased lung vascular permeability (pulmonary capillary leak); pharmacologic blockade of this response in experimental animals and humans has been successful.

Diagnosis

The diagnosis of PE requires a high index of clinical suspicion, as PE is a great *imitator*. The classic triad of dyspnea, chest pain, and hemoptysis occurs in less than 15 per cent of patients, and as many as 20 per cent are entirely asymptomatic. When symptoms occur, their pattern is unpredictable, as demonstrated by large retrospective series (Table 2). The presence of clinical signs of PE is also unreliable, although tach-

TABLE 2. OCCURRENCE OF SYMPTOMS AND SIGNS IN
PATIENTS WITH PULMONARY EMBOLISM

	UPET Trial (1970) n=327	Duke Medical Center (1976) n=1000	PIOPED Trial (1990) n=251
Symptoms			
Dyspnea	83%	77%	79%
Chest or pleuritic pain	70%	63%	58%
Hemoptysis	34%	26%	16%
Altered mental status	59%	23%	
Cough	52%		44%
Syncope		9%	
Classic Triad	14%		
Signs			
Tachycardia	56%	59%	
Fever	43%	43%	
Rales	55%	42%	
Tachypnea	92%	38%	
Thrombophlebitis	32%	23%	
Elevated CVP		18%	
Shock		11%	
Accentuated P_2	50%	11%	
Cyanosis		9%	
Pleural rub		8%	

Abbreviations: UPET = Urokinase Pulmonary Embolism Trial, PIOPED = Prospective Investigation of Pulmonary Embolism Diagnosis, CVP – central venous pressure.

ypnea, tachycardia, and the presence of DVT may often be documented (Table 2). Laboratory tests are nonspecific. Acute arterial hypoxemia is fairly sensitive in that approximately 90 per cent of patients with PE are hypoxemic. The Wacker triad (elevated indirect bilirubin, elevated lactate dehydrogenase, and normal transaminase) was originally thought to be diagnostic, but has fallen into disfavor. Newer serum markers of thrombolysis, including the D-dimer assay and fibrinopeptide A, are promising but require further clinical confirmation. The electrocardiogram is abnormal in 10 to 40 per cent of patients, but usually reveals only nonspecific ST-T changes. The plain chest radiograph is abnormal in 70 to 80 per cent of patients and virtually diagnostic if diminished pulmonary markings (Westermark sign) or pleural-based pulmonary infarctions (Hampton's hump) are present. In the majority of cases, however, the chest film findings are nonspecific and may include a parenchymal infiltrate, atelectasis, and pleural effusion.

Because of the difficulty in establishing the diagnosis of PE on a clinical and laboratory basis, most patients are subjected to one or more specialized confirmatory tests. The most popular objective study is the ventilation-perfusion scintigram (VQ scan), a nuclear medicine scan that utilizes a combination of the techniques of *lung perfusion scanning* and *ventilation scanning*.

Perfusion scanning, introduced in 1964 by Wagner and Sabiston, is performed by the injection of ^{99m}technetium-labeled microspheres or albumin macroaggregates into the venous circulation, which by scintillation counting, allows for visualization of the distribution of pulmonary blood flow within the lungs. The study is enhanced by ventilation scanning in which ^{133}xenon gas is breathed and washed out and a serial image of the ventilated lung segments is obtained. The sequentially derived VQ scans are compared to identify segments ventilated but not perfused and, hence, may represent areas of embolization.

Ventilation-perfusion scanning is dependent on the skill of the operator and adherence to strict criteria for its interpretation. It is most helpful when the chest film is normal and perfusion defects due to other pulmonary processes are unexpected. It is clear from large randomized clinical trials that a completely *normal* VQ scan essentially excludes pulmonary embolism. In addition, a scan interpreted as positive (i.e., "high probability") establishes the diagnosis with 88 per cent certainty. Intermediate- and low-probability scans, however, have an unacceptable specificity, and clinical decisions based on these scans alone are not recommended.

The ultimate standard for the diagnosis of PE is *pulmonary arteriography*, which involves percutaneous advancement of a catheter through the central circulation to the pulmonary arterial tree with selective injection of contrast dye into the pulmonary arteries. The examination is fairly safe, although the requirement for catheterization and dye injection leads to complications in about 5 per cent of patients. Nonetheless, the pulmonary arteriogram is an invaluable diagnostic study and should be obtained when needed as a definitive test.

An algorithm for the diagnosis of PE is shown in Figure 3. Patients who are clinically unstable or who have grossly abnormal chest radiographs precluding accurate assessment with VQ scan should have pulmonary arteriography to establish the diagnosis. If the patient is clinically stable, however, and the chest film is clear, VQ scanning is the method of choice because it is diagnostic in approximately 25 per cent of patients. If the VQ scan is interpreted as being of low or intermediate probability, the patient should proceed to pulmonary arteriogram as previously stated. All patients in whom PE is suspected should eventually undergo venous duplex examination of the lower extremities to detect DVT.

Treatment

An algorithm for treatment of PE is shown in Figure 4. Pulmonary embolism can be clinically classified into *minor, major,* and *massive,* although much overlap oc-

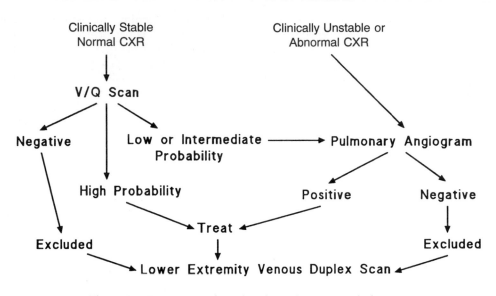

Figure 3. Diagnostic algorithm for pulmonary embolism.

curs. If the degree of pulmonary arterial occlusion is less than 50 per cent and the patient is clinically stable, anticoagulation with heparin is indicated. If there is a major contraindication to anticoagulation (e.g., recent major surgery, gastrointestinal bleeding, recent hemorrhagic stroke, heparin-associated thrombocytopenia), insertion of a transvenous vena caval filter may be considered. Transvenous vena caval filters are devices that are placed percutaneously into the infrarenal vena cava to trap venous thrombi from the legs and pelvis and prevent embolization of the lungs. A variety of filters have been developed, although the largest ex-

perience is reported with the Greenfield filter (Fig. 5) and Bird's Nest filter. The techniques of filter placement have been refined so that the risk of misplacement or failure of insertion is less than 4 per cent. Occlusion of the vena cava from these filters remains a problem and occurs in as many as 5 per cent of patients. Prevention of PE is not universal, as some 4 per cent of patients demonstrate recurrent embolization after the filter is placed. Moreover, these filters may migrate distally or proximally into the heart, the renal veins, or the peritoneal cavity. At present, therefore, placement of a transvenous vena caval filter de-

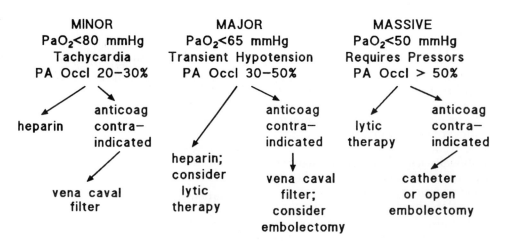

Figure 4. Treatment algorithm for pulmonary embolism.

vice should be reserved for patients who have an absolute contraindication to anticoagulation therapy.

For patients with major or massive PE, thrombolytic therapy should be considered. Although still undergoing trials, thrombolytic therapy can promote immediate dissolution of the embolus with prompt return of pulmonary perfusion. Thrombolysis can be accomplished using one of the thrombolytic agents, including urokinase, streptokinase or *recombinant* tissue-type plasminogen activator (rt-PA). Therapy can be delivered either systemically or directly into the pulmonary artery via selective catheterization, although systemic therapy appears to be superior. The most popular regimen involves the administration of 100 mg rt-PA as a continuous peripheral infusion over a 2-hour period. Thus far, the reported results indicate that this strategy is effective in achieving clot dissolution in over 80 per cent of patients with bleeding complications occurring in less than 5 per cent. Unfortunately, improvements in survival and long-term outcome have not been conclusively demonstrated. In addition, this form of therapy is often not applicable to many postsurgical patients because of the increased risk of bleeding complications at the surgical site. A small group of patients with PE fail to respond to immediate aggressive medical support, and pulmonary embolectomy should be considered. Open surgical embolectomy is currently performed using cardiopulmonary bypass, with a survival rate of about 60 per cent in these critically ill patients. A successful transvenous percutaneous approach to embolectomy has also been described but has not enjoyed widespread acceptance.

Prophylaxis of DVT and PE

Because of the significant morbidity and mortality associated with DVT and PE, considerable attention has been devoted to their prevention. A number of prophylactic regimens have been suggested, although little agreement exists concerning their benefit (Table 3). One of the most important maneuvers is proper patient positioning with the knees higher than the right atrium and the feet higher than the knees (Fig. 6). Too often the patient is incorrectly instructed to simply elevate the legs without attention to the relationship of knees and feet, which may may cause venous pooling and stasis in the calf. In addition, patients should be encouraged to intermittently dorsiflex the ankle for complete emptying of the veins of the calf. An important physical factor in preventing DVT is early mobilization, and every effort should be made to ambulate the patient on the same operative day. Graded *compression* stockings, either thigh-high or knee-high, have been shown to be efficacious in some studies, but many clinicians are convinced that they create a functional tourniquet at the knee and actually

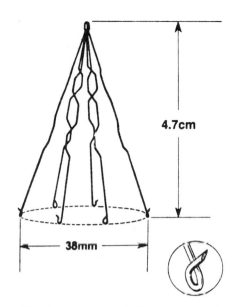

Figure 5. The titanium Greenfield vena caval filter. (From Greenfield LJ, DeLucia A III: Endovascular therapy of venous thromboembolic disease. Surg Clin North Am 72:969–989, 1992, with permission.)

promote thrombosis. *Intermittent pneumatic-compression* (IPC) boots consist of a network of inflatable cuffs that are wrapped around the lower extremities and are sequentially inflated and deflated to stimulate venous flow and the natural fibrinolytic system, but their relative value is questionable. Pharmacologic prophylaxis of DVT and PE is most often accomplished through the use of low-dose heparin (LDH), which is administered in a dose of 5000 U subcutaneously preoperatively and every 8 to 12 hours postoperatively until the patient is ambulatory. While LDH may prevent DVT in certain subsets of general surgical and orthopedic patients, the increased risk of

TABLE 3. POSSIBLE PROPHYLACTIC STRATEGIES FOR DEEP VENOUS THROMBOSIS (DVT) AND PULMONARY EMBOLISM (PE)

Proper patient positioning
Early mobilization
Graded compression stockings
Intermittent pneumatic-compression (IPC) boots
Aspirin
Dihydroergotamine
Iloprost
Low-dose heparin (LDH)
Adjusted-dose heparin
Low-molecular-weight heparin (LMWH)
Dextran 40
Very-low-dose warfarin
Adjusted-dose warfarin
Inferior vena caval interruption

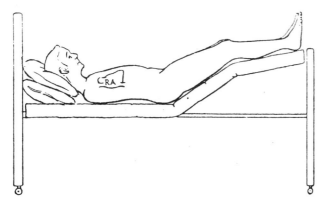

Figure 6. Correct position of lower extremities for prophylaxis of deep venous thrombosis (DVT) and pulmonary embolism (PE). Note the additional bend at the knee: the feet should be higher than the knees and the knees should be higher than the right atrium. (From Sabiston DC Jr: Pulmonary embolism. *In* Sabiston DC Jr [ed]: Textbook of Surgery, ed 14. Philadelphia, WB Saunders Company, 1991, p 1508, with permission.)

hemorrhage at the operative site and the possibility of disseminated intravascular thrombosis syndrome have led most to conclude that routine prophylactic heparin therapy is unwarranted. New forms of heparin, including low-molecular-weight heparin (LMWH), have been developed that may have a limited hemorrhagic effect (less binding of antithrombin III) while retaining their anticoagulant properties (factor Xa inhibition). Effective prophylaxis with LMWH has been reported, but its use is not widespread. Another popular pharmacologic strategy, especially for orthopedic patients, is the use of glucose polysaccharides or *dextrans*. Dextrans increase venous flow velocity, reduce platelet aggregation, and inhibit factor VIII, but have no effect on the bleeding time. The usual dose is 500 ml of dextran 70 twice prior to surgery and once postoperatively. Dextran has been found to be effective in DVT prophylaxis in some series, but the volume expansion required and risk of anaphylaxis has limited its usefulness.

FAT EMBOLISM

The famous German pathologist Zenker first described fat embolism in 1862 found in the pulmonary tissues of patients dying of a variety of injuries. Fat embolism occurs when fat emboli are mobilized from traumatized bone marrow at fracture sites and pass into the bloodstream. It is also thought that chylomicrons are formed from the release of neutral fats and

act as pulmonary emboli following injury. The latter are primarily fat droplets that have toxic effects on tissues. Clinical manifestations of fat embolism generally appear on the second or third day following injury, and are a contributing cause to the respiratory distress syndrome.

A diagnosis of the fat embolism syndrome (FES) is primarily made by manifestations of hypoxia, tachypnea, cyanosis, confusion, petechia, and the appearance of fluffy densities on the chest film. Fat globules may appear in the urine, but this is not necessarily of diagnostic significance. Although serum lipase levels may be elevated, it is not a consistent finding. If FES is of clinical significance, the arterial P_{O_2} is low, generally less than 60 mm Hg on room air. This is associated with an increase in pH and a decrease in P_{CO_2} secondary to hyperventilation. With clinical deterioration, the P_{O_2} falls further with an increasing P_{CO_2} and the development of acidosis.

The treatment of FES is controversial. Clearly, fractures should be stabilized to prevent fat embolism into the venous system. Some have advocated the use of colloids, particularly albumin, and volume expanders, which may be effective. Large doses of steroids (30 mg/kg/day in divided doses) have been recommended on both therapeutic and prophylactic bases. Ventilatory support is of definite value with the addition of positive end-expiratory pressure (PEEP). Therefore, the management of respiratory distress from FES is similar to the management of other forms of hypoxemia.

REFERENCES

Albada J, Nieuwenhuis HK, Sixma JJ: Treatment of acute venous thromboembolism with low molecular weight heparin (Fragmin). Circulation 80:935–940, 1989.

Allison PR: Pulmonary embolism and thrombophlebitis. Br J Surg 54:466–468, 1967.

Barnes RW, Nix ML: Clinical and noninvasive assessment of venous disease as related to pulmonary embolism. J Thorac Imag 4:8–14, 1989.

Cola C, Ansell J: Heparin-induced thrombocytopenia and arterial thrombosis: Alternative therapies. Am Heart J 119:368–374, 1990.

Goldhaber SZ (ed): Pulmonary embolism and deep venous thrombosis. Philadelphia, WB Saunders Company, 1985.

Goldhaber SZ: Thrombolysis for pulmonary embolism. Prog Cardiovasc Dis 34:113–134, 1991.

Goldhaber SZ, Grassi CJ: Management of pulmonary embolism. *In* Sabiston DC Jr (ed): Textbook of Surgery, (update 8). Philadelphia, WB Saunders Company, 1990, pp 115–127.

Goldhaber SZ, Morpurgo M: Diagnosis, treatment, and prevention of pulmonary embolism. Report of the WHO/International Society and Federation of Cardiology Task Force. JAMA 268:1727–1733, 1992.

Greenfield LJ, DeLucia A III: Endovascular therapy of venous thromboembolic disease. Surg Clin North Am 72:969–989, 1992.

47
THE ARTERIAL SYSTEM

JOHN W. HALLETT, Jr., M.D.

Diseases of the arterial system commonly cause disability and death. They are often accompanied by serious coronary heart disease. By the year 2000, nearly 15 per cent of America's population will be over the age of 65, and the prevalence of arterial diseases among this estimated 35 million people will demand thoughtful understanding of the pathophysiology and efficient management of various clinical problems. In contrast, the incidence of arterial trauma continues to increase among younger age groups due to urban violence. An emphasis should be placed on: (1) an understanding of the pathophysiology of the basic types of arterial disease, including stenosis or occlusion, embolic lesions, aneurysms, and arteriovenous fistulas; (2) a knowledge of the diagnostic features, including the history, physical examination, noninvasive diagnostic techniques, and arteriography necessary for recognition and management of various arterial diseases; and (3) a familiarity with the clinical presentations, diagnostic evaluation, and treatment for the various clinical categories of arterial disease. The major clinical categories include acute arterial occlusion of the lower limbs, chronic arterial occlusion of the lower limbs, cerebrovascular disease, aneurysms, aortic dissection, renovascular disease, mesenteric vascular insufficiency, arterial trauma, and circulatory conditions of the upper extremity.

PATHOPHYSIOLOGY

Normal Arterial Anatomy

Arteries must withstand the stress of pulsatile blood flow for many years. Three distinct layers of the arterial wall must remain intact for normal function, and these are the *intima*, *media*, and *adventitia*. The *large*

arteries, such as the aorta, must withstand the greatest stress and thus contain considerable *elastic tissue* in the wall. The *medium-sized* arteries, such as the femoral artery, have less elastic tissue and more *smooth muscle*. Collagen is present in all arteries, but the ratio of collagen becomes dominant as the arteries become smaller.

The arterial system has an abundance of *collateral networks*. These natural bypasses help to maintain viability of the limbs and organs when chronic arterial occlusive diseases obstruct the main arterial pathways. All organs have some degree of collateral circulation, although this varies greatly in different locations. For example, the profunda femoris artery provides excellent collateral flow around an occlusion of the superficial femoral artery. In contrast, the coronary, renal, and retinal arteries have relatively little natural collateral circulation, and acute occlusion of these vessels is usually followed by severe ischemia or infarction. Consequently, such arteries are termed *end-arteries*.

Atherosclerosis

The most common cause of arterial disease is *atherosclerosis*. Pathologically, atherosclerosis is a combination of changes in the intima and media, including focal accumulation of lipids, fibrous tissue, calcium deposits, and, at times, hemorrhage. The development of atherosclerotic lesions is a complex biochemical and cellular process. The gross appearance and developmental sequence may be divided into three major stages. The first stage consists of *fatty streaks* that first appear in childhood and young adult life. Their content is primarily of lipids, and they also have infiltration of macrophages and smooth muscle proliferation. The second stage consists of the development of *fi-*

brous plaques, representing a more permanent lesion. Usually located at arterial bifurcations, fibrous plaques have a lipid core surrounded by a capsule of elastic and collagenous tissue. The most advanced stage is the *complicated plaque*, and necrosis of these plaques may lead to surface ulceration and thromboemboli. Intramural hemorrhage may cause plaque expansion and arterial occlusion. Degeneration of elastic and collagen tissue may cause formation of aneurysms.

Arterial Occlusive Disease

Atherosclerosis (Fig. 1) generally becomes symptomatic by gradual reduction of blood flow to the involved extremity or organ. Symptoms occur when a *critical arterial stenosis* is reached. Generally, blood flow and pressure are not significantly diminished until at least a 75 per cent reduction in the cross-sectional area of a vessel has occurred. This reduced cross-sectional area can be equated to a 50 per cent reduction in diameter of the lumen. The formula for the area of a circle (A = 3.14 × radius^2) defines the relationship between vessel diameter and cross-sectional area.

Arterial Embolic Lesions

One characteristic of atherosclerosis is surface ulceration of an intimal atheroma. Ulcerated plaques

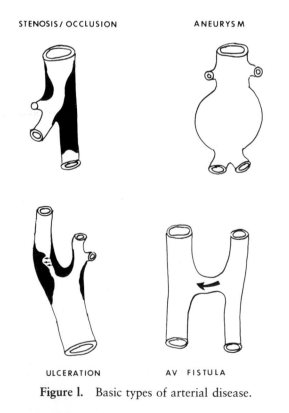

STENOSIS/OCCLUSION ANEURYSM

ULCERATION AV FISTULA

Figure 1. Basic types of arterial disease.

can occur in numerous arterial locations, and from their surface, embolic fragments of plaque material and associated thrombus can pass distally with damage to an organ or an extremity. For example, emboli from ulcerated plaques at the carotid bifurcation can lodge in the brain and cause a transient or permanent stroke.

Aneurysms

An aneurysm is a focal dilation of a vessel and is usually defined as an enlargement of at least 1.5 times the normal. A *true* aneurysm contains all layers of the arterial wall, and a *false* (or pseudo) aneurysm is a local, pulsatile arterial mass without all layers of the arterial wall.

Aneurysms follow degeneration and weakening of the network of protein fibers in the arterial wall, including both elastin and collagen. Although atherosclerosis is commonly associated with arterial aneurysms, recent data indicate a *systemic connective tissue disorder* in many patients. Familial tendencies for aneurysms have been documented repeatedly. Specific genetic defects of collagen and an imbalance of proteolytic and antiproteolytic activity are being identified.

The risk of rupture of an aneurysm is directly related to size of the aneurysm. Stress on the arterial wall increases as the vessel diameter (*d*) enlarges and as wall thickness (*t*) decreases. Wall stress is also proportional to intraluminal pressure (*P*). The simple equation of this phenomenon is Laplace's law, and it emphasizes the importance of blood pressure control in hypertensive patients with aneurysms.

$$\text{Stress} = \frac{P \times d}{t}$$

Arteriovenous Fistula

An arteriovenous (AV) fistula is a direct (noncapillary) connection between the arterial and venous system and encompasses a vast variety of conditions including some that occur in the normal development of the circulation, congenital and acquired malformations, lesions, and iatrogenic shunts. Regardless of the etiology, all AV fistulas cause certain physiologic changes related to the size of the fistula when the fistula occurs between a *large* artery and vein, and it transmits a large volume of blood. Because blood is being shunted directly into the venous circulation, the blood flow is increased. With a large fistula, the cardiac output increases, the heart rate rises, and the diastolic arterial pressure diminishes, usually with an increase in systolic pressure. The blood and plasma volume increase to compensate for the increased volume of blood in the venous circulation. Over time, the artery supplying the fistula usually enlarges and its wall becomes thin. In contrast, the associated vein may also enlarge, but its wall becomes thickened. A long-standing AV fistula may be associated with high-output cardiac failure.

DIAGNOSTIC PRINCIPLES

With a careful history and physical examination most arterial lesions can be correctly diagnosed. Noninvasive tests, including Doppler-derived limb pressures or B mode ultrasonic imaging, are used to document and refine the initial clinical impression. Arteriography is generally reserved for patients requiring more invasive therapy, such as angioplasty or a surgical procedure for which the arterial anatomy must be clearly delineated.

Physical Examination

Most patients have a systemic arterial disorder such as atherosclerosis. Therefore, the initial evaluation should include the entire arterial system to identify signs of other significant arterial disease that may be asymptomatic and unrecognized; for example, an abdominal aortic aneurysm in a patient with claudication. Such an evaluation should include the heart rate and rhythm, bilateral arm blood pressures, auscultation of the neck for carotid bruits and of the heart for arrhythmias, gallops, and murmurs. Additional evaluations to be performed include abdominal palpation for an aortic aneurysm; abdominal auscultation for bruits; palpation of peripheral pulses; auscultation of the femoral region for bruits; and inspection of the upper and lower extremities for ulcers, gangrene, or microembolic phenomena.

Noninvasive Diagnostic Techniques

Although a variety of noninvasive tests are available for the evaluation of arterial disease, some form of Doppler ultrasound is the most useful. A simple hand-held, continuous-wave Doppler can be used to measure upper or lower extremity blood pressures with a standard blood pressure cuff. An *ankle-brachial index* (ABI) is determined by dividing the pressure obtained at the ankle by the brachial arterial pressure (Fig. 2). Normally, the ABI is 1.0 or greater, and a lower ABI indicates arterial occlusive disease. For example, patients who have claudication due to a superficial femoral artery occlusion may have a resting ABI in the 0.6 to 0.8 range. Patients with more severe arterial ischemia such as gangrene of the toes may have an ABI of 0.5 or lower. An important limitation of the ABI is found in diabetic patients with extreme stiffening and calcification of the arterial wall. Because these vessels cannot be compressed by a blood pressure cuff, the ABI may be normal or falsely elevated.

In recent years, duplex ultrasound scanning has combined a real-time B- mode ultrasound *image* with a spectral *waveform*, which allows measurement of blood flow velocity. Duplex scanning has become the preferred method to evaluate arterial stenosis or occlusion in many locations including the carotid, mesenteric, renal, aortic, femoral, and popliteal arteries. With severe stenosis, the duplex spectral waveform shows both turbulence (spectral broadening) and focal arterial narrowing (increased systolic and diastolic velocities) (Fig. 3).

Evaluation of arterial aneurysms can be made by ultrasound, computed tomography (CT), and magnetic resonance imaging (MRI). Ultrasound is the simplest and most accurate method to diagnose and manage aortoiliac, femoral, and popliteal aneurysms. Computed tomographic scanning or MRI are better for evaluating the thoracic or suprarenal aorta.

Recently, *transcutaneous oximetry* (TcPO$_2$) has become a useful method to measure skin-surface oxygen tensions and to assist in the prediction of local healing. In diabetic patients in whom the ABI may not be reliable, a TcPO$_2$ may be more useful to evaluate whether lesions of the foot may heal with good care or whether revascularization is required. Normal TcPO$_2$ is 55 mm Hg or above, while levels less than 40 mm Hg indicate impaired local cutaneous circulation, and skin lesions are unlikely to heal when the TcPO$_2$ is less than 20 mm Hg.

Arteriography

Arteriography involves the injection of a contrast medium into the arterial system to provide a clear image of the arteries prior to an intervention such as angioplasty or operation. Contrast agents are generally iodinated salts in a liquid form. The most common adverse side effects are allergic reactions or nephrotoxicity. Patients with chronic renal failure or diabetes mellitus are more prone to renal complications after arteriography. In selected cases, the contrast medium can be injected into a peripheral vein, with visualization of the arterial system by a *digital subtraction angiogram* (DSA). However, an intravenous DSA may require more contrast material and provides less imaging resolution than conventional intra-arterial angiography.

ACUTE ARTERIAL OCCLUSION OF THE LOWER LIMBS

Acute arterial ischemia follows sudden obstruction of a peripheral artery by either embolism or local thrombosis.

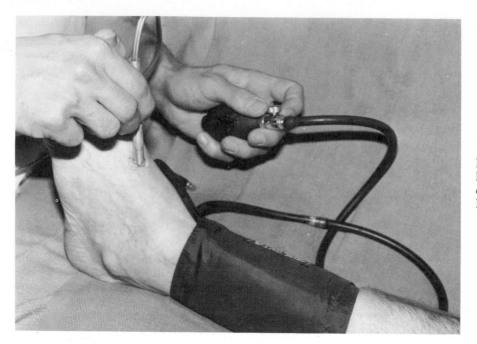

Figure 2. Measurement of an ankle pressure with a blood pressure cuff and handheld continuous-wave Doppler.

Clinical Examination

Acute arterial occlusion should be suspected when a patient presents with a combination of the following "5 Ps":

1. Pain.
2. Pallor (and coolness).
3. Paresthesias.
4. Pulselessness.
5. Paralysis.

Etiology

Embolism consists of a thrombotic, atheromatous, or other material that migrates from a proximal por-

tion of the circulatory system to a more distal site where it obstructs blood flow. The most common causes of arterial embolism are cardiac disease, arterial disease, foreign body, and venous disease. The most frequent cardiac cause of peripheral arterial embolism is atrial fibrillation associated with mural thrombi. Other cardiac disorders include myocardial infarction, ventricular aneurysm, mitral stenosis, prosthetic cardiac valve, bacterial endocarditis, and atrial myxoma. Arterial causes of embolism include thromboemboli from aneurysms or from ulcerated atheromatous plaques. Atheroembolism may cause the *blue toe syndrome*, which is manifest by painful bluish mottling of the feet. An example embolization of foreign body

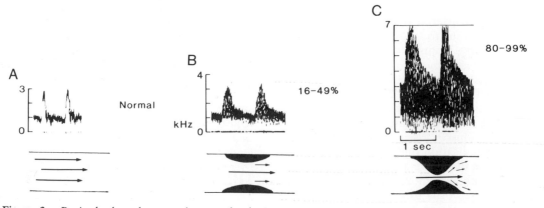

Figure 3. Basic duplex ultrasound spectral velocity patterns. Severe stenosis (>80 per cent) is associated with both disturbed flow (spectral broadening) and increased systolic and diastolic velocities.

is the accidental dislodgment and migration of an arterial catheter or an intravascular bullet from a gunshot wound. Finally, a rare cause of peripheral arterial emboli is a paradoxic embolism caused by the dislodgment of a venous thrombus that passes centrally and across an atrial septal defect or patent foramen ovale into the arterial system.

Peripheral arterial *thrombosis* may also cause acute ischemia and is associated with four common conditions: atherosclerosis, aneurysm, iatrogenic injury, and trauma. The most common cause of arterial thrombosis is an underlying atherosclerotic plaque and associated severe stenosis. Aneurysms of the femoral or popliteal arteries are classically associated with the accumulation of thrombus and eventual occlusion, sometimes with distal thromboembolism. Increasing use of arterial catheterization for coronary and peripheral angiography has caused an epidemic of iatrogenic arterial occlusion at the catheter site. Trauma, especially fracture dislocations of the knee, can cause arterial thrombosis and acute ischemia.

Pathophysiology

When an extremity or organ becomes acutely ischemic, metabolism shifts quickly from aerobic to anaerobic. Anaerobic metabolism is associated with a decrease in cellular concentration of adenosine triphosphate (ATP), an accumulation of lactic acid, and a decrease in the tissue pH. If the tissue is reperfused and reoxygenated within 6 hours, normal cell function is generally restored. If ischemia is prolonged beyond 6 to 8 hours, or extensive extremity thrombus propagation occurs, cellular death begins and is clinically manifested by rising creatine phosphokinase (CPK) muscle enzyme levels and myoglobinuria. After prolonged ischemia, restoration of blood flow can cause a *reperfusion injury* manifested clinically by tense muscle swelling termed *compartment syndrome.*

Clinical Diagnosis

The history can be helpful in ascertaining the possible etiology of the acute arterial occlusion. A chronic history of calf claudication should raise suspicion of a chronic stenosis of the superficial femoral artery complicated by acute thrombosis. A recent myocardial infarction, atrial fibrillation, or a cardiomyopathy make a thromboembolus from the heart more likely. Known aneurysm disease should heighten suspicion of thrombosis of a peripheral femoral or popliteal aneurysm.

On physical examination, the extremity is usually pale and may manifest motor weakness compared to the opposite side. Coolness of the skin and paresthesias to touch are common. An irregular heart beat should call attention to atrial fibrillation and cardiac thromboembolism. The sine qua non of arterial occlusion is absence of peripheral pulses, and the femoral, popliteal, and pedal pulses should be checked. An absent femoral pulse is indicative of a local femoral thromboembolus or a more proximal iliac occlusion. If the popliteal pulse is absent, the presence of an increased contralateral popliteal pulse should raise suspicion that popliteal aneurysm disease is present in both legs. If the foot is paralyzed and no Doppler signals can be heard at the ankle, critically severe ischemia exists, and emergent restoration of blood flow is necessary.

Differential Diagnosis

A careful neurologic and musculoskeletal examination usually differentiates these causes of extremity pain, paresthesias, and paralysis from acute arterial occlusion. Acute deep venous thrombosis can cause acute pain; but the pulses should be palpable.

Diagnostic Evaluation

In acute arterial occlusion, Doppler arterial signals of the affected limb may be diminished or absent. An electrocardiogram may confirm atrial fibrillation or reveal evidence of a myocardial infarction. If the cause of the acute arterial occlusion is unclear, an arteriogram may help to delineate the anatomic location and cause of the acute occlusion.

Treatment

The initial therapy for acute arterial occlusion is intravenous administration of heparin to prevent further thrombus propagation. The usual dose of heparin is a 5000-U bolus followed by approximately 1000 U hourly to maintain the partial thromboplastin time at twice the control value. If an arterial thromboembolus is suspected, the simple solution is a *surgical thromboembolectomy* using a Fogarty balloon catheter introduced by cutdown into the femoral artery. The catheter is passed both proximally and distally. The balloon is inflated, and the catheter is gently withdrawn to retrieve all thromboembolic material. Patients with acute thrombosis of peripheral arterial aneurysms may require a local bypass graft in addition to retrieval of distal thromboemboli by the Fogarty balloon technique. Extensive thrombus propagation into the smaller tibial arteries may require regional infusions of *thrombolytic agents* such as urokinase or *tissue-type plasminogen activator* (t-PA).

Postoperative Management

If the cause of acute arterial occlusion is thrombo-embolism, anticoagulation is usually continued after operation. Long-term warfarin is indicated for atrial fibrillation. Patients who have undergone peripheral bypass grafting for occlusive or aneurysm disease generally do not require long-term anticoagulation. After reperfusion of an acutely ischemic limb, the extremity should be carefully observed for development of tight muscle swelling (compartment syndrome), which may require surgical decompression of the muscle compartments by fasciotomy.

Prognosis

Most acutely ischemic limbs can be saved. The patients at greatest risk for amputation are those with thrombosis of a popliteal aneurysm and/or chronic severe tibial arterial occlusive disease where ischemia has been prolonged greater than 12 to 24 hours and irreversible muscle necrosis has begun.

CHRONIC ARTERIAL ISCHEMIA OF THE LOWER LIMBS

Chronic arterial occlusive disease represents a spectrum of mild to moderate lower extremity walking disability to threatened loss of limb. The most common etiology is atherosclerosis, although other causes must not be overlooked. Clinical manifestation of chronic arterial insufficiency includes muscle pain or tiring with exercise relieved by rest (claudication), pain in the forefoot at rest (ischemic rest pain), ulcers of the foot, gangrene, and pulse deficits.

Etiology and Natural History

As the most common cause of lower extremity arterial disease, atherosclerosis can involve the arteries at any site, including the aortoiliac region, the femoropopliteal segment, and the tibial runoff (Fig. 4). Aortoiliac disease is more common in younger adults (ages 40 to 60) having a strong family history of cardiovascular disease, cigarette smoking, and hyperlipidemia. Combined aortoiliac and femoropopliteal occlusive disease is the natural progression for the same patients who often develop hypertension and adult-onset diabetes mellitus. More distal occlusive disease involving the femoropopliteal and tibial arteries is characteristic of more elderly adults, especially those who have diabetes. Less common causes of chronic arterial occlusive disease include thromboangiitis obliterans (Buerger's disease), popliteal artery muscular entrapment, and cystic adventitial disease of the popliteal artery. These conditions more commonly occur in young adults who present with arterial occlusive disease.

Claudication is associated with a relatively benign prognosis. Annually, only 1 to 2 per cent of these patients progress to amputation, and they are generally those who continue to smoke, have diabetes mellitus, and/or fail to control hyperlipidemia. In contrast, nearly all patients presenting with ischemic rest pain of the foot progress to nonhealing foot ulcers or gangrene within 3 to 6 months.

Pathophysiology

The development of atherosclerosis in the lower extremity is a gradual process occurring over many years and does not become symptomatic until focal atherosclerotic plaques exceed 75 per cent of the cross-sectional diameter. As most of these lesions (e.g., common iliac stenosis or superficial femoral artery stenosis) are focal, good collateral circulation around them generally prevents symptoms at rest. Patients experience claudication with rapid walking or climbing steps or a hill. The symptoms are secondary to acute shifts from aerobic to anaerobic metabolism and the rapid accumulation of lactic acid and other metabolic products. With more extensive occlusive disease, resting baseline cellular metabolism falls below the hypoxic threshold and foot sores can no longer heal or the tissue dies (gangrene).

Clinical Diagnosis

Patients with symptomatic chronic arterial occlusive disease generally present with claudication, ischemic rest pain, or tissue necrosis. Until hemodynamically significant stenosis or occlusion occurs, the patient's only manifestation of peripheral arterial occlusive disease may be diminished peripheral pulses or bruits over plaque sites. Claudication simply means to limp, and it is classically described as a muscle tiring, cramp, or pain that begins with walking a specific distance, is relieved by rest, and occurs again at the same distance. *Pseudoclaudication* due to neurospinal stenosis or musculoskeletal disease may cause back and lower-extremity pain while standing at rest and is often relieved by bending forward while walking. *Ischemic rest pain* is classically defined as forefoot pain that occurs at night while recumbent and is relieved by hanging the foot over the side of the bed. Ischemic rest pain is different from night cramps that occur in the calf muscles. Tissue necrosis includes foot ulcers that are characteristically on the tips of the toe in patients with arterial occlusive disease. Gangrene appears as dark blue or black mummification of a portion of the ex-

TYPE I

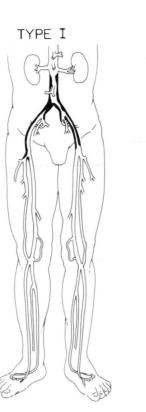

II

III

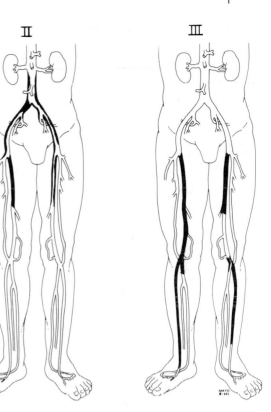

Figure 4. Basic patterns of lower extremity arterial occlusive disease. Type I, aortoiliac disease; type II, multilevel aortoiliac and femoropopliteal disease; type III, femoropopliteal-tibial disease. (From Hallett JW Jr, Brewster DC, Darling RC: Patient Care in Vascular Surgery. Boston, Little, Brown & Co, 1987, with permission.)

tremity and is considered *dry* when not infected and *wet* when there is local maceration, cellulitis, or purulent drainage.

The most important physical sign of chronic arterial occlusive disease is diminution or absence of the femoral, popliteal, or pedal pulses. Localized bruits generally occur over high-grade stenoses, especially in the femoral area or over the distal medial thigh at the level of the adductor magnus tendon where a superficial femoral artery stenosis is commonly found. Some patients have a distinct clinical entity known as *Leriche's syndrome* manifested by bilateral lower-extremity claudication, absent femoral pulses, and impotence due to severe distal aortoiliac arterial occlusive disease, often with complete occlusion.

Differential Diagnosis

Vascular claudication can usually be differentiated from neurogenic or musculoskeletal pain by the history, physical examination, and noninvasive testing. Rest pain can be confused with various types of peripheral neuropathy, but clinical examination is usually distinguishing. If diabetes mellitus is present and the peripheral pulses are palpable, gangrene of the foot over pressure points is more likely due to diabetic neuropathy rather than arterial occlusive disease.

Diagnostic Evaluation

The simplest method to document lower-extremity arterial occlusive disease is measurement of Doppler-derived ABIs at rest and after exercise. An ABI less than 1.0 is suggestive of arterial occlusive disease and confirmatory of severe claudication if the ABI drops significantly with treadmill exercise. When foot sores are present and diabetic medial calcification prevents accurate measurement of an ABI, transcutaneous oximetry is useful in predicting whether ulcers on the foot will heal without revascularization. Before any type of surgical intervention, an arteriogram that usually includes an abdominal aortoiliac view with runoff images of the femoral, popliteal, and tibial arteries is necessary.

Treatment

The initial therapy for mild to moderate claudication is a *medical regimen* including cessation of smoking, modification of hypertension, reduction of hyperlipidemia, and management of the diabetes mellitus with a regular walking program. The walking distance can often be doubled or tripled within 6 weeks by having the patient walk 30 minutes at a comfortable pace at least every other day. The only approved medication for claudication is pentoxifylline, a hemorrheologic agent that reduces blood viscosity by improving red cell membrane flexibility and inhibiting platelet aggregation. About 80 per cent of patients respond to a medical regimen, while 20 per cent need more invasive therapy.

Most patients with incapacitating lower-extremity claudication have arterial occlusion necessitating a *bypass graft*. For severe aortoiliac disease, this includes an aortofemoral bypass, while patients with superficial femoral arterial occlusion generally need a femoropopliteal graft. A few patients have focal iliac or femoropopliteal stenoses amenable to *percutaneous transluminal angioplasty*. Angioplasty may be done by balloons, atherectomy devices, and sometimes supplemented by intravascular expandable stents.

Patients who present with ischemic rest pain, nonhealing sores of the foot, or gangrene generally have extensive arterial occlusion that requires bypass grafting. For severe distal femoropopliteal or tibial arterial occlusive disease, long saphenous vein bypass grafts can be taken distally to the tibial arteries and even to the pedal arteries.

Postoperative Management

Because patients with peripheral arterial occlusive disease often have coronary heart disease, they are generally monitored in an intensive care unit for 12 to 24 hours. Peripheral pulses and Doppler flow must be monitored closely for early thrombosis of grafts. Areas of tissue necrosis or gangrene may require local débridements or amputations.

Prognosis

Patients with stable claudication and compliance with a good medical regimen have a low chance (1 per cent annually) of major amputation. Angioplasty is best for iliac stenosis less than 3 cm in length and is associated with good runoff. Angioplasty of more distal femoral, popliteal, or tibial plaques is associated with a high recurrence rate. Aortofemoral grafts achieve 5- to 10-year patencies of 80 to 90 per cent, while more distal femoral, popliteal, or tibial vein grafts remain patent in 70 to 80 per cent of patients at late follow-up. Vein grafts are preferable to synthetic grafts in the femoral, popliteal, and tibial positions. The leading cause of late death in patients with chronic arterial occlusive disease remains myocardial infarction. Consequently, a careful cardiac evaluation is essential in the preoperative preparation as well as in the long-term surveillance.

EXTRACRANIAL CEREBROVASCULAR DISEASE

Extracranial cerebrovascular disease encompasses occlusive, aneurysmal, or neoplastic lesions of the aortic arch, carotid or vertebral arteries. Such disease may manifest itself as *transient attacks of cerebral ischemia* (TIA), brain infarction (stroke or cerebrovascular accident), pulsatile masses, asymptomatic bruits, or vascular tumors.

Clinical Examination

Extracranial cerebrovascular disease should be suspected when a patient experiences intermittent (TIA) or persistent stroke disturbance in the following neurologic functions: *sight, sensation, strength*, or *speech*. Although rare, masses at the carotid bifurcation may represent as either a *carotid aneurysm* or a *carotid body tumor*. Finally, extracranial cerebrovascular disease may initially be asymptomatic and be manifest by an *asymptomatic cervical bruit*.

Etiology and Natural History

Atherosclerosis causes most extracranial cerebrovascular disease. Stenotic or ulcerated lesions producing TIAs or a stroke are found in the extracranial cerebrovascular vessels in approximately two thirds of patients, while one third of such patients have intracranial or surgically inaccessible disease. The second most common cause of extracranial cerebrovascular disease is *fibromuscular dysplasia* (FMD). This vascular abnormality generally occurs in young or middle-aged women and is frequently associated with hypertension due to concomitant fibromuscular dysplasia of the renal arteries. Aneurysms of the brachiocephalic vessels can be secondary to either atherosclerosis or fibromuscular disease. Finally, *carotid body tumors* or paragangliomas are of neuroendocrine origin, are located in the carotid bifurcation, and usually occur in young to middle-aged adults. Most carotid body tumors have a benign course, although bilateral or familial tumors are more likely to be malignant.

A TIA is a clear warning sign of a future stroke, as approximately one third of such patients suffer a permanent stroke within 5 years, most within 6 to 12 months. Approximately 70 per cent of individuals who have a stroke suffer permanent neurologic dysfunction. Initial mortality for all strokes exceeds 20 per cent, while at least 25 per cent sustain an additional stroke before death. Asymptomatic carotid stenosis greater than 80 per cent is associated with increased risk of future stroke in the range of 3 to 5 per cent per year. Carotid aneurysms rarely rupture but present a risk of thrombosis or thromboembolism, causing a TIA or stroke. Fibromuscular disease, often associated with aneurysms, can cause neurologic symptoms by local dissection, although FMD of the carotid follows a relatively benign course in most patients.

Pathophysiology

The cellular function of the brain is exquisitely sensitive to blood pressure, blood glucose, and arterial oxygen and carbon dioxide tensions. The two anterior carotid arteries and posterior vertebral arteries provide excellent perfusion pressure and depend on the adequacy of collateral circulation via the circle of Willis. Disturbed mentation becomes clinically evident when the blood glucose level falls below 50 mg/dl. Hypoxemia, hypoglycemia, and hypotension can each cause dramatically acute suppression of mental acuity. Hypercarbia causes cerebrovascular dilation.

The pathophysiologic mechanism of transient or permanent cerebrovascular accidents can be either *thromboembolism* or *hypoperfusion.* Ulcerative plaques at the carotid bifurcation (Fig. 5) can release small particles of plaque and thrombus that pass to the brain and cause a TIA or stroke. Thrombotic occlusion of an extracranial artery can cause severe hypoperfusion and cerebral infarction. Other thromboembolic sources of TIA or stroke are the aortic arch and the heart. Cerebral symptoms due to fibromuscular disease may follow acute dissection and occlusion of the carotid artery. Such dissections usually extend to the base of the skull.

Clinical Diagnosis

A careful history is essential in establishing the likely cause of cerebrovascular symptoms and in selecting the initial therapy. A TIA is defined as an acute, focal neurologic deficit causing neurologic disability that lasts less than 24 hours and usually for only a few minutes. The neurologic deficit resolves completely. In contrast, a reversible ischemic neurologic deficit (RIND) is also a focal neurologic deficit that persists more than 24 hours but completely resolves in the next several days or weeks. A RIND implies a small area of severe ischemia or infarction. A stroke or cerebrovascular accident (CVA) is a focal neurologic deficit that presents abruptly and persists beyond 24 hours. The deficit may be permanent or slowly improve over a longer period of time. A *stroke-in-evolution* is defined as a progressing, and sometimes fluctuating, neurologic event. If the cause of the stroke-in-evolution can be clearly identified and corrected, the CVA is often prevented. TIAs, RINDs, or strokes may cause ocular or hemispheric symptoms.

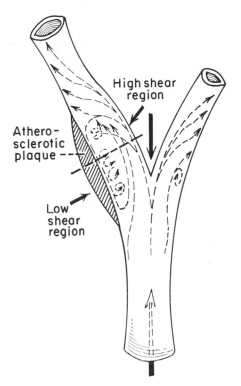

Figure 5. Carotid atherosclerotic plaques causing transient ischemic attacks and strokes occur commonly at the carotid bifurcation where the common carotid divides into the internal and external branches. (From Hallett JW Jr, Brewster DC, Darling RC: Patient Care in Vascular Surgery. Boston, Little, Brown & Co, 1987, with permission.)

Ipsilateral *monocular visual disturbances* are the most common ocular manifestation. Classically, the patient experiences transient monocular blindness described as a curtain or window shade being pulled over the eye and resolving after a few minutes (*amaurosis fugax* or *fleeting blindness*). Occasionally, a patient sustains sudden loss of vision that is usually due to retinal infarction and blindness may be permanent.

Hemispheric symptoms are usually characterized by a motor deficit involving weakness, clumsiness, or paralysis of an arm or leg. A sensory deficit of numbness is often involved. If the patient is right handed, the speech center is usually in the left brain and a left cerebral neurologic deficit may be accompanied by loss or disturbance in speech. In contrast to a TIA or stroke secondary to extracranial cerebrovascular disease, an infarction in the region of small perforating basilar arteries (*lacunar infarction*) is usually associated with hemiplegia *without* cortical signs or sensory signs. Disease of the vertebrobasilar arterial system can cause a myriad of symptoms including lightheadedness, vertigo, ataxia, bilateral visual symptoms, motor and sensory changes of one or both extremities, and drop attacks manifested by sudden loss of motor power in the lower extremities.

A thorough physical examination usually differentiates signs of extracranial cerebrovascular stenosis or occlusion and is essential in documenting baseline neurologic function. *Localized bruits* suggest stenotic lesions, which in the upper chest includes the innominate, proximal left carotid, or left subclavian arteries; in the supraclavicular area, the subclavian artery; and in the midanterior neck, the carotid artery. Decreased or absent pulses at the base of the neck should suggest proximal innominate, left carotid, or left subclavian stenoses or occlusion. An inequality of bilateral arm blood pressures of greater than 10 mm Hg suggests a hemodynamically significant stenosis on the lower side. A funduscopic examination after dilation of the pupils may reveal bright reflective cholesterol plaques termed *Hollenhorst plaques* that cause amaurosis fugax. A thorough baseline neurologic examination is also essential.

Certain features help to distinguish between carotid aneurysm, carotid kinking, and carotid body tumors. Aneurysms generally occur at the carotid bifurcation in the midanterior neck. In elderly hypertensive women, the proximal right carotid artery at the level of the clavicle may be prominent and mistaken for an aneurysm. Such a proximal right common carotid pulsation is usually due to tortuousity of the artery rather than aneurysmal disease. A carotid body tumor is generally palpated at the midanterior neck and is not pulsatile or expansile like an aneurysm. In fact, most carotid body tumors are relatively soft and are without an associated bruit.

Differential Diagnosis

Several intracranial cerebrovascular catastrophes can cause transient or permanent neurologic deficits, including hemorrhagic stroke of the brain, often associated with hypertension and frequently leading to deep coma and death. Subarachnoid hemorrhage from a ruptured berry aneurysm must be suspected in young, otherwise healthy patients who suddenly develop severe headache with rapid onset of a stiff neck or neurologic deterioration. A subdural hematoma causes a mass effect with sudden or insidious onset of increasing lethargy, throbbing headache, and ill-defined neurologic deficits. Such hematomas often occur in elderly patients who fall and injure the head. The evaluation of patients with ocular symptoms must include exclusion of such common conditions as glaucoma or retinal detachment.

Diagnostic Evaluation

The purpose of the diagnostic evaluation is to evaluate the extent of any brain damage and to define any focal lesion that may be amenable to operative correction. A CT or MRI of the brain can usually identify areas of infarction, intracranial hemorrhage, or subdural hematoma. The most common test to evaluate the presence of extracranial carotid stenosis is a duplex ultrasound of the carotids and vertebral arteries. The transesophageal two-dimensional echocardiography is necessary to image the aortic arch and the heart if these sites are suspected as possible sources for thromboemboli. Finally, the definitive test for extracranial cerebrovascular disease is an arteriogram.

Treatment

Anticoagulants or antiplatelet agents have been shown in some studies to reduce the incidence of stroke after TIAs. Initial anticoagulation with intravenous heparin followed by oral anticoagulants (warfarin) is recommended. Aspirin in relatively low doses from 85 to 325 mg daily may suffice to suppress platelet function while minimizing the inhibition of production of prostacyclin by the vascular endothelium. Other important components of medical therapy include treatment of hypertension, elimination of cigarette smoking, and control of hyperlipidemia.

Carotid endarterectomy is highly beneficial for patients with recent hemispheric TIAs or nondisabling strokes and ipsilateral high-grade (70 to 99 per cent) stenosis. The role of carotid endarterectomy for symptomatic patients with moderate stenosis (30 to 69 per cent) or asymptomatic carotid stenosis remains debatable. However, active patients in good health with high-grade (> 80 per cent) carotid stenosis may benefit from carotid endarterectomy. Contraindications to carotid endarterectomy include a recent completed stroke without recovery and internal carotid occlusion.

Symptomatic occlusive lesions of the proximal brachiocephalic arteries in the chest are usually amenable to bypass grafting. Occasionally, proximal vertebral artery stenoses causing debilitating vertebrobasilar symptoms require local endarterectomy or reimplantation of the vertebral artery into the side of the adjacent common carotid artery.

Postoperative Management

The most feared complication of cerebrovascular operations is a perioperative stroke, which should occur in less than 5 per cent of patients. Most postoperative neurologic deficits follow thromboemboli that occur during the operation or thrombosis at the operative site due to technical errors. Patients with an immediate postoperative neurologic deficit are usually returned to the operating room for inspection and correction of any operative site defects. Another common problem following carotid endarterectomy is hypertension requiring intravenous antihypertensives to prevent stroke, cerebral hemorrhage, or myocardial infarction. Myocardial infarction is one of the most common postoperative complications following carotid endarterectomy and is more likely to occur in patients with preexisting coronary heart disease and perioperative hypertension. Neck hematomas also occur more commonly in hypertensive patients. In addition, patients must be examined for signs of cranial nerve injury involving the hypoglossal, vagal, spinal accessory, glossopharyngeal, and superior laryngeal nerves.

Prognosis

Anticoagulation or operative revascularization reduces the occurrence of transient and permanent neurologic deficits by at least 50 per cent compared to untreated patients. For example, approximately 90 per cent of patients undergoing carotid endarterectomy for TIAs due to severe carotid stenosis have no further symptoms or stroke. Late survival is impaired most commonly by coronary events, which are more prevalent in those patients who continue to smoke, have diabetes mellitus, and do not control risk factors such as hypertension and hyperlipidemia.

ANEURYSMS

Although arterial aneurysms are not as prevalent as acute or chronic occlusive disease, the clinical catastrophe of rupture places them in the leading 15 causes of death. Clinical hallmarks include a pulsatile mass in the neck, extremity, or abdomen; sudden pain in the chest, back, or abdomen from a ruptured aneurysm; or shock associated with such pain.

Etiology and Natural History

Aneurysms can generally be classified as being degenerative, inflammatory, mechanical, traumatic, or congenital.

Degenerative Conditions

Atherosclerosis is associated in most patients of aortic or peripheral arterial aneurysms. Because there is a familial tendency in at least 20 per cent of patients with aortic aneurysms, genetic defects of collagen,

elastin, or proteolytic enzyme activity may also have a role. In addition, because aneurysm size is directly related to natural history, rupture risk for thoracic and abdominal aortic aneurysms appears to increase significantly when the aortic diameter exceeds 5 to 6 cm (Fig. 6). Likewise, thromboembolic complications of femoral and popliteal aneurysms occur in at least one third of patients whose aneurysms have exceeded 2 to 3 cm in size.

Less common degenerative causes of aneurysm disease include FMD and cystic medial necrosis. Fibromuscular dysplasia may cause multiple small aneurysms of the renal, mesenteric, or carotid arteries. In contrast, cystic medial necrosis is a common predisposing factor to dissecting aneurysms, especially in patients with hypertension or Marfan's syndrome. This syndrome is characterized by a tall, slender physique, long arms extending nearly to the knees, ocular lens ectopia, and joint and skin laxity. These patients develop aneurysms early in life and have a predilection for sudden death by complication of the aneurysm, such as rupture.

Inflammatory Conditions

Inflammation or infection may cause arterial aneurysms. Prior to the development of penicillin, syphilis was the most common cause of aortic aneurysms, particularly in the ascending aorta. Currently, the most common infected or mycotic aneurysms are the result of either gram-positive or gram-negative bacteremia. *Salmonella* species, *Escherichia coli*, and enterococcus are common examples of bacterial infections. Nonin-

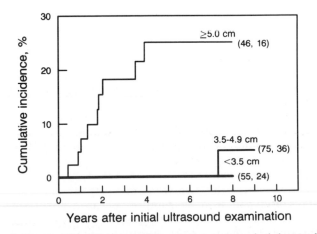

Figure 6. Cumulative incidence of rupture of abdominal aortic aneurysms according to aneurysm diameter at initial ultrasound. (From Nevitt MP, Ballard DJ, Hallett JW Jr: Prognosis of abdominal aortic aneurysms: A population-based study. N Engl J Med *321*:1011, 1989, with permission.)

fectious arteritis, such as giant cell arteritis or polyarteritis nodosa, may also be associated with aneurysmal development. Finally, some so-called inflammatory aneurysms are not associated with particular infectious organisms but appear to be more of an autoimmune response leading to a thick aneurysm wall. In general, infectious or inflammatory aneurysms require both appropriate medical therapy and surgical resection.

Mechanical Causes

This group includes posttraumatic false aneurysms, poststenotic aneurysms distal to a coarctation, and anastomotic false aneurysms associated with breakdown of a suture line with a graft.

Congenital Disorders

These include both the common cerebral berry aneurysm and aneurysms associated with inherited disorders such as Ehlers-Danlos or Marfan's syndromes. In Ehlers-Danlos syndrome, mutations in type III collagen have been identified and multiple areas of aneurysmal dilation are common. The genetic defect in Marfan's syndrome has been identified as diminished amounts of fibrillin, a large glycoprotein associated with the elastic microfibrils and a component of connective tissue.

Pathophysiology

Aneurysms can cause death by rupture, threaten limb viability by thrombosis or thromboembolism, and cause local compressive symptoms of regional nerves or adjacent veins. Although the diameter of the aneurysm is the most important determinant of rupture, the blood pressure and wall thickness are also contributory factors. Hypertension is perhaps the most important physiologic stress that can precipitate aneurysm leakage. Recent evidence also indicates that elevated levels of proteolytic enzymes such as elastase and collagenase are more common in smokers and in patients with ruptured aneurysms. Infectious processes clearly disrupt the structural integrity of aneurysm walls and can lead to rupture. Because aneurysms cause local turbulence, thrombus formation and thromboembolism are the eventual outcome in many peripheral femoral or popliteal aneurysms. Finally, large popliteal aneurysms can (1) compress the adjacent popliteal vein, causing deep venous thrombosis; and (2) cause neurologic symptoms due to tibial nerve pressure.

Clinical Diagnosis

Aneurysms may present in one of three ways: incidental discovery on physical examination, rupture, or thromboembolic events.

Asymptomatic Aneurysms

Many aneurysms are discovered incidentally on routine physical examination. They are also frequently recognized during ultrasounds, plain radiographs, CT or MRI scans, and arteriography for other conditions. During routine physical examination, the examiner should palpate the brachiocephalic, abdominal aorta, femoral, popliteal, and pedal arteries. An aneurysm should be suspected whenever these pulsations feel both enlarged and expansile. The normal abdominal aorta is approximately 2.5 cm in diameter and may be palpated just above or below the umbilicus. The femoral and popliteal arteries are generally less than 1 cm in size. If the popliteal pulse is extremely easy to palpate, a popliteal aneurysm should be suspected.

Rupture

Patients with a ruptured aneurysm generally present with a clinical triad of pain, hypotension, and a pulsatile mass. Rupture of a thoracic aneurysm usually presents with interscapular or low thoracic back pain, while abdominal aneurysms cause sudden severe lumbar back pain that is different than most other backaches previously experienced by the patient. Retroperitoneal hemorrhage may irritate local nerves, causing radiation of pain into the groin or testis. Rare causes of acute abdominal pain and vascular collapse include rupture of visceral artery aneurysms; namely, lesions of the hepatic, splenic, or mesenteric arteries. Rupture of splenic or renal artery aneurysms is more likely to occur in young women of childbearing age.

Thromboembolic Events

It must be emphasized that patients presenting with thromboembolic complications of a femoral or popliteal aneurysm have a 50 per cent chance of a contralateral lower-extremity aneurysm and a 30 to 50 per cent chance of a previously undiagnosed abdominal aortic aneurysm. If the patient presents with acute arterial ischemia of one leg and without a popliteal pulse, the presence of a large bounding popliteal artery in the contralateral lower extremity should raise suspicion of bilateral popliteal aneurysms. An abdominal aortic aneurysm containing loose atheromatous and thrombotic material may also occasionally present with bilateral blue toe syndrome. In the upper extremity, unilateral thromboembolic events to the hand in a younger individual should raise suspicion for a sub-clavian artery aneurysm secondary to thoracic outlet compression syndrome.

Differential Diagnosis

The primary differential diagnosis for a pulsatile mass of the neck, axilla, abdomen, or femoral regions is adjacent lymphadenopathy that transmits the pulse. Aneurysms are generally pulsatile *and* expansile, while adjacent lymphadenopathy is simply pulsatile. An enlarged popliteal mass may represent a Baker's cyst with transmitted pulsation. Severe chest pain and hypotension may be secondary to myocardial infarction or aortic dissection. Likewise, severe abdominal or lumbar back pain with hypotension may be secondary to spontaneous retroperitoneal hemorrhage, especially in patients on long-term anticoagulation, or abdominal apoplexy due to rupture of a smaller mesenteric vessel.

Diagnostic Evaluation

Several radiologic methods are available to confirm aneurysm diagnosis: plain radiographs, ultrasound, CT, MRI, and arteriography. An enlarged mediastinal aortic silhouette on chest radiograph is suspicious of an aneurysm. Likewise, 70 to 80 per cent of abdominal aneurysms have enough calcification in the wall to reveal an aneurysm on a plain abdominal film or on a lumbosacral spine series. Occasionally, an abdominal aortic aneurysm is recognized by calcification seen on an intravenous pyelogram.

Ultrasound is the simplest method to diagnose aneurysms of the neck, abdominal aorta, and femoro-popliteal arteries. Ultrasound permits detection and accurate measurement of intraluminal thrombus. *Computed tomography* is particularly useful for confirming aneurysms that involve the ascending, descending, and thoracoabdominal aorta. A CT scan also assists in differentiating other adjacent problems such as tumors and lymphadenopathy. In a patient with acute thoracic, back, or abdominal pain, a CT scan may also reveal leakage from the aneurysm or dissection of the aorta. *Magnetic resonance imaging* has many of the advantages of both ultrasound and CT scanning and is currently being used to supplement these more traditional forms of imaging. An *arteriogram* is not useful in determining the size of an aneurysm, as intraluminal thrombus may cause a relatively normal appearing lumen. However, arteriography is essential in planning operative intervention when one suspects arterial occlusive disease by physical examination.

Before elective operative intervention for an aneu-rysm, a general medical evaluation is essential, as these patients often have multiple chronic medical problems. In particular, attention should be given to detecting any significant carotid, coronary, or renal disease. At least one third of patients with aneurysms have clinically evident coronary heart disease manifest by angina pectoris, past myocardial infarction, or chronic congestive heart failure. A variety of noninvasive cardiac tests can assess myocardial perfusion (e.g., thallium scanning) and ventricular contractility (echocardiography) in an attempt to classify operative risk.

Treatment

There is no specific medical therapy for arterial aneurysms other than treatment of hypertension for patients who are being followed with small aneurysms or those who have extremely poor health and are not considered appropriate candidates for elective operation. Because small aortic aneurysms (< 5 cm in diameter) are rarely associated with rupture, periodic observation for expansion is appropriate. Approximately one third of small aneurysms eventually enlarge and require elective repair. Asymptomatic femoropopliteal aneurysms greater than 2.5 cm in diameter are associated with more thromboembolic complications and should be electively repaired. Any symptomatic aortic or peripheral aneurysm should be repaired urgently, including those that are painful, tender, or associated with thromboembolic events.

Aortic aneurysms are repaired with interposition prosthetic grafts of Dacron or polytetrafluoroethylene. Such materials are also used for repair of common iliac and femoral aneurysms. In contrast, saphenous vein is the preferable material for repair of popliteal aneurysms or aneurysms of the subclavian arteries. Currently, clinical investigations are underway to ascertain whether selected aortic aneurysms can be durably repaired by passage of collapsible synthetic grafts through femoral artery cutdown into the aorta where the graft can be expanded by inflatable balloons and secured by intravascular metallic stents. This method may eventually be useful in patients with significant aneurysms and serious medical problems.

Postoperative Management

The most common early postoperative complications of aneurysm repair include hemorrhage, graft thrombosis, distal thromboembolization, renal failure, and colon ischemia. For these reasons, patients are initially observed in an intensive care unit. The risk of renal failure has been substantially reduced by better hydration and selective use of pharmacologic agents such as low-dose dopamine and diuretics. Ischemia of the left colon may occur following ligation of the inferior mesenteric artery and exclusion of blood flow into the internal iliac arteries. Ischemia of the colon should be suspected if the patient develops bloody diarrhea in the early postoperative period. Flexible sigmoidoscopy should be performed immediately to ascertain the diagnosis. Milder degrees of colonic ischemia may be treated nonoperatively, but extensive mucosal gangrene requires colonic resection and colostomy.

One of the long-term complications of abdominal aortic aneurysm repair is disturbance of sexual function. Interruption of preaortic sympathetic fibers may cause a failure in ejaculation, although the patient may experience normal penile erection. The possibility of sexual dysfunction, including retrograde ejaculation, should be discussed with the patient preoperatively and again at the first postoperative examination.

Prognosis

The long-term results following aneurysm repair are generally excellent for graft patency. Approximately 5 to 10 per cent of patients who undergo repair of one aneurysm eventually require operation for another aneurysm at some other location in the arterial system. Consequently, long-term surveillance for other aneurysms is recommended and should include a periodic radiograph and abdominal and femoropopliteal ultrasounds. As the most common cause of late death is myocardial infarction, patients should be reminded to report any new angina pectoris or dyspnea on exertion.

AORTIC DISSECTION

Aortic dissection is the most common catastrophe involving the aorta and is associated with an alarmingly high mortality if undiagnosed and untreated. Clinical features include catastrophic tearing chest pain with a difference in upper extremity blood pressures (left arm less than right). The peripheral pulses are decreased, and a murmur of aortic insufficiency is often present.

Etiology and Natural History

An aortic dissection generally begins in the ascending or descending aorta when an *intimal tear* causes a destructive separation of the medial layer of the aorta. A hematoma can spread proximally or distally in the wall of the aorta. At another point from the original intimal tear, the pulsatile hematoma can reenter the true lumen of the aorta. Consequently, blood can be flowing both in the original *true* lumen of the aorta as well as in the dissected pathway, termed the *false lumen.*

Acute dissection occurs most frequently between the ages of 45 and 70, with a male predominance of 3:1. However, 50 per cent of dissections in women under the age of 40 occur during pregnancy. The incidence appears to be greater in patients with Marfan's syndrome or congenital cardiovascular diseases such as coarctation of the aorta and bicuspid aortic valve disease. In addition, dissection also commonly occurs in patients with aortic atherosclerosis. A history of hypertension is extremely common and is present in approximately 80 to 90 per cent of patients with aortic dissection.

The natural history of acute aortic dissection is astonishingly lethal. Early medical series that did not include operative intervention revealed that mortality for acute aortic dissection was 50 per cent at four days, 75 per cent at two weeks, and 90 per cent after 3 months. These dismal results have motivated a more intense investigation of the underlying pathophysiologic mechanisms and have led to a more aggressive approach to both medical and surgical intervention before lethal complications occur.

Pathophysiology

Despite the underlying disease associated with aortic dissection, the primary defect is *destruction of the medial layer* that contains the elastic fibers. Following an intimal tear, pulsatile blood dissects into the aortic media and proceeds for a varying depth and length along the aortic wall. The dissection can extend proximally or distally and can be associated with both obstruction of branches of the aorta or with penetration and rupture of the wall. Tears originating in the ascending aorta may proceed along the entire length of the aorta, whereas those that originate distal to the left subclavian artery dissect distally into the *descending thoracic aorta* and into the abdominal aorta (Fig. 7).

The biologic behavior of dissections depends to a large extent on whether the ascending aorta is involved. Ascending dissection may proceed retrograde to involve coronary arteries and pericardium and to rupture into the mediastinum, leading to death. Retrograde dissection to the coronaries and aortic valve frequently produce aortic insufficiency, a situation poorly tolerated and perhaps associated with cardiac failure and pulmonary edema. In contrast, descending dissections are more commonly complicated by arterial obstruction of circulation to the lower extremity or abdominal organs and occasionally by rupture into the pleural cavity. In general, acute dissection of the ascending aorta is considered to be more dangerous than that originating in the descending aorta.

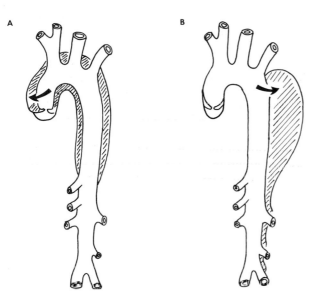

Figure 7. Basic types of aortic dissection. *A*, Dissection originating in ascending aorta. *B*, Dissection originating in descending aorta.

Clinical Diagnosis

Catastrophic tearing pain is the most frequent symptom of acute aortic dissection. The pain is usually located in the upper back, chest, or abdomen, although about one third of patients have some extremity pain. An acute central nervous system neurologic deficit is present in approximately 30 per cent. If the dissection has involved the ascending aorta and affected the aortic valve, dyspnea with associated pulmonary edema may be a chief complaint. Although many of these patients are chronically hypertensive, they may present with shock due to aortic regurgitation and cardiac tamponade from leakage into the pericardium. Chest examination may reveal a murmur of aortic insufficiency, diminished heart sounds, and pulmonary rales. If the dissection involves the left subclavian artery, the blood pressure may be lower in the left arm than in the right arm. Extensive involvement of the distal aorta may diminish lower extremity pulses.

Differential Diagnosis

Differential diagnosis in this group of patients includes myocardial infarction, rupture of the sinus of Valsalva, cerebrovascular accident, leaking thoracic aortic aneurysm, pulmonary embolism, acute surgical abdomen, arterial thrombosis or embolism of the aortic bifurcation, and thrombosis of a peripheral artery.

Diagnostic Evaluation

As severe chest pain is the most common presenting symptom, the primary problem is differentiating acute dissection from acute myocardial infarction or leaking thoracic aortic aneurysm. An electrocardiogram and cardiac enzymes should reveal an acute myocardial infarction. Over 90 per cent of patients with acute aortic dissection have an abnormal chest radiograph, including one or more of the following findings: a dilated aorta, a widened mediastinum with cardiomegaly, pulmonary edema, or a mass effect with or without pleural effusion. Classically, the definitive diagnosis has been made by *aortography*, which usually reveals passage of the contrast column into a true and false lumen and aortic insufficiency when the aortic valve is involved. The diagnosis can also be made by CT, MRI, and transesophageal echocardiography. The essential purpose of these tests is to ascertain whether the dissection involves the ascending aorta, as emergent surgical intervention is more likely in this group than in those where the dissection initially involves only the descending aorta.

Treatment

The initial goal of therapy for acute aortic dissection is to reduce both the mean and systolic arterial blood pressures. Intravenous nitroprusside or one of the newer intravenous β-blockers are the current drugs of choice because of their effectiveness in lowering blood pressure, ease of administration, and rapid control. β-Blockers also help smooth the peak pulse pressure by prolonging the change of pressure over time (dP/dt).

Nearly all patients with ascending aortic dissection are managed surgically with immediate operation in an attempt to avert sudden death from pericardial tamponade, rupture into the mediastinum, or acute aortic insufficiency with cardiac failure. The usual operative approach is a median sternotomy with cardiopulmonary bypass. The goal of operation is to correct the aortic insufficiency, either with aortic valve replacement or, more often, with resuspension of the aortic valve and to graft the ascending aorta, which directs the blood into the true lumen, with obliteration of the false lumen.

Controversy continues over whether acute dissections of the descending aorta should be treated surgically or medically. Indications for immediate operative intervention in this group include failure to control hypertension, continued pain, expansion of any aneurysm, signs or symptoms of rupture, development of a neurologic deficit, or evidence of compromise of major visceral vessels or arteries to the lower extremity. Generally, medical therapy for dissection of the descending aorta is initially chosen in patients in poor general condition.

Postoperative Management

Blood pressure control remains paramount following operation. Patients must also be monitored closely for any signs of progressive ischemia of the abdominal organs (kidneys and gut) or the lower extremities.

Prognosis

Current surgical mortality for patients with acute ascending aortic dissections is in the 5 to 10 per cent range, with long-term survival approaching 60 per cent. The most common cause of late death in patients who are treated medically is subsequent development and rupture of an aortic aneurysm, followed closely by myocardial infarction and stroke. These factors underscore the need for frequent follow-up with imaging studies of the aorta and support the recommendation for operation when the degree of thoracic aortic dilatation reaches 6 cm or when patients develop new symptoms related to recurrent dissection.

RENOVASCULAR DISEASE

Renovascular disease refers to both hypertension and/or renal insufficiency caused by significant stenosis or occlusion of one or both renal arteries. Renovascular hypertension should be suspected when a patient presents with one or both of the following findings: severe, uncontrollable hypertension of recent onset, and rapid progression of previously controlled hypertension. Hypertension in childhood or young adults is also a form of this disease, and a bruit in the hypogastrium or flank is often present. Progressive renal insufficiency follows in association with the hypertension.

Etiology and Natural History

More than 90 per cent of hypertensive patients have *essential hypertension*, defined as an elevation of blood pressure in the absence of an identifiable cause. The remaining 10 per cent may have a surgically correctable lesion. The most common cause of such *secondary hypertension* is renal artery stenosis or occlusion. Atherosclerosis is the most frequent cause of renal artery occlusive disease followed by fibromuscular dysplasia. Less common causes of surgically correctable hypertension include primary hyperaldosteronism, unilateral renal parenchymal disease,

coarctation of the aorta, pheochromocytoma, and Cushing's disease.

Hypertension is the most significant risk factor for the development of atherosclerotic coronary artery disease. Chronic hypertension increases risk of eventual heart failure, stroke, and renal failure. These complications clearly reduce survival compared to age- and gender-matched controls without hypertension.

Pathophysiology

Renovascular hypertension may be caused by (1) unilateral renal artery stenosis with a normal contralateral kidney, or (2) bilateral renal artery stenosis or parenchymal disease. In the case of unilateral renal artery stenosis and a normal contralateral kidney, the diseased kidney receives decreased blood flow, has decreased glomerular filtration, and releases an increased amount of renin from the juxtaglomerular cells of the kidney. Renin generates angiotensin I from the hepatically synthesized enzyme angiotensinogen. *Angiotensin converting enzyme* (ACE) converts angiotensin I to angiotensin II. Angiotensin II is a potent vasoconstricting agent and a secretagogue for aldosterone. Aldosterone leads to sodium retention and subsequent volume expansion. These physiologic effects of aldosterone in addition to the vasoconstrictive activity of angiotensin II potentiate the hypertension. Although renin output from the affected kidney may be high, the renin output from the contralateral kidney may be suppressed. Circulating peripheral renin may be normal or slightly below normal.

Clinical Diagnosis

Several clinical features should heighten suspicion that renovascular disease is causing hypertension or renal insufficiency. Essential hypertension is more prevalent in patients with a longer history of hypertension, in blacks, and in the obese. In contrast, atherosclerotic renovascular hypertension occurs more commonly in older adults and should be suspected whenever hypertension becomes more difficult to control, and it is associated with a rising serum creatinine with abdominal or flank bruits. Fibromuscular hypertension affects younger and middle-aged women and is also frequently accompanied by an abdominal or flank bruit.

Differential Diagnosis

The other causes of surgically correctable hypertension have distinctive clinical features (Table 1). Primary hyperaldosteronism is typically associated with severe hypokalemia. Unilateral parenchymal disease is

TABLE 1. SURGICALLY CORRECTABLE CAUSES OF HYPERTENSION

Renal artery stenosis/occlusion
Renal parenchymal disease
Primary hyperaldosteronism
Pheochromocytoma
Coarctation of the aorta
Cushing's disease

generally recognized by a shrunken kidney seen on intravenous pyelography or ultrasound. Coarctation of the aorta is classically associated with a thoracic bruit and diminished peripheral pulses. Pheochromocytoma presents with manifestations of catecholamine excess including headache, palpitation, diaphoresis, nervousness, and flushing. A myriad of clinical symptoms and signs should suggest Cushing's disease, but the most classic ones include moon facies, a "buffalo hump," truncal obesity, purple striae, and easy bruisability.

Diagnostic Evaluation

Initial laboratory studies include urinalysis, serum electrolytes, blood urea nitrogen, and creatinine. Traditionally, the test for renovascular disease was an intravenous pyelogram (IVP) showing delayed function in the affected kidney. However, the IVP suffers from a sensitivity of approximately 75 per cent and consequently may miss some patients with significant renal artery stenosis. Two *functional* tests for renovascular hypertension are the *captopril test* and *captopril renal scanning*. The captopril test involves oral administration of captopril, an ACE inhibitor, after baseline measurement of plasma renin activity and blood pressure. Renovascular hypertension should be suspected when the postcaptopril plasma renin is excessively high. Some studies indicate that the sensitivity of this test approaches 100 per cent with a specificity in the high 90 per cent range. However, the test is less accurate in the presence of renal failure. Criteria for a positive captopril renal scan include a reduction in glomerular filtration rate and a delay in the time to peak clearing of the radionuclide (e.g., iodohippurate sodium ^{131}I). Complementing these new functional tests are two diagnostic methods of imaging: *duplex Doppler ultrasonography* and *MRI*.

The definitive test for diagnosis of renal artery stenosis or occlusion is an arteriogram, which should be performed when the clinical hallmarks are present and no other cause of secondary hypertension can be identified. Classically, atherosclerotic renal artery stenosis is present at the orifice of the renal arteries and represents an extension of atherosclerotic plaque from the aorta into the renal artery. In contrast, fibromuscular disease tends to involve the mid to distal renal artery,

is described as having a "beaded" appearance, and may involve small branches of the renal artery, including the formation of small aneurysms.

Treatment

Although newer antihypertensive medications may control hypertension in most patients with renal artery stenosis or occlusion, decreased blood flow to the kidney eventually causes loss of parenchyma and progressive renal failure. Generally, high-grade renal artery stenosis or occlusion due to atherosclerosis is best treated by a bypass graft or removal of the plaque by endarterectomy. The most common type of bypass graft is a saphenous vein or synthetic graft from the aorta to the renal artery. In addition to aortorenal bypasses, other methods of renal revascularization currently include hepatorenal, splenorenal, and iliorenal bypasses. Occasionally, a focal atherosclerotic stenosis in the main renal artery can be successfully treated by transcutaneous balloon angioplasty. In contrast, fibromuscular lesions of the main renal artery are effectively treated in many patients by balloon angioplasty. Recent reports indicate that 80 to 90 per cent of patients treated by balloon angioplasty have improvement in hypertension. A small shrunken kidney (< 8 cm in length) associated with chronic renal artery occlusion and high renin output frequently requires nephrectomy to alleviate the hypertension.

Postoperative Management

Until the renin-angiotensin system equilibrates, perioperative hypertension remains the most common problem and generally requires intravenous nitroprusside or β-blockers. Acute renal failure can occur, especially in patients who had preoperative azotemia. Approximately 10 per cent of patients with a preoperative creatinine greater than 3 mg/dl require dialysis in the postoperative period. By the time of discharge, most patients require less antihypertensive medications than were used preoperatively and have improvement in their serum creatinine. One method to assess perfusion of a revascularized kidney is a postoperative renal scan.

Prognosis

Renovascular hypertension is improved in approximately 80 to 90 per cent of patients with a successful revascularization by either balloon angioplasty or operation. Renal function is improved or stabilized in approximately two thirds of patients with pretreatment renal insufficiency. Although patients may not be completely free of antihypertensive medications, at least 70 to 80 per cent take significantly fewer anti-hypertensive medications after successful treatment. Approximately 5 to 10 per cent of patients with atherosclerotic renovascular hypertension and renal insufficiency eventually progress to dialysis. Younger patients with fibromuscular renal artery disease have a 5-year survival similar to the normal population, while patients with atherosclerotic renovascular disease have an impaired 5-year survival in the range of 60 to 70 per cent.

MESENTERIC VASCULAR INSUFFICIENCY

Mesenteric circulatory insufficiency is a relatively uncommon acute or chronic vascular problem, but a highly lethal process when it occurs. Clinical manifestations of acute mesenteric ischemia should be suspected when patients, especially elderly adults, present with sudden, severe, unrelenting abdominal pain with relatively benign physical signs on abdominal examination compared to the severity of the pain. Chronic mesenteric vascular insufficiency is manifested by postprandial abdominal pain (intestinal angina), an epigastric bruit, and weight loss.

Etiology and Natural History

Four causes of acute mesenteric ischemia explain most cases: embolism from the heart, thrombosis of chronic mesenteric atherosclerotic stenoses, nonocclusive vasospastic obstruction, and mesenteric venous thrombosis. Atrial fibrillation is the usual cardiac condition leading to intestinal thromboembolism. Atherosclerotic disease of the mesenteric arteries involves the proximal vessels, is more common in females than males, and is frequently associated with other coronary and aortic atherosclerosis. Nonocclusive mesenteric ischemia is essentially a low-flow circulatory state associated with severely impaired cardiac function, cardiogenic shock, and occasionally vasoconstrictive effects of digitalis and other catecholamines used to support the failing heart. The clinical setting of nonocclusive mesenteric ischemia is often acute myocardial infarction or decompensated chronic heart failure. In contrast, mesenteric venous thrombosis is rare and usually associated with malignancy, chronic liver failure, congestive heart failure, or hypercoagulability.

The natural history of acute mesenteric ischemia from any etiology is bowel infarction and death, if untreated. Even with intervention, 50 to 75 per cent succumb because of delayed diagnosis, infarction of the intestine, and cardiorespiratory complications.

Chronic mesenteric ischemia is due primarily to atheroma of the proximal visceral arteries. Much less common causes are fibromuscular disease, collagen vascular disease, radiation-induced occlusive fibrosis, and extrinsic compression from neural or fibrous bands (celiac compression syndrome). The natural history of these patients is prolonged over months or several years but eventually may end suddenly with acute intestinal infarction.

Pathophysiology

Mesenteric blood flow originates from three main aortic branches: the celiac, superior mesenteric, and inferior mesenteric arteries (Fig. 8). Additional collateral flow is provided by the hemorrhoidal branches of the internal iliac arteries. Consequently, chronic mesenteric ischemia seldom manifests any symptoms unless at least two of these three primary mesenteric arteries are occluded. Food consumption precipitates intestinal angina in patients with mesenteric occlusive disease because digestion increases the demand for mesenteric blood flow by two or three times the baseline levels. Severe occlusive disease prevents this hyperemia, and resulting mucosal ischemia causes hypoxic pain. In contrast, an acute embolus tends to lodge in the more distal superior mesenteric artery and block collateral flow from the pancreaticoduodenal or middle colic collaterals. The affected region of bowel in such embolic cases includes the jejunum, ileum, and the right colon. Infarction usually ensues if adequate perfusion is not restored within 6 to 8 hours.

Clinical Diagnosis

Acute mesenteric ischemia classically presents with sudden severe midabdominal pain that is often accompanied by bowel evacuation (emesis or diarrhea). Initially, the severity of pain is classically out of proportion to relatively benign abdominal physical signs. However, the patient appears acutely distressed. An irregular pulse (atrial fibrillation) should heighten suspicion of a mesenteric thromboembolus. A chronic history of postprandial abdominal pain and weight loss suggests underlying atherosclerotic occlusive disease complicated by acute thrombosis. After several hours, the ischemic bowel may progress to perforation and peritonitis.

Chronic visceral insufficiency causes intestinal angina. This pain is characteristically postprandial, midabdominal, cramping or boring, and with onset 30 to 45 minutes after eating. This is the time period in which postprandial mesenteric blood flow begins to peak. The pain is repeatable with nearly every meal and severe enough that patients develop "food fear" and consequently lose weight. An epigastric bruit is

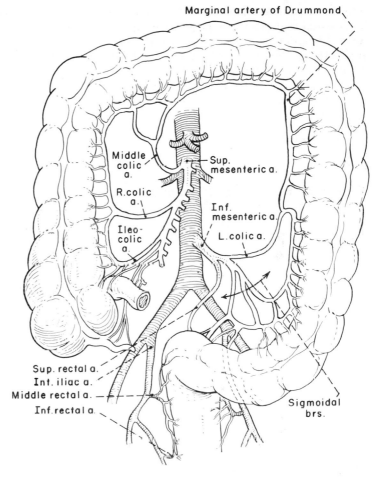

Figure 8. Normal mesenteric arterial circulation. (From Hallett JW Jr, Brewster DC, Darling RC: Patient Care in Vascular Surgery. Boston, Little, Brown & Co, 1987, with permission.)

often audible. Longstanding chronic mesenteric ischemia leads to extreme cachexia, and the patient may be thought mistakenly to have a malignancy.

Differential Diagnosis

The most common causes of acute abdominal pain must be excluded, including acute cholecystitis, a perforated peptic ulcer, appendicitis, and diverticulitis. Likewise, chronic intestinal pain and weight loss have numerous etiologies that must be considered (e.g., peptic ulcer disease, chronic cholecystitis, chronic pancreatitis, pancreatic cancer, chronic inflammatory bowel disease, and other gastrointestinal malignancies).

Diagnostic Tests

The definitive tests for acute mesenteric arterial occlusion is *arteriography*. As the mesenteric arteries originate from the anterior aorta, a lateral aortic view

is essential to visualize the proximal occlusions. Other nonspecific tests compatible with ischemic bowel are leukocytosis with a shift to the left, hyperamylasemia, metabolic acidosis, and other enzyme elevations (e.g., lactate dehydrogenase [LDH]). The usual evaluation for chronic abdominal pain includes upper and lower gastrointestinal tract series, hepatobiliary ultrasound, and abdominal CT scanning. Although duplex ultrasonography may reveal mesenteric artery stenosis or occlusion, an arteriogram is essential to confirmation of mesenteric artery occlusive disease before surgical intervention.

Treatment

Although immediate anticoagulation may prevent propagation of a mesenteric clot, the essential treatment for both acute and chronic mesenteric occlusive disease is *surgical revascularization*. Mesenteric emboli are removed by visceral arteriotomy and Fogarty balloon catheters. Any infarcted bowel is resected.

Chronic proximal atheromatous stenoses or occlusion are treated by aortomesenteric bypass grafts or trans-aortic thromboendarterectomy. Nonocclusive mesenteric artery ischemia with low flow and vasospasm is treated by optimizing cardiac output and intra-arterial vasodilators. Mesenteric venous thrombosis often necessitates segmental resection of the bowel.

Postoperative Management

Patients with acute mesenteric ischemia are generally continued on anticoagulation to prevent recurrent thrombosis. If the bowel has marginal viability at the initial operation, a "second-look" reoperation should be done within 12 to 24 hours to be certain that the remaining intestine is viable, with resection of any necrotic bowel.

Prognosis

Acute mesenteric ischemia has a high surgical mortality if infarction of the bowel has occurred and if the patient has severe underlying cardiovascular disease. Those who suffer arterial thromboembolism have a 10 to 15 per cent chance of recurrence. In contrast, surgical revascularization for chronic mesenteric ischemia relieves intestinal angina in 90 per cent of patients, with return to normal eating and weight. Recurrent mesenteric stenosis eventually affects 10 to 20 per cent, especially patients in whom only one of the mesenteric arteries was revascularized. Consequently, complete mesenteric artery revascularization is recommended for patients with chronic occlusive disease.

ARTERIAL TRAUMA

Arterial trauma includes arterial injuries due to both blunt and penetrating forces that lead to hemorrhage or thrombosis. Arterial injuries should be suspected with external bleeding, an expanding mass (pulsatile or nonpulsatile) adjacent to an injury, and signs of arterial occlusion in the affected extremity (pain, pallor, paresthesias, pulselessness, coolness, and paralysis). Hypotension often follows blunt or penetrating trauma, and a bruit is present in the vicinity of a penetrating injury. Nerve or venous injury may also be present.

Etiology and Natural History

Arterial trauma may follow penetrating trauma, blunt trauma, fracture or dislocation of bones and joints, or iatrogenic injury. *Penetrating* injuries are usually classified as low- or high-velocity trauma.

Low-velocity injuries include stab wounds and gunshot wounds from firearms with a muzzle velocity of less than 2000 feet per second. High-velocity missile injuries are frequently encountered with military weapons or firearms used for large-game hunting. High-velocity bullets cause extensive surrounding soft-tissue damage due to explosive cavitation. *Blunt* injuries are common in pedestrian motor vehicle accidents and following falls. *Fractures* or *dislocations*, particularly those in the area of the knee or elbow, may cause arterial injuries. *Iatrogenic* arterial injuries are currently increasing, often following arterial catheterization, invasive monitoring, thrombolytic therapy, and various types of percutaneous angioplasty.

Pathophysiology

Penetrating injuries may partially or completely transect an artery. Incomplete arterial disruption or laceration may cause considerable hemorrhage, because the vessel is unable to retract and seal as it would with complete transection. Arterial contusion may cause intimal and medial disruption with local thrombosis, which may not initially cause thrombosis, but eventually causes a local false aneurysm that may eventually rupture. A penetrating injury affecting an artery and its adjacent vein may eventually lead to a traumatic arteriovenous fistula. If such a fistula is not recognized immediately, it may become chronic and eventually cause high-output cardiac failure. Bullets may also enter vessels and embolize to distal sites. In general, traumatic arterial thrombosis must be corrected within 6 to 8 hours to avoid serious organ or extremity ischemia.

Clinical Diagnosis

A stab or gunshot wound in any region of the body must initiate the search for an arterial or venous injury. Deceleration injuries from automobile accidents are commonly associated with disruption of the thoracic aorta just beyond the left subclavian artery. Fractures of the arm, elbow, femur, or knee frequently cause arterial damage with thrombosis.

Hypotension is evidence that significant blood loss has occurred. Trauma victims should be completely uncovered and inspected on the front and back of the body for entrance and exit sites when penetrating trauma is suspected. Overt bleeding from penetrating wounds can usually be controlled by point pressure while the remaining examination is completed. An expanding hematoma or a wound in proximity to a neurovascular bundle always suggests the possibility of arterial trauma. Absence of peripheral pulses indicates that thrombosis may have occurred. A continuous bruit is pathognomonic of an arteriovenous fistula. Deformity of an extremity is indicative of a fracture and suggestive of an arterial injury if a large expanding hematoma is present or distal pulses are absent.

Diagnostic Evaluation

When a localized penetrating injury is associated with hemorrhage, an expanding hematoma, or absence of distal pulses, no specific diagnostic tests are necessary, and the patient needs an expeditious surgical exploration. If a hematoma is present at a site of injury, duplex ultrasound can ascertain whether a false aneurysm or arterial venous fistula is present. Arteriography is generally recommended for patients who are at high risk of arterial injury, including those with bilateral first rib resections (subclavian artery), deceleration chest injuries with sternal and rib fractures (torn thoracic aorta), and fracture dislocations of the knee (popliteal artery). If the penetrating injury is not associated with ongoing hemorrhage or expanding hematoma and is accompanied by a normal duplex ultrasound at the site of injury, the patient can generally be observed unless distal pulses subsequently disappear.

Treatment

The initial management of arterial trauma includes general principles of trauma resuscitation, including the "ABCs" (airway, breathing, circulation) (Fig. 9). External bleeding is best controlled by direct pressure from focal finger-tip compression. Intravenous lines are inserted, crystalloid solutions are infused, and blood should be typed and crossmatched. Fractures should be splinted, and dislocations should be reduced as soon as possible. Tetanus prophylaxis and intravenous antibiotics should be administered. Appropriate radiographs in search of fractures should be ordered, and ultrasound or arteriography should be considered.

Although the exact operative approach varies with the specific site of injury, certain principles apply to the management of all arterial injuries. These include a wide operative field, with an uninvolved lower extremity for ready access to a saphenous vein, the best arterial substitute for all but the largest injured arteries. Second, proximal control of the affected artery should be gained before entering large hematomas. Third, damaged arteries should be resected. The distal circulation should be checked for accumulation of thrombus. In general, 1 to 2 cm of artery may be resected and reconstituted by a primary anastomosis. Larger areas of injury require a graft. Finally, all de-

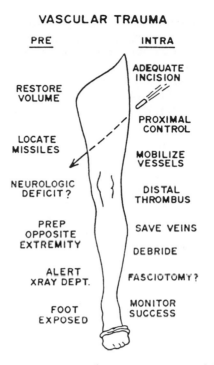

Figure 9. Important considerations prior to and during the operative management of a vascular injury to the lower limb. (From Freeark RJ, Baker WH, Klosak JJ: Arterial injuries. *In* Sabiston DC Jr [ed]: Textbook of Surgery: The Biological Basis of Modern Surgical Practice, ed 14. Philadelphia, WB Saunders Company, 1991, p 1618, with permission.)

vitalized tissue in the area of the injury should be débrided, and if ischemia has been prolonged, a fasciotomy of the distal extremity may be necessary.

Postoperative Management

As many patients with arterial trauma have other injuries, special surveillance is necessary. Peripheral pulses should be monitored frequently for any sign of thrombosis. If fasciotomy has not been performed at the initial operation, the extremity should be monitored carefully for signs of compartment pressure syndrome, including pain, swelling, and tenderness of the distal muscle compartments of the affected limb. If such signs appear, fasciotomies should be performed immediately.

Prognosis

As most patients with arterial trauma are young and otherwise healthy, they usually make a good recovery. Exceptions include patients with prolonged ischemia and those in whom peripheral nerves have been severed. Such patients often have impaired neurologic function and may progress to a syndrome of burning pain in the affected limb, known as *causalgia*.

CIRCULATORY CONDITIONS OF THE UPPER EXTREMITY

In the spectrum of peripheral vascular diseases, arterial problems in the upper extremity, including vasospastic disorders, are relatively uncommon. Clinical manifestations of significant upper extremity ischemia include sudden pain, pallor, paresthesias, pulselessness, and paralysis of the upper extremity; mottled bluish, painful fingertips (microemboli); arm tiring with vigorous exercise ("claudication"); and episodic attacks of pallor, cyanosis, and redness (Raynaud's syndrome).

Etiology and Natural History

The underlying causes of arm ischemia and vasospastic disorders are diverse (Fig. 10). For simplicity, they may be organized into broad groups of emboli, occlusive disease, aneurysms, trauma, and small-vessel vasospastic or arterial occlusive disease. Emboli generally arise from the heart and occasionally from a subclavian aneurysm, which often may be associated with thoracic outlet compression syndromes at the level of the first rib. Although atherosclerotic disease occasionally affects the upper extremity, it is much rarer than atherosclerosis of the lower limbs. Atherosclerotic aneurysms of the subclavian artery are relatively uncommon, and axillary aneurysms are occasionally seen in patients that have used crutches for

many years. The most common form of arterial trauma to the upper extremity is brachial artery injury during cardiac catheterization. Raynaud's syndrome may be either a relatively benign bilateral vasospastic disorder seen in females or a more severe manifestation of collagen vascular diseases.

The natural history of acute or chronic arterial ischemia of the upper extremity is similar to that of the lower limb. Acute occlusion must be treated within 6 to 8 hours to prevent severe limb disability or loss. Poststenotic aneurysms with thoracic outlet syndrome can lead to repetitive thromboemboli to the hand and insidious or sudden loss of hand function. Brachial artery thrombosis following cardiac catheterization may be relatively asymptomatic because excellent collaterals are present around the elbow. However, forearm claudication may occur later if the brachial artery occlusion is not corrected. Raynaud's syndrome, which is not associated with collagen vascular disease, generally follows a relatively benign chronic course. In contrast, Raynaud's syndrome associated with collagen vascular disease is usually associated with occlusion of the small vessels in the hand with nonhealing sores or gangrene.

Pathophysiology

The pathophysiology of acute or chronic arterial occlusive disease of the upper extremity is similar to those conditions already discussed for the lower limb. The pathophysiology of Raynaud's syndrome remains unknown despite more than a century of investigation. Alterations in the sympathetic nervous system, adrenoceptor number and function, and an imbalance in naturally occurring vasoactive peptides such as en-

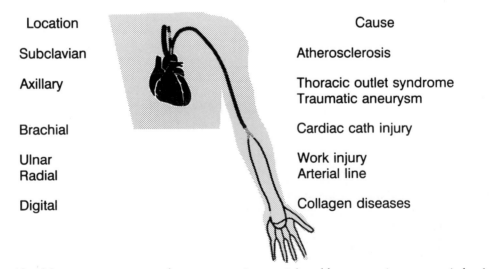

Figure 10. Most common causes of upper extremity arterial problems at various anatomic levels.

dothelin and calcitonin gene-related peptide have been implicated.

Clinical Diagnosis

Patients who present with sudden upper-extremity pain, pallor, and paresthesias may have acute arterial occlusion, which is manifest by loss of pulses and paralysis of motor function. Atrial fibrillation, chronic cardiomyopathy, or a recent myocardial infarction should raise suspicion that this acute occlusion is embolic.

A proximal left subclavian stenosis is a common atherosclerotic lesion and may be associated with exercise-induced heaviness and fatigue of the left upper extremity. An inequality in arm blood pressures (left less than right) should heighten suspicion of a proximal subclavian stenosis or occlusion. If a younger patient complains of arm fatigue and paresthesias of the fourth and fifth finger with elevated exercise, *thoracic outlet compression syndrome* should be suspected. Loss of the radial pulse and a supraclavicular bruit with elevation and abduction of the arm may be present as well as a subclavian aneurysm or a cervical rib.

Patients with Raynaud's syndrome may have relatively normal appearing hands, but exposure to cold or emotional stress may precipitate the triphasic color changes of pallor, cyanosis, and rubor. Benign Raynaud's syndrome is usually bilateral, occurs predominantly in young women, and is not associated with ulceration or gangrene of the fingertips.

Diagnostic Evaluation

Patients who present with acute severe embolic arterial ischemia are generally candidates for immediate thromboembolectomy. If the level of occlusion is unclear and the limb is not severely ischemic, an arteriogram may be helpful. It is also useful for patients who present with chronic arm claudication, nonhealing sores of the hand, or signs of microemboli. Baseline Doppler signal analysis of the brachial, radial, ulnar, and digital arteries, including plethysmographic waveforms, should also be done. Because Raynaud's syndrome may be associated with a collagen vascular disease, serum chemistries, including antinuclear antibodies, rheumatoid factor, and other appropriate tests, should be performed. The most common collagen vascular disease associated with Raynaud's syndrome is *scleroderma*, and approximately 20 per cent of these patients initially present with Raynaud's syndrome. Eventually, 80 per cent of patients with scleroderma have severe Raynaud's syndrome of the hand.

Treatment

Acute arterial ischemia due to emboli necessitates emergent Fogarty thromboembolectomy. Arterial complications of the subclavian artery associated with thoracic outlet compression syndrome necessitates surgical resection of the aneurysm with a vein interposition graft and resection of bony abnormalities including cervical ribs if present and, often, the first rib. Proximal atherosclerotic subclavian occlusive disease generally requires a carotid-to-subclavian artery bypass or reimplantation of the subclavian artery into the side of the common carotid artery. Acute injury of the brachial artery by a catheter should be repaired under local anesthesia. Bypass grafts for proximal occlusive or aneurysmal lesions of the subclavian and axillary arteries have excellent long-term patency.

Benign Raynaud's syndrome is generally treated by avoidance of exposure to the cold, cessation of tobacco use, and warm protection of the hands. Occasionally, patients benefit from vasodilation, usually achieved by a vasodilator such as a calcium channel blocker. Patients incapacitated by Raynaud's syndrome with necrosis of fingertips from collagen vascular disease are difficult to treat, and therapy includes antibiotics, local débridement, and analgesics for nonhealing ulcers or gangrene. Although sympathectomy has been used for severe cases, its role is limited and it is generally not recommended.

Prognosis

The prognosis for acute or chronic occlusive disease of the upper extremity is excellent if therapy is undertaken before acute ischemia has been prolonged and before small vessels of the hand have been filled by recurrent thromboemboli. Females with benign Raynaud's syndrome generally have a chronic but not debilitating course. In contrast, patients with collagen vascular disease and Raynaud's syndrome often suffer severe pain and debilitation of the hands, frequently complicated by tissue loss.

REFERENCES

Gewertz BL, Graham A, Lawrence PF, Provan J, Zarins CK: Diseases of the vascular system. *In* Lawrence PF (ed): Essentials of General Surgery, ed 2. Baltimore, Williams & Wilkins, 1992, pp 328–347.
Hallett JW Jr, Brewster DC, Darling RC: Patient Care in Vascular Surgery, ed 2. Boston, Little, Brown & Co, 1987.
Rutherford RB (ed): Vascular Surgery, ed 3. Philadelphia, WB Saunders Company, 1989.
Sabiston DC Jr: Disorders of the arterial system. *In* Sabiston DC Jr (ed): Textbook of Surgery: The Biological Basis of Modern Surgical Practice, ed 14. Philadelphia, WB Saunders Company, 1991, pp 1523–1664.

48

DISORDERS OF THE LUNG, PLEURA, AND CHEST WALL

I

Pulmonary Function

PETER K. SMITH, M.D.

Respiratory function is significantly altered by the performance of nearly all major surgical procedures. In the presence of preexisting pulmonary disease, these alterations may lead to increased morbidity, respiratory failure, and even death. Mortality is rare with modern anesthetic techniques and postoperative care because of an improved understanding of the basic function of the respiratory system.

CLINICAL EVALUATION OF PULMONARY FUNCTION

The initial evaluation of the preoperative patient includes a complete history and physical examination. Disorders that place the patient at high risk include emphysema, bronchitis, asthma, and allergy. Exposure to environmental pollution, particularly cigarette smoking, should be documented. A history of dyspnea or shortness of breath, particularly with minimal exercise, should alert the physician to potential respiratory failure in the patient who has not yet been categorized by a physician. An insidious reduction of physical activity can mask respiratory dysfunction, and a history of such changes in lifestyle should be actively sought. The chronic production of sputum and any recent change in its degree or character mandate active evaluation. Peripheral or central cyanosis, a rapid respiratory pattern with the use of the accessory muscles of respiration, and the general demeanor of the patient can be revealing. The localized diminution of breath sounds, their character, and the presence of localized or generalized wheezing may indicate potentially reversible causes of respiratory dysfunction. A chest film completes the routine preoperative evaluation. If conditions permit, the pursuit of more detailed information is usually obtained in patients with evidence of significant pulmonary disease or in patients undergoing thoracic or major upper abdominal procedures.

PULMONARY FUNCTION TESTING

Spirometric evaluation allows the estimation of the overall ability to ventilate. These tests are simple to obtain, but they must be carefully interpreted because there are wide variations in the normal population. The results obtained are highly dependent on patient understanding and cooperation.

Static Mechanics

The spirometric measurements of lung volumes and capacities are obtained initially. These subdivisions of the total lung capacity (TLC, liters) are illustrated in Figure 1. The TLC is divided into four lung volumes:

Tidal volume (TV, L). The volume of air inspired during a quiet normal respiration, begun at the end of a normal expiration from the end-tidal point (ETP).

Inspiratory reserve volume (IRV, L). The lung volume between the peak tidal point and the maximal inspiratory point.

Expiratory reserve volume (ERV, L). The lung volume between the ETP and the maximal inspiratory point.

1. Total lung capacity (TLC)
2. Vital capacity (VC)
3. Inspiratory capacity (IC)
4. Functional residual capacity (FRC).

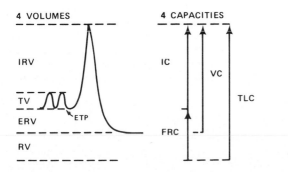

Figure 1. Four volumes and four capacities that subdivide the total lung capacity. For abbreviations and definitions, see text. (From Tisi GM: Pulmonary Physiology in Clinical Medicine, ed 2. Baltimore, Williams & Wilkins, 1983, with permission.)

Residual volume (RV, L). The volume of air remaining in the lung at the maximal expiratory point.

Four lung capacities are defined by spirometry:

Total Lung Capacity (TLC, L). The amount of air in the lungs following maximal inspiration.

Vital Capacity (VC, L). The amount of air that can be expired following a maximal inspiration.

Inspiratory Capacity (IC, L). The amount of air expired from the point of maximal inspiration to the ETP.

Functional Residual Capacity (FRC, L). The amount of air within the lungs at the ETP.

It is apparent that RV is the only volume that cannot be determined from the spirometric tracing. Without a value for RV, TLC and FRC cannot be determined. In practice, RV can be determined by body plethysmography or by gas dilution techniques. Tidal volume and vital capacity can be determined quickly at the bedside with a minimum of equipment and used to follow the progress of therapy perioperatively.

Dynamic Mechanics

The measurement of the ability to move air, through dynamic testing, has proved to be more sensitive in the prediction of postoperative pulmonary dysfunction. Airway obstruction, a primary component of most lung diseases, is measured by recording air flow over time during spirometric testing.

Forced vital capacity (FVC, L). The volume of air that can be forcibly expired with maximal expiratory effort.

Forced expiratory volume—1 second (FEV$_1$, L). The amount of air that can be forcibly expired in first second of the FVC.

Maximal voluntary ventilation (MVV, L). The amount of air that can be breathed in 1 minute during maximal effort, calculated from 15 seconds of actual ventilation.

FEV$_1$/VFC%. The fraction of the FVC maximally expired in 1 second. Other values obtained include the maximal midexpiratory flow rate or the forced expiratory flow rate from 200 ml to 1200 ml below TLC (FEF 200 to 1200), which is less dependent on patient effort.

Arterial Blood Gas

The measurement of the partial pressure of oxygen (PaO$_2$) and carbon dioxide (PaCO$_2$) in arterial blood, as well as the pH, has become an integral part of the evaluation of the pulmonary patient. These values provide direct measures of the patient's ability to support oxidative metabolism. Oxygen combines reversibly with hemoglobin according to the oxyhemoglobin dissociation curve (Fig. 2). The unusual shape of the curve allows the oxygen content of the blood to remain high over a wide range of PaO_2, a range usually easily achieved. Additionally, the steep slope of the curve allows rapid release of oxygen in the tissues at a PaO_2 compatible with oxidative metabolism. Another feature of the curve is the rapid decline in PaO_2 that occurs when the oxygen content is lowered from full saturation. The mixture of desaturated blood with saturated blood, as occurs with a central right to left shunt, results in a stoichiometric alteration of oxygen content. The change in PaO_2 is much more dramatic, following the relatively flat portion of the dissociation curve. The $PaCO_2$ is a direct measure of alveolar ventilation. The normal range is 38 to 42 mm Hg, with values greater than 46 mm Hg indicating significant pulmonary insufficiency.

The arterial pH normally ranges from 7.37 to 7.43, and the pH is maintained by the complex interactions of the blood buffer system, renal compensation, and ventilatory compensation. Acute deviations may be due to hyperventilation, causing a respiratory alkalosis (low $PaCO_2$ and high pH). This is a common clinical finding, caused by the anxiety of arterial puncture. Acidosis that is partially compensated for by hyperventilation (low $PaCO_2$) usually indicates a metabolic abnormality or, more ominously, tissue hypoperfusion. Acidosis accompanied by an elevated $PaCO_2$, perhaps partially compensated by renal retention of bicarbonate, is found in severe respiratory insufficiency.

DISTRIBUTION OF VENTILATION AND PERFUSION

Spirometric evaluation allows the estimation of the overall ability of a patient to ventilate. Of equal importance is the appropriate regional delivery to the inspired gases, coupled with a matching of regional perfusion to ventilation. The distribution of ventilation is determined by many factors. The production of surfactant by terminal airways is important in maintaining small airway and alveolar expansion. Localized infections or secretions, as well as diffuse damage by chronic lung disease, can overwhelm this defense

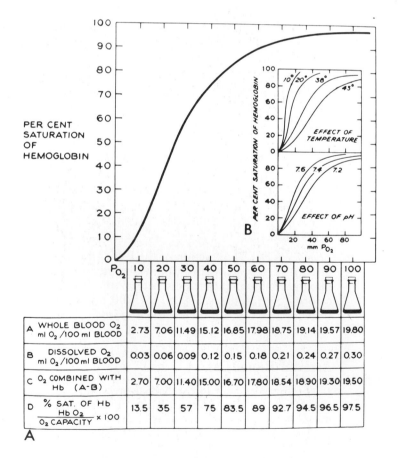

Figure 2. Hemoglobin dissociation curve for hemoglobin. A, The pH is 7.40 at 37°C. B, Effect of changing temperature and pH on the dissociation curve. *Abbreviations*: Hb = Hemoglobin, HbO_2 = oxyhemoglobin. (Data of Severinghaus JW: J Appl Physiol *21*:1108, 1966. From Comroe JH Jr: Physiology of Respiration, ed 2. Chicago, Year Book Medical Publishers, 1974, with permission.)

mechanism and cause regional airway collapse at the lobar, segmental, or even respiratory bronchiole level. Perfusion of nonventilated units leads to venous admixture, which can be viewed as the contamination of arterial blood with venous blood. Ventilation of nonperfused units is wasted ventilation, termed the *physiologic dead space*.

Ventilation

The interaction of the lung and chest wall generates negative intrapleural pressure during all phases of respiration with the exception of forced expiration. The pleural pressure so created varies from -10 cm H_2O at the apex to -2.5 cm H_2O at the base, on average in the upright human. This gradient in pleural pressure depends on the recoil of both chest wall and lung, the phase of respiration, and body position. The intraalveolar pressure is zero with the glottis open, and thus alveolar radius is related to the transmural (pleura–intra-alveolar) alveolar pressure and alveolar compliance. The pleural pressure gradient, therefore, creates a gradient in alveolar size (given uniform alveolar compliance) wherein apical alveoli are larger than basal alveoli. The effect of regional differences in alveolar (and by the same physical principles, airway) size is twofold. The low transmural basal pressure can result in alveolar and airway collapse, and the high apical transmural pressure places the alveoli near the limits of expansion. Studies using radioactive xenon gas have shown that both situations may occur in patients, as illustrated in Figure 3. The volume of the lung at which basilar alveolar and airway closure occurs is termed the *closing volume*. The relations of this volume to the FRC and age are illustrated in Figure 4.

Perfusion

The distribution of perfusion is largely affected by gravitational influences. The systolic pulmonary artery pressure rarely exceeds 30 mm Hg in healthy individuals, which can be insufficient to raise the fluid column (blood) to the apex of the upright lung. Three zones of regional blood flow have been described by West. In the upright individual, *Zone 1* resides in the apex of the lung. Alveolar pressure is greater than both pulmonary artery pressure and pulmonary venous pressure. The alveolar pressure is directly transmitted to the pulmonary capillary resistance vessels, closing them and preventing perfusion altogether. Thus, Zone 1 is ventilated but not perfused, and constitutes a physiologic dead space. *Zone 2*, in the midlung, occurs when the pulmonary artery pressure exceeds alveolar pressure, which exceeds pulmonary venous pressure.

The capillaries behave like flutter valves (Starling resistors), and flow is intermittent throughout the respiratory cycle. Pulmonary venous pressure has no effect on blood flow in this zone, the "vascular waterfall." In *Zone 3*, the lung base, both pulmonary arterial and venous pressures exceed alveolar pressure, and flow thus occurs throughout the respiratory cycle. The magnitude of flow is dependent on the pressure difference between pulmonary artery and pulmonary vein and on the inherent resistance of the pulmonary capillaries modified by the distending pressure of the intraluminal blood. Regional flow is also controlled by the hypoxic vasoconstrictor reflex, which can reduce blood flow to nonventilated lung regions.

REGIONAL MATCHING OF VENTILATION AND PERFUSION

It is apparent that the physical forces controlling regional ventilation and perfusion interact only in the broadest sense and are not generally self-corrective. Pleural pressure changes that would influence ventilation would not necessarily cause a corresponding change in perfusion. Likewise, diminution of pulmonary artery pressure increases the total Zone 1 volume but would not diminish wasted ventilation by the same mechanism. The hypoxic pulmonary vasoconstrictive response is physiologic and compensating, but it is not powerful enough to eliminate the adverse effects of ventilation-perfusion mismatch. In the normal lung, ventilation and perfusion are closely matched, with the preponderance of both ventilation and perfusion distributed to the bases. Commensurate diminution of both ventilation and perfusion occurs in the midlung and apex. Basilar hypoventilation caused by changes in FRC or an elevated closing volume can cause a severe ventilation-perfusion abnormality. The consequences of this abnormality can be striking and are reflected in arterial oxygenation as well as in carbon dioxide content. Ideal matching of ventilation and perfusion permits normal oxygen uptake and carbon dioxide elimination (Fig. 5, Panel I).

Oxygenation

If matching of ventilation and perfusion were ideal, the PaO_2 would be equal to the partial alveolar pressure of oxygen (PAO_2). While one is breathing 100 per cent oxygen, this can be calculated as follows:

$$PAO_2 = PB - (PACO_2 + PH_2O)$$

where PB = barometric pressure, PH_2O = water vapor pressure (corrected for temperature), and $PACO_2$ = alveolar partial pressure of carbon dioxide (in practice, approximately equal to $PaCO_2$). The degree to which

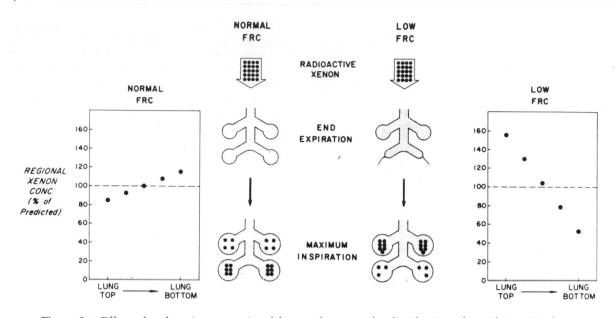

Figure 3. Effect of end-expiratory regional lung volume on the distribution of ventilation. Radioactive xenon was injected at the beginning of inspiration and measured with external counters. An inspiration from normal functional residual capacity (FRC) is distributed preferentially to the lung bottom, as the dependent alveoli are at minimal radius and capable of full expansion while apical alveoli are nearer full expansion. An inspiration from low FRC, where dependent air space is collapsed, results in a reversal of distribution, with the majority of ventilation occurring at the apex. (From Pontoppidan H, Laver MB, Geffin B: Acute respiratory failure in the surgical patient. Adv Surg 4:163, 1970, with permission. Redrawn from data of Milic-Emili J, et al: J Appl Physiol *21*:749, 1966.)

there is a difference between P_{AO_2} and Pa_{O_2} (termed the $P[A-aD_{O_2}]$) reflects the contamination of pulmonary venous blood with mixed venous blood, the result of perfusion of underventilated alveoli (Fig. 5, Panel II). This can be estimated while one is breathing 100 per cent oxygen, allowing easy calculation of P_{AO_2}. The actual magnitude of such mixed venous shunt flow can be calculated.

The product of the cardiac output (QT) and the arterial oxygen content (Ca_{O_2}) yields the amount of oxygen carried in the blood per unit of time. This blood can be viewed as a mixture of blood "shunted" through nonventilated alveoli (QS) and blood ideally perfused through ventilated alveoli (QC). The amount of oxygen carried in each is equal to the product of QS and the oxygen content of mixed venous blood (Cv_{O_2}) and the product of QC and the oxygen content of pulmonary end-capillary blood (Cc_{O_2}).

It follows that:

$$QT*Ca_{O_2} = (QC*Cc_{O_2}) + (QS + Cv_{O_2})$$

and that QT= QC + QS

Solving these two questions yields the "shunt equation," which reflects the fraction of pulmonary flow that is "shunted" past nonventilated alveoli:

$$QS/QT = (Cc_{O_2} - Ca_{O_2})/(Cc_{O_2} - Cv_{O_2})$$

Cc_{O_2} can be calculated from nomograms describing the saturation of hemoglobin at the arterial pH and temperature of the patient, with 100 per cent saturation assumed. Similarly, Ca_{O_2} is calculated from the measured Pa_{O_2} and the hemoglobin content, and Cv_{O_2} from the measured partial pressure of oxygen in mixed venous blood.

Carbon Dioxide

The Pa_{CO_2} is directly related to the magnitude of alveolar ventilation and the rate of carbon dioxide production by oxidative metabolism. The latter is relatively constant, although postoperative shivering may cause a significant increase in Pa_{CO_2}. Ventilation of nonperfused air space causes wasted ventilation, and unless compensated for by increased tidal volume or increased respiratory rate, the Pa_{CO_2} will rise. The two sources of this "dead space" are anatomic and "physiologic." The *anatomic dead space* is that portion of the upper airway that serves to transport respired air and has no intimate contact with the pulmonary capillaries. It is usually fixed in absolute volume (approx-

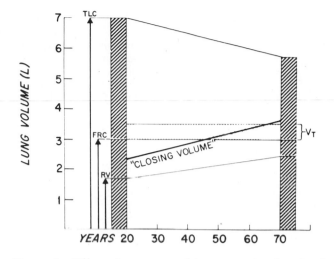

Figure 4. Effect of age on total lung capacity, functional residual capacity (FRC), residual volume, and closing volume. Values are for the normal, supine adult. In the fifth decade, closing volume exceeds the FRC during tidal ventilation, implying airway closure. The resulting ventilation-perfusion abnormality accounts for the hypoxemia seen with increasing age. A decrease in FRC, as seen with surgical incisions, anesthesia, and obesity, would have the effect of moving the tidal volume into the closing volume at a younger age and during a larger proportion of the tidal volume. The resulting ventilation-perfusion abnormality accounts for the hypoxemia seen with age and following surgical procedures. (From Lumb PD: Perioperative pulmonary physiology. *In* Sabiston DC Jr, Spencer FC [eds]: Gibbon's Surgery of the Chest, ed. 4. Philadelphia, WB Saunders Company, 1983. Modified from Pontoppidan H, et al: Acute Respiratory Failure in the Adult. Boston, Little, Brown & Co, 1973, using original data from Bates DV, et al: Respiratory Function in Disease. An Introduction to the Integrated Study of the Lung, ed 2. Philadelphia, WB Saunders Company, 1971; Sorbine et al: Respiration 25:3, 1968 and Leblanc et al: J Appl Physiol 28:448, 1970, with permission.)

imately equal in milliliters to the body weight in pounds) and is usually about one third of the tidal volume. The *physiologic dead space* is that portion of the lung where there is overventilation relative to perfusion. As physiologic dead space increases, minute ventilation must increase to compensate for what can be viewed as an encroachment on the tidal volume (Fig. 5, Panel III).

IMPAIRED DIFFUSION CAPACITY

Oxygen must diffuse across the alveolar and capillary membranes and through the red blood cell membrane (a negligible amount of oxygen is dissolved in plasma). Gas diffusion depends upon distance (in this case, <0.5 μm), solubility of the gas, molecular weight of the gas, and the partial pressure difference across the intervening tissue. Under normal conditions, the partial pressure difference is large (PAO_2 = 105 mm Hg, mixed venous PO_2 = 40 mm Hg). The rapid combination of oxygen with hemoglobin and the steep slope of the oxyhemoglobin dissociation curve tend to maintain this gradient. Thus, only approximately one third of the 0.75-second transit time of the red blood cell is required for near-complete hemoglobin saturation. As a consequence, there is a large margin of safety in diffusion capacity of the normal lung. A large decrease in the pulmonary transit time, as in a septic hyperdynamic state, coupled with air space disease, can severely limit oxygen diffusion.

Carbon dioxide is more than 20 times more soluble in tissue than is oxygen, allowing rapid transport. There is a lower partial pressure difference between the blood (mixed venous PCO_2 = 45 to 50 mm Hg) and the inspired air (PCO_2 = O) than in the case of oxygen. Despite this, the higher molecular weight of carbon dioxide, and the slower reaction rate in the dissolution of carbon dioxide, diffusion impairment leading to hypercapnia is uncommon. The measurement of diffusing capacity for oxygen and carbon dioxide is not possible clinically, but is approximated by the *diffusion capacity of carbon monoxide* (DLCO). The DLCO can be determined rapidly and easily in the pulmonary function laboratory, and has become a routine part of pulmonary function testing.

SPECIFIC PULMONARY DISORDERS

Chronic obstructive pulmonary disease (COPD) is a general term describing a group of patients with respiratory disease, the common denominator being an element of expiratory obstruction. *Bronchitis* is defined as chronic excessive mucus secretion in the bronchial tree and is usually accompanied by productive cough. Peribronchial inflammation and airway narrowing cause outflow obstruction. The FVC, FEV$_1$, and MVV are all decreased. Expiratory obstruction leads to air trapping, with an increase in the TLC and RV. Radioactive scanning techniques demonstrate a predominant overperfusion of underventilated air spaces. As a consequence, hypoxia and hypercapnia are common features. *Emphysema* is characterized as the abnormal enlargement of air spaces distal to the terminal bronchiole, associated with destruction of the alveolar architecture. There is loss of the normal elastic recoil of the lung as well as decreased elastic support of the peripheral airways. The TLC, FRC, and RV are increased. The FVC,

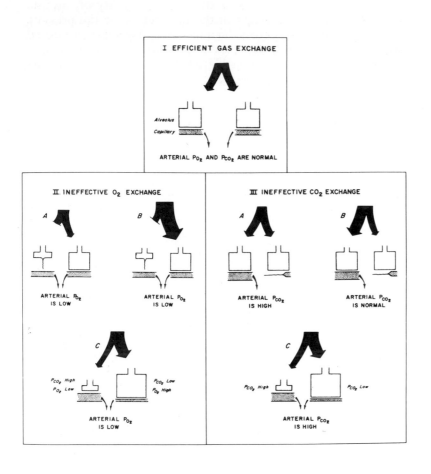

I EFFICIENT GAS EXCHANGE

Alveolus
Capillary

ARTERIAL P$_{O_2}$ AND P$_{CO_2}$ ARE NORMAL

II. INEFFECTIVE O$_2$ EXCHANGE

A

ARTERIAL P$_{O_2}$ IS LOW

B

ARTERIAL P$_{O_2}$ IS LOW

C

P$_{CO_2}$ High   P$_{CO_2}$ Low
P$_{O_2}$ Low   P$_{O_2}$ High

ARTERIAL P$_{O_2}$ IS LOW

III INEFFECTIVE CO$_2$ EXCHANGE

A

ARTERIAL P$_{CO_2}$ IS HIGH

B

ARTERIAL P$_{CO_2}$ IS NORMAL

C

P$_{CO_2}$ High   P$_{CO_2}$ Low

ARTERIAL P$_{CO_2}$ IS HIGH

Figure 5. Effect of changes in ventilation and perfusion on PaO$_2$ and PaCO$_2$. Tidal volume is represented by black arrows, the thickness of the arrows representing changes in magnitude of the tidal volume.

Panel I, The normal lung is represented by two alveoli, each perfused by one half of the cardiac output.

Panel II, A and B, Acute collapse of an alveolus is associated with continued perfusion. Venous admixture results in arterial hypoxemia. An increase in the tidal volume to ventilated-perfused unit is unable to overcome the effect of venous admixture.

Panel II, C, Marked ventilation-perfusion abnormality is present. The left alveolus receives most of the perfusion and little ventilation, the blood remaining poorly oxygenated and with a high PCO$_2$. The reverse is the case for the right alveolus. The result is a decreased PaO$_2$ and an elevated PaCO$_2$.

Panel III, A and B, Continued ventilation to a nonperfused alveolus results in dead space ventilation. Hyperventilation of the perfused alveolus can return PaCO$_2$ to normal, usually requiring an increase in overall respiratory work. Hypotension can increase the amount of Zone 1 lung, increasing this "physiologic" dead space. Pulmonary embolism has a similar effect.

Panel III, C, A marked ventilation-perfusion imbalance induces a smaller dead space volume. (From Laver MB, Austen WG, Wilson RS: Blood-gas exchange and hemodynamic performance. *In* Sabiston DC Jr, Spencer FC [eds]: Gibbon's Surgery of the Chest, ed 3. Philadelphia, WB Saunders Company, 1976, with permission.)

FEV$_1$, and MVV are decreased. There is very little perfusion of nonventilated alveoli, but there is a large amount of physiologic dead space. Consequently, arterial oxygenation is often normal or only mildly depressed and the PaCO$_2$ is usually normal. *Restrictive lung disease* can be caused by many diseases, including fibrothorax, kyphoscoliosis, sarcoidosis, interstitial pneumonitis, infiltrative neoplasms, myasthenia gravis, and cardiogenic pulmonary edema. Pulmonary compliance is decreased, and TLC, VC, and FRC are decreased. The airway size is increased, but the FEV$_1$ may be decreased, particularly in neuromuscular disorders. The FEV$_1$/FVC% is normal, however, when actual airway obstruction is not a component of the lung disease. Ventilation-perfusion abnormalities are common, resulting in hypoxemia. The development of hypercapnia is unusual and reflects the end-stage of restrictive lung disease. The maintenance of normal arterial PCO$_2$ is the result of compensatory hyperventilation, which is achieved at a greatly increased work of breathing.

THE EFFECT OF SURGICAL PROCEDURES ON PULMONARY FUNCTION

The degree of pulmonary dysfunction following operation is directly related to type of procedure and the preoperative status of pulmonary function. For example, operations performed on the extremities generally have little effect on pulmonary function. Thoracic procedures, particularly those involving pulmonary resection, cause severe depression of respiratory function. Abdominal procedures can cause significant respiratory depression, especially with an upper midline incision. Total lung capacity and all the subdivisions of lung capacity are reduced following nonextremity procedures. This reduces the surface area available for gas exchange and promotes airway closure, as the FRC is reduced below the closing volume. The resulting atelectasis, either macroscopic or microscopic, leads to arterial hypoxemia. Atelectasis can also be due to retained secretions, the quality of which may be altered by anesthetic agents. The elimination of these secretions is hampered by diminished cough, caused by pain or narcotic administration. There may be dysfunction of ciliary activity and clearance of microbial agents. Airway closure is also due to postoperative splinting of the chest. The breathing pattern is characteristically altered to accomplish adequate minute ventilation with a lowered tidal volume at an increased respiratory rate. Sighing, a normal mechanism for opening the airways, is virtually eliminated in the early postoperative period. Restriction of the patient to the bed, primarily in the supine position, is also deleterious. Abnormal positioning of the patient during operation can result in pulmonary dysfunction.

PREOPERATIVE EVALUATION OF RISK

Increased age and a smoking history increase the dosing volume. Obesity diminishes the FRC and ERV, such that the end-tidal point approaches the dosing volume. Patients with obstructive pulmonary disease have a diminished ERV. The additive effect of a postoperative decrease in FRC and ERV causes airway closure and atelectasis in patients with these characteristics. Obstructive pulmonary disease is the most important risk factor in surgical patients, the degree of expiratory obstruction being directly related to the risk of postoperative complications. Restrictive lung disease is usually more easily tolerated, despite the fact that lung volumes are decreased postoperatively. This is due to better maintenance of expiratory flow and secretion clearing.

The use of preoperative pulmonary function testing has allowed an approximation of risk based on obstruction. An FEV_1 of greater than 2 L is associated with minimal risk. Increased risk is associated with FEV_1 of from 1 to 2 L. When the FEV_1 is less than 0.8 L, there is moderate risk of severe complications, that risk becoming prohibitive with FEV_1 less than 0.5 L. The 5-year survival of patients with FEV_1 of less than 0.75 L may be as little as 10 per cent, a factor that should be considered in elective surgical procedures. Thoracotomy and pulmonary resection are even less well tolerated. The loss of functional pulmonary tissue and the more direct effects of thoracic incisions tend to depress postoperative pulmonary function more severely. The presence of pulmonary hyperten-

sion and hypercapnia probably contraindicate pulmonary resection. If the FEV_1 is less than 2 L and the MVV less than 50 per cent of predicted, the patient is at increased risk for pulmonary resection and should probably not undergo a pneumonectomy. The quantitative lung scan can be helpful in borderline patients, in whom the removal of nonfunctioning lung tissue may be possible despite limited overall pulmonary function.

PREOPERATIVE PREPARATION

Every effort should be made to convince the patient to cease smoking preoperatively. Ideally, this should be done at least 2 weeks before surgery, although there is marked benefit from cessation for as little as 1 week. The identification of other treatable preoperative conditions is essential. In patients with a productive cough, sputum culture and the institution of appropriate antibiotics are imperative. Patient education and training are very important parts of preoperative preparation. Breathing exercises strengthen the respiratory musculature. Instructions on coughing and deep breathing improve postoperative cooperation. Instruction in the use of prn (as needed) narcotics to allow coughing and deep breathing gives the physician a valuable ally in the titration of these drugs postoperatively. In patients with copious pulmonary secretions, chest percussion and postural drainage may be necessary.

POSTOPERATIVE MANAGEMENT

In general, if preoperative evaluation has been complete, this should be simply a continuation of preoperative therapy. Supplemental oxygen is administered to correct hypoxemia caused by central hypoventilation in the immediate postoperative period. Oxygen therapy is discontinued when it is no longer required, as documented by arterial blood gas determinations or pulse oximetry. The patient is positioned with the head slightly elevated, if possible, and the position in bed changed at frequent intervals. It has been clearly demonstrated that inspiratory exercises, with the encouragement of deep breathing, are the most effective means of minimizing airway closure. Narcotics are administered to minimize postoperative pain and to allow effective coughing. When the cough is ineffective, endotracheal suctioning may be necessary. Early ambulation has proved to be an effective means to prevent postoperative pulmonary complications. Sitting upright and ambulation increase the FRC and lead to improvement in all lung volumes, counteracting the changes induced by surgery. The risk of pulmonary embolism is also reduced.

MEDICAL MANAGEMENT OF BRONCHOSPASM

A variety of therapeutic agents are now available to optimize pulmonary function. An organized approach in the use of these agents is important, as there are many potential drug interactions and serious side effects that may limit therapy.

Adrenergic Agonists and Bronchodilator Aerosol Therapy

β-Agonists are currently the most popular initial bronchodilating agents. The effect of adrenergic agonists is primarily due to direct effects on bronchial smooth muscle, as there is no significant direct sympathetic innervation in the human. The β_2 effects are bronchodilatory and anti-inflammatory by inhibition of mediator release. Mucociliary clearance is also improved. The prototype sympathomimetic drug is epinephrine, but its use has been limited by adverse cardiac effects when given systemically and by poor bioavailability in oral forms. The development of metaproterenol and albuterol has allowed oral dosage and has minimized cardiac or β_1 effects. β_2-Selective agents, such as salbutamol, have been recently introduced.

The effects of adrenergic agents are dose related and show no response plateau. Therapy can be limited by systemic side effects, which include tremor, nervousness, and cardiac arrhythmias. The use of an aerosol administration route allows greater effective dosing with fewer side effects. In acute bronchospasm, the aerosol route may not produce uniform airway distribution, and effectiveness can be delayed. The bronchodilatory effects of the adrenergic agents are probably additive when used in combination with theophylline.

Corticosteroids

Current trends in the management of reactive airway disease include the easy employment of intravenous corticosteroids. Although steroids may adversely affect wound healing, their powerful anti-inflammatory action is of overriding importance, particularly in acute bronchospastic disorders. Intravenous administration is usually accompanied by β-agonist therapy and a short course prescribed in the immediate perioperative period. Patients already receiving chronic steroid therapy for obstructive lung disease should be given perioperative steroids because of adrenal suppression. The introduction of beclomethasone dipropionate has increased the therapeutic efficacy of steroid use, as it is administered by inhalation. Adrenal suppressive effects are not seen with normal prescription. Long-term studies have not shown any adverse histologic effects on the bronchial mucosa.

Anticholinergic, Antimuscarinic Bronchodilators

The primary efferent innervation of the lung is parasympathetic, cholinergic, and excitatory, so that there is a predominant vagal tone causing bronchoconstriction and increased mucus secretion. Atropine has long been recognized as a potent bronchodilator, but its use has been limited by its side effects. Even with aerosol administration, systemic levels are high, causing bladder outlet obstruction, meiosis, and tachycardia. The dangers of inspissation of viscid secretions with chronic anticholinergic therapy may be only a theoretic adverse effect. The introduction of the quaternary ammonium cogeners of atropine, atropine methonitrate, and ipratropium bromide, has resulted in the clinical revival of the anticholinergic agents. These drugs are poorly absorbed after aerosol administration and thus have few systemic effects. They are very potent bronchodilators that act to remove tonic stimulation and interact synergistically with currently available agents. High-dose ipratropium bromide (8 to 12 puffs every 2 hours) is frequently used in patients with severe airway obstruction who are being mechanically ventilated.

Theophylline

Theophylline is a member of the xanthine family. Its mechanism of action is unclear at this time, but it is known to inhibit phosphodiesterase and to specifically antagonize adenosine. Although formerly the most popular initial therapeutic agent for airway obstruction, theophylline has become less frequently used and has assumed an adjunctive role. The specific effects of theophylline preparations include bronchodilatation and pulmonary arterial vasodilatation. An increase in respiratory drive and mucociliary clearance, as well as an inhibition of mast cell mediator release, are also realized.

Bronchodilatation is dose related over a relatively narrow therapeutic drug level range (10 to 20 μg/ml). The maintenance of appropriate serum theophylline levels has been made possible by the development of a clinically available radioimmunoassay. Adverse gastrointestinal effects can be seen with levels greater than 15 μg/ml. Cardiac effects are also seen at higher levels, but no studies have demonstrated adverse effects in the therapeutic range. Intravenous loading with 5.6 mg/kg is indicated in acute bronchospasm, followed by a continuous infusion at a rate dependent on age, smoking habits, and other medical conditions. The possibility that concomitant bronchodilatation and pulmonary arterial dilatation may be distributed in such a way as to worsen ventilation-perfusion matching, and thus lead to hypoxia, should always be considered.

Airway Management

The broad indications for intubation are upper airway obstruction, the need for ventilatory support, and the management of copious secretions. Ventilatory support may be required for hypoventilation, hypoxia, increased work of breathing, or combinations of these features in the clinical setting of *adult respiratory distress syndrome* (ARDS). Some specific indications for intubation and mechanical ventilation are outlined in Table 1, but these criteria should not be viewed as a substitute for clinical evaluation. The decision to intubate a patient in respiratory distress must be made prior to the development of an irreversible clinical state, and early intubation is preferable even if it may prove unnecessary. Intubation should be performed as

an elective procedure if at all possible. In this setting, orotracheal intubation is preferred and is more rapid in experienced hands. A large-bore (at least 8 mm) endotracheal tube is preferred to facilitate suctioning, permit bronchoscopy, and minimize airflow obstruction during weaning from mechanical ventilation.

The safety of prolonged endotracheal intubation has been established for periods of up to 3 weeks. Advances in tube design, particularly the development of thin polyvinyl chloride, large-volume, high-compliance cuffs, have minimized the need for early conversion to tracheostomy. Skilled nursing care and the establishment of respiratory therapy departments have provided the constant surveillance of each patient required for successful long-term intubation. Meticulous attention to adequate humidification, sterile suctioning technique, and frequent culturing of secretions have become routine intensive care practices. If more than 3 weeks of support become necessary, tracheostomy is required. If it is clear from the outset that prolonged intubation will be necessary, tracheostomy should probably be performed 7 to 10 days following intubation, before tracheal mucosal damage becomes severe.

Ventilatory Support

Once airway control is established, mechanical ventilation is usually necessary. There is ample evidence that early aggressive respiratory support can minimize the morbidity of respiratory failure. The goal of ventilatory support is to safely normalize minute volume and the distribution of ventilation and perfusion so as to provide for adequate oxygen delivery and carbon dioxide elimination. All ventilators deliver a mixture of humidified gases under positive pressure, with expiration being a passive process. The most popular ventilators volume-cycle to the expiratory phase, such that the inspiratory phase is accomplished with a controlled volume. By controlling volume, dynamic changes in chest wall compliance during emergence from anesthesia affect airway pressure rather than minute ventilation. Ventilation can be absolutely controlled only in the paralyzed or heavily sedated patient. Respiration can be assisted by means of a variety of ventilatory modes, outlined as follows:

Assisted ventilation (AV). The patient triggers a mechanical inspiration based on the generation of a small detected negative airway pressure.

Intermittent mandatory ventilation (IMV). The patient breathes on his own through the respirator circuit, but receives supplemental ventilation from the respirator at a controlled rate.

Pressure-support (PS) ventilation. A constant inspiratory pressure is used to assist inspiration during IMV,

TABLE 1. GUIDELINES FOR VENTILATORY SUPPORT IN ADULTS WITH ACUTE RESPIRATORY FAILURE[*†]

Data	Normal Range	Indication for Tracheal Intubation and Ventilation
Mechanics		
Respiratory rate	12–20	<35
Vital capacity (ml/kg of body weight[†])	65–75	<15
FEV_1[#] (ml/kg of body weight[†])	50–60	<10
Inspiratory force (cm H_2O)	75–100	<25
Oxygenation		
PaO_2 (mm Hg)	100–75 (air)	<70 (on mask O_2)
$P(A-aDO_2)$ (mm Hg)[§]	25–65	>450
Ventilation		
$PaCO_2$ (mm Hg)	35–45	>55[¶]
V_D/V_T	0.25–0.40	>0.60

[*]From Laver MB, Austen WG: Respiratory function: Physiologic considerations applicable to surgery. *In* Sabiston DC Jr (ed): Davis-Christopher Textbook of Surgery, ed 12. Philadelphia, WB Saunders Company, 1981, with permission. Data from Wilson RS, Pontoppidan H: Crit Care Med 2:293, 1974.

[†]The clinical evaluation of the patient should supersede intubation of a patient based on any single abnormal value. The clinical course of the patient will also modify the above values.

[‡]Ideal weight used if weight is grossly abnormal.

[§]Obtained after 10 minutes of 100 per cent oxygen.

[¶]Except in patients with chronic hypercapnea.

[#]First-second forced expired volume.

a technique that allows ventilator weaning by decreasing inspiratory support rather than by decreasing the IMV rate alone. In all types of pressure-sensitive ventilatory modes, minute ventilation is determined by airway and chest wall compliance as well as patient effort. When these components of airway mechanics are changing or unstable, careful monitoring is essential.

Inverse-ratio mechanical ventilation. In this mode of ventilation, lower mean inspiratory flow rates are employed, such that the time of inspiration exceeds the time permitted for expiration. This is felt to improve gas exchange by more evenly matching the relationship between inspired gas distribution and pulmonary blood flow. It also may reduce the risk of barotrauma by enabling ventilation at a lower peak airway pressure than in conventional ventilation. Inverse ratio ventilation is often employed with pressure-controlled ventilation. A decelerating inspiratory flow pattern is created that has been shown to produce improvement in PaO_2 when compared to volume-controlled ventilation. This combination of inverse-ratio, pressure-controlled ventilation is associated with significant increases in mean airway pressure, however, and the patient must be carefully monitored for cardiac effects and barotrauma.

Continuous positive airway pressure (CPAP). In adults, CPAP is used as pressure support to compensate for the resistive burden of the endotracheal tube during inspiration and to maintain FRC at end expiration.

Positive end-expiratory pressure (PEEP). PEEP is used to maintain FRC in the patient supported for central hypoventilation and therapeutically in respiratory distress syndromes to increase FRC and normalize the ventilation perfusion relationship.

High-frequency ventilation (HFV). Unusually high-frequency ventilation (60 to 100 breaths per minute) at small tidal volumes (3 to 4 ml/kg) are used. This allows for a quiet operative field during pulmonary surgery and can be helpful in cases of barotrauma or bronchopleural fistula by minimizing mean airway pressure.

In addition to providing various modes of ventilation, ventilators provide alarm systems to prevent catastrophic complications. The most important alarm is, of course, represented by the personnel who monitor patients on mechanical ventilator support. The most appropriate response to any of these alarms is an immediate and complete evaluation of the ventilator, its connections, and the patient. Should an easily correctable fault or explanation not be immediately apparent, the ventilator should be disconnected and manual respiration begun until a complete assessment has been made.

CONTROL OF ARTERIAL BLOOD GASES

The control of respiration with a mechanical ventilator permits manipulation of arterial PO_2, PCO_2, and pH that are not possible in any other setting. Arterial PCO_2, reflecting alveolar ventilation, can be lowered by increasing minute ventilation, either by increased tidal volume or by increased respiratory rate. Initial settings of a tidal volume of 10 to 15 ml/kg at a rate of 8 to 12 breaths per minute usually result in a normal PCO_2. When the PCO_2 is too low and the resulting arterial pH is too high, minute ventilation supplied by the ventilator can be decreased in compensation. When spontaneous patient ventilation causes hypocapnia, sedation and increased ventilator control may be necessary. The addition of dead space to the breathing circuit or the addition of carbon dioxide to the inspired gases may also be necessary. The emergence from anesthesia often occurs in the setting of moderate patient hypothermia as a result of the operating room environment. This predictably leads to involuntary shivering and decreased chest wall compliance, which reduces minute ventilation and markedly increases carbon dioxide production. The minute ventilation must be increased, usually by ventilator rate increase, until normothermia is achieved.

The arterial PO_2 can be modified by a variety of maneuvers. Initially, oxygenation can be improved by the administration of oxygen-enriched gases. An arterial oxygen saturation greater than 90 per cent is desirable and must be obtained initially even if the FIO_2 must be increased to 1.0. The ability to maintain oxygenation by this means is limited by the toxic nature of oxygen in concentrations higher than atmospheric. Oxygen toxicity causes a pathologic picture of atelectasis, edema, inflammation, and thickening of alveolar membranes. Bacterial clearance and macrophage function become diminished. The biochemical mechanism of this toxicity appears to be the development of intracellular oxygen radicals and chemically active oxygen metabolites in concentrations exceeding the cellular defense mechanisms. An additional adverse feature of elevated oxygen concentration is the development of venous admixture because of shunting at the alveolar level from atelectasis or edema. At the present time, an absolutely safe level of oxygen supplementation has not been established. It appears that an FIO_2 of 0.4 to 0.5 is well tolerated for prolonged periods. An FIO_2 of 0.6 or greater is hazardous, the hazard increasing directly with increasing oxygen concentration. An FiO$_2$ of 1.0 should not be maintained for more than 48 hours.

In order to improve arterial oxygenation without excessive oxygen administration, other methods are necessary. The use of PEEP has become fundamental in the therapy of respiratory failure in this regard. PEEP has been shown to reduce oxygen requirements by improving ventilation-perfusion matching and by increasing the FRC toward normal in postoperative patients. PEEP should be increased to the highest levels tolerated that also decrease venous admixture. It should be recognized that the effect of PEEP is non-specific, that patients have individual responses to its use, and that certain patients respond to PEEP with an increase in venous admixture. The use of PEEP is limited by dose-related decrease in cardiac output and by barotrauma causing pneumothorax. The cardiac output effect has been shown to be related to a decrease in left heart filling secondary to an increase in right ventricular afterload and to direct effects on the right ventricle that are responsive to volume loading.

WEANING FROM VENTILATORY SUPPORT

Weaning from ventilatory support conceptually begins at the time that it is instituted. Support of nutrition during intubation is imperative, as the respiratory muscles must function at full capacity once the ventilator is discontinued. Once the pathologic process that required support is controlled, the patient should gradually assume more and more responsibility for minute ventilation. This is usually accomplished by gradually decreasing the IMV rate while maintaining approximately 5 cm H$_2$O of PEEP. Minimal support prior to extubation should be 5 cm H$_2$O CPAP or IMV at 2 breaths per minute with 5 cm H$_2$O PEEP. Further reductions in support prior to extubation are in reality unwarranted stress tests. The rate of weaning is determined by the patient's response and by serial arterial blood gas determinations. Pulse oximetry is a useful monitoring technique in this process and has enabled a safe reduction in the number of actual blood gas determinations requested. Slow weaning is required when there has been prolonged intubation to rehabilitate the respiratory musculature. In difficult situations, the use of pressure-support and pressure-control ventilation has allowed successful discontinuation of mechanical ventilation.

A variety of respiratory parameters has been used

to predict the outcome of weaning from mechanical ventilation, including minute ventilation and maximal inspiratory pressure, but these are frequently inaccurate. A recent prospective study has demonstrated that the ratio of respiratory frequency to tidal volume (f/V$_T$) was the most accurate predictor of failure. High values are associated with rapid shallow breathing. Values less than or equal to 105 breaths per minute per liter were most predictive of successful weaning from mechanical ventilation. The cooperation of the patient is essential in the transition to spontaneous ventilation. Occasionally, behavioral modification by a psychotherapist is useful in the chronically supported individual. The final decision to discontinue ventilatory support rests on the measurement of respiratory mechanics, the measurement of arterial blood gases, and observation of the patient on minimal support.

CONCLUSIONS

The management of the pulmonary system in surgical patients requires careful attention to the physiologic principles outlined in this section. With proper selection of patients and attention to preoperative preparation based on a knowledge of the probable postoperative alterations in pulmonary function, excellent surgical results can be obtained. It should always be remembered that if pulmonary resection has not been performed, the alterations in pulmonary physiology that occur following operation are temporary and reversible with appropriate therapy.

REFERENCES

Banner MJ, Kirby RR, McIntyre NR: Patient and ventilator work of breathing and ventilatory muscle loads at different levels of pressure support ventilation. Chest 100(2):531, 1991.
Chan K, Abraham E: Effects of inverse ratio ventilation on cardiorespiratory parameters in severe respiratory failure. Chest 102:1556, 1992.
Newhouse MT: Is theophylline obsolete? Chest 98:1, 1990.
Pesenti A, Pelosi P, Rossi N, Aprigliano M, Brazzi L, Fumagalli R: Respiratory mechanics and bronchodilator responsiveness in patients with the adult respiratory distress syndrome. Crit Care Med 21:78, 1993.
Schnapp LM, Cohen NH: Pulse oximetry. Uses and abuses. Chest 98:1244, 1990.
Yang KL, Tobin MJ: A prospective study of indexes predicting the outcome of trials of weaning from mechanical ventilation. N Engl J Med 324:1445, 1991.

II
Diagnostic Thoracoscopy

JAMES M. DOUGLAS, Jr., M.D.

HISTORIC ASPECTS

The development of thoracoscopy began in 1910 when Jacobaeus used a simple cystoscope to induce pneumothorax and divide pleural adhesions in patients with tuberculosis. Interest in thoracoscopy has increased recently with greater attention being given its use in evaluating patients with malignant diseases. The widespread enthusiasm about video-assisted laparoscopic cholecystectomy in the 1980s introduced added interest in using video-assisted thoracoscopic techniques for the evaluation and treatment of intrathoracic disorders. These techniques are being used to perform many procedures formerly approached by open thoracotomy.

ANATOMIC AND PHYSIOLOGIC CONSIDERATIONS

Thoracoscopy is the technique that allows the visualization of intrathoracic contents by means of transthoracic instrumentation. The complexity of the potential instrumentation used is quite varied. A simple fiberoptic mediastinoscope, a rigid bronchoscope, a flexible bronchoscope, or newer video-assisted laparoscopic instrumentation may be used. Although the simpler instruments allow some procedures to be performed quite well, the newer video-assisted techniques provide the surgeon with expanded capabilities. Satisfactory performance of any of the thoracoscopic procedures requires good patient anesthesia. Although simple procedures can be performed with regional or local anesthesia, the use of general anesthesia is preferred, as it permits optimal patient comfort, improved surgical accessibility, and avoidance of the potential problems of pneumothorax that may occur in the awake patient. Operations on the pleura can generally be performed without specialized ventilatory techniques. However, single-lung ventilation permits a more panoramic view of the intrathoracic structures and enables the surgeon to perform the desired procedures without being limited by the inflated lung. Safe performance of thoracoscopy, particularly with single-lung ventilation, requires close monitoring. Intermittent arterial blood gas analysis supplemented by pulse oximetry and end-tidal carbon dioxide measurements provides optimum monitoring. The degree of monitoring may be determined by the complexity of the planned procedure and the clinical status of the patient. Occasionally, carbon dioxide insufflation of the chest may be required to improve visualization, particularly when single-lung ventilation is not accompanied by adequate collapse of the lung. Care is taken under these circumstances to maintain intrathoracic pressure under 10 mm Hg.

INDICATIONS AND CONTRAINDICATIONS

Diagnostic thoracoscopy may be employed to obtain tissue for biopsy from all intrathoracic structures. The extent to which this can be performed successfully may be limited by intrapleural adhesions, the inability of the patient to tolerate single-lung anesthesia, or instrumentation failure. Successful result also depends on the surgeon's knowledge of the proper sites for instrumentation insertion.

TECHNIQUE

Thoracoscopy can be performed in almost any standard operating position. The most versatile patient positioning is the lateral decubitus orientation, which also permits easy conversion to thoracotomy should the procedure be complicated. The initial passage of instruments into the chest is properly done under direct vision to avoid inadvertent passage into lung parenchyma or mediastinal structures. Subsequent instrumentation placement should be accomplished with visualization through the employed scope. Video-assisted thoracoscopic procedures allow the assistants and operating surgeon to visualize the operative field and work in unison. Care is taken to include all manipulations within view. With these principles, thoracoscopy may be used to obtain a diagnosis of pleural disease, stage malignancies, resect tumors, perform esophageal operations, resect pericardium, and perform many other thoracic surgical procedures once performed through open thoracotomy. Intelligent evaluation of the application of these techniques is re-

quired to ensure that safe, uncompromised patient care is provided.

REFERENCES

Bergqvist S, Nordensteam H: Thoracoscopy and pleural biopsy in the diagnosis of pleurisy. Scand J Respir Dis 47:64, 1966.

Bloomberg AE: Thoracoscopy in perspective. Surg Gynecol Obstet 147:433, 1978.

Jacobaeus HC: The practical importance of thoracoscopy in surgery of the chest. Surg Gynecol Obstet 34:289, 1922.

Page RD, Jeffrey RR, Donnelly RJ: Thoracoscopy: A review of 121 consecutive surgical procedures. Ann Thorac Surg 48:66, 1989.

Wakabayashi A: Expanded applications of diagnostic and therapeutic thoracoscopy. J Thorac Cardiovasc Surg 102:721, 1991.

III
Tracheostomy and Its Complications

PATRICK D. KENAN, M.D.

HISTORY

Tracheostomy for airway support is a technique dating back at least to Galen, but until the 20th century, it was usually reserved for in extremis situations. The procedure was given a semblance of respectability by Jackson in the early 1920s, but was usually done under local anesthesia, often at the bedside, in less than ideal operative conditions. With the advent of the routine use of the endotracheal tube, improved general anesthesia, modern monitoring, and ventilatory assistance, tracheostomy earned the reputation of an operation with reduced risks, low complications, and generally good results.

TECHNIQUES

With an endotracheal airway in place, the patient is flexed at the hips to elevate the upper body, to reduce

venous pressure in the neck. The neck is either in the neutral position or slightly hyperextended, and a vertical or transverse skin incision is made over the upper trachea through the platysma muscle. With lateral retraction, the strap muscles are separated in the midline by Bovie electrodissection (Fig. 1A). The cricoid cartilage is engaged by a hook retractor, and a curved clamp is placed under the thyroid isthmus (Fig. 1B). Division of the isthmus allows exposure of the upper trachea. Triangulated retraction gives tracheal exposure preparatory to entry. Deflation of the cuff of the endotracheal tube permits sharp entry into the trachea by scalpel between the first and second tracheal rings (Fig. 1C), or through a vertical incision through rings 2 through 4. Cautery must never be used to enter the trachea for risk of combustion in the airway, particularly with high delivery of oxygen. Partial withdrawal of the endotracheal tube (Fig. 1D) permits introduction of the tracheostomy tube. With the tube in place

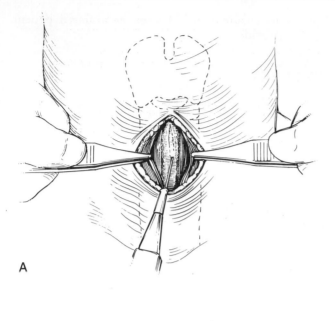

A

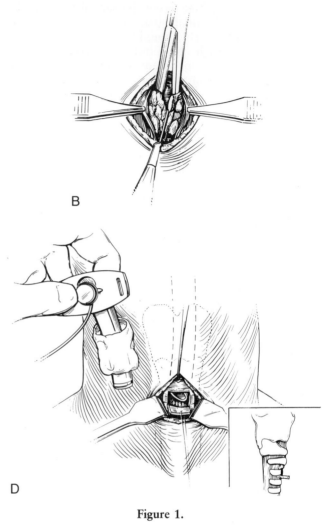

B

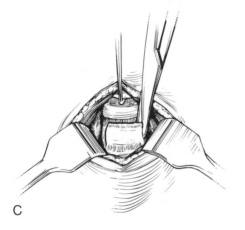

C

D

Figure 1.

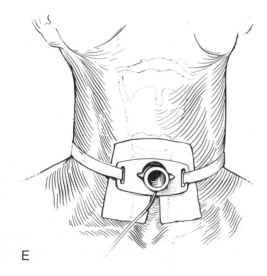

E

(Fig. 1E) and its cuff inflated, the endotracheal tube may be withdrawn when it is obvious that adequate ventilation and gaseous exchange is present through the tracheostomy. The tracheostomy tube is secured by neck straps, sometimes with adjunctive flange sutures, the wound is loosely sutured, and dressed with a pad. Adequate headlight illumination, meticulous attention to sterility, hemostasis, and uninterrupted ventilation are absolute requirements in each tracheostomy and serve to minimize the risk of complications.

Many advocate *cricothyroidotomy*, particularly when rapid entry into the trachea is necessary to secure an adequate airway. In experienced hands, this is an acceptable alternative to the more classical tracheostomy methods, provided no disruption of the cricoid cartilage occurs and that a tube small enough to fit the space is used. The technique may require little more than a vertical stab incision through the cricothyroid membrane into the trachea, with immediate insertion of a small tracheostomy tube. When speed of securing the airway is of utmost importance, cricothyroidotomy is superior, even to oral intubation in most instances.

Changing a tracheostomy tube rarely creates problems of reentry through a well-formed tract, except in children soon after insertion. If a small child's tracheostomy requires changing, it is best done by placing a small-caliber endotracheal tube (ET) through the lumen of the tracheostomy tube, then removing and replacing the tracheostomy over the ET tube. Once a fresh tube is in place, the ET tube is removed and discarded. The technique of extubation (decannulation) deserves comment. In general, a cuffed tube may be changed to an uncuffed tube when mechanical ventilation is no longer needed, and a tube of smaller caliber permits less resistance to breathing around the tube when corked or temporarily occluded. Extubation is best done when a smaller uncuffed tube has been corked fully for at least 24 hours, with demonstration of an adequate airway. A compression dressing is placed at the skin opening on extubation, and the wound is allowed to heal by secondary intention.

COMPLICATIONS

Complications of tracheostomy may occur in both the perioperative period or later, as summarized in Table 1.

MANAGEMENT OF PERIOPERATIVE COMPLICATIONS

Immediate recognition of perioperative complications is essential to effective management. Bleeding, if not controlled intraoperatively, requires ligation of the vessels and occasionally packing of the tracheostomy site postoperatively. Autonomic alterations may be reversed by avoiding excessive tracheal traction, by vasopressors, or other forms of pharmacologic support provided by the anesthesiologist. Prevention of false passages and injury to the recurrent laryngeal nerve or the posterior tracheal wall is possible by adequate visualization, limited entry in anterior trachea, and avoidance of stretching or tearing from a tube that is too large, or prolonged overinflation of the cuff.

Pneumothorax may be prevented by avoiding finger dissection around the trachea and overdistention of the lungs for respiratory support when the airway is restored. A routine posttracheostomy chest film may detect pneumothorax which, if present, may justify placement of a chest tube with suction. Each tracheostomy must be viewed as an open contaminated

TABLE 1. COMPLICATIONS OF TRACHEOSTOMY

Perioperative complications
  Bleeding from vessels, especially of the thyroid
  Autonomic reflexes affecting blood pressure, heart rate, or
    arrhythmias
  False passage through the trachea
  Injury to recurrent laryngeal nerve
  Injury to the posterior tracheal wall or esophagus
  Bronchial obstruction by blood or secretions
  Pneumothorax, pneumomediastinum, and subcutaneous
    emphysema
  Infection in the wound or respiratory tract
  Accidental extubation
  Obstruction by the tube
  Malfunction or rupture of the cuff
Late postoperative complications
  Tracheal obstruction (partial or complete) from stenosis or
    malacia
  Risk of tracheoinnominate arterial hemorrhage
  Tracheal granulations with bleeding or partial obstruction
  Severe scarring or retraction of the skin
  Persistent tracheocutaneous fistula following extubation

wound with a risk of infecting the contiguous airway and introducing sepsis. Infectious complications may be minimized by meticulous wound care, sterile tracheobronchial suctioning, and systemic antibiotics. Good respiratory therapy is essential to avoid significant infection. Accidental extubation and obstruction of the tube may be prevented by avoiding excessive traction on the tracheostomy tube, due to unfavorable linkage to mechanical ventilators, and by appropriate sterile suctioning of the tube or change of inner cannulas. Children may extubate themselves if the arms are not appropriately immobilized. Cuff malfunction or rupture is rare but any cuff may rupture if overinflated or if it impacts upon sharp edges of cartilage. Should cuff malfunction occur, the entire tube must be changed. Every effort must be made to avoid overinflation of cuffs, because rupture may occur and more severe late complications may be induced. If the pressure from a cuff or the tube itself exceeds capillary perfusion pressure, the affected mucosa may become necrotic and cause ulceration, infection, exposure of cartilage, and attendant complications.

MANAGEMENT OF LATE COMPLICATIONS

Severe complications are stenosis and/or malacia following a compromised airway. If either occurs, segmental tracheal resection and reanastomosis may be necessary, with inherent risks of injury to the recurrent laryngeal nerve. At times, serial dilations or endotracheal laser therapy may be useful in treating stenosis but rarely in managing tracheomalacia. Late bleeding from a tracheal stoma may be caused by granulation tissue associated with an open wound and foreign body, but a tracheoinnominate (TI) artery fistula is always possible, and prodromal bleeding may progress to fatal exsanguination unless immediate operation is undertaken. The cause of TI bleeding is usually due to erosion through the tracheal wall from the tip of an oversized tube or from pressure erosion of the cuff of a tube placed too low in the root of the neck. If TI bleeding occurs, only finger tamponade through the stoma, compressing the innominate artery on the underside of the sternum, prevents exsanguination. Tamponade is maintained into the operating room for sternal splitting and ligation of the innominate artery. Scarring, skin retraction, and occasional tracheocutaneous fistula, occur following extubation. Revision of the scar with meticulous layer-by-layer closure corrects these defects.

PREVENTION OF COMPLICATIONS

With rare exceptions, the complications of tracheostomy can be prevented by adherence to proper surgical technique, including adequate headlight illumination, sterility, hemostasis, avoidance of excessive tissue trauma, continuous intraoperative ventilation, adequate monitoring, and conduct of the procedure in the operating room rather than at bedside. The tracheostomy tube must be of correct size, shape, and length to "fit" the patient's tracheal configuration. Avoidance of overinflation of the tracheal cuff is absolutely essential to minimize mucosal damage, necrosis, or sloughing that may lead to stenosis or malacia, or great vessel erosion. Humidified air should be used for days and sometimes weeks. Injury to the cricoid cartilage must be minimized to prevent the risk of an acquired subglottic stenosis.

Finally, it should be emphasized that many complications of tracheostomy can be avoided by endotracheal *intubation* for most forms of airway support, and this is the usual method of assisted ventilation. An endotracheal tube that is too large may create various forms of pressure erosion, particularly in the glottis and subglottis, and the temptation to use large endotracheal tubes for ease of ventilation must be avoided when a smaller tube suffices. Even with routine use of endotracheal intubation for most airway problems, there remains an important role for tracheostomy, especially in situations requiring prolonged ventilatory assistance. A tracheostomy is also more comfortable for the patient than prolonged tracheal intubation.

REFERENCES

Brantigan CO, Grow JB: Cricothyroidotomy: Elective use in respiratory problems requiring tracheotomy. J Thorac Cardiovasc Surg 72:72–81, 1976.

Brantigan CO, Grow JB: Cricothyroidotomy revisited again. Ear Nose Throat J 59:26, 1980.

Grillo HC, Mathison DJ: Tracheotomy and its complications. *In* Sabiston DC Jr (ed): Textbook of Surgery: The Biological Basis of Modern Surgical Practice, ed 14. Philadelphia, WB Saunders Company, 1991.

Jackson C: High tracheotomy and other errors; the chief courses of chronic laryngeal stenosis. Surg Gynecol Obstet 32:392, 1921.

Kenan PD: Complications associated with tracheostomy: Prevention and treatment. Otolaryngol Clin North Am 12:807, 1979.

IV
Pulmonary Infections

RONALD C. HILL, M.D.

Although lung abscesses are declining due to the general use of broad-spectrum antibiotics, premature infants, especially those with congenital defects and other medical problems as well as older patients and those with malignancies, immunosuppressive disorders, history of steroids, postoperative states, and radiation history, may have a more complicated clinical course. Additional etiologies include tuberculosis, mycotic disease, infected cysts, bronchiectasis, pulmonary infarction, tumor, and bronchial obstruction (Fig. 1).

PATHOGENESIS

Aspiration pneumonitis is the most common predisposing factor causing a lung abscess. Although alcoholism is a frequent etiology, other antecedent problems include anesthesia, epilepsy, neurologic and esophageal disorders, dental procedures, and drugs. Anatomically, the superior segment of the right lower lobe is the most frequent location for a lung abscess. However, the posterior segment of the right upper lobe as well as the posterior segment of the right lower lobe may be involved. The patient usually presents with a history of an upper respiratory infection, pleuritic chest pain, and occasionally hemoptysis and weight loss. The chest film may not be very suggestive in the early stages but may become diagnostic with an air-fluid level as areas consolidate and liquefy. Computed tomography (CT) of the chest may be utilized to delineate the disease further (Fig. 1). Because aspiration is one of the more common causes, cultures usually grow anaerobic bacteria. However, in hospital-acquired disease, gram-negative rods may be isolated. Due to the need for urgent diagnosis and institution of antibiotic therapy, cultures may be obtained from transtracheal aspirate, or on occasion, from a small percutaneous needle. However, because of potential problems with these methods, specially designed bronchoscopic protective brushes may be utilized effectively for cultures.

TREATMENT

Penicillin remains the antibiotic of choice in patients with no allergies. Clindamycin as well as other antibiotics may be used in patients who have more resistant organisms or allergies. Bronchoscopy should be performed not only as a diagnostic procedure, but also as a therapeutic procedure to drain the abscess, if possible. If resolution does not occur or complications arise such as empyema, septicemia, or distant spread (brain abscess, bronchogenic), surgical resection may be necessary. Surgical mortality varies from 0 to 11 per cent. In patients who have other systemic diseases, the mortality may be as high as 80 to 90 per cent.

INFECTIONS

Pulmonary infections of the lung include bacterial, viral, and fungal. Cultures are important in order to institute appropriate antibiotic therapy. Bronchoscopy as well as surgical extirpation may be required.

Actinomycosis

Actinomycosis is caused by the anaerobic bacterium *Actinomyces israelii* and is associated with abscess and sinus formation. Cultures must be from the pathologic material of the patient, as it is a normal inhabitant of the oral cavity. This infection is associated with "sulfur granules," the yellow brown granules that drain from the abscesses or sinuses. Penicillin continues to be the drug of choice, and operative therapy may require decortication and drainage of empyema and excision of abscesses and sinus tracts.

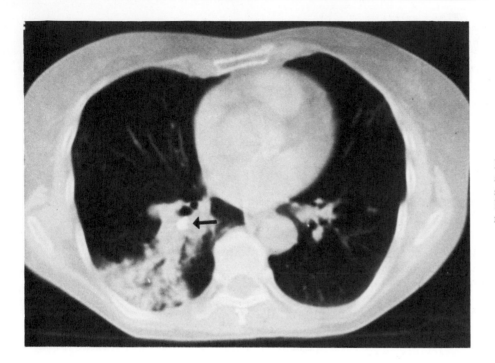

Figure 1. A lung abscess secondary to obstruction of the right superior segmental bronchus by a broncholith requiring segmentectomy.

Nocardiosis

Nocardiosis is caused by *Nocardia asteroides*, both a gram-positive bacterium and a partially acid-fast anaerobic actinomycete. Nocardiosis may mimic other pulmonary infections and is often opportunistic in patients with suppressed immune systems from malignancies, transplantation, or other diseases. Treatment is with trimethoprim sulfamethoxazole, but minocycline may be used as an alternative drug in the allergic patient. If resectable, a cure rate approaching 100 per cent may be obtained.

Pneumocystosis

Pneumocystis pneumonia is caused by *Pneumocystis carinii*, a protozoa that stains similar to fungus with silver methenamine stains. Interstitial plasma cell pneumonia follows and occurs in patients with impaired cellular immunity secondary to drugs, malignancies, or organ transplantation. It is also associated with the acquired immunodeficiency syndrome (AIDS). Actual destruction of pulmonary tissue and spontaneous pneumothoraces may develop. The radiograph usually shows extensive bilateral pneumonitis, with a nodular or granular pattern radiating from the hilum. Diagnosis may be made by transbronchoscopic, percutaneous needle, transthorascopic, or open lung biopsy. Treatment includes the use of either trimethoprim sulfamethoxazole or pentamidine isethionate.

Histoplasmosis

Histoplasmosis is caused by *Histoplasma capsulatum*, a soil-based, nonencapsulated fungus found in pigeon, chicken, and bat droppings, and is endemic in the Mississippi and Ohio river basins. Uric acid found in fowl excreta is a source of nitrogen for this fungus, which grows in areas of high humidity, aerobic conditions, acidic soil, and warm temperatures. Following inhalation of the organism, symptoms may include fever, chills, headaches, cough, and chest pain. The chest film may show diffuse pulmonary infiltration, or scattered nodular densities. Histoplasmin and complement fixation titers may be performed (>1:32 or a fourfold rise in titer). Skin tests are usually nondiagnostic. Histoplasmosis may present as a coin lesion (histoplasmoma) identified by concentric rings of calcification (Figs. 2 and 3). Computed tomography shows satellite lesions. Needle aspiration, bronchoscopic evaluation, or operation may be necessary to make the diagnosis. Histoplasmosis is usually treated in symptomatic patients, and amphotericin B remains the drug of choice for symptomatic patients. One of the major sequelae of histoplasmosis is mediastinal granulomata with fibrosing mediastinitis, which may cause superior vena

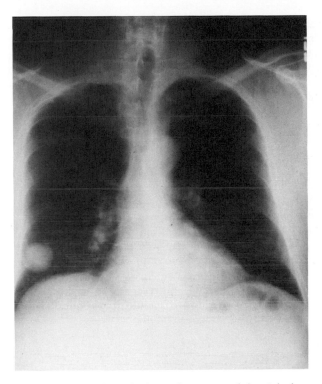

Figure 2. Chest film of a histoplasmoma of the right lower lobe.

caval obstruction plus obstruction of other major veins in the mediastinum and bronchi. Esophageal compression and traction diverticula of the esophagus may result as well. The syndrome may become quiescent with conservative treatment. However, others feel that aggressive treatment with removal of the granulomas may be necessary. Steroids and chemotherapy do not seem to be efficacious.

Coccidioidomycosis

Coccidioidomycosis, caused by the dimorphic fungus *Coccidioides immitis*, is endemic in the southwestern United States (including the San Joaquin Valley), Mexico, and Central and South America. Clinical presentation may range from a relatively mild respiratory disorder associated with red bumps and aching joints known as "valley fever," "desert rheumatism," or "the bumps," to a debilitating disease with extensive dissemination. The diagnosis depends on skin tests and complement fixation tests as well as history. Chest films show infiltrates, cavities, nodules, and/or adenopathy. Although amphotericin B remains a drug of good efficacy, *itraconazole* is also effective in the treatment. Operative therapy may be indicated for diagnosis as well as for patients who do not respond to medical treatment or who present with solitary pulmonary nodules.

North American Blastomycosis

North American blastomycosis is caused by the organism *Blastomyces dermatitidis*, which is a budding yeast endemic in the Mississippi River valley and Africa and South America. It may occur in a cutaneous as well as a pulmonary form. Usually the patient presents with a pneumonic infiltrate and skin lesions. The chest film may show cavitary, nodular, fibrotic, or diffuse lesions. Treatment includes amphotericin B, but ketoconazole has been found to be effective also. Surgical therapy is seldom needed.

Cryptococcosis

Cryptococcus neoformans is a budding yeast in the soil, dust, and pigeon dung. Its thick gelatinous capsule can be demonstrated easily with a mucin carmine stain or India ink preparations of fresh tissue. Although a cause of meningeal disease, cryptococcosis may produce pulmonary lesions as well. Diagnosis is usually made by culture, as the chest film may be nonspecific. Treatment includes the use of amphotericin B or 5-fluorocytosine. Surgical extirpation may be of benefit for resistant disease.

Aspergillosis

Aspergillosis is caused by the fungus *Aspergillus fumigatus*, a filamentous organism with course, septate, fragmented hyphae. Aspergillus is associated with hy-

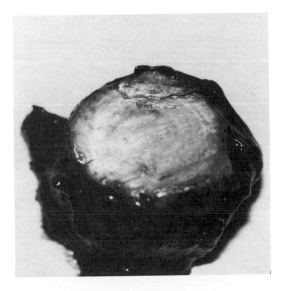

Figure 3. Cut section of the histoplasmoma illustrating the concentric rings of calcification.

persensitivity reactions such as "malt-workers lung" or "farmers' lung." It may invade preexisting pulmonary cavities forming a fungus ball. Patients usually present with chronic lung disease, hemoptysis, and nutritional disorders. In asymptomatic patients, conservative treatment is indicated. However, when hemoptysis is a major problem, surgical removal is recommended if the patient is otherwise able to undergo a surgical procedure. In the high-risk patient, the cavity may be drained and sodium iodide or amphotericin B instilled. Invasive pulmonary aspergillosis occurs in the immunocompromised patient. Medical treatment with iodides, nystatin, hydroxystilbamidine, or amphotericin B has been used, but mortality remains high. Other complications of aspergillosis include empyema (requiring drainage), endocarditis (requiring surgical treatment), and pericarditis.

Candidiasis

Candidiasis is caused by *Candida albicans*, which is an opportunistic organism usually found in the gastrointestinal tract. Systemic infections may occur in patients who are immunosuppressed or who have been on long-term antibiotic therapy. Candida endocarditis may occur and require surgical intervention. Amphotericin B and 5-fluorocytosine are used in conjunction with other treatment modalities.

Miscellaneous Fungal Infections

Mucormycosis is caused by a fungus belonging to the class *Zygomycota*. These organisms have broad nonseptate hyphae and characteristically invade the blood vessels causing thrombosis and infarction. Amphotericin B may be of some help, but most patients have a preexisting immune deficiency and are terminal. Sporotrichosis is caused by *Sporotrichum schenckii*. Although lymphatic and cutaneous involvement is more common, pulmonary manifestations with infiltrates and adenopathy may occur. Treatment with iodides or amphotericin B may be curative. Monosporosis is a mycotic infection caused by *Pseudallescheriasis boydii*, which resides in the soil and may invade preexisting cavities and form a fungus ball-like picture. Chemotherapy is usually ineffective, although ketoconazole and miconazole have been somewhat effective. Local excision is usually the treatment of choice. Paracoccidioidomycosis (South American blastomycosis) is caused by *Paracoccidioides brasiliensis*, a soil inhabitant. It is endemic in Central and South America and may be found in the United States as well. Capillary lesions usually occur, and treatment with sulfonamides is suppressive but not curative. Other effective antibiotics include amphotericin B, ketoconazole, and itraconazole.

REFERENCES

Delarue NC, Pearson FG, Nelems JM, Cooper JD: Lung abscess: Surgical implications. Can J Surg 23:297, 1980.
Diaz M, Puente R, deHoyos LA, Cruz S: Itraconazole in the treatment of coccidioidomycosis. Chest 100:682, 1991.
Eng RH, Bishburg E, Smith SM: Evidence for destruction of lung tissues during *Pneumocystis carinii* infection. Arch Intern Med 147:746, 1987.
Renston JP, Morgan J, DiMarco AF: Disseminated miliary blastomycosis leading to acute respiratory failure in an urban setting. Chest 101:1463, 1992.
Scott SM: Pulmonary infections. *In* Sabiston DC Jr (ed): Textbook of Surgery: The Biological Basis of Modern Surgical Practice, ed 14. Philadelphia, WB Saunders Company, 1991.

V
The Pleura and Empyema

RONALD C. HILL, M.D.

The pleural surface is composed of a serous membrane that covers the lung (*visceral pleura*) and the chest wall (*parietal pleura*). The parietal pleura contains sensory nerve endings and receives its blood supply from the intercostal arteries. The visceral pleura has no sensory nerve endings and receives its blood supply from the bronchial arteries.

PLEURAL EFFUSIONS

Pleural effusions may be divided into either *transudate* or *exudate*, depending on the composition. An exudate is defined as a pleural effusion that has a specific gravity greater than 1.016 and a protein concentration of 3.0 gm/dl. More recently, the ratio between the protein concentration and the *lactate dehydrogenase* (LDH) appears to be the most accurate method in determining the fluid status. Other components include the glucose, presence of malignant cells, red cells, and white cells, amylase level, pH, and lipid levels. Diseases that cause exudates or transudates include congestive heart failure, pulmonary embolism, malignancy, empyema, tuberculosis, rheumatoid arthritis and other collagen-related diseases, chyle, cirrhosis of the liver, pancreatitis, and low albumin states.

Pneumothorax

Pneumothorax is defined as *air within the pleural space* and may occur from various etiologies including iatrogenic, perforated esophagus, ruptured bronchus, rib fractures, trauma, or spontaneous. Spontaneous pneumothorax is secondary to rupture of small subpleural blebs usually located in the apex of the lung. It generally occurs on the right side of young men who smoke. When air has accumulated within the pleural space to the extent that tension occurs, the term *tension pneumothorax* is applied. Mediastinal contents may shift due to the tension causing distortion of the vena cavae and creating partial obstruction of the systemic venous return.

Small pneumothoraces (<20 per cent) may be treated conservatively in asymptomatic patients. Oxygen therapy may speed resolution by increasing the gradient for nitrogen absorption. Larger pneumothoraces, symptomatic pneumothoraces, and tension pneumothoraces should be treated with immediate tube thoracostomy. When patients present with spontaneous pneumothoraces, nonoperative treatment by tube thoracostomy is usually indicated. However, if the air leak persists, if the lung does not fully inflate, or if a recurrence occurs, operation is indicated. Although some have advocated pleurectomy, most feel removal of the blebs and pleural abrasion (*pleurodesis*) is adequate.

HEMOTHORAX

Hemothorax is defined as *the accumulation of blood within the pleural space*. It is associated with trauma, metastatic disease, iatrogenic endeavors, pneumothoraces, and pulmonary neoplasms. Generally, if the hemothorax is small and without associated problems, the treatment is conservative. If, however, a pneumothorax is present or a large hemothorax is present, a chest tube may be necessary to resolve the pneumothorax and evacuate and monitor the blood loss. If the patient continues to bleed at the rate of 200 ml or more for 3 to 4 hours, has complete opacification of one hemothorax, or more than 1000 ml of blood is evacuated immediately, the patient should undergo exploratory thoracotomy. Complications of hemothorax include infection and organization of the blood causing a pleural peel or *fibrothorax*. This may cause restriction in the pulmonary compliance and necessitate its removal (decortication).

CHYLOTHORAX

Chylothorax occurs when chyle accumulates in the pleural space. It may be due to a congenital deformity; a postoperative complication of esophageal, cardiac, or thoracic surgery; traumatic hyperextension of the spine; or penetrating and nonpenetrating injuries to the chest, neck, and abdomen. Other etiologies include malignancies, infections, pseudocysts, cirrhosis, or thrombosis of the jugular and subclavian veins. Non-clotting milky fluid in the pleural space suggests chylothorax. Examination shows a protein content half of that in plasma with predominantly lymphocytes and free microscopic fat. Computed tomography (CT) and possibly lymph angiography may show the chylothorax and the site of leakage, as well as anatomic abnormalities of the thoracic duct system. Treatment includes medium-chain triglyceride diets or total parenteral hyperalimentation to decrease lymph flow. If the effusion is large, tube drainage should be established. If resolution has not occurred after 1 to 4 weeks, surgical intervention may be necessary to either ligate the thoracic duct or close the thoracic duct fistula.

EMPYEMA

Empyema may be caused by pneumonia, pulmonary abscess, esophageal disease, or subphrenic or hepatic abscesses. *Staphylococcus aureus* has become one of the more common bacteria isolated from empyema. Gram-negative bacilli have been increasing in inci-

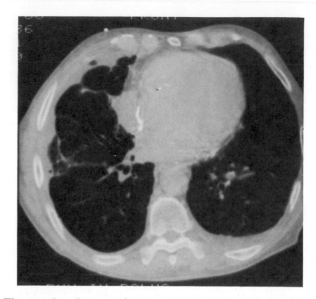

Figure 2. Computed tomography of a malignant mesothelioma.

dence, especially in the elderly, alcoholics, diabetics, and immunocompromised patients. Chest film and CT, along with the patient's clinical picture, usually lead to investigation of the presence of an empyema (Fig. 1). With the current antibiotic use, the fluid may not grow any organisms, but may still be consistent with empyema. Drainage of the pleural space may be accomplished by thoracentesis, tube thoracostomy, rib resection and open drainage with a catheter, or formal thoracotomy and decortication. Reexpansion of the lung should obliterate the space. However, if it cannot

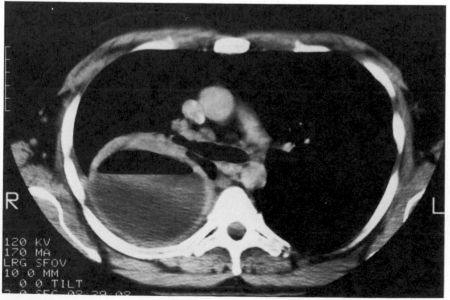

Figure 1. Computed tomography of an empyema prior to drainage.

be fully reexpanded and a space persists, alternatives may be necessary. Thoracoplasty, either Schede or the tailoring type, may be performed. Pleural obliteration with autogenous tissues such as muscle flaps, and omentum, or the utilization of pleural space sterilization with antimicrobial solutions are alternative treatments. Recently, thoracoscopy has been utilized to drain empyemas, and the results remain to be evaluated for long-term effect. If the empyema is associated with a bronchopleural fistula, this complication should be corrected as well.

PLEURAL NEOPLASMS

Pleural neoplasms may be primary or metastatic. Metastatic lesions are associated with breast, pancreas, stomach, and lung primaries. Bloody pleural effusions usually indicate a malignancy. If symptomatic, the malignant effusion may be drained either by thoracentesis or closed tube thoracostomy. Once drained, the pleural space can be sclerosed with agents that create an inflammatory pleuritis and obliterate the pleural space, the agents commonly used being talc and doxycycline. Primary tumors of the pleura may be benign or malignant. Benign mesotheliomas usually arise from the visceral pleura; when symptomatic, signs of pulmonary arthralgias, fever, and clubbing may be present and usually abate with excision of the tumor. Malignant mesotheliomas have been associated with asbestos. Usually the patients have dyspnea and chest pain. Other less common symptoms include pleuritis,

pneumothorax, Horner's syndrome, recurrent laryngeal nerve paralysis, acute paraplegia, or superior vena caval syndrome. The diagnosis is usually made by history, physical examination, and chest film. Computed tomography may show the associated pleural effusions and multiple papillary projections from both the visceral and parietal pleura with incasement of either a portion of, or the entire lung (Fig. 2). If cytologic diagnosis cannot be established by thoracentesis, then either closed or open biopsies may be necessary. Asbestos bodies may be seen on histology. Once the diagnosis has been made, further treatment has been fraught with poor results. Surgical resection, including radical pleurectomy and pneumonectomy, chemotherapy, and radiotherapy have not been shown to have significant differences in survival, which is usually limited to 1 or 2 years following the establishment of the diagnosis.

REFERENCES

Hood RM: Surgical Diseases of the Pleura and Chest Wall. Philadelphia, WB Saunders Company, 1986.

Kittle CF: Current Controversies in Thoracic Surgery. Philadelphia, WB Saunders Company, 1986.

Pairolero PC, Trastek VF: Surgical management of chronic empyema: The role of thoracoplasty. Ann Thorac Surg 50:689, 1990.

Poe RH, Marin MG, Israel RH, Kallay MC: Utility of pleural fluid analysis in predicting tube thoracostomy/decortication in parapneumonic effusions. Chest 100:963, 1991.

Scott SM: The pleura and empyema. In Sabiston DC Jr (ed): Textbook of Surgery: The Biological Basis of Modern Surgical Practice, ed 14. Philadelphia, WB Saunders Company, 1991, pp 1718–1726.

VI
Bronchiectasis

RONALD C. HILL, M.D.

Laënnec first described bronchiectasis in 1819 as changes in the bronchial wall and pulmonary parenchyma usually sparing the upper lobes. Since the advent of antibiotics, the incidence of bronchiectasis has declined greatly, although thoracic surgeons today are occasionally asked to perform procedures on patients with symptomatic bronchiectasis.

ETIOLOGY

Bronchiectasis may be either a congenital or an acquired abnormality. Patients with *situs inversus*, paranasal sinusitis, as well as bronchiectasis (Kartagener's syndrome), have dismotility of the bronchial ciliated cells. Other congenital etiologies include humoral immunodeficiencies, cystic bronchiectasis, cystic fibrosis, and panhypogammaglobulinemia. The acquired disorders are thought to be secondary to infections or trauma. Patients who have aspirated foreign bodies may develop bronchiectasis. Postinfectious causes for bronchiectasis include aspiration pneumonia; tuberculosis; and virulent bacterial and viral infections including pertussis, measles, and influenza. The less common causes for bronchiectasis include carcinoma, bronchitis, abscesses, cystic fibrosis, and rheumatoid arthritis.

PATHOPHYSIOLOGY

Bronchiectasis is usually regional and located in the lower lobes of the lungs; however, when associated with tuberculosis or other granulomatous diseases, it is commonly found in the upper lobes. Bronchiectasis generally affects the medium-size airways, although other airways are not immune from this disorder. The bronchi remain dilated and may extend to the pleura, with very few branching components. There is focal destruction of the bronchial wall, with scar formation

which, in turn, leads to retained secretions and chronic airway inspissation. Although damage to the bronchial wall is common, there may be damage to the surrounding lung tissue, with loss of volume and fibrosis. In the past, bronchiectasis was felt to be either cylindric or saccular. However, in many patients, it is difficult to single out one specific type. A patient may have both types as well as a third type known as a *varicose deformity*. Mucociliary dismotility is not confined to patients with Kartagener's syndrome and other congenital etiologies. Patients with acquired bronchiectasis have also been shown to have abnormal ciliary motility by radioactive studies. Normal ciliary motion has been shown to be cephalad or axial in direction and have a constant velocity. Patients with bronchiectatic changes show different motility patterns, all of which are abnormal. Even though it is not clear as to whether the dismotility is a cause of the bronchiectasis or an effect, most patients have this abnormality. Hemoptysis may occur in patients with bronchiectasis also, most likely secondary to abnormal communications between the bronchial and pulmonary arteries.

DIAGNOSIS

Patients usually present with a history of cough that may be purulent or dry. Because of the inspissated secretions, there may be a foul odor known as *fetor oris*. Also, there may be a history of repeated episodes of pneumonitis, bronchitis, and/or hemoptysis. Physical examination may reveal dullness to percussion as well as rales and rhonchi. The chest film may be unremarkable or may show nonspecific findings such as linear atelectasis. The extent of disease on radiograph tends to correlate with the severity of the bronchiectasis, and increased markings of the bronchial walls, volume loss, and atelectasis of surrounding lung parenchyma and abnormal lung densities may be noted.

In the past, bronchiectasis was diagnosed by bronchography, performed in the nonacute phase, using a contrast agent known as *Lipiodol* (Fig. 1). Currently, computed tomography (CT) scan is used for the diagnosis of bronchiectasis, and bronchography is rarely performed. Indeed, Lipiodol is no longer available. In performing the CT scan, medium thickness (4 to 5 mm) and thin sections (1 to 2 mm) are evaluated. The sensitivity of the CT scan done in this matter is similar to that of bronchography, and CT is easier, less trau-

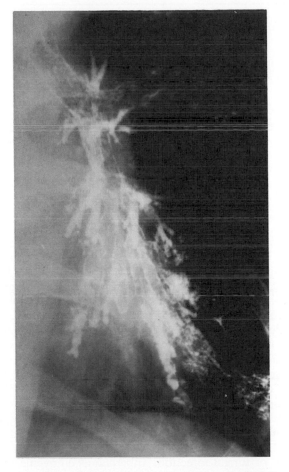

Figure 1. Bronchogram illustrating segmental cylindric and saccular bronchiectasis of the left lower lobe requiring lobectomy.

matic on the patient, and noninvasive. Also, it enables visualization of both lungs simultaneously. Bronchoscopy should be performed to delineate the endobronchial anatomy as well as to obtain bacterial cultures. Foreign bodies and neoplasms may be identified as well. Other studies including pulmonary function studies and arterial blood gases may be required.

TREATMENT

The treatment for bronchiectasis remains conservative if possible. Good postural drainage, as well as antibiotic therapy, can abort the symptoms in most cases. Therapeutic bronchoscopy may be necessary to remove the thicker secretions. Avoidance of smoking and polluted air is important, and pneumococcal and influenza vaccines should be administered. Surgical options should be reserved for those patients who continue to show signs and symptoms of bronchiectasis despite medical therapy. Preservation of lung parenchyma is of utmost importance, and consideration for segmentectomies and lobectomies should be given high priority. If patients have bilateral disease, the most involved side should be treated first to see if there is any improvement prior to treating the opposite side. Patients who undergo surgery and who have limited disease have an excellent prognosis.

REFERENCES

Barker AP, Bardana EJ Jr: Bronchiectasis: Update of an orphan disease. Am Rev Respir Dis *137:969*, 1988.

Glower DD: Bronchiectasis. *In* Sabiston DC Jr (ed): Textbook of Surgery: The Biological Basis of Modern Surgical Practice, ed 14. Philadelphia, WB Saunders Company, 1991, pp 1720–1729.

Hill RC, Sabiston DC Jr: Bronchiectasis. *In* Sabiston DC Jr (ed): Essentials of Surgery. Philadelphia, WB Saunders Company, 1987.

Isawa T, Teshima T, Hirano T, et al: Mucociliary clearance and transport in bronchiectasis: Global and regional assessment. J Nucl Med *31:543*, 1990.

Pang IA, Hamilton-Wood C, Metreweli C: The value of computed tomography in the diagnosis and management of bronchiectasis. Clin Radiol *40:40*, 1989.

Westcott JL: Bronchiectasis. Radiol Clin North Am *29:* 1031, 1991.

VII
Surgical Treatment of Pulmonary Tuberculosis

JON F. MORAN, M.D.

Tuberculosis remains the leading infectious killer in the world, causing 3 million deaths per year. In the early 20th century, while tuberculosis was disappearing rapidly in the United States, Canada, and much of Europe (Fig. 1), it remained a common disease elsewhere. Since 1986, with the epidemic of human immunodeficiency virus (HIV) infection, the incidence of tuberculosis in the United States has been increasing by 5 to 10 per cent annually. Pulmonary tuberculosis represents 90 per cent of all cases of tuberculosis; and less than 3 per cent require surgical treatment. Modern antituberculous drug therapy is very effective, and operative treatment is only required for catastrophic complications or treatment of drug-resistant infections.

Mycobacterium tuberculosis, an aerobic, nonmotile slow-growing bacillus, is responsible for most pulmonary mycobacterial disease. Other mycobacteria, the atypical mycobacteria, can cause pulmonary infection and are more frequently resistant to drug therapy. Runyon classified mycobacteria by their growth characteristics (Table 1). *Mycobacterium avium-intracellulare* and *M. kansasii* are the two atypical species that most often cause pulmonary infection.

PATHOLOGY

The pathologic response within the lung to the various mycobacteria is identical. *Mycobacterium tuberculosis* is a virulent organism requiring a minimal airborne inoculum for infection to occur in normal lungs. Atypical mycobacteria more often invade abnormal lung tissue or compromised individuals. The pneumonic process caused by mycobacteria is characterized by caseous necrosis with formation of a granuloma containing the mycobacteria within a rim of granulation tissue (Fig. 2). The peripheral pneumonic lesion accompanied by hilar nodal enlargement is termed a primary Ghon complex. Most mycobacterial infections are contained at this early stage by the body's own immune response. Miliary tuberculosis occurs rarely from massive hematogenous spread with thousands of 1- to 2-mm (millet-seed-sized) tubercles throughout the body.

Adult pulmonary tuberculosis is the most common form of mycobacterial infection and is called "reinfection" or "postprimary" tuberculosis. Adult tuberculosis begins as a segmental pneumonia in the apical or posterior segment of an upper lobe or the superior segment of a lower lobe (Fig. 3). Bilateral disease is common. The pneumonic infiltrates progress to caseous necrosis with cavity formation when the necrotic area erodes into an adjacent bronchus. Erosion of a cavity into a bronchial vessel may cause severe hemoptysis. A Rasmussen aneurysm, a pulmonary artery aneurysm within or adjacent to a cavity, is found in about 4 per cent of advanced cavitary mycobacterial disease. The visceral and parietal pleura adjacent to the infected area develop an intense inflammatory reaction obliterating the overlying pleural space. Endobronchial tuberculosis may cause bronchostenosis with distal bacterial or fungal infection. Tuberculous empyema may occur from hematogenous or lymphatic seeding of the pleural space or rupture of a cavity into the pleural space.

DIAGNOSIS

An important distinction is made between mycobacterial infection and mycobacterial disease. Infection implies the entrance of an organism into the body without symptoms. The diagnosis of mycobacterial disease depends on the confirmation of active disease by radiographic and bacteriologic studies. Approximately 10 per cent of individuals infected with *M. tuberculosis* develop disease. Symptoms of pulmonary tuberculosis are a chronic cough, easy fatigability, weight loss, hemoptysis, and fever with night sweats. The most frequent radiographic findings in pulmonary tuberculosis are apical infiltrates with frequent cavitation. Current standard tuberculosis skin testing involves the intracutaneous injection of five *tuberculin units* (TU) of *purified protein derivative* (PPD) on the volar aspect of the forearm. This is termed an *intermediate PPD*, and greater than 10 mm of induration after 48 to 72 hours defines a positive test. The intermediate PPD is positive in at least 90 per cent of patients with tuberculosis. The isolation of mycobacterial organisms from the sputum is required to confirm the diagnosis of mycobacterial disease. The presence of acid-fast organisms on smear allows for rapid presumptive diagnosis, though cultures are necessary to document the species of mycobacteria. Approximately 10,000 organisms per milliliter of sputum are required for smear positivity. Mycobacterial cultures require 3 to 6 weeks to grow, and it may be necessary to obtain multiple samples before a positive smear or culture is obtained. Antimycobacterial chemotherapy is often begun as a therapeutic trial while awaiting final cultures. Patients referred for surgical treatment are frequently infected with organisms that are resistant to most antituberculous drugs. Sensitivity testing for a variety of antituberculous drugs is particularly important in patients being considered for operative therapy.

TABLE 1. CLASSIFICATION OF MYCOBACTERIAL SPECIES (RUNYON)

Group I	Photochromogens	*M. kansasii*
Group II	Scotochromogens	*M. scrofulaceum*
Group III	Nonchromogens	*M. tuberculosis*
		M. avium-intracellulare
Group IV	Rapid growers	*M. fortuitum*
		M. chelonei

CHEMOTHERAPY

Chemotherapy for pulmonary mycobacterial infection requires administration of two or three drugs simultaneously to avoid the emergence of drug-resistant organisms. Mycobacteria react differently to drugs, depending upon whether the organisms are *extracellular* or *intracellular*. Extracellular organisms tend to multiply rapidly in the hyperoxic neutral pH environment of the pulmonary cavity. Organisms grow slowly in the environment within macrophages. An effective treatment program halts mycobacterial growth, both intracellularly and extracellularly, causing conversion of the patient to a sputum-negative status within weeks. The most commonly employed antimycobacterial drugs are listed in Table 2. Atypical mycobacterial infections may require the use of other drugs.

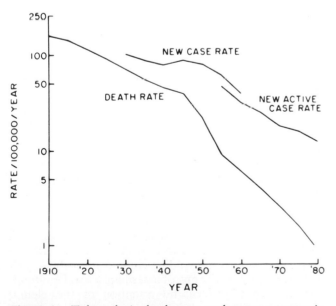

Figure 1. Tuberculosis death rates and new case rates in the United States, 1910–1980. (From Comstock GW: Epidemiology of tuberculosis. Am Rev Respir Dis *125*[Suppl]: 9, 1982, with permission.)

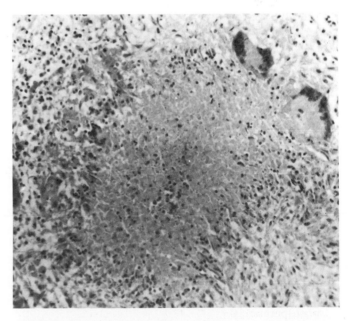

Figure 2. Typical tuberculous granuloma with central caseation and surrounding epithelioid and Langhans giant cells. H & E, X250. (From Dunnill MS: Pulmonary Pathology, ed 2. Edinburgh, Churchill Livingstone, 1987, p 447, with permission.)

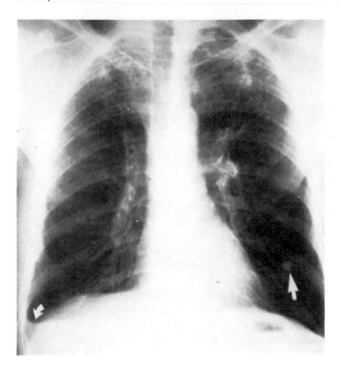

Figure 3. Bilateral apical and posterior segment upper lobe infiltrates typical of adult tuberculosis are seen in this 36-year-old man. Calcified Ghon focus in lingula (*straight arrow*) and blunting of right costophrenic angle (*curved arrow*) are the residua of earlier primary tuberculosis. (From Woodring JH, Vandiviere HM, Fried AM, et al: Update: The radiographic features of pulmonary tuberculosis. Am J Roentgenol *146*:502, 1986, with permission.)

Until recently, it was recommended that chemotherapy be administered continuously for 18 to 24 months. Short-course therapy (6 to 9 months) has been equally effective. The two currently recommended regimens for treatment of pulmonary tuberculosis are: (1) a 6-month course of isoniazid and rifampin with pyrazinamide during the first 2 months; or (2) a 9-month course of isoniazid and rifampin. The primary drug resistance rate for *M. tuberculosis* in the United States is generally 7 to 10 per cent. Although atypical mycobacteria are frequently resistant in vitro to many drugs, four- and five-drug regimens may still be effective. Complications of resectional surgery are reduced in patients who have been converted to sputum-negative status preoperatively. Whenever possible, two or three drugs to which the infecting organism is sensitive should be given perioperatively and for 6 to 9 months postoperatively.

SURGICAL TREATMENT

When an operation is required for pulmonary mycobacterial disease, resection of the diseased portion of the lung is the procedure of choice. Thoracoplasty and other procedures intended to collapse the infected portion of lung are rarely indicated and are of historic interest only. Indications for pulmonary resection in mycobacterial disease are the following:

1. Persistently positive sputum cultures with cavitation following an adequate period of chemotherapy with two or more drugs to which the organism has been proven sensitive.

2. Localized pulmonary disease caused by *M. avium-intracellulare* (or another mycobacterium broadly resistant to chemotherapy).

3. A mass lesion of the lung in an area of mycobacterial infection, requiring resection for diagnosis and treatment of the mycobacterial disease.

4. Massive hemoptysis or recurrent severe hemoptysis, requiring resection of the infected portion of the lung that is the source of the hemorrhage. Pulmonary hemorrhage is a rare but often fatal complication of pulmonary mycobacterial disease. Massive hemoptysis is defined as greater than 200 ml/day. Asphyxiation rather than hypovolemia is the usual cause of death from hemoptysis. The site of bleeding is almost invariably a cavitary lesion. The source of bleeding should be resected on an urgent basis following an episode of massive or recurrent severe hemoptysis, as mortality without resection is high. Tuberculosis remains the most common cause of severe hemoptysis.

5. A bronchopleural fistula secondary to mycobacterial infection that does not respond to tube thoracostomy.

Several special situations may rarely call for surgical treatment of pulmonary mycobacterial disease. Patients severely symptomatic from a destroyed lobe or bronchiectatic area of the lung may benefit from resection, as well as patients with thick-walled cavities who have reactivated or are unreliable in complying with prolonged chemotherapy. A patient with a "trapped lung" following a tuberculous empyema may benefit from decortication with or without resection to allow full expansion of the underlying lung. Children with mycobacterial disease rarely if ever require resection, since chemotherapy is invariably curative in children. Patients referred for operation generally have associated problems that predispose them to complications. Administration of effective antimycobacterial drugs, judicious timing of operation, careful operative technique, and compulsive postoperative care are the important factors in avoiding complications from pulmonary resection for mycobacterial disease. Good pulmonary toilet and careful attention to the pleural drainage system are necessary to assure full reexpansion of the remaining lung to avoid apical space problems. The incidence of bronchopleural fistula after resection for mycobacterial disease is about 3 per cent.

TABLE 2. COMMONLY USED ANTIMYCOBACTERIAL DRUGS

| Drug | Daily Dosage | | Comments |
	Children	Adults	
Isoniazid (INH)	10–20 mg/kg PO or IM	5 mg/kg PO or IM	Bactericidal to both intracellular and extracellular organisms; pyridoxine 10 mg/kg/day as prophylaxis for neuritis
Rifampin (RIF)	10–20 mg/kg PO	10 mg/kg PO	Bactericidal to both intra-cellular and extracellular organisms; colors urine orange; inhibits the effect of oral contraceptives, quinidine, digitalis, corticosteroids, and Coumadin
Pyrazinamide (PZA)	15–20 mg/kg PO	15–30 mg/kg PO	Bactericidal to intracellular organisms; reduces total length of chemotherapy necessary
Streptomycin (SM)	20–40 mg/kg IM	15 mg/kg IM	Bactericidal to extracellular organisms within cavities; limit dose to 10 mg/kg in elderly patients
Ethambutol (EMB)	15–25 mg/kg PO	15–25 mg/kg PO	Bacteriostatic for both intracellular and extracellular organisms

Abbreviations: PO = orally, IM = intramuscularly.

Resectional surgery for mycobacterial disease is now employed in a selected group of problem patients that have failed chemotherapy or have a serious complication such as massive hemoptysis or bronchopleural fistula. Mortality for pulmonary resection of myco-bacterial disease varies from 0 per cent with minimal morbidity when surgical intervention is elective, to 15 per cent or greater when resection is performed as an emergency. The prognosis for long-term survival free of further mycobacterial disease is excellent in opera-tive survivors, with 95 per cent of patients free of dis-ease 5 to 8 years postoperatively.

REFERENCES

Davidson PT, Le HQ: Drug treatment of tuberculosis—1992. Drugs 43(5):651, 1992.
Keers RY: Pulmonary Tuberculosis: A Journey Down the Centuries. London, Balliere Tindall, 1978.
Murray JF: The white plague: Down and out, or up and coming. Am Rev Respir Dis 140(6):1788, 1989.
Pomerantz M, Madsen L, Goble M, Iseman M: Surgical manage-ment of resistant mycobacterial tuberculosis and other mycobac-terial pulmonary infections. Ann Thorac Surg 52(5):1108, 1991.
Snider DE: Mycobacterial diseases. Clin Chest Med 10(3):297–467, 1989.

VIII
Benign Tumors of the Trachea and Esophagus, Including Bronchial Adenomas

JAMES M. DOUGLAS, Jr., M.D.

Malignant tumors of the trachea, bronchi, and esophagus are much more common than benign tumors. However, the benign tumors are important because they may be associated with debilitating symptoms and frequently they must be differentiated from malignant neoplasms. In the trachea, bronchi, and esophagus, benign tumors most commonly become symptomatic as a result of intraluminal obstruction, extraluminal compression, or primary ulceration with bleeding. Oftentimes, these tumors are asymptomatic and are discovered incidentally during other investigations. Although bronchial adenomas are in fact malignant tumors, because of their typically nonaggressive nature, the pertinent characteristics of these tumors are reviewed.

BENIGN TUMORS OF THE TRACHEA AND BRONCHI: GENERAL OVERVIEW

Benign tumors of the trachea and bronchi are usually slow-growing, smooth, rounded masses less than 2 cm in length. As these tumors grow, they may obstruct the airways and cause symptoms such as cough, dyspnea, or wheezing. Overlying ulceration can also cause hemoptysis. Airway obstructive symptoms usually do not occur until more than 75 per cent of the lumen is obstructed. Pedunculated tumors may cause intermittent symptoms as they flip in and out of an obstructed position. Persistent airway obstruction causes distal pulmonary atelectasis and may be complicated by infection. The differentiation between benign and malignant airway tumors cannot be made reliably by radiographic examination. The presence or absence of calcification or the contour of the tumor are not reliable criteria by which to distinguish the biologic characteristics of the tumor. The extent of the tumor can be evaluated by linear tomography, computed tomography (CT), and nuclear magnetic resonance imaging (MRI). For definitive diagnosis of tu-

mors of the trachea and bronchi, laryngoscopic or bronchoscopic biopsy is essential. Caution must be exercised in the biopsy of vascular lesions, and particular attention must be paid to maintenance of the airway to avoid respiratory distress secondary to edema and bronchial constriction.

Most benign tumors of the trachea and bronchi should be treated by either segmental or sleeve resection, particularly when the tumors are sessile. Pedunculated tumors may be removed along with a portion of attached tracheal or bronchial wall. Piecemeal endoscopic removal can be effective but is more prone to cause local recurrence. Squamous papillomatosis is notorious for recurrence and has been treated with laser ablation and bronchoscopic fulguration. Hemangiomas are of interest because of a recognized tendency to regress spontaneously, thereby obviating the need for surgical removal in most patients. The surgical approach to the treatment of proximal airway tumors can be challenging to both the anesthesiologist and the surgeon and may be quite varied depending on the location within the airways. Maintenance of ventilation can require unusual techniques such as distal tracheal intubation or percutaneous transtracheal jet ventilation. Thoracotomy, median sternotomy, transcervical, or combined approaches may be required for exposure of these tumors, and the removal of more than 2 to 3 cm of trachea makes primary reanastomosis unlikely. However, with special mobilization techniques, as much as 6 cm of trachea may be removed and still enable the surgeon to reanastomose the trachea primarily.

BENIGN TUMORS OF THE TRACHEA AND BRONCHI: SELECTED TUMORS

Squamous Papillomatosis

Squamous papillomatosis typically appears as multiple cauliflower-like lesions on the larynx, extending down the trachea and proximal bronchi. On pathologic examination, these tumors are irregular, papillary, or villous processes comprised of branching stalks of loose fibrous tissue covered by thick squamous epithelium budding into the normal respiratory epithelium. Isolated squamous papillomas, which most frequently occur in adults, are composed of squamous epithelium with a core of connective tissue. Squamous papillomas are the most common benign tumors that occur in the trachea, and their etiology is unknown. They are associated with human papilloma virus types VI and XI, and 2 per cent develop malignant transformation. A history of previous radiation therapy increases that risk. Isolated squamous papillomas, most commonly occurring in adults, may have as high as a 50 per cent incidence of malignant change. These tumors frequently present with hoarseness, cough, or recurrent pulmonary infections. The juvenile form tends to regress with age, but in some patients the disease is relentless. Treatment of squamous papillomatosis is notoriously difficult, with recurrence rates as high as 90 per cent. Localized lesions may be surgically resected, but because of the diffuse nature of the disease, laser therapy or bronchoscopic fulguration has most commonly been used, and multiple treatments are usually required. Some success with medical treatment using interferon has been reported.

Hemangiomas

Hemangiomas are the most common tracheal neoplasms occurring in children and most often occur in the subglottic region, whereas in adults they are most often supraglottal or laryngeal. Infants with hemangiomas may be asymptomatic at birth, but 90 per cent are symptomatic by the age of 3 months. Respiratory distress is a prominent symptom and is occasionally misdiagnosed as croup. These tumors have a propensity for regression with time. Consequently, only observation is required in patients without significant symptoms, but tracheostomy and/or surgical excision is occasionally required.

Cartilaginous Tumors

Chondromas are slow-growing, benign lesions of the trachea or bronchi that may develop malignant degeneration. They typically appear as gray to white firm masses composed of cartilage and bone with intact overlying mucosa, and most commonly occur between the ages of 40 and 60 in both sexes. Because of a tendency for local recurrence and the possibility of malignant degeneration, adequate treatment requires complete segmental resection. *Hamartomas* most frequently occur in the bronchi but may occur in the trachea and are composed of varying degrees of cartilage,

fat, lymphoid tissue, or epithelial elements. The most common presentation is that of an asymptomatic solitary pulmonary nodule, and as many as 10 per cent of solitary pulmonary nodules may be hamartomas. Subpleural hamartomas may be easily removed, leaving normal lung parenchyma intact, and proximal endobronchial hamartomas may be treated with sleeve resection. *Tracheobronchopathia osteoplastica* is a distinctive lesion of the trachea appearing as multiple firm nodules on endoscopic examination and is composed of bone and cartilage. Airway obstruction and its consequences may be present, but the condition is most commonly asymptomatic. The peak incidence is about age 50 and the lesion does not occur in children. Significant symptoms are usually best alleviated with bronchoscopic removal.

OTHER BENIGN TUMORS OF THE TRACHEA AND BRONCHI

Fibromas are unusual tumors typically occurring in the cervical trachea of children. They are solitary, well-defined masses composed of fibrous tissue. Local surgical treatment is adequate. A *fibrous histiocytoma* may have benign or malignant characteristics and is most commonly seen in bone but is also an unusual tracheal tumor. *Neurogenic* tumors of the lung are rare and may be particularly difficult to distinguish pathologically as benign or malignant. The benign forms may be treated with local excision only. *Leiomyoma* of the trachea occurs most commonly in the lower third and must be distinguished from malignant leiomyosarcoma. Simple local excision is curative. *Granular cell myoblastoma* most frequently occurs in black women 30 to 50 years of age. Histologically characterized by large foamy cells in syncytial masses containing small, hyperchromatic nuclei and numerous small eosinophilic granules, they may be multiple. Local excision is the treatment of choice. *Lipomas* may occasionally occur in the major airways. Local removal is indicated. *Ectopic thyroid tumors*, comprising approximately 7 per cent of all tracheal tumors, are three times more common in females, and most are associated with goiter. Surgical removal is indicated, with malignant degeneration occurring in approximately 10 per cent.

BENIGN TUMORS OF THE ESOPHAGUS

Benign tumors of the esophagus may be intraluminal, intramural, or extramural. More than 85 per cent of patients with benign esophageal tumors are asymptomatic. However, symptoms may be caused by esophageal obstruction or tumor erosion. Obstruction of the esophagus may cause dysphagia, regurgitation, vomiting, or reflux, and associated aspiration can cause coughing, dyspnea, wheezing, and respiratory infections. Pain or globus can occur. Most symptomatic benign esophageal tumors are pedunculated and intraluminal. Intramural tumors usually are either large or encircle a large portion of the esophageal wall prior to causing symptoms. Extraluminal masses may compress the esophagus or other mediastinal structures and cause predictable problems. The most useful means of diagnosis of esophageal tumors are fiberoptic endoscopy and esophageal contrast studies. These two studies are complimentary and provide information concerning the extent of the tumor, its location, and its pathologic classification. Additionally, fiberoptic endoscopy may be used therapeutically. The overriding concern during the evaluation of esophageal tumors is the differentiation between malignant and benign tumors. Endoscopic biopsy of submucosal and intramural lesions may be nondiagnostic. However, pedunculated mucosal tumors may be diagnosed and treated with endoscopic snare polypectomy techniques. Although surgical removal of benign esophageal tumors may be therapeutic for symptomatic patients, removal is also indicated for asymptomatic lesions to exclude malignancy or prevent future malignant degeneration.

SELECTED BENIGN ESOPHAGEAL TUMORS

Epithelial Tumors

Esophageal polyps are the most common intraluminal benign esophageal lesions, 80 per cent occurring in the cervical region. They are characterized as cylindric intraluminal masses usually attached by an elongated pedicle, and they are composed of fibrovascular tissue. The overlying mucosa is normal. Their pedunculated nature allows movement within the esophagus and is occasionally associated with regurgitation of the tumor into the mouth. Aspiration of these tumors may cause asphyxiation, and the current treatment of choice is endoscopic snare removal.

Squamous cell papilloma comprises approximately 3 per cent of benign tumors of the esophagus. Usually presenting as incidental findings in patients being evaluated for other problems, two thirds occur in the distal esophagus. They are most often single and sessile and are sometimes multiple and pedunculated. The endoscopic appearance may be that of a whitish plaque similar to leukoplakia, or they may be verrucous. This lesion must be distinguished from carcinoma of the esophagus. Histologically, squamous cell papillomas are characterized by finger-like projections with a central core of connective tissue covered with hyperplastic squamous cells. A deep biopsy is required to be certain that a carcinoma is not overlooked. Whenever possible, endoscopic snare removal of this lesion is the treatment of choice. Regular follow-up evaluations should be performed following removal.

Esophageal adenoma is an extremely rare lesion of the esophagus. It is composed of a proliferation of gastric cardia-type glands. Resection is advised for diagnosis and for the prevention of malignant degeneration. Several cystic lesions of the esophagus may present as tumor masses. Inclusion cysts, usually unilocular, smooth, asymptomatic lesions found in the distal esophagus, may be lined by columnar, columnar-ciliated, squamous, or mixed epithelial cells. *Retention cysts* probably occur as a result of obstruction of the long excretory duct arising from the deep esophageal glands, which may be initiated by esophagitis. They may be confused with esophageal varices on endoscopic examination. *Esophageal duplication cysts* are typically extramural, may not connect directly with the esophagus, and appear as mediastinal masses. Their origin is unclear, and they may be associated with symptoms of dysphagia. Endoscopic biopsy would be nondiagnostic; however, endoscopy is required to exclude other pathology. Surgical removal remains the treatment of choice.

Nonepithelial Benign Tumors

Leiomyomas are the most common benign tumors of the esophagus. They are firm, well-circumscribed intramural tumors that present endoscopically as a smooth, mass effect. Biopsy of these tumors endoscopically seldom yields a diagnosis and may be problematic at the time of subsequent surgical removal. On barium swallow examination, these masses appear as smooth tumors projecting into the lumen of the esophagus and form an abrupt angle with the outline of the uninvolved esophagus. They tend to be distributed more commonly in the distal portions of the esophagus. Though many patients are asymptomatic, obstructive symptoms, pain, or bleeding may be associated with these lesions, and excision is the treatment of choice. Although the occasional pedunculated leiomyoma may be removed endoscopically, most require surgical removal, but successful thoracoscopic removal has been described. *Hemangiomas* of the esophagus are rare and usually incidental findings. When symptomatic, surgical resection is indicated. *Lipomas* of the esophagus usually originate in the submucosa and present as polypoid intraluminal masses and are occasionally pedunculated. Treatment is by surgical or endoscopic excision. *Granular cell tumors* of the esophagus are broad-based, polypoid tumors that appear histologically as large polygonal cells containing numerous eosinophilic granules. Their cell of origin has variably been attributed to striated muscle versus Schwann cells. Granular cell tumors have been described in almost every organ, but only 2 per cent involve the esophagus. Multiple tumors have been reported, as have extraesophageal lesions. Symptomatic patients present with dysphagia, but the tumor may also be asymptomatic. Because these tumors arise immediately beneath the squamous epithelium, endoscopic biopsy is frequently diagnostic. Often these specimens show pseudoepitheliomatous hyperplasia and pseudoinvasion, which can be misinterpreted as carcinoma. This appearance is very similar to that seen with breast carcinoma metastatic to the esophagus. Consequently, repeat endoscopy and multiple biopsies should be obtained to exclude metastatic tumors of the esophagus. Because true granular cell tumors are benign and not known to be associated with malignant degeneration, small tumors that are confirmed to be granular cell on biopsy may be treated conservatively with follow-up endoscopy. However, symptomatic or suspicious tumors should be surgically removed.

BRONCHIAL ADENOMAS

Although bronchopulmonary carcinoids, mucoepidermoid tumors, and adenocystic carcinomas of the lung have been grouped together under the term *bronchial adenoma*, each has malignant characteristics and none are completely benign, as the term adenoma implies. Because these tumors most commonly occur in the proximal airways, each may present with similar clinical characteristics. Symptomatic patients may present with wheezing, cough, hemoptysis, or pulmonary infection. Treatment usually requires surgical removal.

Bronchopulmonary Carcinoids

Carcinoid tumors of the lung represent 0.6 to 2 per cent of all lung tumors and 83 per cent of bronchial adenomas. Although the median age of presentation is 55 years, these tumors have been seen at all ages in both sexes, and the pathology is distinctive. Bronchial carcinoids arise from the neuroendocrine argentaffin cells of the bronchial mucosa, also known as Kulchitsky's cells. They are grouped among the *amine precursor uptake and decarboxylation* (APUD) tumors and are known for their ability to produce and store a number of immunoreactive peptide hormones. On electron microscopic examination, neurosecretory granules are characteristic findings. Most carcinoid tumors are slow growing and have a favorable progno-

sis, but about 10 per cent behave aggressively. These "atypical carcinoids" may be distinguished by their more malignant cytologic appearance, including increased nuclear activity, nuclear pleomorphism, and increased cellularity. The tumors generally have few or no secretory granules on electron microscopic examination. Typical and atypical carcinoid tumors appear to be part of a continuum of increasing dedifferentiation of tumors, culminating with small-cell carcinoma. Typical carcinoids have been called Kulchitsky-cell type I tumors, atypical carcinoids, Kulchitsky-cell type II tumors, small-cell carcinomas, and Kulchitsky-cell type III tumors.

Typical carcinoid tumors are generally endobronchial, and patients may present with cough, pneumonia, hemoptysis, or dyspnea. More peripheral tumors are usually asymptomatic, and atypical carcinoids are frequently peripheral. The carcinoid syndrome often described with gastrointestinal carcinoid tumors only occurs with bronchopulmonary carcinoids in about 3 per cent of patients. When present, the syndrome is characterized by episodes of flushing, diarrhea, and other systemic complaints. Cardiac lesions including pulmonary stenosis, tricuspid insufficiency and, rarely, left sided valvular and endocardial lesions are seen. Peripheral carcinoid tumors may be identified on routine radiographic evaluation. The endobronchial lesions may cause distal atelectasis or pneumonia on chest film. Rarely, hyperinflated lung may occur distal to an area of intermittent bronchial obstruction. Linear tomography or CT may reveal endobronchial lesions, but these studies are most helpful for evaluating nodal involvement, local invasion, and distal parenchymal changes. Further staging should include an examination of the liver and adrenals for evidence of metastases. Bronchoscopy is the diagnostic technique of choice, and some carcinoid tumors may be vascular, and caution during biopsy is recommended.

Surgical resection of carcinoid tumors is the treatment of choice, and the extent of resection is determined by the location of the tumor. Because of the low-grade malignancy of these tumors, sleeve resection with sparing of pulmonary parenchyma has been a recommended technique. Nonetheless, lymph node sampling should be performed to evaluate the possibility of metastases. Atypical carcinoids should be treated with more aggressive resection because of their more malignant behavior. For the rare patient in whom pulmonary function may not permit resection, bronchoscopic removal may be required. The prognosis following surgical removal of typical carcinoids is excellent. A 5-year survival of 95 per cent and a 10-year survival of 90 per cent may be expected. Atypical carcinoids have a worse prognosis, with a 5-year survival of 66 per cent and a 10-year survival of 60 per cent.

Adenoid Cystic Carcinoma

Adenoid cystic carcinomas of the bronchus, or cylindromas, are analogous to the tumors of the same name arising from the salivary and lacrimal glands. These tumors are generally more malignant in behavior than typical carcinoid tumors, and represent approximately 12 per cent of all bronchial adenomas. Like carcinoid tumors, they are found in both children and adults in both sexes. Adenoid cystic carcinomas most often arise in the distal trachea or proximal bronchi, and three histologic patterns have been described. The tubular pattern is the most differentiated type and is characterized by single-lumen tubular units with small nests of cells. The cribriform pattern consists of tumor cells arranged in nests or sheets fenestrated by round and oval spaces. The solid form is the most undifferentiated and consists of large cellular nests with no glandular spaces. The adenoid cystic carcinoma may grow submucosally and can extend around perineural lymphatic spaces along the tracheobronchial wall. Because of this tendency, the full extent of the tumor may be misjudged. Symptoms related to this tumor depend on its location and the degree of luminal involvement. Cough, dyspnea, wheezing, or hemoptysis are the typical symptoms.

The definitive diagnosis of adenoid cystic carcinoma may be made on bronchoscopy. Computed tomography is helpful in evaluating the extent of the tumor, whereas plain chest films are rarely diagnostic. Surgical removal is the treatment of choice in all patients with resectable tumors, and nonresectable tumors may be treated with radiation therapy. Occasionally, laser therapy is necessary to open an obstructed airway. Approximately 75 per cent of adenoid cystic carcinomas have lymph node metastases at the time of exploration. Furthermore, only 60 per cent of these tumors are totally resectable at the time of operation. Nonetheless, long-term survival is possible even in the presence of local or distant spread.

Mucoepidermoid Carcinoma

Mucoepidermoid tumors of the lungs constitute 0.2 per cent of all lung tumors, 1 to 5 per cent of all bronchial adenomas, and occur in patients of all ages and both sexes. They may occur in the trachea or proximal bronchi and are pathologically characterized by the presence of squamous or intermediate elements with intracellular bridges or cytoplasmic membranes. The tumors may be characterized as low grade or high grade based on the degree of mitotic activity, cellular necrosis, and nuclear pleomorphism. Microscopically, these tumors resemble adenosquamous cell lung carcinomas, which occur in the periphery and are usually of the high-grade cell type. Symptoms are related to the location of the tumor and degree of luminal involvement. The diagnosis is best obtained by bronchoscopy, and surgical removal remains the treatment of choice, with radiation therapy being of no benefit. The prognosis is generally good, and patients with low-grade tumors have a 5-year survival approaching 100 per cent with therapy. However, high-grade tumors have a 4-year survival of 66 per cent.

REFERENCES

Attar S, Miller JE, Hankins J, et al: Bronchial adenoma: A review of 51 patients. Ann Thorac Surg 40:126, 1985.
Caldarola VT, Harrison EG, Clagett OT, Schmidt HW: Benign tumors and tumor-like conditions of the trachea and bronchi. Ann Otolaryngol 73:1042, 1964.
Gilbert JJ, Mazzarella LA, Feit LJ: Primary tracheal tumors in the infant and adult. Arch Otolaryngol 58:1, 1953.
Herrera JL: Benign and metastatic tumors of the esophagus. Gastroenterol Clin North Am 20(4):775–789, 1991.
Yellin A, Benfield JR: The Pulmonary Kulchitsky Cell (Neuroendocrine) Cancers: From Carcinoid to Small Cell Carcinomas, vol 9. Chicago, Year Book Medical Publishers, 1985.

IX
Carcinoma of the Lung

THOMAS A. D'AMICO, M.D.   DAVID C. SABISTON, Jr., M.D.

Carcinoma of the lung is the most common cause of death by cancer in both men and women. Smoking is definitely the primary etiologic factor in the pathogenesis of lung cancer. The role of oncogenes in the development of carcinoma of the lung has also been recently described. Despite remarkable advances in the understanding of the biology of lung neoplasms, surgical resection offers the best and only opportunity for cure of lung cancer. Radiation therapy and chemotherapy have attained wide use as the therapy for *small-cell lung carcinoma* (SCLC). Graham performed the first successful one-stage pneumonectomy in 1933 in a patient with squamous cell carcinoma. That patient recovered completely and survived for 25 years thereafter, eventually dying of an unrelated disease, and was free of tumor.

PATHOGENESIS

Understanding the molecular biology and the pathogenesis of carcinoma of the lung is critical to its prevention and treatment. A complete description of the pathogenesis must consider known etiologic factors as well as the genetic events that follow the transformation of bronchial epithelial cells to malignant lung cancer cells. Known etiologic agents include cigarette smoking, exposure to workplace carcinogens, and the presence of chronic obstructive pulmonary disease.

Etiology

Tobacco

Evidence linking cigarette smoking and carcinoma of the lung is abundant. Classic retrospective and prospective studies have established a clear relationship between both the duration and the intensity of cigarette use and the incidence of lung cancer. In a study of over 2000 patients with carcinoma of the lung, only 5 per cent were nonsmokers. In a review of 6071 men 45 years of age or older, 805 had carcinoma of the lung, all of whom were smokers. Auerbach, in a landmark postmortem study, examined the entire tracheobronchial tree in 117 men. In this study, 34 died of carcinoma of the lung, and all were smokers. In the remaining 83 patients, four cytologic changes were evaluated in each histologic section: (1) basal cell hyperplasia, (2) stratification, (3) squamous metaplasia, and (4) carcinoma in situ. Auerbach demonstrated in this group of patients that did not die of carcinoma of the lung that the pathologic changes were more frequent in the group that smoked. Moreover, progressive increases in severity of cytologic transformation correlated with the amount of tobacco use.

Other Carcinogens

Passive smoking, considered to account for 25 per cent of carcinoma of the lung in nonsmokers, may increase the risk of cancer by 35 to 53 per cent among nonsmokers who live with smokers. The presence of chronic obstructive pulmonary disease has also been demonstrated to be a predisposing factor in the development of carcinoma of the lung. Other carcinogens include arsenic, cadmium, chromium, radon, and workplace chemicals, such as chromoethyl ether. Most carcinogens act synergistically with cigarette smoke as etiologic agents in the pathogenesis of carcinoma of the lung.

Molecular Biology

Oncogenes

Lung cancer cells exhibit a large number and type of oncogenes, up to 20 genetic lesions per tumor. Genetic transformations involved in the development of carcinoma of the lung include activation of dominant protooncogenes and the inactivation of recessive ("tumor suppressor") oncogenes. Dominant cellular oncogenes cause cellular transformation through inappropriate activation, which reflects a deregulation of their function following a change in one of the alleles. The genes involved effect growth factors, growth factor receptors, membrane proteins associated with signal transduction, and nuclear proteins involved in transcriptional control. Even dominant oncogenes require the cooperation of more that one oncogene to transform normal cells. Point mutations in the *ras* family of protooncogenes occur in approximately 35 per cent of patients with *non–small-cell lung carcinoma* (NSCLC). The presence of the *ras* mutation is associated with shorter overall survival and disease-free survival compared with patients in whom no *ras* mutation has been identified. These *ras* mutations are found in all non–small-cell histologic types; however, they have not been detected in SCLC. Other studies demonstrate that transfecting mutated *ras* genes into SCLC also changes its phenotype to that suggestive of NSCLC.

Transcriptional activation of nuclear protooncogenes (c-*myc*, N-*myc*, L-*myc*) has also been demonstrated. Small-cell lung tumors with c-*myc*–amplified tumors confer a poorer prognosis compared to other small-cell tumors among patients with advanced-stage SCLC. These studies demonstrate a direct relationship between the expression of a particular dominant oncogene and the phenotype of the lung cancer that develops. Recessive oncogenes are characterized by deletion or translocation of DNA from one of the chromosomes and presumably express a recessive mutation on the remaining chromosome. Mutations of the p53 gene, a tumor suppressor gene that normally codes for a nuclear phosphoprotein required to maintain a transformed (malignant) phenotype, are the most common genetic alteration identified in human cancer. Normal p53 negatively regulates cell growth. Mutated forms stimulate cell division and promote malignancy. Mutations in p53 have been found in nearly all cell lines for patients with SCLC and in approximately 75 per cent of cell lines from patients with NSCLC. There has been no association identified between the presence of p53 mutation and survival.

Restrictive fragment length polymorphism analysis has demonstrated 3p, 11p, and 17p allele loss in many cases of carcinoma of the lung. The most prominent lesion occurs in the 3p21 region. This deletion is found in all histologic types of lung cancer, suggesting either a common requirement for development or an early step in the pathogenesis of lung cancer. Also of interest is the deletion localized to the *rb* locus of chromosome 13. While the DNA abnormalities are important, the abnormalities in mRNA expression are even more impressive: the majority of SCLC have absent or dramatically reduced expression of the *rb* gene product.

These findings raise the possibility of correcting the defect by introducing a normal copy of the appropriate gene into the lung cancer cell.

Cell of Origin

Studies with in vitro cultures of SCLC and NSCLC have shown that after long-term tissue culture, small-cell lung cancer can transform into all the non–small-cell histologies. This transformation is accompanied by a change in growth pattern, tumorigenicity, histology, and enzyme content. These studies suggest a common precursor cell in the development of lung cancer and support clinical observations of the transformation of small-cell lung cancer to that of another histologic type. The concept of a pluripotential stem cell also explains the finding that many lung tumors demonstrate two or more histologic patterns when multiple sections are examined.

PATHOLOGIC ASPECTS

Carcinoma of the lung is a pathologically heterogeneous disease. There are 4 *major* pathologic cell types of lung tumors that arise in bronchial epithelium: (1) small-cell (formerly oat cell) carcinoma, (2) adenocarcinoma, (3) squamous cell carcinoma, and (4) large-cell carcinoma. Owing to the difference in therapy, lung cancer is frequently categorized into two broad subtypes: small-cell carcinoma and non–small-cell carcinoma. SCLC is characterized by more rapid growth, greater likelihood of metastases being present at the time of diagnosis, and increased responsiveness to chemotherapy and radiation therapy. The remaining three cell types, together considered NSCLC, represent 75 to 80 per cent of all lung carcinomas and are often discussed collectively because therapeutic approaches to patients with any of these cell types are identical.

A series of progressive pathologic changes have been observed in malignancies arising from bronchial epithelium, particularly squamous cell carcinoma (Table 1). Basal cell proliferation, the initial event, is followed

TABLE 1.   LUNG CANCER: STAGES IN PATHOGENESIS*

Basal cell proliferation
Hyperplasia of goblet cells
Metaplastic stratification of squamous epithelium
Atypical metaplasia
Carcinoma in situ
Infiltration of cancer through basement membrane
Spread to regional lymph nodes
Hematogenous dissemination

*From Linnoila I: Pathology of non–small-cell lung cancer: New diagnostic approaches. Hematol Oncol Clin North Am 4:1027, 1990, with permission.

by hyperplasia of the mucus-secreting goblet cells, metaplasia of the stratified squamous epithelium, and the development of nuclear atypia. Finally, carcinoma in situ develops, which may be followed by invasion through the basement membrane, regional infiltration of lymph nodes, and hematogenous dissemination.

Non–Small-Cell Carcinoma

The major histologic types of NSCLC in the World Health Organization classification are adenocarcinoma, squamous cell carcinoma, and large-cell carcinoma. Other histologic types include adenosquamous carcinoma, bronchoalveolar carcinoma (a subset of adenocarcinoma), bronchial carcinoids, and bronchial gland tumors. There has been a considerable shift in the incidence of histologic types of NSCLC over recent years—adenocarcinomas have been increasing in frequency, and squamous cell carcinomas have become less common. Many pulmonary malignancies demonstrate more than one pattern of histologic differentiation, suggesting the possibility of a pluripotential stem cell. In addition, the development of neuroendocrine cell hyperplasia, which may represent precursor lesions of SCLC, may also be responsible for the production of regulatory peptides that influence the development of NSCLC.

Adenocarcinoma

The most common cell type is adenocarcinoma, occurring in approximately 50 per cent of patients. Adenocarcinomas are usually peripheral lesions and tend to invade the overlying pleura, but may cause bronchial obstruction by local parenchymal or submucosal invasion. While adenocarcinomas may stain for keratin, they also exhibit mucin production, glandular formation, or papillary structures, varying in differentiation patterns from one microscopic field to another. Adenocarcinomas are subdivided histologically into acinar, papillary, and bronchoalveolar forms. Bronchoalveolar patterns originate from alveolar septa and demonstrate no significant desmoplasia or glandular formation. Bronchoalveolar carcinoma may present in two distinct manners, as a solitary pulmonary nodule or as a diffuse infiltrative process, either localized to a particular segment or generalized.

Squamous Cell Carcinoma

Once the most common cell type, squamous cell carcinoma now represents approximately 30 per cent of all lung cancers. Squamous carcinomas occur centrally; grow toward the mainstem bronchus; and invade bronchial cartilage, pulmonary parenchyma, and

lymph nodes. The epithelium in the normal tracheobronchial tree does not contain squamous epithelium. Progressive histologic changes occur in the bronchial mucosa (Table 1) in the development of squamous cell carcinoma. The premalignant changes in the epithelium identify a squamous cell carcinoma as a primary tumor, as opposed to a metastatic lesion. The characteristic histologic features include intracellular and extracellular keratinization, prominent desmosomes, and bundles of intermediate filaments.

Large-Cell Carcinoma

Large-cell carcinomas, peripheral lesions that are unrelated to bronchi, rapidly invade the parenchyma and tend to metastasize early. The diagnosis of large-cell carcinoma is that of exclusion of other cell types. Large-cell carcinomas exhibit no evidence for glandular or squamous differentiation, and are distinguished from small-cell carcinoma by the presence of abundant cytoplasm, distinct borders, and enlarged nuclei containing prominent nucleoli. However, by electron microscopy, many large-cell carcinomas demonstrate aspects of differentiation into adenocarcinoma, squamous carcinoma, or small-cell carcinoma.

Small-Cell Lung Carcinoma

The histologic features of SCLC are quite distinctive. Within the nucleus, the chromatin is uniformly distributed, the nucleoli are unusually small and indistinct, and mitoses are frequent. The cells, which often contain scant cytoplasm, assume a spindle or fusiform shape, arranged in bundles. An important distinguishing characteristic of SCLC is the presence of cytoplasmic neurosecretory granules on electron microscopy. The liver is a frequent site of metastases of SCLC, affecting 15 to 30 per cent of patients at the time of diagnosis. The bone marrow is another common site of metastatic involvement, occurring in 15 to 25 per cent of patients at initial presentation. Other common sites include the brain, cortical bone, and the peritoneum.

Carcinoids

Bronchopulmonary carcinoids, constituting approximately 2 per cent of all lung tumors, are low-grade neoplasms characterized by neuroendocrine features: the presence of neuorsecretory granules by electron microscopy and the production of peptide hormones. Carcinoids are characterized by cellular growth in solid sheets or in mixed patterns of sheets, cords, nests, and trabeculae. Atypical carcinoid tumors, which demonstrate cellular pleomorphism, frequent mitoses, hyperchromatic nuclei, and scant cytoplasm, confer poor prognosis.

CLINICAL MANIFESTATIONS

Most patients with lung cancer present with symptomatic disease, with only 6 per cent asymptomatic at the time of diagnosis. Symptoms relating to carcinoma of the lung are dependent on the anatomic location of the tumor, extension into surrounding structures, metastatic spread, and the systemic effects of paraneoplastic syndromes.

Chest Symptoms

In the thorax, symptoms may follow endobronchial growth, peripheral growth, or regional spread of the primary tumor. Centrally located lesions are associated with cough, stridor, wheezing, hemoptysis, dyspnea, and chest pain. The most common symptom, occurring in up to 75 per cent of patients, is cough, which follows endobronchial erosion and irritation. Peripheral tumors are associated with chest pain, cough, and dyspnea, owing to pleural and chest wall involvement. Large peripheral tumors may undergo cavitation and present as lung abscesses.

Intrathoracic extension of lung tumors may cause involvement of surrounding structures. Involvement of the recurrent laryngeal nerve may be manifested as hoarseness in up to 8 per cent of patients. Dysphagia, indicating involvement of the esophagus, occurs in 1 to 5 per cent of patients. Local extension of a tumor at the apex of the lung and involving the eighth cervical and first thoracic nerves may result in superior sulcus (Pancoast) tumor syndrome, characterized by shoulder and arm pain. Furthermore, paravertebral extension and sympathetic nerve involvement may cause Horner's syndrome, characterized by enophthalmos, ptosis, meiosis, and ipsilateral anhidrosis.

Malignant Pleural Effusion

The pleura is involved in 60 per cent of patients with adenocarcinoma and 34 per cent of those with squamous cell carcinoma. The development of malignant pleural effusion often results in exacerbation of symptoms of chest pain and shortness of breath. Recurrence after aspiration is a poor prognostic sign.

Superior Vena Caval Syndrome

Tumors occurring on the right side or extensive tumor involvement of right mediastinal lymph nodes may cause superior vena caval syndrome, character-
ized by plethoric appearance; distention of the venous drainage of the arm and neck; and edema of the face, neck, and arms. Obstruction usually progresses over a period of time, allowing the development of collateral venous drainage, detectable on physical examination. The possibility of pericardial effusion and pericardial tamponade must be considered owing to the involvement of the heart and pericardium in 15 to 35 per cent of patients with carcinoma of the lung.

Paraneoplastic Syndromes

Paraneoplastic syndromes, symptoms, or findings that are related to the primary tumor or its metastases by hormonal intermediates may accompany carcinoma of the lung. Systemic manifestations of NSCLC include cachexia, parathyroid-like hormone secretion with hypercalcemia, hypertrophic pulmonary osteoarthropathy, and various neurologic syndromes. Weight loss and anorexia occur in up to one third of patients. Noncachectic patients, however, also demonstrate increases in protein turnover, glucose production, and muscular catabolism. Paraneoplastic syndromes are frequently associated with SCLC, more often present at the time of diagnosis than in patients with NSCLC. In addition to weight loss, anorexia, and neuromyopathies, paraneoplastic syndromes may follow tumor elaboration of antidiuretic hormone, adrenocorticotropin, calcitonin, or parathyroid hormone.

DIAGNOSIS AND STAGING

The presence of a solitary pulmonary nodule is common, often leading to the diagnosis of carcinoma of the lung. The differential diagnosis of these lesions also includes tuberculoma, histoplasmoma, blastomycoma, coccidiodomycoma, metastatic carcinoma, and benign pulmonary tumors. The relationship of age to the incidence of malignancy in a solitary pulmonary nodule is shown in Table 2. Staging of lung cancer by thoracic oncologists is essential for estimating prognosis, selecting treatment, and reporting results.

TABLE 2.   INCIDENCE OF MALIGNANCY IN SOLITARY PULMONARY NODULES RELATED TO AGE*

Age (Years)	Malignant
35–44	15%
45–49	26%
50–59	41%
60–69	50%
70–79	70%

*From Sabiston DC Jr: Carcinoma of the Lung. In Sabiston DC Jr, and Spencer FC (eds): Surgery of the Chest, ed 5. Philadelphia, WB Saunders Company, 1990, with permission.

Diagnostic Techniques

The primary objective in the diagnosis and staging of carcinoma of the lung is to identify patients who are candidates to undergo thoracotomy for curative pulmonary resection. A complete history and physical examination are performed, with particular attention to possible manifestations of the primary tumor, regional invasion, distant metastases, and paraneoplastic syndromes. Most importantly, current chest radiographs are reviewed and compared to previous studies.

Chest Films

In the assessment of a patient with carcinoma of the lung, the chest radiograph usually demonstrates a mass, although a pneumonic infiltrate, a pleural effusion, or an elevated diaphragm may also be present. A solitary pulmonary nodule, which may be either a smooth-bordered (coin shaped) lesion or an irregular defect, is the classic radiographic presentation of carcinoma of the lung. Collapse of a pulmonary segment or a lobe distal to an obstructing endobronchial lesion may be manifested as atelectasis. Gross nodal involvement is frequently evident as well. The chest film may also be used to estimate doubling time of the nodule, by comparing its size on previous and recent films. If the doubling time is less than 1 month, the etiology of the nodule is likely to be infectious; if the doubling time is greater than 16 months, it is likely to be benign; and if the doubling time is intermediate between 1 and 16 months, the nodule is more likely to be malignant.

Bronchoscopy

Flexible fiberoptic bronchoscopy is an invaluable adjunct in the diagnosis of carcinoma of the lung. Bronchial biopsy, brushings, washings, and transbronchial aspiration are utilized to establish the diagnosis of malignancy in a majority of cases. Bronchial biopsy is more sensitive than bronchial washing and brushing, especially in patients with SCLC, owing to its submucosal location. When the tumor is bronchoscopically visible, the yield for washings and brushings is approximately 75 per cent, and for biopsy is approximately 85 per cent, for a total yield of 94 per cent. In contrast, bronchoscopy with brushings and washings for nonvisible tumors has a yield of 50 per cent, and bronchoscopy with biopsy has a yield of 60 per cent. The typing accuracy for bronchoscopic biopsy and cytology is only 66 per cent, with most failures occurring with adenocarcinoma and large-cell carcinoma.

Transthoracic Needle Aspiration

Percutaneous aspiration, which may be performed using fluoroscopic, sonographic, or computed tomographic guidance, is useful in the diagnosis of lesions that are not visualized by bronchoscopy. Among two series (3937 patients), correct diagnosis was obtained in 91 per cent of patients, with a false-positive rate of 2.4 per cent, and a false-negative rate of 23 per cent. The indications for transthoracic needle aspiration include pulmonary lesions in patients who are poor candidates for thoracotomy yet require definitive diagnosis, a new pulmonary lesion in a patient with a history of prior malignancy, and a lung mass that is suspicious for small-cell carcinoma.

Computed Tomography

Computed tomography (CT) of the chest is useful in the evaluation of the primary tumor, in assessment of regional lymph node involvement, and in the detection of mediastinal metastases. Computed tomography scans should include the apices of the thorax superiorly and extend inferiorly to include the liver and the adrenal glands. When the primary lesion is centrally located or advanced in size, CT is invaluable in assessing margins and dimensions. In addition to evaluation of the primary tumor, CT is useful in assessing involvement of hilar and mediastinal lymph nodes. It is generally accepted that a maximal diameter of 10 mm is acceptable for considering hilar and mediastinal nodes to be uninvolved, suggesting operability. However, lymph nodes determined by CT scan to be enlarged will contain metastatic tumor in only 70 per cent of cases. Thus, suspected inoperability on the basis of a positive CT scan should be confirmed by direct biopsy, unless evidence is overwhelming. Patients without mediastinal lymphadenopathy on CT who are otherwise operative candidates may proceed to thoracotomy. The false-negative rate with these patients is only 5 per cent.

Magnetic Resonance Imaging

Magnetic resonance imaging (MRI) has also been utilized in the staging of carcinoma of the lung. Magnetic resonance imaging differentiates vascular from solid structures and demonstrates parenchymal, hilar, and mediastinal anatomy in both coronal and sagittal planes without the use of contrast agents or ionizing radiation. Magnetic resonance imaging is limited by long scanning times, motion artifacts, and inferior spatial resolution. Comparative studies of CT and MRI in the evaluation of the primary tumor and nodal involvement demonstrate a slight advantage to CT. The current role for MRI in the staging of carcinoma of

TABLE 3. INTERNATIONAL TNM STAGING SYSTEM FOR LUNG CANCER*

Tumor (T)	
TX	Occult carcinoma (malignant cells in sputum or bronchial washings but tumor not visualized by imaging studies or bronchoscopy)
T1	Tumor ≤3 cm in greatest diameter, surrounded by lung or visceral pleura, but not proximal to a lobar bronchus
T2	Tumor ≥3 cm in diameter, or with involvement of main bronchus at least 2 cm distal to carina, or with visceral pleural invasion, or with associated atelectasis or obstructive pneumonitis extending to the hilar region but not involving the entire lung
T3	Tumor invading chest wall, diaphragm, mediastinal pleura, or parietal pericardium; or tumor in main bronchus within 2 cm of, but not invading, carina; or atelectasis of obstructive pneumonitis of the entire lung
T4	Tumor invading mediastinum, heart, great vessels, trachea, esophagus, vertebral body, or carcina; or ipsilateral malignant pleural effusion
Nodes (N)	
N0	No regional lymph node metastases
N1	Metastases to ipsilateral peribronchial or hilar nodes
N2	Metastases to ipsilateral mediastinal or subcarinal nodes
N3	Metastases to contralateral mediastinal or hilar, or to any scalene or supraclavicular nodes
Distant Metastases (M)	
M0	No distant metastases
M1	Distant metastases

*From Mountain CF: A new international staging system for lung cancer. Chest 89:225S, 1986, with permission.

the lung includes confirmation of spinal cord involvement and nodal staging in patients in whom the use of contrast agents is contraindicated.

Mediastinoscopy

The role of mediastinoscopy in the diagnosis and staging of carcinoma of the lung is controversial. In patients in whom noninvasive staging demonstrates evidence for mediastinal nodal involvement, mediastinoscopy documents involvement in approximately 70 per cent. Mediastinoscopy and biopsy is recommended for patients whose CT scan demonstrates mediastinal lymph nodes greater than 10 mm in diameter, in order to confirm inoperability. However, posterior subcarinal, pericardial, periesophageal, and para-aortic lymph nodes are inaccessible by this technique. Left parasternal mediastinoscopy (Chamberlain procedure) is used for biopsy of enlarged nodes in these areas in some patients with carcinoma of the lung.

Staging of Non–Small-Cell Carcinoma

The TNM staging system, most recently updated by the American Joint Committee on Cancer (AJCC) in 1989, provides a consistent, reproducible description of the anatomic extent of disease at the time of diagnosis. In the TNM system, T represents the primary tumor, and numerical suffixes describe increasing size or involvement; N represents regional lymph nodes with suffixes to describe levels of involvement; and M represents the presence or absence of distant metastases. The TNM categories are illustrated in Table 3. The TNM subsets are subsequently grouped in a

number of stages of disease, to identify groups of patients with similar prognosis and therapy (Table 4 and Fig. 1). The value of the staging system in estimating prognosis is demonstrated by the 5-year survival statistics, illustrated in Table 5.

Staging of Small-Cell Carcinoma

Owing to the tendency for small-cell carcinoma to present with widespread metastases at the time of diagnosis, the TNM staging system has not proved to be prognostically useful. Even patients who present with small primary tumors and no evidence of nodal disease usually have distant metastases. Currently, most thoracic oncologists utilize a staging system that divides patients into two major groups: those with *limited* disease and those with *extensive* disease. Limited disease is considered to be confined to the hemithorax, with or without ipsilateral, mediastinal, hilar, or supraclavicular lymph nodes, and no detectable distant metastases. Extensive disease is characterized by the

TABLE 4. STAGE GROUPINGS FOR CARCINOMA OF THE LUNG*

Occult	TX	N0	M0
Stage I	T1–2	N0	M0
Stage II	T1–2	N1	M0
Stage IIIA	T3	N0–1	M0
	T1–3	N2	M0
Stage IIIB	T4	N0–2	M0
	T1–4	N3	M0
Stage IV	Any T	Any N	M1

*From Mountain CF: A new international staging system for lung cancer. Chest 89:225S, 1986, with permission.

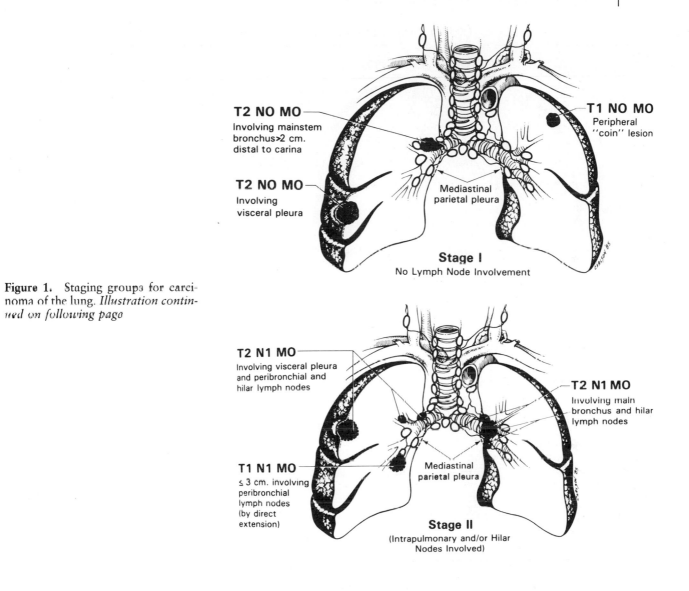

T2 NO MO
Involving mainstem bronchus>2 cm. distal to carina

T2 NO MO
Involving visceral pleura

T1 NO MO
Peripheral "coin" lesion

Mediastinal parietal pleura

Stage I
No Lymph Node Involvement

T2 N1 MO
Involving visceral pleura and peribronchial and hilar lymph nodes

T2 N1 MO
Involving main bronchus and hilar lymph nodes

T1 N1 MO
≤ 3 cm. involving peribronchial lymph nodes (by direct extension)

Mediastinal parietal pleura

Stage II
(Intrapulmonary and/or Hilar Nodes Involved)

Figure 1. Staging groups for carcinoma of the lung. *Illustration continued on following page*

presence of involvement of the contralateral thorax or distant metastases.

SURGICAL MANAGEMENT OF NON–SMALL-CELL CARCINOMA OF THE LUNG

Surgical resection is the standard treatment of all patients with stage I or stage II disease. In addition, a subset of patients with stage III disease, those who are stage IIIA, have been demonstrated to have improved outcome with surgical resection. Every solitary pulmonary nodule should be resected unless the patient's condition contraindicates surgery or the lesion is known to be benign.

Determination of Operability

Criteria for operability must include the medical risk of thoracotomy as well as the risk of removal of the requisite pulmonary tissue. The degree of cardiopulmonary disease, usually a consequence of tobacco use, represents the most significant medical factor in determining the operability and the major cause of postoperative morbidity and mortality. Pulmonary function tests and analysis of arterial blood gases are used to determine the feasibility of pulmonary resection. In particular, most surgeons recognize that patients require a minimal forced expiratory volume at 1 second (FEV_1) of 0.8 to 1.0 L. Estimation of postoperative FEV_1 is based on calculation of preoperative FEV_1 and projected resection of pulmonary paren-

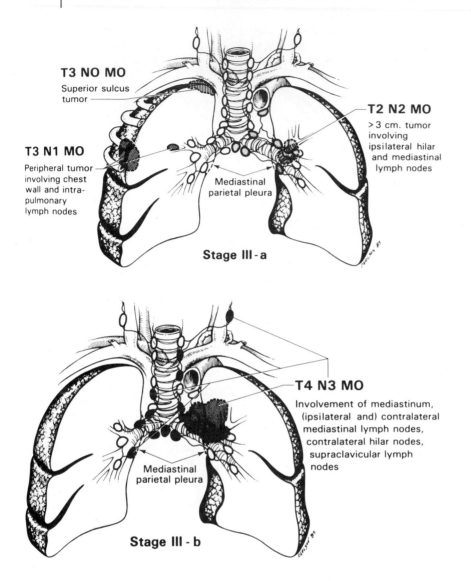

Figure 1. *Continued.* Staging groups for carcinoma of the lung. (From Mountain CF: A new international staging system for lung cancer. Chest *89:*225S, 1986).

chyma. Patients are excluded from surgical therapy if estimated postoperative FEV_1 values fall below the minimum acceptable values.

Surgical Procedures

Intraoperative evaluation of the extent of the tumor, in conjunction with the cardiopulmonary status of the patient, determines the particular surgical procedure employed. Complete resection of the tumor and all grossly involved regional bronchial and mediastinal lymph nodes, including en bloc resection of adjacent structures involved by direct extension of the primary tumor (such as chest wall and pericardium), is undertaken when feasible. Incomplete resection or resection that would leave a patient with an inadequate functional pulmonary reserve should not be performed.

Standard surgical procedures employed in the management of carcinoma of the lung include pneumonectomy, bilobectomy, lobectomy, segmentectomy, and wedge resection. The procedure selected must provide removal of the entire tumor, with adequate margins, while preserving the maximum amount of functional

TABLE 5. FIVE-YEAR SURVIVAL IN NON–SMALL-CELL CARCINOMA ACCORDING TO STAGE*

Stage I	66.7%
Stage II	43.6%
Stage IIIA	22.4%
Stage IIIB	5.4%
Stage IV	5.9%

*From Naruke T, Goya T, Tsuchiya R, et al: Prognosis and survival in resected lung carcinoma based on the new international staging system for lung cancer. J Thorac Cardiovasc Surg 96:440, 1988, with permission.

lung tissue. Posterior thoracotomy, entering the thorax in the fifth or sixth intercostal space, provides adequate exposure in most patients. At thoracotomy, a systematic lymph node dissection is undertaken to ascertain that no hilar or mediastinal metastases are present. Pneumonectomy is usually required for complete removal of lesions involving the main bronchus. In some cases, however, to preserve functional parenchyma, sleeve lobectomy is performed: removal of a portion of the main bronchus or distal trachea and subsequent reanastomosis to more distal uninvolved bronchus to reestablish tracheobronchial continuity. Lobectomy is required for complete resection of most lesions; however, in patients with peripheral stage I or selected stage II (T1,N1) disease, wedge resection may be performed, with no difference in outcome. For all pulmonary resections, the automatic stapling device is routinely employed, reducing the postoperative complication of bronchopleural fistula.

Results of Surgical Resection

Stage I and Stage II

Patients with stage I carcinoma of the lung can expect 3- and 5-year survival rates of approximately 85 and 65 per cent, respectively. The most favorable group of stage I patients, those with T1, N0 disease, experience 5-year survival rates of 75 per cent. Patients with stage II disease experience 5-year survival rates of 40 to 50 per cent. The best survival rates are in patients with T1,N1 disease, with only a single node involved. The rate of recurrence is greater than 50 per cent and most recurrences are distant metastases.

Stage IIIA

Locally advanced carcinoma of the lung, in which the primary tumor is proximal or has invaded adjacent structures or in which mediastinal nodes are involved, is associated with a relatively poor prognosis. However, when surgical resection achieves total removal of the primary tumor and involved lymph nodes, there is a reasonable chance for cure. Patients with stage IIIA carcinoma of the lung who undergo complete resection can expect a 5-year survival of approximately 40 per cent. In the subset of patients with N2 disease, 5-year survival is approximately 30 per cent. Postoperative irradiation does not appear to improve overall survival, although it has improved local control.

Superior Sulcus Tumor

The superior sulcus tumor is a carcinoma of the lung of any histologic subtype, arising at the apex of the upper lobes in the superior sulcus, that may invade the pleura, the brachial plexus, the sympathetic chains, adjacent ribs, or vertebral bodies. Patients with superior sulcus tumor should receive preoperative radiation therapy to the primary tumor, the mediastinum, and the supraclavicular region. Four weeks later, en bloc resection of the lung, chest wall, and mediastinal lymph nodes is performed. Despite the invasive nature of these tumors, 5-year survival of 25 to 30 per cent is expected in patients treated with this regimen.

Multiple Primary Carcinomas of the Lung

In view of the prevalence of carcinoma of the lung in the general population, multiple primary pulmonary malignancies are rare, affecting 1.6 to 3.0 per cent of all patients with lung cancer, and 10 to 25 per cent of those who survive more than 3 years. The most likely explanation is that the overall survival of patients with carcinoma of the lung is poor, so that there may not be enough time for a second primary tumor to develop. Second primary lung carcinomas may be termed synchronous or metachronous. Metachronous lesions are distinguished from metastatic cancer by the following criteria: (1) tumors of different histology; and (2) tumors of the same histology (a) with a time interval of at least 2 years, or (b) demonstrated to arise from carcinoma in situ, or (c) anatomically separate in which lymphatic involvement and extrapulmonary involvement is excluded. In patients in whom a second primary carcinoma of the lung develops, limited surgical resection offers the best treatment, being associated with low operative mortality and prolonged survival. Many studies have shown that patients who appear to be disease free after 5 years may develop second primary lesions, and close lifelong follow-up is required for patients who have undergone resection for carcinoma of the lung.

Surgical Morbidity and Mortality

Optimization of pulmonary status preoperatively and meticulous postoperative care in patients with borderline cardiopulmonary function contribute to minimizing postoperative morbidity and mortality in those who undergo pulmonary resection for carcinoma of the lung. Atelectasis, the most common postoperative complication, is usually managed successfully with postural drainage, chest physiotherapy, and bronchodilators. Failure to clear secretions may progress to lobar collapse, requiring therapeutic bronchoscopy. Air leaks present after pulmonary resection usually resolve spontaneously. Persistence after 7 days may be due to a bronchopleural fistula, which can require surgical exploration. Infection (pneumonia, empyema, sepsis) after thoracotomy is rare but should be aggressively managed. The Lung Cancer Study Group, in a series of 2220 pulmonary resections, has reported an overall 30-day mortality of 3.7 per cent. Mortality increased with the extent of resection: 1.4 per cent for wedge resection or segmentectomy, 2.9 per cent for lobectomy, and 6.2 per cent for pneumonectomy.

ADJUNCTIVE THERAPY IN NON–SMALL-CELL CARCINOMA OF THE LUNG

Radiotherapy

Definitive Radiotherapy

Thoracic irradiation is potentially curative in patients with locoregionally confined disease who are not candidates for surgical resection owing to anatomic unresectability, medical contraindications, or patient refusal. Patients with stage I or II disease should undergo thoracotomy for pulmonary resection whenever possible. Radiotherapy for cure is reserved for patients with stage IIIB disease, selected patients with stage IIIA disease, and patients with medical contraindications to thoracotomy. Important considerations to the application of radiotherapy include tumor extent, volume of normal tissue, and cardiopulmonary reserve. Curative radiotherapy is limited to cases in which the entire tumor volume may be treated with an adequate dosage, with acceptable toxicity. Contraindications to definitive radiotherapy include malignant pleural effusion, distant metastases, inadequate pulmonary reserve, or active pulmonary infection. Current recommendations for definitive irradiation specify conventional fractionation of 200 cGy administered daily, 5 days per week for 6 weeks, for a total of 6000 cGy. Alternatively, split-course irradiation, employing a 3-week interruption in the treatment schedule, allows for better patient tolerance and integration of chemotherapy. Tumor regression, defined as 50 per cent or greater reduction in tumor mass as assessed by the chest radiograph, is accomplished in 50 to 60 per cent of patients who receive radiotherapy for cure. Complete regression is achieved in 20 to 25 per cent of patients. Survival statistics for definitive radiotherapy vary with the clinical stage of the disease. Patients with stage I or II disease who undergo definitive irradiation experience 5-year survival rates of 15 to 20 per cent. For stage III disease, 5-year survival rates of 3 to 10 per cent have been reported, and median survival in most studies ranges from 9 to 12 months.

Adjuvant Radiotherapy

Radiation therapy is an effective adjuvant treatment in many patients with carcinoma of the lung. In patients with squamous cell carcinoma, the first site of recurrence is frequently local. Adjuvant radiotherapy, applied to patients with completely resected stage II or stage III NSCLC, has been shown to decrease local recurrence, but has no significant effect on survival. However, postoperative irradiation may provide a survival advantage in patients who have resection and are found to have metastases to hilar or mediastinal lymph nodes. Thus, the purpose of adjuvant radiotherapy is the prevention of local tumor recurrence, especially when lymph node sampling of the mediastinum at thoracotomy, is incomplete.

Palliative Radiotherapy

Symptoms of cough, chest pain, and dyspnea can be relieved in 60 to 80 per cent of patients, and the clinical signs and symptoms associated with the superior vena caval syndrome are alleviated even more consistently.

Chemotherapy

Approximately 60 per cent of patients with NSCLC have distant metastases at the time of initial diagnosis. Among the patients with apparently resectable disease, 5 per cent are found at operation to have regional spread. The majority of the remainder later prove to have systemic disease. Thus, effective chemotherapy would dramatically improve survival in patients with NSCLC. Chemotherapy has been shown to be only marginally efficacious for the treatment of NSCLC. In contrast to chemotherapy for SCLC, in which many agents have been demonstrated to provide response rates up to 80 per cent, chemotherapy in NSCLC induces tumor regression in a minority of patients.

Despite the limited activity of single chemotherapeutic agents, combinations of agents have been reported to yield response rates of 20 to 50 per cent. Combination chemotherapeutic regimens, most of which include cisplatin and a vinca alkaloid or cisplatin and etoposide, have attained the highest objective response rates. Nevertheless, the clinical value of combination chemotherapy in palliating symptoms or prolonging survival has not been established. Prospective, randomized trials demonstrate that most combination chemotherapeutic regimens containing cisplatin are effective in patients with more advanced resectable disease. Patients with stage IIIA carcinoma of the lung had prolonged recurrence-free survival and overall survival when treated with chemotherapy after complete resection. Patients with stage I or stage II disease did not benefit from chemotherapy following resection.

The treatment of unresectable NSCLC, often complicated by large tumor burden and poor patient performance status, is largely unsuccessful, owing to poor response rates to chemotherapy. Nevertheless, selected patients should be offered the option of treatment with combination chemotherapy. Candidates for chemotherapy include patients with good performance status, minimal weight loss, and minimal bulk disease. Recently, considerable effort has been directed toward the evaluation of preoperative therapy consisting of chemotherapy alone or chemotherapy in combination with radiation therapy, in order to improve survival in marginally resectable patients and to allow resection to be performed in categorically unresectable patients.

MANAGEMENT OF SMALL-CELL CARCINOMA OF THE LUNG

SCLC, more than other solid tumors, behaves as a systemic disease, and the natural history is characterized by a relentlessly progressive course. Locoregional therapy directed toward the primary tumor is ineffective in prolonging survival because the majority of patients present with distant metastases or rapidly relapse with metastatic disease. Multimodal therapy including effective chemotherapy is therefore required for both locoregional control and systemic treatment of SCLC. The goals of therapy are to prolong survival and to alleviate symptoms, while minimizing treatment-associated toxicity. Despite encouraging response rates to aggressive combination chemotherapy, the 2-year survival rate is only 10 per cent.

Chemotherapy

Multiple chemotherapeutic agents are effective in the treatment of SCLC. Cyclophosphamide, an alkylating agent, is the most effective single agent and is commonly employed. Cyclophosphamide achieves a major response rate of up to 40 per cent, and approximately 5 per cent of patients achieve complete remission. Carmustine (BCNU) and lomustine (CCNU), nitrosureas, are also active, achieving response rates of 20 to 30 per cent. Vincristine and vinblastine both have activity as single agents. Vinca alkaloids represent the class of drugs most frequently included in combination chemotherapy, owing to the minor toxicity profile. Etoposide, doxorubicin, and methotrexate are often used in combination regimens. High growth fraction, rapid dissemination, and development of resistance to chemotherapy are problems that have not been overcome. Response

rates of 80 per cent can be achieved for both limited and extensive stages of SCLC. A complete response is achieved in up to 50 per cent of patients with limited disease and in 20 per cent of patients with extensive disease. For patients with limited disease, median survival is greater than 12 months and survival beyond 5 years is attained in 10 to 20 per cent of patients. For patients with extensive disease, median survival is 8 months and survival beyond 5 years is attained in 3 to 5 per cent.

Radiation Therapy

The adjuvant use of radiotherapy in SCLC is being examined in numerous clinical trials. In patients with limited disease, a 5 to 15 per cent improvement in disease-free survival at 2 years has been demonstrated when radiation therapy is added to combination chemotherapy, as well as an increased complete response rate. However, there is no clear survival advantage for patients receiving chemotherapy and radiation therapy, as opposed to chemotherapy alone.

Surgical Resection

Conventional management of SCLC, combination chemotherapy and radiation therapy, can be curative in up to 20 per cent of patients with limited disease at 5 years. With conventional therapy, up to 30 per cent of recurrences are recognized at the primary site, illustrating failure of chemotherapy and radiation therapy to achieve adequate local control. In most surgical series, the rate of recurrence at the primary site is approximately 10 per cent. Thus, complete resection in patients with limited disease may improve local control. Patients subjected to surgical management for SCLC should undergo complete resection, if possible, followed by postoperative chemotherapy and radiation therapy.

Clinical Management of Small-Cell Carcinoma of the Lung

The primary goals in the management of a patient with SCLC are to prolong survival, improve disease-free survival, alleviate symptoms, minimize treatment-associated toxicity, and provide an estimate of prognosis. After ascertaining the histologic diagnosis of SCLC, staging is performed, including thorough neurologic examination and CT evaluation of the chest, abdomen, and brain. For most patients with limited-stage disease, treatment is initiated with six cycles of combination chemotherapy (such as cisplatin/etoposide or cyclophosphamide/doxorubicin/vincristine).

Thoracic radiotherapy is usually employed after three initial cycles of chemotherapy and continued for 4 weeks. Thoracotomy for resection is recommended in patients with stage I SCLC, followed by six cycles of adjuvant chemotherapy. Complete responders are offered prophylactic cranial irradiation. For patients with extensive-stage disease, six cycles of chemotherapy are administered. Therapy for local control is not employed; quality-of-life issues are paramount. Complete responders receive prophylactic cranial irradiation.

REFERENCES

Goodman GE, Livingston RB: Small cell lung cancer. Curr Probl Cancer *13*:1–54, 1989.
Holmes EC: Postoperative chemotherapy for non-small cell lung cancer. Chest *103*:30S, 1993.
Ihde DC, Minna JD: Non-small cell lung cancer. Curr Probl Cancer *15*:61–104, 1991.
Linnoila I: Pathology of non-small cell lung cancer: New diagnostic approaches. Hematol Oncol Clin North Am *4*:1027, 1990.
Sabiston DC Jr: Carcinoma of the lung. *In* Sabiston DC Jr, Spencer FC (eds): Surgery of the Chest, ed 5. Philadelphia, WB Saunders Company, 1990.

X
Thoracic Outlet Syndrome

DAVID B. ROOS, M.D.

The *thoracic outlet syndromes* (TOS) consist of neurovascular symptoms that affect the neck, shoulder, arm, and hand, and are caused by abnormal musculoskeletal tissue compression and irritation of the brachial plexus, subclavian artery, and vein, as these structures traverse the scalene triangle, the thoracic outlet, and the costoclavicular space to supply the upper extremity. The outlet syndromes are divided into three categories: neurologic, venous, and arterial, depending on which of the major structures is predominantly affected by congenital or developmental anomalies of the ribs and scalene muscles. About 96 per cent of patients with TOS have the *neurologic* type, which usually affects patients from their teen years to age 50, with incidence in women predominating 3:1. About 3 per cent are the *venous* type, which is more common in men because of their more strenuous activities in work and sports that contribute to unusual compression of the subclavian vein as it passes through the anterior aperture of the thoracic outlet. The *arterial* type of TOS occurs in only 0.5 to 1 per cent, but it is the most serious and difficult to manage. It occurs in two distinct age groups: in young adults due to external compression of the subclavian artery by a cervical rib (Fig. 1), and in older patients in whom localized degenerative changes of the artery occur from abnormal compression in the posterior compartment of the outlet. The gender incidence is about equal.

ETIOLOGY

Patients who develop thoracic outlet syndromes have underlying congenital anomalies that make them *anatomically susceptible* to develop neurovascular symptoms arising from the thoracic outlet. The most obvious anomaly is a *cervical rib*, which occurs in 0.5 per cent of the population and, again, is three times more common in women. A second bone anomaly associated with TOS is an *elongated transverse process of the C7 vertebra*. An incomplete cervical rib and an elongated C7 process always have a taut fibrous band attaching the tip of the rib or process to the middle third of the first rib. These bands pass under the T1

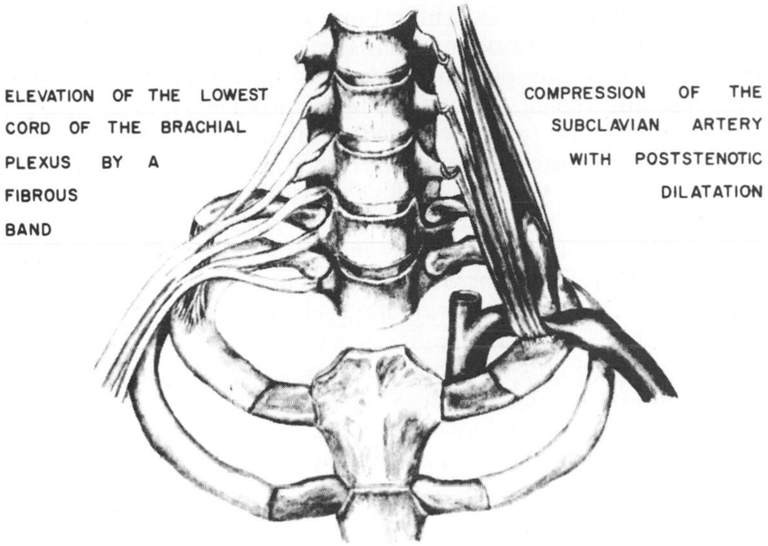

Figure 1. Neurovascular compression due to cervical rib. Schematic illustration of the anatomic relation of a short cervical rib on the right side with *type 1* congenital fibrous band that lies under the brachial plexus. (From Rutherford RB: Vascular Surgery, ed 3, vol 1. Philadelphia, WB Saunders Company, 1989, p 859, with permission.)

ELEVATION OF THE LOWEST CORD OF THE BRACHIAL PLEXUS BY A FIBROUS BAND

COMPRESSION OF THE SUBCLAVIAN ARTERY WITH POSTSTENOTIC DILATATION

nerve and lower trunk of the brachial plexus (Fig. 1). Much more common than the bone anomalies, however, are abnormal *fibromuscular bands* related to the anterior and middle scalene muscles that impinge on the nerves of the brachial plexus or subclavian artery and vein. These anomalies, found in one third of cadaver dissections, are less well appreciated, as they do not show on radiologic studies but are seen clearly during operative procedures. Ten such anomalies in the thoracic outlet at the first rib level and seven anomalies involving the upper nerves of the plexus, C5, C6, and C7 in the neck have been described.

All patients who develop the venous type of TOS, either nonthrombotic intermittent venous congestion of the arm or acute thrombosis of the subclavian-axillary vein, have congenital anomalies compressing the subclavian vein. The anterior scalene muscle usually is found attached farther forward on the first rib than normal, and the subclavius muscle tendon has a much broader insertion on the first rib anterior to and under the vein. These two anomalies may occlude the subclavian vein with elevation of the arm when the muscles contract. Strenuous exertion and lifting produce a strong Valsalva effect that causes slowing or even stopping of venous return from the arm when arterial inflow increases from strenuous effort. Combined with abnormal venous compression in the outlet, such exertion may lead to clotting of the vein, the so-called effort-vein thrombosis or Paget-Schroetter syndrome. Other causes of subclavian-axillary vein thrombosis may be secondary to indwelling catheters from central venous lines or pacemakers, intravenous infusion of irritating medication and radiologic dye, and abnormal coagulation caused by familial or malignancy coa-

gulopathies. These conditions are unrelated to congenital anomalies and differ in etiology and, therefore, in treatment from the *effort-vein thrombosis*. They are not associated with TOS and do not require surgical treatment.

Compression of the subclavian artery severe enough to cause symptoms is usually caused by a cervical rib impinging against the artery, and is aggravated by costoclavicular compression with elevation of the arm. Less commonly, arterial compression may be secondary to callous formation of a fractured clavicle or first rib or by a hypoplastic first rib. These bone anomalies may narrow the lumen of the artery, thus increasing the speed of blood flow through the stenotic segment. When the blood ejects from the restricted area into the normal-sized lumen beyond the cervical rib, blood flow suddenly slows causing turbulence, which increases the lateral pressure of blood against the vessel wall according to the Bernoulli effect. This may cause stretching and degenerative changes of the intima and muscularis, leading to poststenotic dilatation of the artery, perhaps progressing into an aneurysm (Fig. 1). The turbulent blood flow also causes microfissures of the intima, causing platelet deposition, which may progress to mural thrombi. These may dislodge intermittently into the bloodstream causing peripheral emboli and occlusion of the digital vessels of the fingers or larger vessels of the arm and hand.

SYMPTOMS

Symptoms may develop spontaneously, either gradually or suddenly, but in most patients, they are directly related to trauma. The trauma can be chronic repetitive strain from occupations that require use of the arms in raised positions, such as hairdressing, painting, and typing. More commonly, however, it is an acute jerking injury to the neck and shoulders, as in falling on the shoulder or outstretched hand or suffering an acute hyperextension/flexion strain injury of the neck, as in auto accidents. Such injuries cause chronic spasm of neck muscles, and even changes at the cellular level with increased fibrosis and a change from the usual type II fast-twitch muscle fibers to predominant type I slow-twitch fibers, which are in tonic contraction in injured scalene muscles. Thus the altered and contracting scalenes tug, compress, and irritate the nerves of the brachial plexus causing symptoms that spread to the shoulders, upper chest, and down the arms. The neurologic symptoms may be categorized as pain, paresthesias, and paresis. They are usually intermittent, unlike the more persistent though similar complaints caused by cervical disk or carpal tunnel syndromes, because in TOS the compression of the brachial plexus varies with arm activities and positions. Pain is the predominant symptom for which the patient seeks medical attention, although numbness, tingling, weakness, and discoordination of the hand are usually present as well. The pain is a deep aching discomfort in the neck, back of the shoulder, and through the arm interspersed with sharp shooting sensations, often worse at rest than during active use of the extremity.

The pain is described in two different patterns, depending on which nerves of the brachial plexus are most affected (Fig. 2). If the upper nerves, C5, C6, and C7, are especially involved, from anomalies of the scalene muscles and even the plexus itself, the patient feels pain in the front and side of the neck from the clavicle to the ear and mandible, and sometimes through the face up to the temple. It radiates anteriorly into the upper chest and posteriorly into the periscapular region of the rhomboid muscles, along the trapezius ridge and down the *outer* arm, through a *radial* nerve distribution into the forearm, and at times toward the dorsum of the thumb and index fingers. This pattern may simulate the pain and paresthesia description in a patient with a C5–C6 herniated disc.

The pattern of pain emanating from the lower nerves of the brachial plexus, C8 and T1, is quite different. Pain is felt above and below the clavicle, on the back of the shoulder, and from the axilla through the triceps area and inner arm, elbow, and forearm to the ring and small fingers in a typical *ulnar* nerve distribution. As C8 and T1 also contribute to the median nerve as well, the symptoms may spread through the volar forearm to the wrist and into the palm. Occasionally the pain may spread into the upper anterior chest, simulating cardiac angina. Other prominent neurologic symptoms consist of dysesthesias with numbness, tingling, burning, and cold sensation of the hand and fingers. Although these sensations may vary in different patients, they are usually consistent in each patient, with the ulnar nerve involvement being the most common.

As the syndrome progresses, paresis develops with heavy, weak sensation of the entire upper limb and gradual loss of dexterity of the fingers. Muscle atrophy is rare but may involve the intrinsic hand muscles of the interossei, thenar, and hypothenar eminences. Muscle contraction headaches are common in the neurologic type of TOS patient, and they usually radiate up from the back of the neck into the occipital or hemicranial area on the ipsilateral side of the TOS. Patients who have had both report that these headaches may be even more severe than migraine headaches. The differences between the two types of headache are that those associated with TOS are not accompanied by an aura. They may be associated with nausea, but usually not vomiting, they are not relieved by migraine medication, and they may last for days rather than hours, such as occurs with a typical migraine. In some patients, they are the predominant presenting symptom of TOS with the shoulder, arm, and hand symptoms secondary in severity and disability. Their association with TOS is suggested when they regularly occur with an exacerbation of the shoulder, arm, and hand symptoms, and this association is proven when they are relieved by surgical decompression of the brachial plexus.

The venous symptoms of TOS are caused by intermittent, positional occlusion or complete thrombosis of the subclavian vein causing venous congestion of the arm and hand. The patient complains of a heavy, achy, discolored extremity. If symptoms vary, the vein may be severely compressed, but not thrombosed. If symptoms are constant, the subclavian and possibly the axillary vein are clotted. Symptoms worsen with any use of the arm, as the arterial blood flow to the extremity increases with exercise demand, but venous return is blocked producing venous engorgement of the entire extremity. Severe compression of the subclavian artery causes pallor, fatigue, claudication (lameness), and coolness of the arm and hand from ischemia. These symptoms are exaggerated with elevation of the arm, which increases the costoclavicular compression of the artery, and with use of the arm, which causes increased arterial demand that is prevented by the arterial occlusion.

DIAGNOSIS

The diagnosis of TOS may be difficult because of the various symptoms that develop from different lev-

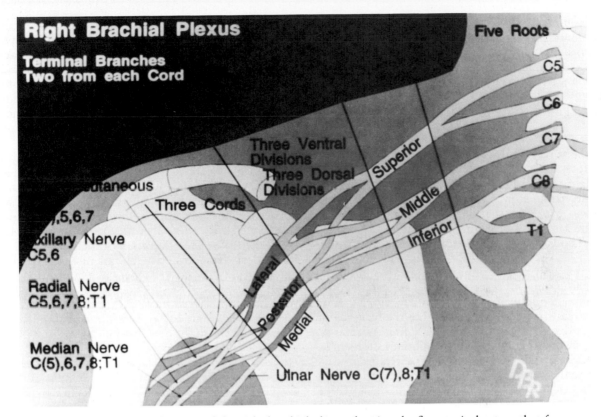

Figure 2. Schematic diagram of the right brachial plexus showing the five cervical nerves that form the cervical plexus and their various branches passing through the axilla and upper arm.

els of the brachial plexus that may be mixed with vascular symptoms of the subclavian vessels and trauma to the musculoskeletal tissues of the neck, shoulder, and arm. Accurate diagnosis depends on a high index of suspicion, familiarity with various TOS symptoms, a detailed history, and a careful physical examination of the neck, shoulder, arm, and hand. Other conditions that may simulate or even coexist with TOS also must be carefully evaluated (Table 1). A thorough physical examination of the neurologic, vascular, and musculoskeletal systems of the neck, shoulder, arm, and hand, and comparison of the two sides for any subtle differences is essential. Tenderness of the nerves of the brachial plexus, the axilla, the cubital tunnel of the inner elbow, and carpal tunnel of the wrist may give important information concerning the level of compression and irritation of the major nerves. Measuring the blood pressure in each arm in the neutral position may detect arterial insufficiency if the pressure in the symptomatic arm is 15 mm Hg less than the asymptomatic limb. Examination of the radial pulse at the wrist in various arm and shoulder positions, so often relied on for diagnosis of TOS, has been found to be worthless in most cases because the predominant symptoms are caused by compression and

irritation of the *nerves*, not by positional arterial compression. Also, most normal, asymptomatic people demonstrate radial pulse deficit with various elevated arm positions. The so-called Adson test is obsolete, unreliable, generally not used by those familiar with the modern concepts of TOS, and is rarely even performed correctly. The true Adson test is performed by palpating the radial pulse with the hand *in the lap and not elevated*, and with the head turned and extended to the ipsilateral side to determine if the pulse is occluded in this unusual neck position. It has no bearing

TABLE 1. DIFFERENTIAL DIAGNOSIS OF THORACIC OUTLET SYNDROME

Cervical disk syndrome
Cervical arthritis
Carpal tunnel syndrome
Ulnar nerve compression at elbow
Orthopedic shoulder problems
Tendinitis
Shoulder sprain
Rotator cuff injury
Spinal cord tumor
Angina pectoris
Multiple sclerosis

on the compression of the brachial plexus by congenital anomalies and is found to be negative in most patients with TOS, but may be positive in some people who have no symptoms (Table 2).

The most reliable clinical test for evaluation of the three types of TOS is the 3-minute elevated arm stress test (EAST) in the "surrender" position (Fig. 3). The arms are placed in the 90-degree abduction external rotation (AER) position with the arms raised 90 degrees, the forearms flexed 90 degrees, and the palms facing forward with the extremity in the frontal plane of the shoulders. The patient is asked to open and close the hands slowly (every 2 seconds) and to describe any symptoms that develop during the 3-minute test. The test position tenses the neck and shoulder muscles and closes the costoclavicular space, thus bringing into play any abnormal compression mechanisms that may affect the brachial plexus and subclavian vessels. Thus all three types of TOS can be tested simultaneously with a simple, painless, brief, noninvasive clinical test at no expense. Normally, a person can perform the stress test with only mild normal fatigue from holding the arms up 3 minutes. In the neurologic type of TOS, the patient feels early, progressive fatigue of the shoulder and arm, tingling in the fingers that spreads through the hand and up the forearm, with the arm progressively getting heavy and aching. The patient has a strong urge to drop the arm to the lap for relief.

In the venous type of TOS, the entire extremity gradually becomes cyanotic from the hand up to the deltoid muscle, and the forearm and wrist veins become distended with progressive aching and heaviness of the arm. In the arterial type, the pulse may be occluded, the hand becomes cadaverically white, and the muscles quickly become exhausted with aching ischemic pain, forcing the arm to drop to the lap. These reactions actually can be a variation of normal from the costoclavicular compression, so the results are of little significance unless they reproduce the same complaints for which the patient seeks relief. This is the simplest and most accurate clinical test available, and the diagnosis of TOS is suspect if it is normal.

After a thorough physical examination of the neck, shoulder, arm, and hand, ancillary tests may be considered. The most common, electromyograms (EMGs), nerve conduction studies, and somatosensory evoked potentials (SEPs), seldom give useful information to establish the diagnosis of the neurologic TOS. The results usually are normal or vaguely abnormal,

almost never specific, and are not worth the great expense and patient discomfort they entail. They may even mislead the physician from the appropriate diagnosis if they are expected to be abnormal for TOS, cubital, or carpal tunnel syndromes, as these studies are normal in most patients suffering from these nerve entrapments. The physician may misinterpret the normal results as "excluding" a significant entrapment syndrome.

Routine use of angiography, including venography of the subclavian veins and arteriography of the arteries, is worthless in 96 per cent of the patients who present with the neurologic type of TOS. These expensive studies are unpleasant for the patient, and are associated with some risk of allergic reactions to the dye used, or perforation of a major vessel. They should be avoided except in patients with specific indications by history and physical examination, which is 4 per cent of all TOS patients with a vascular type of syndrome. However, in a case suspected of venous occlusion, venography is essential and should be performed first with the arm down in the neutral position, then elevated 90 degrees with the hand held behind the skull and elbow in the frontal plane of the shoulders to evaluate the extent of compression of the subclavian vein and collateral vessels accurately. Selective subclavian arteriography using the femoral artery catheter technique is required to demonstrate the type of arterial lesion causing the symptoms in the rare patient with arterial TOS. Atherosclerotic plaque, mural thrombi, poststenotic dilatation, or true aneurysm can be clearly demonstrated, which is essential in planning appropriate surgical treatment.

In examination of the patient with neurologic type of TOS, the strength of the intrinsic muscles of the hand innervated by the ulnar nerves is evaluated with the card pinch test and with finger adduction test against resistance. The extensor muscles of the thumb and wrist are tested for evaluation of the radial nerve, and the thenar muscle strength of the thumbs is tested against resistance to test the motor function of the median innervated muscles. The strength of the biceps, triceps, deltoid, and shoulder shrug muscles also is routinely evaluated against resistance. Sensory function of the ulnar, radial, and median nerves is tested by the simple cotton and pin prick test of both arms and hands. Having the patient tilt the ear to the shoulder and report any symptoms from the opposite brachial plexus on the stretch, then lightly percussing the C5 nerve and superior trunk of the plexus is a simple but accurate clinical test for involvement of the upper nerves of the plexus. Percussion around each shoulder and elbow joint for evidence of localized tenderness indicating inflammatory disease, such as tendinitis or bursitis, and testing the range of motion and tenderness of the cervical spine, and the tendon reflexes of the extremities are routinely performed to evaluate

TABLE 2. ADSON TEST RESULTS IN 250 PATIENTS

Result	Number
Positive on symptomatic side	4 (1.6%)
Positive on asymptomatic side	3 (1.2%)

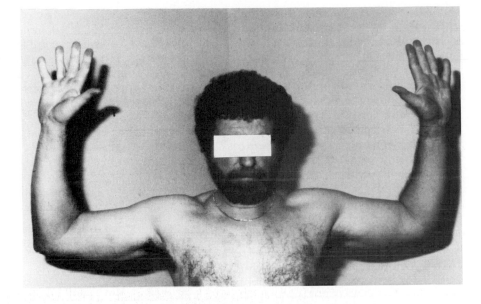

Figure 3. Photograph showing a patient demonstrating the elevated arm stress test (EAST) with the arms in the 90-degree abduction-external-rotation (AER) "surrender" position.

other possible conditions that may accompany or simulate the TOS symptoms (Table 1).

Cervical spine films usually are obtained to evaluate the vertebral bodies, disk interspaces, neural foramina, the C7 transverse processes, and the appearance of the first rib and clavicle. A routine cervical spine series includes the anteroposterior (AP), lateral, and both oblique views of the spine. It affords more meaningful information for TOS evaluation than the much more expensive magnetic resonance imaging (MRI), computed tomography (CT) scans, and myelography, which are of no help in establishing the diagnosis of TOS, although they may be useful in ruling out other conditions when indicated. They are not required in the average case, especially in younger patients who have no clinical evidence of other neurologic conditions from a careful history and physical examination.

MANAGEMENT

Mild symptoms of the neurologic type of TOS may be controlled by having the patient minimize the arm positions and activities known to aggravate their symptoms. Frequent exacerbation of even mild symptoms may cause them to progress and become more resistant to conservative management. If pain, weakness, and dysfunction of the hand worsen, professional treatment is required. Physical therapy with muscle stretching exercises, heat applications, and massage is beneficial for the painful muscle spasms that often are the underlying cause of abnormal compression of the nerves and vessels in the thoracic outlet. However, strenuous exercise with weights, elastic stretch devices, wall push-ups, and cervical traction should be avoided because it increases muscle tension and swelling and actually aggravates the painful spasms that conservative treatment attempts to relieve. Biofeedback techniques to promote muscle relaxation and relief of muscle contraction headaches, along with nonnarcotic analgesics, nonsteroidal anti-inflammatory agents, and muscle relaxants, may help job performance and improve sleep.

If these "conservative" measures adequately control the symptoms enough to permit normal activities, reasonable sleep, and job performance, they should be continued. However, if they fail to control the symptoms satisfactorily or if pain, dysfunction, or swelling worsen, surgical relief should be considered. Decompression of the involved neurovascular structures is the most effective treatment for the severe symptoms of TOS. This includes removal of the first rib, cervical rib, and any fibromuscular anomalies that may contribute to the symptoms of the lower plexus pattern. For upper plexus type of TOS, which affects the C5, C6, and C7 nerves, removal of the entire abnormal anterior scalene muscle through a supraclavicular approach is the operation of choice. If all five nerves of the brachial plexus are significantly involved, the combined operations of a transaxillary first rib resection and supraclavicular anterior scalenectomy may be necessary. The offending structures causing the neurologic compression, the first rib and anterior scalene muscle, are both expendable, as they have no functional or cosmetic significance, and like the appendix or tonsils, they may be removed with no ill effects if they cause significant problems.

Removing the first rib offers several benefits. First, the scissor action with the clavicle compressing the brachial plexus and subclavian vessels is eliminated. Second, the two neck muscles most responsible for brachial plexus compression that triggers regional muscle spasm and muscle contraction headaches (the anterior and middle scalene muscles) are detached from the skeleton and, therefore, relax. Third, removing the rib through the axillary approach permits clear exposure for evaluation and resection of all fibromuscular anomalies affecting the lower plexus and subclavian vessels. Also, an inconspicuous axillary scar remains, which is especially appreciated by female patients.

In a patient with venous type TOS, if the venogram shows patency without thrombosis, transaxillary decompression of the vein by rib and anomalous muscle band resection usually is curative. If venography demonstrates subclavian thrombosis, treatment with the thrombolytic enzyme urokinase (UK) within the first 8 to 10 days is currently the treatment of choice. Urokinase is safer and much more effective than streptokinase (SK) for lysis of fresh clot. Although UK is much more expensive than SK, it requires a shorter infusion period with less chance of systemic bleeding and allergic reactions that can be serious, even fatal, especially with SK. When maximum lysis has been achieved, a completion venogram is performed, again with the arm down and then elevated to shoulder level, to evaluate the postinfusion external compression mechanisms that caused the thrombosis initially and which may continue to affect the subclavian vein. Generally, if the patient has typical TOS effort-vein thrombosis, surgical decompression of the vein and thoracic outlet should be performed before the patient leaves the hospital to minimize the chance of rethrombosis. If this is not accomplished, the fibromuscular anomalies that caused the initial thrombosis remain and rethrombosis may occur anytime, even if the patient is treated with warfarin (Coumadin). Balloon venoplasty of a persistent stenosis seen after thrombolysis is ineffective and should not be performed due to the risk of vein perforation, possible rethrombosis from the effects of the procedure, and predictable failure. Even with persistent stenosis of the vein after thrombolysis, which may be caused by residual mural thrombus, scarred valve, or congenital web, rethrombosis is rare after surgical removal of the *external* compression mechanisms.

If the patient has persistent symptoms of venous insufficiency long after an episode of subclavian vein thrombosis, complete surgical decompression of the thoracic outlet by resection of transaxillary first rib and anomalous fibromuscular tissue may offer considerable improvement of the collateral circulation and the symptoms of chronic swelling and heaviness of the arm. In severe cases of postphlebitic syndrome, if decompression of the outlet does not offer improvement, various bypass or vein reconstruction procedures may be performed.

Treatment of subclavian artery TOS is determined by the severity of the symptoms and selective arteriography. Noninvasive vascular laboratory studies may be used, but are less definitive in this region than dye injection arteriography because the clavicle overlying the artery and vein causes considerable interference with the Doppler ultrasound waves. Mild symptoms require no treatments. If significant arterial insufficiency or emboli of the arm and hand occur from stenosis or occlusion of the artery, routine vascular surgical procedures are indicated, often with graft replacement of the diseased segment. If a cervical rib or band contributed to the arterial compression and disease, it must also be removed to prevent the same fate affecting the repaired vessel.

POSTOPERATIVE CARE

Quiet convalescence with only light use of the arm and hand maintaining full range of motion of the shoulder, elbow, and hand joints is recommended after any of the operations required for the outlet syndromes. Vigorous use, therapy, or exercise should be avoided for approximately 3 months to permit the tissues to heal without strain and stress that may perpetuate the painful muscle spasm and nerve symptoms that the operation is attempting to relieve. Also, energetic treatment in the postoperative period may increase inflammation and serum formation in the operative sites that may evolve into scar tissue and cause severe recurrent nerve entrapment symptoms. Scar tissue entrapment of the brachial plexus is the most common long-term complication of these operations and may become so severe that recurrent symptoms are unresponsive to all types of conservative measures. The only treatment for these symptoms, if they become incapacitating, is reoperation with neurolysis of the involved elements of the brachial plexus. Therefore, the use of hot packs, light massage, and muscle stretching exercises are the preferred techniques of postoperative management, with strict avoidance of vigorous exercises to try to strengthen the previously weakened muscles. Strength is regained quickly after pain and muscle spasms are relieved.

With a careful, accurate clinical diagnosis of TOS and appropriate conservative management, many patients can lead comfortable, productive lives. If symptoms become severe and uncontrollable, specific operative procedures are available that may still offer good to excellent relief in 85 to 90 per cent of patients, with a low rate of complications.

REFERENCES

Adson AW, Coffey JR: Cervical rib: A method of anterior approach for relief of symptoms by division of the scalenus anticus. Ann Surg 85:839, 1927.

Harding A, Silver D: Thoracic outlet syndrome. *In* Sabiston DC Jr (ed): Textbook of Surgery: The Biological Basis of Modern Surgical Practice, ed 14. Philadelphia, WB Saunders Coompany, 1991, pp 1757–1761.

Kunkel JM, Machleder HI: Treatment of Paget-Schroetter syndrome. Arch Surg *124*:1153, 1989.

Machleder HI, Moll F, Verity MA: The anterior scalene muscle in thoracic outlet compression syndrome: Histochemical and morphometric studies. Arch Surg *121*:1141, 1986.

Roos DB: Congenital anomalies associated with thoracic outlet syndrome: Anatomy, symptoms, diagnosis and treatment. Am J Surg *132*:771, 1976.

Roos DB: The place for scalenectomy and first rib resection in thoracic outlet syndrome. Surgery *92*:1077, 1982.

XI
Congenital Deformities of the Chest Wall

DAVID C. SABISTON, Jr., M.D.

A number of lesions that involve the chest wall are amenable to surgical therapy. The results of surgical treatment for benign neoplasms are excellent but are less than optimal for malignant tumors. The congenital malformations are generally followed by excellent postoperative therapeutic and cosmetic results.

CONGENITAL MALFORMATIONS

Pectus Excavatum ("Funnel Chest")

Of the severe deformities of the chest wall, the most frequent is *pectus excavatum*. This deformity ranges from a very mild and barely noticeable disorder to one that is quite severe (Fig. 1). Often termed "funnel chest," it is primarily a deformity of the costal cartilages, which curve posteriorly rather than joining the sternum in the normal position. The sternum is secondarily depressed, thus reducing the distance between the posterior surface of the sternum and the anterior surface of the vertebral column (Fig. 2).

Clinical manifestations may be absent, or there may be varying degrees of respiratory insufficiency, especially with exercise. Few patients with this disorder become competitive athletes and thus have some intolerance to exercise. The *cosmetic* effects of this deformity are appreciable, and the vast majority of children become quite sensitive to their problem by the time school begins. Moreover, continuing psychological difficulties persist if the condition is not corrected. Although it has been suggested that spontaneous correction is possible, it rarely occurs.

For significant pectus excavatum, surgical correction is generally indicated. The operation involves subperichondrial resection of all the costal cartilages with total separation of the sternum from surrounding structures except for the manubrium. A posterior wedge osteotomy is also performed at the sternomanubrial joint, and the sternum is overcorrected with a wedge of cartilage placed in the osteotomy. This procedure was developed, refined, and advocated by Ravitch and is quite successful. The results are usually very good.

Pectus Carinatum ("Pigeon Breast")

A less common deformity than pectus excavatum is *pectus carinatum*, characterized by an unusual prominence of the sternum (Fig. 3). The sternum bulges anteriorly as a result of the positions of the costal cartilages. Management of this condition is by resection of the costal cartilages subperichondrially with freeing of the sternum in a manner quite similar to that for pectus excavatum. The results are generally quite

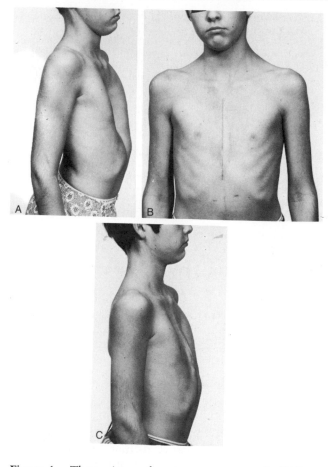

Figure 1. Three views of pectus excavatum. *A,* Oblique view demonstrating severe pectus deformity. *B,* Postoperative view illustrating correction of defect. *C,* Postoperative oblique view illustrating correction of defect. (From Sabiston DC Jr: Disorders of the chest wall. *In* Sabiston DC Jr [ed]: Essentials of Surgery. Philadelphia, WB Saunders Company, 1987, p 1013, with permission.)

good, and the patient's psychological health usually returns to normal.

Poland's Syndrome

Poland's syndrome consists of variable absence of the costal cartilages, pectoral muscles, and portions of the ribs. It is a part of a spectrum of anomalies in which syndactylism, absent phalanges, and other anomalies occur. Surgical correction can be achieved in this malformation but is more complicated than pectus excavatum or pectus carinatum.

Sternal Clefts

Sternal clefts are congenital lesions usually obvious at birth. There are three principal types: (1) those in-

volving the manubrium and gladiolus to the third or fourth intercostal space, (2) distal clefts involving the lower third or half of the sternum, and (3) the complete sternal cleft. A Type I lesion involving the manubrium and upper sternum is shown in Figure 4. This deformity can be effectively corrected as shown in Figure 5. The distal sternal defect may be associated with ectopia cordis, and an operation may be required in the first few months of life. Both diaphragmatic and pericardial defects are associated with this lesion and can be appropriately closed. *Complete sternal cleft* is rare and may be associated with a ventral abdominal or diaphragmatic defect. Prosthetic material may be required to close these lesions.

NEOPLASMS OF THE STERNUM AND RIBS

The chest wall is the site of a variety of benign and malignant neoplasms. They may occur in the sternum, ribs, and diaphragm and may be primary, metastatic, or the result of direct invasion of the chest wall from either a bronchogenic or breast neoplasm. Primary tumors arising in the chest wall account for approximately 8 per cent of all intrinsic bone tumors.

Benign Neoplasms

The more common *benign* neoplasms of the chest wall include chondromas, osteochondromas, bone cysts, fibrous dysplasia, and eosinophilic granuloma. Some lesions present with the appearance of a mass, at times tender, and show few clinical signs or symptoms to suggest the specific type of neoplasm. The chondroma is the most common benign tumor of the chest wall with most appearing in the ribs and a minority in the sternum. En bloc excision with a 4-cm margin around the lesion is the appropriate operation. The same type of treatment applies to osteochondromas as well as bone cysts and eosinophilic granuloma. In a study of 53 primary chest wall tumors, 26 were benign, with 49 occurring in the ribs and four in the sternum. All the patients with benign neoplasms were treated by excision with no recurrence or mortality. In general, it is not possible to distinguish benign neoplasms from malignant ones occurring in the chest wall *unless* cortical destruction and involvement of soft tissues are visualized. Therefore, in the management of benign as well as malignant lesions, all neoplasms should be considered malignant until proven otherwise. Wide excision with a 4-cm margin is appropriate and provides for the largest number of patients to become long-term survivors.

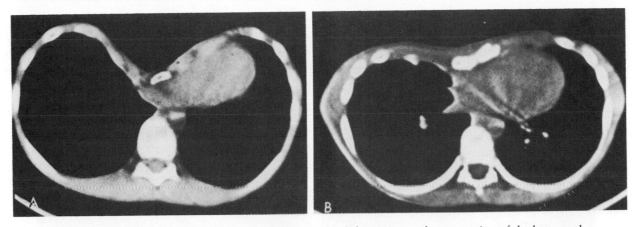

Figure 2. Pectus excavatum CT scan showing (*A*) the deformation and compression of the heart and (*B*) striking relief by operation. (From Ravitch MM: *In* Sabiston DC Jr [ed]: Textbook of Surgery, ed 13. Philadelphia, WB Saunders Company, 1986, p 2082, with permission.)

Malignant Tumors

Malignant tumors may outnumber benign tumors in lesions arising in the chest wall. *Chondrosarcoma* is generally the most common malignant lesion and appears as a lobulated, smooth, firm mass often showing

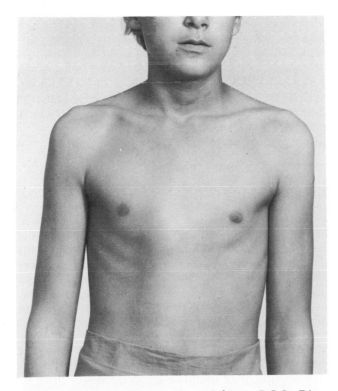

Figure 3. Pectus carinatun. (From Sabiston DC Jr: Disorders of the chest wall. *In* Sabiston DC Jr [ed]: Essentials of Surgery. Philadelphia, WB Saunders Company, 1987, p 1015, with permission.)

destruction of the cortex on the radiograph. It should be removed by radical en bloc dissection. *Ewing's tumor* is best evaluated by chest and bone films that show evidence of destruction or lysis of bone with a diffuse, expanded bone lesion with little periosteal reaction in some of the patients. Both surgical excision and radiation and chemotherapy are employed. Lymphomas are also managed primarily by chemotherapy and radiation. Another primary malignant lesion is *plasmacytoma*, and radical excision, with or without radiation, is necessary. Clinical features suggesting that a neoplasm is malignant include recent and rapid increase in size, invasion of surrounding structures, and distant metastases. Although diagnostic biopsy has been reported, most today believe that initial wide excision of the neoplasm is the most appropriate treatment. In a series of 27 malignant primary tumors of the chest wall, the overall 5-year survival was 33 per cent and the 10-year survival 18 per cent. Other malignant neoplasms include osteogenic sarcoma, neurosarcoma, fibrous sarcoma, liposarcoma, and angioplastic sarcoma.

Neoplasms arising in other structures may metastasize to the chest wall by extension of metastases or blood-borne deposits. In general, surgical intervention in such lesions is palliative and should be done only to establish the diagnosis or for uncontrollable discomfort. Although some neoplasms are amenable to radiotherapy, those that are radioresistant include chondrosarcoma, osteogenic sarcoma, neurosarcoma, fibrosarcoma, liposarcoma, angiosarcoma, and anaplastic neoplasms. The radiosensitive malignant tumors include Ewing's sarcoma, reticulum cell sarcoma, plasma cell myeloma, Hodgkin's disease, and lymphosarcoma.

In one series of 100 patients with chest wall tumors, metastases were present in 32 instances, including 12

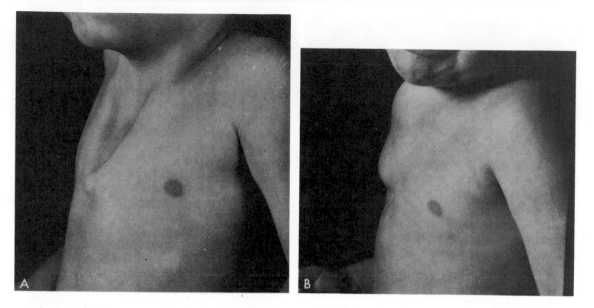

Figure 4. Cleft sternum. *A*, At rest. *B*, During forced expiration. Superior clefts of the sternum are variously V- or U-shaped. The appearance of the child as he cries explains the term "ectopia cordis," although the heart is actually not misplaced. In the newborn, defects of this kind can be corrected by direct apposition of the sternal halves. In this child, closure of the defect was made possible by sliding chondrotomies on either side. (From Sabiston DC Jr: J Thorac Surg *35*:118, 1958, with permission.)

from sarcomas, nine from the breast, four from the kidney, three from the lung, three from other genito-urinary sources, and one from the thyroid gland. The value of en bloc resection of the chest wall for patients with bronchogenic carcinoma has been demonstrated.

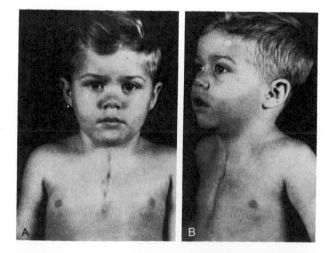

Figure 5. Correction of sternal cleft. *A*, Postoperative photograph. *B*, Postoperative photograph (oblique). (From Sabiston DC Jr: Disorders of the chest wall. *In* Sabiston DC Jr [ed]: Essentials of Surgery. Philadelphia, WB Saunders Company, 1987, p 1017, with permission.)

More controversial, however, is radical resection in patients with breast cancer metastatic to the chest wall. Skin ulceration was present in 11 of 14 cases of breast cancer, and these were treated with excision and palliation. Wide radical chest wall resection with immediate reconstruction, including the use of flaps and chest wall muscles as well as omentum and prosthetic materials (e.g., Prolene or polytetrafluoroethylene patch [PTFE] patch), is effective for many malignant lesions.

Neoplasms of the Diaphragm

Among the *benign* tumors of the diaphragm are fibromas, lipomas, mesotheliomas, angiofibromas, and neurogenic tumors. In addition, congenital cysts of the diaphragm occur. Considerably more common have been malignant lesions, primarily metastatic, from neighboring structures such as the esophagus, lung, liver, and colon. Retroperitoneal malignant neoplasms may also extend to the diaphragm. Primary malignant lesions include fibrosarcomas and neurofibrosarcomas. Symptoms may be elusive and the lesions are generally diagnosed by radiography. Computed tomography has also become quite useful in the diagnosis of these lesions. The management of benign lesions is simple excision; for malignant primary lesions, wide removal with replacement by fascia lata or prosthetic material is required. Radiotherapy and chemotherapy are infrequently indicated. It has been reported that of the primary tumors of the diaphragm, the malignant lesions predominate in 60 per cent while the remaining 40 per cent of neoplasms are benign.

REFERENCES

Pairolero PC, Arnold PG: Chest wall tumors: Experience with 100 consecutive patients. J Thorac Cardiovasc Surg *90*:367, 1985.

Piehler JM, Pairolero PC, Weiland LH, Offord KP, Payne WS, Bernatz PE: Bronchogenic carcinoma with chest wall invasion: Factors affecting survival following en bloc resection. Ann Thorac Surg *34*:684, 1982.

Ravitch MM: Congenital deformities of the chest wall and their operative corrections. Philadelphia, WB Saunders Company, 1977.

Sabiston DC Jr: The surgical management of congenital bifid sternum with a partial ectopia cordis. J Thorac Surg *35*:118, 1958.

XII
Extracorporeal Membrane Oxygenation

JAMES R. MAULT, M.D.

Since the first successful application of cardiopulmonary bypass (CPB) by Gibbon in 1953, artificial replacement of the heart and lungs has been performed on a routine basis during cardiac surgery. In 1975, Bartlett used a modified CPB system for several days to treat a newborn infant with severe respiratory failure. This adaptation of CPB for long-term support of patients with severe but potentially reversible respiratory and/or cardiac failure is called *extracorporeal membrane oxygenation* (ECMO). The major differences between ECMO and standard CPB are shown in Table 1. ECMO is a supportive therapy that supplements or replaces a patient's gas exchange and hemodynamic requirements for days or weeks. By removing exposure to the toxic levels of oxygen and barotrauma required for conventional mechanical ventilation, ECMO permits resolution of respiratory failure under optimal conditions. While the principles of extracorporeal circulation, gas exchange, and oxygen delivery are similar for all ages and sizes of patients,

the pathophysiology of acute respiratory failure is significantly different between newborn infants and older patients. In recent years, ECMO has become the standard of care for support of neonates with severe respiratory failure. ECMO has recently been applied to children and adults, although characterization and standardization of indications and techniques for these patient populations are ongoing.

INDICATIONS AND PATIENT SELECTION

The most important criterion of patient selection for ECMO is the reversibility of the underlying disease process. In this regard, neonates often experience severe but reversible forms of acute respiratory failure due to aspiration of meconium, congenital diaphragmatic hernia, neonatal sepsis, or respiratory distress syndrome. In each of these conditions, the common pathophysiologic mechanism is persistent pulmonary hypertension of the newborn (PPHN). In the neonatal lung, severe pulmonary vasoconstriction occurs under conditions of hypoxia, hypercarbia, and acidosis. The resultant elevation in pulmonary vascular resistance can cause right-to-left shunting of blood flow away from the lungs and through the ductus arteriosus and foramen ovale. As the neonate becomes more hypoxemic and acidotic, this negative cycle perpetuates. Standard therapy for PPHN consists of mechanical ventilation, induced respiratory alkalosis, and various pharmacologic agents. However, approximately 2 to 5 per cent of neonates fail to respond to this therapy and are considered for ECMO.

ECMO is indicated for patients with acute respiratory failure that is refractory to maximal levels of conventional therapy. In evaluating a patient for ECMO, the *oxygenation index* (OI) is used to objectively assess the severity of respiratory failure. It is calculated as follows:

$$OI = \left\{ \frac{\text{mean airway pressure} \times F_{IO_2}}{P_{aO_2}} \right\} \times 100$$

In the neonatal population, when treated by conventional management alone, neonates with an OI of 25 have a predicted mortality of greater than 50 per cent, and an OI of 40 defines a mortality of approximately 80 per cent. Currently, patients are considered candidates for ECMO if the OI is greater than 40 on maximal conventional therapy in three of five measurements obtained over a 4-hour period. Prior to initiation of ECMO, cerebral and cardiac abnormalities must be excluded by echocardiography and cranial ultrasonography. Due to the risk of intracerebral hemorrhage, newborns under 34 weeks' gestation or less than 2.0 kg are usually excluded from ECMO. In addition, mechanical ventilation with inspired oxygen concentrations greater than 60 per cent for longer than 10 days is a contraindication to ECMO due to the likelihood of irreversible lung injury.

THE ECMO CIRCUIT

ECMO is performed by draining venous (deoxygenated) blood, pumping it through an artificial lung where carbon dioxide is removed and oxygen is added, and returning the blood to the circulation via an artery (venoarterial ECMO) or a vein (venovenous ECMO). The differences between venoarterial (VA) and venovenous (VV) ECMO are contrasted in Table 2. In VA ECMO, the functions of both the heart and the lungs are partially or totally replaced. Deoxygenated blood is drained from the right atrium via cannulation of the right internal jugular (RIJ) or femoral vein while oxygenated blood is pumped back into the circulation via the right common carotid artery. ECMO candidates who are hemodynamically unstable and require cardiovascular support in addition to gas exchange are placed on VA ECMO.

VV ECMO provides gas exchange but no cardiac support. Venous drainage and infusion cannulae are placed into the right atrium or vena cava via the RIJ or femoral veins. Alternatively, a double-lumen catheter may be positioned in the right atrium through the RIJ vein for both drainage and infusion. In either case, blood is drained from and returned to the venous circulation at the same rate. With VV ECMO, systemic oxygenation saturations are slightly lower than with VA ECMO due to a recirculation fraction. Most patients with acute respiratory failure who are hemodynamically stable are initially placed on VV ECMO. If hemodynamic instability develops, cannulation can be easily converted to VA ECMO.

The components of a standard ECMO circuit are illustrated in Figure 1. Deoxygenated blood drains passively into a distensible silicone bladder that operates as the control point of a servo-regulated roller pump. If the pump flow exceeds the passive venous return, the bladder collapses and the roller pump automatically slows down or stops until it reexpands. Blood is then pumped through a silicone-coated membrane lung designed to function for long durations. After passing through a countercurrent heat exchanger, the warmed, oxygenated blood is then returned to the patient via the arterial or venous circulation. A tubing bridge is created between the drainage and perfusion catheters to allow recirculation of the blood during priming and weaning. Heparin and fluids are infused into the circuit immediately before the bladder.

TABLE 1. COMPARISON OF ECMO TO STANDARD CARDIOPULMONARY BYPASS

	ECMO	Cardiopulmonary Bypass
Setting	Respiratory and/or cardiac failure	Intraoperative cardiac surgery
Location	Extrathoracic	Intrathoracic
Vascular access	Venoarterial or venovenous	Venoarterial only
Blood reservoir	No	Yes
Bubble traps	No	Yes
Blood pump	Roller or centrifugal	Roller
Artificial lung	Silicon-coated membrane oxygenator	Membrane oxygenator
Temperature	Normotheric only	Normothermic or hypothermic
Duration	Days to weeks	Hours

TABLE 2.   COMPARISON OF VENOARTERIAL AND VENOVENOUS ECMO

	Venoarterial ECMO	Venovenous ECMO
Organ support	Gas exchange and cardiac output	Gas exchange only
Pulse contour	Reduced pulsatility	Normal pulsatility
CVP	Unreliable	Reliable
PA pressure	Unreliable	Reliable
Circuit SvO$_2$	Reliable	Unreliable
Circuit recirculation	None	15–50%
Arterial oxygen saturation	≥95%	80–95%
Carbon dioxide removal	Sweep gas flow dependent	Sweep gas flow dependent
Ventilator settings	Minimal	Moderate

Abbreviations: CVP = central venous pressure, PA = pulmonary artery, S$\bar{v}$O$_2$ = mixed venous oxygen saturation, ECMO = extracorporeal membrane oxygenation.

PATIENT MANAGEMENT DURING ECMO

Gas Exchange

Upon initiation of ECMO support, immediate improvement of the patient's condition is usually noted. Cyanosis quickly resolves, and ventilator settings are reduced to minimal levels to provide lung rest and optimal conditions for pulmonary recovery. All aspects of gas exchange are now controlled by the mixture and flow of a "sweep" gas circulated through the membrane lung of the ECMO circuit. The concentration of oxygen in the sweep gas determines the patient's arterial PO$_2$, while the flow rate of sweep gas determines the carbon dioxide removal and arterial PCO$_2$. With VA ECMO, systemic arterial oxygen saturations range from 95 to 100 per cent, while VV ECMO ranges from 80 to 95 per cent saturation due to recirculation.

Oxygen Delivery

The pump flow rate of the ECMO circuit is determined by the oxygen delivery requirements of the patient. Typical blood flow rates are 100 to 150 ml/kg/min in neonates and 80 to 120 ml/kg/min in children. Blood flow during VA ECMO is usually 80 per cent of the total cardiac output, resulting in a diminished but observable pulse pressure. The exact flow rate is best managed by continuous, in-line monitoring of the mixed venous oxygen saturation (S$\bar{v}$O$_2$). An S$\bar{v}$O$_2$ of 75 per cent or greater indicates adequate oxygen delivery. Inadequate oxygen delivery, as indicated by a falling S$\bar{v}$O$_2$, is treated by increasing the circuit blood

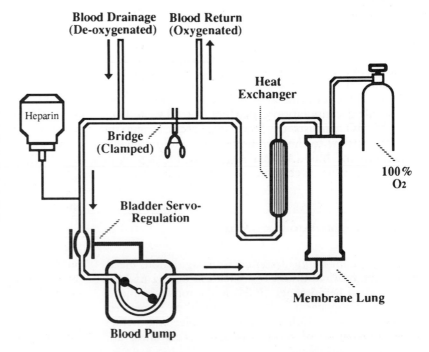

Figure 1.   ECMO circuit schematic. Deoxygenated blood drains passively to a distensible bladder. If negative pressure occurs within the bladder, the roller pump is automatically shut off. After passing through the membrane lung, oxygenated blood is circulated through a countercurrent heat exchanger and back to the patient. Heparin is delivered into the circuit immediately before the bladder.

flow. During VV ECMO, blood is drained and returned to the venous circulation at the same rate and thus has no influence on cardiac output or hemodynamics. Because of recirculation of oxygenated blood, the pump flow for total respiratory support with VV ECMO is 20 to 50 per cent higher than VA ECMO for the same patient. Also, with recirculation, $S\bar{v}O_2$ is less reliable during VV ECMO. Throughout the ECMO course, oxygen delivery is optimized by maintaining a hematocrit of 40 per cent.

Anticoagulation

Due to the high surface area and thrombogenicity of the ECMO circuit, a continuous heparin infusion of 15 to 60 U/kg/hr is required during ECMO. The activated clotting time (ACT) is measured hourly, and the heparin infusion is titrated to maintain an ACT of 160 to 180 seconds. Platelet transfusions are required on a daily basis to maintain a count of 150,000/mm^3.

Weaning From ECMO

ECMO support is usually maintained for 4 to 7 days. Indications of lung recovery include an increasing $S\bar{v}O_2$ and systemic PO_2, or decreasing PCO_2 while ECMO flow and ventilator settings are constant. Other signs of improvement are noted by increased pulmonary compliance and a normalizing chest radiograph. Upon documenting significant improvement in native respiratory function during VA ECMO, blood flow is gradually reduced over a period of hours. When the native lung and heart can provide adequate oxygen delivery and gas exchange at 20 per cent of the baseline VA ECMO flow, a brief trial off bypass (cannulae clamped, bridge open) is attempted on moderate ventilator settings. If this is successful, VA ECMO is restarted and the patient is prepared for the sterile decannulation procedure. A trial wean from VV ECMO consists of decreasing and capping the sweep gas flow to the membrane lung without changing the pump blood flow. If the native lungs provide adequate gas exchange, VV ECMO can be discontinued.

COMPLICATIONS OF ECMO

Due to continuous systemic anticoagulation, bleeding is the most common complication during ECMO. Intracranial hemorrhage (ICH) is the most significant bleeding complication and occurs in 10 to 15 per cent of ECMO cases. Other locations of bleeding include the gastrointestinal tract, vascular access sites, and

TABLE 3. OUTCOME OF ECMO FOR RESPIRATORY FAILURE*

	N	Survival (%)
Newborn infants (84 centers)	**8020**	**81**
Meconium aspiration syndrome	2997	93
Respiratory distress syndrome	982	84
Primary pulmonary hypertension	1008	83
Neonatal sepsis	1197	76
Congenital diaphragmatic hernia	1543	58
Other causes	293	76
Children (63 centers)	**567**	**48**
Trauma, aspiration	61	59
Infection	201	49
Respiratory distress syndrome	152	45
Other causes	153	47
Adults (11 centers)	**90**	**33**
Bacterial pneumonia	11	9
Viral pneumonia	10	70
Respiratory distress syndrome	23	52
Lung transplantation	11	27
Other respiratory	12	25
Postcardiac surgery	23	13

*Data from the ECMO Registry Report of the Extracorporeal Life Support Organizations, Ann Arbor, MI, July 1992.

pericardial tamponade. Bleeding complications are best managed by titrating heparin to a lower ACT target of 160 seconds and aggressively maintaining a platelet count greater than 150,000/mm^3. ECMO is usually discontinued in response to confirmed ICH or uncontrollable bleeding. Other complications encountered during ECMO include seizures, hemolysis, hyperbilirubinemia, renal insufficiency, cardiac arrhythmias, pulmonary hypertension, and sepsis. Technical complications occur in approximately one fifth of ECMO applications but have had no measurable effect on outcome.

OUTCOME AND FUTURE OF ECMO

As part of its charter, the Extracorporeal Life Support Organization (ELSO) maintains an international registry of all patients treated with ECMO. Hospital survival rates for all neonates, children, and adults supported by ECMO for acute respiratory failure through July 1993 are listed in Table 3. In the neonatal population, 8020 patients have been treated at 84 centers since 1975. Results are consistently better in neonates with meconium aspiration, respiratory distress syndrome, or idiopathic PPHN, as compared with neonatal sepsis and congenital diaphragmatic hernias. A recent prospective, randomized trial of ECMO also supports its use for treatment of neonates with severe respiratory failure. Long-term follow-up studies have documented approximately 25 per cent of ECMO survivors as having some residual neurologic or pulmonary deficit. The remaining 75 per cent of ECMO survivors are normal, healthy individuals.

Over the next decade, the indications and techniques for the use of ECMO in children and adults are apt to become clearly defined. Bleeding, the major complication of ECMO, is substantially reduced or eliminated by new surface technology that will allow ECMO to be performed with little or no systemic anticoagulation. These and other technologic developments will expand the use of ECMO to other settings such as the emergency room and cardiac catheterization laboratory.

REFERENCES

Bartlett RH, Gazzaniga AB, Toomasian J, et al: Extracorporeal membrane oxygenation (ECMO) in neonatal respiratory failure: 100 cases. Ann Surg 204:236–245, 1986.

Bartlett RH: Extracorporeal life support for cardiopulmonary failure. Curr Probl Surg 27:623–705, 1990.

Heiss K, Manning P, Oldham KT, et al: Reversal of mortality for congenital diaphragmatic hernia with ECMO. Ann Surg 209: 225–230, 1989.

O'Rourke PP, Crone RK, Vacanti JP, et al: Extracorporeal membrane oxygenation and conventional medical therapy in neonates with persistent pulmonary hypertension of the newborn: A prospective randomized study. Pediatrics 84:957–963, 1989.

Toomasian JM, Snedecor SM, Cornell RG, Cilley RV, Bartlett RH: National experience with extracorporeal membrane oxygenation for newborn respiratory failure: Data from 715 cases. Trans ASAIO 34:140–147, 1988.

XIII
The Mediastinum

R. DUANE DAVIS, Jr., M.D.   DAVID C. SABISTON, Jr., M.D.

The mediastinum is an important anatomic division of the thorax. Its anatomic borders include the thoracic inlet superiorly, the diaphragm inferiorly, the sternum anteriorly, the vertebral column posteriorly, and the mediastinal parietal pleura laterally. It is the site of many localized disorders and is also involved in a number of systemic diseases. The localized disorders include infections, hemorrhage, emphysema, aneurysms, and many primary tumors and cysts. Systemic diseases include metastatic neoplasms, granulomatous, and other general inflammatory disorders. Because many mediastinal tumors and cysts occur in characteristic locations, the mediastinum has been divided artificially into three subdivisions to facilitate localizing specific types of lesions: the *anterosuperior*, *middle*, and *posterior* (Fig. 1). The anterosuperior mediastinum is anterior to the pericardium and the pericardial reflection over the great vessels. The posterior mediastinum is posterior to the pericardium and the

pericardial reflection. The middle mediastinum is contained within the pericardial sac.

The contents of the anterosuperior mediastinum include the thymus gland, the aortic arch and its branches, the great veins, lymphatics, and fatty areolar tissue. The middle mediastinal contents include the heart, pericardium, phrenic nerves, tracheal bifurcation and main bronchi, the hila of each lung, and lymph nodes. The posterior mediastinum contains the esophagus, vagus nerves, sympathetic nervous chain, thoracic duct, descending aorta, the azygous and hemiazygos systems, paravertebral lymphatics, and fatty areolar tissue (Fig. 2). Lesions that originate in the esophagus, great vessels, trachea, and heart may present as a mediastinal mass, or may cause symptoms related to compression or invasion of adjacent mediastinal structures. Although these lesions are discussed in the sections covering the specific organ system of origin, they are relevant in the differential diagnosis of the various primary mediastinal disease processes. Mediastinal disorders present in a myriad of different clinical settings. Symptoms may be related to local involvement of adjacent structures, tumor-secretory factors, or immunologic factors. In addition, many patients are asymptomatic and the disorder is identified on routine chest films. Advances in diagnostic imaging, pathologic identification, and therapeutic interventions have reduced patient morbidity and increased survival and quality of life.

HISTORIC ASPECTS

Prior to the introduction of endotracheal anesthesia and methods of closed pleural drainage, the risk of producing a pneumothorax and subsequent cardiopulmonary insufficiency limited surgical interventions within the mediastinum. The initial procedures were performed through various sternal splitting exposures

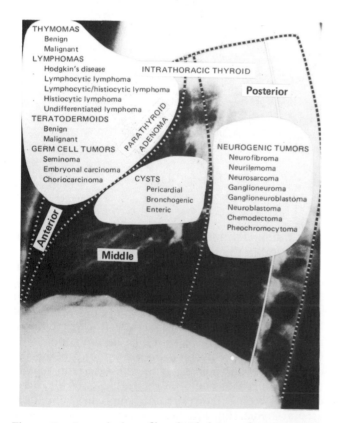

Figure 1. Lateral chest film divided into three anatomic subdivisions with the tumors and cysts that occur most frequently in each region. (From Davis RD Jr, Sabiston DC Jr: The mediastinum. *In* Sabiston DC Jr [ed]: Textbook of Surgery: The Biological Basis of Modern Surgical Practice, ed 14. Philadelphia, WB Saunders Company, 1991, p 1772, with permission.)

that did not violate the pleural spaces. In 1893, Bastianelli excised a dermoid cyst from the anterior mediastinum after resecting the manubrium. In 1897, Milton reported the first use of a median sternotomy approach to remove two caseous lymph nodes from the anterior mediastinum of a young male with mediastinal tuberculosis. The introduction of endotracheal anesthesia made possible the safe performance of transpleural operations. Harrington in 1929 and Heuer and Andrus in 1940 reported the first series of patients documenting the safety and efficacy of the transpleural approach to a variety of mediastinal diseases. In 1939, Blalock introduced the surgical treatment of myasthenia gravis when he reported the excision of the thymus in a young woman with this condition. Subsequently, the patient had a marked amelioration of symptoms. In the 1950s and 1960s, Kaplan and associates introduced megavoltage radiation therapy and pioneered the treatment of Hodgkin's disease and other radiosensitive tumors. More recently, a number of groups have contributed to the management of many malignant diseases with chemotherapeutic agents. Significant improvements in survival and cure have been achieved, particularly in the treatment of lymphomas and germ cell tumors.

MEDIASTINAL EMPHYSEMA

Air within the mediastinum produces *mediastinal emphysema* or *pneumomediastinum*. The source of the air may be from the esophagus, trachea, bronchi, neck, or abdomen. Common causes of pneumomediastinum include penetrating wounds and perforations of these structures, blunt trauma that causes fractured ribs or vertebrae, and barotrauma. High airway pressures created by compressive forces to the thorax, particularly when the glottis is closed and mechanical ventilation in noncompliant lungs or in patients with exacerbations of bronchospastic disease may rupture alveoli or blebs within the pulmonary parenchyma. While dissection of air through the visceral pleura causes a pneumothorax, dissection of air along vascular structures into the hilum and mediastinum creates pneumomediastinum. Mediastinal emphysema may also be caused by intra-abdominal air dissecting through the diaphragmatic hiatus. The clinical manifestations of pneumomediastinum include substernal chest pain that may radiate into the back and crepitance in the region of the suprasternal notch, chest wall, and neck. With increasing pressure, the air can dissect into the neck, face, chest, arms, abdomen, and into the retroperitoneum. Frequently, pneumomediastinum and pneumothorax occur simultaneously. Auscultation of the precordium may reveal a characteristic crunching sound that is accentuated during systole. Only rarely

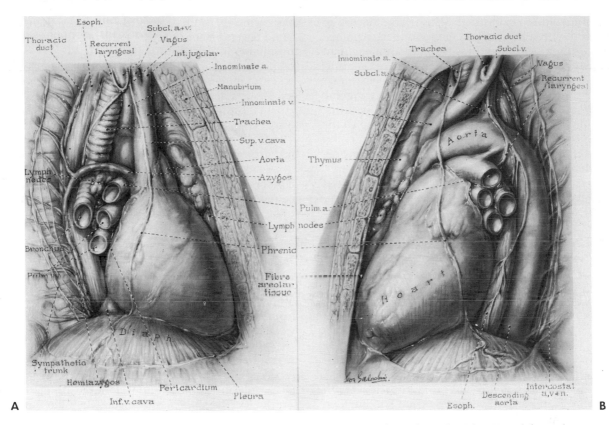

Figure 2. The anatomic structures of the mediastinum as seen from the right side (*A*) and from the left side (*B*). (From Sabiston DC Jr: The esophagus and mediastinum. *In* Cooke RE, Levin S [eds]: The Biologic Basis of Pediatric Practice. New York, McGraw-Hill, 1968, with permission.)

does sufficient pressure develop to cause compression of venous structures and impair venous return. With impairment of venous return, clinical manifestations similar to the *superior vena caval syndrome* occur including cyanosis, prominence of neck and upper extremity veins, dyspnea, and in severe cases, circulatory failure. The diagnosis of pneumomediastinum is confirmed by the presence of air in the mediastinum on chest films or computed tomography (CT) scans. Treatment is directed toward identifying the source of air and correcting the cause when possible. Contrast studies of the esophagus and bronchoscopy are the best initial studies to evaluate the esophagus, trachea, and major bronchi. Perforations of these structures require urgent surgical treatment. Spontaneous mediastinal emphysema and pneumomediastinum secondary to barotrauma usually respond to conservative measures that treat bronchospasm and minimize further barotrauma without sequelae, and surgical decompression is rarely necessary. In patients with pneumomediastinum and pneumothorax, tube thoracostomy is indicated in the affected pleural space. Patients with pneumomediastinum secondary to barotrauma contin-

uing to require high levels of pressure support may require bilateral tube thoracostomies as prophylaxis against development of tension pneumothorax.

HEMORRHAGE

Mediastinal hemorrhage is most frequently caused by blunt or penetrating trauma, thoracic aortic dissection, rupture of aortic aneurysm, or surgical procedures within the thorax. Penetrating trauma to the thorax or cervical region may cause lacerations of major veins or arteries. Most mediastinal hemorrhage associated with blunt trauma is due to rupture of small mediastinal veins, but the possibility of aortic injury should be evaluated with arch aortography when mediastinal widening is present. Over 90 per cent of aortic transections occur immediately distal to the origin of the left subclavian artery. Iatrogenic causes of mediastinal hemorrhage include laceration of great vessels during placement of catheters or pacing leads, erosion of indwelling vascular devices, and erosion of tracheostomy tubes, usually into the innominate artery. Spontaneous mediastinal hemorrhage occurs in association with a mediastinal mass, sudden sustained hypertension, altered hemostasis due to anticoagulant therapy, thrombolytic therapy, uremia, hepatic insufficiency or hemophilia, and transient, sharp increases in intrathoracic pressure, which occur during coughing or vomiting. The clinical presentation varies with the underlying etiology. Retrosternal pain radiating to the back or neck is common. With increased accumulation of blood in the mediastinum, signs and symptoms develop related to compression of mediastinal structures, primarily the great veins, including dyspnea, venous distention, cyanosis, and cervical ecchymosis due to blood dissecting into soft tissue planes. Sufficient accumulation of blood causes mediastinal tamponade manifested by tachycardia, hypotension, reduced urinary output, equalization of right- and left-sided cardiac filling pressures, and diastolic collapse of the right ventricle. The chest film is the initial diagnostic intervention. Usual findings include mediastinal widening, loss of the normal aortic contour, and displacement of anatomic structures. Patients in extremis due to mediastinal hemorrhage or tamponade require immediate operative intervention without further diagnostic evaluation.

Arteriography is urgently indicated in patients with mediastinal hemorrhage following trauma. Computed tomography scanning, magnetic resonance imaging (MRI), transesophageal echocardiography, or arteriography are indicated in patients with possible aortic dissections. Therapy is directed toward evacuation of existing clot and repair of the underlying process. In patients with mediastinal hemorrhage that occurs spontaneously or in association with iatrogenic injury, conservative management with invasive monitoring in an intensive care unit usually is successful. Evidence of continued bleeding or development of tamponade requires operative exploration.

SUPERIOR VENA CAVAL OBSTRUCTION

A number of benign and malignant processes may cause obstruction of the superior vena cava (SVC) leading to *superior vena caval syndrome*. The syndrome develops when there is increased pressure in the venous system draining into the superior vena cava, leading to the characteristic features of the syndrome: edema of the head, neck, and upper extremities; distended neck veins with dilated collateral veins over the upper extremities and torso; cyanosis; headache; and confusion. Initially, symptoms are noted and remain more prominent when the patient is in a recumbent position. Although most patients develop symptoms slowly, pathologic processes that cause rapid or sudden occlusion produce striking clinical presentations. Rapid development of cerebral edema and intracranial thrombosis leads to coma and death.

The pathologic cause of the superior vena caval obstruction may be compression, invasion, or thrombosis. Malignant lesions represent over 75 per cent of patients. Bronchogenic carcinoma, usually of the right upper lobe, is the most common lesion. Malignant germ cell tumors, thymomas, lymphomas, primary mediastinal carcinomas, and metastatic involvement of mediastinal lymph nodes are other common malignant etiologies. Benign processes implicated include mediastinal granulomatous diseases, particularly histoplasmosis and tuberculosis, idiopathic mediastinal fibrosis, mediastinal goiter, bronchogenic cyst, teratoma, pleural calcification, and thoracic aortic aneurysm. Although it has become more common to encounter superior vena caval obstruction secondary to indwelling catheters or trauma to the vessel, the superior vena caval syndrome rarely results. The syndrome infrequently occurs in children. However, when it does, it mostly occurs following cardiac procedures, particularly after atrial level repairs for transposition of the great vessels. Other significant causes of childhood superior vena caval syndrome include mediastinal neoplasm (most are non-Hodgkin's lymphomas), ventriculoatrial shunts, and mediastinal fibrosis.

Contrast-enhanced CT scanning or MRI is the basis of the diagnostic evaluation, confirming the diagnosis of obstruction of the SVC, identifying the relative level of the anatomic obstruction, and assisting in the differential diagnosis. Venous angiography is required in patients considered for surgical bypass to determine the patency of the tributary veins.

Because the malignant processes responsible for the superior vena caval syndrome are usually not surgically resectable, a percutaneous needle biopsy technique is often used to establish a histologic diagnosis. Attempts to obtain a histologic diagnosis are made prior to the initiation of empiric therapy because the alteration of the morphology following therapy precludes making a diagnosis in over 40 per cent of patients. Open biopsy in patients able to tolerate anesthesia may be necessary to establish a diagnosis. However, these patients are at an increased risk for cardiorespiratory compromise during general anesthesia. The most useful types of therapy include radiation, corticosteroids, and multiagent chemotherapy. The optimal therapeutic regimen is dependent on the histologic diagnosis. In patients in whom the syndrome develops rapidly or when neurologic symptoms are present, therapy may be necessary on an emergency basis. The rate of success in the treatment of a number of the malignant causes of the superior vena caval syndrome has improved, particularly with the lymphomas and germ cell tumors. Even when treating obstruction secondary to bronchogenic carcinoma, at least transient decompression can usually be obtained.

Surgical bypass of obstructing lesions is appropriate in a few highly selective patients. Of particular importance for success is the presence of adequate flow through either of the innominate veins. In conditions where longstanding superior vena caval obstruction has been present with collateral development, the innominate veins are usually thrombosed, making them unsuitable for revascularization. Occasional long-term survival is possible in patients able to undergo complete resection and SVC reconstruction.

Superior vena caval syndromes that are caused by benign disease usually respond to medical therapy that consists of diuretics, upright positioning, and fluid restriction until collateral channels develop, permitting clinical regression.

MEDIASTINITIS

Infection of the mediastinal space is a serious and potentially fatal process. Etiologic factors responsible for the development of acute mediastinitis include perforation of the esophagus due to instrumentation, foreign bodies, penetrating or, more rarely, blunt trauma; spontaneous esophageal disruption (Boerhaave's syndrome); leakage from an esophageal anastomosis; tracheobronchial perforation; and mediastinal extension from an infectious process originating in the pulmonary parenchyma, pleura, chest wall, vertebrae, great vessels, or neck. Currently, mediastinitis occurs most frequently following median sternotomy for open heart cardiac operations. Superficial wound infections occur in approximately 4 per cent of patients following cardiac operations. In 1 to 2 per cent of patients, the infection involves the mediastinum. Risk factors for the development of mediastinitis include prolonged operation, lengthy cardiopulmonary bypass, reexploration for postoperative bleeding, dehiscence, external cardiac massage, postoperative cardiogenic shock, and the use of bilateral internal mammary arteries for coronary artery bypass grafting, especially in elderly patients or in patients with diabetes mellitus.

Mediastinitis is manifested by fever, tachycardia, leukocytosis, and pain that may be localized to the chest, back, or neck, although in some patients the clinical course remains indolent for long periods. When mediastinitis is secondary to esophageal perforation following instrumentation, the pain is most frequently localized to the neck because the most common site of perforation is at the level of the cricopharyngeal muscle. In these cases, subcutaneous emphysema is almost invariably present. Postoperative mediastinitis usually presents between 3 days and 3 weeks following the operation, although occasionally

delayed manifestations may occur months later. Clinical indications of postoperative mediastinitis include wound erythema, drainage, pain, unstable sternum, spiking fevers, and leukocytosis. The lateral chest film is useful in evaluating for air-fluid levels, abnormal soft tissue densities, and sternal dehiscence. Computed tomography may be useful when mediastinal gas is present, indicating the presence of gas-forming organisms or distinct abscess. Computed tomography also may identify associated or contiguous infections such as an empyema, subphrenic abscess, or cervical soft tissue infection. Water-soluble contrast studies of the esophagus and esophagoscopy are important in evaluating a potential esophageal perforation or disruption. In patients with penetrating or blunt trauma, the use of both procedures has been necessary to minimize the number of overlooked esophageal injuries. Similarly, bronchoscopy is the optimal procedure to evaluate potential tracheobronchial disruption.

Treatment of mediastinitis requires correction of the inciting cause and aggressive supportive therapy. After obtaining cultures, appropriate antimicrobial coverage should be initiated with modification after culture reports and sensitivities are available. In patients with mediastinal infections in continuity or communication with empyema, subphrenic abscess, or neck abscess, drainage of the empyema with tube thoracostomy or percutaneous drainage of the abscess in conjunction with appropriate antimicrobial therapy is frequently successful. Similarly, mediastinitis associated with catheter sepsis can often be treated with removal of the catheter and antimicrobial therapy. However, in patients with mediastinitis secondary to most other etiologies, thorough débridement of necrotic and infected tissue is necessary in conjunction with surgical drainage. When costal cartilage is infected, it is necessary to excise the cartilage back to bleeding bone. Delays in establishing the diagnosis and subsequently initiating therapy, especially when the etiologic factor involves esophageal or tracheobronchial disruption, are associated with sharp increases in morbidity and mortality.

Postoperative mediastinitis following median sternotomy has been successfully treated with a number of different techniques. The simplest approach involves incision, débridement, and drainage of the involved area in conjunction with local irrigation with antibiotics or antiseptic agents and wound care using dressings soaked in dilute povidone-iodine, Dakin's solution, or acetic acid. Delayed closure is possible, although an unstable sternum is the usual result. Improved results have been obtained after thoroughly débriding all affected tissue by using closed irrigation systems. Depending on the severity of the infection, the wound can either be closed or left open after the placement of large-bore drainage tubes through which continuous irrigation with antibiotic solution or diluted povidone-iodine is done. The tubes are removed gradually to minimize residual dead space.

The best results have been obtained using a variety of tissue flaps to obliterate dead space and to provide immediate coverage of the heart, bypass grafts, and great vessels following effective surgical control of the wound. Débridement of infected and necrotic sternum, cartilage, and soft tissue in conjunction with wound care is often necessary to provide a clean wound to optimize results. This therapy has further reduced morbidity and mortality, usually results in a good long-term functional result, and has significantly reduced the duration of hospitalization. The pectoralis major and rectus abdominis muscles have been the most commonly used tissue flaps. Because the rectus abdominis flap is based on the superior epigastric artery, this flap is only useful when the internal mammary artery remains viable. The omentum may be rotated into the sternum using either the left or right gastroepiploic vessels as blood supply.

Although chronic mediastinitis may be due to an indolent bacterial infection, more frequently chronic infections are granulomatous processes that follow tuberculosis or mycotic infections. Active infection necessitates treatment with antituberculosis or antifungal agents. With progressive cases of chronic infection, the granulomatous process within the mediastinal lymph nodes may compress adjacent structures, such as the venae cavae, trachea, bronchi, or esophagus. Of the mycotic infections, histoplasmosis has the greatest predilection for severe involvement of the mediastinal lymph nodes. Rarely, surgical decompression, excision, or bypass is necessary in addition to medical therapy to treat the resultant obstruction.

PRIMARY NEOPLASMS AND CYSTS

A large number of neoplasms and cysts arise from multiple anatomic sites in the mediastinum and present with a host of clinical signs and symptoms. The natural history varies from those that are asymptomatic to those with benign slow growth causing minimal symptoms, to aggressive, invasive neoplasms that are often widely metastatic, and rapidly lead to death. A classification of primary mediastinal tumors and cysts is shown in Table 1. Although some differences in the relative incidence of neoplasms and cysts exist in some series, the most common mediastinal masses are neurogenic tumors (20 per cent), thymomas (19 per cent), primary cysts (21 per cent), lymphomas (13 per cent), and germ cell tumors (10 per cent). Mediastinal masses are most frequently located in the anterosuperior mediastinum (54 per cent), with the posterior (26 per cent) and middle mediastinum (20 per

TABLE 1. CLASSIFICATION OF PRIMARY MEDIASTINAL TUMORS AND CYSTS*

Neurogenic tumors	Mesenchymal tumors
Neurofibroma	Fibroma/fibrosarcoma
Neurilemoma	Lipoma/liposarcoma
Neurosarcoma	Leiomyoma/
Ganglioneuroma	leiomyosarcoma
Neuroblastoma	Rhabdosarcoma
Chemodectoma	Xanthogranuloma
Paraganglioma	Myxoma
	Mesothelioma
Thymoma	Hemangioma
Benign	Hemangioendothelioma
Malignant	Hemangiopericytoma
	Lymphangioma
Lymphoma	Lymphangiomyoma
Hodgkin's disease	Lymphangiopericytoma
Lymphoblastic	
Large cell diffuse growth	Endocrine tumors
pattern	Intrathoracic thyroid
T immunoblastic sarcoma	Parathyroid adenoma/
B immunoblastic sarcoma	carcinoma
Sclerosing follicular cell	Carcinoid
Germ cell tumors	Cysts
Teratodermoid	Bronchogenic
Benign	Pericardial
Malignant	Enteric
Seminoma	Thymic
Nonseminomas	Thoracic duct
Embryonal	Nonspecific
Choriocarcinoma	
Endodermal	Giant lymph node hyperplasia
	Castleman's disease
Primary carcinomas	
	Chondroma
	Extramedullary hematopoiesis

*From Davis RD Jr, Sabiston DC Jr: The mediastinum. *In* Sabiston DC Jr [ed]: Textbook of Surgery: The Biological Basis of Modern Surgical Practice, ed 14. Philadelphia, WB Saunders Company, 1991, p 1775, with permission.

cent) being less frequently involved. Many of the mediastinal lesions occur in characteristic sites within the mediastinum. In the anterosuperior mediastinum, the most frequent neoplasms are thymoma (31 per cent), lymphoma (23 per cent), and germ cell tumor (17 per cent). Posterior mediastinal lesions are usually neurogenic tumors (52 per cent), bronchogenic cysts (22 per cent), and enteric cysts (7 per cent). Middle mediastinal masses are usually pericardial cysts (35 per cent), lymphomas (21 per cent), and bronchogenic cysts (15 per cent). Because of the characteristic location of many mediastinal masses, the site of the mass establishes a useful differential diagnosis that aids in planning the diagnostic evaluation and possible operative procedure. In addition, the location of the mass explains some typical symptoms because of compression or invasion of adjacent mediastinal structures. Anterosuperior mediastinal masses are most likely to produce the superior vena caval syndrome, middle mediastinal masses are most likely to cause tamponade, and posterior mediastinal masses are most likely to cause spinal cord compression syndromes. The common symptoms related to mechanical involvement with mediastinal structures are listed in Table 2.

Malignant neoplasms represent 25 to 42 per cent of mediastinal masses. Lymphomas, thymomas, germ cell tumors, primary carcinomas, and neurogenic tumors are the most common. The relative frequency of mediastinal mass malignancy varies with the anatomic site in the mediastinum. Anterosuperior masses are most likely malignant (59 per cent), relative to middle mediastinal masses (29 per cent) and posterior mediastinal masses (16 per cent). The relative percentage of lesions that are malignant also varies with age (Fig. 3). Patients in the second through fourth decades have a greater proportion of malignant mediastinal masses. This period corresponds with the peak incidence of lymphomas and germ cell tumors. In contrast, in the first decade of life, a mediastinal mass is most likely benign (73 per cent).

The incidence of various mediastinal masses varies in infants, children, and adults. In children with mediastinal masses neurogenic tumors (35 per cent), lymphomas (25 per cent), germ cell tumors (11 per cent), and primary cysts (16 per cent) are diagnosed most frequently. The neurogenic tumors in children most commonly originate from sympathetic ganglion cells, gangliomas, ganglioneuroblastomas, and neuroblastomas. In contrast, neurilemomas and neurofibromas are the most common neurogenic tumors in adults. The childhood lymphomas are usually of a non-Hodgkin's variety. The germ cell tumors are most frequently benign teratomas. Pericardial cysts and thymomas are uncommon in children.

The clinical presentation varies in patients with a mediastinal mass from those who are asymptomatic (the diagnosis is made by routine chest film), to those with symptoms related to mechanical effects of invasion or compression, and to those who have systemic symptoms. These systemic symptoms may be vague and nonspecific, or they may be characteristic for a specific neoplasm, such as the relationship between myasthenia gravis and thymoma.

Of patients with a mediastinal mass, 56 to 65 per cent are symptomatic at presentation. Patients with a benign lesion are more often asymptomatic (54 per cent) than are patients with a malignant neoplasm (15 per cent). The absence of symptoms is associated with a benign histologic diagnosis: 76 per cent of asymptomatic patients have a benign lesion; in contrast, 62 per cent of symptomatic patients have a malignant neoplasm. The most common symptoms are chest pain, cough, and fever. Myasthenia gravis occurs in over 40 per cent of patients with thymomas. Infants most likely present with symptoms or findings (78 per

TABLE 2. CLINICAL MANIFESTATIONS OF ANATOMIC COMPRESSION OR INVASION BY NEOPLASMS OF THE MEDIASTINUM*

Vena caval obstruction
Pericardial tamponade
Congestive heart failure
Dysrhythmias
Pulmonary stenosis
Tracheal compression
Esophageal compression
Vocal cord paralysis
Horner's syndrome
Phrenic nerve paralysis
Chylothorax
Chylopericardium
Spinal cord compressive syndrome
Pancoast's syndrome
Postobstructive pneumonitis

*From Davis RD Jr, Sabiston DC Jr: The mediastinum. *In* Sabiston DC Jr [ed]: Textbook of Surgery: The Biological Basis of Modern Surgical Practice, ed 14. Philadelphia, WB Saunders Company, 1991, p 1776, with permission.

cent) because of the relatively small space within the mediastinum. Paralleling the relative percentages of malignant neoplasms within the different anatomic regions, tumors of the anterosuperior mediastinum are most likely to cause symptoms (75 per cent) relative to the posterior mediastinum (50 per cent) and the middle mediastinum (45 per cent).

Symptoms related to compression or invasion of mediastinal structures, such as the superior vena caval syndrome, Horner's syndrome, hoarseness, and severe

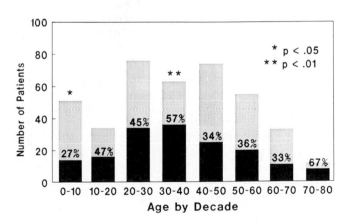

Figure 3. Age distribution and incidence of malignancy relative to age. The largest number of patients with a mediastinal mass were in the third through fifth decades. The fourth decade had a significantly greater proportion of malignant disease. The first decade had a significantly lower proportion of malignant disease. (From Davis RD Jr, Oldham HN Jr, Sabiston DC Jr: Primary cysts and neoplasms of the mediastinum: Recent changes in clinical presentation, methods of diagnosis, management, and results. Ann Thorac Surg 44:229, 1987, with permission.)

pain, are more indicative of a malignant histologic diagnosis, although patients with a benign lesion, on occasion, present in this manner. A number of primary mediastinal lesions produce hormones or antibodies that cause systemic symptoms that may characterize a specific syndrome (Table 3). Examples of these syndromes include *Cushing's syndrome*, caused by ectopic production of adrenocorticotropic hormone (ACTH), most frequently by carcinoid tumors; *thyrotoxicosis*, caused by mediastinal goiter; *hypertension* and a *hyperdynamic* state caused by pheochromocytoma; and hypercalcemia secondary to a mediastinal parathyroid adenoma.

In other syndromes, the pathophysiology is not as well understood, such as the association of large mesenchymal tumors with episodic hypoglycemia, presumably related to production of circulating factors capable of insulin-like action or of provoking insulin release (Doege-Potter syndrome). Autoimmune mechanisms have been implicated in the association of myasthenia gravis and red cell aplasia with thymoma. Associations that remain largely unexplained include osteoarthropathy and neurogenic tumors, pain after ingestion of alcohol and the cyclic Pel-Ebstein fevers of Hodgkin's disease, and the opsomyoclonus syndrome and neuroblastoma.

Diagnostic Evaluation

The goal of the diagnostic evaluation in a patient with a mediastinal mass is a precise histologic diagnosis so that optimal therapy can be performed. The preoperative evaluation of a patient with a mediastinal mass should achieve the following: (1) differentiate a primary mediastinal mass from masses of other etiologies that have a similar radiographic appearance; (2) recognize associated systemic manifestations that may impact on the patient's perioperative course; (3) evaluate for possible compression by the mass of the tracheobronchial tree, pulmonary artery, or superior vena cava; (4) ascertain whether the mass extends into the spinal column; (5) determine if the mass is a nonseminomatous germ cell tumor; (6) assess the likelihood of resectability; and (7) identify significant factors of medical comorbidity and optimize overall medical condition.

The initial diagnostic intervention should be a careful history and physical examination. The recognition of associated systemic syndromes with many mediastinal neoplasms is necessary to avoid potentially serious intraoperative and postoperative complications. Although most systemic syndromes listed in Table 4 may be of little consequence regarding the planned surgical management, the association of myasthenia gravis, malignant hypertension, hypogammaglobulinemia, hypercalcemia, and thyrotoxicosis with medi-

astinal neoplasms markedly impact on appropriate management.

The posteroanterior and lateral chest films provide important information: size of the lesion, its location within the mediastinum, displacement and alteration of anatomic structures in the mediastinum and adjacent regions, and the relative density of the mass with regard to whether the lesion is cystic or solid, and the presence and pattern of calcifications. Information regarding the anatomic location of the mediastinal mass narrows the differential diagnosis. Computed tomo-

TABLE 3.   SYSTEMIC SYNDROMES CAUSED BY MEDIASTINAL NEOPLASM HORMONE PRODUCTION*

Syndrome	Tumor
Hypertension	Pheochromocytoma, chemodectoma, ganglioneuroma, neuroblastoma
Hypoglycemia	Mesothelioma, teratoma, fibrosarcoma, neurosarcoma
Diarrhea	Ganglioneuroma, neuroblastoma, neurofibroma
Hypercalcemia	Parathyroid adenoma/carcinoma, Hodgkin's disease
Thyrotoxicosis	Thyroid adenoma/carcinoma
Gynecomastia	Nonseminomatous germ cell tumors

*From Davis RD Jr, Sabiston DC Jr: The mediastinum. *In* Sabiston DC Jr [ed]: Textbook of Surgery: The Biological Basis of Modern Surgical Practice, ed 14. Philadelphia, WB Saunders Company, 1991, p 1778, with permission.

TABLE 4.   SYSTEMIC SYNDROMES ASSOCIATED WITH MEDIASTINAL NEOPLASMS*

Tumor	Syndrome
Thymoma	Myasthenia gravis
	Red blood cell aplasia
	White blood cell aplasia
	Aplastic anemia
	Hypogammaglobulinemia
	Progressive systemic sclerosis
	Hemolytic anemia
	Megaesophagus
	Dermatomyositis
	Systemic lupus erythematosus
	Myocarditis
	Collagen vascular disease
Lymphoma	Anemia, myasthenia gravis
Neurofibroma	von Recklinghausen's disease
Carcinoid	Cushing's syndrome
Carcinoid, thymoma	Multiple endocrine adenomatosis
Thymoma, neurofibroma, neurilemoma, mesothelioma	Osteoarthropathy
Enteric cysts	Vertebral anomalies
Hodgkin's disease	Alcohol-induced pain
	Pel-Ebstein fever
Neuroblastoma	Opsomyoclonus
	Erythrocyte abnormalities
Enteric cysts	Peptic ulcer

*From Davis RD Jr, Sabiston DC Jr: The mediastinum. *In* Sabiston DC Jr [ed]: Textbook of Surgery: The Biological Basis of Modern Surgical Practice, ed 14. Philadelphia, WB Saunders Company, 1991, p 1779, with permission.

graphic imaging with contrast should be obtained in the majority of patients with a mediastinal mass. In patients with a contraindication to the use of contrast dye, MRI is useful. Accurate anatomic information regarding the relationship of the mass to surrounding structures is provided. Considerable information can be obtained regarding the relative invasiveness and malignant nature of the mediastinal mass. Tumor disruption of fat planes; irregularity of pleural, vascular, or pericardial margins by tumor; and infiltration into muscle or periosteum is useful information for differentiating tumor compression from invasion. Computed tomography more accurately predicts resectability of a neoplasm than unresectability. Additional information obtained using CT includes the presence of chest wall invasion, differentiation of multiple masses from a single large mass (useful in differentiating lymphomas from other common solitary lesions), and possible extension from a posterior mediastinal mass into the spinal column. These posterior mediastinal masses should be further evaluated with CT myelography or MRI.

Computed tomography or MRI reliably differentiates mediastinal tumors from mediastinal masses that are of a cardiovascular etiology such as aneurysms, dilations, and abnormal locations of cardiac or vascular structures, and may appear on chest film as a mediastinal mass (Table 5). Similarly, abnormalities of the spinal column, such as meningoceles, are differ-

entiated from neurogenic tumors and other posterior mediastinal masses. This differentiation is particularly important in patients with neurofibromatosis who are at a greater risk for the development of both meningoceles and neurofibromas. Also differentiated are other entities that may resemble a mediastinal mass including esophageal lesions (such as esophageal diverticula, tumor, hiatal hernia, and achalasia), diaphragmatic herniations, pancreatic pseudocysts, herniations of peritoneal fat, mediastinitis, and a number of primary pulmonary parenchymal lesions and infections.

Several mediastinal masses can be diagnosed preoperatively using these imaging modalities due to their characteristic location, appearance, and attenuation values. For example, pericardial cysts usually occur at the cardiophrenic angle with smooth, circumscribed borders and near-water attenuation values. Despite the accuracy of CT imaging, emphasis must remain on establishing the precise histologic diagnosis to avoid mistreating a potentially curable neoplasm. Using CT, the correct preoperative diagnosis is made in only approximately 68 per cent of patients.

Serologic evaluation is indicated in certain patients. Alpha-fetoprotein (αFP) and beta-human chorionic gonadotropin (β-HCG) serologies should be obtained in male patients with an anterosuperior mediastinal mass in the second through fifth decades. A positive test is indicative of a nonseminomatous germ cell tu-

TABLE 5. MEDIASTINAL MASSES DUE TO CARDIOVASCULAR LESIONS*

Mediastinal Location	Systemic Venous System	Pulmonary Arterial System	Pulmonary Venous System	Systemic Arterial System
Anterior				Aortic stenosis (poststenotic dilation) Ascending aortic aneurysm
Middle	Superior vena caval aneurysm Azygous vein enlargement	Pulmonary valve stenosis Idiopathic dilation of the pulmonary trunk Congenital absence of the pulmonary valve Pulmonary embolism Pulmonary arterial hypertension Anomalous left pulmonary artery	Pulmonary venous varix Pulmonary venous confluence Partial anomalous pulmonary return to the superior vena cava	Aortic stenosis Right aortic arch Transverse arch aortic aneurysm Aneurysm/fistula of the coronary artery
Posterior				Coarctation and pseudo-coarctation Descending aortic aneurym Tortuous innominate artery
Superior	Aneurysms of the innominate veins Persistent left superior vena cava Hemiazygous vein enlargement	Aneurysm of the ductus	Partial anomalous pulmonary venous return to the innominate vein Total anomalous pulmonary venous return (supracardiac)	Cervical aortic arch Coarction of the aorta Transverse arch aortic aneurysm

*From Davis RD Jr, Sabiston DC Jr: The mediastinum. *In* Sabiston DC Jr [ed]: Textbook of Surgery: The Biological Basis of Modern Surgical Practice, ed 14. Philadelphia, WB Saunders Company, 1991, p 1781, with permission.

mor, and appropriate treatment with *cis*-platinum–based chemotherapy may be initiated without surgical exploration.

Measurement of urinary excretion of vanillylmandelic acid (VMA) and catecholamines should be performed in patients with a mediastinal mass and history of significant hypertension or hypermetabolism. This enables the initiation of appropriate perioperative adrenergic blockers in patients with hormonally active intrathoracic pheochromocytoma, paraganglioma, and neuroblastoma, limiting perioperative complications secondary to episodic catecholamine release.

Asymptomatic patients with contrast-enhancing lesions in the superior mediastinum should be evaluated with an ^{131}I scan. Careful observation without excision using serial CTs to evaluate for growth is indicated in an *asymptomatic* patient with a positive scan indicative of a thyroid lesion and no identifiable active thyroid tissue elsewhere.

Increased success has been reported in making a cytologic diagnosis preoperatively by using fine-needle biopsy techniques (22-gauge needle), with low morbidity and almost zero mortality. Fluoroscopic visualization is usually used to guide the biopsy. Because they permit better localization of the mass and improved placement of the needle, CT and echocardiography have increased the sensitivity of the technique. Although a precise histologic diagnosis is not always possible, a cytologic diagnosis of benign or malignant can be made in 80 to 90 per cent of patients. Complications related to the procedure include: pneumothorax in 20 to 25 per cent of patients with approximately 5 per cent requiring tube thoracostomy; hemoptysis in 5 to 10 per cent, with rare occurrences of significant hemorrhagic complications; and tumor seeding along the needle tract, which is a theoretical but extremely rare complication. An increased sensitivity in obtaining a precise histologic diagnosis has been reported using cutting needle techniques (16-gauge needle) without an apparent increase in morbidity (23 per cent incidence of pneumothorax). Needle biopsy techniques are particularly useful for evaluating patients with small-cell carcinoma or metastatic carcinoma because of the possibility of obviating a thoracotomy or other invasive procedure to establish a histologic diagnosis. The use of electron microscopy to examine the cellular ultrastructure and immunohistochemical staining has increased the sensitivity of the various needle biopsy techniques.

Some tumors with marked associated desmoplastic changes are rarely diagnosed using a needle biopsy, such as nodular-sclerosing Hodgkin's lymphoma. Additionally, needle biopsy rarely provides adequate tissue for precise immunotyping, which is necessary to determine optimal therapy, particularly with the non-Hodgkin's lymphomas. Poorly differentiated malig-

nant tumors of the anterosuperior mediastinum, particularly thymomas, lymphomas, germ cell tumors, and primary carcinomas, can have remarkably similar cytologic and morphologic appearances. Diagnoses based on examination of frozen sections are therefore frequently incorrect, and similarly, therapeutic decisions based on frozen section examination may be in error. To establish an accurate diagnosis, it may be necessary to use special staining and immunostaining techniques and electron microscopy of multiple sections of the tumor, in addition to light microscopy. The characteristic ultrastructural features as evaluated by electron microscopy are shown in Table 6. Monoclonal antibodies for surface antigens specific to a cell line of origin and for tumor-secretory products can be useful in establishing a precise diagnosis. Immunotyping of non-Hodgkin's lymphomas has allowed accurate subtyping of these lesions, which has been important in predicting natural history and optimal therapy.

Although surgical excision is not essential for the treatment of a number of malignant neoplasms, the optimal therapeutic regimen often requires precise histologic subclassification. Because needle biopsy techniques do not usually produce sufficient tissue for this purpose, more invasive procedures are often required. Mediastinoscopy and mediastinotomy are useful for incisional biopsy of lesions in the anterosuperior mediastinum. Median sternotomy and anterolateral thoracotomy for anterosuperior masses and posterolateral thoracotomies for middle and posterior mediastinal masses allow for better exposure, a better evaluation of the resectability of the mass, and, when possible, resection of the mass.

Although most patients with a mediastinal mass can undergo general anesthesia with minimal risk, patients, particularly children, with a large anterosuperior or middle mediastinal mass are at an increased risk

TABLE 6. ULTRASTRUCTURAL CHARACTERISTICS OF MEDIASTINAL TUMORS*

Tumors	Ultrastructure
Carcinoid	Dense core granules, fewer tonofilaments and desmosomes
Lymphoma	Absence of junctional attachments and epithelial features
Thymoma	Well-formed desmosomes, bundles of tonofilaments
Germ cell	Prominent nucleoli, even chromatin, scant desmosomes, rare tonofilaments
Neuroblastoma	Neurosecretory granules, synaptic endings

*From Davis RD Jr, Sabiston DC Jr: The mediastinum. *In* Sabiston DC Jr [ed]: Textbook of Surgery: The Biological Basis of Modern Surgical Practice, ed 14. Philadelphia, WB Saunders Company, 1991, p 1780, with permission.

for life-threatening cardiorespiratory compromise intraoperatively due to compression by the mass of the tracheobronchial tree, pulmonary artery, or superior vena cava. Exacerbation of superior vena caval obstruction or extrinsic airway compression occurs during general anesthesia. Patients with posture-related dyspnea and superior vena caval syndrome are at increased risk. Useful techniques for identifying patients who have significant airway compromise but who are asymptomatic include CT imaging, in which a reduction in tracheal cross-sectional area of more than 35 per cent is indicative of an increased risk with general anesthesia, and pulmonary flow mechanics, in which reductions in peak expiratory flow serve as a sensitive indicator of functional airway compression. In patients with airway compression or superior vena caval obstruction, the risk of general anesthesia is prohibitive, and attempts to obtain a histologic diagnosis should be limited to needle biopsies or open procedures done under local anesthesia. Occasionally, benign tumors, usually teratomas in young children and infants, may produce this situation. In patients with large mediastinal masses who have increased anesthetic risk but in whom histologic diagnosis is needed before therapy or for whom complete excision is the preferred treatment, recommendations for anesthetic management include: (1) fiberoptic evaluation of the tracheobronchial system for evidence of severe extrinsic compression, (2) induction of anesthesia in a semi-Fowler's position with the ability to change to the lateral or prone positions, (3) use of long endotracheal tubes to allow advancement of the tube beyond the site of obstruction, (4) standby rigid bronchoscopy to allow reestablishment of an adequate airway, (5) avoidance of muscle relaxants and use of spontaneous ventilation when possible, (6) lower extremity intravenous intubation to provide access to the systemic venous circulation if a sudden superior vena caval obstruction should occur, and (7) standby cardiopulmonary bypass with bilateral groin preparation.

Neurogenic Tumors

Neurogenic tumors are the most common neoplasm in the collected series, comprising 21 per cent of all primary tumors and cysts. These tumors are usually located in the posterior mediastinum and originate from the sympathetic ganglia (ganglioma, ganglioneuroblastoma, and neuroblastoma), the intercostal nerves (neurofibroma, neurilemoma, and neurosarcoma), and the paraganglia cells (paraganglioma). Although the peak incidence occurs in adults, neurogenic tumors comprise a proportionally greater percentage of mediastinal masses in children (35 per cent). Whereas most neurogenic tumors in adults are benign,

a greater percentage of neurogenic tumors are malignant in children.

Many of these tumors are found in asymptomatic patients on routine chest films. When present, symptoms are usually caused by mechanical factors such as chest and back pain due to compression or invasion of intercostal nerve, bone, and chest wall; cough and dyspnea due to compression of the tracheobronchial tree; and Pancoast's syndrome and Horner's syndrome due to involvement of the brachial and the cervical sympathetic chain. Approximately 10 per cent of neurogenic tumors have extensions into the spinal column. These tumors are termed dumbbell tumors because of their characteristic shape due to the relatively large paraspinal and intraspinal portions connected by a narrow isthmus of tissue traversing the intervertebral foramen. Although 60 per cent of patients with a dumbbell tumor have neurologic symptoms related to spinal cord compression, the significant proportion of patients without symptoms underscores the importance of evaluating all patients with a posterior mediastinal mass for possible intraspinal extension. Computed tomography, MRI, and vertebral tomography are useful for indicating enlargement of the foramen, erosion of bone, and intervertebral widening. If these findings are present, CT with myelography or MRI is indicated to evaluate the presence and extent of the intraspinal component. A single-stage approach with excision of both the thoracic component and the intraspinal component is recommended by most series. Symptoms with some neurogenic tumors may be systemic and related to production of neurohormonal agents. Production of catecholamine by paragangliomas and neuroblastomas causes the constellation of symptoms that are characteristic of pheochromocytomas: hypertension, which is often severe and episodic, sweating, headaches, and palpitations. Production of vasoactive intestinal polypeptide by ganglioneuromas and neuroblastomas causes a syndrome of abdominal distention and profuse watery diarrhea.

The most common neurogenic tumor is the *neurilemoma*, which has a defined capsule and is well circumscribed. The cell of origin is the perineural Schwann cell, and the peak incidence is in the third through fifth decades. *Neurofibromas* originate as a proliferation of all the elements of the peripheral nerve. These tumors are poorly encapsulated, and surgical excision effects a cure.

Neurosarcomas originate by malignant degeneration from neurilemoma or neurofibroma in addition to developing de novo. Although they usually occur in adults, these tumors sometimes are seen in children with neurofibromatosis. Although surgical excision is optimal therapy, these are aggressive, rapidly growing tumors that invade vital structures early, often precluding surgical removal. Adjuvant therapies are minimally beneficial.

Ganglioneuroma, ganglioneuroblastoma, and *neuroblastoma* originate from the sympathetic chain and are composed of ganglion cells and nerve fibers. These tumors differ in terms of differentiation of the ganglion cells. Ganglioneuromas are composed of mature cells, neuroblastomas are composed of immature cells, and ganglioneuroblastomas are composed of a mixture of cells. These tumors occur in infancy and childhood and are initially located in the paravertebral gutter. Ganglioneuromas are well encapsulated, and surgical excision provides cure.

Ganglioneuroblastomas are differentiated into two histologic patterns: *composite,* which is characterized by predominantly mature ganglion cell with focal areas of primitive neuroblasts and is associated with a high incidence of metastatic disease; and *diffuse,* which is characterized by a mixture of mature and immature neuroblasts and is associated with metastatic disease in less than 5 per cent of patients. Ganglioneuroblastoma and neuroblastoma are staged as follows: stage I, well-circumscribed, noninvasive tumor; stage II, tumor invasion locally without extension across the midline; stage III, tumor spread across the midline; and stage IV, tumor with metastasis. Mediastinal neuroblastomas comprise 10 to 20 per cent of all neuroblastomas. These are highly invasive lesions that have frequently metastasized at the time of diagnosis. Regional lymph nodes, bone, brain, liver, and lung are common sites of metastases. Patients are usually symptomatic, most commonly with cough, dyspnea, dysphagia, back or chest pain, and symptoms related to recurrent pulmonary infections. A variety of paraneoplastic syndromes have been reported including "pheochromocytoma syndrome" due to catecholamine secretion, profuse watery diarrhea and abdominal pain related to vasoactive intestinal polypeptide (VIP) production, and the opsoclonus-polymyoclonus syndrome, an unexplained symptom complex characterized by cerebellar and truncal ataxia with rapid, darting eye movements (dancing eyes) that is possibly related to an autoimmune mechanism. The immunobiology of neuroblastomas is unique. Well-documented cases of spontaneous regression or maturation of tumor have been reported. In vitro, this can be stimulated by VIP hormone or retinoids.

In patients with ganglioneuroblastoma, stage I and II disease is treated with surgical excision, with 5-year survival of almost 90 per cent, while patients with stage III or IV disease, composite morphology, or age greater than 3 years are treated with multiagent chemotherapy. In patients with neuroblastomas, therapy is determined by the stage of the disease: stage I is treated with surgical excision; stage II, with excision and radiation therapy; and stages III and IV with mul-

timodality therapy using surgical debulking, radiation therapy, and multiagent chemotherapy, as well as a second-look exploration to resect residual disease when necessary. Children less than 1 year of age have an excellent prognosis even when widespread disease is present. However, with increasing age and extent of involvement, the prognosis worsens. Interestingly, mediastinal neuroblastomas appear to have a better prognosis than tumors occurring elsewhere. In patients with neuroblastomas resistant to therapy or in those who relapse, ablative chemotherapy with autologous bone marrow transplantation has been attempted with some success.

Mediastinal paragangliomas are rare tumors representing less than 1 per cent of all mediastinal tumors and less than 2 per cent of all *pheochromocytomas.* Although most are found in the paravertebral sulcus, an increasing number of middle mediastinal paragangliomas occur in the branchial arch structures, coronary and aortopulmonary paraganglia, the atria, and islands of tissue in the pericardium. As compared to tumors of the adrenal medulla, mediastinal paragangliomas are less likely to be functionally active and rarely produce epinephrine. Catecholamine production causes the classic constellation of symptoms associated with pheochromocytomas including periodic or sustained hypertension, often accompanied by orthostatic hypotension, hypermetabolism manifested by weight loss, hyperhidrosis, palpitations, and headaches. Measurement of elevated levels of urinary catecholamines or their metabolites, the metanephrines and VMA, usually establishes the diagnosis. Tumor localization has improved remarkably through the use of CT and metaiodobenzylguanidine (^{131}I-MIBG) scintigraphy, particularly when the tumors are hormonally active. Hormonally active tumors may be located with an 85 per cent sensitivity using the ^{131}I MIBG scan. When appropriate, surgical resection, is the optimal therapy after a preoperative course with an α-adrenergic antagonist. In patients with tumors involving the middle mediastinum, cardiopulmonary bypass may be necessary to enable resection. Differentiation of benign from malignant tumors is determined by the patient's clinical course. Although 50 per cent of tumors appear malignant morphologically, metastatic disease develops in only 3 per cent of patients. Approximately 10 per cent of patients have multiple paragangliomas.

Thymoma

Thymoma is the most common neoplasm of the anterosuperior mediastinum. While thymomas are rare in the first two decades, they occur throughout adulthood, with a peak incidence in the third through fifth decades. Patients are usually symptomatic at presentation, and symptoms may be related to local mass effects causing chest pain, dyspnea, hemoptysis, cough, and the superior vena caval syndrome. Thymomas frequently are associated with systemic syndromes presumably caused by immunologic mechanisms, and the most common is myasthenia gravis. However, many other syndromes have been associated with thymomas including red cell aplasia, pure white cell aplasia, aplastic anemia, Cushing's syndrome, hypogammaglobulinemia and hypergammaglobulinemia, dermatomyositis, systemic lupus erythematosus, progressive systemic sclerosis, hypercoagulopathy with thrombosis, rheumatoid arthritis, megaesophagus, and granulomatous myocarditis.

Thymomas are histologically classified by either the predominance of epithelial or lymphocytic cells (lymphocytic, epithelial, mixed, and spindle) or by the morphologic resemblance to cortical or medullary epithelium. Unfortunately, a wide variance in the cellular composition often is present within the tumor and a consistent relationship is not present between the microscopic appearance and biologic behavior, either with tumor invasiveness or association with systemic syndromes. The differentiation between benign and malignant disease is determined by the presence of *gross* invasion of adjacent structures, metastasis, or microscopic evidence of capsular invasion. Fifteen to 65 per cent of thymomas are benign. The relative percentage is partially related to early surgical treatment of myasthenia gravis; if thymectomy is performed early in the course of myasthenia gravis, a greater percentage of thymomas are benign.

Whenever possible, the therapy for thymoma is surgical excision with protection of vital structures. Even with well-encapsulated thymomas, extended thymectomy with eradication of all accessible mediastinal fatty-areolar tissue should be performed to ensure removal of all ectopic thymic tissue, an approach that lowers the number of recurrences. The best operative exposure is obtained using a median sternotomy. Because many thymomas are radiosensitive, the placement of surgical clips to outline the anatomic extent of disease aids in the determination of optimal radiation portals.

Staging of thymoma is as follows: stage I, tumor is well encapsulated without evidence of gross or microscopic capsular invasion; stage II, tumor exhibits pericapsular growth into adjacent mediastinal fat, pleura, or pericardium; stage III, tumor invades adjacent organs or intrathoracic metastasis is present; and stage IV, extrathoracic metastatic spread, which occurs uncommonly. The adjunctive use of radiation therapy with a dose of 3500 to 5000 rad is the recommended treatment for stage II and III disease. Preoperative radiation therapy is useful when superior vena caval obstruction is present or when extensive invasion is man-

ifested by CT or MRI. Occasionally, tumors that are not resectable on initial exploration become resectable following therapy. In patients with stage IV disease or recurrent disease unresponsive to therapy, multiagent chemotherapy (CHOP, CAP-doxorubicin, cyclophosphamide, and *cis*-platinum) has been used. The prognosis for patients with thymoma is dependent on clinical stage; 5-year survival is as follows: stage I, 85 to 100 per cent; stage II, 60 to 80 per cent; stage III, 40 to 70 per cent; and stage IV, 15 to 50 per cent.

Myasthenia Gravis

Myasthenia gravis occurs in 10 to 50 per cent of patients with thymoma, and the incidence increases with age. In males over 50 and females over 60, the incidence appears to be greater than 80 per cent, but it is clear that most patients with myasthenia gravis do not have thymoma. The incidence is 10 to 42 per cent depending on the specific medical center. Males with myasthenia gravis are 1.8 to 2 times more likely than females to have a thymoma. Because of the significant association between thymoma and myasthenia gravis, an evaluation of the mediastinum with CT or MRI is recommended in all patients with myasthenia gravis.

The diagnosis of myasthenia gravis is usually confirmed by a transient increase in muscle strength following the administration of a short-acting anticholinesterase inhibitor such as edrophonium (Tensilon). Electromyographic testing is also used to make the diagnosis and to follow the course of the disease quantitatively. An abnormal loss of muscle contraction strength following multiple stimulations (usually 3 to 5/sec) of the appropriate motor nerve constitutes a positive test. The surgical management of thymoma is discussed in a later section.

In patients with myasthenia gravis, perioperative management is extremely important to prevent complications. Discontinuation of anticholinesterase inhibitors decreases the amount of pulmonary secretions and prevents inadvertent cholinergic weakness. This is usually possible with the routine use of plasmapheresis within 72 hours of thymectomy. Plasmapheresis is very effective in controlling generalized weakness in most patients. Also, careful attention to the maintenance of pulmonary function with chest physiotherapy, endotracheal suctioning, and bronchodilators is the goal of postoperative management. The decision to extubate the patient is based on evidence of adequate respiratory mechanics (e.g., vital capacity >15 ml/kg and expiratory pressures >40 cm H_2O) rather than evidence of adequate ventilation as determined by analysis of arterial blood gases. Currently, the presence of myasthenia gravis is not an adverse predictor of survival, and prognosis is determined by stage of the tumor.

Germ Cell Tumors

Mediastinal germ cell tumors are both benign and malignant neoplasms thought to originate from primordial germ cells that fail to complete the migration from the urogenital ridge and remain in the mediastinum. Although these lesions are identical histologically to germ cell tumors originating in the gonads, they are not considered to be metastatic from primary gonadal tumors. They are classified as teratomas and teratocarcinomas, seminomas, embryonal cell carcinomas, choriocarcinoma, and endodermal cell (yolk sac) tumors.

Teratomas are neoplasms comprised of multiple tissue elements derived from the three primitive embryonic layers foreign to the area in which they occur. The peak incidence is in the second and third decades of life, without a sex predisposition. These tumors are located most commonly in the anterosuperior mediastinum, although 3 to 8 per cent occur in the posterior mediastinum. Symptoms, when present, are related to mechanical effects and include chest pain, cough, dyspnea, or symptoms related to recurrent pneumonitis. If a communication between the tumor and the tracheobronchial tree develops, the pathognomonic finding of a cough productive of hair or sebaceous material may result. Hematogenous infection of the cystic component of the tumor may cause symptoms of hemoptysis and recurrent infections due to contiguous spread. Unusual presentations include recurrent pericarditis or pericardial tamponade following invasion or rupture into the pericardium. Rupture into the pleural space may cause respiratory distress due to the markedly irritative nature of the cyst fluid. However, with the greater use of routine chest films, patients are diagnosed more frequently while asymptomatic with smaller tumors.

Although rare, the diagnosis of these tumors can be made by the identification on imaging study of well-formed teeth. Despite occasional characteristic appearances using various imaging techniques, the diagnosis usually depends on microscopic examination.

The *teratodermoid* (dermoid) cyst is the simplest form and is comprised predominantly of derivatives of the epidermal layer, including dermal and epidermal glands, hair, and sebaceous material. Teratomas are histologically more complex. The solid component of the tumor contains well-differentiated elements of bone, cartilage, teeth, muscle, connective tissue, fibrous and lymphoid tissue, nerve, thymus, mucous and salivary glands, lung, liver, or pancreas. Malignant tumors are differentiated from benign by the presence of primitive or embryonic tissue. Therefore, the diagnosis and therapy rely on surgical excision. For those benign tumors of such large size or that have involvement with adjacent mediastinal structures such that complete resection is impossible, partial resection has led to resolution of symptoms, frequently without relapse.

Malignant germ cell tumors also occur predominantly in the anterosuperior mediastinum and represent approximately 4 per cent of the primary tumors and cysts in the collected series. Unlike the benign teratomas, there is a marked male predominance, with peak incidence in the third and fourth decades of life. Most patients are symptomatic with chest pain, cough, dyspnea, and hemoptysis, and the superior vena caval syndrome occurs commonly. The chest film usually demonstrates a large anterior mediastinal mass that is often multilobulated, with frequent evidence of intrathoracic spread of disease. Computed tomography and MRI are most helpful in defining the extent of involvement and providing a means of following response to therapy and diagnosing relapses. These images are also useful in determining impingement on vital structures that may contraindicate general anesthesia. The malignant germ cell tumors are divided into seminomas and nonseminomas due to the marked radiosensitivity of the former and relative insensitivity of the latter. Serologic measurement of αFP and β-HCG is useful in making this differentiation. Seminomas rarely produce β-HCG (7 per cent) and never produce αFP. In contrast, over 90 per cent of nonseminomas secrete one or both of these hormones. All patients with choriocarcinoma and some patients with embryonal cell tumors have elevated levels of β-HCG, a hormone secreted by the syncytiotrophoblast. Alpha-fetoprotein is most commonly elevated in patients with embryonal cell carcinomas and yolk sac tumors.

Seminomas comprise 50 per cent of malignant germ cell tumors. Unlike other malignant germ cell tumors, seminomas usually remain intrathoracic with local extension to adjacent mediastinal and pulmonary structures. Although metastatic spread occurs first through lymphatics, hematogenous spread with extrathoracic involvement may develop late in the course of disease. Bone and lung are the most common sites of metastatic spread, although liver, brain, spleen, tonsil, and subcutaneous tissue also can be involved. Therapy is determined by the stage of the disease. Occasionally, excision is possible without injury to vital structures (22 per cent) and is recommended when possible. Adjuvant therapy is unnecessary. In disease limited to the thorax, adequate tissue is obtained at biopsy to establish the diagnosis. The basis of therapy is megavoltage radiation to a shaped mediastinal field including the supraclavicular and neck regions (sites of initial lymphatic spread of disease). When cervical lymph nodes are involved, the field is expanded to incorporate the axilla, the site of subsequent lymphatic spread. A dosage of 4500 to 5000 rad (midplane dosage) is usually given over a 6-week course. In patients with extrathoracic disease, relapse following appropriate therapy, or sufficient intrathoracic disease to preclude the likelihood of a complete response using radiation therapy alone, *cis*-platinum–based multiagent chemotherapy has successfully induced remission in most patients.

Malignant nonseminoma tumors include choriocarcinoma, embryonal cell carcinoma, malignant teratoma, and yolk sac (endodermal cell) tumors, of which 40 per cent are a mixture of tissue types. Characteristically, these tumors have extensive intrathoracic involvement and frequently have metastasized outside of the thorax. Frequent sites of metastatic disease include brain, lung, liver, bones, and the lymphatic system, particularly the supraclavicular nodes. Chest wall involvement is common.

A number of chromosomal abnormalities are associated with an increased incidence of germ cell tumors, including Klinefelter's syndrome, trisomy 8, and 5q deletion. Additionally, mediastinal but not testicular germ cell tumors are associated with the development of rare hematologic malignancies such as acute megakaryocytic leukemia and malignant histiocytosis, as well as other hematologic abnormalities including the myelodysplastic syndrome and idiopathic thrombocytopenia (ITP) refractory to treatment.

The local invasiveness of these tumors and frequent metastases usually preclude surgical resection of all disease at the time of diagnosis. Initially, operative intervention is necessary to establish the histologic diagnosis. Therapy may be initiated without open biopsy in males with an anterosuperior mass and elevated levels of αFP or β-HCG with a cytologic diagnosis of a malignancy. Multiagent chemotherapy including *cis*-platinum is the basis of therapy. Other agents to which these tumors respond include vinblastine, bleomycin, methotrexate, etoposide, and doxorubicin. After the tumor hormones have become normal, operative exploration with removal of as much residual disease as possible is indicated. The presence of residual disease following reexploration portends an extremely poor prognosis. Using surgical resection as an adjuvant to multiagent chemotherapy, complete responses in 20 to 80 per cent of patients have been reported.

A subset of these tumors also contains malignant tissue that is not germ cell in origin, but adenocarcinoma or sarcoma. Malignant teratomas or other germ cell tumors with mature differentiated teratoma within the primary are most commonly involved. Despite response of the germ cell component to chemotherapy, there is usually progression of the non–germ cell component and the overall prognosis is poor.

Lymphoma

Although the mediastinum is frequently involved in patients with lymphoma sometime during the course of the disease (40 to 70 per cent), it is infrequently the sole site of disease at the time of presentation. Only 5 to 10 per cent of patients with Hodgkin's and non-Hodgkin's lymphomas present solely with symptoms due to local mass effects, such as mediastinal involvement. Patients are usually symptomatic, with chest pain, cough, dyspnea, hoarseness, and the superior vena caval syndrome being the most common clinical manifestations. Lymphomas also can cause a clinical pattern compatible with pulmonary stenosis and pulmonary embolism by encasement of the pulmonary artery. Nonspecific systemic symptoms of fever and chills, weight loss, and anorexia are frequently noted and are important in the staging of patients with Hodgkin's lymphoma. Symptoms characteristic of Hodgkin's lymphoma include chest pain after consumption of alcohol and the cyclic fevers that were first described by Pel and Ebstein.

Characteristically, these tumors occur in the anterosuperior mediastinum or in the hilar region of the middle mediastinum. Computed tomography and MRI are useful in delineating the extent of disease, determining invasion into contiguous structures, differentiating the lesions from cardiovascular abnormalities, aiding the selection of radiation portals, and following the response to therapy and diagnosing relapse. Also, differentiation from thymomas and germ cell tumors, which usually are solitary masses, is possible because lymphomas usually are comprised of multiple involved nodes that appear as separate masses by CT. Therapy is based on radiation therapy and chemotherapy depending on the stage of disease and the histologic subclassification of the tumor. The surgeon's role is to provide adequate tissue for histologic diagnosis and to assist in pathologic staging, a process frequently requiring staging exploratory laparotomy. Although extrathoracic lymph nodes are frequently involved and available for biopsy, when the sole site of involvement is the mediastinum, a needle biopsy is often unsuccessful because larger tissue samples are needed to make a histologic diagnosis, particularly with nodular sclerosing lesions. Thoracotomy, mediastinoscopy, or mediastinotomy may be necessary to obtain sufficient tissue.

The *Hodgkin's lymphomas* are subdivided by histologic appearance into nodular sclerosing, lymphocyte predominant, mixed cellularity, and lymphocyte depleted. Mediastinal involvement is most common with nodular sclerosing (55 to 75 per cent) and lymphocyte predominant (40 per cent). Stage IA and IIA disease, as defined by the Ann Arbor classification, is treated with megavoltage external beam radiation with a total dose of 4500 rad. Ten-year survival greater than 90 per cent has been reported. Patients with stage IIb, III, and IV disease are usually treated with chemotherapy, and those with higher grade tumor, advanced stage of disease, persistence of an abnormal erythrocyte sedimentation rate (ESR), extensive mediastinal disease, and advanced age (>50 years) are at an increased risk of relapse. Patients with mediastinal disease greater than 35 per cent of the cardiothoracic diameter are often treated with multiagent chemotherapy due to the high relapse rate, although no survival benefit has been shown over treating patients with relapses using salvage chemotherapy. Following treatment, most patients with mediastinal disease have residual mediastinal abnormalities. Treatment with additional chemotherapy or radiation should be reserved for biopsy-confirmed relapse.

Non-Hodgkin's lymphomas are usually either of lymphoblastic morphology (60 per cent) or large cell morphology with a diffuse pattern of growth (40 per cent). In 40 to 80 per cent of patients with lymphoblastic lymphoma, the mediastinum is involved. Although all ages may be afflicted, the peak incidence is in the second and third decades of life. Lymphoblastic lymphoma is characterized by: (1) advanced stage of disease at presentation with 91 per cent of patients having stage III or IV disease, (2) early bone marrow involvement with frequent development of leukemia, (3) tumor cells that exhibit T-lymphocyte antigens, (4) early metastatic spread to the leptomeninges, and (5) initial responsiveness to radiation therapy uniformly followed by relapse. The best results have been obtained using aggressive chemotherapy in conjunction with CNS prophylaxis. The large cell lymphomas of diffuse growth pattern (DHL) are a heterogeneous group differing in the cell type of origin, clinical presentation, natural history, and response to therapy. The DHL tumors can be subclassified into at least three diseases: T-immunoblastic sarcoma, B-immunoblastic sarcoma, and sclerosing variants of follicular cell lymphoma. The T-immunoblastic sarcomas are characterized by morphologic appearance similar to peripheral T-cell lymphomas, slight female predominance, smaller, more confined masses that usually remain intrathoracic, and a higher incidence of causing the superior vena caval syndrome. In comparison, the B-immunoblastic and sclerosing follicular cell lymphomas are more aggressive tumors with more extensive intrathoracic and extrathoracic involvement The peak incidence is in the third and fourth decades with no clear gender predisposition. Therapy is based on doxorubicin-containing chemotherapeutic protocols.

Thyroid Neoplasms

Although substernal extension of a cervical goiter is common, totally intrathoracic thyroid tumors are rare and comprise only 1 per cent of all mediastinal masses and 0.8 per cent of excised thyroids. These tumors arise from heterotopic thyroid tissue, which occurs most commonly in the anterosuperior mediastinum but may also occur in the middle mediastinum between the trachea and esophagus as well as in the posterior mediastinum. Although there may be a demonstrable connection with the cervical gland, usually a fibrous connective tissue band, a true intrathoracic thyroid gland derives its blood supply from thoracic vessels.

The peak incidence is in the sixth and seventh decades, and females are more commonly affected. Symptoms related to tracheal compression are often present such as dyspnea, cough, wheezing, and stridor, or esophageal compression manifested by dysphagia. Rarely, symptoms are related to thyrotoxicosis. On chest film, these lesions appear as sharply circumscribed, dense masses, occurring more frequently on the right. Intrathoracic goiters are contrast-enhancing lesions when visualized by CT. Although some of these neoplasms are functionally inactive and are not identified by the radioactive iodine (^{131}I) scan, it is usually diagnostic.

Most of these tumors are adenomas, but carcinomas have been reported. If the lesion is identified as the sole functioning thyroid tissue and the patient is asymptomatic, surgical exploration and excision is not indicated. In these patients, frequent follow-up radiographic examinations are indicated to evaluate changes in the size or nature of the lesion. Otherwise, these lesions should be resected due to the propensity to enlarge and compress adjacent structures. Because of thoracic derivation of the blood supply, intrathoracic thyroid tumors should be approached through the thorax. Substernal extensions of a cervical goiter are excised using a cervical approach.

Parathyroid Tumors

Although 10 per cent of parathyroid glands occur in the mediastinum, they are usually accessible through a cervical incision. A sternotomy incision is necessary to excise a hyperfunctioning parathyroid gland in approximately 2.5 per cent of all patients and 15 per cent of those with a mediastinal gland. These adenomas are usually located in the anterosuperior mediastinum. The inferior parathyroids are usually associated with the thymus due to the common embryogenesis from the third branchial pouch. The superior parathyroid glands and the lateral lobes of the thyroid gland are derived from the fourth branchial pouch. Because they migrate with the lateral lobes of the thyroid gland to a paraesophageal position, they are found in the posterior mediastinum when they migrate further caudad.

The clinical manifestations of mediastinal parathyroid tumors are similar to those that occur with tumors of the cervical region. The symptoms are related to the excess secretion of parathyroid hormone causing the hyperparathyroid syndrome. Most frequently, the mediastinal adenoma is excised following a negative exploration of the cervical region through the existing cervical incision. Usually, the vascular supply to the adenoma extends from cervical blood vessels. Mediastinal exploration using a median sternotomy is indicated in those patients with persistent hyperparathyroidism producing severe biochemical or metabolic disease following an unsuccessful cervical exploration in which four normal glands have been identified. In these patients, preoperative localization using CT, MRI, thallium and technetium scanning, venous angiography with selective sampling, and selective arteriography, is indicated and is successful in approximately 75 per cent of patients.

Parathyroid carcinomas are usually hormonally active. Patients differ in clinical presentation in that they often have higher serum calcium levels and manifest more severe symptoms of hyperparathyroidism. When possible, surgical resection is the optimal therapy.

Unlike parathyroid adenomas and carcinomas, parathyroid cysts are usually not hormonally active. These cysts are defined by the presence of parathyroid cells identifiable within the cyst wall. Because these lesions are frequently larger than adenomas, symptoms related to local mass effects are more common, as is visualization on chest film. Surgical excision yields a cure.

Mediastinal carcinoid tumors arise from cells of Kulchitsky located in the thymus. Occurring more often in males, these tumors usually are located in the anterosuperior mediastinum. Due to their origin from APUD cells, they may be hormonally active and have been most frequently associated with Cushing's syndrome with production of ACTH. These tumors are not associated with the carcinoid syndrome but may occur as a variant of the multiple endocrine neoplastic (MEN) syndromes.

In patients with hormonally inactive tumors, symptoms are related to local effects of the mass causing chest pain, dyspnea, cough, and the superior vena caval syndrome. Hormonally inactive carcinoids tend to be larger and frequently are invasive locally. In addition, metastatic spread to mediastinal and cervical lymph nodes, liver, bone, skin, and lungs occurs in most patients. Although carcinoids may be difficult to differentiate from other anterosuperior mediastinal tumors, they are characterized by the ultrastructural findings of dense core neurosecretory granules. Positive immunohistochemical staining for ACTH of these granules also is characteristic. Surgical removal when possible is the preferred treatment. Consistent benefit using radiation therapy and multiagent chemotherapy has not been documented.

Mediastinal mesenchymal tumors originate from the connective tissue, striatal and smooth muscle, fat, lymphatic tissue, and blood vessels present within the mediastinum, giving rise to a diverse group of neoplasms. Relative to other sites in the body, these tumors occur less commonly within the mediastinum. Mesenchymal tumors comprised 7 per cent of the primary masses in the collected series, with no apparent difference in incidence between sexes. The soft tissue neoplasms include lipomas, liposarcomas, fibrosarcomas, fibromas, xanthogranulomas, leiomyomas, leiomyosarcomas, benign and malignant mesenchymomas, rhabdomyosarcomas, and mesotheliomas. These tumors have a similar histologic appearance and generally follow the same clinical course as the soft tissue tumors found elsewhere in the body, with 55 per cent malignant. Surgical resection remains the primary therapy, as poor results have been obtained using radiation and chemotherapy.

Similarly, the mesenchymal tumors derived from blood and lymph vessel are common elsewhere in the body, but rare in the mediastinum. Although they occur anywhere in the mediastinum, the most frequent location is in the anterosuperior mediastinum. They include the capillary, cavernous, and venous hemangiomas; hemangioendotheliomas; hemangiopericytomas; lymphangiomas; and the derivatives of lymphangiomas. Symptoms are related to the size and invasiveness of the lesion. Occasionally, hemorrhage into the lesion may lead to a rapid increase in the size. Significant compression and obstruction of mediastinal structures may result, causing a variety of clinical manifestations of which respiratory failure is the most dramatic. Rupture of hemangiomas into the pleural space may cause exsanguination, and rupture into the mediastinum may cause tamponade. Lymphangiomas are usually diagnosed in children, frequently cause symptoms due to obstruction of the trachea (including stridor, dyspnea, recurrent pulmonary infection, and tachypnea), and usually occur in the anterosuperior mediastinum as an extension of cervical lesion. Their growth is by proliferation of endothelium-lined buds that spread along tissue planes. The local ingrowth of vessels and fibrous reaction to the endothelial buds prevent easy surgical removal due to the lack of well-defined tissue planes. However, because radiation therapy and sclerotherapy have not been successful, operative resection is the optimal treatment.

Giant lymph node hyperplasia was initially described by Castleman in 1954. Although the mediastinum was the site of disease in the initial report and in most patients, these tumors may develop wherever lymph nodes are present. Although usually located in the anterosuperior mediastinum, they also are found in the posterior mediastinum and at the pericardiophrenic angle where they may be confused with neurogenic tumors and pericardial cysts, respectively. The tumors most frequently appear as single, well demarcated lesions. Two distinct histologic entities exist: (1)

hyaline vascular—characterized by small hyaline follicles and interfollicular capillary proliferation, representing 90 per cent of Castleman's tumors, and (2) plasma cell—characterized by large follicles with intervening sheets of plasma cells. While patients with the hyaline vascular type are most often asymptomatic, those with the plasma cell type often exhibit systemic symptoms including fever, night sweats, anemia, and hypergammaglobulinemia. Surgical excision effects cure, although resection of the hyaline vascular type may be associated with significant hemorrhage due to extreme vascularity.

Multicentric Castleman's disease is characterized by generalized lymphadenopathy with morphologic features of giant lymph node hyperplasia. Patients are most often symptomatic with fever, chills, weight loss, and hepatosplenomegaly, and exhibit disordered immunity and autoimmune phenomena. Unlike the benign clinical course of classic Castleman's disease, multicentric disease is a much more malignant disease, with frequent deaths following infectious complications. It has also been reported in association with HIV infection.

Chondromas are rare tumors that occur in the posterior mediastinum originating from the primitive notochord. Males are affected twice as frequently as females, with the peak age of incidence in the fifth through seventh decades. Chest pain, cough, and dyspnea are the most common symptoms. Spinal cord compression may follow extension into the spinal canal. Radical surgical excision is the only effective therapy, but most patients develop distant metastases, with a mean survival of approximately 17.5 months. Extramedullary hematopoiesis occurs at all ages, usually a result of altered hematopoiesis. In the adult, this is typically due to massive hemolysis, myelofibrosis, spherocytic anemia, or thalassemia. These lesions appear as bilateral, asymmetric paravertebral masses. Surgical resection is unnecessary unless there is invasion or compression of mediastinal structures. Radiation therapy can produce rapid shrinkage of these masses.

Primary Cysts

Primary cysts of the mediastinum comprise 20 per cent of the mediastinal masses in the collected series. These cysts can be bronchogenic, pericardial, enteric, or thymic, or may be of an unspecified nature. More than 75 per cent of patients are asymptomatic, and these lesions rarely cause morbidity. However, due to the proximity of vital structures within the mediastinum, with increasing size, even benign cysts may cause significant morbidity. In addition, they should be differentiated from malignant tumors.

Bronchogenic cysts are the most common primary cysts of the mediastinum, comprising 6.3 per cent of primary mediastinal masses and 34 per cent of cysts. They originate as sequestrations from the ventral foregut, the antecedent of the tracheobronchial tree. The bronchogenic cyst may lie within the lung parenchyma or the mediastinum. The cyst wall is composed of cartilage, mucous glands, smooth muscle, and fibrous tissue with a pathognomonic inner layer of ciliated respiratory epithelium. When bronchogenic cysts occur in the mediastinum, they are usually located proximal to the trachea or bronchi and may be just posterior to the carina. Rarely, a true communication between the cyst and the tracheobronchial tree exists, and an air-fluid level may be observed on the chest film.

Two thirds of patients with bronchogenic cysts are asymptomatic. In infants, they may cause severe respiratory compromise by compressing the trachea or the bronchus. Compression of the bronchus may cause bronchial stenosis and recurrent pneumonitis. Tumors located below the carina are sometimes not well visualized using standard roentgenography, and may require CT to be imaged. Surgical excision is recommended in all patients to provide definitive histologic diagnosis, alleviate symptoms, and prevent the development of associated complications. Malignant degeneration has been reported, as well as the presence of a bronchial adenoma within the cyst wall.

Pericardial cysts are the second most frequently encountered cysts within the mediastinum and comprise 6 per cent of all lesions and 33 per cent of primary cysts. These cysts classically occur in the pericardiophrenic angles, with 70 per cent at the right pericardiophrenic angle, 22 per cent on the left, and the remainder in other sites in the pericardium. In patients with a characteristic CT appearance of a pericardial cyst (i.e., pericardiophrenic location, near-water attenuation value, and smooth borders), management may utilize needle aspiration and follow-up with serial CT rather than surgical excision. Surgical excision of pericardial cysts is indicated primarily for diagnosis and to differentiate them from malignant lesions.

Enteric cysts (duplication cysts) arise from the posterior division of the primitive foregut, which develops into the upper division of the gastrointestinal tract. They are found less frequently than bronchogenic or pericardial cysts and comprise 3 per cent of the mediastinal masses in collected series. They are most frequently located in the posterior mediastinum, usually adjacent to the esophagus. These lesions are composed of smooth muscle with an inner epithelial lining of esophageal, gastric, or intestinal mucosa. When gastric mucosa is present, peptic ulceration with perforation into the esophageal or bronchial lumen may occur, producing hemoptysis or hematemesis. Erosion into the lung parenchyma may cause hemorrhage and lead to lung abscess formation. Gastric mucosa within enteric cysts may be visualized using ^{99m}Tc scanning. Usually, enteric cysts have an attachment to the esophagus and may be embedded within the muscularis layer.

Symptoms are usually due to compression of the esophagus causing obstruction, commonly presenting as dysphagia. Compromise of the tracheobronchial tree with symptoms of cough, dyspnea, recurrent pulmonary infections, and chest pain may also occur. Most enteric cysts are diagnosed in children, who are also more likely to be symptomatic.

When enteric cysts are associated with anomalies of the vertebral column, they are termed *neuroenteric cysts.* Such cysts may be connected to the meninges, or, less frequently, a direct communication with the dural space may exist. In patients with neuroenteric cysts, preoperative evaluation for potential spinal cord involvement is mandatory. Computed tomography and myelography are useful in delineating the vertebral deformities, extension into the spinal column, and the possibility of a connection with the dural space. Rarely, multiple mediastinal enteric cysts may occur, or there may be an association with a duplication of the abdominal portion of the alimentary tract. In the latter, there may be a transdiaphragmatic connection between abdominal and mediastinal components. Treatment is surgical excision, providing a definite histologic diagnosis as well as alleviating symptoms and preventing potential complications.

Thymic cysts may be inflammatory, neoplastic, or congenital lesions. Congenital cysts are thought to originate from the third branchial arch and are not usually related to thymomas. These cysts are defined by the presence of thymic tissue within the cyst wall. An apparent increase in the incidence of thymic cysts following treatment of malignant anterior mediastinal neoplasms has been reported.

Nonspecific cysts include those lesions in which a specific epithelial or mesothelial lining cannot be identified and may originate in any of the aforementioned cysts by the destruction of the inner epithelial lining by an inflammatory or digestive process. Other causes include postinflammatory cysts and hemorrhagic cysts.

REFERENCES

Davis RD Jr, Oldham HN, Sabiston DC Jr: Primary cysts and neoplasms of the mediastinum: Recent changes in clinical presentation, methods of diagnosis, management, and results. Ann Thorac Surg 44:229, 1987.

Davis RD Jr, Sabiston DC Jr: The mediastinum. *In* Sabiston DC Jr (ed): Textbook of Surgery: The Biological Basis of Modern Surgical Practice, ed 14. Philadelphia, WB Saunders Company, 1991.

Ginsberg RJ: Evaluation of the mediastinum by invasive techniques. Surg Clin North Am 67:1025, 1987.

King RM, Telander RL, Smithson WA, et al: Primary mediastinal tumors in children. J Pediatr Surg 17:512, 1982.

Nakahara K, Ohno K, Hashimoto J, Maeda H, Miyoshi S, Sakurai M, Monden Y, Kawashima Y: Thymoma: Results with complete resection and adjuvant postoperative irradiation in 141 consecutive patients. J Thorac Cardiovasc Surg 95:1041, 1988.

Verley JM, Hollman KH: Thymoma: A comparative study of clinical stages, histologic features, and survival in 200 cases. Cancer 55:1075, 1985.

XIV
Surgical Disorders of the Pericardium

JAMES M. DOUGLAS, Jr., M.D.

ANATOMY AND PHYSIOLOGY OF THE PERICARDIUM

The parietal pericardium is a connective tissue sac composed of collagen and elastic fibers with an inner serous layer of mesothelial cells. This sac encompasses the heart and fuses with the great arteries, pulmonary veins, and venae cavae. The visceral pericardium is on the surface of the heart and consists of a thin layer of fibrous tissue covered by mesothelial cells. The visceral and parietal pericardium become continuous at the level of the great vessels. The parietal pericardium is anchored anteriorly to the sternum and xiphoid process, posteriorly to the vertebral column, and inferiorly to the diaphragm. The arterial blood supply arises from small branches off of the aorta, internal mammary artery, and musculophrenic arteries. Parasympathetic innervation arises directly from the vagus, the left recurrent laryngeal nerve, and the esophageal plexus, with sympathetic innervation from the stellate and first dorsal ganglia and from the aortic, cardiac, and diaphragmatic plexuses. The phrenic nerves course along the lateral aspect of the pericardium prior to terminating at the diaphragm. Pain perception, particularly to the anterior surface of the parietal pericardium, appears to travel along afferent fibers entering the spinal cord at levels C4 and C5. The pericardial space, which normally completely separates the visceral and parietal pericardium beyond its attachments to the great vessels, typically contains 10 to 50 ml of ultrafiltrated fluid. Under normal conditions, the volume of pericardial fluid is maintained relatively constant by means of lymphatic drainage to the thoracic duct and the right lymphatic duct in the right pleural space. With its inelastic nature and its multiply fixed points, the pericardium stabilizes the heart, modulates transmural pressures, and limits cardiac distention. However, the presence of the pericardium does not appear to be essential, as is illustrated by the fact that congenital absence of the parietal pericardium has not been associated with significant functional cardiac impairment.

ACUTE PERICARDITIS

Acute inflammation of the pericardium may be caused by viral, fungal, or bacterial infections, including tuberculosis. Other causes include uremia, acute myocardial infarction, neoplasia, rheumatic diseases, drugs, and postpericardiotomy syndrome. Clinically, the patient most often complains of chest pain exacerbated by deep inspiration, coughing, or lying in the supine position. The pain may be lessened upon leaning forward. On physical examination, the presence of a pericardial friction rub, classically of three components, is pathognomonic of acute pericardial inflammation. The presence of the rub may be fleeting and difficult to detect.

The electrocardiogram may show characteristic findings, and four stages are typically present in the evolution of the electrocardiographic diagnosis of pericarditis. Stage one is characterized by diffuse ST segment elevation in all leads with the exception of a VR and V_1. In stage two, which develops several days following stage one, the ST segments are normal and the T waves are flattened. In stage three, the T-wave inversion returns but is not associated with the loss of R-wave voltage and the appearance of Q waves, as seen during the evolution of myocardial infarction. Finally, the fourth stage, which occurs weeks or months later, is characterized by a reversion of the T waves to normal. Echocardiography may provide confirmation of the diagnosis by revealing pericardial thickening and effusion.

Treatment of acute pericarditis should include specific treatment of infectious or neoplastic causes or discontinuation of inciting drugs. Nonsteroidal anti-inflammatory agents or corticosteroids may be given when pericarditis is not due to infection. Surgical treatment is reserved for hemodynamic complications occurring as a result of pericardial effusion and/or constriction.

PERICARDIAL EFFUSION

Pericardial effusion may be associated with nearly all forms of pericardial disease. The fluid may be characterized as serous, serosanguinous, sanguinous, purulent, fibrinous, or fibrinopurulent, and the presence of the fluid itself may or may not be symptomatic, depending upon its volume and rapidity of accumulation. The acute accumulation of 200 ml of fluid around the normal heart is associated with definite signs of embarrassment, while a liter or more of fluid accumulating over weeks or months may have no detectable hemodynamic compromise. Additionally, underlying cardiac abnormalities increase the sensitivity of the heart to external compression. The diagnosis of a pericardial effusion is rarely made on physical examination, although muffled heart sounds are suggestive. After the accumulation of at least 250 ml of fluid, the chest film may reveal an enlarged cardiac silhouette or, with large effusions, a "water bottle" shape, and the QRS voltage on the electrocardiogram may be reduced. Nonetheless, the diagnostic procedure of choice is echocardiography, as this study may detect as little as 20 ml of pericardial fluid and allows the distribution and character of the fluid to be determined. Pericardial effusions require surgical treatment only in the setting of hemodynamic compromise. However, diagnostic pericardiocentesis may be required to guide medical therapy. When direct therapy is indicated, simple pericardiocentesis, a pericardial window, or a total pericardiectomy may be required.

CARDIAC TAMPONADE

Whenever external compression of the heart impairs diastolic filling and reduces stroke volume from the ventricles, cardiac tamponade is present. Occurring most often as a result of the accumulation of fluid within the pericardium, its development depends on both the volume and the rapidity of fluid accumulation. Cardiac tamponade may develop following a host of diseases involving the pericardium. Malignancies, infections, rheumatic diseases, postpericardiotomy syndrome, uremia, and hypothyroidism in association with pericardial effusion may cause cardiac tamponade, and acute cardiac tamponade may be caused by hemopericardium following trauma, acute aortic dissection, or myocardial rupture. Symptomatic cardiac tamponade can cause dyspnea, tachycardia, and hypotension. Chronic tamponade is frequently associated with the development of ascites and peripheral edema, and the patient may have signs of conges-

tive heart failure or acute cardiogenic shock. The classic physical finding is a pulsus paradoxus, defined as an inspiratory decrease of aortic systolic pressure greater than 10 mm Hg. The jugular venous pressure is elevated and usually associated with jugular venous distention, the cardiac impulse may be difficult to palpate, and the heart sounds may be distant. The electrocardiogram may show changes of electrical alternans characterized by a change in R-wave amplitude from beat to beat. The diagnosis of cardiac tamponade can be confirmed by echocardiography. However, when the clinical diagnosis is evident and the patient is in extremis, emergency subxiphoid pericardiocentesis may be required. Frequently, the removal of only a small amount of fluid produces significant hemodynamic improvement. More definitive therapy is then dictated by the underlying cause.

CONSTRICTIVE PERICARDITIS

Many diseases of the pericardium, including viral pericarditis, uremic pericarditis, rheumatic diseases, hemopericardium, bacterial pericarditis, and previous cardiac surgery, may be followed by the development of scar tissue and accumulation of fluid that constricts the heart. In the past, tuberculosis was the most common cause of constrictive pericarditis. The pericardial scarring typically involves both the atria and the ventricles, although the degree of involvement may be asymmetric. This scarring causes a restriction of diastolic filling of the heart and causes an elevation and equilibration of the diastolic pressures in all cardiac chambers. Cardiac catheterization reveals the characteristic early diastolic dip in pressure followed by a plateau waveform in both the right and left ventricular pressure tracings, commonly termed the *square root sign*. The normal respiratory changes and intrathoracic pressure are not transmitted to the pericardial space, and consequently, systemic and right atrial pressures do not fall with inspiration. This contrasts with the findings seen in cardiac tamponade. Hemodynamic compromise is caused primarily by an impairment of diastolic function, with systolic function being normal in most cases. However, myocardial systolic function may also be impaired due to myocardial fibrosis, atrophy, or obstruction to coronary blood flow. Most patients with constrictive pericarditis present with symptoms of dyspnea and fatigue. Physical findings include pedal edema, jugular venous distention, hepatomegaly, and ascites. Rarely, a pericardial knock may be auscultated. The chest film is nonspecific, although some cardiomegaly and occasionally calcification of the pericardium may be seen. The electrocardiogram reveals generalized T-wave inversion and occasional atrial fibrillation, and a low QRS voltage may be found. Echocardiography may be helpful by demonstrating a thickened pericardium, abnormal ventricular septal movement, or other more subtle findings. Computed tomographic (CT) scans and nuclear magnetic resonance imaging (MRI) may also be useful.

The most reliable diagnostic technique remains cardiac catheterization. The finding of equalization of the intracardiac end-diastolic pressures and the square root sign are characteristic. The right atrial pressure is elevated, although severe pulmonary hypertension is unusual, and the left ventricular end-diastolic pressure is usually normal. The findings in restrictive cardiomyopathy may be very similar to constrictive pericarditis. When right ventricular systolic hypertension is present and the left ventricular diastolic pressure exceeds the right ventricular diastolic pressure at rest by more than 5 mm Hg, restrictive cardiomyopathy is likely. Occasionally, endocardial biopsy may be necessary to differentiate chronic constrictive pericarditis from restrictive cardiomyopathy.

Constrictive pericarditis is characteristically progressive and severely disabling. Although medical therapy with diuretics and vasodilators may be helpful, definitive treatment requires pericardiectomy, and a total pericardiectomy by a median sternotomy appears to be the treatment of choice, although patients have also been successfully treated through a left anterior thoracotomy approach. Rarely, bilateral thoracotomy with a transverse sternotomy has been used, as this incision can be associated with significant morbidity. Patients with constrictive pericarditis are typically quite ill, and the in-hospital mortality is approximately 10 per cent. In one large study, the 5-year survival was 75 per cent and, at 10 years, was approximately 65 per cent. The most important independent predictor of mortality is increasing right ventricular end-diastolic pressure. Furthermore, radiation-induced pericarditis had the worst prognosis and the least favorable postoperative improvement.

SPECIFIC PERICARDIAL DISEASES

Tuberculous Pericarditis

Tuberculous pericarditis occurs in approximately 1 to 2 per cent of cases of tuberculosis and probably arises from blood-borne infection, although some cases may be caused by retrograde lymphatic spread or direct invasion from infected lung, pleura, or mediastinal lymph nodes. The disease begins with an early stage of fibrinous pericarditis and progresses to the slow development of a pericardial effusion. Patients present with malaise, fever, sweats, and a cough. The classic friction rub of pericarditis may not be present. Early diagnosis and treatment of this disease is important to avoid the complications of severe systemic infection and late constrictive pericarditis. Peri-

cardiocentesis may reveal acid-fast bacilli during the effusive stage. Triple drug therapy and early pericardial drainage or pericardiectomy should be considered in all patients. In its chronic form, tuberculous pericarditis causes a calcific, constricted pericardium that must be treated surgically. Operative approach may be through a left anterior thoracotomy, although a median sternotomy is often preferred.

Uremic Pericarditis

Uremic pericarditis occurs in approximately 50 per cent of patients with untreated renal disease and approximately 20 per cent of patients on hemodialysis. The development of uremic pericarditis appears to be unrelated to the absolute level of the blood urea nitrogen (BUN) and serum creatinine, and it occurs less often in patients on peritoneal dialysis. Symptomatic patients should initially be treated with daily dialysis, which allows recovery in approximately half. Short courses of steroids or nonsteroidal anti-inflammatory agents may be added, particularly for the treatment of chest pain and fever. Pericardiocentesis should be performed for treatment of hemodynamic compromise. In patients with significant hemodynamic instability, an anterior pericardiectomy for drainage is mandatory. Additionally, patients who develop an enlarging effusion or an effusion unresponsive to 10 days of medical therapy should be considered for anterior pericardiectomy.

Purulent Pericarditis

Bacterial infection of the pericardium is most commonly caused by *Staphylococcus* or gram-negative organisms in adults, and *Haemophilus influenzae* or *Staphylococcus* species in children. It may follow direct contamination from injury or contiguous pneumonic or subdiaphragmatic infection, and blood-borne infection may cause purulent pericarditis. Symptoms commonly include chest pain and fever, and the sudden accumulation of fluid may cause cardiac tamponade. Respiratory distress, anorexia, or abdominal discomfort may occur, particularly in children. Purulent pericarditis is diagnosed by pericardiocentesis. Treatment should consist of appropriate antibiotic therapy and aspiration of the purulent fluid, and pericardiectomy should be performed for cardiac tamponade or persistent fever. Additionally, some authors have recommended early pericardiectomy when the bacterial organism is *Haemophilus influenzae*. Early aggressive drainage by means of a subxiphoid pericardial window and insertion of a tube has also been advocated.

Postpericardiotomy Syndrome

The postpericardiotomy syndrome, a malady occurring usually 2 to 4 weeks following surgical intervention within the pericardium, is characterized by symptoms of fever and chest pain and is associated with pericardial and pleural effusions. Other symptoms include dyspnea, nonproductive cough, fatigue, and body aches, and severity varies from a very mild symptom complex to severe, incapacitating malaise. The syndrome occurs to some extent in approximately 10 to 40 per cent of patients following cardiac operation and is thought to be due to an autoimmune reaction directed against the epicardium. The association between elevated anti–heart antibody titers and elevated antiviral titers suggests that viral infection may somehow trigger the symptom complex. Treatment of postpericardiotomy syndrome primarily involves the use of anti-inflammatory agents, and steroid therapy may be required for severe cases. Occasionally, thoracentesis or pericardiocentesis is necessary when pleural or pericardial fluid accumulation becomes symptomatic. Constrictive pericarditis can also occur following cardiac operations and may not be associated with a previous postpericardiotomy syndrome. Pericardiectomy is required for recurrent symptomatic effusions or constrictive pericarditis.

Neoplastic Pericarditis

Cardiac involvement occurs in approximately 10 per cent of patients with malignancies, and neoplastic disease is present within the pericardium in 85 per cent. Carcinoma of the lung and breast, melanoma, leukemia, and lymphoma are the most common neoplasms associated with cardiac metastases. Pericardial spread may be associated with increasing pericardial effusions. The diagnosis is most easily confirmed with samples of the pericardial tissue, although 28 per cent of malignant pericardial effusions have positive cytologic examinations. Pericardial effusions secondary to malignant diseases have an extremely high mortality, with only 20 per cent of patients with malignant pericarditis surviving 1 year.

Symptomatic patients may initially be treated with pericardiocentesis. However, recurrent or large effusions are best treated with a pericardial window, most often via the subxiphoid approach. Although the recurrence rate is probably lower when pericardiectomy is performed through a left anterior thoracotomy, the generally poor prognosis in these patients and the less invasive nature of the subxiphoid approach appear to make it preferable. Experience is also being gained with a thoracoscopic approach to creating a pericardial window with drainage of the fluid into the left chest.

SURGICAL TECHNIQUES

The diagnosis of pericarditis and its complications involves a number of techniques of varying complexity and effectiveness. *Pericardiocentesis* is primarily employed as a diagnostic test or temporizing method for treatment of cardiac tamponade. This technique is sometimes done in a blind fashion using a subxiphoid needle insertion approach. Electrocardiographic, fluoroscopic, and echocardiographic monitoring has been used in an effort to decrease the likelihood of complications. For more chronic drainage of thin effusions, catheter insertion over a guidewire may be employed for several days of drainage. More definitive treatment of pericardial effusion, particularly when effusion is recurrent and secondary to malignant disease, can be accomplished by means of a *subxiphoid pericardial window* and placement of mediastinal tube. This approach provides tissue for diagnostic studies and allows excellent drainage of most effusions. Although this technique is quite effective, a greater degree of pericardial excision along with drainage of fluid into the pleural space can be accomplished by means of a left anterior thoracotomy. Recurrence of the effusion is less likely to occur with this approach, and it may be preferable in patients who have a good prognosis. Excision of a large amount of pericardium and drainage into the left chest can also be accomplished by means of a thoracoscopic approach, and experience is rapidly being gained with this technique. For the treatment of constrictive pericarditis, radical pericardiectomy through a median sternotomy is probably the treatment of choice. Care is taken at the time of operation to release the pericardium over the left ventricle prior to the right ventricle to avoid pulmonary vascular congestion. A median sternotomy allows excision of pericardium from the ventricles, atria, and venae cavae. Cardiopulmonary bypass is usually unnecessary, although it may be required in complex cases. Some authors advocate a left anterior thoracotomy because of the excellent exposure of the pericardium surrounding the left ventricle. However, access to the pericardium overlying the atria and vena cava is poor through this approach. A *transsternal, bilateral thoracotomy* approach has also been employed but is generally avoided because of the associated morbidity.

REFERENCES

Frame JR, Lucas SK, Pederson JA, Elkins RC: Surgical treatment of pericarditis in the dialysis patient. Am J Surg 146:800, 1983.

Hawkins JW, Vacek JL: What constitutes definitive therapy of malignant pericardial effusion? "Medical" versus surgical treatment. Am Heart J 118:428, 1989.

Morgan RJ, Stephenson LW, Woolf PK, Edie RN, Edmunds LH Jr: Surgical treatment of purulent pericarditis in children. J Thorac Cardiovasc Surg 85:527, 1983.

Seifert FC, Miller DC, Oesterle SN, et al: Surgical treatment of constrictive pericarditis: Analysis of outcome and diagnostic error. Circulation 72(3 pt 2):II-264–II-273, 1985.

Spodick DH: The normal and diseased pericardium: Current concepts of pericardial physiology, diagnosis, and treatment. J Am Coll Cardiol 1:240, 1983.

49

THE HEART

I

CONGENITAL CARDIAC DISORDERS:
Patent Ductus Arteriosus, Coarctation of
the Aorta, Interruption of the Aortic Arch,
Aortopulmonary Window, Anomalies of the
Aortic Arch, Pulmonary Artery Sling,
Atrial Septal Defects, and Ventricular
Septal Defects

J. WILLIAM GAYNOR, M.D.

PATENT DUCTUS ARTERIOSUS

Anatomy and Physiology

The ductus arteriosus is a normal fetal structure that extends from the main or left pulmonary artery to the descending aorta distal near the origin of the left subclavian artery. The size of the ductus is variable, between 5 and 10 mm in length and a few millimeters to 1 to 2 cm in diameter. In utero blood ejected by the right ventricle flows almost exclusively through the ductus to the lower extremities and placenta, bypassing the high-resistance pulmonary circulation.

Closure of the ductus occurs at birth during the transition from the fetal to the adult circulation. The lungs expand and the arterial oxygen saturation increases with the first breath, causing a decrease in the pulmonary vascular resistance and an increase in pulmonary blood flow. Closure occurs within the first 10 to 15 hours of life after constriction of the smooth muscle layer, which causes apposition of intimal cushions in the wall of the ductus and is mediated by various substances that constrict (oxygen) or dilate (certain prostaglandins) ductal smooth muscle. The sensitivity of the ductal smooth muscle to these substances is dependent on gestational age and is lower in premature infants. Anatomic closure by fibrosis is usually complete 2 to 3 weeks following birth, producing the ligamentum arteriosum connecting the pulmonary artery to the aorta. Persistent patency of the ductus may occur as an isolated lesion or may be associated with other congenital anomalies. Final closure may occur at any age but is uncommon after 6 months. In infants with complex congenital heart disease, the pulmonary or systemic blood flow may be dependent on the patency of the ductus, and decompensation may occur if the ductus closes. Infusions of prostaglandin to dilate the ductus in these patients often produces dramatic clinical improvement. Persistent patency of the ductus causes a left-to-right shunt of blood with pulmonary congestion and left ventricular volume overload. With a large nonrestrictive ductus, the level of pulmonary vascular resistance is important in determining the severity of shunting. Shunting occurs throughout systole and diastole, producing diastolic hypotension and may impair perfusion of the brain, heart, lower extremities, and abdominal organs.

Incidence and Natural History

Isolated patent ductus arteriosus (PDA) occurs approximately once in 2500 to 5000 live births. The incidence increases with prematurity and with decreasing birth weight. PDA is not a benign entity, although prolonged survival has been reported. In the preantibiotic era, 40 per cent of patients with PDA died of bacterial endocarditis and many of the remainder died of congestive heart failure. Patients surviving to adulthood with a PDA may develop pulmonary hypertension with reversal of shunting. Premature infants with PDA often have associated problems of prematurity that are aggravated by the left-to-right shunting. Congestive heart failure often results and responds poorly to medical management. Young children with persistent patency of the ductus may show growth retardation.

Clinical Manifestations and Diagnosis

The signs and symptoms of PDA depend on the size of the ductus, the pulmonary vascular resistance, the age at presentation, and associated anomalies. Full-term infants usually do not become symptomatic until

pulmonary vascular resistance falls at 6 to 8 weeks of life allowing a significant left-to-right shunt. Premature infants have less smooth muscle in the pulmonary arteries, thus pulmonary vascular resistance decreases earlier and symptoms may develop in the first week of life.

A hemodynamically significant ductus usually presents with congestive heart failure characterized by tachycardia, tachypnea, and poor feeding. The physical examination reveals a hyperdynamic circulation with a hyperactive precordium and bounding peripheral pulses. The systolic blood pressure is usually normal, but diastolic hypotension may be present.

Auscultation reveals a systolic or continuous murmur, often called a *machinery murmur*, in the pulmonic area that radiates toward the middle third of the clavicle. However, absence of the characteristic murmur does not exclude the presence of a PDA, especially in premature infants. Hepatomegaly may be present; however, cyanosis is not present in uncomplicated isolated PDA.

The diagnosis of PDA can often be made noninvasively, and the physical examination alone may be almost diagnostic. The chest film shows cardiomegaly, and pulmonary congestion may be seen. In older infants, children, and adults, the electrocardiogram (ECG) may show left ventricular hypertrophy. Two-dimensional echocardiography with color flow Doppler imaging is very useful to demonstrate the ductus, reveal the direction of shunting, and evaluate associated anomalies. Cardiac catheterization should be reserved for older patients and those with atypical findings or pulmonary hypertension. Patients with a moderate-sized PDA may remain asymptomatic until the second or third decade of life. The earliest sign may be dyspnea on exertion followed by increasing congestive heart failure. A small PDA usually causes no symptoms or growth retardation. A systolic or continuous murmur is present. The ECG and chest film are usually normal. Rarely patients with a PDA present with bacterial endocarditis as the first clinical manifestation.

The development of pulmonary hypertension in a patient with PDA is a serious prognostic sign. Pulmonary hypertension occasionally may be encountered in children who are under 2 years of age with a nonrestrictive PDA and greatly increased pulmonary blood flow. However, significant pulmonary hypertension is usually noted in older patients with patent ductus arteriosus. The elevated pulmonary pressures may be secondary to increased blood flow and can normalize after surgical closure of the PDA. However, in some patients irreversible pulmonary vascular changes occur and pulmonary hypertension persists following closure of the PDA.

The presence of a PDA in a child or adult is sufficient indication for closure because of the increased mortality and risk of endocarditis. In symptomatic patients, closure should be undertaken when the diagnosis is made. In asymptomatic children, intervention can be postponed but should be performed in the preschool years. Older patients should have the ductus closed when the diagnosis is made.

Management

The operation is done through either a left anterior or posterior thoracotomy. Careful dissection is mandatory to avoid damage to the recurrent laryngeal nerve. The ductus is mobilized, and the aortic arch and descending aorta are identified. After the ductus has been mobilized, it may be either obliterated by multiple suture ligation (Fig. 1) or divided (Fig. 2). In neonates, single or double ligation is usually the procedure of choice. Closure of the ductus in neonates by applying one or two surgical clips has also been successful.

Surgical closure of a PDA may be complicated by hemorrhage, pneumothorax, chylothorax, recurrent laryngeal nerve damage, phrenic nerve paralysis, and infection. Great care must be taken when dissecting or placing clamps on the ductus, as the ductal tissue may be friable and a tear can cause hemorrhage that is difficult to control. The incidence of recurrent ductal patency should approach zero following division or multiple suture ligation. In recent years, there has been increasing interest in the nonoperative closure of a PDA using a double umbrella device. Transcatheter techniques are potentially useful in patients who are poor candidates for operation. This technique is being utilized with increasing frequency for routine closure of a PDA; however, the exact role for transcatheter closure of PDA has not been determined.

Results

Surgical closure of an isolated PDA has become a very safe procedure, and the operative mortality approaches zero even in critically ill neonates. In premature infants, hospital mortality and long-term results depend primarily on associated pulmonary disease, coexistent anomalies, and the degree of prematurity. The mortality is increased, and long-term results are less satisfactory in patients with severe pulmonary hypertension and right-to-left shunting. Most patients with a PDA become functionally normal with a normal life expectancy after closure.

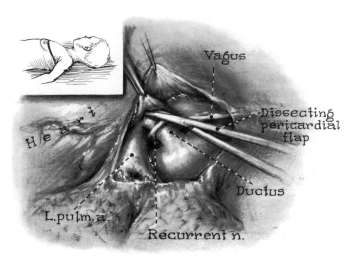

Figure 1. Operative treatment of PDA by ligation. (From Sabiston DC Jr, Spencer FC: Surgery of the Chest, ed 5. Philadelphia, WB Saunders Company, 1990, p 1132, with permission.)

COARCTATION OF THE AORTA

Anatomy

Coarctation of the aorta is defined as a narrowing that diminishes the aortic lumen, producing an obstruction to the flow of blood. The lesion may be a definite localized obstruction or diffusely narrowed segment, which is termed tubular hypoplasia. The most common site for isolated coarctation is at the site of the insertion of the ductus (or ligamentum) arteriosus. Externally, the aorta appears to be sharply con-

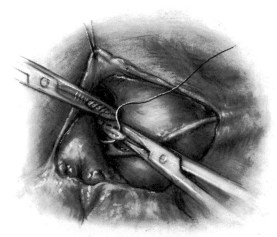

Figure 2. Treatment of PDA by division. (From Sabiston DC Jr, Spencer FC: Surgery of the Chest, ed 5. Philadelphia, WB Saunders Company, 1990, p 1132, with permission.)

stricted, and internally there is an obstructing diaphragm on the posterior wall that is usually more marked than is apparent by the external appearance. Tubular hypoplasia most often involves the aortic isthmus (the segment of aorta between the left subclavian artery and the insertion of the ductus). Anomalies that occur commonly with coarctation of the aorta include bicuspid aortic valve, ventricular septal defect, PDA, and various mitral valve disorders. The hypertension that occurs with coarctation is caused by multiple mechanical and renal factors. In experimental coarctation, hypertension can be eliminated by transplanting one kidney to the neck (proximal to the obstruction) with contralateral nephrectomy, suggesting that diminished renal perfusion is a factor. However, studies of renal blood flow and the renin-angiotensin system in patients with coarctation have yielded conflicting results.

Incidence and Natural History

Coarctation of the aorta represents 5 to 10 per cent of congenital heart disease. The age at presentation and the mode of presentation depend mainly on the location of the coarctation and the associated anomalies. When the coarctation occurs in a preductal position, there is an increased incidence of other cardiac defects and the patients usually present in infancy with congestive heart failure. Paraductal and postductal coarctation are usually isolated obstructions that have a low incidence of associated defects.

Coarctation of the arch does not seriously alter the normal fetal circulation and, therefore, does not provide a stimulus to the development of a collateral circulation in utero. Infants with a severe narrowing may appear normal at birth and have palpable femoral pulses because a PDA allows blood to flow past the obstructing shelf. Symptoms develop as the PDA closes, producing significant aortic obstruction. Older children and adults often present with unexplained hypertension or complications of hypertension. Some patients may be entirely asymptomatic for many years and lead an active life. Presenting complaints include headache, visual disturbances, and exertional dyspnea. Rarely, patients present with a cerebrovascular accident, aortic rupture, dissecting aneurysm, or bacterial endocarditis. The natural history of untreated coarctation of the aorta depends on the age at presentation and associated anomalies. Symptomatic infants have a higher mortality depending on the severity of coarctation and the presence of associated defects. Patients surviving until adulthood without treatment have a decreased life expectancy. In the preantibiotic era the most common causes of death were spontaneous rupture of the aorta, bacterial endocarditis, and cerebral hemorrhage.

Diagnosis

The diagnosis of coarctation can usually be made clinically. Infants with coarctation are irritable, tachypneic, and feed poorly. A systolic murmur may be heard over the left precordium and posteriorly between the scapula. The femoral pulses are usually not palpable. Hypotension, oliguria, and severe metabolic acidosis may be present. Findings include hypertension, a systolic pressure gradient between the arms and legs, and a systolic murmur. In older children and adults, there may be evidence of collateral circulation. The collateral circulation involves branches of the subclavian arteries that are proximal to the obstruction including the internal mammary, thyrocervical, and costocervical arteries, which form connections with the intercostal arteries and other arteries below the obstruction. A systolic pressure gradient is usually present between the arms and legs. The ECG in infancy may show right, left, or biventricular hypertrophy. In older children and adults, it may be normal or show evidence of left ventricular hypertrophy. The chest film may reveal cardiomegaly with left ventricular hypertrophy. In infants with heart failure, extreme cardiomegaly and pulmonary congestion may be present. Erosions on the underside of the ribs (rib-notching) secondary to the enlarged tortuous intercostal vessels are almost pathognomonic. Two-dimensional echocardiography with color flow Doppler imaging is the most useful diagnostic modality to visualize the obstruction and evaluate associated anomalies. Cardiac catheterization is usually not required preoperatively in patients with isolated coarctation.

Management

Nonsurgical therapy has only a small role in the management of patients with coarctation, and the presence of a coarctation is generally sufficient indication for surgical correction. The major questions are the timing and method of repair. Symptomatic infants usually require urgent intervention, although a few improve with conservative medical treatment of congestive heart failure and can then undergo elective surgical correction. Infusion of prostaglandin E_1 can reopen and maintain patency of the ductus arteriosus in many critically ill neonates with coarctation, improving perfusion of the lower body and allowing surgical correction to be accomplished under more optimal conditions. The timing of elective repair of coarctation in asymptomatic patients is perhaps the most important determinant of surgical outcome. Repair in late childhood or adulthood, although providing relief of some symptoms, has an increased incidence of persistent hypertension with its morbidity. The current trend is for elective repair at an early age in symptomatic and asymptomatic infants to prevent the development of complications.

Surgical Procedures

The classical method of repair is resection of the area of obstruction via a left thoracotomy with primary end-to-end anastomosis. To obtain an optimal result, it is absolutely necessary to resect the entire constricted segment and construct the anastomosis without tension. Even in infants with tubular hypoplasia, the aorta is elastic and can usually be mobilized sufficiently to allow primary repair. In the early years of cardiac surgery, the results of primary anastomosis, especially in infants, were unsatisfactory, and other techniques were developed including prosthetic patch aortoplasty and the subclavian flap repair. Patch aortoplasty is highly effective in relieving the aortic obstruction with a low incidence of restenosis and persistent hypertension. The area of constriction is incised longitudinally, the obstructing shelf is excised, and a prosthetic patch is used to enlarge the lumen. However, the use of prosthetic material may predispose to infection, and there are reports of aneurysms and pseudoaneurysms following patch aortoplasty. The subclavian flap aortoplasty is performed via a left thoracotomy. The left subclavian artery is mobilized and ligated at its first branch. A longitudinal incision is then made through the region of the coarctation and continued onto the subclavian artery, creating a flap. The posterior obstructing shelf is resected, and the flap of subclavian artery is turned down to repair the aorta and relieve the obstruction. In recent years, there has been renewed interest in repair by extended resection of the area of constriction and creation of a wide anastomosis that extends on to the underside of the aortic arch to completely relieve the obstruction.

Correction of coarctation may be complicated by hemorrhage, chylothorax, recurrent nerve paralysis, infection, and suture line thrombosis. The most dreaded complication of coarctation repair is paraplegia, which occurs in 0.5 to 1 per cent of patients. Poor collateral circulation, anomalous origin of the right subclavian artery, distal hypotension during the period of aortic crossclamping, and reoperation all may predispose to paraplegia. This complication is rarely seen in neonates undergoing repair of coarctation and is more common in older patients and those undergoing reoperation.

Results

The results of surgical correction depend on the age at repair, the type of repair used, and the associated anomalies. Operative mortality in neonates has decreased to 5 to 10 per cent and is lower in older children. The mortality is very low in patients with isolated coarctation. As a prospective randomized trial of the various repair techniques has not been performed, long-term results cannot be accurately compared. Coarctation repair should be individualized on the basis of the anatomy, clinical condition, and associated anomalies. In recent years, percutaneous transluminal balloon angioplasty was introduced as an alternative therapy for coarctation, and the initial results were encouraging. However, reports soon followed of aneurysmal dilatation after balloon angioplasty of previously unoperated coarctations. Dilatation of recurrent stenosis has been more successful, and there have been fewer reports of aneurysm formation. The long-term results of balloon angioplasty in terms of recoarctation and aneurysm formation are not yet known. The results of angioplasty for recoarctation appear to be better than for native coarctation and may be associated with less mortality and morbidity than reoperation.

Recoarctation usually manifests as persistent hypertension or an arm/leg pressure gradient. The arm/leg pressure gradient should be measured in the immediate postoperative period to differentiate residual stenosis secondary to an inadequate repair from true recoarctation. The causes of recoarctation include failure of growth of the anastomosis and failure to adequately resect the area of constriction. Reoperation is indicated if significant hypertension is present and a pressure gradient can be demonstrated. Some patients with a technically excellent repair may not have complete resolution of hypertension. The cause of persistent hypertension is unclear but is related to the age at repair and the duration of preoperative hypertension. As has been emphasized, the long-term prognosis of many patients is determined primarily by the associated anomalies.

INTERRUPTION OF THE AORTIC ARCH

Complete absence of a segment of the aortic arch without any anatomic connection between the proximal and distal segments is termed *interruption of the aortic arch* (IAA). This is a rare anomaly that constitutes less than 1.5 per cent of congenital heart disease. IAA may be an isolated defect but is usually associated with ventricular septal defect and PDA. IAA may be associated with a wide variety of complex cardiac anomalies and is often found coexistent with truncus arteriosus or aortopulmonary window. In IAA type A, the interruption occurs distal to the subclavian artery; in type B, between the left subclavian and left common carotid; and with type C, between the left common carotid and innominate arteries. IAA type B is the most common type of IAA and is frequently found in association with DiGeorge's syndrome (absence of the third and fourth pharyngeal pouches). The etiology of IAA is unclear. The prognosis of uncorrected interruption of the aortic arch is poor, with a mean age at death of 4 to 10 days. Approximately 90 per cent of infants with IAA die in the first year of life unless they undergo surgical correction.

Most infants with IAA present with congestive heart failure. Lower body perfusion is maintained by right-to-left shunting through a PDA. When the PDA closes, perfusion of the lower body essentially ceases and infants become anuric, severely acidotic, and the femoral pulses become nonpalpable. However, with an infusion of prostaglandin E_1, it is possible to restore and maintain ductal patency and to stabilize these patients.

The physical examination is not specific for IAA, and there are no characteristic murmurs. The ECG is not useful, and the chest film reveals an enlarged heart with pulmonary congestion. Echocardiography is particularly useful for accurate diagnosis of IAA and in evaluating associated anomalies. In infants with type B IAA, there is a high incidence of DiGeorge's syndrome and great care must be taken to avoid hypocalcemia. Because of the immunologic defect, these patients should receive irradiated blood products to prevent the development of graft-versus-host disease. Various procedures have been used to palliate or correct IAA. The ultimate goal is restoration of aortic continuity and correction of associated anomalies. Repair of IAA is most commonly performed using cardiopulmonary bypass with profound hypothermia and circulatory arrest for the arch repair. Aortic continuity is restored by direct anastomosis of the proximal and distal aortic segments, and associated defects are repaired.

AORTOPULMONARY WINDOW

Aortopulmonary windows (APW) are rare congenital heart defects caused by abnormal septation of the truncus arteriosus into the aorta and pulmonary artery. An APW is usually a single large defect beginning a few millimeters above the aortic valve on the left lateral wall of the aorta. A defect may occasionally be found more distally overlying the origin of the right pulmonary artery. The APW allows a large left-to-right shunt that causes pulmonary hypertension and congestive heart failure. Irreversible pulmonary vascular disease may occur at an early age. The clinical course is thought to be similar to that of untreated patients with a large ventricular septal defect.

Infants with APW usually present with congestive heart failure, growth retardation, and recurrent pulmonary infections. The physical examination reveals a systolic murmur and occasionally a continuous murmur similar to a PDA. APW must be differentiated from PDA, persistent truncus arteriosus, and ventricular septal defect with aortic regurgitation. Two-dimensional echocardiography can be used to visualize the defect. However, cardiac catheterization and retrograde arteriography may be necessary to provide accurate visualization of the defect. It is necessary to document the presence of separate aortic and pulmonary valves to confirm the diagnosis. The location of the coronary ostium must be carefully demonstrated before surgical intervention, as a coronary artery may occasionally arise from the pulmonary artery.

The presence of an APW is sufficient indication for repair. The preferred technique is transaortic closure using cardiopulmonary bypass and direct suture or patch closure. Simple ligation should not be done because of the risk of hemorrhage from the friable tissues. The transaortic approach is preferred to the transpulmonary method because it allows better visualization of the defect and the coronary ostia. In some patients, separation of the aorta and pulmonary artery by division of the defect with patch closure of the defects in both vessels may be utilized. Operative mortality is low for repair of isolated APW. Long-term results are good if there are no associated anomalies.

ANOMALIES OF THE AORTIC ARCH

Vascular rings are developmental anomalies of the aorta and great vessels that encircle and may constrict the esophagus and trachea. The natural history of vascular rings is obscured by the wide spectrum of anomalies and the range of symptoms. Vascular rings should be suspected in any infant with stridor, dysphagia, recurrent respiratory tract infections, difficulty feeding, and failure to thrive. Afflicted infants most commonly present with respiratory difficulties and stridor, which may be exacerbated by feeding. Hyperextension of the neck tends to reduce the constriction, and respiratory distress may occur if the neck is flexed. The physical examination is usually nondiagnostic, although signs of associated cardiovascular defects may be found. The plain chest film may be normal, show pneumonia, or occasionally show compression of the air-filled trachea. The barium esophagogram is a particularly valuable study. The combination of posterior compression of the esophagus with anterior tracheal compression is almost pathognomonic for a vascular ring. However various other diagnostic modalities such as angiocardiography, echocardiography, and bronchoscopy may be required in some patients.

Although a few patients with constricting rings may improve with growth, the long-term prognosis of medical therapy is poor. Despite the wide spectrum of anomalies, the principles of surgical therapy are simple. Surgical intervention should be undertaken at the time of diagnosis and is designed to divide the vascular ring, relieve the constriction, and preserve circulation to the aortic branches. The most common anomaly with a true vascular ring is persistence of the right and left fourth aortic arches forming a double aortic arch. The right posterior arch is usually larger with a left descending aorta and left ductus arteriosus. Occasionally the arches are of equal size. Partial atresia of an arch may be present. Patients with double aortic arch usually present early in infancy and are severely symptomatic. The diagnosis can easily be made from a barium esophagogram. Repair is undertaken by a left thoracotomy, and the small anterior arch divided at its junction with the descending aorta so that the left carotid and subclavian arteries arise from the ascending aorta. Other commonly seen anomalies of the aortic arch include right aortic arch, aberrant origin of the right subclavian artery from the descending aorta, and anomalous origin of the innominate artery.

PULMONARY ARTERY SLING

Pulmonary artery sling is a rare cardiac anomaly occurring when the left pulmonary artery arises aberrantly from the right esophagus causing compression of the distal trachea and right bronchus. Infants with a pulmonary artery sling often present with respiratory symptoms at birth, and most are symptomatic by 1 month of age. A barium esophagogram may be diagnostic and show anterior pulsatile compression of the esophagus. Bronchoscopy is particularly useful for evaluation of associated tracheobronchial anomalies, including the presence of complete cartilaginous rings of the trachea.

Surgical intervention is indicated in any patient with pulmonary artery sling and symptoms of respiratory obstruction. The recommended procedure is division of the anomalous artery with anastomosis to the main pulmonary artery. In some patients, the management of associated tracheobronchial anomalies may be a difficult problem requiring resection of a stenotic segment. If complete tracheal rings are present, an anterior tracheoplasty with autologous pericardium may be necessary.

ATRIAL SEPTAL DEFECTS

Defects in the atrial septum may occur as isolated anomalies or as part of more complex congenital heart disease. Secundum atrial septal defects (ASD) are among the most common cardiac malformations. ASDs may vary widely in size and location, and oc-

casionally multiple defects may be present. The foramen ovale is a normal opening that normally seals after birth but may be patent in 15 to 20 per cent of adults. A secundum ASD occurs in the midportion of the atrial septum in the region of the fossa ovalis and may extend to involve the orifice of the inferior vena cava. Sinus venosus defects occur high in the atrial septum at the junction of the superior vena cava and right atrium and are frequently associated with anomalous drainage of the pulmonary veins of the right upper lobe. The ostium primum ASD (partial atrioventricular canal defect) is caused by a deficiency in the atrioventricular septum and may be associated with anomalies of the mitral valve (cleft anterior leaflet). Partial anomalous drainage of the pulmonary veins may be seen in all types of ASD.

Pathophysiology and Natural History

An ASD allows a shunt of blood between the right and left atria. The direction of the shunt is dependent on the compliance of the two ventricles and the size of the defect. Because the left ventricle is thicker and less compliant than the right ventricle, an isolated ASD causes a shunt of oxygenated blood from the left atrium to the right atrium, increasing pulmonary blood flow. Although the pulmonary blood flow may be two to three times greater than systemic blood flow, pulmonary hypertension is uncommon in patients with isolated secundum ASD. Many patients with ASD are asymptomatic; however, there may be growth retardation and an increased susceptibility to respiratory tract infections in children. Symptoms may increase with age. The average life expectancy of patients with isolated ASD is decreased and is estimated to be approximately 40 years. The natural history of patients with an ostium primum ASD is worse secondary to mitral valve insufficiency. Pulmonary hypertension may occur in 15 to 20 per cent of patients with ASD.

Diagnosis

If symptoms are present, they most commonly are exertional dyspnea, fatigue, and palpitations. Atrial fibrillation may occur in adults with uncorrected ASD. Cyanosis occurs very rarely. The physical examination reveals a soft systolic murmur at the left sternal border with fixed splitting of the second heart sound. In patients with an ostium primum ASD, a murmur of mitral insufficiency may be present, and the chest film may show mild cardiac enlargement. The most useful test for diagnosis of an isolated defect is echocardiography, which can define the extent of the defect and evaluate associated anomalies. Cardiac catheterization is only rarely necessary and should be reserved for patients with associated anomalies or possible pulmonary hypertension.

Management

Although many patients with an ASD are asymptomatic at the time of diagnosis, operation is recommended if the pulmonary blood flow is more than 1.5 time the systemic blood flow. In children who are asymptomatic, operation is undertaken when they are 4 or 5 years of age, before they enter school. In adults, the procedure should be performed at the time of diagnosis.

The operation is usually performed through a median sternotomy, although a right thoracotomy may be used for cosmetic purposes in females. The patient is placed on cardiopulmonary bypass using bicaval cannulation, and the heart arrested with cardioplegia. A right atriotomy is performed and the anatomy assessed. Care must be taken to define the orifices of all pulmonary veins to exclude associated partial anomalous pulmonary venous drainage. In many patients with isolated secundum defects, closure can be performed by direct suture (Fig. 3). However, some prefer to close these defects with a patch of autologous pericardium or prosthetic material (Fig. 3). If partial anomalous pulmonary venous drainage is present, the defect should be closed with a patch to divert the pulmonary venous drainage across the ASD into the left atrium. In patients with ostium primum defects, anomalies of the mitral valve are common and may require repair.

Results

In most patients without pulmonary hypertension, the mortality for enclosure of an isolated secundum ASD should be less than 1 per cent, and the long-term results are excellent. The risk of operation is slightly higher in patients with ostium primum defects and has been reported to be between 2 and 5 per cent. The most important factor affecting long-term survival is the degree of insufficiency of the mitral valve. Worsening insufficiency of the mitral valve may occur despite an apparently adequate repair and may require reoperation for mitral valve repair replacement.

VENTRICULAR SEPTAL DEFECTS

Ventricular septal defects (VSD) are defects in the interventricular septum between the right and left ventricles. A VSD may occur as an isolated anomaly or as part of a complex cardiac defect. The septum between the right and left ventricles has three muscular components, termed the inlet septum, the apical trabecular septum, and the infundibular septum. There is also a fourth portion, the membranous septum, that is located near the anterior-septal commissure of the tricuspid valve. The tricuspid and mitral valves normally attach at different levels on the ventricular septum so that a portion of the membranous septum is situated between the right atrium and left ventricle and is termed the atrioventricular septum.

Muscular VSDs are defects that are completely surrounded by muscular tissue. Defects that occur in the region of the membranous septum are termed perimembranous VSDs. Perimembranous VSDs are related to the anterior septal commissure of the tricuspid valve. The bundle of His may be closely related to the inferior margin of perimembranous VSDs. Perimembranous VSDs may extend into the inlet or outlet portions of the ventricular septum. Most muscular VSDs occur in the trabecular septum and may be either single or multiple. VSDs may also be located in the infundibular septum and are termed subarterial when the aortic and pulmonary valve annulae form part of the rim of the defect. Associated anomalies include PDA, coarctation of the aorta, and congenital valvar or subvalvar aortic stenosis.

Physiology

A VSD causes a left-to-right shunt of blood across the ventricular septum. VSDs of approximately the size of the aortic orifice (or larger) are considered to be large defects and cause systemic levels of right ventricular pressure. Smaller VSDs may be restrictive (produce resistance to flow) and produce lesser elevations of right ventricular pressure. The magnitude of shunt across the VSD depends on the size of the defect and the pressure gradient across the defect. Small defects are restrictive, and shunting may occur only when there is a large pressure differential during systole. When a defect is large, shunting may occur throughout the entire cardiac cycle. A large left-to-right shunt increases pulmonary blood flow and may cause cardiac failure. If a VSD is not corrected, the increased pulmonary blood flow may cause severe pulmonary vascular disease.

Natural History

VSDs with large left-to-right shunt and increased pulmonary blood flow may cause severe congestive heart failure, and growth retardation at an early age. The risk of pulmonary vascular disease depends on the size of the defect and the magnitude of left-to-right shunting. Some VSDs close spontaneously, and this

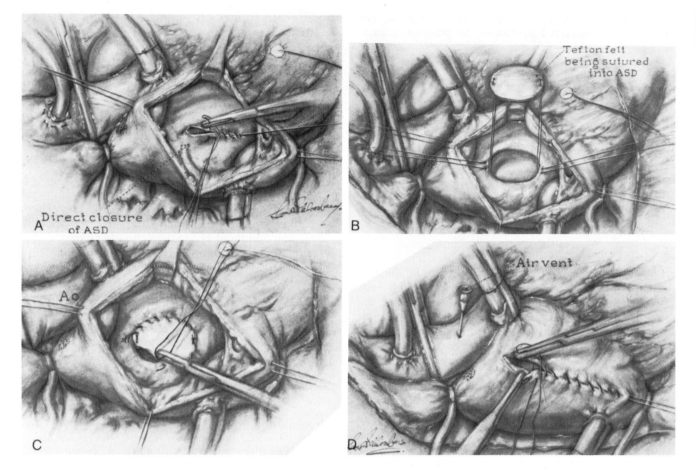

Figure 3. A secundum ASD (*A*) can be closed primarily with a continuous-suture technique (*B*) with a patch of prosthetic material or pericardium such that the sutures are placed around the entire rim of the defect (*C*). Before completing the ASD suture line, one evacuates air from the left atrium by filling it with saline. The atriotomy is then repaired (*D*). A needle vent to allow any air ejected by the left side of the circulation to escape from the aorta should be placed before one allows the heart to resume normal sinus rhythm. (From Ebert PA: Atlas of Congenital Cardiac Surgery. New York, Churchill Livingstone, 1989, with permission.)

must be considered when making decisions concerning the timing of operative therapy. Although severe pulmonary vascular disease is uncommon in infants less than 2 years of age, irreversible pulmonary vascular changes can occur in young infants. In some patients with perimembranous VSDs, the defect is closely related to the aortic valve, and aortic insufficiency may develop secondary to prolapse of a valve cusp.

Diagnosis

The physical findings of VSDs depend on the size of the defect and degree of shunting. Patients with a small VSD may have only a systolic murmur. If there is a large defect and a large left-to-right shunt, a diastolic murmur may be present secondary to congestive heart failure. If the pulmonary vascular resistance is elevated, the shunt may be bidirectional or reversed (right to left) and no murmur may be present. In patients who have reversal of the shunt secondary to increased pulmonary vascular resistance, cyanosis may be present. The chest film in patients with a large VSD shows cardiomegaly with increased pulmonary vascularity. The most useful test is echocardiography, which permits accurate definition of the location of the defect, the direction of shunting, and evaluation of associated anomalies. Cardiac catheterization may be required in some patients to assess the pulmonary vascular resistance.

Management

The timing of operative repair depends on the size of the VSD, the presence of symptoms, and the age of the patient. Infants with a large VSD may have severe heart failure with growth retardation, and repair is indicated at the time of diagnosis. In infants who are asymptomatic, repair may be postponed because of the possibility that spontaneous closure may occur. In older patients with a large VSD, the possibility of pulmonary vascular disease must be considered when planning surgical correction. Cardiac catheterization and measurement of the pulmonary vascular resistance is indicated in these patients. If significant elevation of the pulmonary vascular resistance with reversed shunting (Eisenmenger syndrome) has developed, operation may not be advisable. Patients with moderate or small VSDs that do not cause significant pulmonary hypertension may be asymptomatic and may be observed for several years in the hope that the VSD will close spontaneously. If there is no change, closure should be undertaken.

Operative Technique

Closure is the preferred treatment for all patients with an isolated significant VSD. In previous years, pulmonary artery banding to decrease pulmonary blood flow was used in some small infants with a significant VSD. However, advances in neonatal cardiac surgery make primary closure the preferred technique. Repair is performed through a median sternotomy using cardiopulmonary bypass. Most VSDs may be approached through the right atrium, although a right ventriculotomy may be necessary for some infundibular and muscular defects. The VSD should be repaired using a prosthetic patch. Because of the proximity of the conduction system of the heart to the borders of the VSD, great care must be taken with placement of sutures to avoid the creation of complete heart block.

Results

The mortality for primary repair of isolated VSD should be very low even in neonates. In older patients, the presence of significant pulmonary vascular disease adversely affects the operative mortality. Closure of an isolated VSD should permit a normal, or almost normal, life expectancy.

REFERENCES

Backer CI, Ilbawi MN, Idriss PS, DeLeon SY: Vascular anomalies causing tracheoesophageal compression. J Thorac Cardiovasc Surg 97:725, 1989.

Bender HW Jr: Diagnosis and correction of anomalous pulmonary venous return. Ann Thorac Surg 45:346, 1988.

Binet JP, Langlois J: Aortic arch anomalies in children and infants. J Thorac Cardiovasc Surg 73:428, 1977.

Blackstone EH, Kirklin JW, Bradley EL, DuShane JW, Appelbaum A: Optimal age and results in repair of large ventricular septal defects. J Thorac Cardiovasc Surg 72:661, 1976.

Dunn JM, Gordon I, Chrispin AR, deLeval MR, Stark J: Early and late results of surgical correction of pulmonary artery sling. Ann Thorac Surg 28:230, 1979.

Hoffman JIE, Randolph AM: The natural history of ventricular septal defects in infancy. Am J Cardiol 16: 634, 1965.

John S, Muralidharan S, Jairaj PS, et al: The adult ductus: Review of surgical experience with 131 patients. J Thorac Cardiovasc Surg 82:314, 1981.

Lansman S, Shapiro ASJ, Schiller MS, et al: Extended aortic arch anastomosis for repair of coarctation in infancy. Circulation 74(suppl I):37, 1986.

Palder SB, Schwartz MZ, Tyson KRT, Marr CC: Management of patent ductus arteriosus: A comparison of operative versus pharmacologic treatment. J Pediatr Surg 22:1171, 1987.

CONGENITAL CARDIAC DISORDERS:
Disorders of Pulmonary Venous Connection, Tetralogy of Fallot, Double Outlet Right Ventricle, Tricuspid Atresia

HENRY L. WALTERS, III, M.D.   ALBERT D. PACIFICO, M.D.

DISORDERS OF THE PULMONARY VENOUS CONNECTION

Disorders of the connections of the pulmonary veins to the left atrium can be either total or partial. *Total anomalous pulmonary venous connection* (TAPVC) is present when none of the pulmonary veins connect to the left atrium, but connect directly to the right atrium or indirectly to one of its systemic venous tributaries. In contrast, *partial anomalous pulmonary venous connection* (PAPVC) is present when some, but not all, of the pulmonary veins of one or both lungs drain directly into the right atrium or into one of its major tributaries.

An examination of the associated embryology is essential to an understanding of the anatomy of these disorders. The lung develops as an outpouching from the ventral surface of the primitive foregut. Early in its development, the venous drainage of this primitive lung bud is to a plexus of veins termed the *pulmonary venous plexus*. This plexus initially does not drain to the primitive left atrium, but to the systemic veins, which in normal development eventually drain into the right atrium. At approximately 4 weeks' gestation, a structure termed the *common pulmonary vein* sprouts from the back of the primitive left atrium and merges with the pulmonary venous plexus, thereby introducing the pulmonary venous drainage to the left atrium for the first time. This venous confluence is absorbed into the primitive left atrial wall to form the four pulmonary veins. During this time, the connection of the pulmonary venous plexus to the systemic veins dissolves and leaves the pulmonary venous drainage solely committed to the left atrium. Disorders

in this normal developmental process produce the wide variety of pathology seen in total and partial anomalous pulmonary venous connection.

Total Anomalous Pulmonary Venous Connection

Brief History

The first pathologic description of this disorder was made in 1798 by Wilson. While it was partially surgically corrected for the first time by Muller in 1951, it was Lewis and Varco who, in 1956, performed the first successful total correction. During the same year, Burroughs and Kirklin performed the first repair using cardiopulmonary bypass.

Morphology

In TAPVC, it is the abnormal pathway that the pulmonary venous drainage takes to eventually arrive at the right atrium that serves as the basis for the classification of its morphology. Hence, the morphology is divided into four basic types: supracardiac (45 per cent), cardiac (25 per cent), infracardiac (25 per cent), and mixed (5 per cent) (Fig. 1).

In TAPVC, the pulmonary veins nearly always drain into a common chamber termed a *common pulmonary venous sinus* (CPVS) or *confluence*. This chamber is located behind (posterior to) the left atrium, which is itself located on the back (posterior surface) of the heart. The CPVS, an extrapericardial structure that can be oriented either vertically or horizontally, exists

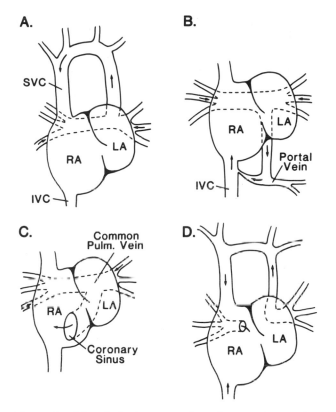

Figure 1. Morphologic types of total anomalous pulmonary venous return. *A*, Supracardiac. *B*, Infracardiac. *C*, Cardiac. *D*, Mixed. (Adapted from Fyler DC, Nadas AS: Total anomalous pulmonary venous return. *In* Avery ME, First LR [eds]: Pediatric Medicine. Baltimore, Williams & Wilkins, 1989, p 370, with permission.)

because the common pulmonary vein is not incorporated into the developing left atrium. As a result, the pulmonary venous drainage follows an alternate, sometimes circuitous pathway to the heart. This roundabout pathway forms when the connections of the pulmonary venous system to the systemic veins, which normally dissolve, remain intact.

In the *supracardiac* type of TAPVC, the pulmonary veins empty into the CPVS, which drains into the right atrium through a systemic vein such as the azygous vein, the right-sided superior vena cava or, more commonly (66 per cent), a left-sided superior vena cava. This left-sided superior vena cava, also called the *vertical vein*, flows into the innominate vein and down into the right atrium by way of the right-sided superior vena cava. In the *cardiac* type, the CPVS drains into the right atrium through the coronary sinus (80 per cent) or joins the right atrium directly (20 per cent). In the *infracardiac* type, the CPVS drains below the diaphragm directly into one of the systemic veins such as the inferior vena cava, the portal vein, the ductus

venosus, a gastric vein, or a hepatic vein. The *mixed* type combines two or more of the above kinds of pulmonary venous drainage. For example, the left upper lobe pulmonary vein might drain into a left superior vena cava, while the remainder of the pulmonary venous drainage connects directly to the coronary sinus. In all forms of TAPVC, the ultimate destination of the total pulmonary venous drainage is the right atrium.

An interatrial communication, either a patent foramen ovale or an atrial septal defect (ASD), coexists in all patients who survive the neonatal period because it provides the only avenue for blood to reach the left side of the heart. Approximately 25 to 50 per cent of patients have an associated patent ductus arteriosus. Other associated cardiac anomalies are rare.

Pathophysiology and Clinical Presentation

The obligatory mixing of systemic and pulmonary venous blood at the right atrial level produces the variable degrees of cyanosis that characterize this disorder. Pulmonary venous obstruction occurs in 60 to 75 per cent of all patients and usually consists of a stenosis of the vein connecting the CPVS to the systemic venous system. In order of decreasing frequency, pulmonary venous obstruction occurs in nearly all infracardiac types, in many supracardiac types, and in only a few of the cardiac types. This frequent obstruction of pulmonary venous blood flow causes serious pulmonary venous hypertension, which leads to dangerous degrees of pulmonary arterial and right ventricular hypertension.

The presentation of a child with TAPVC depends on the degree of pulmonary venous obstruction. Severe pulmonary venous hypertension causes marked respiratory distress due to pulmonary edema, marked cyanosis due to low pulmonary blood flow, and severe right heart failure. These neonates are critically ill, and without prompt surgical intervention at least 80 per cent die within the first year of life—most within the first 3 months. Patients without pulmonary venous obstruction (25 to 40 per cent) often go undetected in the neonatal period and present later in infancy with symptoms similar to an ASD, except for the presence of mild cyanosis. In this group of patients, pulmonary vascular disease due to pulmonary overcirculation develops more rapidly than in patients with isolated ASDs. Approximately 50 per cent die within the first year of life, and few survive infancy.

Diagnosis

The chest radiograph of patients with severe pulmonary venous obstruction shows diffuse pulmonary edema. In patients without obstruction, the chest radiograph shows an enlarged heart and increased pulmonary vascularity due to exuberant pulmonary blood flow. The electrocardiogram (ECG) is nonspecific. Two-dimensional echocardiography shows right ventricular diastolic volume overload, paradoxic ventricular septal motion to the left due to right ventricular hypertension, and an echo-free space posterior to the left atrium representing the CPVS. Cardiac catheterization and cineangiography provide the diagnosis in almost all cases by demonstrating the anomalous pulmonary venous pathway and documenting the presence of pulmonary venous obstruction.

Treatment and Results

Because of the critical clinical condition and dismal survival of unoperated patients with the obstructed form of TAPVC, emergent surgical intervention is indicated following diagnosis. In the nonobstructed forms, operation should be undertaken in early infancy to prevent the early development of pulmonary vascular disease. In critically ill neonates, the initial medical management should be guided by arterial and central venous pressure monitoring. Treatment includes sedation, paralysis, and endotracheal intubation using mechanical hyperventilation with 100 per cent oxygen to lower pulmonary vascular resistance. These measures increase pulmonary blood flow and lessen the associated profound cyanosis. Acidosis and hypoglycemia should be vigorously corrected, and cardiac output maximized with proper treatment of the volume status and the administration of appropriate inotropic agents.

The surgical approach to the infracardiac and supracardiac types of TAPVC requires the use of low-flow, hypothermic cardiopulmonary bypass and/or circulatory arrest with hypothermic, enriched, hyperkalemic, dilute, sanguineous cardioplegia. The proper surgical approach requires minimal disturbance of the irritable myocardium and immediate decompression of the hypertensive pulmonary vascular circulation after the institution of cardiopulmonary bypass by ligation of the patent ductus arteriosus and incision of the CPVS. The incised CPVS, which lies just behind (posterior to) the left atrium, is anastomosed to the posterior wall of this chamber to provide an unobstructed flow of pulmonary venous blood.

The postoperative course of these critically ill neonates is rarely straightforward. Pulmonary vascular hypertension often persists into the postoperative period, complicating management and necessitating prolonged periods of mechanical ventilatory and inotropic support. Extracorporeal membrane oxygenation is sometimes necessary as a life-saving adjunct to postoperative care. The results of surgical management have improved over time, with some centers reporting early postoperative mortality of 10 to 20 per cent or less.

Patients with TAPVC to the coronary sinus are usually unobstructed and are operated on electively in early infancy. The principles of cardiopulmonary bypass and myocardial protection are the same; however, the case can usually be performed with low-flow, hypothermic cardiopulmonary bypass alone and does not usually involve the use of total circulatory arrest. The roof of the coronary sinus is incised into the left atrium to provide unobstructed pulmonary flow into this chamber, and the resulting ASD is closed with a patch of autologous pericardium. The hospital mortality for the unobstructed forms of TAPVC is less than 5 per cent, and long-term results are excellent.

Partial Anomalous Pulmonary Venous Connection

Morphology

The most common variant of PAPVC is the *sinus venosus syndrome*. This disorder consists of a sinus venosus ASD (located just beneath the superior vena cava) with the venous return from the right upper and middle lobes draining to the superior vena cava (SVC) or to the SVC–right atrial junction. Less common is the scimitar syndrome, in which all or part of the venous return of the right lung drains into a vertically oriented vein that descends parallel to the right pericardial border to empty into the inferior vena cava near its junction with the right atrium. This syndrome is usually associated with a hypoplastic right lung and pulmonary artery and may or may not be associated with an ASD or pulmonary sequestration. Other forms of PAPVC include: (1) the right superior pulmonary vein connecting to the SVC without an ASD, (2) the right pulmonary veins connecting directly to the right atrium with or without an ASD, (3) the left pulmonary veins connecting to a left vertical vein that drains into the innominate vein, and (4) various forms of bilateral PAPVC.

Pathophysiology and Clinical Presentation

The pathophysiology is determined by the combined effect of the left-to-right shunt due to the PAPVC and the ASD (if present). If the left-to-right shunt is small (<1.5 to 1), the patient typically remains asymptomatic. In the presence of a large left-to-right shunt (>1.8 to 1), signs and symptoms of pulmonary overcirculation, such as tachypnea, frequent respiratory infections, and palpitations, develop. Rarely, patients with neglected disease present with cyanosis due to right-to-left shunting secondary to the development of pulmonary vascular disease.

The natural history of untreated sinus venosus syndrome is similar to that of ASD; right heart failure due to pulmonary vascular disease develops in the fourth through sixth decades. Patients with untreated scimitar syndrome with a large left-to-right shunt also have a natural history similar to those with ASD if there is no associated right lung pathology. When right lung pathology is present, pulmonary infection and hemoptysis dominate the clinical picture.

Diagnosis

In patients with a large left-to-right shunt, the chest radiograph shows an enlarged right heart with prominent pulmonary vascular markings. Patients with the scimitar syndrome demonstrate a crescentic shadow resembling a scimitar parallel to the right heart border. The ECG shows an incomplete right bundle branch block and a clockwise frontal loop. While two-dimensional echocardiography can usually diagnose the sinus venosus syndrome, cardiac catheterization and cineangiography should be performed if there is doubt about the diagnosis, if there are associated major cardiac anomalies, or if one of the less common forms of PAPVC is suspected.

Treatment and Results

Principles of surgical treatment involve closure of the ASD with autologous pericardium to direct the pulmonary venous return from its entrance into the right atrium through the ASD and into the left atrium. The operative mortality is less than 1 per cent, and the long-term results are excellent.

TETRALOGY OF FALLOT

Tetralogy of Fallot (TOF), the most common cyanotic congenital cardiac anomaly, is characterized by a ventricular septal defect (VSD), right ventricular outflow tract obstruction (RVOTO), an overriding aorta, and right ventricular hypertrophy. Its embryogenesis includes underdevelopment of the right ventricular outflow tract and anterior displacement of the portion of the interventricular septum that lies directly beneath the pulmonary valve. This condition was first palliated by Blalock in 1945 when he developed the first systemic–to–pulmonary artery (Blalock-Taussig) shunt. Lillehei performed the first complete correction of TOF in 1954 using cross-circulation.

Morphology

The VSD is typically large and is usually located in the interventricular septum near the junction of the septal and anterior leaflets of the tricuspid valve (perimembranous location), just below the aortic valve. Multiple VSDs are rare. The *right ventricular outflow tract* (RVOT) is obstructed to varying degrees and at varying levels due to hypoplasia and hypertrophied muscle bundles. Most patients have a small pulmonary annulus; 75 per cent have some degree of pulmonary valve stenosis that contributes to the RVOTO. Pulmonary atresia occurs in 15 to 20 per cent. The main pulmonary artery and its branches can be hypoplastic, stenotic, maldistributed, or a combination of these. The reduction in pulmonary blood flow caused by the RVOTO stimulates the development of aortic branches that serve as collateral vessels to the lung. Right ventricular hypertrophy, a secondary response to the chronic pressure overload imposed by the RVOTO, worsens over time. The aorta arises to varying degrees from the right ventricle and overrides the interventricular septum. Associated anomalies include ASD, right aortic arch (25 per cent), anomalous coronary artery branching (especially left anterior descending from the right coronary artery, 5 per cent), atrioventricular canal defect, absent pulmonary valve, and persistent left superior vena cava.

Pathophysiology and Clinical Presentation

Because the VSD is usually nonrestrictive, the pathophysiology of the disorder depends on the degree of RVOTO. With severe RVOTO there is predominantly right-to-left shunting across the VSD, producing cyanosis and progressive polycythemia. In most patients with TOF, the cyanosis becomes apparent clinically within the first 6 months of age. Moderate RVOTO produces bidirectional shunting and less severe cyanosis. Mild RVOTO produces predominantly left-to-right shunting, the so-called pink tetralogy, and the potential for the development of congestive heart failure due to pulmonary overcirculation.

Early and profound cyanosis with acidosis occurs in neonates with TOF and pulmonary atresia when, shortly after birth, the ductus arteriosus begins to close, thereby eliminating the only source of pulmonary blood flow. Only an infusion of prostaglandin E_1 reverses this process to allow stabilization of the neonate until a systemic–to–pulmonary artery shunt can be performed electively. Infants with TOF characteristically squat. By raising the peripheral vascular resistance, this maneuver increases left ventricular afterload, which reduces the magnitude of right-to-left shunting across the VSD, thereby lessening cyanosis temporarily. *Tet spells* are produced when a spasm of the RVOT causes increased right-to-left shunting, a sudden decrease in oxygen saturation, increased cyanosis, and sometimes neurologic injury or death.

The natural history of TOF is unfavorable if not treated surgically. Approximately 50 per cent of patients die by 2 years of age, and only 5 to 10 per cent live to age 21. The consequences of chronic and severe cyanosis are the sequelae of progressive polycythemia: pulmonary emboli, infarction, and abscesses as well as cerebral vascular accidents and brain abscesses.

Diagnosis

The chest radiograph usually reveals a normal heart size and diminished pulmonary vascular markings. The right ventricular hypertrophy gives the heart the characteristic *coeur en sabot* or *boot-shaped* appearance. The upper mediastinal shadow is narrow due to the small size of the pulmonary artery. The ECG shows right axis deviation and right ventricular hypertrophy.

Although the diagnosis of TOF can be made reliably by either two-dimensional echocardiography or cardiac catheterization, both methods complement each other. Echocardiography accurately demonstrates the VSD with its size, location, and direction of shunting; shows the overriding aorta; defines and characterizes the RVOTO; and estimates chamber pressures and obstructive gradients. Cardiac catheterization with cineangiography measures chamber pressures and obstructive gradients more accurately, measures saturation data, and calculates shunts. It also more clearly demonstrates branch pulmonary artery size and distribution, the presence of multiple VSDs, the anatomy and significance of collateral bronchopulmonary circulation, the coronary anatomy, the size and function of the ventricles, and the anatomy of the branches of the aortic arch.

Treatment and Results

Surgical treatment options include either early primary complete repair or palliation (with a systemic-to-pulmonary artery shunt) followed by complete repair at a later date. The most commonly performed shunt is a Blalock-Taussig shunt or a modification thereof. This procedure creates a reliable source of pulmonary blood flow by connecting the subclavian artery to the pulmonary artery either directly or by means of a polytetrafluoroethylene tube graft (Gore-Tex, W.L. Gore and Associates, Inc., Flagstaff, AZ). Complete repair includes the elimination of any previous shunts, closure of the VSD, relief of the RVOTO, and the correction of any associated anomalies.

The indications for and timing of complete repair are controversial. Some advocate complete repair in early infancy, citing as advantages: (1) the avoidance of shunt-related complications, (2) avoidance of the

need to obliterate the shunt at the time of complete repair, (3) elimination of the long-term effects of cyanosis, and (4) elimination of the long-term effects of right ventricular hypertension and hypertrophy. Our policy has been to perform complete repair on symptomatic patients (clinically significant cyanosis or "tet spells") or on patients with anatomically threatening RVOTO, regardless of age. In asymptomatic patients with favorable anatomy, we recommend primary repair between 3 and 6 months of age. In patients with surgically significant coronary artery anomalies, multiple VSDs, significant pulmonary artery hypoplasia or pulmonary atresia, we elect to perform palliative systemic-to-pulmonary artery shunts, when indicated, and delay complete repair until 1 to 3 years of age.

The results of surgical therapy for TOF are gratifying. Most survivors live unrestricted and productive lives with normal exercise tolerance. In some series, the surgical mortality is 1 to 5 per cent, with a 20-year survival of 90 per cent.

DOUBLE OUTLET RIGHT VENTRICLE

Double outlet right ventricle (DORV) represents a wide and complex spectrum of congenital cardiac malformations that lie morphologically between simple *ventricular septal defect* and transposition of the great arteries with VSD. In this disorder, both great arteries arise entirely or in large part from the right ventricle, usually in association with a VSD. DORV represents between 1 and 2 per cent of all congenital cardiac malformations and may coexist with a wide variety of other cardiac lesions. The first successful repair of this disorder was performed in 1956 by Kirklin at the Mayo Clinic.

Morphology

DORV is present when more than 50 per cent of each great artery arises from the morphologic right ventricle. We prefer to modify this definition in the case of TOF-type defects where all of the pulmonary artery and greater than 90 per cent of the aorta must arise from the right ventricle to be called DORV. The morphology of DORV is best described in terms of (1) the relationship of the VSD to the great vessels, (2) the orientation of the great vessels to each other, (3) the presence or absence of pulmonary stenosis, and (4) the connection of the atria to the ventricles.

There are four possible relationships of the VSD to the great vessels: *subaortic*, *subpulmonary*, *doubly committed*, or *noncommitted*. A *subaortic* VSD is the most common (60 per cent) and is located immediately beneath the aortic valve in the perimembranous position. A *subpulmonary* VSD occurs 30 per cent of the time and is located directly beneath the pulmonary valve. DORV in association with a subpulmonary VSD is usually called a *Taussig-Bing malformation*. In the remainder of cases, the VSD is either *doubly committed* (located directly beneath both the aortic and pulmonary valves) or *noncommitted* (located in a position far removed from both the aortic and pulmonary valves). On rare occasions, either no VSD (incompatible with life) or multiple VSDs exist.

The relationships of the great vessels to each other can vary and are best described by the position of the aorta in relation to the pulmonary artery. The most common relationships are with the aorta to the *right* of the pulmonary artery and either posterior (normal), side by side, or anterior to it. Less commonly, the aorta may lie to the left and anterior to the pulmonary artery. Because of its effect on the clinical presentation of the patient, the presence or absence of pulmonary stenosis is critical to the description of DORV. Pulmonary stenosis occurs in 35 per cent of all cases of DORV, most commonly in association with a subaortic VSD, and may be valvular, subvalvular, or both. In 90 per cent of the cases of DORV, the right atrium connects to the right ventricle and the left atrium connects to the left ventricle (atrioventricular concordance—normal anatomy). Occasionally the connection may be reversed (atrioventricular discordance).

Pathophysiology and Clinical Presentation

In the absence of other major cardiac anomalies, the clinical presentation of patients with DORV depends upon the relationship of the VSD to the great arteries and the presence or absence of pulmonary stenosis. Cyanosis is produced in these patients either by restriction to pulmonary blood flow or by streaming. Congestive heart failure is caused by the unrestricted pulmonary blood flow created by a large VSD without pulmonary stenosis.

For example, patients with a subaortic VSD associated with pulmonary stenosis present similarly to patients with TOF with cyanosis and the absence of congestive heart failure. A subaortic VSD without pulmonary stenosis produces a clinical picture similar to that of an isolated, large VSD. The patient is acyanotic due to the streaming of saturated left ventricular blood through the subaortic VSD into the aorta and is prone to the development of congestive heart failure due to the unrestricted pulmonary blood flow. In the presence of a subpulmonary VSD (Taussig-Bing malformation), which usually has no pulmonary stenosis, the unrestricted flow of saturated left ventricular blood into the pulmonary artery produces early and severe congestive heart failure. Desaturated right ventricular blood streams into the aorta, producing marked cyanosis. This latter condition mimics the clinical presentation of transposition of the great arteries with VSD.

Diagnosis

The chest radiograph findings are varied and nonspecific and depend primarily on the amount of pulmonary blood flow and the presence of associated major cardiac anomalies. Cineangiography is the "gold standard" for diagnosis and should be examined carefully for at least eight findings: (1) the size and relationship of the VSD to the great arteries, (2) the presence or absence of multiple VSDs, (3) the relationship of the great arteries to each other, (4) the presence or absence of pulmonary stenosis and the level(s) at which it occurs, (5) the size and adequacy of the ventricles, (6) the anatomy and function of the atrioventricular valves, (7) the relationship of the atria to the ventricles (concordant or discordant), and (8) other associated cardiac anomalies. Two-dimensional echocardiography more clearly defines atrioventricular valve abnormalities and more accurately characterizes the location and boundaries of the VSD with its relationship to the great arteries.

Treatment and Results

The timing of surgical intervention depends on the symptomatic state of the patient and the anatomy of other cardiac anomalies associated with the DORV itself. The anatomy determines the ultimate surgical approach, which dictates the optimal age for definitive repair. The clinical state of the patient dictates the need for initial palliative procedures. The principal part of the corrective operation for DORV is the tunnel repair; the VSD is connected to a great artery by creating a tunnel within the right ventricle.

DORV and a subaortic or doubly committed VSD can usually be repaired by creating an intracardiac tunnel connecting the left ventricle (via the VSD) to the aorta using a synthetic patch. Those without pulmonary stenosis should be repaired by 6 to 12 months of age (or sooner if medically refractory congestive heart failure occurs) because of the early development of pulmonary vascular disease. When pulmonary stenosis is present in this form of DORV, it can usually be relieved by intracardiac muscular resection, the use of a pulmonary transannular patch, or a combination of both. Management of this subset is similar to the surgical management of patients with TOF, and repair is generally advised before 1 year of age. A definitive repair is performed prior to this time if the patient develops significant cyanosis and if an intracardiac repair can be accomplished with confidence. A palliative systemic–to–pulmonary artery shunt is created first if the eventual need for an extracardiac conduit is anticipated. Survival in this overall group of patients is excellent (97 per cent at 10 years).

Patients with a subpulmonary VSD (Taussig-Bing malformation) physiologically resemble those with transposition of the great arteries with VSD. Patients without pulmonary stenosis are repaired most commonly with an intracardiac tunnel connecting the VSD to the pulmonary artery, thereby creating anatomic transposition of the great arteries. An arterial switch procedure is added to connect the left ventricle to the aorta and the right ventricle to the pulmonary artery. These patients develop severe congestive heart failure and/or pulmonary vascular disease early in life and require surgical intervention within the first 3 months of life. When pulmonary stenosis is present in this group of patients, a palliative systemic–to–pulmonary artery shunt is sometimes needed to treat severe cyanosis. A definitive repair, performed at 2 to 3 years of age, involves closure of the VSD to the aorta and placement of a valved extracardiac homograft conduit from the right ventricle to the pulmonary artery.

Patients with DORV, noncommitted VSD, and absent pulmonary stenosis ultimately require repair using a valved extracardiac homograft conduit or a modification of the Fontan procedure. They are usually palliated with a pulmonary artery banding when congestive heart failure develops. Definitive repair can be accomplished at 1 to 4 years of age depending on the procedure.

TRICUSPID ATRESIA

Tricuspid atresia is a congenital cardiac anomaly marked by the failure of development of the right atrioventricular valve, causing a lack of communication between the right atrium and the hypoplastic right ventricle. The only outlet from the right atrium is an interatrial communication, such as an atrial septal defect or a patent foramen ovale. This anomaly is almost always associated with a ventricular septal defect. It accounts for 1 to 5 per cent of all congenital heart defects and is the third most common condition causing cyanosis besides TOF and transposition of the great arteries. The exact embryogenesis of this disorder is controversial. Blalock, in 1945, performed the first palliative procedure (systemic–to–pulmonary artery shunt) for this disorder, and Fontan and Beaudet reported the first "corrective" procedure in 1971.

Morphology

The morphology is based on three factors: (1) the association of the great arteries with the ventricles (ventriculoarterial connection), (2) the presence or absence of pulmonary outflow obstruction, and (3) the size of the ventricular septal defect (Fig. 2). Type 1 defects are the most common (70 per cent) and consist solely of those with concordant (normal) ventriculoarterial connection. Most of type 1 defects (75 per cent) have obstruction to pulmonary blood flow. Fifteen per cent are unobstructed, and 10 per cent have atresia (absence) of the pulmonary valve. Type 2 (27 per cent) and type 3 (3 per cent) defects consist of those hearts with discordant (transposed) ventriculoarterial connections. Within the type 2 group of patients, 65 per cent have no obstruction to pulmonary outflow, while 35 per cent do. In all types of tricuspid atresia, the pulmonary outflow obstruction may occur at the level of the VSD, the level of the pulmonary valve, the level of the main or branch pulmonary arteries, or a combination of any of these. In those patients with discordant ventriculoarterial connections, subaortic stenosis can occur due to narrowing of the VSD or due to muscular obstruction within the subaortic, rudimentary right ventricle. An interatrial communication of some kind is always present to provide an outlet for right atrial blood.

Pathophysiology and Clinical Presentation

In most patients with tricuspid atresia, desaturated blood from the superior vena cava, inferior vena cava, and coronary sinus flows into the right atrium from whence it passes into the left atrium through the interatrial communication. From there, it flows into the left ventricle and is ejected into the great vessel directly communicating with the left ventricle (as long as that great vessel is not atretic). At the same time the desaturated blood is also ejected from the left ventricle through the VSD into the hypoplastic right ventricle and into the great vessel communicating therewith (again, as long as that great vessel is not atretic).

If the interatrial communication is restrictive, the patient presents with signs of right heart failure (due to right atrial hypertension), low cardiac output (due to poor left ventricular filling), and cyanosis (due to low pulmonary blood flow). In general, patients without obstruction to pulmonary blood flow appear acyanotic with congestive heart failure. In contrast, patients with obstruction to pulmonary blood flow are usually cyanotic and not in congestive heart failure. If pulmonary atresia is present, the only source of pulmonary blood flow is usually from a patent ductus arteriosus. As the patent ductus arteriosus closes shortly after birth, the patient becomes critically hypoxic and acidotic. Over time the VSD in patients with tricuspid atresia can become smaller, thereby creating subvalvular obstruction beneath the great artery that arises from the hypoplastic right ventricle. If there is

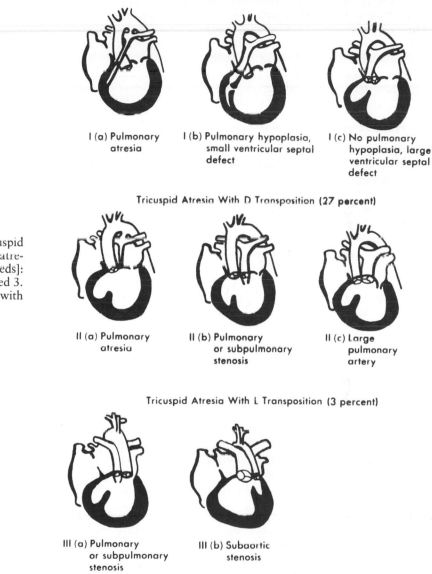

Tricuspid Atresia With No Transposition (69 percent)

I (a) Pulmonary atresia

I (b) Pulmonary hypoplasia, small ventricular septal defect

I (c) No pulmonary hypoplasia, large ventricular septal defect

Tricuspid Atresia With D Transposition (27 percent)

II (a) Pulmonary atresia

II (b) Pulmonary or subpulmonary stenosis

II (c) Large pulmonary artery

Tricuspid Atresia With L Transposition (3 percent)

III (a) Pulmonary or subpulmonary stenosis

III (b) Subaortic stenosis

Figure 2. Morphologic types of tricuspid atresia. (Adapted from Vlad P: Tricuspid atresia. In Keith JD, Rowe RD, Vlad P [eds]: Heart Disease in Infancy and Childhood, ed 3. New York, Macmillan, 1978, p 521, with permission.)

ventriculoarterial concordance (normal), cyanosis ensues due to a progressive reduction in pulmonary blood flow. With ventriculoarterial discordance (transposition), low cardiac output may occur due to progressive subaortic obstruction. Without some form of surgical intervention, most patients with tricuspid atresia die from the consequences of either reduced or unrestricted pulmonary blood flow before they reach 1 year of age.

Diagnosis

The ECG usually shows evidence of an atrial abnormality manifested by notched P waves with a taller

initial peak. The chest radiograph findings are nonspecific. While the heart size is usually normal, it may be enlarged in the presence of congestive heart failure. Although the lung fields are usually clear, they may appear congested in the presence of increased pulmonary blood flow. Two-dimensional echocardiography and cardiac catheterization with cineangiography are complementary in diagnosing this disorder. It is important to identify the following features: (1) the absence of the tricuspid valve, (2) hypoplasia of the right ventricle, (3) the size and function of the left ventricle, (4) the size of the interatrial communication with the measurement of any pressure gradients across it, (5) the size and location of the VSD, (6) the ventriculoarterial connection, (7) the presence or absence of pulmonary or aortic obstruction, (8) the presence or absence of atrioventricular valve abnormalities, (9) the size and distribution of the pulmonary arteries with their associated pressure and pulmonary vascular resistance, (10) the systemic oxygen saturation, and (11) any associated abnormalities.

Treatment and Results

Palliative measures are sometimes necessary prior to performing a corrective procedure. Neonates with marked cyanosis due to obstruction to pulmonary blood flow should be treated with prostaglandin E_1 to maintain patency of the ductus arteriosus until a systemic artery–to–pulmonary artery shunt (i.e., Blalock-Taussig shunt) can be performed. Patients with unrestricted pulmonary blood flow may require a palliative pulmonary artery banding to forestall the development of congestive heart failure and pulmonary vascular disease. Patients with a restrictive interatrial communication must undergo a balloon atrial septostomy or surgical atrial septectomy.

The usual procedure for this disorder is a modification of the Fontan procedure known as a total cavopulmonary connection. This involves connection of the superior and inferior vena cavae or, alternatively, the right atrium itself to the pulmonary artery. In this way, desaturated blood flows passively through the pulmonary circulation without the assistance of an intervening pumping chamber. The procedure, although not *anatomically* corrective is *physiologically* corrective, as the desaturated blood flows to the lungs, and the saturated blood is ejected by the left ventricle to the body.

At times the modified Fontan procedure is performed in two separate stages. First, an anastomosis of the end of the superior vena cava to the side of the right pulmonary artery (bidirectional cavopulmonary shunt) is performed. This directs the superior vena caval portion of the systemic venous return passively into the pulmonary circuit. Later, the inferior vena caval return is baffled into the pulmonary circulation to complete the total cavopulmonary connection. The first stage may be performed as early as 6 months of age, and the second stage or the performance of the entire procedure in one stage may be performed as early as 12 months of age.

Several factors may adversely affect the passive flow of desaturated blood through the pulmonary circuit and, hence, the outcome of any cavopulmonary connection. These include: (1) small size of the superior vena cava; (2) stenoses of any of the suture lines or baffles; (3) hypoplastic, stenotic, or maldistributed pulmonary arteries; (4) high pulmonary vascular resistance and pulmonary artery pressure; (5) poor left ventricular function with high left ventricular end-diastolic pressure; (6) mitral stenosis or regurgitation; and (7) refractory arrhythmias.

Greater than 90 per cent of postoperative survivors of a total cavopulmonary connection are in functional class 1 to 2. While most patients do have a below-normal response to exercise testing, they usually lead unrestricted and productive lives. Long-term complications can include protein-losing enteropathy, chronic pleural and pericardial effusions, arrhythmias, thrombus formation, and cerebral infarction.

REFERENCES

Gustafson RA, Murray GF, Warden HE, Hill RC, Rozar GE Jr: Early primary repair of tetralogy of Fallot. Ann Thorac Surg 45: 235, 1988.

Kirklin JW, Pacifico AD, Blackstone EH, Kirklin JK, Bargeron LM Jr: Current risks and protocols for operations for double outlet right ventricle. J Thorac Cardiovasc Surg 92:913, 1986.

Pacifico AD (Guest Editor): Seminars in Thoracic and Cardiovascular Surgery (vol 2, no 1): Surgical Management of Classical Tetralogy of Fallot. Philadelphia, WB Saunders Company, 1990.

Sade RM, Fyfe DA: Tricuspid atresia: Current concepts in diagnosis and treatment. Pediatr Clin North Am 37(1):151, 1990.

Sano S, Brawn WJ, Mee RB: Total anomalous pulmonary venous drainage. J Thorac Cardiovasc Surg 97:886, 1989.

CONGENITAL CARDIAC DISORDERS:
Truncus Arteriosus, Transposition of the Great Arteries, Aortic, Pulmonary, Mitral, and Tricuspid Valve Disease

ERLE H. AUSTIN, III, M.D.

TRUNCUS ARTERIOSUS

Truncus arteriosus is characterized by a single arterial trunk that arises from a single semilunar (truncal) valve that overrides a large ventricular septal defect and emanates from the heart and gives rise to the aorta and pulmonary artery (Fig. 1A). Although truncus arteriosus represents only 2 per cent of congenital heart defects, its recognition is important because survival is unlikely without intervention. Current surgical techniques permit physiologic correction, with excellent long-term survival and functional status.

Anatomy

During the fifth week of normal gestation, two opposing ridges appear in the conus of the developing heart and fuse to form a truncoconal septum separating the aortic and pulmonary channels. In truncus arteriosus, the two ridges fail to fuse, leaving a single channel overlying a large defect in the interventricular septum. Truncus arteriosus was classified by Collett and Edwards according to how the pulmonary arteries come off of the truncus with 90 per cent of patients either type I or type II. In type I, a single main pulmonary artery arises from a single orifice near the base of the truncus and divides into left and right branch pulmonary arteries. In type II, the left and right pulmonary arteries arise separately but close together in the posterior aspect of the truncus. In type III the left and right pulmonary arteries arise from individual orifices that are widely separated from each other. Type IV, in which the blood supply to the lungs is derived from bronchial collaterals, is now recognized as a severe form of pulmonary atresia with ventricular septal defect. In most patients, the truncal valve has three leaflets, although four leaflets are not unusual. Myxomatous thickening of these leaflets may cause significant truncal valve incompetence (20 per cent) or stenosis (10 per cent). Thymic atresia and DiGeorge syndrome are important associated conditions.

Pathophysiology

In truncus arteriosus, both ventricles eject blood into the common trunk, and this admixture of saturated and desaturated blood is distributed to the systemic and pulmonary circulations. The pattern of flow depends on the relative resistances in the systemic and pulmonary vascular beds. At birth, pulmonary vascular resistance is close to systemic levels, causing a relatively equal distribution of blood to the pulmonary and systemic circulations. By 3 to 4 weeks of life, however, when pulmonary vascular resistance drops, the increase in pulmonary blood flow causes ventricular volume overload and congestive heart failure. At this stage, infants may die from progressive heart failure or begin to counteract the high pressure and high volume blood flow by developing obstructive pulmonary vascular disease. These infants often improve clinically as pulmonary blood flow decreases but subsequently develop cyanosis and become unsuitable candidates for repair because of irreversible pulmonary hypertension.

Clinical Features

In the absence of surgical intervention, the prognosis for infants with truncus arteriosus is poor, with only 30 per cent surviving to 3 months of age. The prognosis is worse if there is severe truncal valve insufficiency or stenosis. The typical infant with truncus

A

B

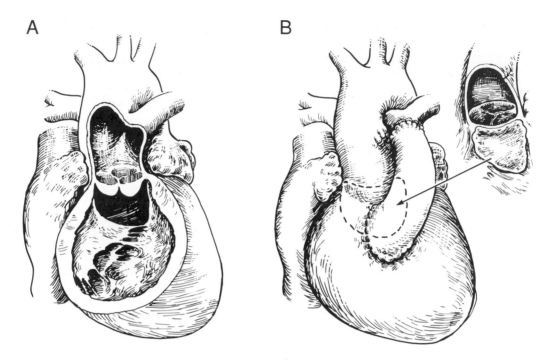

Figure 1. *A,* Truncus arteriosus. A single arterial trunk straddles a large ventricular septal defect and gives rise to the aorta and pulmonary arteries. *B,* Surgical repair includes patch closure of the ventricular septal defect, separation of the pulmonary arteries from the arterial trunk, and establishment of right ventricular–to–pulmonary artery continuity with an allograft-valved conduit.

arteriosus presents at 3 to 4 weeks of age with symptoms of tachypnea, irritability, and poor feeding. Cyanosis is unusual at this stage because of high pulmonary blood flow. On physical examination, the heart appears hyperdynamic and a loud holosystolic murmur is present at the lower left sternal border. A wide pulse pressure produces prominent peripheral pulses. Electrocardiography indicates biventricular hypertrophy and a normal axis. Cardiomegaly, increased pulmonary vascular markings, and an absent main pulmonary artery segment are seen on chest radiography. A right-sided aortic arch may be present. In most patients, definitive diagnosis can be made with two-dimensional echocardiography. The presence of a single large artery and semilunar valve overriding a large ventricular septal defect is diagnostic. The origin of the pulmonary artery and the presence of truncal insufficiency or stenosis can usually be determined by this technique. Cardiac catheterization, however, should also be performed to definitively discern the pulmonary artery and aortic arch anatomy and to determine the pulmonary vascular resistance. In the very young infant, the pulmonary vascular resistance should be only mildly elevated (2 to 4 Woods units), but resistance greater that 8 Woods units precludes operative repair. Truncal valve insufficiency and/or

stenosis should be thoroughly evaluated at catheterization.

Management

In view of the poor natural history of this defect, its presence is an indication for surgical repair. Bilateral pulmonary artery banding, once used to palliate these infants, is no longer recommended. At the time of diagnosis, measures to ameliorate the degree of congestive heart failure including digitalis, diuretics, and ventilatory support are employed to stabilize these infants. At one time, these measures were vigorously applied to permit these infants to reach 6 months of age before repair. Many such infants, however, deteriorate before that time, forcing emergency correction under less than ideal circumstances. Consequently, most medical centers currently recommend primary repair at the time of diagnosis. Physiologic repair of truncus arteriosus includes separating the main pulmonary artery or pulmonary branches from the truncus, closing the ventricular septal defect with a Dacron patch, and establishing right ventricular to pulmonary continuity with a valved conduit (Fig. 1B). Currently, antibiotic-preserved or cryopreserved aortic allografts are preferred for this purpose. Because the conduit employed is, by necessity, small and because the patients are expected to grow, reoperation is necessary to insert a larger conduit. In most patients, conduit replacement is not required until 3 to 4 years of age, at which time a significantly larger conduit can be placed.

Results

The earliest experiences with surgical correction of truncus arteriosus were obtained in patients who had survived to 2 years of age before operation. In this group, hospital mortality was approximately 25 per cent. Of the operative survivors, 70 per cent were alive 10 years after repair. Most of these patients were New York Heart Association (NYHA) Class I or II. More recent experience with surgical repair in neonates and infants in the first months of life indicates that a hospital mortality of 10 per cent can now be achieved. Although reoperation for conduit replacement is inevitable with this approach, hospital mortality for the second procedure is less than 1 per cent.

TRANSPOSITION OF THE GREAT ARTERIES

In transposition of the great arteries, the aorta arises from the right ventricle, and the pulmonary artery arises from the left ventricle. As a result, desaturated systemic venous blood is pumped to the systemic arterial circulation and oxygenated pulmonary venous return is pumped back to the lungs. Without some communication between these two parallel circulations, transposition of the great arteries would be incompatible with life. Most infants born with this defect, however, survive the first hours of life by limited mixing of saturated and desaturated blood through a patent foramen ovale and a ductus arteriosus. Before the availability of techniques to diagnose and treat these infants, transposition of the great arteries caused more cardiac-related deaths within the first 2 months of life than any other congenital heart lesion. Today, appropriate recognition and management permits long-term survival for almost 90 per cent.

Anatomy

In transposition of the great arteries, the atria are connected to their appropriate ventricles (atrioventricular concordance), but the ventricles give rise to inappropriate great vessels (ventriculoarterial discordance). The aorta, as it emanates from the right ventricle, is usually anterior and slightly to the right of the pulmonary artery, which arises from the left ventricle (Fig. 2A). Two thirds of infants born with

transposition of the great arteries have no other significant cardiac defects other than a patent foramen ovale or an atrial septal defect. Approximately 20 per cent have a ventricular septal defect, and 5 per cent have a ventricular septal defect associated with some form of left ventricular outflow tract obstruction.

Pathophysiology

The anatomic malformation of transposition of the great arteries converts the normal sequential relationship of the pulmonary and systemic circulations into a parallel one. Access of desaturated blood from the body to the lungs and of saturated blood from the lungs to the body can only occur if the two circulations are allowed to communicate. Potential sites for mixing of the two circulations include a patent foramen ovale or an atrial septal defect, a ventricular septal defect, or a patent ductus arteriosus. The degree of hypoxia depends on the adequacy of mixing between the two circulations. The preferable defect is a large atrial septal defect that allows unrestricted bidirectional shunting at low pressure. A ventricular septal defect or patent ductus arteriosus may provide satisfactory mixing, but the high-pressure pulsatile flow from these lesions is more likely to cause excessive pulmonary blood flow causing congestive heart failure and early pulmonary vascular obstructive disease. In transposition of the great arteries, the right ventricle is the systemic ventricle and must generate adequate pressure to maintain systemic perfusion. The left ventricle is the pulmonary ventricle and, in the absence of left ventricular outflow tract obstruction or a large ventricular septal defect, the left ventricle needs to generate only enough pressure to overcome pulmonary vascular resistance. At birth, pulmonary vascular resistance is high and left ventricular pressure is very close to systemic. However, within weeks of birth, pulmonary vascular resistance decreases and left ventricular pressure drops accordingly.

Clinical Features

Transposition of the great arteries occurs in about 1 in 3000 births, representing 5 to 10 per cent of patients born with congenital heart defects. It is more common in males by a factor of 2:1. Survival without treatment depends on the presence or absence of associated defects. Infants with transposition of the great arteries and an intact ventricular septum have the worst prognosis, with 80 per cent survival at 1 week and less than 20 per cent survival at 2 months of life. Early survival is better in infants with transposition of the great arteries and ventricular septal defect, but only 30 per cent are alive at 1 year. Untreated patients

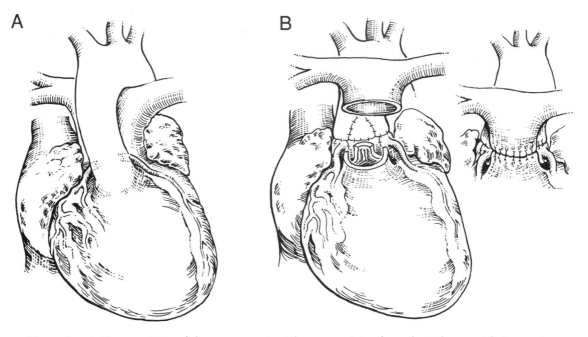

Figure 2. *A,* Transposition of the great arteries. The aorta arising from the right ventricle is anterior to the pulmonary artery that arises from the left ventricle. *B,* The arterial switch procedure. The aorta and pulmonary artery are surgically transposed. The origins of the two coronary arteries are transferred to the posterior great vessel.

with transposition of the great arteries, ventricular septal defect, and left ventricular outflow tract obstruction have the best early survival, with 70 per cent surviving to 1 year. As with prognosis, the presentation of symptoms varies with the degree of mixing. Infants with poor mixing present with severe cyanosis in the first hours of life. Aside from the cyanosis, physical examination is often unremarkable. Arterial blood gases demonstrate a low PaO_2 (<40 mm Hg) that does not improve on 100 per cent inspired oxygen. As the infant worsens, the PaO_2 decreases. When the pH begins to decrease from the metabolic acidosis of tissue hypoxia, the situation becomes increasingly critical. Infants with good mixing, such as those with large ventricular septal defects, may not present until 2 to 4 weeks of life, when the normal postnatal decrease in pulmonary vascular resistance causes a large left-to-right shunt. The left ventricle becomes volume overloaded, and congestive heart failure follows. These infants may exhibit only mild cyanosis, but present with tachypnea, poor feeding, and hepatomegaly. A loud systolic murmur is often present. Once suspected, the diagnosis of transposition of the great arteries can be made reliably and noninvasively with two-dimensional echocardiography. This technique accurately depicts the abnormal position and connection of the great arteries. Associated abnormalities, including atrial septal defect, ventricular septal defect, patent ductus arteriosus, and left ventricular outflow tract obstruction,

can also be identified. Cardiac catheterization with angiocardiography also provides definitive diagnosis and is employed at most institutions to confirm the echocardiographic diagnosis as well as provide early stabilization using the technique of balloon atrial septostomy.

Management

Early recognition of transposition of the great arteries is important in the cyanotic newborn, since medical therapy has little to offer. Balloon atrial septostomy, introduced by Rashkind in 1966, is performed at the time of cardiac catheterization with a balloon-tipped catheter that is inserted into the femoral vein and fluoroscopically guided across the patent foramen ovale into the left atrium. The balloon is then inflated and rapidly pulled back into the right atrium, tearing a 1- to 1.5-cm hole in the interatrial septum. The improvement in mixing that occurs from this procedure increases systemic arterial saturations to greater than 60 per cent and reverses any developed acidosis. Most infants palliated with balloon atrial septostomy rapidly stabilize, permitting the performance of a surgically corrective procedure on a more or less elective basis. Although anatomic correction by surgical transposition of the great arteries back to their appropriate ventricle is intuitively the most definitive treatment for this defect, early attempts at this procedure were uniformly unsuccessful. For over 25 years, physiologic correction of transposition of the great arteries has been achieved by redirecting the incoming venous circulations at the atrial level. With this redirection, the desaturated systemic venous return from the venae cavae is directed to the mitral valve and pumped by the left ventricle to the lungs. The oxygenated pulmonary venous return is directed to the tricuspid valve and pumped by the right ventricle to the systemic circulation. The two operations that accomplish this physiologic correction are known as the *Senning* and the *Mustard* procedures. The Mustard operation employs a piece of pericardium as the intra-atrial baffle, whereas the Senning procedure uses flaps of atrial tissue to achieve the same effect. Historically, infants with transposition of the great arteries were initially palliated with balloon atrial septostomy and returned at between 3 and 12 months of age to undergo one of these procedures. Choice of atrial redirection operation used was usually related more to the experience and results at the particular medical center than to clear superiority of one technique over the other.

Improvements in surgical and anesthetic techniques in the last 10 to 15 years have renewed interest in anatomic correction of transposition of the great arteries (Fig. 2B). Since the first successes with the arterial switch procedure were reported by Jatene in 1976, increasing experience has transformed this technique into the procedure of choice for most patients with transposition and intact ventricular septum and transposition with ventricular septal defect. Success of the arterial switch in patients with intact ventricular septum requires that it be performed within the first 2 weeks of life while left ventricular pressure is still nearly systemic. For the small group of patients with transposition of the great arteries, ventricular septal defect, and left ventricular outflow tract obstruction, the arterial switch procedure is contraindicated. Most of these patients do not require operation as infants and can be followed until 4 to 5 years of age when a definitive procedure can be performed. The most common procedure for this combination of defects, the *Rastelli* operation, involves the creation of an intraventricular tunnel from the left ventricle through the ventricular septal defect to the aorta. An externally placed valved conduit directs flow from the right ventricle to the main pulmonary artery.

Results

Early and late results using either the Senning or Mustard technique have been good, and the operative mortality has been 5 per cent or less, with 5-year survival ranging from 85 to 90 per cent and 20-year survival in excess of 75 per cent. Both atrial redirection techniques, however, have demonstrated some early

and late problems. Obstruction of either pulmonary or venous return has been observed in 5 to 10 per cent of patients, many requiring reoperation. Atrial dysrhythmia is particularly common, with the incidence increasing with time. Disturbingly, sudden death has occurred in some patients many years after what appeared to be an excellent result from an atrial redirection operation. Current assessment of the arterial switch procedure suggests that it is a significant improvement over the Senning and Mustard procedures. Most neonatal cardiac surgeons now perform this procedure with an operative survival of 95 per cent. Follow-up of these patients indicates 5-year survival of greater that 95 per cent, and virtually all survivors are fully active without limitations. Atrial dysrhythmias have been rare, and the only significant postoperative complication has been the occasional development of supravalvular pulmonary stenosis. The incidence of this problem, however, appears to be decreasing with increasing experience with the technique. For those patients who undergo the Rastelli procedure for transposition of the great arteries, ventricular septal defect, and left ventricular outflow tract obstruction, the hospital mortality is currently less than 5 per cent. Ten-year survival is approximately 80 per cent, and over 75 per cent of patients are in NYHA Class I functional status. Reoperation is sometimes required to replace an outgrown or obstructed right ventricular–to–pulmonary artery conduit.

CONGENITAL LESIONS OF THE AORTIC VALVE

Aortic Stenosis

Congenital aortic stenosis refers to a group of malformations that cause obstruction of blood flow from the left ventricle to the aorta. Although stenosis occurs most commonly at the level of the aortic valve, obstructive lesions also occur above and below the valve. Aortic stenosis is one of the most common congenital heart defects, representing 5 to 10 per cent of congenital cardiac anomalies.

Anatomy

From a pathologic standpoint, congenital aortic stenosis is separated into valvular, subvalvular, and supravalvular subtypes. These lesions usually appear in isolated form but can occur in combination. Additionally, 20 to 25 per cent of patients with aortic stenosis have associated defects including coarctation of the aorta, patent ductus arteriosus, ventricular septal defect, or pulmonary stenosis. Isolated valvular aortic stenosis is the most common subtype, representing 70 to 80 per cent. In these patients, the valve leaflets are thickened, with varying degrees of fusion at the commissures (Fig. 3, top). In the most typical case, the right and left coronary cusps are completely fused, creating a bicuspid valve. The degree of fusion at the remaining two commissures dictates the amount of obstruction. Discrete subaortic stenosis is the next most common subtype, accounting for 10 to 20 per cent of patients. In these patients, a fibrous ring of tissue exists several millimeters below the aortic valve (Fig. 3, middle). In severe cases, the subaortic ring can resemble a long narrow tunnel of fibromuscular tissue. Supravalvular aortic stenosis, the least common subtype, most commonly displays an "hourglass" appearance, with a normal diameter at the base of the valve and marked narrowing at the top of the valve commissures (Fig. 3, bottom).

Pathophysiology

Aortic stenosis, regardless of the level of obstruction, causes systolic left ventricular hypertension and a compensatory concentric increase in left ventricular mass. Systolic function may be preserved by this hypertrophy, but left ventricular compliance is decreased and higher end-diastolic pressures are required to achieve adequate ventricular filling. When the hypertrophy is severe, the combination of high systolic wall tension and increased myocardial mass may cause subendocardial ischemia. Symptoms of congestive heart failure develop as left ventricular end-diastolic pressure rises. Symptoms of angina or syncope begin to occur during exertion when myocardial oxygen demands are increased. The degree of hypertrophy correlates with the severity of stenosis, which is graded on the basis of the pressure gradient measured across the obstruction. For mild stenoses, the systolic outflow gradient is less than 50 mm Hg. In moderate stenoses, the gradient is between 50 and 75 mm Hg. Any gradient greater than 75 mm Hg represents severe stenosis.

Clinical Features

Symptoms are unusual in infants and children with mild to moderate aortic stenosis, most often discovered by the presence of a loud systolic murmur. Progression to severe stenosis, however, can cause chest pain, syncope, heart failure, and sudden death. The presentation of aortic stenosis in the neonate or young infant differs considerably from that in the older child. The neonate presents with rapidly progressive heart failure and quickly deteriorates and dies within the first days or weeks of life if the stenosis is not relieved. The diagnosis of aortic stenosis is suggested by the presence of a systolic ejection murmur and evidence

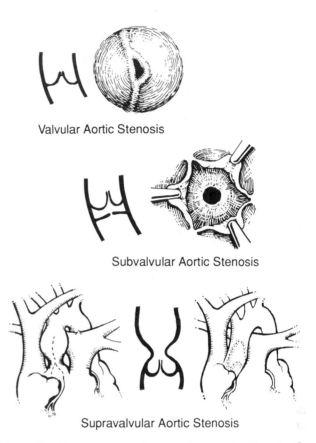

Valvular Aortic Stenosis

Subvalvular Aortic Stenosis

Supravalvular Aortic Stenosis

Figure 3. Types of congenital aortic stenosis. *Top*, Leaflet thickening and fusion at the valve commissures cause stenosis at the level of the valve. *Middle*, A fibrous or fibromuscular ring several millimeters below the aortic valve creates subvalvular aortic stenosis. *Bottom*, An "hourglass" appearance is typical of supravalvular aortic stenosis. Repair of this defect includes insertion of an inverted Y-shaped patch.

of severe left ventricular hypertrophy on electrocardiography. Heart size on chest radiography is usually normal in children but may be markedly enlarged in newborns in congestive heart failure. Two-dimensional echocardiography can definitively identify the stenosis and characterize the level. Doppler ultrasound measurement of flow across the stenosis can estimate the extent of obstruction, but cardiac catheterization is usually required to reliably measure the pressure gradient.

Treatment

Treatment is dictated by the manner of presentation, the magnitude of the outflow gradient, and the type of stenotic lesion. In the case of the neonate or young infant with valvular aortic stenosis and congestive heart failure, urgent relief of the valvular obstruction is indicated. For older children with isolated valvular aortic stenosis, operation is reserved for those with gradients that exceed 75 mm Hg. Since the degree of stenosis is more rapidly progressive in children with supra-aortic stenosis and discrete subaortic stenosis, operation is indicated at gradients of 50 mm Hg or above in these two groups. The surgical procedure performed depends, of course, on the form of stenosis being relieved. All procedures are performed using cardiopulmonary bypass and direct exposure of the aortic valve. In the case of valvular aortic stenosis, a valvotomy is performed by sharply dividing the fused commissures to within 1 mm of the aortic wall. Repair of supra-aortic stenosis requires incision into one or more of the sinuses of Valsalva and inserting one or more patches of pericardium or Dacron to eliminate the hourglass configuration (Fig. 3, bottom). For discrete subaortic stenosis, the obstructing diaphragm is easily seen beneath the cusps of the aortic valve (Fig. 3, middle). The fibrous ridge is excised, taking care not to damage the anterior leaflet of the mitral valve or the bundle of His. Replacement of the aortic valve with a prosthetic device is rarely necessary at initial operation in children with aortic stenosis. Prosthetic valves with outer diameters smaller than 17 mm pose excessively high transvalvular gradients. Thus, in the unusual circumstance when aortic valve replacement becomes necessary in a small child, enlargement of the aortic valve annulus may be required to permit prosthetic valve insertion. Favorable early results are currently being obtained in children undergoing aortic valve replacement with aortic valve allografts.

Results

For children older than 1 year of age, the hospital mortality for aortic valvotomy and repairs of supravalvular and subvalvular subaortic stenosis is less than 1 per cent. However, for newborns and infants younger than 1 year of age, the hospital mortality is over 50 per cent in many series. More recent experience suggests that the current hospital mortality for neonates undergoing open valvotomy for critical aortic stenosis is in the range of 15 to 25 per cent. Long-term survival is good for operative survivors, as over 90 per cent are alive 10 years after the initial operation. Reoperation for restenosis or development of aortic valve insufficiency or bacterial endocarditis is required in less than 10 per cent in the first 10 years. However, up to 40 per cent of these patients may come to reoperation by 20 years.

AORTIC ATRESIA

In aortic atresia, the aortic valve is imperforate and the ascending aorta is hypoplastic (Fig. 4). This con-

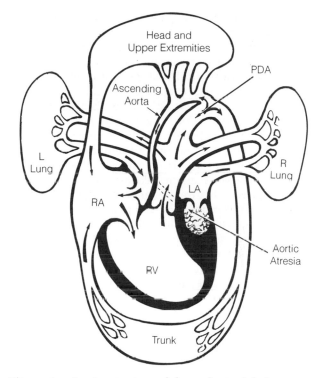

Figure 4. Aortic atresia and hypoplastic left heart syndrome. The right ventricle functions as a single ventricle. Systemic and coronary blood flow are dependent upon a widely patent ductus arteriosus.

dition is almost always associated with mitral atresia or mitral valve hypoplasia and a very small or non-existent left ventricle and is most often referred to as the *hypoplastic left heart syndrome*. Initial survival is possible, as pulmonary venous return crosses the foramen ovale to mix with systemic venous return and pass through the tricuspid valve into the right ventricle, which serves as a single systemic ventricle. Blood from the right ventricle is then pumped to the lungs via the branch pulmonary arteries and to the systemic arterial circulation via the ductus arteriosus. Delivery of blood to the coronary circulation requires retrograde flow down the hypoplastic ascending aorta. Survival, however, is short in these infants, as the natural closure of the ductus arteriosus eliminates blood delivery to the coronary and systemic circulations. Recognition of aortic atresia and hypoplastic left heart syndrome has become important in recent years as surgical techniques have evolved that can salvage some of these infants. Furthermore, this complex defect represents at least 5 per cent of infants born with congenital heart disease. Without treatment, these patients die within the first 1 to 2 weeks of life.

Infants with aortic atresia and hypoplastic left heart syndrome are usually full-term babies who present in the newborn period with mild cyanosis, respiratory distress, and tachycardia. Diagnosis can be made reliably with two-dimensional echocardiography. Immediate institution of prostaglandin E_1 is mandatory to maintain ductal patency and adequate systemic and coronary perfusion until a surgical procedure can be performed. The operation most commonly performed for aortic atresia and hypoplastic left heart syndrome, the *Norwood procedure*, is designed to stabilize the infant until pulmonary vascular resistance falls to normal and a single ventricle operation of the *Fontan* type can be performed. In the Norwood procedure, the ductus arteriosus is eliminated and right ventricular output is directed to the underside of the aortic arch. The interatrial septum is completely removed to allow unrestricted mixing of pulmonary and systemic venous returns, and a small systemic–to–pulmonary artery shunt provides controlled blood flow to the lungs. The hospital mortality for this procedure is 35 per cent in experienced hands, and significant mortality may occur between this procedure and the Fontan operation, which imposes its own hospital mortality of approximately 15 per cent. Because of the high mortality of the Norwood-Fontan approach and its requirement for staged procedures, some centers offer cardiac transplantation to newborns with aortic atresia and hypoplastic left heart syndrome. Assuming an appropriate donor heart can be located, operative mortality for cardiac transplantation has been less than 20 per cent in this group, and 1- to 5-year survival has been excellent. While there is much enthusiasm for this approach, the limited supply of suitable donor hearts prevents many patients from receiving this form of treatment.

CONGENITAL AORTIC REGURGITATION

Aortic valve regurgitation is the least common congenital lesion of the aortic valve. It is most commonly caused by a bicuspid valve that is usually competent in infancy and early childhood but gradually becomes incompetent as the larger of the two leaflets prolapses below the smaller one. Most patients are relatively asymptomatic males in their teens or early twenties who become aware of vigorous contractions in their chests or pulsations in their necks. A high-pitched aortic diastolic murmur is present on physical examination. The diagnosis of aortic regurgitation can often be made reliably by physical examination, but two-dimensional echocardiography provides reliable confirmatory information. The degree of regurgitation and the response of the left ventricle to the regurgitation is determined at cardiac catheterization. Most patients with aortic regurgitation can be managed for many years with medical therapy that includes digi-

talis and afterload-reducing agents. The best time for valve replacement for aortic regurgitation is controversial, but most authorities feel that aortic valve replacement should be performed before congestive heart failure develops. Regular echocardiographic assessment is indicated to identify any significant functional change that would warrant proceeding to valve replacement. Should valve replacement become necessary, porcine valve prostheses should be avoided in the young because the durability of these valves is limited in younger age groups. A mechanical valve is the valve of choice for most young patients but does pose a constant threat of thromboembolism and requires lifelong anticoagulation. Should patient compliance or activity introduce a major concern with regard to anticoagulation, an allograft aortic valve may be a better alternative.

CONGENITAL LESIONS OF THE PULMONARY VALVE

Malformations of the right ventricular outflow tract and pulmonary valve are inherent in certain complex congenital heart defects, such as tetralogy of Fallot and pulmonary atresia with ventricular septal defect. The present discussion is limited to those defects in which the primary pathology is limited to the pulmonary valve.

Pulmonary Stenosis and Intact Ventricular Septum

Pulmonary stenosis and intact ventricular septum is one of the most common congenital heart defects, occurring in 10 per cent of patients with congenital heart disease. It is characterized by obstruction to flow from the right ventricle to the pulmonary circulation and occurs most frequently at the level of the pulmonary valve. Morphologically, the leaflets of the pulmonary valve are fused, creating a doming effect with a small opening at the apex (Fig. 5). The hemodynamic effect of this lesion depends on the severity of the stenosis. When the stenosis is severe, the pressure in the right ventricle may equal or exceed that in the left ventricle. In these patients, significant right ventricular hypertrophy develops and the resultant increase in right ventricular end-diastolic pressure elevates the right atrial pressure. Right atrial pressures over 15 mm Hg may cause right-sided heart failure, with hepatomegaly, ascites, pleural effusion, and peripheral edema. If an atrial septal defect or a patent foramen ovale is present, right-to-left shunting at the atrial level can produce severe systemic arterial desaturation. Most patients with pulmonary stenosis and intact ventricular

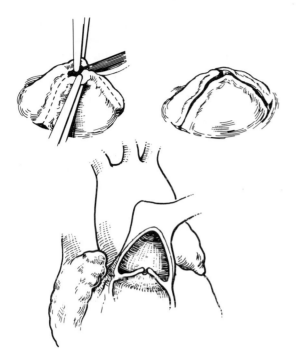

Figure 5. Pulmonary stenosis with intact ventricular system. Fusion of the valve leaflets creates a dome-shaped appearance. Open valvotomy permits precise separation of the valve leaflets at the commissures.

septum are asymptomatic throughout childhood and are discovered when a loud systolic murmur is noted. When the condition presents in the newborn, however, the infant is critically ill, tachypneic, and usually severely hypoxic from right-to-left shunting at the atrial level. Diagnosis in the child or young adult is suggested by the characteristic murmur, a prominent pulmonary knob, and left pulmonary artery on chest radiograph and right ventricular hypertrophy on electrocardiography. In the critically ill neonate, radiographic evidence of clear lung fields and a large cardiac silhouette should suggest the diagnosis. In both children and neonates, two-dimensional echocardiography can provide the definitive diagnosis. The diagnosis of critical pulmonary stenosis and intact ventricular septum in the neonate is sufficient indication for intervention, as virtually all such infants die without treatment. For the older infant, child, or young adult with pulmonary stenosis and intact ventricular septum, however, intervention is reserved for patients with right ventricular pressures that exceed 75 mm Hg. Patients with right ventricular pressures between 50 and 75 mm Hg should undergo periodic electrocardiography and echocardiography to identify any evidence of progressive right ventricular hypertrophy.

Relief of valvular pulmonary stenosis can be per-

formed by surgical procedure or using percutaneous balloon valvotomy. Currently, balloon valvotomy is the technique of choice for most children with isolated pulmonary stenosis. The procedure involves fluoroscopically guiding a percutaneously introduced angioplasty catheter across the pulmonary valve orifice and rapidly inflating the balloon. In most patients, this procedure causes a clean split at the valve commissures and a marked reduction in the transvalvular gradient. Open pulmonary valvotomy on cardiopulmonary bypass continues to be the preferred technique in most medical centers for relief of critical pulmonary stenosis in the neonate. Direct exposure of the stenotic valve permits precise opening of the valve commissures (Fig. 5). Should the pulmonary annulus be hypoplastic, the annulus can be enlarged with a diamond-shaped patch of pericardium. Not uncommonly, a systemic–to–pulmonary artery shunt is also constructed to assure adequate oxygenation in these severely compromised infants. The results of pulmonary valvotomy in children with pulmonary stenosis and intact ventricular septum, using either open or percutaneous techniques, have been excellent, with a procedural mortality of less than 1 per cent. Long-term survival and functional status approach that of the normal population. For neonates with critical pulmonary stenosis and intact ventricular septum, operative mortality is approximately 10 per cent and survival at 5 years exceeds 75 per cent.

Pulmonary Atresia and Intact Ventricular Septum

In pulmonary atresia with intact ventricular septum, the right ventricular outflow tract is totally occluded, with pulmonary blood flow dependent upon patency of the ductus arteriosus. This malformation is present in 1 per cent of patients born with congenital heart disease. In this condition, the pulmonary valve may appear as an imperforate membrane between a normal-sized main pulmonary artery and a patent but hypertrophied infundibulum. In more severe cases, the valve and infundibulum are both atretic and the tricuspid valve and right ventricle are markedly hypoplastic. Infants with pulmonary atresia and intact ventricular septum usually present on the first day of life with cyanosis that becomes progressively worse as the ductus closes. Definitive diagnosis is made by two-dimensional echocardiography. Prostaglandin E$_1$ is begun once the diagnosis is suspected in order to reverse ductal closure and stabilize the infant for operation. The only effective treatment for this condition is surgical, and the procedure employed must be tailored to the specific morphology. When the atretic segment is limited to a membrane and the right ventricle approaches normal size, an open excision of this membrane is performed using cardiopulmonary bypass. A transannular pericardial patch is placed if the annulus or infundibulum is narrowed. In addition, a systemic–to–pulmonary artery shunt is created. Establishing continuity between the right ventricle and pulmonary artery permits right ventricular growth so that by the time the patient is 1 to 2 years of age, shunt closure is possible and a two-ventricle repair achieved. In patients in whom the tricuspid valve and right ventricle are severely hypoplastic, initial operation is limited to a systemic-to-pulmonary artery shunt to provide adequate pulmonary blood flow until 1 to 2 years of age, when a single ventricle repair (the Fontan operation) can be performed. By tailoring the operation to the size of the tricuspid valve and right ventricle, patients with pulmonary atresia and intact ventricular septum can be managed with a hospital mortality of 20 per cent and a 2-year survival of 60 per cent. Long-term survival is expected to be best for those children that ultimately come to a two-ventricle repair.

Congenital Pulmonary Valve Insufficiency

Isolated congenital pulmonary valve insufficiency is an uncommon condition that occurs as a consequence of abnormal development of the pulmonary valve cusps or from idiopathic dilatation of the pulmonary trunk. Since the right ventricle is a low-pressure pump, it readily adapts to the volume load of pulmonary valve regurgitation. Most patients are asymptomatic children or young adults who are discovered to have a diastolic murmur on routine physical examination or a dilated pulmonary arterial trunk on a routine chest radiograph. As an isolated lesion, pulmonary valve insufficiency is well tolerated and requires no medical or surgical therapy. Heart failure can develop, however, should an increase in pulmonary arterial pressure occur from another disease process such as emphysema or left ventricular failure.

CONGENITAL LESIONS OF THE MITRAL VALVE

Congenital abnormalities of the mitral valve are rare, occurring in less than 0.5 per cent of patients with congenital heart disease. Hemodynamically significant mitral stenosis or insufficiency follow abnormal development of one or more components of the mitral apparatus. In the typical case of congenital mitral stenosis, the two papillary muscles arise close to one another, the chordae tendineae are shortened, and the interchordal spaces are reduced or obliterated. In an extreme form of this condition, called the *parachute mitral valve*, all of the chordae insert on a single

eccentric papillary muscle. Some patients with congenital mitral stenosis have a supravalvular ring of fibrous tissue. The supravalvular ring and parachute mitral valve may coexist with subaortic stenosis and coarctation of the aorta as components of *Shone syndrome*. Congenital mitral insufficiency is more likely to be caused by developmental anomalies of the valve leaflets. A cleft in the anterior leaflet and hypoplasia of the posterior leaflet are two such examples. Patients with congenital mitral stenosis present in infancy or early childhood with symptoms of dyspnea, orthopnea, and paroxysmal nocturnal dyspnea. An apical middiastolic murmur with presystolic accentuation may be heard on auscultation. Chest radiography shows left atrial enlargement, cardiomegaly, and pulmonary venous congestion. Two-dimensional echocardiography with Doppler interrogation usually provides a definitive diagnosis. Once a diagnosis is made, surgical relief of the stenosis is indicated, as survival past 5 years of age is unlikely without treatment. At operation, all effort is made to repair the valve rather than replace it. The repair must be tailored to the varied pathology but may include excision of a supravalvular ring, leaflet incisions at commissural sites, and splitting of fused chordae and papillary muscles. Patients with congenital mitral insufficiency become symptomatic several years later than those with congenital mitral stenosis. An apical holosystolic murmur radiating to the axilla is a characteristic physical finding. Diagnosis is also made reliably with two-dimensional echocardiography. If symptoms are mild or moderate, the patient is treated with digitalis and afterload-reducing agents so that when operation does become necessary, an adult-sized valve prosthesis can be inserted, should valve replacement be required. Nevertheless, when symptoms are severe, operation is performed in an effort to repair the valve. Techniques to narrow a dilated mitral annulus, suture a cleft leaflet, or shorten elongated chordae tendineae can often produce a competent mitral valve. Should valve replacement become the only alternative for congenital mitral valve disease, a mechanical prosthesis should be employed because porcine valve prostheses degenerate rapidly in the young. If the mitral annulus is too small for the smallest available prosthesis (17 mm), the replacement device can be seated in the left atrium above the annulus. In such a case, the patient can be expected to outgrow this valve and need at least one more operation to insert a larger prosthesis.

CONGENITAL LESIONS OF THE TRICUSPID VALVE

Congenital abnormalities of the tricuspid valve are rare. Other than tricuspid atresia, the most significant developmental abnormality of the tricuspid valve is Ebstein's anomaly.

Ebstein's Anomaly

Described by Wilhelm Ebstein in 1866, this congenital heart defect is characterized by an abnormal tricuspid valve with a large sail-like anterior leaflet attached to the atrioventricular junction and two smaller leaflets displaced below this junction and adherent to the right ventricular wall. The portion of the valve orifice displaced into the right ventricle creates an intermediate zone that is functionally right atrium but anatomically right ventricle (*atrialized right ventricle*) (Fig. 6). This structural derangement usually causes marked tricuspid insufficiency and may, in some patients, cause tricuspid stenosis. This rare anomaly (<1 per cent of congenital heart defects) is secondary to incomplete development of the posterior and septal leaflets of the tricuspid valve during embryogenesis. The effect of Ebstein's anomaly on hemodynamics is determined by the degree of incompetence and stenosis of the tricuspid valve and by the amount of right ventricle that is taken over by the "atrialized" segment. When tricuspid incompetence and/or stenosis is severe and right ventricular function is diminished, right atrial and systemic venous pressure is elevated and peripheral edema may follow. A patent foramen ovale or atrial septal defect, present in most patients with Ebstein's anomaly, permits right-to-left shunting with resultant cyanosis and possible paradoxic embolism. Atrial dysrhythmias are common in these patients and often accentuate the hemodynamic consequences of the malformation. The natural history of Ebstein's

anomaly depends on the patient's age at presentation. When it presents in the newborn, cyanosis and congestive heart failure are noted within the first 2 to 3 days of life, and without treatment most of these infants die within days of presentation. Patients who present as older infants, children, or young adults have a much more favorable prognosis, with symptoms usually limited to mild exercise intolerance and occasional palpitations from episodes of supraventricular tachyarrhythmia. These patients lead relatively normal lives during their first three decades, with some patients living into their sixties before being diagnosed. When symptoms of heart failure become prominent or heart size exceeds a cardiothoracic ratio of 0.60, prognosis abruptly worsens.

The diagnosis of Ebstein's anomaly should be suspected in newborn infants with severe right heart failure, cyanosis, and marked cardiomegaly. The child or young adult is more likely to present with mild dyspnea and fatigue and episodes of cyanosis and/or palpitations. Right bundle branch block and enlarged P waves are typical electrocardiographic findings. Five per cent also have electrocardiographic evidence of Wolff-Parkinson-White (WPW) syndrome. Supraventricular arrhythmias, including atrial flutter and fibrillation, are common and are not necessarily related to the accessory bypass tracts of WPW. The chest radiograph usually demonstrates marked cardiomegaly. Definitive diagnosis of Ebstein's anomaly is made by two-dimensional echocardiography. This technique depicts the distinctive appearance of the tricuspid valve and permits evaluation of the size and function of the right ventricle and right atrium; assesses the degree of tricuspid insufficiency; and identifies the presence, size, and effect of any interatrial communication.

Management of patients with Ebstein's anomaly must be individualized in view of the spectrum of clinical presentation. Neonates who present in extremis must be intubated, started on prostaglandin E_1, and stabilized in preparation for a procedure to exclude the right ventricle from the circulation and provide pulmonary blood flow with a systemic-to-pulmonary artery shunt. Survivors of this procedure become candidates for the single-ventricle Fontan operation at 12 to 24 months of age. Patients diagnosed beyond the neonatal period can usually be followed with minimal medical intervention other than antibiotic prophylaxis for dental or endoscopic procedures and appropriate antiarrhythmic medication for tachyarrhythmias. When these patients begin to experience increasing symptoms of congestive heart failure and/or cyanosis, show evidence of progressive cardiomegaly, or develop complications of right-to-left shunting, operation becomes indicated. Closure of any interatrial communication and repair of the tricuspid valve is the preferred technique for Ebstein's anomaly. Valvuloplasty techniques for this malformation involve plication of the

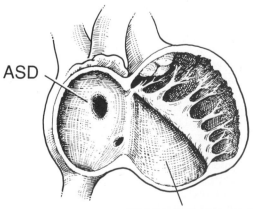

Figure 6. Ebstein's anomaly. Abnormal development of the posterior and septal leaflets of the tricuspid valve causes an intermediate zone of "atrialized" right ventricle. An atrial septal defect (ASD) that permits right-to-left shunting is commonly present.

atrialized portion of the right ventricle and reduction of the circumference of the tricuspid annulus. When anatomic variation prevents satisfactory repair, tricuspid valve replacement is performed using a mechanical prosthesis for children and young adults and a porcine bioprosthesis for older adults. Division of accessory atrioventricular bypass tracts can be performed at the time of valve repair or replacement. Hospital mortality for tricuspid valve repair or replacement is 5 to 10 per cent. Ten-year postoperative survival is over 80 per cent, with most patients returning to NYHA Class I or II after operation.

REFERENCES

Adams FH, Emmanouilides GC, Riemenschneider TA (eds): Moss' Heart Disease in Infants, Children, and Adolescents. ed 4, Baltimore, Williams & Wilkins, 1989.
Ebert PA: Atlas of Congenital Cardiac Surgery. New York, Churchill Livingstone, 1989.
Kirklin JW, Barrett-Boyes BG: Cardiac Surgery: Morphology, Diagnostic Criteria, Natural History, Techniques, Results, and Indications, ed 2. New York, Churchill Livingstone, 1993.
Perloff JK: The Clinical Recognition of Congenital Heart Disease, ed 3. Philadelphia, WB Saunders Company, 1987.
Sabiston DC Jr (ed): Textbook of Surgery: The Biological Basis of Modern Surgical Practice, ed 14. Philadelphia, WB Saunders Company, 1991.

II
ACQUIRED CARDIAC CONDITIONS: Coronary Artery Disease and Ventricular Aneurysms

R. DUANE DAVIS, Jr., M.D.   DAVID C. SABISTON, Jr., M.D.

Atherosclerotic coronary artery disease remains the leading cause of death in the United States, with over 500,000 deaths annually. Approximately 3 per cent of Americans (7 million) have symptomatic coronary artery disease, of which 1.5 million experience a myocardial infarction each year. The incidence and mortality rates have declined since the 1960s, with a particularly notable decrease in the number of sudden deaths. These trends probably reflect both changes in therapy and prevention of disease by altering known risk factors. However, due to the growth and the aging of the population, the prevalence, mortality, and economic cost of coronary artery disease continue to escalate.

ANATOMY

The right and left main coronary arteries are the first branches of the aorta, arising from the anterior and posterior sinuses of Valsalva. The length of the left main coronary artery is usually 10 to 20 mm. It courses between the left atrial appendage and the pulmonary artery to reach the left atrioventricular groove where it usually bifurcates into the *left anterior descending* (LAD) artery and the *left circumflex artery* (LCA) (Fig. 1). The LAD proceeds distally over the interventricular septum, extending around the apex into the posterior interventricular groove. Branches of the LAD include septal perforators, which are 7 to 8 cm in length and course along the *right ventricular* (RV) side of the anterior septum; diagonal branches, which course obliquely across the *left ventricle* (LV) free wall; and right ventricular free wall branches, some of which communicate with the infundibular branches of the *right coronary artery* (RCA) to form the arterial circle of Vieussens, an important route of collateral flow. The left circumflex artery arises from the left main artery at a 90-degree angle and continues in the left atrioventricular groove. Branches to the LV from the circumflex artery, termed *marginal arteries*, course over the lateral and inferior surface of the heart.

The RCA courses anteriorly in the right atrioventricular groove (Fig. 2). At the acute margin of the heart where the vessel turns posteriorly toward the crux of the heart, the acute marginal branch artery arises and courses toward the apex of the heart. At the crux of the heart, the RCA gives rise to the artery to the *atrioventricular* (AV) node in 90 per cent of cases before bifurcating into the *posterior descending artery* (PDA) and right posterolateral artery. Dominance of the coronary arterial system is defined by which system provides the PDA. The PDA arises solely from the RCA in 75 per cent of patients (right dominance), solely from the left circumflex in 10 per cent (left dominance), and in 15 per cent of patients, the RCA and left circumflex are in continuity (codominance). The PDA courses in the posterior interventricular groove providing branches to the RV, LV, and perforating branches to the septum. Proximal branches of the RCA and left circumflex arteries provide circumflex branches to the atria.

The LAD and its branches provide the blood supply to the anterior two thirds of the septum, the anterior LV free wall, and a portion of the RV free wall. The lateral LV wall is supplied by the first diagonal and marginal branches of the LAD and circumflex arteries, respectively. The posterior portion of the LV is supplied by the terminal marginal branches of the LV and, when present, posterolateral branches of the RCA in right-dominant systems. The specialized conduction system is supplied in a variable manner. The *sinoatrial* (SA) node is supplied by a proximal branch of RCA in 55 per cent, and from a branch of the left main or circumflex arteries in the remainder. The AV node artery arises from the PDA. The His bundle and proximal bundle branches are supplied by the AV node ar-

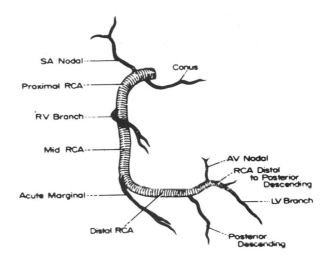

Figure 2. Normal right coronary artery anatomy seen from a left anterior oblique orientation. (From Franch RH et al: Techniques of cardiac catheterization including coronary arteriography. *In* Hurst JW [ed]: The Heart, ed 5. New York, McGraw-Hill Book Company, 1982, with permission.)

tery. The distal bundle branches and Purkinje system are supplied by septal perforators off the LAD. The anterolateral papillary muscle of the LV is supplied by branches of the LAD and circumflex arteries and the posteromedial papillary muscle by terminal branches of the RCA or circumflex arteries.

The venous drainage of the heart is via superficial and deep vessels. The superficial veins conduct most of the venous blood and accompany the respective coronary arteries. The surface veins enter into the coronary sinus or the anterior cardiac vein, both of which drain into the right atrium. The deep veins communicate with both the atrial and ventricular cavities by thebesian veins and sinusoidal channels.

NORMAL PHYSIOLOGY

Coronary blood flow provides oxygen and metabolic substrate to generate chemical energy. This energy is converted into mechanical energy for cardiac contraction for maintenance of blood pressure and blood flow. Coronary perfusion also removes the byproducts of metabolism. Because the heart is required to perform a tremendous amount of mechanical work to sustain life, coronary perfusion and myocardial oxygen consumption are much greater relative to other organs. The normal coronary blood flow is between 0.6 and 0.9 ml/gm of myocardium per minute, and myocardial oxygen consumption is normally 0.8 to 0.15 ml oxygen per gram. Because the heart relies almost exclusively on *aerobic* metabolism to generate its energy requirements, the measurement of oxygen con-

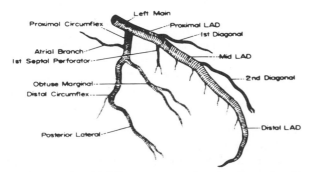

Figure 1. Normal left coronary artery anatomy seen from a right anterior oblique orientation. (From Franch RH et al: Techniques of cardiac catheterization including coronary arteriography. *In* Hurst JW [ed]: The Heart, ed 5. New York, McGraw-Hill Book Company, 1982, with permission.)

sumption provides an accurate measure of myocardial energy use. The major determinants of myocardial oxygen consumption are the development of systolic wall tension, heart rate, and contractility. The energy requirements to maintain cellular integrity and electrical activity are relatively small, accounting for approximately 20 per cent of energy usage. The myocardial energy expenditure for mechanical work has two components: (1) *internal energy*, which is the energy utilized during the isovolumic phase of cardiac contraction, or *pressure work*, and (2) *external energy*, which is the energy utilized during the ejection phase of the cardiac cycle, or *stroke work*. Importantly, the energy requirements of performing pressure work are much greater than performing stroke work.

Coronary perfusion is closely associated with myocardial oxygen consumption. Because the myocardium extracts much of the available oxygen in blood in the capillaries, actually 75 per cent during basal conditions and more than 90 per cent with stress, a significant increase in myocardial oxygen consumption requires additional myocardial perfusion. The coronary circulation has a remarkable ability to vasodilate rapidly, and coronary blood flow can be increased three- to sixfold over basal conditions. Although normal capillary density is 4000 capillaries per square millimeter of myocardium, precapillary sphincters through these beds are dependent on myocardial needs. In addition, the epicardial vessels and the transmural vessels are capable of vasoregulation. The coronary circulation also demonstrates characteristics of autoregulation, maintaining relatively constant coronary flow when coronary perfusion pressure is in the range of 60 to 130 mm Hg. Coronary blood flow shows phasic characteristics relative to the cardiac cycle. The majority of LV perfusion occurs during diastole, as it follows the transmission of compressive forces occurring with the development of wall tension upon the intramural coronary vessels during systole. Resistance to flow is greater during systole. Because wall tension development is less in the RV, systolic flow is proportionally greater in the RV compared to the LV. Myocardial wall tension also affects myocardial blood flow within the myocardium. Because wall tension and the degree of shortening is greater in the subendocardium as compared to the subepicardium, both myocardial oxygen consumption and resistance due to transmitted compressive forces are greater in the subendocardium. To enable more flow to the subendocardium, the normal ratio of subendocardial to subepicardial flow is 1.25. The subendocardial vasculature is therefore relatively vasodilated. The subendocardium has a limited vasodilator reserve and is subsequently more susceptible to ischemia.

Coronary vascular resistance is altered by a number of neurogenic, metabolic, and hormonal factors. Stimulation of α_1- and α_2-adrenergic receptors induce coronary vasoconstriction. Conversely, β-adrenergic stimulation induces vasodilatation. Although the tight coupling of coronary blood flow to myocardial oxygen consumption has been well demonstrated, the mechanisms have not been completely elucidated. Adenosine, a degradation product of adenine nucleotides that is released during ischemia or hypoxia, is a potent vasodilator. Oxygen has a direct effect on precapillary sphincters: decreased oxygen tension induces vasodilatation. The endothelium is important in regulating coagulation and coronary resistance, and it produces a number of vasoactive substances that are predominantly vasodilators. In addition, the endothelium transduces responses to a number of neurohumoral agents (Table 1). *Prostacyclin* (PGI$_2$) and *endothelial-derived relaxing factor* (EDRF), a nitric oxide analog, appear to be the most important vasodilators released by the endothelium. EDRF induces smooth muscle relaxation. It is released in response to acetylcholine, bradykinin, histamine, serotonin, and adenosine diphosphate (ADP). The vasodilatory and anticoagulant activity of the intact endothelium is in direct opposition to those of activated platelets. Importantly, in processes that injure the endothelium, such as atherosclerosis and hypercholesterolemia, paradoxic vasoconstriction and procoagulant activity occur.

PATHOLOGIC ANATOMY

Coronary atherosclerosis is a progressive process that occurs as a response to injury. The earliest manifestation of atherosclerosis is the fatty streak that may be present in children and occurs in the same locations as the advanced lesions of atherosclerosis. It is comprised of lipid-laden macrophages and smooth muscle cells within the intima. Progression of this process is manifest by proliferation of the smooth muscle cells and macrophages. The advanced lesion of atherosclerosis, the fibrous plaque, is grossly yellow-white and protrudes into the lumen. The plaque consists of a dense layer of connective tissue, smooth muscle cells, macrophages, and lymphocytes. Beneath the fibrous cap are lipid-laden macrophages and smooth muscle cells. Necrosis of these cells leads to deposition of cholesterol crystals and calcification. Fissures form in the plaques, particularly those eccentrically located, and complicated plaques can rapidly increase in size by accumulating blood within the fissure or by clot formation due to the exposure of the markedly thrombogenic material within the plaque. These complicated plaques are associated with acute transmural myocardial infarction when the plaque causes coronary oc-

TABLE 1.   IMPORTANT SUBSTANCES PRODUCED BY OR ACTING THROUGH VASCULAR ENDOTHELIUM*

Vasodilator	Vasoconstrictor	Anticoagulant/Antithrombotic/Antiplatelet	Procoagulant
Produced by endothelium			
Adenosine	? Endothelin	Adenosine	Collagen
EDRF	Peptidoleukotrienes	EDRF	FVIII–VWF complex
EDHF		Glycosaminoglycans	Fibronectin
Peptidoleukotrienes		Plasminogen activator	Plasminogen inhibitors
PGE_2		PGE_1, PGE_2	
PGE_2		PGI_2	
$PGF_{1\alpha}$		Thrombomodulin	
PGI_2		Tissue factor	
Acts through endothelium			
Acetylcholine	Angiotensin	Heparin	
ADP	Vasopressin		
Bradykinin			
Catecholamines			
Histamine			
Peptidoleukotrienes			
Serotonin			

*From Dinerman JL, Mehta JL: Endothelial, platelet and leukocyte interactions in ischemic heart disease: Insights into potential mechanisms and their clinical relevance. J Am Coll Cardiol 16: 207, 1990, with permission.

Abbreviations: ADP = adenosine diphosphate, EDHF = endothelium-derived hyperpolarizing factor, EDRF = endothelium-derived relaxing factor, FVIII = coagulation factor VIII, PG = prostaglandin, VWF = von Willebrand factor.

clusion and unstable angina when subtotal obstruction occurs.

The anatomic distribution of atherosclerotic lesions is not uniform throughout the coronary vasculature. The lesions occur most frequently in the proximal large coronary arteries, usually in association with branching vessels. In patients undergoing coronary arteriography, involvement of the LAD is most common, followed by the RCA and the circumflex arteries. Approximately 5 to 10 per cent involve the left main artery, and most patients have more than one vessel involved. Approximately 40 per cent have three vessels involved, 30 per cent have two vessels involved, and 25 per cent have single-vessel disease. Quite important is the fact that 80 to 90 per cent have disease amenable to surgical bypass.

ISCHEMIC PATHOPHYSIOLOGY

Impairment in blood flow may be secondary to fixed obstructive lesions or due to vasospasm, often in conjunction with relatively insignificant atherosclerotic lesions. Stenosis of the arterial lumen in greater than 75 per cent of the cross-sectional area causes a critical resistance that effectively limits flow. Although flow through a critical stenosis may be adequate during steady-state conditions, increases in myocardial oxygen consumption or decreases in perfusion pressure cause ischemia. Maximally vasodilated vessels distal to a critical stenosis are therefore unable to further augment flow. Subendocardial tissues located distal to a critical stenosis are particularly susceptible to ischemia.

Ischemia is associated with a rapid cessation of contractile function. Regions of ischemic myocardium are either akinetic (noncontractile) or dyskinetic (paradoxically bulge outward during systole). Ischemic myocardium does not relax normally and is less compliant, and restoration of blood flow does not immediately restore systolic or diastolic function to the baseline. This delay in return to function is referred to as stunning. The duration of *stunning* is proportional to the duration and severity of ischemia.

Myocardial cell death occurs as early as 20 minutes after the onset of ischemia, and cell death occurs as a wave-front phenomenon. Subendocardial cell death occurs first, usually within 60 minutes following total cessation of flow, and extends across the myocardial cell wall to the subepicardium after 4 to 6 hours, which emphasizes the importance of early restoration of myocardial blood flow to salvage myocardial tissue. Transmural infarcts are associated with complete occlusions of the coronary artery. Subendocardial infarction is more commonly associated with significant stenoses in two or more coronary arteries. Unlike other arterial beds, the human heart has a marginal ability to develop collaterals, and they usually develop in association with stenoses greater than 90 per cent. The presence of adequate collaterals limits both the size of a myocardial infarction and the development of a ventricular aneurysm.

CLINICAL PRESENTATION

The most common presentation of coronary artery disease is *angina pectoris*. Anginal chest pain is usually located retrosternally and is often described as pressure, tightness, or a sense of strangling. The symptoms of angina were originally described by Heberden in 1759. He said:

> But there is a disorder of the breast marked with strong and peculiar symptoms, considerable for this kind of danger belonging to it, and not extremely rare, which deserves to be mentioned more at length. The seat of it, and sense of strangling, and anxiety with which it is attended, may make it not improperly be called angina pectoris.
>
> They who are afflicted with it, are seized while they are walking (more especially if it be up a hill, and soon after eating), with a painful and most disagreeable sensation in the breast, which seems as if it would extinguish life, if it were to increase or to continue; but the moment they stand still, all this uneasiness vanishes.
>
> In all other respects, the patients are, at the beginning of this disorder, perfectly well, and in particular have no shortness of breath, from which it is totally different. The pain is sometimes situated in the upper part, sometimes in the middle, sometimes at the bottom of the os sterni, and often more inclined to the left than to the right side. It likewise very frequently extends from the breast to the middle of the left arm. The pulse is, at least sometimes, not disturbed by this pain, as I have had opportunities of observing by feeling the pulse during the paroxysm. Males are most liable to this disease, especially such as have passed their fiftieth year.
>
> After it has continued a year or more, it will not cease so instantaneously upon standing still; and it will come on not only when the persons are walking, but when they are lying down, especially if they lie on their left sides, and oblige them to rise up out of their beds. In some inveterate cases, it has been brought on by the motion of a horse, or a carriage, and even by swallowing, coughing, going to stool, or speaking, or any disturbance of mind . . .
>
> *The termination of the angina pectoris is remarkable. For if no accident intervene, but the disease go on to its height, the patients all suddenly fall down, and perish almost immediately. Of which indeed their frequent faintnesses, and sensation as if all the powers of life were failing, afford no obscure intimation.*

Anginal equivalents such as dyspnea, palpitation, and breathlessness may occur. The typical anginal episode lasts between 10 seconds and 30 minutes, and pain lasting longer than 30 minutes is characteristic of unstable angina or myocardial infarction. In patients who have fixed coronary artery stenoses, angina may occur with a surprisingly reproducible amount of activity. A circadian rhythm exists: anginal threshold is lower and infarct incidence is higher in the morning. The severity of angina is graded by the activity required to induce symptoms. The New York Heart Association (NYHA) classification system is as follows: Class I, symptoms occurring with strenuous activity;

Class II, symptoms occur that slightly limit ordinary activity; Class III, symptoms markedly limit ordinary activity; and Class IV, symptoms occur with any activity or occur at rest. Higher NYHA classification correlates with increasing severity of anatomic disease, as well as with an increased risk of myocardial infarction and cardiac death.

A small percentage of patients never have symptoms associated with ischemic episodes. Most patients who have typical anginal episodes also have episodes of silent ischemia. Furthermore, as many as 25 per cent of myocardial infarctions are silent. Patients who suffer silent ischemia or myocardial infarction are more likely to have diabetes mellitus and hypertension.

Coronary artery disease (CAD) may also cause unstable angina. Unstable angina is defined as angina occurring at rest, new-onset Class IV angina, postinfarction angina, or crescendo angina, the progression in NYHA classification over a short time. In particular, postinfarction angina and rest angina are associated with the presence of complicated atherosclerotic plaques, with greater cardiac morbidity.

An important percentage of patients experience an *acute myocardial infarction* (AMI) or sudden cardiac death as the initial manifestation of CAD. However, most patients with an AMI have an increase in the frequency and severity of anginal episodes prior to the AMI. In patients with an AMI, the symptoms of chest pain are usually greater in severity and the duration is usually longer than 30 minutes. Symptoms of LV failure such as dyspnea and breathlessness may be predominant, particularly in elderly patients with AMI. The amount of myocardium infarcted affects the clinical presentation: 15 per cent is associated with a decrease in LV ejection fraction and elevated ventricular filling pressures; 25 per cent is associated with overt symptoms of congestive heart failure; and more than 40 per cent is associated with cardiogenic shock (systolic blood pressure < 90 mm Hg with inadequate cardiac output).

In patients with CAD, the physical examination is often unremarkable. Evidence of impaired LV compliance may be manifest by the presence of a fourth and, more specifically, a third heart sound. In such patients, rales may also be present. Although the resting electrocardiogram (ECG) is often normal, inverted T waves and alterations in the ST segments may be present, particularly during anginal episodes or during stress testing. Persistent ST segment elevation or depression and the development of Q waves is indicative of an AMI. Exercise testing using ECG, echocardiography, and nuclear cardiography is useful in assessing the functional significance in a patient with CAD. Although stress testing may be used as a screening technique for the presence of CAD, false-negative and false-positive responses occur. Importantly, exercise testing provides useful information regarding prognosis. Patients with early positive studies are likely to have severe coronary artery disease and are more apt to suffer AMI and cardiac death, and the LV ejection fraction measured during exercise is a powerful predictor of survival (Fig. 3).

Cardiac catheterization and coronary arteriography are required to diagnose the presence and anatomic severity of CAD. The relative amount of myocardium at risk and the degree of ventricular impairment present can be assessed allowing determination of prognosis and optimal therapy. In addition, this anatomic map is crucial before embarking on revascularization by catheter dilation or other techniques or for bypass grafting.

MANAGEMENT

Optimal management of patients with CAD requires an assessment of the patient's relative risk for an adverse myocardial event such as AMI, sudden death, as well as the severity of the symptoms. The natural history of patients with CAD is such that with increasing amounts of myocardium at risk due to stenosis of the

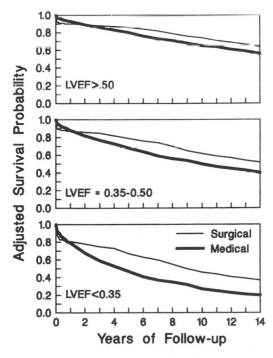

Figure 3. (From Muhlbaier LH, Pryor DB, Rankin JS, et al: Observation comparison of event-free survival with medical and surgical therapy in patients with coronary artery disease. Circulation 86(suppl. II):II–198, 1992, with permission.)

supplying coronary artery, survival is decreased. Survival is best with single-vessel disease and diminishes with increasing vessel involvement (two-vessel > three-vessel > left main) (Fig. 4). Obstructions occurring proximally in a coronary artery are associated with impaired survival compared with those occurring distally. The specific coronary artery involved also has important prognostic significance, as survival is worst with LAD involvement and best when the RCA is diseased. Additional risk is imparted by an increase in the severity of symptoms, impaired LV function, and by ischemia that is inducible by low levels of exercise.

Differences in survival based on the form of treatment have been demonstrated in certain groups of patients with CAD. A significant survival advantage in patients treated with *coronary artery bypass grafting* (CABG) has been demonstrated in a number of randomized clinical trials in the following groups: (1) patients with greater than 75 per cent stenosis of the left main artery; (2) those with three-vessel or two-vessel disease with proximal LAD involvement, and in association with either moderate to severe anginal symptoms (NYHA Class III or IV), impaired LV ejection fraction (LVEF <50 per cent), or easily inducible ischemia with exercise. CABG is recommended as therapy in these patients, although some may be amenable to treatment with *percutaneous transluminal coronary angioplasty* (PTCA). CABG is indicated in patients with anginal symptoms refractory to medical management, particularly when the anatomy is not appropriate for PTCA.

Patients who are assessed to have low risk for coronary events are appropriately managed medically. Modification of known risk factors associated with CAD should be initiated, including cessation of tobacco use, control of hypertension, reduction of serum lipids, and, when appropriate, weight reduction. Success in correcting these risk factors has been shown to decrease the incidence of AMI and to lead to regression of atherosclerosis. In patients undergoing CABG, graft patency is also improved.

The primary agents effective in either reducing the frequency of anginal episodes, or preventing AMI or cardiac death include nitrates, β-blockers, calcium channel blockers, and aspirin. Usually, nitrates are first selected for treatment and can be short- or long-acting, administered topically, orally, or intravenously. They are useful in terminating anginal episodes (usually sublingual tablets) or preventing anginal episodes. Nitrates reduce myocardial oxygen consumption by reducing preload and afterload and increase myocardial perfusion by a non–endothelium-dependent vasodilatation. The development of early tolerance limits the utility of nitrates.

β-blockers, including atenolol, metoprolol, nadolol, and propanolol, effectively decrease the frequency of

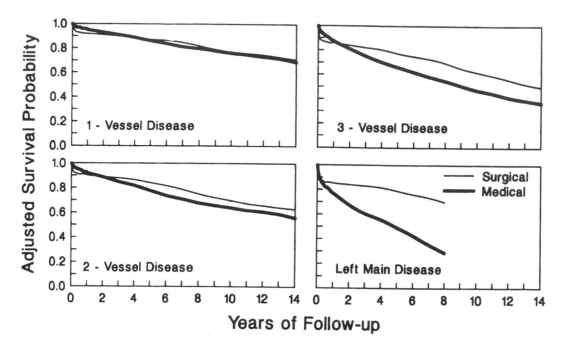

Figure 4. (From Muhlbaier LH, Pryor DB, Rankin JS, et al: Observation comparison of event-free survival with medical and surgical therapy in patients with coronary artery disease. Circulation *86*(suppl. II):II–198, 1992, with permission.)

anginal episodes, prevent reinfarction after AMI, and decrease the incidence of sudden death. They act primarily by decreasing myocardial oxygen consumption through a decrease in heart rate, as well as a decrease in myocardial contractility and in blood pressure, but their use is limited by bradycardia, heart block, ventricular failure, and bronchospasm. Calcium channel blockers, including nifedipine, verapamil, and diltiazem, are effective in limiting the frequency of anginal episodes. However, the use of these agents has not demonstrated any advantage in survival in patients with coronary artery disease, particularly following AMI or in patients with ventricular failure. Aspirin reduces the incidence of AMI and prolongs bypass graft patency through antiplatelet activity.

UNSTABLE ANGINA

Patients with unstable angina initially should be managed medically. Factors that increase myocardial oxygen consumption, such as hyperthyroidism, anemia, dysrhythmias, and infection, should be sought and treated. Patients should be admitted to the hospital and placed on bed rest. Measurement of myocardial isoenzymes (creatine phosphokinase [CPK] with Mb band) should be performed to exclude AMI. Nitrates, β-blockers, aspirin, and heparin are the basis of therapy. The latter two agents are effective due to

the strong association of complicated plaques with platelet aggregation or thrombi and the development of unstable angina. Early coronary arteriography is indicated in patients with persistent angina. Approximately 80 per cent of patients have multivessel or left main occlusive disease. The incidence of adverse myocardial events is increased during the initial months following presentation, particularly in those with multivessel disease, rest pain, complex lesion morphology, intracoronary thrombi, ischemia demonstrated during Holter monitoring, or in the elderly. In patients with persistent angina, institution of an *intra-aortic balloon pump* (IABP) is efficacious. Revascularization using PTCA or CABG is frequently indicated, although the risk of a periprocedural myocardial infarction or mortality is approximately twice that of an elective procedure.

ACUTE MYOCARDIAL INFARCTION

In 1912, Herrick initially made the observation that AMI was associated with thrombosis of the coronary artery. Subsequently, it has been shown that 90 per cent of transmural infarcts are associated with a totally occluded related vessel. Recent clinical evidence has reinforced the importance of obtaining myocardial reperfusion as early as possible, and intravenous thrombolytics, including streptokinase, tissue-type plasminogen activator (t-PA), and anisoylated plasminogen streptokinase activator complex (APSAC), achieve patency of the related vessel in as many as 85 per cent. Thrombolytics have been shown to decrease mortality, decrease infarct size, and preserve ventricular function. The benefit is greatest when given early after onset of pain. Less benefit is achieved when given more than 6 hours after the onset of pain. Importantly, the adjuvant use of heparin and aspirin has limited the reocclusion and reinfarction rates. Complications of thrombolytics include allergic reactions, hypotension and, most frequently, bleeding, usually at sites of vascular puncture. Intracranial hemorrhage occurs in 0.5 per cent of patients. Patients who do not achieve reperfusion with thrombolytics have a contraindication to thrombolytic therapy or have recurrent ischemia benefit from reperfusion using PTCA. Unfortunately, less than 25 per cent of patients with AMI receive thrombolytic therapy due to delays in presentation after the onset of pain and delays in diagnosis.

All patients with presumed AMI should be admitted for cardiac monitoring. Serial cardiac isoenzymes (CPK with Mb isoenzyme fraction) should be obtained to help assess the size of the infarct. Control of pain is achieved using short-acting nitrates, analgesics, usually morphine, and β-blockers. Invasive monitoring using *pulmonary artery* (PA) catheters is indicated in patients with AMI with hypotension, which is resistant to volume administration, heart failure, or who require pressors or an IABP. Pulmonary artery catheters are also indicated in those with mechanical complications of AMI, including postinfarction *ventricular septal defects* (VSD) and ischemic mitral regurgitation. At many centers, cardiac catheterization and coronary arteriography are obtained in most patients after AMI. Patients with a low risk for a subsequent cardiac event, as demonstrated by normal ventricular function and absence of ischemia during hospitalization and at a predischarge submaximal stress test, can be managed medically with good results. The use of aspirin and β-blockers has been shown to decrease reinfarction rates. Patients at a high risk for subsequent cardiac events should undergo cardiac catheterization. Patients with multivessel disease in which the proximal LAD is involved have a survival benefit with revascularization.

Mechanical complications of AMI occur due to tearing of myocardial tissue. Such complications include rupture of the ventricular free wall, ventricular septal defect, and rupture of a papillary muscle, which causes severe mitral regurgitation. Echocardiography can establish the diagnosis. These complications occur less frequently in patients treated with thrombolytics, and more frequently in those on corticosteroids or nonsteroidal anti-inflammatory drugs (NSAIDs). Patients are usually elderly. The mortality in patients treated medically with these complications exceeds 90 per cent.

Rupture of the ventricular free wall causes hemopericardium and tamponade and accounts for 10 per cent of hospital deaths due to AMI. Pericardiocentesis confirms the diagnosis and provides temporary hemodynamic relief. Urgent surgical therapy with ventricular reconstruction can lead to survival.

A postinfarction VSD is manifest clinically by the new onset of a harsh holosystolic murmur usually associated with a thrill. Hemodynamic compromise with ventricular failure occurs early. In addition to color-flow echocardiography, a right heart catheterization demonstrating an oxygen saturation step-up at the level of the right ventricle establishes the diagnosis. Except in moribund patients, correction of the VSD by patch closure and bypass grafting should be performed. Rarely, the patient may be stable and the operation can be delayed, allowing the infarct tissue to heal, as better results are obtained in these patients, with survival approaching 90 per cent. However, in most patients, urgent operation is needed. Use of an IABP provides a degree of hemodynamic support. Survival following surgical correction is approximately 50 to 75 per cent.

Rupture of a papillary muscle leads to severe mitral regurgitation, with rapid development of pulmonary edema and hypotension. A holosystolic murmur is usually present, and echocardiography is diagnostic. Unlike postinfarction VSD, papillary muscle rupture is often associated with a limited size of infarction. Frequently, local circumflex or RCA disease is present. IABP use provides hemodynamic support. Early operative therapy with mitral valve repair when possible, or mitral valve replacement in conjunction with bypass grafting, is indicated. Survival is reported as approximately 50 to 70 per cent.

Left Ventricular Aneurysm

Left ventricular aneurysms (LVA) develop as a complication in 10 to 30 per cent of patients with an acute transmural infarct. These aneurysms usually develop in association with an acutely occluded coronary artery with poor collateral flow. Due to the increased use of thrombolytic agents and PTCA to achieve reperfusion, the incidence of LVA is decreasing. An LVA is comprised of a transmural fibrous scar with minimal remaining myocardium. The region of the LVA during ventricular systole is either akinetic (noncontractile) or, more commonly, dyskinetic (paradoxic outward motion). The subendocardial surface is smooth rather than manifesting the typical trabecular pattern. In most patients with LVA, mural thrombus is present. Frequently, the epicardium is densely adherent to the aneurysm. In patients with an LVA, the location is anteroapical or anterolateral in 85 to 90 per cent and inferoposterior (near the base of the heart) in 5 to 10 per cent. Lateral wall aneurysms are infrequent. Over 50 per cent of patients with LVA have multivessel CAD. The LAD is involved in over 90 per cent and is occluded in approximately 80 per cent. In patients with inferoposterior aneurysms, the posterolateral papillary muscle is often involved, which causes mitral insufficiency. In addition, a significant proportion of posterior aneurysms are false aneurysms, which are contained ruptures of the myocardium by the surrounding pericardium.

Patients with an LVA most frequently have symptoms of angina or those related to ventricular failure, such as dyspnea and orthopnea, which may progress to respiratory failure. In 15 to 30 per cent of patients with LVA, symptoms related to ventricular dysrhythmias, such as recurrent sudden death, syncope, and paroxysmal episodes of heart failure, are prevalent. Although most have mural thrombus, thromboembolic episodes are relatively infrequent.

Myocardial oxygen consumption is increased in patients with LVA. The presence of an LVA indicates a loss of myocardium that requires the remaining myocardium to augment its function to maintain overall cardiac performance. Systolic stroke work is lost due to pooling of blood into the dyskinetic portion to the LVA during systole. Most importantly, the LV chamber develops generalized dilation. Myocardial wall stress is directly proportional to the radius of the curvature of the LV chamber (law of Laplace) and is therefore increased with an LVA. Because of these factors that increase myocardial oxygen consumption, the amount of myocardial ischemia is increased in patients with CAD and an LVA. Similarly, these factors also impair systolic and diastolic function, causing the symptoms of heart failure. In patients with a posterior aneurysm, mitral insufficiency is common and further impairs ventricular performance.

Survival in patients with LVA treated medically is approximately 50 per cent at 5 years. If the function of the nonaneurysmal LV is impaired, survival decreases to 35 per cent at 5 years. In patients with a large LVA who are symptomatic, repair is indicated. Left ventricular aneurysm repair is usually done in conjunction with bypass grafting of associated critical coronary artery stenoses. However, the aneurysm-related occluded coronary artery is often not bypassed due to lack of viable myocardium in its region of distribution. The LVA is repaired while on cardiopulmonary bypass. After the aneurysm is opened and all mural thrombus is removed, the aneurysm wall may be excised and the defect closed primarily, usually using large felt strips to buttress the repair. When primary closure of the ventricular defect would leave an inadequate LV chamber, a patch of synthetic material is used to close the defect and the aneurysm wall is closed over the patch (Fig. 5).

In-hospital mortality following LV aneurysmectomy is 5 to 10 per cent, with most deaths occurring due to acute myocardial failure and low cardiac output syndrome. Factors that increase the risk of mortality include poor ventricular function in the nonaneurysmal myocardium, older age, symptoms of congestive heart failure, higher NYHA functional class, elevated left ventricular end-diastolic pressure (LVEDP), and significant ventricular dysrhythmias. Approximately 80 per cent of patients have marked improvements in their symptoms. Although most patients who have a large LVA repaired show improvements in LVEF as well as lower LV end-systolic and -diastolic pressures and volumes, relief of symptoms may occur without objective improvements in ventricular function. Long-term survival in patients with an LVA is better following resection, 65 per cent at 5 years, than when treated medically, 50 per cent at 5 years. However, survival is less than in patients with similar CAD without LVA.

SURGICAL MANAGEMENT

Prior to operation, the patient's medical condition should be optimized. Coexisting abnormalities in the pulmonary and renal systems are common. Cessation of tobacco use, treatment of bronchospasm and bronchitis, and management of pulmonary edema reduce postoperative pulmonary complications. Serum blood urea nitrogen (BUN) and creatinine should be monitored, and these levels should be stable and not increasing prior to operation, particularly after the administration of contrast dye. Sources of ongoing infection should be identified and treated prior to operation. Assessment of the extracranial cerebral arteries using Doppler ultrasound or angiography should be performed in patients with neurologic symptoms such as transient ischemic attacks or a prior cerebral vascular accident, particularly if recent. In patients with symptomatic carotid occlusive disease, carotid endarterectomy prior to or simultaneous with CABG may be considered.

Importantly, cardiac ischemia and hemodynamic instability should be controlled when possible. Nitrates, β-blockers, calcium channel blockers, and heparin are continued until operation. Preoperative use of the IABP may be necessary to reverse ischemia or hemodynamic lability.

Surgical Procedure

Although a number of indirect procedures were devised to treat coronary artery disease in the first half

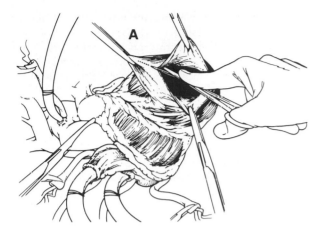

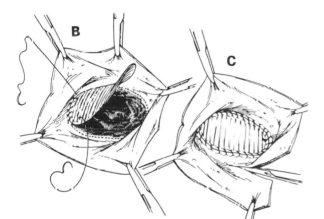

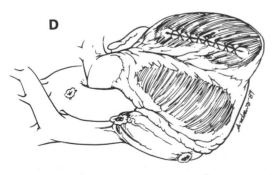

Figure 5. Steps for aneurysmectomy and reconstruction of the left ventricle. *A,* The aneurysm is opened and any mural thrombus carefully and completely removed. *B,* The fibrous rim of the aneurysm is identified from within the aneurysm and is closed using a patch fashioned to approximate the size of the defect. *C,* The remaining aneurysm sac is trimmed. *D,* The aneurysm sac is closed over the repair, usually without buttresses or pledgets. (From Colley DA: Ventricular endoaneurysmorrrhaphy: Results of an improved method of repair. Texes Heart Inst J 16:72, 1989. Drawn by Bill Andrews.)

of this century, the first effective and direct approach to treat coronary artery disease was the coronary endarterectomy, performed initially in 1956 by Bailey and subsequently modified by Longmire. However, endarterectomy is applicable to only a minority of patients and the long-term patency rates are poor. The first coronary artery bypass was performed by Sabiston in 1962 using a reversed saphenous vein. Although this patient succumbed to a perioperative *cerebrovascular accident* (CVA), later clinical success by Favalaro and Johnson in the late 1960s demonstrated the clinical efficacy of CABG.

Coronary artery bypass grafting is usually performed using a median sternotomy to expose the mediastinum, heart, and great vessels. The conduits used to bypass the coronary artery obstruction are most commonly the internal mammary artery, as a tissue pedicle, or a segment of saphenous vein. The saphenous vein is reversed with the distal vein anastomosed to the ascending aorta (Fig. 6) and the proximal end anastomosed to the coronary artery beyond the obstruction (Fig. 7). The proximal end of the internal mammary artery is left in continuity with the subclavian artery, and the distal end is anastomosed to the coronary artery (Fig. 8), usually the LAD. These anastomoses are performed while the patient is on cardiopulmonary bypass. The coronary artery anastomoses

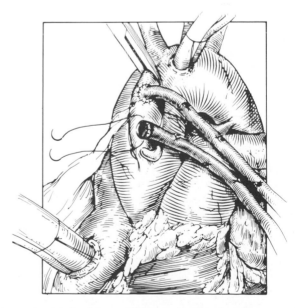

Figure 6. Method for performing proximal saphenous vein anastomoses to the aorta. A portion of the aorta is excluded using a partial occlusion clamp, and the vein grafts are anastomosed to circular aortotomies with running 6-0 polypropylene sutures. (Modified from Ochsner JL, Mills NL: Coronary Artery Surgery. Philadelphia, Lea & Febiger, 1978, with permission.)

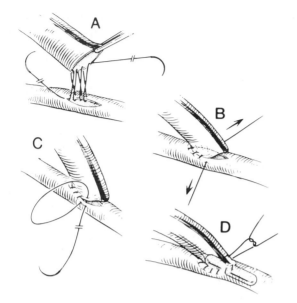

Figure 7. A standard method for distal vein graft anastomosis using a running suture technique. (From Sabiston, DC Jr: The coronary circulation. In Sabiston DC Jr [ed.]: Textbook of Surgery, ed 13. Philadelphia, WB Saunders Company, 1986, with permission.)

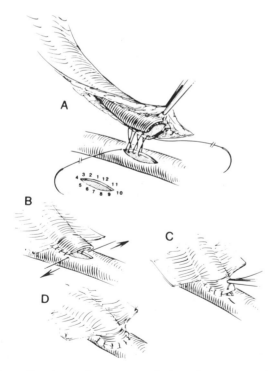

Figure 8. A running suture technique for constructing distal internal mammary artery anastomoses. (From Sabiston DC Jr: The coronary circulation. In Sabiston DC Jr [ed.]: Textbook of Surgery, ed 13. Philadelphia, WB Saunders Company, 1986, with permission.)

are done after the ascending aorta is occluded and after the heart is arrested by delivery of a potassium cardioplegic solution. Although different techniques are available for myocardial protection while blood flow is interrupted, most centers use cold cardioplegia with topical hypothermia of the heart. By cooling the heart to <10°C and inducing diastolic arrest, myocardial energy expenditure is reduced 100-fold. This approach provides a motionless heart and a dry field. All coronary arteries larger than 1.5 mm in diameter and with greater than a 60 per cent stenosis are bypassed. Emphasis is placed on complete revascularization. Following completion of the bypass grafts, assurance of hemostasis around the anastomoses, and placement of temporary epicardial pacing wires, the patient is weaned from cardiopulmonary bypass. The mediastinum and opened pleural spaces are drained with large-bore chest tubes.

Postoperative Care

Following CABG, patients are managed in an intensive care unit and are mechanically ventilated in the early postoperative period. Arterial blood pressure, ECG, *central venous pressure* (CVP), chest tube output, urinary output, and often pulmonary artery pressure are continuously recorded. Periodic measurement of arterial blood gases (PO_2, PCO_2, and pH), as well as serum hemoglobin, and blood electrolytes is obtained. In patients with a pulmonary artery catheter, cardiac output and *pulmonary capillary wedge pressure* (PCWP) periodically are determined. The use of an oximetric PA catheter allows continuous reading of the systemic venous oxygen concentration (SvO_2). Appropriate tissue perfusion is manifest by a cardiac index greater than 2, SvO_2 greater than 70 per cent, absence of acidosis, and an adequate urine output. Causes of inadequate tissue perfusion include hypovolemia, dysrhythmias, myocardial dysfunction, and mechanical causes of obstruction. Hypovolemia may represent ongoing bleeding and peripheral vasodilatation, which accompanies the increase in body temperature and fluid loss through leaky capillary beds. Central venous pressure and PCWP measurements will be low. Treatment is with volume replacement.

Mechanical causes of venous obstruction include tension pneumothorax and cardiac tamponade. Tension pneumothorax is manifest by absence of breath sounds, hyperresonance to percussion, tracheal shift, and elevated peak ventilator pressures. Although a chest film confirms the diagnosis, a high level of suspicion in a patient who is hemodynamically unstable is an indication for tube thoracostomy. Cardiac tamponade is manifest by decreasing systemic perfusion in association with an elevated and equalized left and right heart filling pressures (PCWP and CVP), increased heart rate, and a widened mediastinum demonstrated by chest film. Often, tamponade develops in patients who initially have significant mediastinal bleeding that subsequently decreases dramatically, and reexploration of the mediastinum with evacuation of hematoma and blood is indicated urgently. Postoperative myocardial dysfunction is more commonly observed in patients with a low preoperative LVEF, unstable angina, acute myocardial infarction, as well as the 3 to 5 per cent of patients in whom an intraoperative myocardial infarction occurs. Systemic perfusion is supported through the use of inotropic agents, with dopamine, dobutamine, epinephrine, and amrinone being the most frequent. Mechanical assistance of myocardial function using the IABP and, less frequently, ventricular assist devices may be indicated.

Blood loss from the mediastinum, as measured by the output of the chest tube, usually is in the range of 500 to 1250 ml. Abnormalities of the coagulation system, particularly platelet dysfunction, due to the use of cardiopulmonary bypass are common and may require treatment with blood components. Approximately 2 to 3 per cent of patients require reoperation to control excessive bleeding.

Atrial and ventricular dysrhythmias frequently complicate postoperative care. Identification and correction of reversible causes, including hypoxia, hypokalemia, hypomagnesemia, myocardial ischemia, and hyperthyroidism, should be performed initially. In patients who are hemodynamically compromised, cardioversion or defibrillation is indicated. Atrial dysrhythmias, such as premature atrial contractions, atrial fibrillation, and atrial flutter, occur in 20 to 35 per cent of patients following CABG. The ventricular response rate can be controlled using intravenous digoxin and verapamil, and pharmacologic conversion can be achieved using procainamide, quinidine, calcium channel blockers, β-blockers, and type Ic antiarrhythmics. Rapid atrial pacing is useful in converting atrial flutter, and cardioversion may be necessary after initiating drug therapy. Ventricular dysrhythmias, including multifocal *premature ventricular contraction* (PVC), ventricular tachycardia, and fibrillation may occur after CABG. In patients not requiring cardioversion, pharmacologic therapy is initiated, usually in the following order: lidocaine, procainamide, bretylium, and esmolol. Persistent ventricular dysrhythmias are indicative of myocardial ischemia and infarction, which may be due to graft occlusion.

Pulmonary complications include atelectasis, pneumonia, and respiratory insufficiency requiring prolonged mechanical ventilation. Preoperative *chronic obstructive pulmonary disease* (COPD), bronchitis, tobacco use, pulmonary edema, and pulmonary hypertension increase the risk of these complications. Renal insufficiency, manifest by oliguria and a rising serum creatinine and BUN, is associated with low cardiac output syndrome, preoperative renal insufficiency, and prolonged duration of cardiopulmonary bypass. Maintenance of adequate cardiac output, low-dose dopamine (1 to 3 μg/kg/min), avoidance of nephrotoxic agents, and limitation of fluid and potassium are initial therapeutic measures. Dialysis may be required, and peritoneal dialysis and continuous low-flow hemodialysis cause less hemodynamic instability than intermittent hemodialysis.

The most common infectious complications involve the urinary and respiratory systems. Superficial infection of the sternotomy wound occurs in approximately 3 per cent of patients, and half have deep infections involving the sternum and soft tissues of the mediastinum. Predisposing factors include diabetes mellitus, use of both internal mammary arteries, the low cardiac output syndrome, presence of infection at another site, and obesity. Untreated, overwhelming sepsis or exsanguination from the anastomotic leaks or from other cardiovascular structures frequently follow. Clinical manifestations of mediastinitis include fever, leukocytosis, periwound cellulitis, and usually sternal instability. Treatment requires antibiotics and débridement of infected and necrotic tissue. The use of vascularized tissue pedicles of muscle or omentum to obliterate the mediastinal space has reduced morbidity, mortality, and length of hospital stay.

Results

The mortality is approximately 3 per cent in large series of patients undergoing CABG. It is significantly increased by advanced age, incomplete revascularization, reoperative CABG, preoperative hemodynamic instability, unstable angina, female sex, and impaired ventricular function as measured by LVEF, particularly in those patients with mitral regurgitation or symptoms of congestive heart failure. In patients without significant risk factors, the mortality approaches 1 per cent. Long-term survival at 5, 10, and 15 years is approximately 90, 75, and 65 per cent, respectively. Long-term survival is adversely affected by low ejection fraction, particularly as measured during exercise, advanced age, diabetes mellitus, and by not using the internal mammary artery for grafting.

Early after CABG, rates of relief of anginal symptoms and freedom from myocardial infarction are excellent, approximately 85 and 95 per cent at 5 years, respectively. After 5 years, recurrence of angina and myocardial infarction rates increase. At 10 years the rates are 60 and 80 per cent respectively. The increase in myocardial events reflects progression of atherosclerosis in the coronary vasculature and the progressive loss of bypass grafts, particularly those using saphenous vein. The 1-year patency rate of bypass grafts using internal mammary artery and saphenous vein is 95 and 90 per cent, respectively. Graft patency at 10 years remains good (85 per cent to 90 per cent) using the internal mammary artery. The patency rate of grafts using saphenous vein begins to decrease after 4 years and is only 50 to 60 per cent after 10 years.

CABG significantly improves both myocardial function and patient performance. Exercise tolerance is markedly improved in patients after CABG, and remains better than patients treated medically as many as 10 years following operation. Regional wall function and exercise ejection fraction are both improved within 2 weeks following operation. Similar improvements in diastolic function as measured by ventricular compliance occur following CABG.

ROLE OF PTCA

Since the introduction of PTCA by Gruntzig in 1977, PTCA has become the most commonly used invasive therapy in the treatment of CAD. With improving technology, PTCA is now performed with greater initial success and fewer complications. It has been applied in a wider realm of clinical situations. Treatment of a wider range of atherosclerotic plaques, both with regard to anatomic locations and the complexity of the plaque, has occurred, but the nature of the plaque and its anatomic location affects the rate of success and complications (Table 2). Good risk lesions that are proximally located, short in length, concentric, and without calcification can be dilated with success rates of approximately 95 per cent. Major early complications include those at the vascular access site, including bleeding and thrombosis, and those at the site of dilation, primarily dissection, which causes vessel occlusion in 4 to 7 per cent of patients undergoing PTCA. Although 50 per cent of these occluded vessels can be reopened by repeat PTCA, sometimes in conjunction with placement of an intravascular stent, the other 50 per cent of patients require an emergency bypass procedure if evidence of myocardial ischemia is present. In patients requiring emergency operation, the placement of a perfusion catheter across the site of occlusion with side holes proximal and distal to the occlusion allows continuous myocardial perfusions, with a subsequent better survival rate and fewer myocardial infarctions. However, the mortality is approximately 5 per cent, twice the rate of an elective procedure. Importantly, the rate of myocardial infarction is 30 per cent, and the long-term complication of recurrent stenosis at the angioplasty site remains a substantial limitation. At 6 months, 30 to 40 per cent of patients develop restenosis, although only 20 to 25 per cent experience recurrent ischemic symptoms. Unfortunately, no effective therapy has yet been

TABLE 2. LESION-SPECIFIC CHARACTERISTICS OF TYPE A, B, AND C LESIONS*

Type A Lesions (high success, >85%; low risk)	
• Discrete (<10 mm length)	• Little or no calcification
• Concentric	• Less than totally occlusive
• Readily accessible	• Not ostial in location
• Nonangulated segment, <45 degrees	• No major branch involvement
• Smooth contour	• Absence of thrombus

Type B Lesions (moderate success, 60 to 85%; moderate risk)	
• Tubular (10 to 20 mm length)	• Moderate to heavy calcification
• Eccentric	• Total occlusions <3 months old
• Moderate tortuoisity of proximal segment	• Ostial in location
• Moderately angulated segment, >45 degrees, <90 degrees	• Birfurcation lesions requiring double guidewires
• Irregular contour	• Some thrombus present

Type C Lesions (low success, <60%; high risk)	
• Diffuse (>2 cm length)	• Total occlusion >3 months old
• Excessive tortuosity of proximal segment	• Inability to protect major side branches
• Extremely angulated segments >90 degrees	• Degenerated vein grafts with friable lesions

*From Ryan TJ, Faxon DP, Gunnar RM, et al: Guidelines for percutaneous transluminal angioplasty: A report of the American Cardiology/American Heart Association task force on assessment of diagnostic and therapeutic cardiovascular procedures. J Am Coll Cardiol 12:529, 1988, with permission.

†Although the risk of abrupt vessel closure is moderate, in certain instances the likelihood of a major complication may be low as in dilation of total occlusions less than 3 months old or when abundant collateral channels supply the distal vessel.

established to lower the restenosis rate. Treatment of these obstructive lesions with PTCA is as effective as an initial PTCA with comparable success and restenosis rates.

The indications for PTCA include the presence of a critical coronary artery stenosis (>75 per cent), which affects perfusion to a moderate to large amount of myocardium, causing significant ischemia. The ischemia can be manifest by angina or infarction or by noninvasive means such as ECG monitoring. Contraindications to PTCA include left main lesions or equivalent lesions in which vessel occlusion would cause cardiogenic failure, poor-risk lesions (type C lesions in Table 2) in patients with acceptable alternative therapies, and diffuse coronary artery disease in patients amenable to CABG. Advantages of PTCA relative to CABG include decreased initial cost and hospitalization, quicker and easier patient convalescence after the procedure, and a greater ability to repeat the procedure or apply operative therapy subsequently. However, the significant restenosis rate following PTCA requires a greater number of additional invasive procedures and is associated with a higher rate of cardiac events than those patients treated with CABG.

Unfortunately, prospective randomized trials comparing PTCA with CABG or medical therapy are not yet available. Although the relative roles of PTCA and CABG are controversial, currently most patients with symptomatic single-vessel or two-vessel coronary artery disease amenable to angioplasty are treated initially with PTCA, whereas patients with symptomatic three-vessel disease are treated with CABG. Additionally, PTCA of culprit lesions appears warranted in patients with AMI who have either a contraindication to thrombolytic therapy or fail to achieve vessel patency after thrombolytic therapy. In patients with AMI in whom thrombolytic therapy is successful in restoring vessel patency, early PTCA of the residual atherosclerotic plaque is associated with less satisfactory results and more complications as compared to delayed PTCA. A more rational approach to the treatment of patients with coronary artery diseases should be forthcoming following the data obtained from ongoing clinical trials.

REFERENCES

Califf RM, Harrell FE, Lee KL, Rankin JS, Hlatky MA, Mark DB, Jones RH, Muhlbaier LH, Oldham HN, Pryor DB: The evolution of medical and surgical therapy for coronary artery disease: A 15-year perspective. JAMA 261:2077, 1989.

Dinerman JL, Mehta JL: Endothelial, platelet and leukocyte interactions in ischemic heart disease: Insights into potential mechanisms and their clinical relevance. J Am Coll Cardiol 16:207,1990.

Franch RH, et al: Techniques of cardiac catheterization including coronary arteriography. *In* Hurst JW (ed): The Heart, ed 5. New York, McGraw-Hill Book Company, 1982.

Lee KL, Pryor DB, Pieper KS, Harrell FE, Califf RM, Mark DB, Hlatky MA, Coleman RE, Cobb FR, Jones RH: Prognostic value of radionuclide angiography in medically treated patients with coronary artery disease. Circulation 82:1705, 1990.

Muhlbaier LH, Pryor DB, Rankin JS, Smith LR, Mark DB, Jones RH, Glower DD, Harrell FE, Lee KL, Califf RM, Sabiston DC: Observational comparison of event-free survival with medical and surgical therapy in patients with coronary artery disease. Circulation 86(suppl II):II-198, 1992.

Ochsner JL, Mills NL: Coronary Artery Surgery. Philadelphia, Lea & Febiger, 1978.

Ryan TJ, Faxon DP, Gunnar RM, et al: Guidelines for percutaneous transluminal angioplasty: A report of the American Cardiology/American Heart Association task force on assessment of diagnostic and therapeutic cardiovascular procedures. Circulation 78:486-502, 1988.

Sabiston DC Jr: The coronary circulation. The William F. Rienhoff, Jr lecture. Johns Hopkins Med J 134:314, 1974.

Sabiston DC Jr (ed): Textbook of Surgery: The Biological Basis of Modern Surgical Practice, ed 14. Philadelphia, WB Saunders Company, 1991.

ACQUIRED CARDIAC CONDITIONS:
Surgical Procedures for Cardiac Arrhythmias, Pacemakers, Cardiac Arrest, and Management of the Patient with Heart Disease

T. BRUCE FERGUSON, Jr., M.D.

SURGICAL PROCEDURES FOR ARRHYTHMIAS

In this section, the anatomic principles unique to the types of arrhythmia ablation currently performed as well as the status of surgical intervention for supraventricular and ventricular arrhythmias is presented.

Anatomic Principles

Anatomy of the Mature Conduction System

The sinoatrial node is a spindle-shaped structure, the head of which extends toward the interatrial groove, while the tail extends toward the orifice of the inferior vena cava. It is generally agreed that preferential conduction (but not discrete anatomic) pathways exist for the spread of excitation from the sinus to the atrioventricular (AV) node. Well-oriented atrial muscle tracts comprised of fibers that course in parallel are located in the intra-atrial septum. Activation of adjacent myocardium along these bands as broad wavefronts explains the preferential conduction known to occur in the atrium.

There are no gross anatomic landmarks to indicate the locations of the AV node and bundle of His. These structures are contained within the triangle of Koch, which is bounded by the anulus of the tricuspid valve inferiorly, the tendon of Todaro superiorly, and a line drawn between the coronary sinus and the tricuspid anulus posteriorly. The apex of the triangle is the central fibrous body of the heart and the supra-anular portion of the membranous intraventricular septum. The node is usually far removed (anteriorly) from the coronary sinus, and the transitional cell zones extend backward and superiorly from the compact node, but are contained within the boundaries of the triangle.

The compact AV node becomes the penetrating bundle at the apex of the triangle and passes into the ventricular septum beneath the attachment of the tendon of Todaro to the central fibrous body, just posterior to the membranous septum. The nonbranching and branching bundles are sandwiched between the muscular ventricular septum and the membranous septum. Branching of the bundle takes place on the muscular septum beneath the commissure between the right coronary and noncoronary cusps of the aortic valve. Importantly, the compact node, penetrating bundle, and branching bundle form a continuous axis of cells that courses the length of the muscular ventricular septum. The atrial component lies above the anulus, the penetrating bundle passes through the anulus, and branching bundles lie beneath the anulus fibrosis of the heart.

Supraventricular Tachycardias

For localization of *accessory atrioventricular connections*, the heart can be sectioned in the horizontal plane at the level of the AV groove and divided into the left free wall, the right free wall, the posterior septal, and the anterior septal spaces. The posterior and anterior septal spaces are epicardial spaces that abut onto the atrial septum posteriorly and anteriorly. The two fixed boundaries defining these spaces are the left and right fibrous trigones of the skeletal structure of the heart. However, the fibrous skeleton of the heart is not entirely horizontal. The tricuspid anulus is more apical in position than is the mitral anulus. As a result, the anterior part of the central fibrous body extends into the ventricles beneath the attachment of the tricuspid valve. For this reason, radiofrequency (RF) ablation of right-sided pathways is feasible from the atrial septum above the tricuspid valve, while ablation of left-sided pathways is performed from beneath the mitral valve anulus.

The AV groove between the left fibrous trigone and the right fibrous trigone (the anterior portion of the central fibrous body) lies in the horizontal plane and represents the site of continuity between the anterior leaflet of the mitral valve and the aortic valve anulus. This is the only area in the AV groove where atrial muscle is not in juxtaposition to ventricular muscle, and for this reason, accessory atrioventricular pathways are not found between the left and right fibrous trigones.

Accessory pathways are thought to be congenital remnants of atrial tissue directly connecting the atrial and ventricular muscle and producing abnormal atrioventricular activation. The success of electrophysiologic identification of the accessory pathway potentials and the results with radiofrequency ablation suggest that most accessory pathways are juxta-anular. Those pathways that are not able to be ablated by the RF technique are probably disparate in location from the true anulus.

The electrophysiologic substrate for AV *nodal reentrant tachycardia* is the presence of "dual AV nodal conduction pathways," one fast and one slow, through the AV node or the perinodal tissues. Histologic analysis of the AV nodal and perinodal tissue has not identified the anatomic correlate of the electrophysiologic substrate for AV nodal reentrant tachycardia. The recent experience with surgical and RF ablation suggests that perinodal tissue, either posterior to the compact node (most commonly) or anterior to the node is involved. From an anatomic point of view, *ectopic or automatic atrial tachycardias* can originate from foci occurring anywhere within the left or right atrial tissue or atrial septum. In addition, multiple foci may be present, some of which may be latent and become manifest only at some interval following ablation.

The anatomic substrate for *atrial fibrillation and flutter* has been elucidated in the past several years through a combination of experimental and clinical intraoperative mapping studies. Atrial flutter most likely occurs on the basis of a single macroreentrant circuit in the right atrial tissue that is dependent on fixed anatomic obstacles (e.g., the venae cavae or surgical incisions) to create areas of conduction block. Intraoperative localization of the reentrant circuit responsible for the flutter has been possible using sophisticated multipoint computerized mapping.

Experimental studies have also confirmed that atrial fibrillation is due to intra-atrial reentry, in which multiple reentrant wavelets in the atrium are maintained by the inhomogeneity of tissue refractoriness in atrial myocardium. This uneven refractoriness slows the activation wavefront in some areas but not in other areas, producing uneven conduction that causes a single wavefront to be dissociated into multiple reentrant waves. No discrete anatomic structure or abnormality has been definitively associated with this arrhythmia. Further studies confirm that as atrial size increases, there is an increase in the number of wavefronts during atrial fibrillation and in the duration of atrial fibrillation. As the cycle lengths decrease and become more variable, various regions of the atria become completely dissociated from each other.

Ventricular Tachycardias

Ventricular tachycardia in infants and children is usually nonischemic in origin and is most often associated with a cardiomyopathy, prior procedures for congenital heart defects, and cardiac tumors. In patients with *diffuse cardiomyopathy*, due to patchy myocardial fibrosis, angiographic and hemodynamic data usually indicate some type of abnormal myocardial contractility associated with recurrent tachycardia. Ventriculography demonstrates diffuse dilatation of both ventricles. This same finding on ventriculography may also be present in cases of *idiopathic ventricular tachycardia*, due to repeated bouts of tachycardia. However, in this latter entity, there is no pathologic evidence of primary cardiac disease. *Arrhythmogenic right ventricular dysplasia* (ARVD) is a congenital myopathy remarkable pathologically for transmural infiltration of adipose tissue. Anatomically, this causes weakness and aneurysmal bulging of three pathologic areas of the right ventricle: the *infundibulum*, *apex*, and *posterior basilar region*. Ventriculography demonstrates diffuse dilatation of the right ventricle, with a significant reduction in contractility and marked delay in right ventricular emptying. Ventricular bulges or frank aneurysms are seen in one or all of the three pathologic areas. *Cardiac tumors* can be localized to the left or right ventricle or septum in association with isolated arrhythmogenic tissue, or they can diffusely involve cardiac muscle and conduction tissue. Localized tumors may be epicardial, intramyocardial, or on the endocardial surface of the heart. Patients with *congenital heart defects*, especially tetralogy of Fallot, may develop ventricular arrhythmias long after the corrective procedure. The occurrence of these arrhythmias appears to be in part related to the hemodynamic result achieved with the operative procedure. Some of these arrhythmias have been shown to originate from the right ventriculotomy site.

Ventricular tachyarrhythmias in adults are most commonly secondary to *ischemic coronary artery disease*. In most patients, there is progression of acutely ischemic tissue to cell death, leaving a fibrous scar in place of the injured myocardium. The interlacing anisotropic pattern of the remaining scar and normal myocardium may harbor local areas of slow conduction, unidirectional block, uneven refractoriness, and nonuniform repolarization, the electrophysiologic substrates for the development of reentrant circuits associated with ventricular aneurysm formation. Both microreentrant and macroreentrant circuits have been demonstrated to occur. These same substrates are also produced by the application of tension and/or compression forces by the most prevalent anatomic correlate of ischemic ventricular tachycardia, that of *ventricular aneurysm*. Most commonly, these occur in the anteroapical position secondary to occlusion of flow in the left anterior descending coronary artery, but they also occur posteriorly (inferiorly) in the distribution of the posterior descending coronary artery.

Surgical Treatment for Supraventricular Arrhythmias

Accessory AV Connections

Currently, candidates for surgical ablation of accessory pathways include patients with recurrent reciprocating tachycardia who are poorly controlled on medical therapy or who have developed significant toxicity to an otherwise successful medical regimen and who (1) have failed attempted RF ablation or (2) have concomitant cardiac disease requiring surgical intervention. Patients with symptomatic arrhythmias due to less common and more complicated accessory atrioventricular connections (atrio-His, nodoventricular, and fasciculoventricular fibers) should undergo operation if they are resistant or intolerant to medical therapy and fail RF ablation.

The location of the pathway(s) is determined from the preoperative electrophysiologic data and from intraoperative epicardial mapping. In decreasing order of frequency, accessory pathways are located in the left free wall, posterior septal, right free wall, and anterior septal positions. Approximately 20 per cent of patients in surgical series have multiple (two to four) pathways.

Since 1981, an *endocardial technique* and an anatomically based operation for division of all accessory pathways has been available. The principles of this operative approach are (1) accurate intraoperative localization of the pathway(s) to one of the four anatomic areas in the horizontal plane, (2) appreciation that the location of the pathway in the vertical plane may be variable, (3) appreciation that the endocardial dissection technique divides the ventricular insertion of the pathway without affecting the atrial insertion of the pathway, (4) complete dissection of the appropriate anatomic space(s) in every patient regardless of the location of the pathway within that space as determined by intraoperative mapping, (5) appreciation that certain pathways may exist as "broad bands" and that when the ventricular insertion site is located at the junction of two anatomic areas (e.g., left paraseptal region), complete dissection of both anatomic spaces should be performed, and (6) that isolation of the atrial rim of tissue above the anulus of the valve is necessary to prevent a juxta-anular pathway from retrogradely activating the atrium.

Surgical intervention following a failed RF ablation attempt does not seem to be more difficult or associated with increased morbidity, provided that the RF technique used places the ablation catheter below the anulus of the mitral valve and that excessive energies are not used on the right side of the heart. Direct RF ablation of the left atrial side of the AV groove has caused complete destruction of normal tissue planes and injury to circumflex coronary and coronary sinus vessels. Excessive application of RF energy to the right atrial septum has likewise caused obliteration of normal tissue planes. Placement of a recording catheter in the coronary artery for mapping purposes has been associated with early development of severe atherosclerotic coronary disease.

AV Nodal Reentrant Tachycardia

Currently, the initial ablative treatment of choice is RF, and surgical intervention is reserved for failed RF ablation or when concomitant surgery is performed. The exposure for the discrete cryosurgical procedure is through the right atrium. A nitrous oxide cryoprobe with a 3-mm tip is used to place cryolesions along the borders of the triangle of Koch. When the cryolesion approaches the nodal tissue, the AV interval prolongs in a nearly linear manner. When block occurs, cryothermia is terminated instantly and the AV interval shortens back to baseline. Used in this way, the cryoprobe acts as a "reversible knife." Electrophysiologically, this procedure probably "silently" eliminates the slow pathway (regardless of whether it is anterior or posterior to the nodal tissue). The AV prolongation and heart block are produced after elimination of the alternative pathway of conduction due to proximity of the cryolesion to the remaining pathway for AV conduction.

Automatic (Ectopic) Atrial Tachycardias

Accurate preoperative localization is particularly important in patients with automatic atrial tachycardias if surgical ablation of the focus is contemplated, because (1) general anesthesia frequently suppresses the ectopic focus, (2) intraoperative mapping without sophisticated computerized multipoint systems can be prohibitively difficult and time consuming, and (3) ectopic tachyarrhythmias are not inducible by standard programmed stimulation techniques.

If the tachycardia focus can be localized, a variety of techniques have been advocated for surgical treatment, including cryoablation, wide excision with pericardial patch repair, or a combination of cryoablation and resection.

Foci on the left atrium tend to be near the entrance of the pulmonary veins, and localized isolation procedures have met with limited success. In these instances, the ectopic foci should be excluded from the remainder of the heart using the left atrial isolation procedure. Postoperatively, these patients remain in normal sinus rhythm despite the presence of an incessant tachycardia confined to the left atrium. This therapy is preferable to the other therapeutic alternative, that of elective His bundle ablation and pacemaker insertion. Right atrial tachycardias are usually confined to the body of the right atrium and may be multifocal. If the arrhythmia circuit or focus cannot be localized at operation, a right atrial isolation procedure should be performed, which isolates the body of the right atrium while leaving the atrial pacemaker complex in continuity with the atrial septum and ventricles.

Surgical Treatment For Ventricular Arrhythmias

Nonischemic Tachycardias

Nonischemic tachycardias usually arise in the right ventricular free wall or septum and in general are extremely resistant to medical therapy. Localized surgical isolation techniques are usually employed for tachycardias arising in the right ventricular free wall, while multipoint map-guided cryoablative techniques are used for arrhythmias localized to the septum. In certain patients with ARVD, intraoperative mapping has suggested that the entire right ventricular free wall may be arrhythmogenic, giving rise to multiple morphologic types of tachycardia. In the past, surgical isolation of the entire right ventricular free wall has been performed. However, postoperative right ventricular dilatation has occurred in these patients, and currently, cardiac transplantation in a suitable patient with this arrhythmia is the most feasible surgical approach.

Ventricular tachycardia in association with the long QT interval syndrome frequently presents as *torsades de pointes*. Medical therapy consists of β-adrenergic blockade, and this recently has been coupled with permanent atrial or ventricular pacing. Implantation of an *implantable cardioverter defibrillator* (ICD) in patients with a history of life-threatening arrhythmias is now recommended. In refractory cases, cardiac transplantation should be considered.

Ischemic Ventricular Tachycardia

Important concepts in the optimal surgical treatment of refractory ischemic ventricular tachycardia are listed below.

1. Evaluation for surgical intervention should be made prior to the institution of amiodarone therapy. This is true for patients considered for either direct surgery or ICD implantation. The depressant effect of amiodarone on left ventricular function is aggravated by ischemic cardioplegic arrest in most patients; moreover, complications from the pulmonary toxicity effect of the drug can significantly complicate either operative procedure.

2. For direct surgical intervention, the patient should have a sufficient amount of left ventricular function remaining after aneurysmectomy to survive operative intervention. In other words, the function of the nonaneurysmal portion of the ventricle should be normal or near normal. Ejection fraction is not an accurate predictor of operative mortality in patients with aneurysms.

3. If the patient has a prohibitive degree of left ventricular dysfunction, implantation of an ICD should be considered if the patient meets the standard indications for ICD therapy. Patients who do not meet these criteria should be started on amiodarone.

4. If the patient's tachycardia is uncontrolled on amiodarone or with an ICD, cardiac transplantation should be considered. If the patient is not a transplant candidate, "salvage" ventricular tachycardia surgery is the only therapeutic option available.

5. If the patient's left ventricular function is acceptable for surgery, and there is a sustained ventricular tachycardia that can be mapped intraoperatively, direct surgical intervention should be undertaken.

A number of different surgical techniques for direct surgical intervention for ventricular tachycardias have been described. Our current technique involves intraoperative mapping using a 160-channel computerized mapping system. The results of the preoperative electrophysiologic study and this intraoperative map "guide" the surgical resection and cryoablation procedure. With the heart in the normothermic beating state and preferably during ventricular tachycardia, the ventricle is opened through the infarct or aneurysm and all of the associated endocardial fibrosis is resected except that which extends onto the base of the papillary muscles. Endocardial cryolesions are applied with a 1.5-cm nitrous oxide cryoprobe to the site(s) of origin of the tachycardia(s) as determined by the intraoperative mapping, thus ablating the myocardium deep to the visible fibrosis in the event that this tissue is involved in the tachycardia circuit. These techniques are applicable to both anterior and posteroinferior infarct/aneurysms. If coronary artery bypass grafting or other procedures are required, they are performed after completion of the antiarrhythmic portion of the procedure.

The standard approach for ICD implantation is through a left anterior thoracotomy, although multiple different implant techniques have been described. The patches are placed in the extrapericardial position, and either endocardial or epicardial rate-sensing leads are used. After demonstration of adequate sensing parameters, morphology characteristics, and defibrillation thresholds, the generator pocket is created below the left rectus sheath in the upper left abdominal wall. A median sternotomy approach is used for patients requiring concomitant coronary artery bypass grafting or valve replacement. Recently, nonthoracotomy systems using endocardial electrodes and a subcutaneous patch array have undergone clinical investigation. While these systems are associated with higher initial defibrillation thresholds and their stability over time remains to be determined, in selected patients they are apt to be beneficial in the future. Algorithms to determine which patients should receive which type of systems are being developed.

The operative and long-term follow-up results for ventricular tachycardia surgery argue strongly against routine implantation of the ICD device and performance of coronary bypass surgery as the primary therapeutic modality for ventricular tachycardia in patients who are otherwise candidates for a map-directed, wide-resection/cryoablative procedure as described above. The ICD device provides a viable therapeutic option for patients in whom performance of ventricular tachycardia surgery has been fraught with an excessive mortality; namely, patients with extreme degrees of ventricular dysfunction. Judicious selection of patients for ICD implantation has reduced the operative mortality for patients undergoing direct procedures, without increasing prohibitively the mortality for ICD implantation. This selection process has thereby reduced the overall operative mortality for ventricular tachycardia procedures.

As technologic advances continue with implantable defibrillators, it is anticipated that the fourth and fifth generations of these devices that combine defibrillation, antitachycardia pacing, single and/or dual chamber bradycardia support, and tiered therapy will all be contained in a device that can be safely implanted without a thoracotomy. These ICDs will become the standard of therapy of ischemic and nonischemic ventricular tachycardia/ventricular fibrillation (VT/VF) that is not amenable to surgical cure with the direct procedures described above.

Surgical Results

Division of Accessory Pathways

In over 300 patients operated upon for the Wolff-Parkinson-White (WPW) syndrome and/or other accessory pathways since 1981, the incidence of successful surgical correction of the WPW syndrome using the techniques described is 100 per cent with the initial operation, with an operative mortality for elective, uncomplicated cases of 0.5 per cent. There have been no early or late recurrences following surgery using the endocardial technique.

AV Nodal Reentry

The discrete cryosurgical procedure has been performed on 37 patients at our institution to date. In all cases, postoperative electrophysiologic study has demonstrated the persistence of only a single AV conduction pathway, and the reentrant tachycardia could not be induced. There have been no instances of permanent heart block and no late recurrences.

Automatic Atrial Tachycardias

If the ectopic focus can be adequately localized in the operation room, the operative procedures for isolation and/or ablation of the arrhythmia should be uniformly successful. The left atrial isolation procedure has been performed on six patients, and the right atrial isolation procedure has been performed on three patients. There have been no adverse sequelae from these operations to date.

Ischemic Ventricular Tachycardias

The long-term success rate in our series of patients operated upon for ischemic ventricular tachycardia is 87 per cent at 9 years, and these data agree with the other published large series. Essentially, all of this experience was gained prior to the advent of ICD therapy. The effect of the availability of ICD therapy has been to exclude the less optimal candidates for direct surgery from this pool, which reduces the operative mortality for direct VT surgery to 4 to 5 per cent for anterior aneurysms and 6 to 7 per cent for posterior aneurysms. Importantly, the application of ICD therapy to the patients who are not optimal candidates for direct surgery has not increased the operative mortality or morbidity for this procedure. In follow-up, patients with ICD implants have a very low incidence of arrhythmia-related death and long-term survival is more related to underlying ventricular function.

Surgical Management of Atrial Fibrillation

The "ideal" procedure for atrial fibrillation accomplishes three goals: (1) restoration of sinus rhythm, (2) restoration of atrial transport function, and (3) decrease or elimination of the risk of thromboembolism by eliminating passive stasis of blood in either or both atria.

The Maze Procedure

The experimental and clinical investigations that have been performed over the past 10 years have led to the development of the *Maze procedure*. The intraoperative mapping data acquired in humans suggested that the only effective operation would be one that would prevent the circuits from forming at all; that is, the space between the incisions needed to be small enough to prevent the short cycle lengths associated with the fibrillation circuits from closing back on themselves, establishing the reentrant mechanism. In addition, the operation would permit sinus depolarization and maintain normal AV synchrony, and would restore atrial transport function. These last two characteristics theoretically would decrease or eliminate the incidence of thromboembolism.

The complete description of the operation has been published elsewhere. After completion of the Maze procedure, the distances between the incisions, the nonconduction fibrous skeleton of the heart, and the fixed anatomic obstacles of the right and left atrium are such that reentrant circuits cannot form because the circuit becomes extinguished by one of these excisions or obstacles before a reentrant loop can be established. The only sustained conduction pathway originates from the sinus nodal area, proceeds anteriorly around the right atrial tissue, enters the atrial septum anteriorly, and depolarizes the AV nodal tissue. This anterior atrial depolarization carries across to the anterior left atrium and around posteriorly to depolarize the tissue beneath the pulmonary veins. Thus, normal AV conduction is maintained and the entire atrium is depolarized in sequential fashion after this operative procedure.

Surgical Results

At the time of this publication, 60 patients have undergone the Maze procedure since September 1987, with intermediate-term (> 6 months) follow-up available in 34. The indications for surgery included arrhythmia intolerance in 56 per cent (19 of 34), drug intolerance in 29 per cent (10 of 34), and transient ischemic attack in 15 per cent (5 of 34). In all patients, the Maze procedure has prevented the occurrence of atrial fibrillation and restored AV conduction. Because a number of patients have underlying sick sinus syndrome, dual-chamber pacemakers have been implanted in approximately 40 per cent of patients for atrial chronotropic support. Atrioventricular conduction has been intact in all patients. Finally, atrial contraction has been demonstrated in all patients postoperatively by either dynamic magnetic resonance imaging (MRI) or echocardiography. Thus the Maze operation, based on intermediate-term follow-up data, appears to approach the "ideal" procedure for the cure of atrial fibrillation.

Summary

Ablative therapy for arrhythmias is in a continual state of evolution. Currently, surgical intervention for accessory atrioventricular connections and AV nodal reentrant tachycardias is reserved for those patients who fail RF ablative therapy. It is possible that RF therapy may be successful in a number of patients with ectopic atrial tachycardias as well. The complexity and variability of ventricular tachyarrhythmias and the associated diseases (e.g., coronary artery disease, ventricular aneurysms) make surgical therapy the option of choice in most patients. The effect of the availability of the ICD devices has impacted positively on the mortality for direct surgery for ventricular tachycardia, and ICD therapy continues to be expanded to different patient populations with ventricular tachyarrhythmias and sudden cardiac death. The Maze procedure provides an experimentally and clinically verified treatment for patients with chronic or paroxysmal atrial fibrillation. Further clinical experience and longer follow-up are necessary to determine if the risk of thromboembolism is decreased in this patient population as well.

CARDIAC PACEMAKERS

The implantable cardiac pacemaker was first developed in 1960 by Chardack and associates, using a single-chamber device that paced the ventricle asynchronously and was implanted through a left thoracotomy incision. In the ensuing 30 years, the developments in pacing have clearly prolonged life and improved the quality of life. At the present time, technologic developments in pacing are proceeding at a remarkable rate, such that current devices are implanted completely transvenously, are capable of more than ten different pacing modes, pace both the atria and ventricles synchronously, and are less than one tenth the size of the original devices. With the rapid developments in microcomputer technology, these advances are certain to continue well into the next century.

Electrophysiology of Cardiac Pacing

Automaticity is a property of certain cells in the atrial tissue under normal conditions, specifically the *sinoatrial* (SA) nodal tissue and the AV nodal tissue. These specialized cells of the cardiac conduction tissue are capable of spontaneous depolarization and are responsible for initiation of the cardiac impulse under normal conditions. Different cells within the sinoatrial pacemaker complex appear to dominate at different degrees of cholinergic and sympathetic stimulation, corresponding to the normal chronotropic responsiveness of cardiac tissue. Activation of atrial tissue occurs as a result of the myocardial cell-to-cell syncytium and is more rapid in some areas than others. Decremental conduction is a normal property of AV nodal tissue, and the AV node is the location of both normal and pathologic forms of second- and third-degree heart block. The ventricles are activated after conduction of the impulse through the bundle of His, the bundle branches, and the Purkinje fibers to the cell-to-cell syncytium of ventricular myocardium.

Myocardial cells can also be depolarized by artificially applied electrical stimuli. The stimulus must have sufficient strength to bring a critical number of ventricular or atrial cells to threshold. When an activation wavefront is initiated by an artificial stimulus, it propagates throughout the myocardium in the manner of a normal cardiac impulse. This unique property of myocardial tissue forms the basis for artificial cardiac pacing.

Current Pacing Technology

Endocardial pacing leads consist of one (unipolar) or two (bipolar) electrode wires insulated with a polyurethane or silicon external coating. The electrode is the uninsulated tip that comes in contact with the myocardial tissue. In unipolar systems the cathode (negative) is in contact with the myocardial tissue and the circuit is completed by making the pacemaker the anode (positive). In bipolar systems, the cathode is in contact with the myocardium and the anode is a second electrode located approximately 1 cm farther proximal on the electrode wire. The exposed tip of the electrode is usually made of platinum, iridium, nickel alloys, or activated carbon. Porous or solid platinum-iridium electrode tips are the most commonly used. Steroid-eluting electrode tips have also been developed, the concept being that chronic leakage of a small amount of steroid at the tip over time minimizes the tissue reaction at the electrode-myocardial interface and causes lower chronic pacing thresholds.

Epicardial electrodes are screwed into the epicardium of the ventricle or hooked into the atrial myocardial tissue. They may be either unipolar (single electrode) or two may be placed adjacent to one another for a bipolar configuration. Epicardial electrodes generally must be placed at the time of the cardiac surgical procedure or, if done separately, through a thoracotomy or subxiphoid approach. Endocardial electrode placement is preferred when possible.

Endocardial transvenous electrodes are passed into the appropriate chamber of the heart using a system of stylet guidewires. Attachment of the lead electrode tip to the myocardial tissue is accomplished either actively or passively. Active-fixation leads have a tiny screw mechanism that "actively" attaches the tip to the heart tissue. Passive-fixation lead tips consist of three or more tines of polyurethane or silicon that are designed to insinuate themselves into the trabeculations of the apical right ventricular endocardium or the atrial trabeculations in the atrial appendage.

The ability to capture the myocardial tissue and to sense the patient's intrinsic electrical activity affects the size of the electrode tip. The larger tip provides a greater surface area for sensing, while a smaller tip produces lower thresholds because of higher current density. Typical electrode surface areas for pacing are 8 to 10 mm^2.

Pulse generators contain the power source for the pacing system as well as the computerized microchip circuitry that properly times the sensing and pacing functions of the device and provides for telemetry of on-line and stored information. Current solid-state power cells have a dry, crystalline electrolyte between the anode and cathode, most commonly lithium and iodine, respectively. Electrical current is produced by ionization of the anode, causing migration of positively charged metallic ions (lithium) through the electrolyte toward the cathode (iodine) to form a lithium-iodide electrolyte barrier. The higher the resistance in the electrolyte conductor, the longer the life expectancy of the power cell. Currently, most dual-chamber pacemakers last 7 to 10 years depending upon the degree of pacemaker dependence of the patient.

The "brains" of modern pacemakers are integrated in circuitry embedded on microchips that function essentially as microcomputers. These systems contain central processing units; some memory capability; and input-output circuits that perform all pacing, sensing, and timing functions. As with most small computers, reprogramming can be done by software rather than hardware changes. The most dramatic advances in pacing technology that are apt to occur over the next decade will be in the area of memory storage and on-line telemetry of electrophysiologic information.

These advances in microchip technology have permitted the interface of pacing with physiology over the past 8 years, leading to the development of "activity" pacemakers. These devices have sensors that monitor physiologic response in an on-line manner. This information is used by the device to provide physiologic chronotropic support for the patient to meet the physiologic demands of the activity being performed. The two most commonly implanted pacemakers at Washington University use a piezoelectric crystal attached to the posterior aspect of the generator that senses the increased activity of the chest wall skeletal muscle associated with patient activity and translates it into an increase in the rate output of the device. When the activity ceases, the rate of the pacemaker gradually slows back down to the baseline resting level. Other physiologic sensors include those that monitor minute ventilation, temperature, QT interval, and oxygen saturation. Currently under investigation are devices that incorporate multiple physiologic sensors with auto-programming functions to mimic exactly the normal conduction system in terms of chronotropic function.

The size of pacing devices continues to decline. Most dual-chamber pacemakers weigh less than 30 gm and are less than 4 mm thick, without a loss in the expected longevity of the device. The smallest single-chamber device available is only slightly larger than a quarter. In the future, truly "smart pacemakers" will incorporate pacing, sensing, physiologic, and telemetry information into an integrated package; will monitor the overall integrity of the recipient's physiologic state; and will adjust itself accordingly.

Indications for Cardiac Pacing

With the advent of this technology, the indications for cardiac pacing have grown from complete heart block, which was the first indication, to a large number of relatively complicated supraventricular and ventricular conduction disturbances. The final decision regarding pacemaker implantation should ideally be made in conjunction with the primary care provider, a cardiology and/or electrophysiology consultant, and the implanting physician.

Selection of the Type of Pacing System

Given the variability of certain of the underlying arrhythmias, and the multiprogrammability of the devices, the options for pacing in the present era are multiple and complex and require a great deal of expertise to maximally benefit the individual patient.

Pacemaker Implantation

In adults, most devices are implanted using a subclavian approach. At Washington University, where approximately 300 new devices are implanted each year, greater than 98 per cent are performed using this technique. The leads are introduced into the left or right subclavian vein beneath the clavicle and advanced under fluoroscopic control into the atrium or ventricle. After positioning, the pacing, sensing, and impedance characteristics of the lead are tested using a *pacing system analyzer*. Because these thresholds change over the first 6 weeks following implant, low-pacing thresholds and high-sensing thresholds at implant are necessary. The lead or leads are connected to the generator, which is implanted in a pocket on the anterior chest wall. The subxiphoid or anterior thoracotomy approach is used for epicardial ventricular lead implantation in adults with difficult endocardial pacing problems and occasionally in children. However, with advances in technology, even small infants who require pacing for congenital conduction defects can usually undergo transvenous implantation of a device, and the leads are positioned so as to permit growth of the child. Complications of pacemaker insertion include pneumothorax, hemorrhage, perforation, infection, and device failure. These are infrequent and readily treatable when they occur.

Follow-Up of Pacemaker Patients

Given the complexity of pacemakers today, adequate follow-up is absolutely mandatory and has gone beyond the scope of many practitioners not actively involved in electrophysiologic cardiovascular disease. Following implant, all patients undergo a complete pacemaker system evaluation. All devices are multi-programmable, using a radiofrequency induction coil to communicate with the device. The sensing and pacing characteristics of the generator are fine tuned to provide an adequate safety factor for pacing and sensing. In patients with activity devices, the activity mode is activated and the parameters are set. Follow-up after discharge is usually by pacemaker-telephone telemetry, where the basic characteristics of the pacemaker system can be determined over a special telephone connection. Occult problems with programming, generator end-of-life, or changes in the underlying rhythm can readily be detected with these simple yet effective devices. The complexity of the current pacemaker systems requires that most patients return to the pacemaker center for a complete evaluation once or twice annually.

Temporary Cardiac Pacing

Most commonly, temporary cardiac pacing is used following all types of open heart surgery, both in adults and in children. Temporary atrial and ventricular pacing wires are placed at the time of the operation and brought out through the skin, and these wires are removed prior to discharge. Until recently, only single-chamber (VVI or AAI) or atrially committed dual-chamber (DVI) devices were available for temporary pacing in this setting. While helpful in restoring atrioventricular synchrony, the committed pacing of the atrium in the setting of the atrial ectopy that frequently occurs following open heart surgery undoubtedly resulted in "creation" of the substrate for atrial fibrillation and flutter. More recently, the dual-chamber pacing technology developed for permanently implantable devices has been applied to temporary pacing. These new temporary pacemakers have an atrial sensing circuit capable of detecting the patient's intrinsic atrial rhythm(s) and inhibiting the atrial output of the device when appropriate. Use of these devices may decrease the incidence of supraventricular arrhythmias in the postoperative period in many cardiac surgical patients.

Summary

Rapid advances in pacing technology will continue to impact on the quality of life of many patients with cardiovascular disease. A truly "smart" device, which seemed fanciful 30 years ago, now seems to be a virtual certainty early in the next century.

CARDIAC ARREST

Over the past 15 years, advances in *cardiopulmonary resuscitation* (CPR) and *emergency cardiac care* (ECC) have dramatically improved the survival for certain patients with profound circulatory collapse and cardiac arrest. However, the magnitude of this problem remains great. Although declining over the past several decades, the mortality due to cardiovascular disease approaches nearly 1 million individuals annually, with approximately 500,000 of these deaths due to coronary artery disease (CAD), and most due to sudden death. Some 45 per cent of all heart attacks occur in people under the age of 65, and approximately 65 per cent of sudden deaths due to CAD occur outside the hospital and usually within 2 hours of the onset of symptoms. Thus, sudden death due to CAD is the most prominent medical emergency in this country. Implementation of the basic principles of CPR and ECC can profoundly effect survival in these patients. In addition, these techniques are applicable to victims of trauma (particularly in pediatric and young adult patients), drowning, electrocution, suffocation, and drug intoxication.

Basic Life Support

The major objective of *basic life support* (BLS) is to provide oxygen to the brain and heart until appropriate, definitive medical treatment can restore normal cardiac and ventilatory action. This objective is accomplished by preventing respiratory or circulatory arrest or insufficiency through prompt recognition and intervention and supporting the ventilation of a victim of respiratory arrest with rescue breathing or the ventilation and circulation of a victim of cardiac arrest with CPR. *Advanced cardiac life support* (ACLS) constitutes that definitive medical treatment. For cardiac arrest, the highest hospital discharge rate has been achieved in patients in whom CPR was initiated within 4 minutes of arrest and ACLS within 8 minutes. Thus, rapid assessment and response is essential for survival.

BLS Sequence

Because most adults (80 to 90 per cent) with sudden atraumatic cardiac arrest are found to be in ventricular fibrillation at the time the initial ECG is obtained, early defibrillation coupled with early bystander CPR has been shown to significantly increase the chance for survival.

1. Rapid and accurate assessment of the situation is critical, to include determination of unresponsiveness, breathlessness, and pulselessness. If head or neck trauma has been sustained, movement of the patient is contraindicated unless absolutely necessary to prevent further injury.

2. Since rapid defibrillation is essential, the BLS guidelines currently recommend activating the emergency medical system (EMS) *before* beginning CPR by calling 911 or the local emergency telephone number. Information such as the location, the calling phone number, the number of victims involved, how many of the victims need assistance, the layperson's diagnosis, and the aid being given to the victims is generally requested.

3. Once the EMS system has been activated, the person administering BLS must position the patient in the supine position on a flat surface. The head, neck, and torso should remain in the same plane. The airway should be assessed by opening the victim's mouth and removing all foreign debris. In the absence of a neck injury, the head tilt–chin lift maneuver is performed by placing the palm of one hand on the forehead of the patient to push the head down, while pull-

ing up on the underside of the chin with the other hand. This elevates the lower jaw (and the tongue) off the posterior pharynx. In this position, the rescuer is capable of determining breathlessness by listening to the open mouth for airway movement and observing at the chest for respiratory inspiration and expiration. If stable spontaneous respirations are resumed, the victim should be placed in the *recovery position* (on the side with the head supported) in the absence of head or neck trauma. This position helps to maintain an open airway.

If ventilation is not present or cannot be sustained by the victim, rescue breathing should be performed. The rescuer's exhaled air contains enough oxygen to supply the acute needs of the victim. Two initial slow breaths are administered, followed by 10 to 12 breaths per minute. Adequate ventilation (800 to 1200 ml volume) is indicated by *chest wall movement* and *audible exhalation*. Mouth-to-mouth breathing is preferred. If ventilation through the victim's mouth is impossible, mouth-to-nose rescue breathing is recommended. Mouth-to-barrier device breathing is becoming more common in the present environment. Two broad categories of barrier devices are available. Mask devices have a one-way valve so that exhaled air does not enter the rescuer's mouth, while face shields do not have an exhalation valve and air often leaks around the shield.

For one-rescuer CPR, a pause for ventilation should be taken after every 15th chest compression. For two-rescuer CPR, a pause for ventilation should be taken after every fifth compression. Exhalation is passive and occurs during chest compressions.

4. Pulselessness is determined by palpation of the carotid artery. Pressure should not be applied for longer than 5 to 10 seconds. Chest compressions in the pulseless patient consist of a series of rhythmic applications of pressure over the lower half of the sternum. While the exact mechanism of forward blood flow is controversial and may be variable, a generalized increase in intrathoracic pressure or direct compression of the heart has a role. The patient must be horizontal, or blood flow to the brain is further compromised. The proper compression technique involves locked elbows, with the rescuer's shoulders directly over his or her own hands. Compression of the average adult sternum should be over a distance of 1.5 to 2 inches. If possible, palpation of the carotid pulse during compression should be performed. Arterial compression during chest compression is maximal when the duration of compression is 50 per cent of the compression-release cycle. A target rate of 80 to 100 compressions per minute is necessary. Higher rates (120 compressions per minute) have been advocated as well.

5. For a single rescuer, after four cycles of compressions and ventilation (15:2 ratio), the rescuer should reevaluate the patient by palpating for a carotid pulse and observing for an effective ventilatory effort. If these are not present, CPR should be reinstituted until the EMS technicians arrive. For two rescuers, the same compression rate and assessment parameters should be obtained. When the compressor becomes fatigued, the two individuals should exchange positions as rapidly as possible. The generated pulse of the compressions should be monitored frequently by the ventilating rescuer.

The major complication of rescue breathing is gastric distention resulting from volume and rate excesses. Distention can promote regurgitation and aspiration, particularly if the stomach was full at the time of the arrest. Rib and/or sternal fractures, pneumothoraces, and lung lacerations are the major complications of chest compressions. All of these complications can be minimized with careful attention to the details outlined above.

6. Airway obstruction may be caused by intrinsic and extrinsic obstruction. Foreign-body obstruction should be suspected in any victim who suddenly stops breathing, becomes cyanotic, and falls unconscious for no apparent reason. Although this usually occurs during eating, in the pediatric age group, it may result from ingestion of any number of foreign objects. Partial or complete obstruction is possible. Persistent partial obstruction and complete obstruction should precipitate activation of the EMS service. Rapid evacuation of the obstructing material from the posterior pharynx is essential for survival. The so-called Heimlich maneuver (subdiaphragmatic abdominal thrusts) elevates the diaphragm, forcing air from the lungs and creating an artificial cough that expels the foreign material. Each individual thrust should be administered with the intent of relieving the obstruction. If the patient is standing or sitting, the maneuver should be performed from behind, with the rescuer's fists grasped over the victim's abdomen. With the victim supine, the rescuer sits astride the victim's knees and delivers the thrusts beneath the xiphoid with the base of the palms of the hand. If the patient is unconscious, a finger may be used to clear the posterior pharynx of foreign material. If the victim passes from consciousness to unconsciousness during the attempted resuscitation, an oral evacuation should be performed at that point.

7. The new guidelines contain additional recommendations regarding disease transmission during CPR. The layperson who performs CPR, whether on an adult or a pediatric victim, is most likely to do so in the home, where 70 to 80 per cent of respiratory and cardiac arrests occur. Because of the concern about disease transmission between victim and rescuer, the guidelines established by the Centers for Disease

Control and the Occupational Safety and Health Administration should be followed. For health care workers, guidelines include the use of barriers (latex gloves) and mechanical ventilation equipment (bag-valve masks and other masks capable of diverting expired air from the rescuer). Rescuers who have an infection should not perform mouth-to-mouth resuscitation if circumstances allow other immediate or effective methods of ventilation. The probability of infection with hepatitis B virus (HBV) or human immunodeficiency virus (HIV) is minimal. Transmission of HBV and HIV between health care workers and patients has been documented as a result of blood exchange or penetration of the skin by blood-contaminated instruments, and transmission of HBV and HIV infection during mouth-to-mouth resuscitation has not been documented. HBV-positive saliva has not been shown to be infectious, even to oral mucous membranes. In addition, saliva has not been implicated in the transmission of HIV after bites, percutaneous inoculation, or contamination of cuts and open wounds with saliva from HIV-infected patients.

Advanced Cardiac Life Support

Advanced cardiac life support includes (1) BLS, (2) the use of adjunctive equipment and special techniques for establishing and maintaining effective ventilation and circulation, (3) ECG monitoring and arrhythmia recognition, (4) establishment and maintenance of intravenous (IV) access, (5) therapies for emergency treatment of patients with cardiac and respiratory arrests (including stabilization in the postarrest phase), and (6) treatment of patients with suspected acute myocardial infarction (MI).

Airway Management

With respiratory arrest, a number of adjuncts for oxygenation delivery, including ventilatory devices and airway control, are available for ACLS. In essentially all circumstances, 100 per cent oxygen should be administered during the resuscitation effort. Masks, bag-valve devices, oxygen-powered manually triggered devices, and automatic transport ventilators (ATVs) have been demonstrated to be effective in certain circumstances. Of these, the ATVs have a number of advantages to alternative methods of ventilation in both unintubated and intubated patients. Oropharyngeal and nasopharyngeal airways should be used when possible for patients who are not intubated. The indications for endotracheal intubation include (1) inability of the rescuer to ventilate the unconscious patient with conventional methods, (2) inability of the patient to protect her or his airway (coma, areflexia, cardiac arrest), (3)

cardiac arrest with ongoing chest compressions, or (4) inability of a conscious patient to ventilate adequately. Endotracheal intubation should always be performed by a trained individual, and the maximum interruption of ventilation during CPR should be 30 seconds. Gentle pressure should be applied to the lateral aspects of the cricoid cartilage and maintained until the endotracheal tube cuff is inflated. Careful auscultation of the epigastrium and documentation of airway movement during the first gentle manual breaths is mandatory to exclude esophageal intubation. A selected tidal volume of 12 to 15 ml/kg should be delivered at 12 to 15 ventilations per minute. This ventilatory effort should not be synchronized with chest compressions. Each breath should be delivered over 2 seconds. Endotracheal suctioning should be performed if possible after establishment of the airway.

Assessment, Monitoring, and Vascular Access

There are no good prognostic guidelines to assess the efficacy of ongoing CPR efforts. In patients for whom arterial pressure monitoring is available, optimizing diastolic and myocardial perfusion pressure during CPR is indicated.

As most deaths are caused by electrical derangements of the heart, ECG monitoring should be established immediately. "Quick-look" defibrillator paddles can be used initially to avoid delay in the resuscitation. At a minimum, it should be possible to recognize: (1) sinus tachycardia, (2) sinus bradycardia, (3) premature atrial complexes, (4) paroxysmal supraventricular tachycardia (PSVT), (5) atrial flutter and fibrillation, (6) junctional rhythms, (7) atrioventricular block of all degrees, (8) premature ventricular complexes (PVCs), (9) ventricular tachycardia including torsades de pointes, (10) ventricular fibrillation, and (11) asystole. Distinction between rapid, wide complex supraventricular tachycardias and VT can be difficult. If the patient is pulseless, in shock, or in congestive heart failure, such rhythms should always be assumed to be VT and managed accordingly.

Vascular access during a cardiac arrest must be deferred for basic CPR, defibrillation, and airway management. During ongoing chest compressions, a peripheral (antecubital or external jugular) vein should be cannulated. Medications require 1 to 2 minutes to reach the central circulation when given by a peripheral vein and should be given rapidly and followed by a bolus of intravenous fluid. If spontaneous circulation cannot be restored, a central (internal jugular or subclavian) vein should be cannulated. However, early defibrillation should take priority over central venous access if defibrillation is indicated. Upper thoracic access is preferred, as little cephalad blood flow occurs from below the diaphragm during CPR.

Endotracheal medication administration (epinephrine, lidocaine, atropine) can be useful in those situations when vascular access hasn't been established. Drug dosages at 2 to 2.5 times the recommended IV dosage should be diluted in 10 ml of saline or distilled water, injected down a catheter passed beyond the tip of the endotracheal tube directly onto the tracheal mucosa, and followed by several rapid insufflations of the lungs to aerosolize the medication and facilitate its dispersion. Interosseous administration of drugs is an excellent alternative, particularly in pediatric patients. Somewhat higher than recommended intravenous drug dosages should be administered.

Drugs Used in ACLS

OXYGEN. As mentioned above, 100 per cent oxygen should be administered regardless of the cause of the hypoxemia.

IV FLUIDS. Volume expansion is critical in many noncardiac conditions requiring ACLS (ruptured blood vessel, shock due to volume loss). Crystalloid solutions (0.9 per cent NaCl or Ringer's lactate) or colloid solutions (6 per cent hetastarch, human serum albumin) are used most commonly in out-of-hospital settings. Blood products should be administered, if possible, after crossmatch. Unless specifically indicated, normal saline should be used for maintenance of line patency, as D_5W may cause hyperglycemia, which has been shown to worsen neurologic prognosis in patients suffering a cardiac arrest.

Drugs for Control of Cardiac Arrhythmias

The toxic-to-therapeutic balance of *lidocaine* is delicate, and recent data indicate that routine prophylactic use of lidocaine in patients suspected of having an MI is not indicated. However, therapeutic administration is indicated with determination of drug levels and lowering of the dose at 24 to 48 hours is recommended. Intravenous *procainamide* is recommended when an allergy to lidocaine is present or when lidocaine fails to suppress ventricular ectopy or restore a regular rhythm. Blood levels of procainamide and the N-acetyl metabolite should be closely monitored. The drug has well-documented proarrhythmic effects, particularly in patients with prolongation of the QT interval. In these patients procainamide is contraindicated. *Bretylium tosylate* is recommended in the treatment of (1) resistant VT and VF unresponsive to defibrillation, epinephrine, and lidocaine; (2) recurrent VT/VF after the above therapy; (3) hemodynamically stable VT that is not controlled by lidocaine and procainamide; and (4) wide-complex tachycardias that are not controlled by lidocaine and adenosine.

Within 4 hours of thrombolytic therapy for acute MI, *β-blockade* may reduce the rate of nonfatal reinfarction and recurrent ischemia. Atenolol, metoprolol, and propranolol reduce the incidence of VF in post-MI patients not receiving thrombolytic agents. *Atropine sulfate* is useful for symptomatic bradycardia and asystole, reversing cholinergic-mediated depression of heart rate, hypotension, and vascular resistance. Atropine should be used very cautiously in the setting of acute MI. The only indication for *isoproterenol* in ACLS is for refractory torsades de pointes and immediate temporary control of hemodynamically significant bradycardia in cardiac transplant recipients. *Verapamil and diltiazem* may terminate reentrant supraventricular arrhythmias that require AV-nodal conduction as part of the reentrant circuit. They also may control the ventricular response rate in patients with atrial fibrillation, flutter, or multifocal atrial tachycardia.

Adenosine is the agent of choice for diagnosing (and terminating) supraventricular arrhythmias. The endogenous purine nucleoside depresses sinoatrial and AV-nodal impulse formation and conduction. If the arrhythmia is not due to reentry involving the AV node or sinus node (e.g., flutter, fibrillation, ectopic atrial tachycardia, or ventricular arrhythmias), adenosine administration does not terminate the arrhythmia but may cause transient heart block, which may help clarify the underlying rhythm problem. The half-life of adenosine is less than 5 seconds, and the drug produces no intrinsic cardiac or hemodynamic compromise. *Magnesium deficiency* is associated with cardiac arrhythmias, symptoms of cardiac insufficiency, and sudden cardiac death. In addition, magnesium infusion may reduce the incidence of postinfarction ventricular arrhythmias.

Drugs for Pharmacologic Hemodynamic Resuscitation

The following drugs utilized in ACLS either affect peripheral vascular tone or augment the myocardial inotropic and/or chronotropic response.

The beneficial effect of *epinephrine* during cardiac arrest is due to its α-adrenergic receptor–stimulating properties, which act to increase myocardial and cerebral blood flow during CPR. 1 mg (10 ml of a 1:10,000 solution) is administered IV every 3 to 5 minutes during resuscitation. Some controversy exists regarding *low-dose* versus *high-dose* initial administration. Currently, however, the initial 1-mg dose is recommended, followed by a 5-mg dose if the initial dose fails. The pharmacologic effects of *norepinephrine, dopamine, dobutamine,* and *amrinone* in ACLS are similar to those for perioperative cardiovascular system support.

Retrospective and prospective studies have not demonstrated a benefit to the use of *calcium* in cardiac arrest. Theoretically, high levels of intracellular calcium may be detrimental. Thus, during ACLS, calcium chloride (10 per cent solution, 2 to 4 mg/kg) should only be given in the setting of hyperkalemia and hypocalcemia or after multiple blood transfusions or calcium channel blocker toxicity.

Digitalis preparations have very limited use in the setting of ACLS. *Intravenous nitroglycerin* is an effective adjunct in the treatment of unstable angina and congestive heart failure in the setting of acute myocardial infarction. In combination with dobutamine, considerable improvement in hemodynamic performance can be achieved with reduction in the risk of ischemic damage. The pharmacologic effects of nitroglycerin are primarily dependent on the patient's intravascular volume status and less on the dosage; 30 to 40 µg/min produces venodilation, while 150 to 500 µg/min produces arteriolar dilatation.

Laboratory and clinical data indicate that *sodium bicarbonate* administration (1) does not improve the ability to achieve defibrillation during CPR; (2) shifts the oxyhemoglobin saturation curve to the left, inhibiting oxygen release; (3) induces hyperosmolarity and hypernatremia; (4) produces paradoxic acidosis due to production of carbon dioxide (which diffuses into myocardial and cerebral cells, thereby depressing function); and (5) may inactivate simultaneously administered catecholamines. During CPR, carbon dioxide generated in tissues is not cleared well by low blood flow. The mainstay of acid-base balance during cardiac arrest is adequate alveolar ventilation and prompt restoration of tissue perfusion, beginning with effective CPR. Adrenergic responsiveness, the ability to defibrillate, the ability to restore spontaneous circulation, and short-term survival are not effected by low pH. Administration of bicarbonate may be beneficial in hyperkalemia or drug overdose (tricyclic antidepressant or phenobarbital). An initial dose of 1 mg/kg, followed by half of the initial dose every 10 minutes thereafter, is recommended.

Defibrillator Therapy

The recommended energy for initial defibrillation attempts is 200 joules (J), for the second shocks 200 to 300 J, and a third shock of 360 J. Again, the most important determinant of survival in adult out-of-hospital arrest is rapid defibrillation, and the defibrillation attempts should be undertaken as soon as the equipment arrives on the scene. The initial energy for cardioversion of hemodynamically significant atrial fibrillation and flutter is 100 J, delivered synchronously. Stepwise increases in energy are made if the initial attempts fail. There is no evidence that attempting to defibrillate "asystole" is successful; however, multiple leads should be checked to assure that a single recording lead is not missing the recording of fine VF.

Temporary Pacing During ACLS

Temporary pacing should be initially attempted transcutaneously during ACLS because of the speed with which it can be instituted. The Zoll transcutaneous pacing system, in development for over 20 years, provides the capability for this type of temporary pacing. Indications for emergent pacing include hemodynamically unstable bradycardia, bradycardia with malignant escape rhythms unresponsive to pharmacologic therapy, and occasionally to terminate supraventricular or ventricular arrhythmias. In patients dependent on pacing, once the situation is stabilized temporary transvenous leads can be placed.

MANAGEMENT OF THE PATIENT WITH HEART DISEASE

Patients with a significant history of cardiac disease undergoing surgical procedures require careful preoperative preparation and close surveillance during and after operation. Their management is based on a thorough understanding of physiologic principles and pharmacologic interventions to maintain cardiovascular homeostasis. Clinical pharmacology has progressed to the point that specific drugs can now alter virtually any parameter of cardiac physiology.

Clinical Physiology

Preoperative surgical risk related to cardiovascular disease must be carefully assessed in all patients before surgical intervention. A history of recent myocardial infarction (<3 months), congestive heart failure, angina, poorly controlled hypertension, rhythm disturbances, and pulmonary or renal problems must be fully evaluated prior to surgical intervention if at all possible. Confirmation of these findings on physical and laboratory examinations should suggest additional preoperative work-up. The indications, dosages, and efficacy of chronic drug therapy for these diseases should be assessed, and dosages altered if necessary prior to surgery.

Once the patient comes to the operating room, perioperative cardiac performance is assessed by (1) evaluation of clinical signs, including peripheral pulses, capillary refill, and skin temperature; (2) peripheral perfusion assessment by measurement of peripheral oxygenation; (3) electrocardiographic monitoring; (4) hemodynamic measurements, including central venous, systemic, and pulmonary arterial pressures;

(5) systemic and pulmonary vascular resistances; and (6) cardiac output. A cardiac index (stroke volume times heart rate divided by body surface area) of 2 L/min/m^2 is considered adequate for maintenance of cerebral, coronary, and systemic perfusion. Based on these measurements, heart rate, afterload, preload, and contractility are controlled to optimize cardiac performance.

Afterload is the impedance to ventricular emptying that results from increasing arteriolar resistance. In the postoperative patient, this is most often due to hypertension. A greater afterload increases the work of the heart and thus myocardial oxygen consumption during the critical period during and following operation. *Preload* is the volume of blood available to fill the ventricles during diastole. On the basis of the Frank-Starling relationship, preload determines cardiac performance at the myocardial level on a beat-to-beat basis. The status of the peripheral venous capacitance and pulmonary arterial systems has a major role in determining preload. *Contractility* describes the vigor with which the heart contracts during each beat. It is largely determined by the level of endogenous or exogenous catecholamines acting on the cardiovascular system. The contractile state of the heart can be increased only with a concomitant increase in myocardial oxygen consumption.

Autonomic receptors on the heart, lungs, kidneys, and vascular smooth muscle are classified as α (or excitatory) or β (or inhibitory) according to their response to catecholamine stimulation. The vessels that cause increased arteriolar resistance (afterload) and venous capacitance (preload) contain α- and β-receptors, as do myocardial (contractility) and conduction (heart rate) tissues in the heart. Specific agonist and antagonist drugs can alter all four aspects of myocardial function by interaction at these vascular receptor sites (Table 1).

The Peripheral Cardiovascular System

In the perioperative patient, it is useful to group the venous and arteriolar vascular beds, the lungs, and the kidneys as one system involved in the regulation of intravascular volume. Pharmacologic agents that affect the peripheral cardiovascular system are listed in Table 2.

Antihypertensive and Vasodilating Agents

Peripheral vasodilator agents are used perioperatively to control hypertension and to optimize cardiac performance by altering afterload and preload. *Sodium nitroprusside* is given intravenously, and a hemodynamic response is noted rapidly following administration or termination of the drug. It acts on both the arteriolar and venous systems, augmenting stroke volume by increasing preload and decreasing afterload by α-blockade at the arteriolar level. It is metabolized to thiocyanate, which can be toxic after prolonged administration of high levels of the drug. *Chlorpromazine*, a phenothiazine, is a quick-acting (within 15 minutes) vasodilator useful in the treatment of acute postoperative hypertension. Its action is due to a combination of central and peripheral α-blockade effects. *Hydralazine* is a fast-acting agent that causes arteriolar and venous dilatation in 15 to 30 minutes following intramuscular (IM) or IV administration. It is also thought to have a positive inotropic effect, causing a significant increase in cardiac output with a relatively small drop in filling pressure. This effect, however, along with the resulting reflex tachycardia, increases myocardial oxygen consumption. *Prazosin* is a direct antagonist of the vascular α_1-receptor that dilates both the arteriolar and the venous peripheral systems and is useful in weaning patients from nitroprusside. *Clonidine* is a central nervous system (CNS) adrenergic inhibitor that reduces sympathetic outflow from vasopressor centers in the brain, and has the advantage of maintaining cardiac reflexes intact. Abrupt withdrawal preoperatively can precipitate hypertensive crises, but this agent can be useful in the postoperative period and should be restarted as soon as possible in patients who are taking it preoperatively. *Phentolamine* temporarily blocks both α_1- and α_2-receptors and is used as an arteriolar vasodilator. Its primary indications are for hypertensive crises and during anesthesia for pheochromocytoma surgery. *Nitrates* (topical, oral, and IV) are antianginal agents, have systemic vasodilating properties, and increase venous capacitance. Their major effect is pulmonary vasodilation, and thus they are useful in patients with pulmonary congestion. *Calcium channel blockers*, specifically nifedipine and verapamil, are mildly potent vasodilators that act through blockade of Ca^{++} entry into vascular smooth muscle cells. They also have antianginal effects, and electrophysiologic effects through their action on the sinoatrial and atrioventricular nodal tissue, and they are useful in weaning patients from nitroprusside in the postoperative period.

Vasoconstrictive Agents

Phenylephrine is a rapid-acting arteriolar and venous vasoconstrictor, and effect mediated by α_1 stimulation. It is used primarily to increase peripheral vascular resistance in postoperative cardiac patients. *Norepinephrine* is occasionally used as a vasoconstrictive agent in prolonged resuscitation efforts or during cardiopulmonary bypass when the systemic vascular

TABLE 1.   SPECIFIC AGONIST AND ANTAGONIST DRUGS THAT ALTER MYOCARDIAL INFARCTION

Effector Organ	Receptor Type	Agonist	Antagonist

Cardiac
  Conduction
  Myocardium
	β_1
	  Heart rate
	  Contractility
		Isoproterenol
		Epinephrine
		Dopamine
		Dobutamine
		Norepinephrine
			Propranolol
			Atenolol
			Metaprolol
			Esmolol

Arterioles	α_1, α_2 (vasoconstrictor)	Norepinephrine Epinephrine Dopamine Phenylephrine	Prazocin Phentolamine
	β_2 (vasodilator)	Isoproterenol Dopamine Dobutamine Epinephrine	Propranolol
Pulmonary	β_2 (bronchodilator)	Terbutaline Metaproterenol Isoproterenol Epinephrine	Propranolol
Renal	Dopaminergic (vasodilator)	Dopamine	

resistance cannot be supported by phenylephrine alone.

Angiotensin-Converting Enzyme (ACE) Inhibitors

Captopril inhibits the formation of angiotensin II, a potent vasoconstrictor. Used as an afterload-reducing agent in the treatment of heart failure, it has been shown to increase myocardial oxygen demand to a lesser degree than either prazosin or hydralazine. It has been successfully used to control hypertension in postoperative coronary bypass patients with residual myocardial dysfunction, acting to increase forward cardiac output with minimal increase in oxygen demand. However, due to renal excretion, it cannot be used in patients with elevated serum creatinine.

Enalapril is a recently available ACE inhibitor for IV administration that is useful in controlling postoperative hypertension, particularly in patients with abnormal ventricular function. Abrupt withdrawal can precipitate severe hypertension; therefore, these agents should be maintained throughout the perioperative period or alternative agents substituted in appropriate circumstances.

Diuretics

In the postoperative patients, diuretics are used to decrease total body water, thereby acting to decrease preload. *Furosemide* is a rapid-acting loop diuretic, with an effect lasting 2 to 3 hours following intravenous injection. Its action is kaliuretic, and potassium must be rigorously replaced in the postoperative patient to prevent arrhythmias. Furosemide is used to remove excess fluid accumulated following cardiopulmonary bypass and is used as a pulmonary vasodilator and is effective in acute pulmonary edema. *Ethacrynic acid* is also a loop agent, usually reserved for patients not responding to initial diuretic therapy. *Metolazone* is an oral thiazide diuretic, given in combination with intravenous loop agents to stimulate diuresis in patients developing acute renal failure postoperatively.

Pulmonary Bronchodilators

Because the pulmonary vasculature is innervated with α- and β-adrenoreceptors, agents used to treat bronchoconstriction in the immediate postoperative period can have significant cardiac side effects. *Metaproterenol* is a β_2-agonist bronchodilator used as an aerosolized inhaler for bronchial constriction (wheezing). Cardiovascular side effects including tachycardia can be minimized by adjusting the dosage. *Aminophylline* is an intravenous xanthine dilator, the drug used for initial treatment of significant postoperative bronchoconstriction. Cardiac side effects include tachycardia, decreased coronary blood flow, and increased myocardial oxygen extraction.

The Central Cardiovascular System

The heart itself constitutes the central cardiovascular system, which can be separated into *vascular*, *functional*, and *electrophysiologic* components. Optimal care of surgical patients requires knowledge of the

TABLE 2. PHARMACOLOGIC AGENTS THAT AFFECT THE CARDIOVASCULAR SYSTEM

The Peripheral Cardiovascular System
Vasodilating agents
  Sodium nitroprusside
  Chlorpromazine
  Hydralazine
  Prazocin
  Clonidine
  Phentolamine
  Nitrates
  Calcium channel blockers
Vasoconstrictor agents
  Phenylephrine
  Norepinephrine
Angiotensin II inhibitors
  Captopril
  Enalapril
Diuretics
  Furosemide
  Ethacrinic acid
  Metolazone
  Diamox
Pulmonary bronchodilators
  Metaproterenol
  Aminophylline

The Central Cardiovascular System
Vascular component
  Nitrates
  β-Adrenergic receptor blocking agents
  Calcium-channel blocking agents
Functional component
  Cardiac glycosides
  Adrenoreceptor agonists
    Dopamine
    Dobutamine
    Isoproterenol
    Epinephrine
    Norepinephrine
  Phosphodiesterase inhibitors
    Amrinone
  Calcium chloride or gluconate
  Cardiac assist device: intra-aortic balloon pump
Electrophysiologic component
  Supraventricular arrhythmias
    Bradycardia
      Atropine
      Isoproterenol
      Temporary pacing
    Sinus tachycardia
      β-blocking agents
      Neostigmine
      Lopressor
    Atrial fibrillation and flutter
      Digoxin
      β-blocking agents
      Verapamil
      Procainamide
      Quinidine
  Ventricular arrhythmias
    Ventricular premature complexes, tachycardias
      Lidocaine
      Procainamide
      Bretylium

multiple pharmacologic agents that affect each component (Table 2).

Vascular Component

Myocardial ischemia follows when oxygen demand exceeds oxygen supply, usually because of limitations of coronary blood flow. Surgical procedures constitute a significant stress in patients with cardiac disease, and proper management of antianginal medication in patients undergoing noncardiac operation is essential. Most patients with coronary artery disease undergoing bypass grafting are maintained on a combination of nitrates, β-blockers, and calcium antagonists.

Nitroglycerin (NTG) causes relaxation of all types of smooth muscle of the vascular system, and it is a potent coronary vasodilator. Relief of angina results from decreased wall tension with decreased ventricular volume (preload) and intraventricular pressure, which causes a decreased myocardial oxygen requirement. Patients with known or suspected coronary artery disease should be maintained on intravenous NTG during the perioperative period to prevent precipitation of angina.

β-Adrenergic receptor blocking agents block the principal β-receptor site on the heart. Diminished heart rate, blood pressure, contractility, and an increased diastolic perfusion time result, which decreases the myocardial oxygen requirements. Propranolol, nadolol, timolol, and pindolol are noncardioselective agents, while atenolol and metoprolol are cardioselective and are used preferentially in patients with severe pulmonary disease. Rebound effects from abrupt withdrawal of the drug should be avoided.

Calcium channel blocking agents such as nifedipine, verapamil, and diltiazem inhibit the slow inward current, are potent coronary vasodilators, and diminish myocardial oxygen consumption. They are particularly useful in patients with chronic obstructive pulmonary disease in whom β-blockade is not possible. However, they may unmask hypovolemia and cause significant hypotension after mild volume loss. Nifedipine is the drug of choice for vasospastic angina.

Functional Component

Myocardial contractility can be altered in the perioperative period by two types of agents, the *cardiac glycosides* and *β₁-receptor agonists*. The $β_1$-receptors normally respond to norepinephrine, released by the cardiac sympathetic nerves. With chronic cardiac failure the norepinephrine stores in these nerve endings are depleted and the heart becomes less responsive to endogenous catecholamine stimulation. However, the receptors remain intact and responsive to exogenously administered agents.

CARDIAC GLYCOSIDES. Digitalis is the only oral inotropic drug available for routine use. The inhibition of the Na/K adenosine triphosphatase pump at the sarcolemmal level is thought to increase cytosolic calcium concentration and thereby increase the contractile state. Maintenance of postoperative therapeutic drug levels is important for patients with cardiac disease undergoing noncardiac procedure. Digitalis products have recently been implicated with an increased risk of death in patients taking this drug for arrhythmia control and, therefore, should be used judiciously. Digitalis toxicity requires prompt diagnosis and treatment.

ADRENORECEPTOR AGONISTS. Across the pharmacologic spectrum, the sympathomimetic amines directly affect all four adrenoreceptor sites. These agents should be used only when it becomes necessary to support the failing circulation, because they uniformly increase myocardial oxygen consumption.

Dopamine is a catecholamine agent with a broad-action spectrum. It is an intermediate compound in the synthesis of epinephrine and norepinephrine and stimulates release of norepinephrine from the cardiac nerve endings. In low doses, it acts on β_1-receptors of the heart, producing positive chronotropic and inotropic responses. At medium doses, β_2-receptors in the periphery are stimulated, producing vasodilatation; but with high doses, vasoconstriction occurs, with stimulation of peripheral α_1-receptors. At low doses, specific dopaminergic receptors in the renal vascular bed are stimulated to increase renal blood flow and diuresis.

Dobutamine is a synthetic analog of dopamine and produces a relatively stronger inotropic (from direct β_1 stimulation) than chronotropic response. Conversion from dopamine to dobutamine may circumvent dopamine-induced tachycardia. In addition, in many patients there is a peripheral vasodilatory response due to a predominance of a β_2 effect over a mild peripheral α_1-agonist effect. As dobutamine does not rely on release of norepinephrine for its inotropic effect, it may be relatively more useful in patients with chronic heart failure who require support. It also decreases wall stress in the myocardial wall and is thus useful in patients with coronary artery disease.

Isoproterenol acts on the cardiac β_1- and peripheral β_2-receptors, causing vasodilatation, tachycardia, and increased contractile force. However, myocardial oxygen consumption increases out of proportion to the increase in contractility, limiting the drug's effectiveness. It is used for right-sided heart failure and for the drug's chronotropic effect in patients with sustained sinus bradycardia, particularly heart transplant recipients.

Epinephrine acts on all receptor sites at relatively low concentrations, increasing contractility and causing α-mediated vasoconstriction. Medium-dose epi-nephrine is useful in patients with inadequate peripheral vascular tone and near-adequate myocardial function. It is combined with dopamine or dobutamine to treat significant postoperative myocardial failure. Its use in ECC is described above.

Norepinephrine acts predominantly on the α-receptor in the periphery and the β_1-receptors on the heart. However, the increase in peripheral resistance causes a significant increase in myocardial oxygen consumption without augmentation of cardiac output. Its use is usually limited to patients with refractory cardiovascular collapse.

Amrinone is a phosphodiesterase type III inhibitor and acts by increasing cyclic adenosine monophosphate (cAMP) levels. It causes strong inotropic effects as well as direct arterial and venous vasodilatory effects, while having essentially no effect on heart rate. The peripheral vasodilatory effect can be variable, however. Long-term administration is associated with a nonimmunologically mediated thrombocytopenia.

Calcium. Augmentation of Ca^{++} availability to the contractile apparatus within the myocyte is the final common pathway of positive inotropic stimulation of the heart. Intravenous injection of calcium chloride or gluconate causes a positive inotropic response without increasing ventricular or altering peripheral vascular tone.

Cardiac Assist Devices. The intra-aortic balloon pump is used to treat medically uncontrollable angina in preoperative patients scheduled for *coronary artery bypass grafting* (CABG) and to facilitate discontinuation of *cardiopulmonary bypass* (CPB) in patients who are difficult or impossible to wean from CPB without such assistance. The pumping mechanism augments diastolic coronary perfusion and diminishes afterload with each beat.

Electrophysiologic Component

Arrhythmias in the perioperative surgical patient can be caused by multiple factors, including underlying cardiac disease, induction and reversal of anesthesia, electrolyte imbalance, and hypoxia. Each of these factors must be considered and corrected if present, whenever supraventricular and ventricular arrhythmias appear in postoperative patients.

In terms of therapy, investigators have classified antiarrhythmic compounds into four classes based on their effect on the action potential. Class I agents (lidocaine, quinidine, procainamide, disopyramide, phenytoin, mexiletine, aprindine, tocainide, and encainide) act on the fast sodium current. Class II agents (β-antagonist drugs) alter sympathetic activity. Class III agents (amiodarone and bretylium) affect repolarization and widen the action potential duration. Class

IV agents (calcium channel blocking drugs) affect the slow inward current.

Supraventricular Arrhythmias

Bradycardia due to excessive vagal parasympathetic input to the sinoatrial (SA) node can be treated with atropine; isoproterenol; or pacing by epicardial, esophageal, or transcutaneous leads in patients following surgical procedures. *Sinus tachycardia* increases myocardial oxygen requirements at rates much greater than 100 to 105 beats per minute, and the short diastolic filling time may compromise cardiac function. The rapid rate may be slowed by careful propranolol infusion or by neostigmine, an anticholinesterase agent. If hypertension is present, labetalol may also be carefully titrated to control the rate and blood pressure. *Atrial fibrillation and flutter* occurs in as many as 35 to 40 per cent of patients undergoing open heart procedures and in a number of patients with underlying cardiac disease who are subjected to general surgical procedures. Treatment depends on the degree of associated hemodynamic instability and the ventricular response rate.

Specific Therapies

PERIOPERATIVE ATRIAL FIBRILLATION AND FLUTTER

Digoxin slows conduction through the AV node, probably because of parasympathetic stimulation. Digitalization usually slows the ventricular response without additional antiarrhythmic agents. Correction of hypokalemia and hypoxia is important, because both conditions can exacerbate digitalis toxicity.

Intravenous propanolol slows conduction through the AV node and suppresses atrial ectopic foci, but bradycardia and cardiodepression are important deleterious side effects of such therapy. Intravenous esmolol is an ultra-short-acting cardioselective agent for intravenous use; its pharmacologic effect is dissipated within 30 minutes, and it is effective for β-blockade in the coronary care unit setting as well as perioperatively. β-Blockade is useful in cases of supraventricular tachycardia secondary to digitalis toxicity.

Intravenous verapamil converts rapid fibrillation to sinus rhythm in 10 to 15 per cent of patients by inhibiting calcium-mediated conduction in AV nodal tissue. Intravenous diltiazem has recently become available for maintenance infusion of calcium channel blockage until conversion to oral therapy can be achieved. These agents have no effect on ventricular arrhythmias. Concomitant propranolol therapy or digitalis toxicity are absolute contraindications to intra-

venous verapamil therapy, because complete heart block can occur.

Procainamide acts on both atrial and ventricular arrhythmias. In atrial fibrillation, it acts to suppress atrial ectopy once conversion to sinus rhythm has occurred. The N-acetyl metabolite also has antiarrhythmic properties, and serum levels of both drugs should be monitored. *Quinidine*, the prototype Class I antiarrhythmic agent, is used to suppress atrial and ventricular ectopy and to maintain sinus rhythm following chemical or electrical cardioversion. The mechanism of atrial flutter differs from that of fibrillation, but the treatment is similar. In cardiac patients who have temporary pacing wires in place, rapid atrial pacing often entrains the atrial focus, with conversion to a sinus rhythm. Atrial fibrillation does not respond to rapid atrial pacing. In both fibrillation and flutter, synchronized electrical cardioversion is used when significant hemodynamic instability is present.

VENTRICULAR ARRHYTHMIAS

The use of antiarrhythmic agents in the perioperative setting is similar to their use in ACLS. All patients exhibiting ventricular ectopy in the perioperative period should be treated with lidocaine. However, prophylactic therapy can no longer be supported due to the recognition of the proarrhythmic effects of antiarrhythmic agents. As mentioned, intravenous procainamide can also be used. However, for patients with persistent ectopy, oral suppressive therapy with quinidine or procainamide may be necessary. *Bretylium* is effective in managing ventricular fibrillation refractory to lidocaine and to electrical defibrillation, and its use is limited to refractory arrhythmias present during cardiac arrest. Tachycardia or fibrillation is immediately treated by defibrillation at 200, 300, and 360 J if necessary.

Clinical Therapy

Bradycardia should be treated with atropine, isoproterenol, or where feasible with temporary pacing to augment cardiac output. Postoperative hypertension is treated by afterload reduction. Restoration of adequate preload with volume replacement using colloid and crystalloid constitutes the initial therapy for hypotension. Blood or blood products are administered when indicated by the hematologic profile. Carefully planned and monitored peripheral vasoconstriction may be necessary to augment peripheral vascular resistance. Addition of afterload reduction to a volume-restored vascular space decreases the resistance to ventricular outflow and, thus, overall cardiac work. Using this combination of rate augmentation, volume replacement, and afterload reduction, an adequate cardiac output can be achieved in most patients with minimal increase in myocardial oxygen consumption. This rationale is particularly important following cardiac operation and when a major noncardiac surgical procedure is performed in a patient with underlying cardiac disease.

With adequate cardiac output, excess extravascular volume can be drawn into the vascular space and diuresis can be stimulated with diuretics or with low-dose dopamine acting on receptors in the kidney. Despite the above measures, however, adequate cardiac performance cannot be achieved in some patients. This may be due to reversible myocardial injury or to systemic processes affecting the heart, such as sepsis. The addition of sympathomimetic amines is indicated to augment contractility and to assure adequate perfusion of peripheral organ systems at adequate levels of perfusion pressure. All of these agents increase the work of the heart, augmenting myocardial oxygen consumption, and therefore should be used judiciously. Dobutamine or dopamine is usually the first agent of choice for a primary cardiac problem, alone or in combination with nitroprusside for afterload reduction. Alternatively, amrinone can be added to provide both afterload reduction and contractility support. If performance continues to be inadequate despite midrange dosages of these drugs, an additional inotropic agent, usually epinephrine, is initiated. The failing left ventricle can be additionally supported by insertion of an intra-aortic balloon pump. Isoproterenol can be added to support the right side of the circulation, and prostaglandin E_1 can be added for selective pulmonary vasodilation.

The use of this selective strategy, based on assessment and reassessment of adequate cardiac performance and optimization of each of the four components of cardiac function individually and then collectively, usually provides a therapeutic scheme to permit adequate perfusion of the heart and other organ systems even in very sick surgical patients.

Atrial fibrillation and flutter is treated initially by correction of the possible precipitating factors and etiologic conditions. A rapid ventricular response is controlled with digitalization. Rate response can also be controlled, and conversion to sinus rhythm can be attempted with intravenous verapamil, diltiazem, or β-blockade. Procainamide can be added to maintain sinus rhythm once conversion has occurred. The same sequence is used for atrial flutter with the added option of rapid atrial pacing in patients with postoperative temporary pacing wires in place. Immediate control and suppression of ventricular premature complexes and tachycardia are obtained with intravenous lidocaine, procainamide, or bretylium. Heart block in cardiac patients can be treated with temporary atrioventricular sequential pacing. Hemodynamic instability due to atrial or ventricular dysrhythmias

is immediately treated with cardioversion or defibrillation.

After the acute postoperative phase, patients can be gently weaned from cardiovascular system support and antiarrhythmic therapy in most cases. If continued support or therapy is necessary, conversion to oral agents can be easily accomplished during this weaning phase. Often, these oral agents can be discontinued by the time of the first or second postoperative visit, when the patient has fully recovered from the effects of the operation. A thorough understanding of these principles facilitates management of the cardiovascular system in surgical patients to ensure minimal morbidity and maximal recovery of cardiac function postoperatively.

REFERENCES

ACC/AHA Guidelines for Permanent Pacemaker Implantation. Circulation (in press).

Anderson RW, Visner MS: Shock and circulatory collapse. In Sabiston DC, Spencer FC (eds): Gibbon's Surgery of the Chest, ed 5. Philadelphia, WB Saunders Company, 1990.

Centers for Disease Control: Guidelines for prevention of transmission of human immunodeficiency virus and hepatitis B virus to health-care and public safety workers. MMWR 38(suppl 6):1–37, 1989.

Cox JL, Boineau JP, Schuessler RB, Ferguson TB Jr, Lindsay BD, Cain ME, Corr PB, Kater KM, Lappas DG: A review of surgery for atrial fibrillation. J Cardiovasc Electrophysiol 2:541–561, 1991.

Emergency Cardiac Care Committee and Subcommittees, American Heart Association: Guidelines for cardiopulmonary resuscitation and emergency cardiac care. JAMA 268:2171–2298, 1992.

Ferguson TB, Cox JL: Temporary external DDD pacing following cardiac surgery. Ann Thorac Surg 51:723–732, 1991.

Ferguson TB Jr, Cox JL: Surgical treatment of cardiac arrhythmias. In Chatterjee K, Cheitlin MD, Karliner J, Parmley WW, Rapaport E, Scheinman MM (eds): Cardiology. An Illustrated Text/Reference. Philadelphia, Lippincott/Gower, 1991.

Ferguson TB, Cox JL: Cardiac arrhythmia disturbances. In Shires GT, Barrie PS (eds): Surgical Intensive Care. Boston, Little, Brown & Co, 1993.

Ferguson TB Jr, Cox JL: Antiarrhythmic surgery: Ventricular arrhythmias. In Horowitz LN (ed): Current Management of Arrhythmias. Philadelphia, BC Decker, 1990, pp 382–391.

Ferguson TB Jr, Cox JL: Complications related to the surgical treatment of supraventricular and ventricular cardiac arrhythmias. In Waldhausen JA, Orringer MB (eds): Complications in cardiothoracic surgery. St. Louis, Mosby Year Book Publishers, 1990.

Ferguson TB Jr, Cox JL: Surgical therapy for patients with supraventricular tachycardia. In Scheinman MM (ed): Cardiology Clinics. Philadelphia, WB Saunders Company, 1990, pp 535–556.

Jackman WM, Wang X, Friday KJ, Roman CA, Moulton KP, Beckman KJ, McClelland JH, et al: Catheter ablation of accessory atrioventricular pathways (Wolff-Parkinson-White syndrome) by radiofrequency current. N Engl J Med 324:1605–1611, 1991.

Katz AM: Physiology of the Heart. New York, Raven Press, 1977.

Kette F, Weil MH, von Planta M, Gazmuri RJ, Rackow EC: Buffer agents do not reverse intramyocardial acidosis during cardiac resuscitation. Circulation 81:1660–1666, 1990.

Lau C-P: The range of sensors and algorithms used in rate adaptive cardiac pacing. PACE 15:1177–1211, 1992.

Malik M: How a computer computes: Hardware- and software-based pacemakers. PACE *15*:1212–1214, 1992.

Moses HW, Taylor GJ, Schneider JA, Dove JT (eds): A Practical Guide to Cardiac Pacing, ed 2. Boston, Little, Brown & Co, 1987.

Opie LH: The Heart-Physiology, Metabolism, Pharmacology and Therapy. London, Grune & Stratton, 1985.

Saksena S, Goldschlager N (eds): Electrical therapy for cardiac arrhythmias: Pacing, antitachycardia devices, catheter ablation. Philadelphia, WB Saunders Company, 1990.

Smith PK: Postoperative care in cardiac surgery. *In* Sabiston DC, Spencer FC (eds): Gibbon's Surgery of the Chest, ed 5. Philadelphia, WB Saunders Company, 1990.

Waldo AL, MacLean WAH: Diagnosis and Treatment of Cardiac Arrhythmias Following Open Heart Surgery. Mt. Kisco, NY, Futura Publishing Company, 1980.

ACQUIRED CARDIAC CONDITIONS: Aortic, Mitral, and Tricuspid Valve Disease and Hypertrophic Cardiac Myopathy

DONALD D. GLOWER, Jr., M.D.

ACQUIRED DISORDERS OF THE AORTIC VALVE

Aortic Stenosis

Pathophysiology

The aortic valve normally consists of three equal-sized leaflets termed the *right*, *left*, and *noncoronary cusps*. Congenital aortic stenosis may present early in life with a unicuspid or dome-shaped valve, or congenital bicuspid aortic stenosis may become symptomatic in the sixth to eighth decades as the bicuspid valve becomes progressively stenotic (Fig. 1). In adults, rheumatic aortic stenosis may produce leaflet fibrosis, fusion, and calcification, and degenerative aortic stenosis may develop from progressive valvular calcification.

Longstanding aortic stenosis causes increased left ventricular systolic pressure, compensatory left ventricular hypertrophy, and decreased left ventricular diastolic compliance. After a long asymptomatic phase, patients may develop angina from impaired myocardial blood flow, exercise induced syncope, and ultimately congestive heart failure, often with left ventricular dilation and decreased ejection fraction. Symptoms occur when the normal aortic valve area of 3 to 4 cm² becomes less than 1 cm², and severe aortic stenosis occurs when the mean left ventricular–to–aortic pressure gradient reaches 50 to 60 mm Hg or when calculated aortic valve area is less than 0.8 cm². Survival after onset of symptoms is generally 1 to 5 years (Fig. 2).

Diagnosis

Physical examination in aortic stenosis reveals a systolic murmur at the base of the heart radiating into the carotid arteries. The severity of aortic stenosis may be assessed using Doppler echocardiography and a modified Bernoulli equation:

$$\Delta_{pk} = 4V^2$$

where Δ_{pk} is the peak ventriculoaortic gradient and V is the maximal blood flow velocity (m/sec) across the valve. In addition, cardiac catheterization may allow direct measurement of the ventriculoaortic gradient

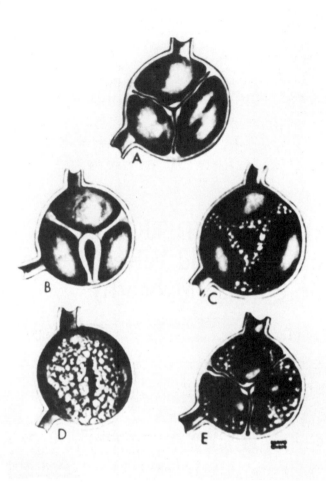

Figure 1. Forms of aortic stenosis. *A*, Normal aortic valve. *B*, Congenital aortic stenosis. *C*, Rheumatic aortic stenosis. *D*, Calcific aortic stenosis. E, Calcific senile aortic stenosis. (From Brandenburg R, et al: Valvular heart disease—when should the patient be referred? Pract Cardiol 5:50, 1979, with permission.)

and calculation of effective aortic valve area (AVA) using the Gorlin formula:

$$AVA(cm^2) = Q/(44.5 \sqrt{\Delta_{mean}})$$

where Δ_{mean} is the mean systolic ventriculoaortic gradient (mm Hg) and Q is the cardiac output (ml/min) per systolic ejection period (sec/min). A simplified Gorlin formula is:

$$AVA = cardiac\ output\ (L/min)\ \sqrt{\Delta_{mean}}$$

Treatment

Indications for intervention in aortic stenosis include onset of angina, syncope, or congestive heart failure, or, in an asymptomatic patient, onset of ven-

tricular dilation. Intervention generally requires aortic valve replacement, with an operative mortality of 2 to 8 per cent and a 5-year survival of 80 to 85 per cent. Symptoms resolve in most patients after aortic valve replacement, and ventricular dilation and hypertrophy may resolve over several months. Percutaneous aortic balloon valvuloplasty may provide some short-term (6 months) improvement of symptoms in patients who are not candidates for aortic valve replacement.

Aortic Insufficiency

Pathophysiology

Aortic insufficiency may be caused by congenital malformation of the aortic valve, rheumatic fever with valve thickening and retraction, myxoid degeneration of the valve as in Marfan's syndrome or connective tissue disease, infective endocarditis with bacterial destruction of leaflets, blunt trauma, aortic dissection with prolapse of aortic valve leaflets, and severe aortic dilation (annuloaortic ectasia) preventing coaptation of the leaflets. Aortic insufficiency represents a volume overload of the left ventricle, with resultant left ventricular dilation and eccentric hypertrophy. Congestive heart failure may develop, along with left ventricular dilation, and some patients may experience angina.

Diagnosis

Physical examination generally reveals a diastolic murmur, and examination may occasionally reveal a mid-diastolic rumble (Austin-Flint murmur), Corrigan's hammer pulse, and head bobbing with each systole. Aortic insufficiency may be diagnosed using either Doppler echocardiography or cardiac catheterization to demonstrate diastolic flow across the aortic valve. Aortic insufficiency is graded on a scale of 1+ to 4+ or as mild, moderate, or severe.

Management

Intervention for aortic insufficiency generally requires aortic valve replacement. Some patients with aortic insufficiency due to aortic dissection or focal leaflet damage may undergo aortic valve repair. The indications for aortic valve replacement include onset of congestive heart failure or angina, or, in an asymptomatic patient, onset of left ventricular dilation. Mortality from aortic valve replacement for aortic insufficiency is from 4 to 6 per cent.

Choice of Valve Prosthesis

Aortic valve prostheses may be classified as either mechanical prostheses (St. Jude, Medtronic-Hall,

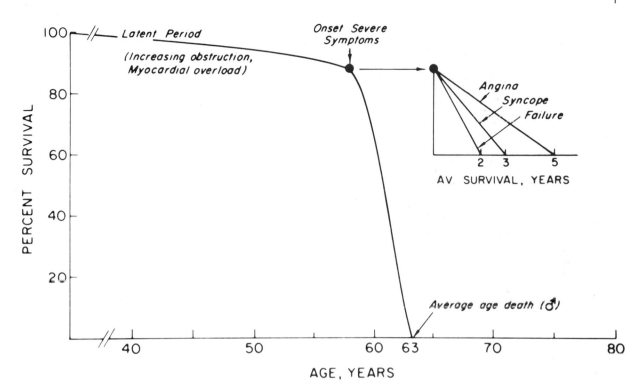

Figure 2. The natural history of medically treated stenosis. (From Ross RS, Braunwald E: Circulation *37*(suppl V):V-61, 1968, with permission.)

Bjork-Shiley) or *bioprotheses* (Carpentier-Edwards, Hancock, human homograft). Mechanical valves have a greater durability (10 to 20 years) relative to bioprostheses (5 to 12 years), but mechanical valves generally require anticoagulation with Coumadin to prevent thromboembolism. Anticoagulation with Coumadin is associated with a 1 to 5 per cent per patient-year complication and a roughly 1 per cent per patient-year mortality. Bioprostheses have a low thromboembolic rate (0.1 to 0.5 per cent per patient-year) and normally do not require anticoagulation. The durability of porcine bioprostheses (Carpentier-Edwards, Hancock) may be less in patients under the age of 35, and the long-term viability of homograft valves may be greater than 10 years.

MITRAL AND TRICUSPID VALVE DISEASE

Normal Physiology

Embryologically, the mitral valve is quadricuspid, but the adult mitral valve is composed of two leaflets, the *anterior leaflet* and the *posterior leaflet*. Each leaflet is attached to both the anterior and posterior papillary muscles by thin, fibrous chordae tendineae. The anterolateral papillary muscle generally receives blood supply from the left anterior descending or circumflex coronary systems, while the posterior medial papillary muscle is generally perfused from the posterolateral branches of the right coronary artery. The tricuspid valve apparatus is similar to that of the mitral valve except that three leaflets are present: *anterior, posterior,* and *septal*. Both mitral and tricuspid valves serve to allow blood flow from the atria into the ventricles during diastole and to prevent return of blood into the atria during ventricular systole. Most diastolic ventricular filling occurs during the rapid filling phase, actually before left ventricular pressure reaches its diastolic minimum.

Mitral Stenosis

Pathophysiology

The most common etiology of mitral stenosis is rheumatic fever. Acute inflammatory infiltrates characterize early valvular lesions in rheumatic fever with later development of fibrous tissue, leaflet fusion and thickening, frequent leaflet calcification, and shortening and fusion of the chordae. The development of severe mitral stenosis occurs at least 2 years after an episode of rheumatic fever and commonly follows an asymptomatic latent phase of 20 years or more. Obstruction of the mitral valve produces elevation of left atrial pressure with atrial dilation, onset of atrial fibrillation, and, often, embolism of atrial thrombus. As left atrial pressure rises, pulmonary artery pressure also increases and may ultimately progress to pulmonary hypertension. Pulmonary venous congestion produces symptoms of dyspnea that may initially be effort related and may eventually progress to occurring during rest or while lying flat. Cardiac output may be reduced due to impairment of left ventricular filling.

Diagnosis

Progressive exertional dyspnea, orthopnea, and easy fatigability are the most frequent symptoms of mitral stenosis. Dysphagia or hoarseness may follow left atrial encroachment on the left recurrent laryngeal nerve or esophagus. Physical examination may include cachexia, sallow mitral facies, ruddiness of the cheeks, peripheral cyanosis, jugular venous pulsation, irregular pulse, peripheral edema, hepatojugular reflux, pulmonary rales, and a sternal right ventricular heave. Early mitral stenosis may accentuate the first heart sound and also produce an opening snap, and the pulmonary component of the second heart sound may be accentuated by pulmonary hypertension. The most characteristic auscultatory finding in mitral stenosis is a diastolic rumbling murmur appreciated at the left ventricular apex.

Electrocardiogram may demonstrate an accentuated p-mitrale, atrial fibrillation, and right ventricular hypertrophy, and the chest film may show left atrial enlargement with prominence of the left atrial appendage, elevation of the left mainstem bronchus, ovoid double density through the central cardiac shadow, posterior displacement of the left atrium, engorgement of superior pulmonary veins, and Kerly B lines. Echocardiography may show thickening of the mitral valve and subvalvular apparatus, along with an increased blood velocity through the mitral valve orifice during diastole. Cardiac catheterization is indicated in patients over the age of 35 or in the presence of angina to demonstrate coronary anatomy. Cardiac catheterization calculating from the Gorlin formula may also assess mitral or tricuspid regurgitation, pulmonary artery pressures, thermodilution cardiac output, mean diastolic mitral gradient, and mitral valve orifice area. Mitral valve orifice area is normally 3 cm^2/m^2 of body surface area, and significant mitral stenosis correlates with a calculated area of 1 cm^2/m^2.

Therapy

The natural history of mitral stenosis involves a latent asymptomatic period of approximately 20 years, followed by progression of symptoms to total inca-

pacity over the next 7 years. Ten-year survival with symptomatic mitral stenosis may be as low as 34 per cent, with the most common causes of death being congestive heart failure in 62 per cent, thromboembolism in 22 per cent, and infectious endocarditis in 8 per cent. Onset of atrial fibrillation in patients older than 40 years is associated with emboli in one half of patients. For these reasons, the indications for correction of mitral stenosis include New York Heart Association (NYHA) Class III or IV congestive heart failure, the onset of atrial fibrillation (even if asymptomatic), worsening pulmonary hypertension, an episode of systemic embolization, and infectious endocarditis in the presence of significant valvular obstruction. Class II congestive heart failure in patients over the age of 40 with undesirable limitation in lifestyle should also be considered for interventional therapy.

Mitral stenosis may be corrected surgically by closed mitral commissurotomy without using cardiopulmonary bypass, by open mitral commissurotomy on cardiopulmonary bypass, and by mitral valve replacement. Closed mitral commissurotomy involves separation of fused mitral commissures using either a finger or a mechanical dilator. Closed mitral commissurotomy is seldom performed today because open commissurotomy can correct valvular pathology more precisely and permits direct visualization of possible left atrial thrombus. Open mitral commissurotomy involves the use of cardiopulmonary bypass to expose the mitral valve to separate fused mitral commissures under direct vision, and to repair any other valvular abnormalities. Symptoms of 95 per cent of patients are reduced to Class I or II after open commissurotomy, but recurrent symptoms or reoperation may occur after 8 to 10 years (Fig. 3).

Mitral valve replacement requires cardiopulmonary bypass (Fig. 4). Mechanical valves have a greater durability, from 10 to 20 years, but require the use of anticoagulation with Coumadin. Recent studies suggest that with modern mechanical prostheses such as the St. Jude valve the prothrombin time may be maintained at 1.4 to 1.5 times normal values. Bioprostheses in the mitral valve position have a disadvantage of less durability from 7 to 10 years but have a lower incidence of thromboembolism without anticoagulation in patients with normal sinus rhythm. Anticoagulation using Coumadin is indicated in patients with a bioprosthesis and atrial fibrillation to reduce the incidence of thromboembolism. The failure rate of bioprostheses may be increased in patients under the age of 30 and in patients with chronic renal failure. Percutaneous balloon mitral valvotomy, introduced in 1984, appears to provide hemodynamic and symptomatic relief comparable to that provided by open or closed mitral commissurotomy. Early data do suggest,

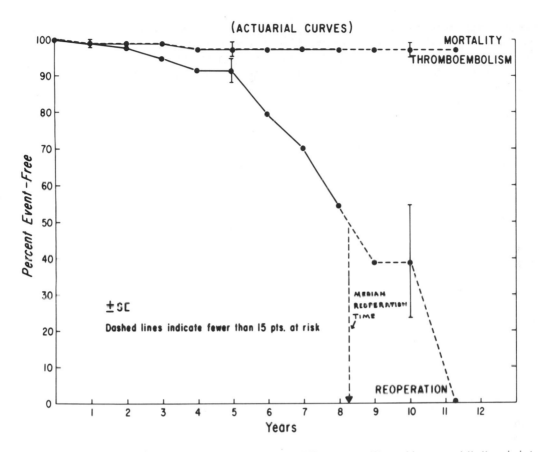

Figure 3. Late results after open commissurotomy in 100 patients. (From Housman LB, Bonchek L, Lambert L, et al: Prognosis of patients after open mitral commissurotomy: Actuarial analysis of late results in 100 patients. J Thorac Cardiovasc Surg 73:742, 1977, with permission.)

however, that recurrent symptoms may present somewhat earlier than after surgical commissurotomy.

Mitral Regurgitation

Pathophysiology

Mitral regurgitation may be caused by dysfunction of the mitral valve annulus, the valve leaflets, the chordae tendineae, the papillary muscles, or the ventricular wall, with 40 per cent following rheumatic heart disease with fibrosis and fusion of the chordae tendineae and fibrosis and calcification of leaflets. It may also be idiopathic in association with calcification of the valvular and subvalvular apparatus. Myxomatous degeneration of the mitral valve may produce elongation of the chordae tendineae, redundancy of the leaflets, and mitral valve prolapse, ultimately with rupture of weakened chordae in severe cases. Leaflet or chordal rupture may also follow trauma or infective endocarditis. Posterior wall myocardial infarction may produce mitral regurgitation by posterior annular dila-

tion, papillary muscle elongation, loss of papillary muscle shortening, and papillary muscle rupture.

Mitral regurgitation elevates left atrial pressure and may secondarily produce pulmonary arterial hypertension, right ventricular failure, functional tricuspid regurgitation, and atrial fibrillation. It represents a volume load on the left ventricle with resultant increases in diastolic left ventricular pressure, left ventricular dilation, and eccentric hypertrophy of the left ventricle. Because of the low afterload that the left atrium represents to the left ventricle, left ventricular ejection fraction may initially increase, but ejection fraction generally falls after onset of left ventricular dilation. Untreated, patients ultimately expire from biventricular cardiac failure, low cardiac output, and pulmonary edema. As with mitral stenosis, systemic embolization and bacterial endocarditis may also occur.

Diagnosis

Most symptomatic patients exhibit exertional dyspnea and orthopnea along with easy fatigability and

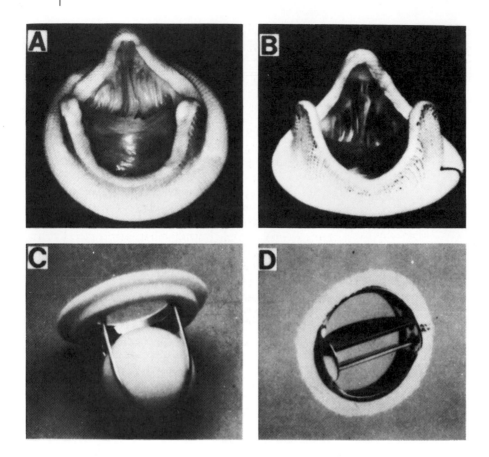

Figure 4. Commonly used prosthetic mitral valves. *A,* Hancock valve (Extracorporeal Medical Specialties, Inc., Anaheim, CA). *B,* Carpentier-Edwards valve (American Edwards Laboratories, Santa Ana, CA). *C,* Starr-Edwards 6120 valve (American Edwards Laboratories, Santa Ana, CA). *D,* St. Jude Medical valve (St. Jude Medical, St. Paul, MN). (From Rankin JS: Mitral and tricuspid valve disease. *In* Sabiston DC Jr [ed]: Textbook of Surgery: The Biological Basis of Modern Surgical Practice, ed 14. Philadelphia, WB Saunders Company, 1991, p 2041, with permission.)

ultimate cardiac cachexia. Physical examination may reveal an irregular pulse, a right ventricular sternal heave, and an apical, holosystolic murmur radiating to the axilla and back. The electrocardiogram may show left ventricular hypertrophy or biventricular hypertrophy with a p-mitrale or atrial fibrillation. Chest radiograph typically demonstrates left atrial enlargement, cephalization of pulmonary flow, and Kerly B lines. Biventricular and atrial enlargement may produce cardiomegaly. Cardiac catheterization demonstrates prominent left atrial v-waves due to ejection of blood into the left atrium during systole, and the presence of severe pulmonary hypertension indicates a worse overall prognosis. Cardiac catheterization may assess cardiac output by thermodilution, and the severity of mitral regurgitation may be graded from left ventriculography. Echocardiography may better define abnormalities of the mitral valve apparatus itself while also quantifying the severity of mitral regurgitation.

Therapy

The natural history of mitral regurgitation is highly variable depending upon the etiology of the valvular lesion. Rheumatic or myxomatous mitral regurgitation may have a protracted course until the onset of congestive heart failure when clinical status deteriorates more rapidly. The severity of congestive heart failure symptoms have not been as closely related to survival as has left ventricular dilation. Thus, indications for surgical intervention include significant limitation of lifestyle due to congestive heart failure, NYHA Class III or IV congestive heart failure, progression of pulmonary hypertension, onset of atrial fibrillation, or onset of left ventricular dilation. A highly accelerated clinical course may be present with mitral regurgitation due to infective endocarditis, trauma, or ruptured chordae tendineae, with rapid progression to pulmonary edema and cardiogenic shock. Under these conditions, operation should be performed as expeditiously as possible given the patient's overall condition.

Interventional management of mitral regurgitation involves operative mitral valve repair or mitral valve replacement. For regurgitant mitral valves, many techniques of valvular repair have been described to correct annular dilation, ruptured chordae, chordal elongation or fusion, leaflet perforation, and leaflet prolapse. In-hospital mortality for mitral valve replacement or repair in mitral regurgitation ranges from 3 to 10 per cent or more, depending on the patient's condition and the urgency of operation.

Tricuspid Valve Disease

Pathophysiology

Tricuspid valve dysfunction may be either functional or organic. *Functional* tricuspid regurgitation is generally caused by right ventricular dilation and enlargement of the tricuspid annulus. *Organic* tricuspid valve regurgitation may be produced by rheumatic fever, congenital malformations, papillary muscle rupture, trauma, Marfan's syndrome, infective endocarditis, carcinoid tumor, or cardiac tumors due to abnormalities of the valve leaflets and chordae. Tricuspid stenosis is generally rheumatic in origin but may also follow carcinoid syndrome, congenital defects, or cardiac tumors.

Diagnosis

Common symptoms of tricuspid stenosis or regurgitation include fatigue, weakness, and pedal edema. Physical examination may reveal jugular venous distention, an enlarged or pulsatile liver, a tricuspid opening snap, a holosystolic murmur of tricuspid regurgitation, or a diastolic rumble of tricuspid stenosis. Electrocardiogram may demonstrate atrial enlargement or atrial fibrillation, and chest radiograph may show cardiomegaly with prominence of the right atrial shadow. Tricuspid regurgitation may be quantified as *mild*, *moderate*, or *severe*, either by Doppler echocardiography or by cardiac catheterization. In tricuspid stenosis, echocardiography may demonstrate increased velocity of flow across the stenotic valve, and cardiac catheterization can directly measure the mean diastolic gradient across the tricuspid valve, with 3 mm Hg producing symptoms and 5 mm Hg representing significant tricuspid stenosis.

Therapy

Significant tricuspid stenosis requires tricuspid valve replacement, generally performed using bioprosthetic valves due to the relatively high incidence of mechanical valve thrombosis in the tricuspid position. Tricuspid regurgitation may require tricuspid valve replacement or may be amenable to tricuspid annuloplasty if the tricuspid regurgitation is functional due to annular dilation. Total excision of the tricuspid valve without replacement may be a reasonable alternative in drug addicts with tricuspid valve endocarditis and a high likelihood of recurrent valve infection.

SURGICAL TREATMENT OF HYPERTROPHIC CARDIOMYOPATHY

Pathophysiology

Hypertrophic cardiomyopathy is characterized by asymmetric septal hypertrophy and microscopic disorganization of muscle bundles, and 25 per cent of patients may have dynamic systolic subaortic obstruction caused by contact between the mitral valve and the ventricular septum (Fig. 5). The dynamic subaortic obstruction may occur spontaneously and may be augmented by increased contractility, decreased arterial pressure, or decreased ventricular volume. Most patients have diastolic dysfunction evidenced by impaired relaxation, decreased compliance, and impairment of diastolic filling, which may be improved by calcium channel blockers and aggravated by atrial fibrillation with loss of the atrial kick. Myocardial ischemia may occur and produce chest pain in the absence of coronary artery disease due to high left ventricular pressures, increased myocardial oxygen demand, and abnormalities in small-vessel coronary flow. Mitral regurgitation may also occur and may correlate with the degree of left ventricular outflow tract obstruction and systolic anterior motion of the mitral valve leaflets.

Clinical Features

Hypertrophic cardiomyopathy may present at any age from infancy to senescence, with morphologic abnormalities typically appearing by 20 years of age and symptoms often appearing by age 40. Hypertrophic cardiomyopathy is more common in males and is familial in 60 per cent of patients with an autosomal-dominant genetic transmission. Symptoms of hypertrophic cardiomyopathy may include dyspnea, chest pain, presyncope, and syncope, all of which correlate poorly with the nature and severity of underlying pathophysiologic mechanisms. Sudden death occurs with an incidence of 2 to 3 per cent per patient-year and is thought to result primarily from arrhythmias.

Diagnosis

Physical examination may reveal an S_4 gallop in most patients and a systolic murmur in a minority of patients. Electrocardiogram is usually abnormal in symptomatic patients and may demonstrate atrial fibrillation, left ventricular hypertrophy, or ST segment and T-wave abnormalities. Echocardiography may demonstrate asymmetric septal hypertrophy, systolic anterior motion of the mitral valve, mitral valve regurgitation, subvalvular stenosis, and impaired diastolic performance. Cardiac catheterization may simi-

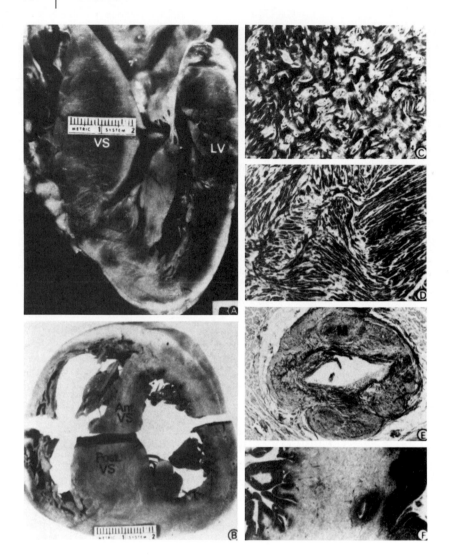

Figure 5. Pathologic features of hypertrophic cardiomyopathy. *A,* Heart specimen sectioned longitudinally demonstrating asymmetric septal hypertrophy with wall thickening primarily in the anterior septum, which bulges into the left ventricular outflow tract. *B,* Specimen with hypertrophy primarily in the posterior ventricular septum. *C,* Disordered cellular architecture with adjacent myocytes arranged at perpendicular or oblique angles. *D,* Bundles of hypertrophied cells with a disorganized, interwoven arrangement. *E,* Intramural coronary with narrowed lumen and medial hypertrophy. *F,* Extensive transmural scarring of the septum. (From Maron BJ, Bonow RO, Cannon RO, Leon MB, Epstein SE: Hypertrophic cardiomyopathy: Interrelations of clinical manifestations, pathophysiology, and therapy. N Engl J Med *316*:780, 1987, with permission.)

larly demonstrate most of these features in addition to identifying the presence of coronary artery disease. In the catheterization laboratory, dynamic subvalvular outflow obstruction may be elicited by administration of amyl nitrate or during a postextrasystole (Brockenbrough maneuver). A resting or elicited subvalvular aortic gradient over 50 mm Hg is considered to be significant.

Natural History and Operative Treatment

The natural history of hypertrophic cardiomyopathy is extremely variable, with many patients remaining asymptomatic until midlife. Onset of atrial fibrillation may acutely exacerbate symptoms in some patients. Medical therapy is effective in controlling symptoms in most patients, with β-blockers and cal-

cium channel blockers being the mainstays of medical therapy, and amiodarone is used for selected patients with nonsustained ventricular tachycardia.

Operative intervention is reserved for patients with symptoms unresponsive to medical therapy and with a resting gradient over 50 mm Hg across the subvalvular ventricular outflow tract or with significant mitral regurgitation. The two primary surgical treatments for hypertrophic cardiomyopathy are septal myotomy-myectomy and mitral valve replacement. Septal myotomy-myectomy removes a strip of obstructing septal muscle at the point of contact with the mitral valve. Mitral valve replacement has also been effective, particularly in patients with severe mitral valve disease or previous septal myotomy. The operative mortality for either procedure is 5 to 8 per cent with complications such as ventricular septal defect, complete heart block, and aortic or mitral valve damage occurring in less than 5 per cent. Long-lasting symptomatic relief occurs in 70 per cent up to 25 years postoperatively.

REFERENCES

Alpert JS: Chronic aortic regurgitation. *In* Dalen JE, Alpert JS (eds): Valvular Heart Disease, ed 2. Boston, Little, Brown & Co, 1987, p 283.

Blanchard DG, Ross J Jr: Hypertrophic cardiomyopathy. Prognosis with medical or surgical therapy. Clin Cardiol *14*:11, 1991.

Block PC, Tuzcu FM, Palacios IF: Percutaneous mitral balloon valvotomy. Cardiol Clin 9:271, 1991.

Cosgrove DM, Stewart WJ: Mitral valvuloplasty. Curr Probl Cardiol *14*:359–415, 1989.

Craver JM, Weintraub WS, Jones EL, Guyton RA, Hatcher CA Jr: Predictors of mortality, complications, and length of stay in aortic valve replacement for aortic stenosis. Circulation 78:85–90, 1988.

Crumbley AJ, Crawford FA Jr: Long-term results of aortic valve replacement. Cardiol Clin 9:353, 1991.

Horstkotte D, Loogen F: The natural history of aortic valve stenosis. Eur Heart J 9(suppl E):57, 1988.

Kratz J: Evaluation and management of tricuspid valve disease. Cardiol Clin 9:397, 1991.

Maron BJ, Bonow RO, Cannon RO, Leon MB, Epstein SE: Hypertrophic cardiomyopathy: Interrelations of clinical manifestations, pathophysiology, and therapy. N Engl J Med *316*:780 (part I), 844 (part II), 1987.

McIntosh DL, Maron BJ: Current operative treatment of obstructive hypertrophic cardiomyopathy. Circulation 78:487, 1988.

Morrow AG: Hypertrophic subaortic stenosis. J Thorac Cardiovasc Surg 76:423, 1978.

Rankin JS: Mitral and tricuspid valve disease. *In* Sabiston DC Jr (ed): Textbook of Surgery: The Biological Basis of Modern Surgical Practice, ed 14. Philadelphia, WB Saunders Company, 1991, pp 2026–2043.

Rankin JS, Hickey MS, Smith LR, Muhlbaier L, Reves JG, Pryor DB, Wechsler AS: Ischemic mitral regurgitation. Circulation 79(suppl I):I-116, 1989.

Whitman GJR, Harken AH: Acquired disorders of the aortic valve. *In* Sabiston DC Jr (ed): Textbook of Surgery: The Biological Basis of Modern Surgical Practice, ed 14. Philadelphia, WB Saunders Company, 1991, pp 2011–2018.

Yun KL, Miller DC: Mitral valve repair versus replacement. Cardiol Clin 9:315, 1991.

ACQUIRED CARDIAC CONDITIONS: Cardiac Assist Devices and the Artificial Heart

MARK P. ANSTADT, M.D.

HISTORY

More than 40 years have been invested in the development of devices for mechanical circulatory support. Not surprisingly, many early concepts remain fundamental in the current technology. Probably the best example is the advent (by Dennis in 1951) and successful application (by Gibbon in 1954) of the pump-oxygenator, which evolved into the most common method of circulatory support used today, *cardiopulmonary bypass* (CPB). While CPB is primarily used during cardiac procedures, the concept of prolonged circulatory support emerged from its application.

The discovery that increasing diastolic blood pressure has salutary effects on coronary blood was first observed by the Kantrowitz brothers, who experimentally delayed the arrival of systolic pressures to the coronary arteries by an interposed rubber conduit. Diastolic augmentation was later applied by wrapping a hemidiaphragm around the descending thoracic aorta and stimulating this skeletal muscle to compress the aorta during diastole by Kantrowitz in 1959. Harken postulated that aspiration of arterial blood during systole followed by its reinfusion during diastole could diminish cardiac work without compromising coronary perfusion. A device subsequently developed by Clauss and associates achieved *diastolic counterpulsation* by withdrawing and reinfusing blood via arterial cannulae. Modern pulsatile ventricular assist devices, synchronized with the cardiac cycle, use this principle. In these devices, blood is withdrawn from the atrium or ventricle for more effective ventricular unloading. The most practical approach to diastolic augmentation was reported in 1962 by Clauss and co-workers, who described the inflation and deflation of latex balloons in the thoracic aorta. This method of intravascular volume displacement has matured into the modern *intra-aortic balloon pump* (IABP).

While these important concepts evolved, other efforts were directed toward complete cardiac replacement. In 1957, Kolff and Akutsu reported the first successful use of a *total artificial heart* (TAH). Flexible pumps molded from the natural heart and contained within a common rigid housing were regulated by air pressure to maintain the canine circulation for 90 minutes. Subsequent TAH designs separated the right and left ventricles for independent control of the pulmonary and systemic circulations. Thrombogenic tendencies were reduced by newer materials and pump designs. By the early 1970s, calves, which proved to be better models than dogs for the TAH because of their larger size and CPB tolerance, were being successfully supported for days. During the same time, the first human application of the TAH was reported. In the 1980s, a TAH became commercially available with some features (air-powered, flexible-pump diaphragms) reflecting Kolff's first design.

PHYSIOLOGIC CONSIDERATIONS

Generally, the underlying problem necessitating circulatory support is pump failure secondary to myocardial ischemia or valvular disease. Assist devices are ordinarily employed on a temporary basis with two therapeutic goals. First, an assist device improves blood flow and arterial pressure to ensure adequate organ perfusion. Second, the device modulates hemodynamics to reduce cardiac work and promote myocardial recovery.

To recognize how assist devices benefit the failing

heart, an understanding of cardiac physiology during normal and pathologic states is necessary. These principles, while pertinent to both the systemic and pulmonary circulations, are best characterized for the *left ventricle* (LV).

Normally, the LV operates within a narrow range of *end-diastolic volumes* (EDV). Changes in EDV due to fluctuations in venous return are accommodated by LV distention. The EDV just prior to cardiac contraction is termed *preload* and regulates the force of myocardial contraction in a compensatory manner known as the *Frank-Starling relationship*. Stretching the functional units of cardiac muscle (the sarcomeres) causes the number of cross-bridge attachments between the thick (myosin) and thin (actin) filaments to increase, which strengthens cardiac contraction. Therefore, preload affects cardiac work by establishing the LV wall tension prior to systole.

Because blood flow only occurs when the LV pressure exceeds arterial pressure, termed *afterload*, the heart's predominant burden is to develop adequate LV wall tension during systole. This energy requirement is the primary hemodynamic determinant of myocardial oxygen consumption as delineated by the *time-tension index* (TTI) (Fig. 1). In contrast, myocardial oxygen delivery correlates with the *diastolic pressure time index* (DPTI), which represents the driving force for coronary blood flow. The balance between myocardial oxygen supply and demand, or the DPTI:TTI ratio, is termed the *endocardial viability ratio* because of the endocardium's notable susceptibility to ischemia. Conditions that unfavorably alter this critical balance may become life threatening if not corrected.

Myocardial ischemia due to coronary artery disease is the leading cause of cardiovascular morbidity and mortality. Severe ischemia depresses ventricular function, causing cardiac distention as pump failure progresses. The increased EDV may cause some compensatory improvements; however, these salutary responses become less adequate as cardiac pathology worsens. If LV distention continues to progress, the optimal wall tension for actin and myosin interactions is surpassed, which further decreases contractility. These conditions lead to reduced ventricular compliance exhibited by marked elevations in end-diastolic pressures. Deleterious effects of ventricular distention are amplified by coincident increases in energy demands during systole. The LV wall tension necessary to develop a given systolic pressure increases in proportion to EDV, as described by the law of Laplace. Therefore, these conditions set in motion a cycle that places increasing demands on an already compromised heart. Further hemodynamic deterioration merely worsens myocardial ischemia, which initiated this vicious cycle.

Before considering a mechanical device, cardiac failure should be treated with appropriate medical management. Volume should be adjusted to optimize preload as determined by monitored filling pressures. Inotropic agents are then used to augment contractility; however, this benefit must be weighed against the associated increase in myocardial oxygen consumption. Vasodilators counter these negative effects through afterload reduction, but caution must be exercised to avoid jeopardizing coronary perfusion pressure. Additional therapies are directed toward correcting the underlying pathology. When these measures fail to restore adequate hemodynamics, mechanical circulatory support should be considered.

THE IABP

When circulatory support is thought necessary, the IABP is the most appropriate initial therapy. The device can be instituted relatively easily and assists the failing heart by lowering myocardial oxygen demand and improving perfusion pressure. The IABP avoids technical complexity and invasiveness, while it improves common features of cardiac failure.

IABP support helps correct imbalances between myocardial oxygen supply and demand in the failing heart. This process is accomplished, not by actually pumping blood, but by merely displacing intravascular volume (Fig. 2). The IABP occupies (inflation) and vacates (deflation) space within the central aorta during diastole and systole, respectively. Two favorable hemodynamic changes result. First, mean diastolic blood pressure increases due to aortic volume displacement during balloon inflation. Second, afterload is reduced by the sudden vacancy of aortic volume caused by balloon deflation just prior to systole. Diastolic augmentation, the term adopted to describe these hemodynamic alterations, is somewhat misleading. Although increased diastolic pressures improve myocardial perfusion, the failing heart most benefits from decreased myocardial oxygen demand caused by afterload reduction.

Another feature of the IABP is its easy insertion. Balloon insertion simply requires cannulation of the common femoral artery by surgical exposure or percutaneous techniques. Catheters of increasing size are then passed over a guidewire until the balloon and an introducer sheath can be accommodated. The balloon is advanced until its tip lies just below the left subclavian artery, placing the balloon's proximal portion above the renal arteries (Fig. 2). Deviations from this location may cause aortic trauma if the balloon tip extends into the aortic arch, or renal artery occlusion when the balloon is not advanced sufficiently. A chest radiograph should be obtained following IABP insertion to confirm its position.

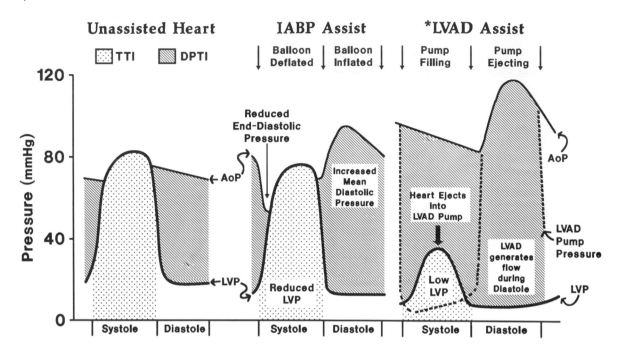

Figure 1. Hemodynamic determinants of myocardial oxygen demand (time tension index [TTI]) and delivery (diastolic pressure time index [DPTI]) are illustrated for the unassisted heart, and during intra-aortic balloon pump (IABP) and left ventricular assist device (LVAD) therapies. *Abbreviations*: AoP = aortic pressure, LVP = left ventricular pressure (* hemodynamic alterations representative for synchronized, LVAD counterpulsation).

Once the IABP is properly inserted, balloon pumping must be carefully synchronized with the cardiac cycle. Balloon inflation should coincide with cardiac diastole, and deflation with cardiac systole (Fig. 1). If balloon inflation is too prolonged, the heart may experience periods of increased afterload, which would be counterproductive. Conversely, inordinately abbreviating balloon inflation diminishes its desired effects. Therefore, the operator sets the initial inflation and deflation parameters manually to optimize the hemodynamic results. A computer system then synchronizes the settings to the patient's electrocardiogram (ECG) signal. Less commonly, the IABP is triggered by a pacemaker signal or an arterial pressure tracing.

Aberrant cardiac rhythms and rapid heart rates are common clinical conditions that reduce the IABP's efficacy. Arrhythmias can be so severe that synchronous support is not possible, in which case a fixed rate independent of the heart's rhythm is used. Tachycardia presents yet another problem because the IABP can fill and empty only at a limited rate. When rates exceed 100 beats per minute, the drive system is generally set to augment every other heartbeat (1 to 2 mode). Unfortunately, this setting not only reduces the effectiveness of support, but also abruptly increases afterload with each unassisted heartbeat, which may be harmful.

Complications that may occur during IABP support include limb ischemia, infection, bleeding, and thromboembolic phenomena. Thrombogenicity is inherent to all blood contacting devices and necessitates anticoagulation. While anticoagulation reduces thrombosis and embolic sequelae, it increases the risk of bleeding and contributes to the frequent formation of hematomas at the balloon insertion site. Hematomas predispose to wound infections, caused by the balloon catheter's persistent violation of the skin barrier. The most common complication of IABP support, however, is limb ischemia distal to the insertion site. Factors that contribute to this problem include balloon catheter obstruction, underlying atherosclerosis, and/or thrombus formation in the vicinity of the insertion site.

Because IABP therapy is associated with potentially serious complications, it should be reserved for patients who have few other options. Patients suffering cardiogenic shock who do not adequately respond to pharmacologic measures clearly fall into such a category. Unfortunately, the appropriate regimen of inotropic agents and vasopressors used before contemplating IABP support remains controversial. Following cardiac surgery, however, general criteria have been established to determine the need for IABP support (Table 1). Some of these criteria apply to other clinical

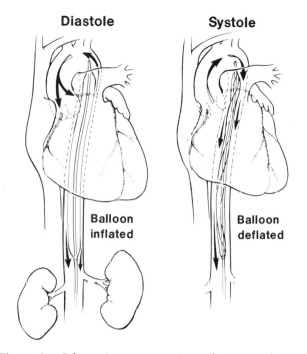

Diastole   **Systole**

Balloon inflated   **Balloon deflated**

Figure 2. Schematic representation of a properly positioned intra-aortic balloon pump. Arrows indicate blood displacement. During cardiac diastole, balloon inflation displaces blood volume toward the coronary circulation. During cardiac systole, balloon deflation reduces resistance to forward flow.

settings in which IABP support is utilized (Table 2). The only distinct contraindication for IABP therapy is aortic insufficiency, which is exacerbated by increased diastolic pressure.

In the past, cardiogenic shock secondary to myocardial infarction was the major indication for IABP support. Currently, in these circumstances, IABP therapy is reserved for patients with surgically correctable complications that contribute to their condition (Table 2). Otherwise, massive myocardial infarction carries a poor prognosis for which IABP support can offer little

TABLE 1. GENERAL CRITERIA FOR IABP SUPPORT FOLLOWING CARDIAC SURGERY

Inability to separate from CPB despite multiple interventions after 30 minutes
Inadequate hemodynamics despite maximal inotropic support including:
    Persistent hypotension (systolic blood pressure <70 mm Hg)
    Low cardiac index (< 2.0 L/min/m^2)
    Elevated left atrial pressure (> 20 mm Hg)
    High peripheral vascular resistance (> 2500 dynes/sec/cm^{-5})
Requirement of inotropic agents at deleterious levels
Persistent malignant ventricular arrhythmias

Abbreviations: IABP = intra-aortic balloon pump, CPB = cardiopulmonary bypass.

TABLE 2. INDICATIONS FOR IABP SUPPORT

Postcardiotomy cardiogenic shock (most commonly, inability to separate from CPB)
Cardiogenic shock secondary to myocardial infarction in addition to:
    Postinfarction ventricular septal defect
    Postinfarction papillary muscle rupture with mitral regurgitation
Myocardial ischemia refractory to medical therapy including:
    Unstable angina
    Refractory ventricular tachyarrhythmias
Postoperative cardiogenic shock
Preoperative prophylaxis (less common)
Failed coronary angioplasty with myocardial ischemia (preoperative)

Abbreviations: IABP = intra-aortic balloon pump, CPB = cardiopulmonary bypass.

benefit. Today, the largest subpopulation of IABP recipients is comprised of patients undergoing cardiac surgery who can either not separate from cardiopulmonary bypass or experience cardiac failure during the postoperative period. In fact, the IABP is used in approximately 2 to 12 per cent of all cardiac operations in the United States.

IABP support is continued until cardiac recovery permits reduction and/or discontinuation of inotropic agents. Weaning is then accomplished by either reducing the balloon rate or inflation volume so that progressively less assistance is provided. When cardiac function appears adequate, the IABP is temporarily turned off or "fluttered." The patient's hemodynamic stability is monitored, and a decision is made to either resume support or remove the device. Fortunately, most patients who receive an IABP can be weaned from the device, and over 50 per cent survive to leave the hospital. These results are remarkable when one considers that most of these patients would die if IABP therapy were unavailable.

VENTRICULAR ASSIST DEVICES

When IABP therapy is inadequate, a variety of ventricular assist devices (VADs) can be instituted for more effective circulatory support. Unlike the IABP, VADs are true blood pumps that function as temporary substitutes for the left (LVAD), right (RVAD), or even both ventricles (BiVAD). Unfortunately, VADs are relatively complex and expensive and, depending on the particular device, installation can be technically difficult. Furthermore, complications frequently occur that can lead to significant morbidity and mortality. For these reasons, appropriate use of VADs not only requires surgical skill, but careful clinical judgment to balance a complex array of potential risks against the possible therapeutic benefit.

Access to the cardiovascular system is fairly similar

among the VAD systems. LVAD cannulation techniques are most common due to the predominance of LV failure. In these circumstances, a cannula is positioned in either the left atrium or ventricle for delivering blood to the LVAD pump (Fig. 3A and B). Blood is returned via a separate cannula usually placed in the ascending aorta (alternate sites include the femoral artery). Biventricular support is accomplished by adding a second pump that receives blood from the right atrium and returns it through the pulmonary artery. Less commonly, right ventricular failure predominates so that only an RVAD is required.

It is important to understand that nearly all forms of cardiac failure affect both the left and right ventricles to some degree. Because the right ventricle (RV) is usually subject to less injury and has the added luxury of a relatively low work load, RV failure usually responds adequately to inotropic agents and volume loading. For this reason, either an IABP or LVAD is frequently sufficient when the need for mechanical circulatory support arises. Nevertheless, RV function must be carefully assessed during LVAD support; significant right ventricular failure that remains unrecognized is associated with a high mortality.

The various forms of cardiac failure may appear relatively simple when contrasted with the broad assortment of VADs conceived for their treatment. While a detailed description of each device is beyond the scope of this text, discussion of the more common features provides a basis for selecting an appropriate VAD. One important distinction used to categorize these devices is their generation of either *pulsatile* or *nonpulsatile flow*.

Nonpulsatile VADs are generally easier to use and less expensive. These systems employ either a roller or centrifugal pump identical to those used in standard cardiopulmonary bypass circuits. Use of such devices avoids the exhaustive regulatory restraints placed on other VAD systems and makes them comparatively less expensive and more widely available. As an example, *extracorporeal membrane oxygenation technology* (ECMO), which provides life-saving therapy for select forms of lung injury, exclusively employs nonpulsatile systems. A more detailed discussion of ECMO appears in another chapter.

Unlike nonpulsatile pumps that generate continuous flow, pulsatile VADs oscillate flow in a manner that more closely mimics the normal hemodynamic state. Generally, pulsatile VADs squeeze blood from fabricated ventricles using either motorized pusher plates or hydraulically actuated, flexible sacs. Because these designs cause less hemolysis, they have been used with greater success for long-term support (weeks to months) compared with nonpulsatile pumps. However, clinical experience has demonstrated little difference between pulsatile and nonpulsatile systems when

shorter periods of support are required (hours to days). For these reasons, implantable pulsatile VADs are being developed for long-term support, whereas the nonpulsatile VADs have remained extracorporeal and are primarily intended for short-term support. The most intricate totally implantable VADs are powered via the transfer of electrical energy across the skin (Fig. 4). Implantable systems should reduce infection rates and permit patient ambulation. These two issues become more significant as support durations increase. While other distinctions exist between VADs, they impart little objective influence on device selection when the need for circulatory support arises.

Ventricular assist devices should only be instituted after fluid replacement, inotropic agents, and IABP support prove inadequate. Hemodynamic criteria similar to those for IABP therapy (Table 1) are combined with clinical indicators of end-organ compromise (e.g., decreased urine output and poor oxygen delivery) to predict the need for VAD support. Because the culprit is ordinarily predominant left ventricular failure, LVADs usually provide sufficient hemodynamic support. Arterial pressures and organ perfusion improve as the device reinstates normal flow. In addition, LVADs significantly reduce blood volume entering the LV chamber. Therefore, the heart pumps less blood, further reducing its energy expenditure. Oxygen demands are also diminished by the lower myocardial wall tension paralleling preload reduction.

The ultimate decrease in cardiac work is achieved when a pulsatile LVAD provides synchronous counterpulsation. In this situation, the heart pumps blood into the filling LVAD, and the LVAD pumps during cardiac diastole. The TTI is thereby markedly reduced due to the low resistance (afterload) offered by the LVAD pump. DPTI is also optimized by the augmented diastolic pressures of LVAD counterpulsation. Unfortunately, synchronous LVAD support has proven difficult to achieve in most clinical settings due to technical problems with device timing. Most pulsatile systems are, instead, operated in a nonsynchronous, *fill-to-empty* mode. A sensor detects when the pump is full and signals the drive system to empty. As a result, the pump is completely washed during each cycle, which has the advantage of reducing blood stagnation and the likelihood of thrombus formation within the pump.

After LVAD support is initiated, hemodynamic parameters are reassessed. Preload should be increased to optimize VAD filling. With these maneuvers, the LVAD can sometimes unmask RV failure. While left atrial filling pressures are kept low through LVAD support, central venous pressures rise due to the RV's inability to accept accompanying increased venous return. If the situation persists despite pharmacologic therapy, the patient should be converted to BiVAD support

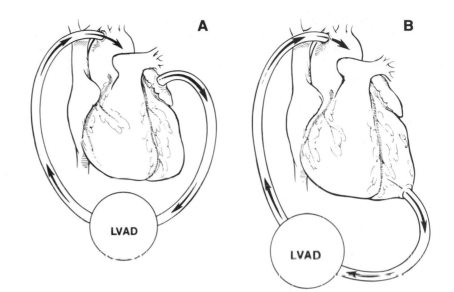

Figure 3. Two common configurations for a left ventricular assist device (LVAD). Arrows indicate the direction of blood flow. The LVAD receives blood from either a left atrial cannula (*A*) or a left ventricular cannula (*B*). Blood is pumped by the LVAD into the ascending aorta.

without hesitation. Less commonly, initial hemodynamics indicate predominant RV failure, in which case an RVAD in combination with inotropic agents and/or an IABP is usually sufficient therapy.

The largest group of VAD recipients is comprised of patients who either cannot separate from cardiopulmonary bypass or deteriorate in the intensive care unit shortly after cardiac surgery. Unfortunately, the mortality of postcardiotomy VAD recipients is over 50 per cent. The critical status of these patients and the complications of VAD support contribute significantly to their poor outcome. However, those who are weaned from VAD support and survive generally enjoy a good quality of life.

Patient outcome is best when VAD support is brief, which, in part, reduces the chance of device-related complications. For these reasons, cardiac function should be periodically assessed within the first 24 hours by briefly turning the VAD off. When the heart shows signs of improvement, VAD flows are gradually decreased. As with IABP therapy, inotropic agents should be reduced before VAD support is discontinued. Patients who successfully separate from VAD support normally require 2 to 5 days of assisted circulation for adequate myocardial recovery. Patients who require more than 1 to 2 weeks of support are presumed to have irreversible myocardial damage and should be considered for cardiac transplantation.

Bridging to cardiac transplantation represents the second most common use for VADs. These VAD recipients must meet the same strict selection criteria as any other patient considered for cardiac transplantation. The exclusion of relatively ill patients and the benefit of transplant therapy explain why this category

of VAD recipients do best overall. Because one distinct problem during bridge to transplant support is the potentially long and indefinite wait for a donor heart, patients expected to have relatively extended waiting periods (e.g., patients with a large body habitus, O-negative blood types, and/or a high panel reactive antibody test) may be better served by totally implantable VADs.

Unlike the bridge-to-transplant setting, the postcardiotomy VAD setting presents the dilemma of appropriate patient selection. Although hemodynamic inclusion criteria can guide this decision process, a great deal of uncertainty still exists.

The issue of patient selection becomes even more important when cost and complications are considered. While the technology is itself expensive, VADs demand significant additional expenses for installation and patient care. Some of the more complex systems require specially trained teams for implantation. In addition, technically successful VAD implantations are frequently followed by complications that cause significant morbidity and mortality, prompted by the blood contact required to artificially pump blood. Anticoagulants must be used to prevent thrombus formation and associated embolic sequelae, which promotes bleeding, the most common problem during VAD support, and frequently requires reoperation. Other serious complications in order of frequency include renal failure, biventricular failure (during LVAD support), infection, and thromboembolism.

New biomaterials may reduce complication rates by curtailing the problems of blood contact. Heparin bonding, now being used in some nonpulsatile devices, fixes the heparin molecule directly to artificial surfaces.

The thromboresistant coating decreases the requirement for systemic anticoagulation. Textured blood-contacting surfaces may also reduce the need for anticoagulation and represent another remarkable advancement. Such a material, employed in a pulsatile VAD (Thermocardiosystems, Houston, TX), has been demonstrated to promote fibrin deposition with the formation of a "pseudoendothelium" on the VAD's blood interface. This biologic shield appears securely fastened to the VAD surface and has not yet caused detectable emboli. These and other new technologies should markedly improve the efficacy of VAD therapy.

THE TOTAL ARTIFICIAL HEART

Total replacement of the heart was first envisioned by Julien-Jean-Cesar La Gallois in 1812, but realistic work on the TAH concept did not begin until the 1950s. A number of novel devices have since been developed. These elegantly engineered pumps meet anatomic constraints for implantation and provide effective circulatory support, but their intended role for permanent cardiac replacement continues to be questioned. Currently, the TAH is only used for bridging

patients to cardiac transplantation, a role shared by VADs. Total artificial hearts differ from VAD systems because they inhabit the space generally occupied by the native heart and must provide total biventricular support. Each device consists of two blood pumps that, when taken individually, have characteristics mimicking pulsatile VADs. However, the pumps are molded together so they can fit inside the chest.

As with VADs, the TAH drive systems exist in two general forms. External drive systems power pneumatic TAHs via drive lines tethered to the patient, one example of which is the most frequently used TAH, the Jarvik heart. Because percutaneous drive lines have proven to be a source of inevitable infection, another type of TAH is currently being developed that incorporates totally implantable drive systems that utilize energy transfer technology previously described for their VAD counterparts (Fig. 4). Totally implantable TAHs should reduce the chance of infection, a critical criterion for long-term support. Unfortunately, implantations will become more technically demanding when these devices reach fruition.

As with some VADs, surgical implantation of the TAH requires that the patient first be placed on cardiopulmonary bypass; and, unlike any VAD implantation, the heart is excised in a manner similar to that used for cardiac transplantation. Care is made to preserve the patient's atria, aortic root, and pulmonary trunk, which facilitates anastomoses of these structures to the TAH. Specially designed cuffs are sewn to each atria. The cuffs come either fixed to the TAH inlet ports or snap-on following their anastomosis to the atria. The aorta and pulmonary artery are coupled to the TAH via large vascular grafts. After completing the necessary surgical anastomoses, the surgeon must remove all air from the TAH before turning on the drive system to prevent air emboli.

Initial experience with the TAH as a permanent form of cardiac replacement has been discouraging. Serious septic and thromboembolic complications were the cause of death in the only five patients who received a permanent Jarvik TAH. Although outcome may improve with totally implantable systems, use of the TAH for permanent support remains experimental. On the other hand, the TAH has been generally accepted as a bridge to cardiac transplantation. In particular, transplant candidates with irreversible biventricular failure for whom the likelihood of receiving a donor heart is poor may best be bridged with a TAH.

Patients who receive TAHs as a bridge to transplantation have outcomes significantly worse than those receiving VADs for similar purposes. One possible explanation for this difference is that TAH recipients generally have devices implanted for longer periods, subjecting them to a greater risk for developing complications. Clinical experience also indicates that this

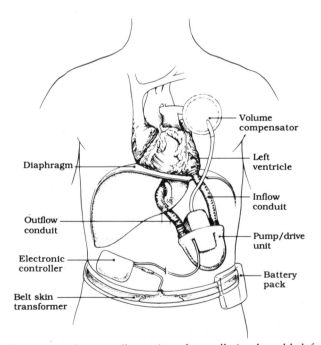

Figure 4. Schematic illustration of a totally implantable left ventricular assist device. All components, including the drive system, are implanted within the patient's body. Electrical energy is transferred across the skin to power the drive unit. (Photo courtesy of Baxter Healthcare Corporation, Novacor Division).

Labels in figure:
- Volume compensator
- Left ventricle
- Inflow conduit
- Pump/drive unit
- Battery pack
- Diaphragm
- Outflow conduit
- Electronic controller
- Belt skin transformer

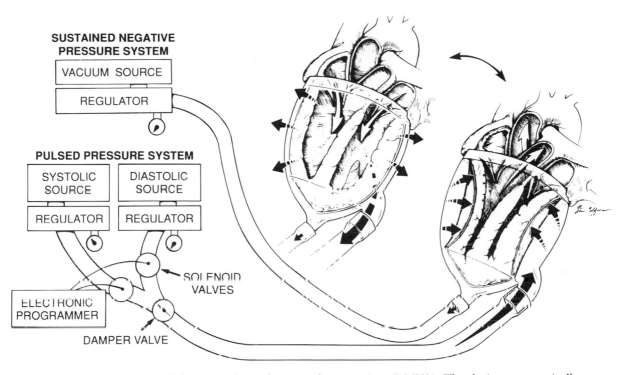

SUSTAINED NEGATIVE PRESSURE SYSTEM

VACUUM SOURCE

REGULATOR

PULSED PRESSURE SYSTEM

SYSTOLIC SOURCE

DIASTOLIC SOURCE

REGULATOR

REGULATOR

SOLENOID VALVES

ELECTRONIC PROGRAMMER

DAMPER VALVE

Figure 5. Diagram of direct mechanical ventricular actuation (DMVA). The device pneumatically actuates the ventricles into systolic (*right*) and diastolic (*left*) configurations, which provides total circulatory support without contacting the blood. (From Anstadt MP, Anstadt GL, Lowe, JE: Direct mechanical ventricular actuation: A review. Resuscitation *21*:8, 1991, with permission.)

increased risk is inherently associated with the TAH. The complications that accompany TAH support essentially parallel those described for VADs, except they generally occur at a slightly greater frequency and do not include biventricular failure. Determining factors responsible for the greater frequency of complications during TAH support should aid in improving patient outcome.

The TAH is more expensive and more technically difficult to use than existing BiVADs, which may be equally effective and less prone to complications. Newer, totally implantable TAHs will likely be used experimentally in patients with irreversible end-stage cardiomyopathies who are not candidates for transplantation. If successful, these devices may revitalize the TAH as a permanent form of cardiac replacement.

OTHER CONCEPTS

Three unique methods of circulatory support currently undergoing clinical investigation deserve mention. The first is a small archimedean screw that rotates in a narrow cylindric housing to generate unidirectional, nonpulsatile flow. The pump diameter is 7 mm, which enables it to lie across the aortic valve

with its inlet and outlet ports positioned in the left ventricle and ascending aorta, respectively. A long cable, fed through the aorta, exits the femoral artery to communicate with a rotor system that rapidly spins the pump's screw (25,000 rpm). The principal limitations are that the device can only provide partial LV support and that it requires anticoagulation.

Two other methods exist that do not require anticoagulation because they avoid blood contact. In one method, termed *dynamic cardiomyoplasty*, transformed, fatigue-resistant skeletal muscle is wrapped around the heart and electrically stimulated to augment the heart during systole. One problem is that the skeletal muscle needs electrical stimulation ("preconditioning") for weeks before it becomes fatigue resistant. Furthermore, the operation required to wrap the muscle around the heart is not well tolerated in severely ill patients. The method may significantly benefit select patients who require chronic circulatory support.

Unlike cardiomyoplasty, *direct mechanical ventricular actuation* (DMVA) is another non–blood contacting method that can immediately provide total circulatory support (Fig. 5). DMVA employs a "heart cup" that is attached by vacuum to encompass both ventricles. Within the cup, a pneumatically regulated diaphragm compresses and dilates the ventricular chambers. Clinically, DMVA has been successfully applied as a bridge to cardiac transplantation. The device has also supported a patient who was suffering from life-threatening, viral myocarditis for 1 week after which normal cardiac function returned. It has not been determined whether prolonged support using DMVA injures the heart. Irrespectively, the device's greatest potential may be its unique ability to provide rapid resuscitative support.

SUMMARY

A number of devices are available for treating cardiac failure. Overall, the IABP remains the mainstay of therapy when circulatory support is required. When the IABP proves inadequate, VADs and the TAH offer life-saving potential, but are attended by significant morbidity and mortality. The primary goal of these devices is to allow recovery of the patient's cardiac function or bridge to other therapies such as cardiac transplantation. Development of feasible methods for permanent circulatory support or cardiac replacement remains a difficult challenge, and problems inherent to blood contact appear to be the single most important obstacle to the advancement of these technologies.

REFERENCES

Anstadt MP, Anstadt GL, Lowe JE: Direct mechanical ventricular actuation: A review. Resuscitation 21:7–23, 1991.

Chitwood WR Jr: Intra-aortic balloon counterpulsation: Physiology, indications, and techniques. In Sabiston DC Jr (ed): Textbook of Surgery: The Biological Basis of Modern Surgical Practice, ed 14. Philadelphia, WB Saunders Company, 1991, pp 2116–2126.

Pierce WS: The artificial heart. In Sabiston DC Jr, Spencer FC (eds): Surgery of the Chest, ed 5, vol II. Philadelphia, WB Saunders Company, 1990, pp 1965–1978.

Richenbacher WE, Olsen DB, Gay WA Jr: The artificial heart. In Sabiston DC Jr (ed): Textbook of Surgery: The Biological Basis of Modern Surgical Practice, ed 14. Philadelphia, WB Saunders Company, 1991, pp 2126–2132.

Sarnoff SJ, Braunwald E, Welch GH Jr, Case RB, Stainsby WN, Macruz R: Hemodynamic determinants of oxygen consumption of the heart with special reference to the tension-time index. Am J Physiol 192:148–156, 1958.

Wolvek S: The evolution of the intra-aortic balloon: The datascope contribution. J Biomat Appl 3:527–543, 1989.

INDEX

Note: Page numbers in *italics* indicate illustrations; page numbers followed by t indicate tables.

ISBN 0-7216-5019-8

90069